ANTIEPILEPTIC DRUGS

Third Edition

ANTIEPILEPTIC DRUGS

Third Edition

Editors

René H. Levy, Ph.D.
Departments of Pharmaceutics and Neurological Surgery
University of Washington Schools of Pharmacy and Medicine
Seattle, Washington

F. E. Dreifuss, M.B., F.R.C.P., F.R.A.C.P.
Department of Neurology
University of Virginia School of Medicine
Charlottesville, Virginia

Richard H. Mattson, M.D.
Department of Neurology
Yale University School of Medicine
West Haven Veterans Administration
Medical Center
New Haven, Connecticut

Brian S. Meldrum, M.B., Ph.D.
Department of Neurology
Institute of Psychiatry
University of London
London, England

J. Kiffin Penry, M.D.
Department of Neurology
Bowman Gray School of Medicine
Wake Forest University
Winston-Salem, North Carolina

Associate Editor

B. J. Hessie
Rockville, Maryland

Raven Press ⬥ New York

Raven Press, 1185 Avenue of the Americas, New York, New York 10036

Made in the United States of America

Library of Congress Cataloging-in-Publication Data

Antiepileptic drugs / editors, René H. Levy . . . [et al.] ; associate
 editor, B. J. Hessie.—3rd ed.
     p.   cm.
   Includes bibliographies and indexes.
   ISBN 0-88167-539-3
   1. Epilepsy—Chemotherapy.   2. Anticonvulsants.
   [DNLM: 1. Anticonvulsants.   2. Epilepsy—drug therapy. QV 85
 A628]
 RC374.C48A58   1989
 616.8′53061—dc20
 DNLM/DLC
 for Library of Congress   88-42524
                                                                    CIP

The material contained in this volume was submitted as previously unpublished material, except in the instances in which credit has been given to the source from which some of the illustrative material was derived.

Great care has been taken to maintain the accuracy of the information contained in the volume. However, neither Raven Press nor the editors can be held responsible for errors or for any consequences arising from the use of the information contained herein.

Materials appearing in this book prepared by individuals as part of their official duties as U.S. Government employees are not covered by the above-mentioned copyright.

9 8 7 6 5 4 3 2

Preface

This third edition of *Antiepileptic Drugs* maintains the successful format of the previous editions, but has been thoroughly revised to emphasize advances in the chemotherapy of the epilepsies that have taken place since the publication of the second edition in 1982. A modern view of the development of antiepileptic drugs is one of these important advances. The development of drugs by structural analogy is the traditional approach, and a relatively successful one. We can enhance the search for new antiepileptic drugs, however, by exploiting our knowledge of the pathophysiology of epilepsy. The door to this approach was unlocked by the discovery of the anticonvulsant effect of valproate, which is thought to be the result of its influence on neurotransmitter activity. This new volume marks the watershed between the empirical development of antiepileptic drugs and a more rational development based on putative mechanisms of epileptogenesis.

The belief that anticonvulsant activity of a chemical compound is limited to specific structural features, as in barbiturates and hydantoins, is abandoned forever. We now believe that a wide variety of chemical structures can yield potent anticonvulsant activity. This theory is illustrated in the section on potential antiepileptic drugs, which contains seven new and structurally unrelated chemical entities. We also believe that in the age of molecular biology and biotechnology-based pharmaceuticals, advances in basic mechanisms of drug action and in drug development should proceed *pari passu*. In this edition, the chapter on mechanisms of antiepileptic drug action precedes the other chapters in each of the major drug sections.

In the last decade, the evolution of analytical methodology led to an understanding of the pharmacokinetics of antiepileptic drugs and to their more rational use through the application of pharmacological principles. The refinement of the classifications of epileptic seizures and syndromes of the epilepsies has spawned the concept of specificity of drugs for particular seizure types, in which the pharmacological mode of action is related to the etiology of the seizures. Consequently, new chapters have been added to address the issues of selection, use, and discontinuation of antiepileptic drugs.

This third edition, like its predecessors, seeks to "present in a single source all of the recent advances in knowledge concerning the antiepileptic drugs as well as an in-depth review of basic pharmacologic data from both animals and man." At the same time, it points the way to improved care of patients with seizure disorders, thereby exerting the influence of research on treatment and finally ending the era of empiricism in epilepsy.

The Editors

Preface to the Second Edition

When *Antiepileptic Drugs* was first published a decade ago, as a compilation of the available information concerning all aspects of drug therapy for the epilepsies, it was obvious that our knowledge of the mechanisms of action of antiepileptic drugs was incomplete and that the therapeutic application of the existing information was inadequate.

During the past 10 years, however, many of the gaps in our knowledge of the antiepileptic drugs have been filled and the clinical management of the epilepsies has improved. Many factors are responsible for these advances. Improved techniques of video monitoring and telemetered electroencephalography allowed better determination of the seizure type. Rapid technological developments in the quantification of antiepileptic drugs in biological fluids by gas-liquid chromatography, high-pressure liquid chromatography, and homogeneous enzyme immunoassay permitted the correlation of drug concentration with clinical response. With this information, it was then possible to establish the pharmacokinetic profiles of individual patients in various clinical situations.

Simultaneously with the clinical studies, basic research on the epilepsies provided new insights into the mechanisms that cause and regulate seizure activity in the central nervous system and into the ways that antiepileptic drugs alter these mechanisms. Such basic studies are exemplified by exploration of the role of neurotransmitters in the regulation of neuronal activity and investigation of ionic channels, the gating process, and ion transport across neuronal membranes.

Without a doubt, however, the key factor in the advances in our knowledge and use of the antiepileptic drugs is the dedicated efforts of investigators throughout the world to provide better care for patients with epilepsy. It is impossible to cite each individual who has contributed to these advances, but special recognition should be given to the National Institute of Neurological and Communicative Disorders and Stroke, the Epilepsy Foundation of America, the International League Against Epilepsy, and the organizers of the Workshops on the Determination of Antiepileptic Drugs in Body Fluids.

The aim of this second edition duplicates that of the original work, namely, to "present in a single source all of the recent advances in knowledge concerning the antiepileptic drugs as well as an in-depth review of basic pharmacologic data from both animals and man." With an up-to-date presentation of this information on both old and new drugs and the addition of current findings on the mechanisms of action of antiepileptic drugs, this new volume offers a thorough treatment of the pharmacological approach to the epilepsies.

Notwithstanding the recent advances mentioned above, the drug therapy of epilepsy is still wanting. It is our hope that this book will enhance our basic and clinical understanding of the antiepileptic drugs for the good of patients with epilepsy. We hope, too, that it will serve to stimulate future investigations in this field.

Acknowledgments

The editors are grateful for the concerted actions of the many dedicated persons who helped to bring this volume to fruition. They include, first of all, the authors, whose signal contributions and enthusiastic cooperation made this work possible, and last but not least, the staff of Raven Press, particularly Kathey Alexander, who lent invaluable assistance at every stage of the developmental and publication process.

Contents

Introduction   xxiii
JAMES J. CEREGHINO

GENERAL PRINCIPLES

1   Drug Absorption, Distribution, and Elimination   1
RENÉ H. LEVY AND JASHVANT D. UNADKAT

2   Biotransformation   23
EMILIO PERUCCA AND ALAN RICHENS

3   Toxicology   49
GABRIEL L. PLAA

4   Principles of Antiepileptic Drug Action   59
ROBERT L. MACDONALD AND BRIAN S. MELDRUM

5   Experimental Selection, Quantification, and
Evaluation, of Anticonvulsants   85
EWART A. SWINYARD, JOSE H. WOODHEAD,
H. STEVE WHITE, AND MICHAEL R. FRANKLIN

6   Selection of Antiepileptic Drug Therapy   103
RICHARD H. MATTSON

7   How to Use Antiepileptic Drugs   117
ROGER J. PORTER

8   Discontinuation of Antiepileptic Drugs   133
J. CHRISTINE DEAN AND J. KIFFIN PENRY

PHENYTOIN

9   Mechanisms of Action   143
ROBERT J. DE LORENZO

10   Chemistry and Methods of Determination   159
ANTHONY J. GLAZKO

11   Absorption, Distribution, and Excretion   177
DIXON M. WOODBURY

12 Biotransformation   197
    THOMAS R. BROWNE AND TSUN CHANG

13 Interactions with Other Drugs   215
    HENN KUTT

14 Clinical Use   233
    B. J. WILDER AND ROGELIO J. RANGEL

15 Toxicity   241
    E. H. REYNOLDS

    OTHER HYDANTOINS

16 Mephenytoin and Ethotoin   257
    HARVEY J. KUPFERBERG

    PHENOBARBITAL

17 Mechanisms of Action   267
    JAMES W. PRICHARD AND BRUCE R. RANSOM

18 Chemistry and Methods of Determination   283
    SVEIN I. JOHANNESSEN

19 Absorption, Distribution, and Excretion   293
    ROBERT S. RUST AND W. EDWIN DODSON

20 Biotransformation   305
    GAIL D. ANDERSON

21 Interactions with Other Drugs   313
    HENN KUTT

22 Clinical Use   329
    MICHAEL J. PAINTER

23 Toxicity   341
    RICHARD H. MATTSON AND JOYCE A. CRAMER

    OTHER BARBITURATES

24 Methylphenobarbital and Metharbital   357
    MERVYN J. EADIE

PRIMIDONE

25 Chemistry and Methods of Determination   379
    HELMUT SCHÄFER

26 Absorption, Distribution, and Excretion   391
    JAMES C. CLOYD AND ILO E. LEPPIK

27 Biotransformation and Mechanisms of Action   401
    BLAISE F. D. BOURGEOIS

28 Interactions with Other Drugs   413
    RICHARD W. FINCHAM AND
    DOROTHY D. SCHOTTELIUS

29 Clinical Use   423
    DENNIS B. SMITH

30 Toxicity   439
    ILO E. LEPPIK AND JAMES C. CLOYD

CARBAMAZEPINE

31 Mechanisms of Action   447
    ROBERT L. MACDONALD

32 Chemistry and Methods of Determination   457
    HENN KUTT

33 Absorption, Distribution, and Excretion   473
    PAOLO L. MORSELLI

34 Biotransformation   491
    J. W. FAIGLE AND K. F. FELDMANN

35 Carbamazepine Epoxide   505
    BRADLEY M. KERR AND RENÉ H. LEVY

36 Interactions with Other Drugs   521
    WILLIAM H. PITLICK AND RENÉ H. LEVY

37 Clinical Use   533
    PIERRE LOISEAU

38 Toxicity   555
    LENNART GRAM AND PEDER KLOSTERSKOV JENSEN

VALPROATE

39 Mechanisms of Action 567
RUGGERO FARIELLO AND MICHAEL C. SMITH

40 Chemistry and Methods of Determination 577
HARVEY J. KUPFERBERG

41 Absorption, Distribution, and Excretion 583
RENÉ H. LEVY AND DANNY D. SHEN

42 Biotransformation 601
THOMAS A. BAILLIE AND ALBERT W. RETTENMEIER

43 Interactions with Other Drugs 621
RICHARD H. MATTSON AND JOYCE A. CRAMER

44 Clinical Use 633
BLAISE F. D. BOURGEOIS

45 Toxicity 643
FRITZ E. DREIFUSS

ETHOSUXIMIDE

46 Mechanisms of Action 653
JAMES A. FERRENDELLI AND
KATHERINE D. HOLLAND

47 Chemistry and Methods of Determination 663
TSUN CHANG

48 Absorption, Distribution, and Excretion 671
TSUN CHANG

49 Biotransformation 679
TSUN CHANG

50 Clinical Use 685
ALLAN L. SHERWIN

51 Toxicity 699
FRITZ E. DREIFUSS

OTHER SUCCINIMIDES

52 Methsuximide 707
THOMAS R. BROWNE

TRIMETHADIONE

53 Trimethadione 715
HAROLD E. BOOKER

BENZODIAZEPINES

54 Mechanisms of Action 721
WILLY HAEFELY

55 Diazepam 735
DIETER SCHMIDT

56 Clonazepam 765
SUSUMU SATO

57 Nitrazepam 785
AGOSTINO BARUZZI, ROBERTO MICHELUCCI, AND
CARLO ALBERTO TASSINARI

58 Clorazepate 805
ALAN J. WILENSKY AND PATRICK N. FRIEL

59 Clobazam 821
SIMON DAVID SHORVON

60 Lorazepam 841
RICHARD W. HOMAN AND HAL UNWIN

OTHER ANTIEPILEPTIC DRUGS

61 Sulfonamides and Derivatives: Acetazolamide 855
DIXON M. WOODBURY

62 Bromides 877
FRITZ E. DREIFUSS

63 Paraldehyde 881
LAWRENCE A. LOCKMAN

64 Progabide 887
PAOLO L. MORSELLI AND RAFFAELE PALMINTERI

65 Adrenocorticotropic Hormone (ACTH) 905
O. CARTER SNEAD III

POTENTIAL ANTIEPILEPTIC DRUGS

66 Oxcarbazepine   913
    MOGENS DAM

67 Gabapentin   925
    B. SCHMIDT

68 Vigabatrin   937
    ALAN RICHENS

69 Lamotrigine   947
    LENNART GRAM

70 Stiripentol   955
    PIERRE LOISEAU

71 Flunarizine and Other Calcium Entry Blockers   971
    C. D. BINNIE

72 Felbamate   983
    ILO E. LEPPIK AND NINA M. GRAVES

    Appendix   *991*

    Author Index   *995*

    Subject Index   *997*

Contributors

GAIL D. ANDERSON, PH.D.
Research Associate, Department of Pharmaceutics, and Assistant Professor of Pharmacy Practice, University of Washington School of Pharmacy, Seattle, Washington 98195

THOMAS A. BAILLIE, PH.D.
Associate Professor of Medicinal Chemistry, Univeristy of Washington School of Pharmacy, Seattle, Washington 98195

AGOSTINO BARUZZI, M.D.
Institute of Clinical Neurology, University of Bologna School of Medicine, 40123 Bologna, Italy

PROF. COLIN D. BINNIE
Consultant Clinical Neurophysiologist, The Maudsley Hospital, London SE5, England

HAROLD E. BOOKER, M.D.
Professor of Neurology, University of Cincinnati College of Medicine; and Chief of Neurology, Veterans Administration, Medical Center, Cincinnati, Ohio 45220

BLAISE F. D. BOURGEOIS, M.D.
Section of Epilepsy and Clinical Neurophysiology, Department of Neurology, The Cleveland Clinic Foundation, Cleveland, Ohio 44095

THOMAS R. BROWNE, M.D.
Professor and Vice Chairman, Department of Neurology, Boston University School of Medicine; and Associate Chief, Neurology Service, Veterans Administration Medical Center, Boston, Massachusetts 02130

JAMES J. CEREGHINO, M.D.
Chief, Epilepsy Branch, Division of Convulsive, Developmental, and Neuromuscular Disorders, National Institute of Neurological Disorders and Stroke, National Institutes of Health, Bethesda, Maryland 20892

TSUN CHANG, M.S.
Director, Pharmacokinetics/Drug Metabolism, Parke-Davis Pharmaceutical Research Division, Warner Lambert Company, Ann Arbor, Michigan 48105

JAMES C. CLOYD, PHARM.D.
Associate Professor, Department of Pharmacy Practice, and Clinical Pharmacist, Comprehensive Epilepsy Program, University of Minnesota College of Pharmacy, Minneapolis, Minnesota 55455

JOYCE A. CRAMER, B.S.
Project Director, Epilepsy Research, West Haven Veterans Administration Medical Center; and Associate in Research, Deparment of Neurology, Yale University School of Medicine, New Haven, Connecticut 06516

MOGENS DAM, M.D., Ph.D.
Associate Professor, University Clinic of Neurology, Hvidovre Hospital, DK-2650 Hvidovre, Copenhagen, Denmark

J. CHRISTINE DEAN, M.D.
Research Assistant, Department of Neurology, Bowman Gray School of Medicine, Wake Forest University, Winston-Salem, North Carolina 27103

ROBERT J. DE LORENZO, M.D., Ph.D., M.P.H.
Professor and Chairman of Neurology, and Professor of Pharmacology, Medical College of Virginia, Richmond, Virginia 23298

W. EDWIN DODSON, M.D.
Professor of Pediatrics and Neurology, St. Louis Children's Hospital, St. Louis, Missouri 63110

FRITZ E. DREIFUSS, M.B., F.R.C.P., F.R.A.C.P.
Professor of Neurology, and Director, Comprehensive Epilepsy Program, University of Virginia School of Medicine, Charlottesville, Virginia 22908

MERVYN J. EADIE, M.D., Ph.D., F.R.A.C.P.
Professor of Clinical Neurology and Neuropharmacology, University of Queensland; and Neurologist, Department of Medicine, Royal Brisbane Hospital, Herston, Brisbane, Australia 6029

JOHANN W. FAIGLE, Ph.D.
Senior Research Associate, Research Department, Pharmaceuticals Division, CIBA-GEIGY Limited, CH-4002 Basel, Switzerland

RUGGERO G. FARIELLO, M.D.
Chairman and Professor of Neurology, Department of Neurological Science, Medical College of Rush University, Chicago, Illinois 60612

KARL F. FELDMANN Ph.D.
Senior Staff Scientist, Research Department, Pharmaceuticals Division, CIBA-GEIGY Limited, CH-4002 Basel, Switzerland

JAMES A. FERRENDELLI, M.D.
Professor of Pharmacology and Neurology, Washington University School of Medicine, St. Louis, Missouri 63110

RICHARD W. FINCHAM, M.D.
Professor of Neurology and Director, Epilepsy Clinic, University of Iowa College of Medicine, Iowa City, Iowa 52242

MICHAEL R. FRANKLIN, Ph.D.
Professor of Pharmacology and Toxicology, University of Utah College of Pharmacy, Salt Lake City, Utah 84112

PATRICK N. FRIEL, B.S.
Research Scientist, Regional Epilepsy Center, University of Washington School of Medicine, Seattle, Washington 98104

ANTHONY J. GLAZKO, Ph.D.
Parke-Davis Pharmaceutical Research Division (Retired), Warner-Lambert Company, Ann Arbor, Michigan 48105

LENNART GRAM, M.D.
Chief Neurologist, Dianalund Epilepsy Hospital, DK-4293 Dianalund, Denmark

NINA M. GRAVES, Pharm. D.
Assistant Professor of Pharmacy, University of Minnesota College of Pharmacy, Minneapolis, Minnesota 55414

WILLY HAEFELY
Pharmaceutical Research Department, F. Hoffmann-La Roche and Company, Limited, CH-4002 Basel, Switzerland

KATHERINE D. HOLLAND, B.S.
Departments of Pharmacology and Neurology, and Neurological Surgery, Washington University School of Medicine, St. Louis, Missouri 63110

RICHARD W. HOMAN, M.D.
Director, Regional Epilepsy Center, Veterans Administration Medical Center; and Associate Professor, Department of Neurology, University of Texas Southwestern Medical Center, Dallas, Texas 75235

PEDER KLOSTERSKOV JENSEN, M.D.
Medical Department, CIBA-GEIGY Limited, CH-4002 Basel, Switzerland

SVEIN I. JOHANNESSEN, Ph.D.
Director of Research, The National Center for Epilepsy, N-1301 Sandvika, Norway

BRADLEY M. KERR, Ph.D.
Senior Fellow, Department of Pharmaceutics, University of Washington School of Pharmacy, Seattle, Washington 98195

HARVEY J. KUPFERBERG, Ph.D.
Chief, Preclinical Pharmacology Section, Epilepsy Branch, Division of Convulsive, Developmental, and Neuromuscular Disorders, National Institute of Neurological Disorders and Stroke, National Institutes of Health, Bethesda, Maryland 20892

HENN KUTT, M.D.
Associate Professor of Neurology and Pharmacology, Cornell University Medical Center, New York, New York 10021

ILO E. LEPPIK, M.D.
Professor of Neurology, and Director of Research, Comprehensive Epilepsy Program, University of Minnesota Medical School, Minneapolis, Minnesota 55414

RENÉ H. LEVY, Ph.D.
Professor and Chairman, Department of Pharmaceutics, and Professor of Neurological Surgery, University of Washington Schools of Pharmacy and Medicine, Seattle, Washington 98195

LAWRENCE A. LOCKMAN, M.D.
Associate Professor of Pediatric Neurology, University of Minnesota Medical School, Minneapolis, Minnesota 55455

PIERRE LOISEAU, M.D.
Professor of Neurology, Bordeaux University, France, 33076 Bordeaux, France

KENNETH G. LLOYD, Ph.D.
Department of Clinical Research, Laboratoire d'Etudes et de Recherches Synthelabo—(L.E.R.S.), F-75013 Paris, France

ROBERT L. MACDONALD, M.D., Ph.D.
Professor of Neurology and Physiology, University of Michigan Medical Center, Ann Arbor, Michigan 48104

RICHARD H. MATTSON, M.D.
Chief, Neurology Service, West Haven Veterans Administration Medical Center; and Professor of Neurology, Yale University School of Medicine, New Haven, Connecticut 06510

BRIAN S. MELDRUM, M.B., Ph.D.
Professor in Experimental Neurology, Institute of Psychiatry, University of London, London SE5 8AF, England

ROBERTO MICHELUCCI, M.B., Ph.D.
Institute of Clinical Neurology, University of Bologna School of Medicine, 40123 Bologna, Italy

PAOLO LUCIO MORSELLI, M.D.
Director, Department of Clinical Research, Laboratoire d'Etudes et de Recherches Synthelabo—(L.E.R.S.), F-75013 Paris, France

MICHAEL J. PAINTER, M.D.
Chief, Division of Child Neurology, and Associate Professor of Pediatrics and Neurology, University of Pittsburgh School of Medicine, Pittsburgh, Pennsylvania 15213

RAFFAELE PALMINTERI
Department of Clinical Research, Laboratoire d'Etudes et de Recherches Synthelabo—(L.E.R.S.), F-75013 Paris, France

J. KIFFIN PENRY, M.D.
Professor of Neurology and Associate Dean for Development and Research, Bowman Gray School of Medicine, Wake Forest University, Winston-Salem, North Carolina 27103

EMILIO PERUCCA, Ph.D.
Division of Clinical Pharmacology, Department of Internal Medicine and Therapeutics, University of Pavia, Pavia, Italy 27100

WILLIAM H. PITLICK, Ph.D.
Associate Director, Department of Health and Human Services, and Research Resources Officer, National Institutes of Health, Bethesda, Maryland 20892

GABRIEL L. PLAA, Ph.D.
Professor of Pharmacology, University of Montreal Faculty of Medicine, Montreal, Quebec, Canada, H3C 3J7

ROGER J. PORTER, M.D.
Deputy Director, National Institute of Neurological Disorders and Stroke, National Institutes of Health, Bethesda, Maryland 20892

JAMES W. PRICHARD, M.D.
Professor of Neurology, Yale University School of Medicine, New Haven, Connecticut 06510

ROGELIO J. RANGEL, M.D.
Postdoctoral Fellow in Neurology, Veterans Administration Medical Center and University of Florida College of Medicine, Gainesville, Florida 32611

BRUCE R. RANSOM, M.D., PH.D.
Department of Neurology, Yale University School of Medicine, New Haven, Connecticut 06510

ALBERT W. RETTENMEIER, M.D.
Institut für Arbeits–und Sozialmedizin der Universität Tübingen, D-7400 Tübingen, Federal Republic of Germany

E. H. REYNOLDS, M.D.
Consultant Neurologist, Department of Clinical Neurology, Maudsley and King's College Hospitals, London SE5 9RS, England

ALAN RICHENS, PH.D., F.R.C.P.
Professor of Pharmacology and Therapeutics, University of Wales College of Medicine, Heath Park, Cardiff CF4 4XN, Wales

ROBERT S. RUST, JR., M.D.
Instructor in Pediatrics and Neurology, Washington University School of Medicine, and Fellow, The McDonnel Center for Studies of Higher Brain Function, St. Louis, Missouri 63110

SUSUMU SATO, M.D.
Chief, EEG Laboratory, National Institute of Neurological Disorders and Stroke, National Institutes of Health, Bethesda, Maryland 20892

DR. RER NAT HELMUT SCHÄFER
Desitia Arzneimittel Gmbh, D-2000 Hamburg 63, Federal Republic of Germany

BERND SCHMIDT, M.D., PH.D.
Hasenbuckweg 14, D-7801 Wittnau, Federal Republic of Germany

DIETER SCHMIDT, M.D.
Ludwig – Maximilians Universitat Munchen, Klinikum Grosshadern, Neurologische Poliklinik, 8090 Munchen 70, Federal Republic of Germany

DOROTHY D. SCHOTTELIUS, PH.D.
University of Iowa Colleges of Pharmacy and Medicine, Iowa City, Iowa 52242

DANNY D. SHEN, PH.D.
Associate Professor, Department of Pharmaceutics, University of Washington School of Pharmacy, Seattle, Washington 98195

ALLAN L. SHERWIN, M.D., PH.D.
Professor of Neurology, McGill University, Montreal Neurological Institute, Montreal, Quebec, Canada H3A 2B4

SIMON DAVID SHORVON, M.D.
Senior Lecturer in Neurology, Consultant Neurologist, Institute of Neurology, National Hospital for Nervous Diseases, and Chalfont Centre for Epilepsy, London WC1N 3BG, England

DENNIS B. SMITH, M.D.
Director, Oregon Comprehensive Epilepsy Program; and Clinical Professor of Neurology, Oregon Health Sciences University, Portland, Oregon 97210

MICHAEL C. SMITH, M.D.
Assistant Professor of Neurology, Department of Neurological Science, Medical College of Rush University, Chicago, Illinois 60612

O. CARTER SNEAD, III, M.D.
Professor, Pediatrics and Neurology, and Member, Neuropsychiatry Research Program, School of Medicine, University of Alabama at Birmingham, Birmingham, Alabama 35233

EWART A. SWINYARD, Ph.D. D.Sc.
Emeritus Professor of Pharmacology, College of Pharmacy, University of Utah College of Pharmacy, Salt Lake City, Utah 84112

CARLO ALBERTO TASSINARI, M.D.
Professor of Neurological Clinics, Institute of Clinical Neurology, University of Bologna School of Medicine, 40123 Bologna, Italy

DAVID THOMASSEN, Ph.D.
Research Fellow, Laboratory of Chemical Pharmacology, National Institutes of Health, Bethesda, Maryland 20891

JASHVANT D. UNADKAT, Ph.D.
Assistant Professor of Department of Pharmaceutics, University of Washington School of Pharmacy, Seattle, Washington 98195

D. HAL UNWIN, M.D.
Instructor, Department of Neurology, University of Texas Health Sciences Center, Dallas, Texas 75235

H. STEVE WHITE, Ph.D.
Research Assistant Professor, Department of Pharmacology and Toxicology, University of Utah College of Pharmacy, Salt Lake City, Utah 84112

B. J. WILDER, M.D.
Chief, Neurology Service, Veterans Administration Medical Center; and Professor of Neurology, University of Florida College of Medicine, Gainesville, Florida 32611

ALAN J. WILENSKY, M.D., Ph.D., F.R.C.P.(C)
Attending Neurologist, Epilepsy Center; and Associate Professor, Departments of Neurological Surgery and Medicine (Neurology), University of Washington School of Medicine, Seattle, Washington 98104

DIXON M. WOODBURY, Ph.D.
Professor of Pharmacology, Division of Neuropharmacology and Epileptology, University of Utah College of Medicine, Salt Lake City, Utah 84132

JOSE H. WOODHEAD, B.S.
Senior Research Specialist, Department of Pharmacology and Toxicology, University of Utah College of Pharmacy, Salt Lake City, Utah 84112

Antiepileptic Drugs, Third Edition, edited by
R. Levy, R. Mattson, B. Meldrum,
J. K. Penry, and F. E. Dreifuss.
Raven Press, Ltd., New York © 1989.

Introduction

James J. Cereghino

Although advances in basic neuroscience research have elucidated the anatomic pathways of seizures, the metabolic aspects of epileptogenesis, and the cellular mechanisms of seizure genesis and spread, the ultimate cause of epilepsy is not known and the search for a cure continues. Over the centuries, many substances and concoctions were used for the control of epilepsy (33,34), but the best early hope was offered by the recognition of bromide's antiepileptic properties in the mid-1800s (22,23,30) and by the synthesis and clinical application of phenobarbital in 1912 (19). For half a century, potassium bromide was the mainstay of treatment for epilepsy until it was replaced by phenobarbital. Both substances were generally considered valuable remedies, but were not ideal. Reports of variable seizure control were often tempered by reports of serious side effects of bromides (18) and fear of habituation with the hypnotic phenobarbital (10,17).

MODERN DRUGS FOR EPILEPSY

The search for better antiepileptic drugs continued into the late nineteenth and early twentieth centuries, with phenobarbital-related substances holding the most promise (1,20,24,26,35). Not until the discovery of the anticonvulsant effect of diphenylhydantoin (phenytoin) in the late 1930s (25,29), however, was there a major breakthrough in the pharmacotherapy of epilepsy. Persons confined to epilepsy colonies could now rejoin the community, and pharmacologists were encouraged to screen other nonsedative compounds for anticonvulsant activity.

The next breakthrough occurred with the introduction of trimethadione in 1946. Originally studied as an analgesic, trimethadione was systematically evaluated in a battery of tests and found to prevent pentylenetetrazol-induced seizures in rats (31) and to be most effective against absence seizures in humans. This discovery brought about the first recognition that better definition of seizure patterns could result in more specific, less toxic treatment of convulsive disorders. Until then, the epilepsies were simply classified according to etiology: those caused by brain lesions (i.e., symptomatic, organic, lesional, structural) and those caused by the brain's predisposition to seizures (i.e., cryptogenic, idiopathic, essential, genetic). New classifications were proposed in the 1960s, when it was recognized that epilepsies caused by brain lesions could diffusely involve the brain, such as the encephalopathy of Lennox-Gastaut syndrome, and that idiopathic epilepsies could be associated with partial seizures, such as the rolandic spikes of benign childhood epilepsy (2). Virtually all controlled clinical trials of new antiepileptic drugs now utilize either the clinical and electroencephalographic classification of

TABLE 1. *Antiepileptic drugs marketed in the United States*

Year introduced	International nonproprietary name	U.S. trade name	Company
1912	phenobarbital	Luminal	Winthrop
1935	mephobarbital	Mebaral	Winthrop
1938	phenytoin	Dilantin	Parke-Davis
1946	trimethadione	Tridione	Abbott
1947	mephenytoin	Mesantoin	Sandoz
1949	paramethadione	Paradione	Abbott
1950	phenthenylate[a]	Thiantoin	Lilly
1951	phenacemide	Phenurone	Abbott
1952	metharbital	Gemonil	Abbott
1952	benzchlorpropamide[b]	Hibicon	Lederle
1953	phensuximide	Milontin	Parke-Davis
1954	primidone	Mysoline	Ayerst
1957	methsuximide	Celontin	Parke-Davis
1957	ethotoin	Peganone	Abbott
1960	aminoglutethimide[c]	Elipten	Ciba
1960	ethosuximide	Zarontin	Parke-Davis
1968	diazepam[d]	Valium	Roche
1974	carbamazepine	Tegretol	Geigy
1975	clonazepam	Clonopin	Roche
1978	valproate	Depakene	Abbott
1981	clorazepate[d]	Tranxene	Abbott

[a] Withdrawn from the market in 1952.
[b] Withdrawn from the market in 1955.
[c] Withdrawn from the market in 1966.
[d] Approved by FDA as an adjunct.

epileptic seizures (8) or the classification of the epilepsies and epileptic syndromes (9), or both.

Spurred on perhaps by the marketing of diphenylhydantoin in 1938, antiepileptic drug development in the late 1940s to the early 1960s made rather startling progress, with the introduction of 12 new drugs, compared with four from 1912 to 1946 (Table 1). The succinimides (phensuximide, methsuximide, and ethosuximide) were an important group of drugs introduced during this period (5), and except for phensuximide, still have a place in antiepileptic therapy.

HIATUS IN DRUG DEVELOPMENT

From 1961 through 1973, no new antiepileptic drugs were marketed in the United States, although nearly fifty drugs or chemical agents were being used or experimentally evaluated for the treatment of epilepsy (21). Only diazepam was approved as adjunct therapy in 1968. Although carbamazepine was marketed in Switzerland in 1963, valproate was released in France in 1967, and clonazepam was marketed in Europe in 1973, there was no enthusiasm for these drugs in the United States. Therapy was often inadequate, but there seemed to be a general impression that better use of the available drugs was the solution to the problem, and many physicians seemed reluctant to try new drugs for their patients even though the familiar ones were not entirely satisfactory. Drug development lagged also from restrictions and costs imposed by new drug testing regulations of the U.S. Food and Drug Administration (FDA) calling for proof of not only the safety of new drugs but also their efficacy (11,16). The history and impact of these regulations have been reviewed in previous editions of this book (3,4). Furthermore, physicians were not well-acquainted with the controlled clinical trials that are essential for the rational development of new drugs for epilepsy, even though as early as 1868

Clouston (6) had called for controlled collaborative trials of bromide. In addition, the pharmacokinetics of drug response were poorly understood.

RENEWING THE SEARCH FOR NEW DRUGS

The situation began to change in the mid-1960s. With the support and encouragement of the then newly established Epilepsy Branch of the National Institute of Neurological Diseases and Stroke (NINDS), the scientific community applied rapidly emerging scientific concepts and technology to the development of new antiepileptic drugs. Guidelines for testing new drugs were advocated by the International League Against Epilepsy (27) and issued by the FDA both as general considerations (12,13) and specifically for antiepileptic drugs (14,15). Revised drug testing guidelines have been proposed (7). The importance of therapeutic drug monitoring to assessment of drug efficacy was emphasized, and methods of determining drugs in body fluids were expanded and refined as potential new drugs were developed.

In 1968, the first controlled clinical trials of several drugs with anticonvulsant properties were initiated by the Epilepsy Branch of NINDS. Experience gained in these trials contributed ultimately to the approval of carbamazepine, clonazepam, valproate, and clorazepate for use in epilepsy in the United States. In 1975, the search for drugs with greater potency and less toxicity than existing drugs began formally with the establishment of the NINDS Antiepileptic Drug Development Program (28). More than 12,000 compounds have been screened since the program's inception. The preclinical testing phase of the program includes toxicologic evaluation of drugs judged to have a favorable anticonvulsant and toxicity profile. Those compounds that show promise as potential new drugs are considered for controlled clinical trials in co-partnership with the pharmaceutical sponsor. An interest in new trial designs has emerged.

A MOLECULAR APPROACH

Consideration is now being focused on the concept that the development of new therapies for epilepsy must be based on knowledge of the molecular and cellular events responsible for the disorder. While such an approach is laudable, it is hampered by lack of knowledge of how existing antiepileptic drugs work and of how seizures are produced. A modest understanding of neuronal events underlying a seizure exists, but details at the molecular level are unknown. Synaptic events relating to inhibition and excitation are beginning to be understood, but the full range of neurotransmitters has probably not been identified. The problem with the current methods of screening for antiepileptic drugs was succinctly stated by Schmidt (32), who said, "The 'ideal' antiepileptic might not even be an anticonvulsant." That is, the current screening tests might fail to discover the antiepileptic effects of drugs that do not protect against experimentally induced convulsions. While awaiting a better understanding of epileptogenesis at the molecular level and its relation to site of drug action, it might be useful to concentrate on the development of new rapid, reproducible, and relatively inexpensive preclinical screening procedures. Examples of such procedures are the kindling and *in vitro* methods, involving neuron cultures and brain slices.

FUTURE OF ANTIEPILEPTIC DRUG DEVELOPMENT

The past decade has seen the better use and testing of antiepileptic drugs through the application of advances in basic neuroscience and new knowledge from neuropharmacology and pharmacokinetics, yet much remains to be done. Improvements are needed in clinical trial methodology, including more rapid determination of drug efficacy and testing of more representative populations. Only in recent years has the distinction been made between epileptic seizures and the epilepsies, and more experience is needed to determine if using the classification of the epilepsies and epileptic syndromes might be a better means of assessing the clinical efficacy of new drugs. It is not known if antiepileptic drugs slow or stop the progression of epilepsy, that is, have a preventive function, or if they simply suppress seizures. As more is learned about mechanisms of drug action, effects of both acute direct suppression and chronic prevention may be found. Antiepileptic drugs traditionally have acted directly on the brain after crossing the blood-brain barrier. Neurologic drugs are now being developed that act in the gut to produce, for example, effects that influence brain neuropeptides. Perhaps in the future, antiepileptic drugs will act by modulating neurotransmitters or some other molecular chemical substance by an action outside the central nervous system.

REFERENCES

1. Blum, E. (1932): Die bekamptung epileptischen anfalle und ihrer filgeerscheinungen mit Proximal. *Dtsch. Med. Wochenschr.,* 58:696–698.
2. Cereghino, J. J. (1989): Treatment implications from classification of seizures and the epilepsies. In: *Epilepsy: Current Approaches to Diagnosis and Treatment,* edited by D. B. Smith, Raven Press, New York.
3. Cereghino, J. J., and Penry, J. K. (1972): General principles. Testing of anticonvulsants in man. In: *Antiepileptic Drugs,* edited by D. M. Woodbury, J. K. Penry, R. P. Schmidt. Raven Press, New York.
4. Cereghino, J. J., and Penry, J. K. (1982). General principles. Testing of antiepileptic drugs in humans: clinical considerations. In: *Antiepileptic Drugs, Second Edition.* edited by D. M. Woodbury, J. K. Penry, and C. E. Pippenger, pp. 141–158. Raven Press, New York.
5. Chen, G., Portman, R., Ensor, C. R., and Bratton, A. C. (1951): The anticonvulsant activity of α-phenylsuccinimide. *Arch. Int. Pharmacodyn. Ther.,* 152:115–120.
6. Clouston, T. S. (1868/69): Experiments to determine the precise effect of bromide of potassium in epilepsy. *J. Ment. Sci.,* 14:305–321.
7. Commission on Antiepileptic Drugs of the International League Against Epilepsy (1989): Guidelines for clinical evaluation of antiepileptic drugs. *Epilepsia,* 30 (*in press*).
8. Commission on Classification and Terminology of the International League Against Epilepsy (1981): Proposal for revised clinical and electroencephalographic classification of epileptic seizures. *Epilepsia,* 22:489–501.
9. Commission on Classification and Terminology of the International League Against Epilepsy (1989): Proposal for revised classification of epilepsies and epileptic syndromes. *Epilepsia,* 30 (*in press*).
10. Dercum, F. X. (1916): Epilepsy with special reference to treatment. *J. A. M. A.,* 67:247–253.
11. *Drug Amendments Act of 1962.* Public Law 87-781, 21, USC 355.
12. FDA (1977): *General Considerations for the Clinical Evaluation of Drugs.* HEW Publication No. (FDA)77-3040.
13. FDA (1977): *General Considerations for the Clinical Evaluation of Drugs in Infants and Children.* HEW Publication No. (FDA)77-3041.
14. FDA (1977): *Guidelines for the Clinical Evaluation of Anticonvulsant Drugs (Adults and Children).* HEW Publication No. (FDA)77-3045.
15. FDA (1980): *Guidelines for the Clinical Evaluation of Anticonvulsant Drugs (Adults and Children).* HHS Publication No. (FDA)81-3110.
16. *Federal Food, Drug, and Cosmetic Act of 1938.* Public Law 717, 75th Congress.
17. Grinker, J. (1920): Experiences with Luminal in epilepsy. *J. A. M. A.,* 75:588–592.
18. Hammond, W. A., and Cross, T. M. B. (1874): *Clinical Lectures on Diseases of the Nervous System.* D. Appleton, New York.
19. Hauptmann, A. (1912): Luminal bei Epilepsie. *Munch. Med. Wochenschr.,* 59:1907–1909.
20. Heyde, W. (1932): Uber proximal-und Luminawirkung bei Schweren epileptischen erkrankugen. *Klin. Wochenschr.,* 50:696–698.
21. Livingston, S. (1966): *Drug Therapy for Epilepsy.* Charles C Thomas, Springfield, IL.
22. Locock, C. (1857): Discussion of paper by E. H. Sieveking. Analysis of fifty-two cases of epilepsy observed by the author. *Lancet,* 1:527–528.
23. Locock, C. (1857): Discussion of paper by E. H. Sieveking. Analysis of fifty-two cases of epilepsy observed by the author. *Med. Times Gazette,* 14:524–526.
24. Maillard, G., and Renard, G. (1925): Un nouveau traitement de l'épilepsie: la phenylmethylmalonyluree (Rutonal). *La Presse Med.,* 1:315–317.
25. Merritt, H. H., and Putnam, T. J. (1938): Sodium diphenylhydantoinate in the treatment of convulsive disorders. *J. A. M. A.,* 111:1068–1073.

26. Peasky, E. (1919): Nirvanol bei Epilepsie. *Med. Klin. Berl.,* 15:364.
27. Penry, J. K. (1973): Principles for clinical testing of antiepileptic drugs. *Epilepsia,* 14:451–458.
28. Porter, R. J., Cereghino, J. J., Gladding, G. D., Hessie, B. J., Kupferberg, H. J., Scoville, B., and White, B. G. (1984): Antiepileptic drug development program. *Cleve. Clin. J. Med.,* 51:293–305.
29. Putnam, T. J., and Merritt, H. H. (1937): Experimental determination of the anticonvulsant properties of some phenyl derivatives. *Science,* 85:525–526.
30. Radcliffe, C. B. (1860): Gulstonian lectures for 1860. On the theory and therapeutics of convulsive diseases, especially of epilepsy. Lecture III (concluded). *Lancet,* 1:614–618.
31. Richards, R. K., and Perlstein, M. A. (1946): A new experimental drug for treatment of convulsive and related disorders. I. Pharmacological aspects. II. Clinical investigations. *Arch. Neurol. Psychiatr.,* 55:164–165.
32. Schmidt, R. P. (1969): Discussion of paper by J. G. Millichap. Relation of laboratory evaluation to clinical effectiveness of antiepileptic drugs. Symposium on Laboratory Evaluation of Antiepileptic Drugs, Salt Lake City, Utah, May 13–14, 1968. *Epilepsia,* 10:326–328.
33. Swinyard, E. A. (1982): Introduction. In: *Antiepileptic Drugs, Second Edition,* edited by D. M. Woodbury, J. K. Penry, C. E. Pippenger, pp. 1–10. Raven Press, New York.
34. Swinyard, E. A., and Goodman, L. S. (1972): Introduction. In: *Antiepileptic Drugs,* edited by D. M. Woodbury, J. K. Penry, and R. P. Schmidt. Raven Press, New York.
35. Weese, H. (1932): Zur pharmakologie des Prominal. *Dtsch. Med. Wochenschr.,* 58:696.

Antiepileptic Drugs, Third Edition, edited by
R. Levy, R. Mattson, B. Meldrum,
J. K. Penry, and F. E. Dreifuss.
Raven Press, Ltd., New York © 1989.

1

General Principles

Drug Absorption, Distribution, and Elimination

René H. Levy and Jashvant D. Unadkat

INTRODUCTION

Most modern textbooks of pharmacology include a chapter on pharmacokinetics in the section covering general principles. However, the relevance of pharmacokinetics to various drug classes is not uniform. In that regard, antiepileptic drugs occupy a privileged position. For example, some of the fundamental concepts of pharmacokinetics were developed to understand the disposition characteristics of phenytoin, a drug with a narrow therapeutic range that also exhibits Michaelis-Menten kinetics. Also, a glance at the table of contents of this text will show that many of the chapters describing each of the major antiepileptic drugs treat their pharmacokinetic aspects.

This chapter covers the basic determinants of drug disposition in the human body. The approach selected emphasizes mechanisms of pharmacokinetic phenomena (distribution, clearance) rather than their mathematical description. Wherever possible, references to specialized textbooks or review articles are given to avoid detailed derivations.

DEFINITIONS AND TERMINOLOGY

One of the main objectives of pharmacokinetics is to describe and interpret quantitatively the time course of levels of a drug and its metabolites in the intact organism. Several definitions of pharmacokinetics have been proposed. Some definitions are quite broad in that they include not only the kinetics of absorption, distribution, and elimination but also the kinetics of pharmacological response, sometimes referred to as pharmacodynamics. The term drug disposition is used to refer to all the processes that account for the fate of a drug in the body. Elimination is understood as referring to drug disappearance by all routes and includes metabolism (or biotransformation) as well as excretion of drug in its unchanged form by any route.

The growth of knowledge in pharmacokinetics has enabled a clearer distinction to be made between linear and nonlinear pharmacokinetic phenomena. Nonlinearities exist with respect to dose and time. Kinetic linearity with respect to dose has been defined as direct proportionality of transfer (e.g., elimination rate) to concentrations. This definition implies that all distribution and elimination processes are first order. Kinetic linearity with respect to time includes the notion of constancy of all rate constants and pharmacokinetic parameters with respect to time. Since pharmacokinetics seek to describe and interpret quantitatively the time course of drug and metabolite levels, it is necessary to use mathematical representations or models. These models vary in degree of complexity, depending on the characteristics of the system they emphasize, and involve one or more compartments. Traditionally, the fate of drugs in the body was conceived of in terms of compartmentalized systems in which compartments are theoretical concepts resulting from specific kinetic behaviors. Such examples are the classic one- and two-compartment models in which each compartment represents an average, rather than an exact, state. Recently, multicompartment models have appeared that emphasize the physiological and anatomical bases of individual compartments. The parameters used in these models are blood flow through organs, tissue-to-plasma distribution coefficients, and extracellular spaces. Such multicompartment physiological models allow a description of tissue concentrations and have been applied to a few drugs, antineoplastic agents in particular.

LINEAR PHARMACOKINETICS

Kinetics After Intravenous Administration

Although few drugs are commonly administered intravenously, an examination of this route of administration makes possible a logical presentation of the concepts of clearance, extraction ratio, volume of distribution, and biological half-life. This is so because administration of an intravenous bolus dose is equivalent to instantaneous absorption and, consequently, intravenous kinetics essentially reflect the processes of distribution and elimination.

One-Compartment Model

The one-compartment model is applicable to drugs for which the kinetics of distribution are rapid compared with the ki-

netics of elimination from the body.[1] In this model, the body is represented as a single compartment of volume V. Distribution is so rapid that there is no visible distribution phase. However, rapid distribution does not imply uniform distribution (as explained below). The first-order rate constant, K, is equal to the sum of several rate constants corresponding to individual processes of elimination (metabolism and excretion). C and A represent drug concentration and amount, respectively, at any time t, and D refers to the dose of drug injected as a bolus at $t = 0$. In quantitative terms, first-order elimination means that at any time $t > 0$, drug concentration decreases in a monoexponential fashion according to

$$C = C_0 e^{-Kt} \qquad [1]$$

Several notions are contained in this relationship: at time zero, C has a value of C_0; the decrease in concentration is largest at the beginning, when concentrations are high, and smaller as time increases and concentrations decrease (Fig. 10); what is constant in an exponential process is the relative rate of decrease of concentration (it is equal to K).

A semilogarithmic ($\log_{10}$) plot of concentration versus time is linear (intercept = C_0 and slope = $K/2.3$). In the special case where $C = \frac{1}{2}C_0$, equation 1 yields a relationship useful in defining the biological half-life, $T_{1/2}$

$$T_{1/2} = \frac{0.693}{K} \qquad [2]$$

$T_{1/2}$ is the time required for blood concentration of the drug to decrease by one-half. This relationship shows that the larger the elimination rate constant, the smaller the half-life.

---

[1] The gastrointestinal tract, as well as the urine, sweat, and expired air, are considered to be outside the body in a pharmacokinetic sense.

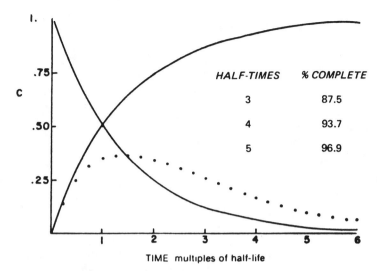

HALF-TIMES	% COMPLETE
3	87.5
4	93.7
5	96.9

TIME multiples of half-life

FIG. 1. Time course of decrease (i.v. bolus) and increase (i.v. infusion) in blood levels as a function of drug half-life (smooth curves). The filled circles represent the time course of blood concentration following a single oral dose. (From ref. 10, with permission.)

Physiological Basis for Drug Distribution and Elimination

Volume of Distribution

At time zero, immediately after injection of the dose of drug, the amount of drug in the body A_0 is equal to the administered dose. Similarly, at that time, the concentration has a value C_0 (which is also apparent in equation 1 when $t = 0$). The volume of distribution can then be determined from the ratio:

$$V = \frac{D}{C_0} = \frac{A}{C} \qquad [3]$$

For drugs exhibiting one-compartment behavior, the volume of distribution is the ratio of amount of drug in the body to blood drug concentration at any time. It is defined as an apparent volume of body fluids in which the drug would be distributed at a concentration equal to that of blood. Although it was traditionally emphasized that this volume is apparent and lacks physiological meaning, it was shown by Gillette (13) that this volume can be related to real body spaces. It can be defined in terms of plasma volume, V_P, and extravascular space (plus erythrocyte volume), V_T, as given by

$$V = V_P + V_T \frac{f}{f_t} \qquad [4]$$

where f represents the fraction of drug unbound in plasma and f_t the fraction of drug unbound in tissues. This approach to volume of distribution has several ramifications. Qualitatively, it shows that the volume of distribution is a function of the drug's affinity for binding to plasma proteins as well as to tissue constituents. Consequently, intersubject variability in volume of distribution can be attributed to individual variation in body size and composition as well as variation in drug binding. This approach is especially useful to explain changes in drug distribution in pathophysiological states where drug binding might be altered, such as in hypoalbuminemia and in uremia. For example, an increase in f (or decrease in binding) should produce an increase in V as long as the other variable,

f_t, is not affected. This is, in fact, the case for phenytoin in uremia. However, the decrease in V of digoxin in uremia is attributed to an increase in f_t larger than the increase in f.

Clearance Concepts.[2]

Clearance is one of the basic determinants of drug disposition, therefore an understanding of clearance concepts is paramount. Clearance emerges as a pharmacokinetic parameter not simply because it represents a mathematical quantity but primarily because it reflects a physiological (and, in some cases, an anatomical) reality. There exist several clearance terms; in order to analyze them in a relatively simple fashion, a few assumptions become necessary. In particular, let us assume that drug elimination occurs only by metabolism through the liver and that the latter behaves as a "well-stirred" organ, such that free drug concentration in the liver is equal to that in the hepatic venous blood. The pharmacokinetic description of clearance takes into consideration the following anatomical and physiological facts: drug is brought to the liver by the portal vein and the hepatic artery and leaves the organ by the hepatic vein. It diffuses from plasma water to reach metabolic enzymes in the smooth endoplasmic reticulum. Therefore, *a priori*, there are at least three major parameters to consider in quantifying drug elimination by the liver: (a) blood flow through the organ, Q, which reflects transport of drug to the organ; (b) degree of protein binding expressed as free fraction of drug in blood, f, which affects access of the drug to the metabolic enzymes; and (c) intrinsic ability of hepatic enzymes to metabolize the drug once it has reached the metabolic enzymes.

The ability of liver enzymes to metabolize

a drug, independent of the limitations of liver blood flow and drug binding in blood, is measured as a clearance term, the intrinsic clearance, Cl'. It is defined as the volume of liver water cleared of drug per unit time. Its relationship to enzyme parameters (maximum velocity, V_{max}, and Michaelis constant, K_m) is a direct one, as seen from the Michaelis-Menten equation under first-order conditions (substrate concentration much smaller than K_m):

$$Cl' = \frac{V_{max}}{K_m} \qquad [5]$$

V_{max} has units of amount per time, and K_m has units of concentration; the ratio has units of volume per time. The net organ clearance or hepatic clearance, Cl_H, is a result of the interplay among these three parameters, as shown in the following relationship:

$$Cl_H = \frac{Q \cdot f \cdot Cl'}{Q + f \cdot Cl'} \qquad [6]$$

The terms Cl_H, Q, and Cl' have units of flow or volume per time, whereas f is a fraction and it is therefore unitless. Cl_H is the apparent volume of blood cleared of drug per unit time. Intuitively, it should be apparent that the maximum clearance that a drug could have should be equal to the total volume of blood reaching that organ per unit time, i.e., blood flow through the organ.

Thus, it is reasonable to compare the actual hepatic clearance of a drug to hepatic flow. In fact, the ratio of Cl_H to Q is an important drug parameter and is called the extraction ratio, E. Its minimum value is 0 for a drug that is not metabolized in the liver, and its maximum value is 1 when Cl_H = Q. The above relationship shows that E is equal to zero when $f \cdot Cl'$ is 0. When $f \cdot Cl'$ is very small relative to Q, hepatic clearance becomes equal to $f \cdot Cl'$, and all flow terms disappear from equation 6 (Fig. 2). In such a case, clearance is called flow independent. It is also referred to as restrictive

---

[2] For additional information on clearance concepts consult Pang and Rowland (26,27), Rowland et al. (31), and Wilkinson and Shand (46).

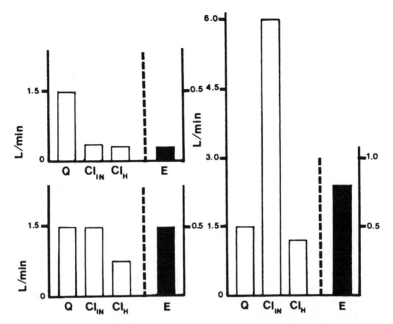

FIG. 2. Relationship between intrinsic clearance (Cl_{in}) and blood flow (Q) and its consequences on hepatic clearance (Cl_H) and extraction ratio (E). The three cases presented illustrate drugs with extraction ratios of 0.10, 0.50, and 0.80.

clearance because it is limited by the free fraction of drug in blood. The product $f \cdot Cl'$ is also a clearance term. Its relationship to Cl' is as follows: whereas Cl' refers to elimination of drug from plasma water in free form, $f \cdot Cl'$ refers to elimination of drug in the free plus bound form. When $f \cdot Cl'$ is much larger than Q (intrinsic ability of liver enzymes is very large), the extraction ratio ($f \cdot Cl'/Q + f \cdot Cl'$) approaches unity, and hepatic clearance approaches hepatic flow. In such a case, clearance is called flow dependent or flow limited (Fig. 2).

Thus, to each drug molecule metabolized by the liver, we can attach an extraction ratio. Drugs can be compared to one another and classified according to their extraction ratios. Most of the antiepileptic drugs in clinical use belong to the low-extraction-ratio category, E < 0.2. Examples of drugs with medium or high extraction ratios are lidocaine, propranolol, and meperidine.

When the liver is not the sole organ re-

sponsible for drug elimination from the body, overall elimination is dependent on the drug systemic clearance, Cl_s, which is defined as the volume of blood cleared of drug from the systemic circulation per unit time. Clearance terms are additive. For example, when a drug is eliminated by hepatic metabolism and renal excretion of unchanged drug, Cl_s is given by:

$$Cl_s = Cl_H + Cl_R \qquad [7]$$

where Cl_R is the renal clearance.

The determination of Cl_s is linked to the calculation of area under the curve (AUC). When a dose, D, of drug is administered intravenously and blood samples are measured for several half-lives, the area under the blood concentration–time curve, AUC_{iv}, can easily be calculated. Systemic clearance is equal to the ratio D_{iv}/AUC_{iv}. Systemic clearance and AUC_{iv} are inversely proportional to each other; although AUC is a measure of drug presence in the body, it also reflects the inability of the eliminating organs to remove a drug; a large AUC is a direct consequence of a low ability of the body to remove a drug.

Relationship Among Clearance, Volume of Distribution, and Half-Life

In the early pharmacokinetic literature, the half-life of a drug was often used as an index of the body's ability to remove a drug. However, for the majority of drugs, half-life and clearance cannot be used interchangeably for that purpose. Relative to clearance and volume of distribution, half-life is a dependent parameter. Individual organ clearances constitute direct measures of the abilities of those organs to eliminate a drug. Independently, a particular value of volume of distribution results from a binding interaction between the drug molecule and tissue constituents and plasma proteins. The more extensive the tissue binding (the lower the f in equation 4), the larger the volume of distribution. Half-life is a result of all these phenomena of distribution and elimination and therefore reflects both processes.[3] Quantitatively, the relationship among these three parameters is:

$$T_{1/2} = \frac{0.693 \ V}{Cl_s} \qquad [8]$$

This relationship shows that the larger the volume of distribution, the longer the half-life. Independently, the larger the clearance, the smaller the half-life. Half-life is dependent on systemic clearance and volume of distribution, whereas clearance and volume are independent of each other and independent of half-life. This approach to the relationship among these three parameters is essential to the understanding of

---

[3] It appears that the confusion in the early literature arose from the fact that clearance was calculated as the product of $K \times V$. Clearance was erroneously interpreted as being dependent on K and V.

changes in kinetic parameters in disease states.

Kinetics After Oral Administration

Qualitative Aspects

The oral route represents the most frequent mode of drug administration, especially since it enables the use of solid dosage forms (tablets, capsules). A number of reviews in the field of biopharmaceutics have discussed the factors that affect drug absorption from the gastrointestinal tract (3,28). Each dosage form should be considered as a drug delivery system which releases the drug in a definite pattern, eventually determining the rate and extent of absorption or bioavailability. The drug must be in solution before it can cross the gastrointestinal membranes and be absorbed. A tablet, for example, must first disintegrate into small particles in order to increase the surface area of drug exposed to gastrointestinal fluids and enhance the dissolution rate. For certain drugs, the processes of disintegration and/or dissolution can become rate limiting. These processes are affected by physicochemical variables, such as salt and crystalline form, and manufacturing variables, such as nature of lubricants, binders, and compression pressure. Physiological variables such as gastric emptying time can also become significant. From the stomach to the duodenum and jejunum, there is an increase in pH and a very large increase in surface area of contact for absorption. Gastric emptying and the accompanying increase in pH are especially significant for drug absorption from enteric-coated tablets. Once in solution, drug molecules are absorbed, mostly by passive diffusion and, less frequently, by facilitated diffusion. When the drug is ionizable, absorption of drug in solution is governed by the pH partition hypothesis and diffusion of the un-ionized species.

Quantitative Aspects

Rate of Absorption

The data accumulated to date on gastrointestinal absorption indicate that for many drugs, absorption behaves like a first-order process in spite of the fact that a number of variables influence this process. The gastrointestinal tract behaves as a single compartment in which the amount of drug decreases at a rate controlled by a first-order absorption rate constant, k_a. A typical oral curve is shown in Fig. 1. The shape of this curve is a direct consequence of the fact that absorption and elimination rates vary over time. The rate of change of amount of drug in the body at any time is equal to the absorption rate minus the elimination rate. At time zero, all of the initial dose, D, is in the gastrointestinal tract. The absorption rate (which is equal to the product of k_a and the amount of drug in the gastrointestinal tract) is at its maximum, since that amount is equal to the total dose. In the body, the elimination rate is equal to the product of the elimination rate constant, K, and the amount of drug in the body A. At time zero, there is no drug in the body, and, consequently, the elimination rate is equal to zero and is at its minimum. Thus, the amount of drug in the body increases rapidly at first since the absorption rate is much larger than the elimination rate. As time increases, the amount of drug in the gastrointestinal tract decreases, and therefore the absorption rate decreases. Simultaneously, in the body the amount of drug increases, and the elimination rate (which is proportional to that amount) increases. There comes a time when the elimination rate reaches a value equal to the absorption rate. At that time, the amount of drug in the body is at its maximum (peak time). At times longer than peak time, the absorption rate continues its decrease toward zero, and the elimination rate also decreases. For the majority of drugs, k_a is larger than K, and the absorption rate becomes negligible shortly after peak time. In this latter phase, drug disappearance in the body reflects only the kinetics of elimination. Consequently, a semilogarithmic plot of concentration versus time is linear in its terminal phase, and the elimination half-life can be determined from that portion of the curve.

In some cases, k_a is smaller than K, and absorption becomes the rate-limiting step during the apparent "elimination" phase. This situation results from the fact that, absorption being slow, the majority of the dose is still in the gastrointestinal tract at peak time. The half-life determined in the terminal phase is the half-life of absorption. This phenomenon is encountered with drugs with slow dissolution rate characteristics and is taken advantage of in the design of sustained-release formulations. The time course of drug amount (or concentration) can be described quantitatively by a biexponential equation (see Appendix). Dose, k_a, and K are three independent variables which determine the value of A at any time. Increasing dose yields increasing peak concentrations (in a proportional fashion), with no change in time course of absorption, k_a, or in elimination half-life. Decreasing the absorption rate constant results in lower peak height and longer peak time. Decreasing the elimination rate constant produces a higher peak concentration and delayed peak times.

Extent of Absorption

The fraction of a dose of drug reaching the systemic circulation, or availability (also called bioavailability), is an important pharmacokinetic parameter (37). Before appearing in the systemic circulation, a drug must cross three different barriers: the gastrointestinal lumen, the intestinal wall, and the liver. Each of these barriers tends to decrease the systemic availability. In the gastrointestinal tract, the dosage form must release the drug (i.e., in the case of a tablet, the processes of disintegration and dissolution must leave the total dose dissolved in the gastrointestinal fluids). Loss of drug can occur through a number of degradation reactions, enzymatic and nonenzymatic (acid hydrolysis), and complexations. The relationship between drug permeability through the intestinal membrane and gastrointestinal transit time must be optimal to enable drug transfer on the mucosal side. Metabolism by enzymes in the intestinal wall must also be avoided. The fraction of dose appearing in the portal circulation, F_G, must then cross the liver where it is subject to the so-called "first-pass effect." The fraction of F_G that is lost by metabolism during the first pass through the liver is equal to the extraction ratio, E. The fraction $F_L = 1 - E$ represents the metabolic availability across the liver. The systemic availability, F, is equal to the product $F_G \cdot F_L$ since F_L can openly operate on the fraction of the dose, F_G, that reaches the liver.

$$F = F_G \cdot F_L \qquad [9]$$

The component F_L of bioavailability is metabolic in nature and cannot be altered by modifications of the dosage form. A drug with an extraction ratio of 0.4 has a maximum bioavailability of 0.6. If 10% of the administered dose is lost prior to appearance in the portal vein, the systemic availability is $F = 0.9 \times 0.6 = 0.54$. Loss of drug by first-pass metabolism is not of consequence among antiepileptic drugs, since they have low extraction ratios. On the other hand, drugs such as aspirin, lidocaine, propranolol, and propoxyphene exhibit significant first-pass effects. The bioavailability, F, is determined by comparison of areas under the curve following oral $[(AUC)_o]$ and intravenous $[(AUC)_{iv}]$ administration of drug (with dose correction, if the intravenous and oral doses are different).

$$F = \frac{[(AUC)_o]}{[(AUC)_{iv}]} \times \frac{D_{iv}}{D_o} \qquad [10]$$

This determination is based on the rationale that it is the same systemic clearance that operates on the dose, D_{iv}, to yield AUC_{iv}, and on the amount, FD_o, to yield AUC_o. The constancy of clearance between the two experiments is an assumption. This assumption can be avoided by using newer methods of determination of bioavailability involving the use of stable, isotopically labeled species. Both studies are performed simultaneously, but each route involves a different isotopic label. This approach is not widespread because blood samples have to be assayed by mass spectrometry to distinguish between the two isotopic masses.

Oral Clearance

The relationship between the determinants of hepatic elimination (blood flow, intrinsic clearance) and the rate and extent of drug bioavailability requires further elaboration. The determination of bioavailability is based on the relationship

$$AUC_o = \frac{FD_o}{Cl_s} \qquad [11]$$

Another clearance term, the apparent oral clearance, Cl_o, which relates D_o and AUC_o, is defined such that

$$AUC_o = \frac{D_o}{Cl_o} \qquad [12]$$

Assuming that the total dose reaches the portal circulation (i.e., $F = F_L = 1 - E$), the term Cl_o can be written as

$$Cl_o = \frac{Cl_s}{F} = \frac{QE}{1 - E} \qquad [13]$$

From the relationship that defines hepatic

clearance as a function of Q and Cl′ (equation 6), it can be shown that

$$f \cdot Cl' = \frac{QE}{1 - E} \qquad [14]$$

and therefore, $Cl_o = f \cdot Cl'$. Thus, the apparent oral clearance of a drug is its intrinsic clearance. This finding has several consequences, especially in assessing the effects of disease states on drug kinetics.

Kinetics of Urinary Excretion

Since the kidney, like the liver, is an organ of drug elimination, mass balance consideration shows that renal clearance, Cl_R, is the ratio of urinary excretion rate (dA_e/dt where A_e refers to amount of drug in urine) and plasma concentration:

$$Cl_R = \frac{dA_e/dt}{C} = \frac{k_e A}{C} = k_e V \qquad [15]$$

where k_e is the rate constant for urinary excretion.

From a knowledge of the value of renal clearance of a drug, inferences can be made as to the mechanisms of renal excretion. Since the value of glomerular filtration rate is equal to 120 mL/min, a renal clearance of 60 mL/min indicates that tubular reabsorption is prevalent. Similarly, a renal clearance larger than 120 mL/min reflects the presence of active secretion.

The proportionality between excretion rate and blood concentration indicates that the excretion rate of a drug will also be governed by the drug's biological half-life. For example, a semilogarithmic plot of excretion rate versus time will be linear with a slope equal to $-K/2.3$. Another consequence of the constancy of renal clearance is the fact that the fraction of a dose excreted unchanged in urine is constant and represents a property of the drug. It is equal to the ratio of excretion-rate constant to elimination-rate constant (k_e/K).

Urinary excretion studies present some practical advantages over blood-level studies. Foremost, they are noninvasive. Also, urinary concentrations are much higher than plasma concentrations and thus easier to assay analytically. However, little use has been made of urinary excretion data in therapeutic drug monitoring.

Multiple-Dose Kinetics

Plateau Principle: Constant-Rate Intravenous Infusion

This principle can be stated in general terms as follows: if the rate of input into a system is constant (zero order), and the rate of output is exponential (first order), the content of the system will accumulate until a steady state is reached. In pharmacokinetics, when a drug is infused at a constant rate, it will eventually reach a steady state or plateau level in blood and tissues. As long as the infusion is maintained, the plateau level is maintained.

Why is a steady state achieved? This question is best answered by comparing the elimination rate to the infusion rate, R, as time increases. At time zero, the amount of drug in the body, A, is equal to zero, and the elimination rate, KA, which is proportional to A, is also equal to zero. Since the infusion rate has a finite value, A begins to increase rapidly. As A increases, the elimination rate, KA, increases. Eventually, KA approaches the value of R, and when KA equals R, A cannot increase further, and a steady state is achieved (A_{ss}). What factors control the value of the steady state? The answer to this question emerges after equating infusion and elimination rates, i.e.,

$$R = KA_{ss} \qquad [16]$$

The amount and concentration at steady state, C_{ss}, are given by:

$$A_{ss} = \frac{R}{K} \qquad [17]$$

$$C_{ss} = \frac{R}{KV} = \frac{R}{Cl_s} \qquad [18]$$

Steady-state drug concentration is directly proportional to the infusion rate, and the constant of proportionality between C_{ss} and R is the reciprocal of clearance. If R is doubled, C_{ss} is also doubled, but, as will be explained further, this does not imply that steady state is reached sooner. Although it is apparent that C_{ss} is also inversely proportional to Cl_s, this notion is not emphasized since Cl_s is not a parameter that can be varied for a given drug.

When is steady state achieved? The rate at which steady state is achieved is determined solely by the elimination rate constant of the drug as shown in the following relationship:

$$C = C_{ss}(1 - e^{-Kt}) \qquad [19]$$

By simple substitutions of values of t equal to multiples of the half-life, we find that $C = 0.5 \, C_{ss}$ at $t = T_{1/2}$, $C = 0.75 \, C_{ss}$ at $t = 2T_{1/2}$, and $C = 0.875 \, C_{ss}$ at $t = 3T_{1/2}$ (Fig. 1). Steady state is practically achieved (97%) after five biological half-lives. Thus, when the infusion rate is doubled, drug concentration at any time is also doubled, but the rate at which steady state is achieved is unchanged. In one half-life, concentration is equal to half of the new steady state.

These notions have several applications in the therapeutic management of patients receiving drugs such as lidocaine that are commonly administered by prolonged constant-rate intravenous infusion. In particular, it is relatively simple to calculate an infusion rate by multiplying the desired steady-state concentration with the value of clearance ($R_o = C_{ss} \cdot Cl_s$). Also, when it is necessary to achieve a steady state rapidly, it is possible to combine the constant-rate infusion with an intravenous bolus dose.

Multiple Dosing

The plateau principle described above is also applicable in the case of discontinuous mode of administration as long as elimination is first order and the rate of drug administration is constant. The latter is the case with a fixed-dose, fixed-time schedule in which the administered dose, D, and the dosing interval, τ, are constant. The dosing rate is equal to the ratio D/τ in the case of intravenous administration and FD/τ for oral dosing. Since drug administration is discontinuous, the steady-state situation is characterized by a maximum, a minimum, and an average drug amount or concentration ($\overline{C}_{ss}$). The relationship that defines $\overline{C}_{ss}$ is essentially the same as that derived for the infusion case:

$$\overline{C}_{ss} = \frac{FD}{Cl_s \tau} \qquad [20]$$

$\overline{C}_{ss}$ is proportional to the dose (also called maintenance dose) and inversely proportional to the dosing interval. The rate of rise of drug concentration toward the steady state is governed by the drug's biological half-life (consistent with the plateau principle). In one half-life, $\overline{C} = 0.5 \, \overline{C}_{ss}$, and in five half-lives, $\overline{C} = 0.97 \, \overline{C}_{ss}$. A number of complex equations have been derived to describe drug concentration at any time during the period of drug accumulation (12,43). However, such concentrations can be simply determined by addition; i.e., the concentration at any time is equal to the sum of the remaining concentrations from all previous doses.

If steady state needs to be achieved rapidly, a loading dose (D_L) can be administered at the first dose. D_L can be obtained by multiplying D by the multiple dose factor [$1/(1 - e^{K\tau})$ for intravenous dosing and $1/(1 - e^{-K\tau})(1 - e^{-k_a})$ for oral dosing]. Alternatively, it can be approximated from the product of the desired steady-state concentration and the volume of distribution ($\overline{C}_{ss} \cdot V$).

The above notions can be used to derive dosage regimens for new drugs or to understand the rationale behind established dosing schedules for old drugs. The frequency of drug administration depends on two parameters: the width of the therapeutic range of the drug and the value of the biological half-life. In cases in which the therapeutic range is narrow (digoxin, phenytoin), there are at least two possibilities: (a) if the half-life is long (longer than 24 hr, digoxin), the dosing interval will be shorter than the half-life (τ = 24 hr or 12 hr or even 8 hr), and oscillations will be less than 50% (the amount of drug in the body at steady state is much larger than the maintenance dose); (b) if the half-life is short (less than 6 hr, lidocaine), the oscillations associated with dosing intervals of 6 to 8 hr are not tolerable (in light of the therapeutic range), and the drug is best administered by constant-rate intravenous infusion. In cases in which the therapeutic range is wide (antibiotics), oscillations are of less concern, and a convenient dosing interval can be selected almost independent of the drug's half-life. If the half-life is short (less than 6 hr), a significant fraction of the dose will be eliminated between doses (A_{ss} is only slightly larger than D). If the half-life is relatively long (over 24 hr), the oscillations between maximum and minimum during the dosing interval would be minimal (A_{ss} is much larger than D). In this latter case, it would take several days to achieve steady state, and a loading dose would be indicated.

Multicompartment Models

For the majority of drugs, the assumption of instantaneous distribution is unrealistic. Drug distribution requires a finite time during which drug elimination also takes place. This is seen clearly after intravenous bolus injection. Drug disappearance from blood (or plasma) is rapid at first, mostly because drug is leaving plasma to enter tissues. This first phase is often referred to as the distributive phase, whereas the slower phase is called the elimination phase. The most commonly used multicompartment model is the two-compartment model which distinguishes between accessible body fluids and highly perfused organs (heart, liver, kidney, brain) and poorly perfused tissues (fat, muscle). Several types of two-compartment models have been derived. Also, three- and four-compartment models have been used. These models generally contain first-order or elimination (input is variable) rate constants. Such models yield differential equations that, when integrated, are of a polyexponential nature (43). The mathematical complexity of such systems is beyond the scope of this chapter, and the reader is referred to several textbooks in which multicompartment systems have been adequately described (11). However, it is important to retain the notion that there are model-dependent and model-independent pharmacokinetic parameters. For example, the relationship between clearance and area under the curve is model independent. Therefore, independently from the polyexponential nature of a given curve, the area under that curve can be determined by the trapezoidal rule, and clearance can be determined. Volume of distribution, on the other hand, is a model-dependent parameter (2). These basic parameters have the same properties as described previously in the case of a one-compartment model.

Kinetics of Drug Metabolites

In humans, the majority of therapeutically useful drugs are eliminated, at least in part, by biotransformation. A given molecule can lead to many (in some cases 50 or more) metabolites. From a clinical point of view, only the efficacious and/or toxic metabolites are of interest. Examples of parent-metabolite pairs among antiepileptic drugs are primidone-phenobarbital, carbamazepine–carbamazepine-10,11-epoxide, and diazepam-nordiazepam. Also, some metabolites devoid of efficacy or toxicity can influence the therapeutic outcome of a drug by interacting pharmacokinetically with the parent drug (e.g., inhibition of phenytoin metabolism by its hydroxy metabolite in the rat). From a drug disposition point of view, it is important to describe all the metabolite conversions that take place once a drug enters the body. In spite of the relevance of this topic, the literature on the kinetics of genesis and elimination of metabolites is relatively limited. As pointed out by Gillette (14), urinary profiles of metabolites do not reflect the "past history" of metabolism in blood or plasma. This section emphasizes the time course of metabolites in blood.

The following discussion is based on a number of assumptions: (a) metabolism of the parent drug occurs only in the liver; (b) the liver behaves as a homogeneous, well-stirred compartment; (c) parent drug and metabolite have low hepatic extraction ratios; and (d) all processes are first order. The basic model considered is shown in Fig. 3.

Area and Steady-State Relationships

The following mass balance relationship holds at all times:

Rate of change of amount of metabolite

$$= \text{Formation rate} - \text{Elimination rate} \quad [21]$$

$$= C \cdot Cl_f - C_m \cdot Cl_m$$

where C and C_m represent parent drug and metabolite blood concentrations; Cl_f is the formation clearance (intrinsic) of the metabolite considered; and Cl_m is the elimination clearance (intrinsic) of the metabolite. Integration of this relationship from time 0 to infinity yields a relationship between areas under the curve of parent drug (AUC) and metabolite (AUC_m):

$$\frac{AUC_m}{AUC} = \frac{Cl_f}{Cl_m} \quad [22]$$

Since, by definition, the sum of $Cl_f + Cl_R$ is equal to the total clearance of parent drug, Cl_s, it follows that the fraction of dose metabolized, f_m, is equal to the ratio of Cl_f/Cl_s. Therefore, the area ratio above can also be expressed as

$$\frac{AUC_m}{AUC} = f_m \frac{Cl_s}{Cl_m} \quad [23]$$

It has been shown that the same relationships hold with average steady-state concentrations of parent drug ($\overline{C}_{ss}$) and metabolite ($\overline{C}_{mss}$) (19).

$$\frac{\overline{C}_{mss}}{\overline{C}_{ss}} = \frac{f_m Cl_s}{Cl_m} \quad [24]$$

These relationships indicate that when a parent drug yields a polar metabolite with a clearance larger than that of its precursor ($Cl_m > Cl_s$), that metabolite will yield an area under the curve smaller than that of

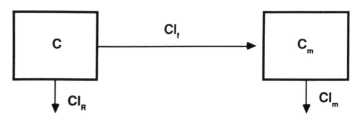

FIG. 3. The basic model for determining the kinetics of drug metabolites in the blood. C and C_m represent parent drug and metabolite concentrations; Cl_f is the formation clearance (intrinsic) of the metabolite considered; Cl_m is the elimination clearance (intrinsic) of the metabolite and Cl_R is the clearance of parent drug by all other routes.

the parent drug. Also, its steady-state concentration will be lower than that of its precursor. Conversely, a metabolite with a clearance lower than that of its precursor ($Cl_m < Cl_s$) will tend to accumulate, yielding high metabolite-to-parent-drug concentration ratios. Thus, a high metabolite-to-parent-drug concentration ratio does not simply reflect a high fraction metabolized. The above relationships also show that in order to determine the fraction of dose of a drug metabolized to a particular metabolite, a knowledge of the clearance of this metabolite is needed. This, in turn, requires administration of the metabolite by a systemic route. The above principles and relationships are independent of the number of metabolites formed.

Kinetic Relationships

The time course of metabolite concentration following a single intravenous dose of parent drug (monoexponential decay) is analogous to that of an oral dose of a drug. The relationship describing concentration of metabolite as a function of time is also biexponential (see Appendix), depending on the elimination rate constants of the parent drug (K) and metabolite (K_m). When the half-life of the metabolite is shorter than that of the parent drug ($K_m > K$), the disappearance of the metabolite is rate-limited by that of the parent drug (the slower). In such a case, the true metabolite half-life cannot be obtained (unless the metabolite is administered separately). When the half-life of the metabolite is longer than that of the parent drug ($K_m < K$), the disappearance of the metabolite is slower than that of the parent drug. The half-life of the metabolite can be determined from data on metabolite concentration following administration of the parent drug (after several half-lives of decay of the parent drug).

Pharmacokinetics in Disease States[4]

Many of the developments in the field of clinical pharmacokinetics have been based on the finding that the pharmacokinetic properties of several drugs are altered in specific pathological states involving the two main organs responsible for drug elimination, the kidney and liver. This section includes the mechanisms of modifications in pharmacokinetic parameters in renal and hepatic disease.

Drug Kinetics in Renal Disease

The early contributions in this area were made by Kunin (18) and Dettli (7,8). The effects of renal disease on the pharmacokinetic behavior of a given drug are related to the drug class to which it belongs. There are three drug classes: type A, drugs eliminated completely by renal excretion; type B, drugs eliminated by hepatic or other nonrenal routes; and type C, drugs eliminated by both renal and nonrenal routes.

Dettli (7) proposed a linear relationship between the elimination rate constant, K, and a measure of glomerular filtration rate such as the clearance of creatinine, Cl_{cr}

$$K = R\,Cl_{cr} + k_{nr} \qquad [25]$$

where k_{nr} is the rate constant for drug elimination by nonrenal routes and R is the slope of the plot of K versus Cl_{cr}. The latter is equal to zero for type A drugs.

When such a relationship has been established for a given drug, a new dosing regimen can be calculated as a function of the degree of renal failure using the computed value of K. The new maintenance dose is reduced proportionately to the reduction in K. Alternatively, a new dosing interval (inversely proportional to the elimination rate constant) can be used. Dosing nomograms

---

[4] The volumes edited by Benet (1) and Evans et al. (9) are recommended reading on this subject.

have been developed for a number of drugs, including gentamicin, kanamycin, and digoxin.

However, Dettli's approach does not take into consideration that renal failure can affect drug elimination by nonrenal routes, as is the case with procainamide. Elimination of metabolites with efficacious or toxic properties is also affected. For example, *N*-acetyl procainamide, a metabolite of procainamide with antiarrhythmic properties, is eliminated primarily by renal excretion. Finally, renal disease has been associated with a reduction in the plasma protein binding of many drugs. An increase in plasma free fraction[5] is expected to produce an increase in plasma clearance (with no change in intrinsic clearance) (equation 6) and an increase in volume of distribution (equation 4). An example that has been extensively studied is phenytoin. Phenytoin free fraction, which is normally around 6% to 10%, increases in uremic patients to reach values as high as 30%. Gugler et al. (16) compared phenytoin steady-state concentrations (C_{ss}), total clearance (Cl_s), and free concentration (Cf_{ss}) in a group of normal subjects (N) and in hypoalbuminemic patients (P) with the nephrotic syndrome: C_{ss} values were 6.8 and 2.9 μg/mL in groups N and P, respectively; corresponding Cl_s values were 0.022 and 0.048 liter/kg·hr; Cf_{ss} values were not significantly different at 0.69 and 0.59 μg/mL, respectively; f values were 0.10 and 0.19 in the two groups. These findings were reanalyzed and explained by pharmacokinetic theory (20). The latter predicts that if the free fraction of a drug with low extraction ratio is increased, the C_{ss} will decrease, but Cf_{ss} will remain unchanged:

$$C_{ss} = \frac{R}{Cl_s} = \frac{R}{f \cdot Cl'} \qquad [26]$$

---

[5] Although the same symbol is used for plasma and blood free fractions, it should be noted that they are related by the blood-to-plasma concentration ratio: free fraction in blood = free fraction in plasma/(blood concentration/plasma concentration).

When f increases, total clearance increases (proportionately), and C_{ss} decreases accordingly. But since $Cf_{ss} = fC_{ss}$, it can be seen that Cf_{ss} is independent of a change in f:

$$Cf_{ss} = \frac{R}{Cl'} \qquad [27]$$

This is in fact the case for phenytoin in patients with the nephrotic syndrome. The increase in clearance in accordance with the increase in free fraction is seen by computing the intrinsic clearance for both groups: 0.22 and 0.25 liter/kg·hr for the N and P groups, respectively. The decrease in C_{ss} with the lack of difference in Cf_{ss} is compatible with the pharmacokinetic rationale provided. These findings suggest that in such instances, monitoring free drug levels would be of interest.

Drug Kinetics in Hepatic Disease

There are at least five categories of liver disease that have been examined with respect to their effects on drug disposition: (a) chronic liver disease, (b) acute hepatitis, (c) drug-induced hepatotoxicity, (d) cholestasis, and (e) hepatic neoplastic disease. The most significant alterations in drug disposition occur in chronic liver disease. A rational understanding of these alterations must be based on physiological models of hepatic elimination that identify the basic determinants of clearance as free fraction in blood (or plasma), intrinsic clearance, and blood flow (5,32,45).

In cirrhotic patients, albumin levels are frequently lower than normal. For several drugs that are highly bound to albumin (diazepam, phenytoin, phenylbutazone, propanolol), the low albumin levels result in a decrease in extent of binding and an increase in free fraction in plasma. As explained previously in the section on hepatic clearance, the consequences of an increase in free fraction in plasma depend on the extraction ratio of the drug. If the latter is high, clearance is independent of free fraction and limited mostly by blood flow. If the extraction ratio is low, an increase in free fraction should result in a concomitant increase in hepatic clearance. This is the case for tolbutamide, amobarbital, and phenytoin. However, intrinsic clearance of free drug may also be affected by the disease state, and the effect on the total clearance is a resultant of the effects of hepatic disease on its components.

In the discussion on volume of distribution, it was pointed out that an increase in plasma free fraction is expected to result in an increase in volume of distribution if tissue binding remains unaltered. This has been shown to be the case for several drugs (diazepam, clorazepam, chlordiazepoxide, and valproic acid). In the cases of phenytoin and tolbutamide in viral hepatitis, it was also suggested that tissue binding was decreased. Consequently, the volume of distribution remained unchanged.

The ultimate effect on drug half-life is a resultant of the changes in clearance and volume of distribution (as shown by equation 8). This is illustrated in the case of tolbutamide. It was found that tolbutamide half-life was decreased in acute viral hepatitis (47). This was totally explained by an increase in plasma clearance, since volume of distribution was unchanged. However, the intrinsic ability of the liver to eliminate the drug was not significantly altered, since all the increase in clearance could be accounted for by an increase in free fraction in plasma.

Although decreases in intrinsic clearance of free drug would be expected in hepatic disease, such occurrences are not systematically found. For example, the intrinsic clearances (free) of theophylline and diazepam were decreased in cirrhotic patients, whereas those of lorazepam and oxazepam were not affected. Similarly, in viral hepatitis, the intrinsic clearances of phenytoin, tolbutamide, warfarin, oxazepam, and lor-

azepam are not affected, whereas those of antipyrine, diazepam, chlordiazepoxide, and hexobarbital are decreased. As was the case for free fraction, decreases in intrinsic clearances of free drug will primarily influence the clearances of drugs with low extraction ratios. In addition, decreases in intrinsic clearance are expected to yield higher oral bioavailabilities for drugs with medium and high extraction ratios (examples are chlormethiazole, labetalol, and pentazocine).

Hepatic blood flow appears to be decreased in chronic liver disease, but is not significantly altered in viral hepatitis. Changes in hepatic blood flow are expected to affect the total clearances of drugs with medium and high extraction ratios. Blood flow probably plays a role in the decreases in clearances observed with lidocaine and propranolol.

Influence of Age on Drug Kinetics

Most of our knowledge of the effect of age on drug disposition has been acquired in the last few years. Although significant differences in drug kinetics have been found among various age groups, no unifying theory is available. Often these differences are drug specific, and it is necessary to examine a number of examples in order to obtain a picture of age effects on drug disposition. One book (24) and three reviews on the subject have been published (17,25,41).

Newborn, Young Infant, and Child

The plasma protein binding of several drugs is generally reduced in newborns. Such a generalization cannot be extended to infants. Newborns have a lower total plasma protein concentration and high levels of free fatty acids, both of which are compatible with higher free fractions than in adults. For example, phenytoin free fraction in newborn is double the adult value and even larger in hyperbilirubinemia. Interestingly, phenytoin volume of distribution is also approximately twice the adult value. In infants (3–24 months), phenytoin binding approaches adult values. In the case of diazepam, plasma free fraction in newborns is also increased, but the volume of distribution is slightly lower than in adults. This is attributed to the lower body lipid content in neonates. Although phenobarbital is not extensively bound in adults (f = 0.5–0.6), its free fraction is slightly increased in the neonate with a corresponding increase in volume of distribution.

Hepatic microsomal activity is reduced in the neonate. Very few clearances have been reported in the literature. However, the half-lives of several drugs including phenobarbital, phenytoin, and valproic acid are longer in the neonate. The patterns of change in drug elimination in the first months of life are drug specific. For phenobarbital, half-life decreases during the first 2 to 4 weeks and remains shorter in infants than in adults. Similarly, diazepam half-life decreases from values of 40 to 400 hr in premature newborns to 8 to 14 hr in infants, whereas adult values range between 20 and 30 hr.

For most antiepileptic drugs, the ratio of steady-state drug level to dose is lower in children than in adults. This reflects the fact that clearance is generally larger in this age group than in adults. In many cases (e.g., carbamazepine), there appears to be a gradual increase in this ratio from the newborn to the adolescent and the adult.

Drug Disposition in the Aged

A body of data has accumulated indicating that the metabolism of some drugs is impaired with increased age (6,30,39,40). Several possible explanations of these observations have been advanced: decreased intrinsic ability to metabolize drugs, selective mortality (rapid metabolizers die

sooner), and resistance to environmental enzyme inducers. For example, the studies of Vestal and Wood (41) illustrate the effects of increasing age on basic kinetic parameters. These authors examined three model compounds with different extraction ratios: antipyrine (low), indocyanine green (high), and propranolol (medium). For antipyrine, the mean plasma clearance was 39% lower in the older age group (48–68 yr) than in the younger age group (21–37 yr). Volume of distribution was significantly smaller in the older group. As a result, there was no significant difference in half-life between the groups. Also, with respect to antipyrine clearance, there was no age group difference among nonsmokers, whereas younger smokers exhibited a twofold larger clearance than older smokers. For indocyanine green, systemic plasma clearance was 46% larger in the younger group. However, there was no age effect in volume of distribution. Consequently, indocyanine green half-life was longer (40%) in the younger group.

The age effect for propranolol paralleled that observed for indocyanine green. Systemic clearance was significantly larger in the younger than in the older group. There was no difference in volume of distribution, and half-life differences reflected the clearance effect. Calculated intrinsic clearances were different between the two age groups only for smokers. Apparent liver blood flow was 24% lower in the older group. The decrease in intrinsic clearance with age manifests itself also in the form of a reduced first-pass effect when propranolol is given orally.

Pharmacokinetics in Pregnancy

Several drugs exhibit a classic pattern of altered pharmacokinetics during pregnancy: at a constant dosing rate, steady-state levels are lower during pregnancy than after delivery or relative to preconception values. Typically, plasma levels decrease by 30% to 50% in a significant proportion of the patients. This phenomenon is prevalent among antiepileptic drugs (22). Several mechanisms have been proposed to account for altered drug disposition during pregnancy. Decreased bioavailability and/or compliance have been suspected but there are no strong experimental findings to support these hypotheses. Plasma protein binding is decreased since albumin concentration decreases from 35 g/liter to 24–30 g/liter in the first half of pregnancy. The decrease in plasma binding is compatible with a decrease in total drug concentration. However, some studies with phenytoin have shown that unbound concentration is decreased during pregnancy. The evidence supporting an increase in metabolic clearance is also limited and therefore the phenomenon of increased drug clearance during pregnancy warrants further investigation. Practically, therapeutic monitoring of drugs with narrow therapeutic ranges is indicated during pregnancy.

NONLINEAR PHARMACOKINETICS

This topic is of particular relevance in the clinical pharmacology of antiepileptic drugs since they exhibit both types of nonlinearities observed in pharmacokinetics: dose dependency and time dependency.

Dose-Dependent Kinetics

Dose dependence results from dependence of rates of transfer or metabolism on concentration. Pharmacokinetically, this results in concentration (or dose) dependence of basic parameters such as free fraction or intrinsic clearance. Thus, plots of area under the curve and steady-state concentration versus dose become nonlinear (Fig. 4), and half-life and the time to reach steady state become dose dependent. Phenytoin is the classic example of a drug exhibiting a decreased clearance with increasing dose as the result of saturable metabolism (38). Valproic acid, on the other hand, exhibits increases in clearance and volume of distribution because of increases in free fraction with increasing dose (4).

From a theoretical point of view, it is of interest to review the relationship between linear and nonlinear behavior of clearance in Michaelis-Menten kinetics. The rate of metabolism, V, is assumed to be dependent on plasma concentration according to the relationship

$$V = \frac{V_{max}C}{K_m + C} \qquad [28]$$

where V_{max} and K_m are as previously defined. For phenytoin, V_{max} values range between 100 and 1,000 mg/day, and K_m values between 1 and 15 µg/mL. When concentration is less than $0.1\ K_m$, V becomes proportional to C in a first-order fashion. The ratio V_{max}/K_m is the clearance and is dose independent. When concentration is much higher than K_m, V becomes equal to V_{max} and is constant and maximum. With concentrations around K_m, V is concentration dependent as described by the above nonlinear relationship.

For a steady state to be achieved, the rate of drug administration, R, has to equal the rate of elimination; i.e.,

$$R = \frac{V_{max}C_{ss}}{K_m + C_{ss}} \qquad [29]$$

From this relationship, it is possible to express C_{ss} as a function of dosing rate

$$C_{ss} = \frac{R \cdot K_m}{V_{max} - R} \qquad [30]$$

When R is smaller than $0.1\ V_{max}$, C_{ss} is proportional to R, the constant of proportionality being the reciprocal of clearance (kinetics are linear). When R is smaller than V_{max} (but larger than $0.1\ V_{max}$), the increase in steady-state concentration is more than proportional to the increase in R (Fig. 4).

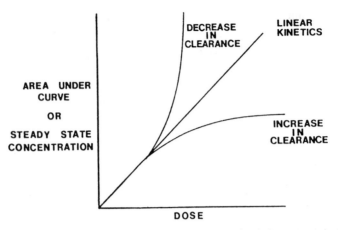

FIG. 4. Relationship between area under the curve or steady-state concentration and dosing rate, illustrating two types of dose dependencies. In linear kinetics, the clearance is constant.

As R approaches V_{max}, C_{ss} increases asymptotically. When R is equal to or larger than V_{max}, a steady state is not achieved. Similarly, the time to reach a fraction of steady state increases with R.

In nonlinear kinetics, clearance and half-life have limited utility. The useful parameters are V_{max}, K_m, and volume of distribution. An extensive body of literature describes methods of determination of V_{max} and K_m for phenytoin and their applications to epileptic patients; the reader may wish to consult reviews (23,38).

Nonlinearity in plasma protein binding results in increases in total clearance for drugs with low extraction ratios (Fig. 4). Increases in dosing rate result in less than proportional increases in steady-state concentration. However, as shown in equation 26, free concentration should increase in proportion to the dose. In such increases, therapeutic monitoring of free levels proves very useful.

Time-Dependent Kinetics

The time dependencies reported in the literature to date can be classified into two categories: (a) physiologically induced time dependency (chronopharmacokinetics); and (b) chemically induced time dependency (21). Both types of time dependencies are found among antiepileptic drugs.

Chronopharmacokinetics[6]

This type of time dependence is related to the fact that rhythms are a fundamental property of most physiological functions. The word chronopharmacokinetics has been used to describe rhythms in drug absorption, distribution, and elimination. Chronovariability in absorption-elimination parameters (such as peak concentration and peak time) has been observed for many different drugs: phenacetin, acetaminophen, antipyrine, chlorazepate, β-methyldigoxin, indomethacin, theophylline, carbamazepine, and clonazepam in rhesus monkeys. Daily variations in enzymatic metabolic activity were also observed with a variety of substrates in rodents. Plasma free fractions of phenytoin and valproic acid were found to vary in a reproducible fashion over a diurnal phase in normal volunteers. Also, several examples have illustrated the fact

---
[6] References to the examples cited can be found in Levy (20).

that the diurnal rhythm in urinary pH influences the excretion of weak acids (salicylic acid, sulfonamides) and bases (amphetamine).

Chemically Induced Time Dependence

Auto- and heteroinduction of drug clearance represent typical examples of this type of time dependence. The time course of change in drug clearance is assessed by following the time course of decreases (addition of inducer) or increases (removal of inducer) in steady-state blood levels. Many examples of such changes have been reported using pharmacokinetic models of induction. Warfarin levels were followed after addition and/or removal of several inducers, dichloral phenazone, antipyrine, amylobarbital, and quinalbarbitone. The time course of autoinduction of carbamazepine was found to be faster in rhesus monkeys (1.5–2 days) than in healthy humans (3 weeks) or epileptic children (3–5 weeks). The decrease in clonazepam levels following the addition of carbamazepine was found to be faster in rhesus monkeys than in humans. The induction of valproic acid and ethosuximide clearances by carbamazepine was also examined in rhesus monkeys and humans.

This second type of time dependence generally has more clinical significance than chronopharmacokinetic phenomena because of the extent of the changes in drug levels. However, chronovariability in pharmacokinetic parameters should be taken into consideration in experimental designs of pharmacokinetics studies.

POPULATION PHARMACOKINETICS AND INDIVIDUALIZATION OF DOSING REGIMENS

An ultimate aim of most pharmacokinetic studies is to design a safe and efficacious dosing regimen of drug for the patient. This individualization of therapy is particularly important for drugs with a narrow therapeutic window, such as the antiepileptics. In order to individualize drug therapy, the average value of the pharmacokinetic parameters of the drug in the patient population must first be estimated. Moreover, whenever possible, the factors responsible for the interindividual variability in the disposition of the drug must be identified. These factors include, but are not necessarily limited to, those already discussed such as age and disease state. Once these parameters have been obtained, therapy with the drug can be initiated and the dosing regimen can subsequently be individualized based on monitoring drug level and adverse effects.

Estimates of the average population pharmacokinetic parameters and their variability (called the population pharmacokinetic parameters) for the patient population of interest can be obtained by one of two methods. The first (called the Two-Stage approach) involves conducting (intensive sampling) pharmacokinetic studies in a large number of patients (20–30) drawn from the population of interest. The pharmacokinetic parameters of the drug in each individual are then estimated and the population pharmacokinetic parameters arrived at by estimating the mean and the covariances of the parameters. The second method is a relatively new approach called Nonlinear Mixed Effect Modeling (NONMEM) (36). This method utilizes routinely collected data (called sparse data) from a relatively large number of patients (for example one to two drug levels from 50–100 patients). This type of data may be collected during routine monitoring of drug levels or they may be collected during phase III/IV efficacy trials of the drug. It is because such data can be used that the NONMEM approach can be much more cost effective when compared with the Two-Stage approach. There are several other advantages to the NONMEM approach. First, the

NONMEM approach has been shown to provide more accurate estimates of the variability of the parameters when compared with the Two-Stage approach (35). Second, the plasma concentration data utilized by the NONMEM approach can be obtained at a random time during the dosing interval. Third, data for each patient need not all be obtained during one dosing interval. The reader is referred to some excellent reviews (34,44) for an in-depth discussion of these two approaches.

There have been several practical applications of the NONMEM approach to individualization of therapy (34). An example of interest here is phenytoin. Sheiner and Beal (35) have obtained estimates of V_{max} and K_m for phenytoin from routinely collected data. Vozeh et al. subsequently showed the utility of these parameters in individualizing phenytoin therapy using the Bayesian approach (see below) in the form of an orbit plot (42). However, this approach can only be used for patients who are representatives of the population used to construct the plot. This could cause a problem if populations differ, as they do for phenytoin, in the manner in which they handle the drug. To elucidate these differences, Grasela et al. (15) investigated the population pharmacokinetics of phenytoin in several populations at different geographical locations, and of varying age, gender, and body size. They found that V_{max} is not influenced by gender, age, height, or location, but is significantly influenced by body weight (V_{max}[mg/day] = 32 × [weight] 0.6) of the patient. The value of K_m is affected by age but in a discontinuous fashion (Table 1).

The use of routinely collected data to derive population pharmacokinetic parameters is a powerful technique that is useful for both new and existing drugs. It can provide useful information as to factors which are important in determining interindividual variability in pharmacokinetics. Last, but not least, population pharmacokinetic pa-

TABLE 1. *Estimates of* K_m

Race	Age (years)	Mean K_m(mg/L)
European	>15	5.7
European	<15	3.2
Japanese	>15	3.8
Japanese	<15	2.2

Data from Grasela et al., ref. 15.

rameters are essential if Bayesian forecasting is to be used in predicting individual dosing regimens.

Bayesian Forecasting of Individual Dosing Regimens

Bayesian forecasting is essentially a sophisticated nomogram based on sound statistical theory. To illustrate the utility and basis of this technique let us consider the phenytoin nomogram proposed by Rambeck et al. (29). This nomogram seeks to predict a steady-state dosing regimen for phenytoin based on prior estimates of the population pharmacokinetic parameters V_{max} and K_m, and a single steady-state plasma concentration. In doing so, they propose that the K_m be fixed to the population estimate and the V_{max} be estimated from the single plasma concentration. Once values of both V_{max} and K_m are available, clearance and the steady-state dose of phenytoin for a target drug concentration can be computed. An assumption made in using this nomogram is that the K_m of the individual is identical to the average K_m of the population. Of course, this assumption is incorrect. The advantage of the Bayesian approach is that such an assumption is not made in forecasting when estimates of the population pharmacokinetic parameters and their (co)variances are avaiable. For example, if K_m variances are available, the Bayesian approach utilizes the information on the variability of the parameter within the population to predict the dosing regimen. For example, if K_m of the population is much more variable than V_m, the Bayesian approach will use this information and will try to hold the estimate of K_m close to that of the population mean while obtaining the best estimate of K_m from the single plasma concentration observation. As further steady-state plasma concentration observations are made, the Bayesian approach will move away from the population estimates and use the data obtained from the patient to refine the estimate of the patient's pharmcokinetic parameters (for further detail, see ref. 33).

REFERENCES

1. Benet, L. Z., ed. (1976): *The Effect of Disease States on Drug Pharmacokinetics.* American Pharmaceutical Association, Washington.
2. Benet, L. Z., and Galeazzi, R. L. (1979): Noncompartmental determination of the steady-state volume of distribution. *J. Pharm. Sci.,* 68:1071–1074.
3. Blanchard, J., Sawchuk, R. J., and Brodie, B. B., eds. (1979): *Principles and Perspectives in Drug Bioavailability.* S. Karger, Basel.
4. Bowdle, T. A., Patel, I. H., Levy, R. H., and Wilensky, A. J. (1980): Valproic acid dosage and plasma protein binding and clearance. *Clin. Pharmacol. Ther.,* 28:486–492.
5. Branch, R. A., and Shand, D. G. (1976): Hepatic drug clearance in chronic liver disease. In: *The Effect of Disease States on Drug Pharmacokinetics,* edited by L. Z. Benet, pp. 77–86. American Pharmaceutical Association, Washington.
6. Crooks, J., O'Malley, K., and Stevenson, I. H. (1976): Pharmacokinetics in the elderly. *Clin. Pharmacokinet.,* 1:280–296.
7. Dettli, L. (1970): Multiple dose elimination kinetics and drug accumulation in patients with normal and impaired renal function. In: *Advances in the Biosciences. Vol. 5,* edited by G. Raspe, pp. 39–54. Pergamon Press, New York.
8. Dettli, L. C. (1974): Drug dosage in patients with renal disease. *Clin. Pharmcol. Ther.,* 16:274–280.
9. Evans, W. E., Schentag, J. J., and Jusko, W. J., eds. (1980): *Applied Pharmacokinetics: Principles of Therapeutic Drug Monitoring.* Applied Therapeutics, San Francisco.
10. Fingl, E. (1972): Absorption, distribution, and elimination: Practical pharmacokinetics. In: *Antiepileptic Drugs,* 1st edition, edited by D. M. Woodbury, J. K. Penry, and R. P. Schmidt, pp. 7–21. Raven Press, New York.
11. Gibaldi, M., and Perrier, D. (1982): Multicompartment models. In: *Pharmacokinetics,* edited by M. Gibaldi and D. Perrier, pp. 45–111. Marcel Dekker, New York.
12. Gibaldi, M., and Perrier, D. (1982): Multiple dosing. In: *Pharamacokinetics,* edited by M. Gibaldi and D. Perrier, pp. 113–144. Marcel Dekker, New York.
13. Gillette, J. R. (1971): Factors affecting drug metabolism. *Ann. N.Y. Acad. Sci.,* 179:43–66.
14. Gillette, J. R. (1977): The phenomenon of species variations; problems and opportunities. In: *Drug Metabolism—From Microbe to Man,* edited by D. V. Parke and R. L. Smith, pp. 147–168. Taylor and Francis, London.
15. Grasela, T. H., Sheiner, L. B., Rambeck, B., Boenigk, H. E., Dunlop, A., Mullen, P. W., Wadsworth, J., Richens, A., Ishizaki, T., Chiba, K., Miura, H., Minagawa, K., Blain, P. G., Mucklow, J. C., Bacon, C. T., and Rawlins, M. (1983): Steady-state pharmacokinetics of phenytoin from routinely collected patient data. *Clin. Pharmacokinet.,* 8:355–364.
16. Gugler, R., Shoeman, D. W., Huffman, D. H., Cohlmia, J. B., and Azarnoff, D. L. (1975): Pharmacokinetics of drugs in patients with the nephrotic syndrome. *J. Clin. Invest.,* 55:1182–1189.
17. Hilligoss, D. M. (1980): Neonatal pharmacokinetics. In: *Applied Pharmacokinetics: Principles of Therapeutic Drug Monitoring,* edited by W. E. Evans, J. J. Schentag, and W. J. Jusko, pp. 76–94. Applied Therapeutics, San Francisco.
18. Kunin, C. M. (1967): A guide to the use of antibiotics in patients with renal disease. A table of recommended doses and factors governing serum levels. *Ann. Intern. Med.,* 67:151–158.
19. Lane, E. A., and Levy, R. H. (1980): Prediction of steady state behavior of metabolite from dosing of parent drug. *J. Pharm. Sci.,* 69:610–612.
20. Levy, G. (1976): Clinical implications of interindividual differences in plasma protein binding of drugs and endogenous substances. In: *The Effect of Disease States on Drug Pharmacokinetics,* edited by L. Z. Benet, pp. 137–151. American Pharmaceutical Association, Washington.
21. Levy, R. H. (1982): Time-dependent pharmacokinetics. *Pharmac. Ther.,* 17:383–397.
22. Levy, R. H., and Yerby, M. S. (1985): Effects of pregnancy on antiepileptic drug utilization. *Epilepsia,* 26 (Suppl. 1):552–557.
23. Ludden, T. M. (1980): Phenytoin. In: *Applied Pharmacokinetics: Principles of Therapeutic Drug Monitoring,* edited by W. E. Evans, J. J. Schentag, and W. J. Jusko, pp. 315–318. Applied Therapeutics, San Francisco.
24. Morselli, P. L. (1977): *Drug Disposition During Development.* Spectrum Publications, New York.
25. Morselli, P. L., Franco-Morselli, R., and Bossi, B. (1980): Clinical pharmacokinetics in newborns and infants: Age-related differences and therapeutic implications. *Clin. Pharmacokinet.,* 5:485–527.
26. Pang, K. S., and Rowland, M. (1977): Hepatic clearance of drugs. I. Theoretical considerations of a "well-stirred" and a "parallel tube" model. *J. Pharmacokinet. Biopharm.,* 5:625–653.
27. Pang, K. S., and Rowland, M. (1977): Hepatic clearance of drugs. II. Experimental evidence for acceptance of the "well-stirred" model over the

"parallel tube" model using lidocaine in the perfused rat liver *in situ* preparation. *J. Pharmacokinet. Biopharm.*, 5:665–680.

28. Prescott, L. F., and Nimmo, W. S., eds. (1981): *Drug Absorption: Proceedings of the Edinburgh International Conference.* ADIS Press, Sydney, Australia.

29. Rambeck, B., Boenigk, H. E., Dunlop, A., Mullen, P. W., Wadsworth, J., and Richens, A. (1979): Predicting phenytoin dose—A revised nomogram. *Ther. Drug Monitor.* 1:325–333.

30. Richey, D. P., and Bender, D. (1977): Pharmacokinetic consequences of aging. *Ann. Rev. Pharmacol. Toxicol.*, 17:49–65.

31. Rowland, M., Benet, L. Z., and Graham, G. G. (1973): Clearance concepts in pharmacokinetics. *J. Pharmacokinet. Biopharm.*, 1:123–136.

32. Rowland, M., Blaschke, T. F., Meffin, P. J., and Williams, R. L. (1976): Pharmacokinetics in disease states modifying hepatic and metabolic function. In: *The Effect of Disease States on Drug Pharmacokinetics,* edited by L. Z. Benet, pp. 53–75. American Pharmaceutical Association, Washington.

33. Sheiner, L. B. (1984): Methods for drug dosage individualization: Past, present and future. In: *Pharmacokinetics,* edited by L. Z. Benet, G. Levy, and B. L. Ferraiolo, pp. 295–314. Plenum Press, New York.

34. Sheiner, L. B., and Beal, S. B. (1984): The population approach to pharmacokinetic data analysis: Rationale and standard data analysis methods. *Drug Metabolism. Rev.,* 15:153–171.

35. Sheiner, L. B., and Beal, S. B. (1980): Evaluation of methods for estimating population pharmacokinetic parameters. I. Michaelis-Menten model: Routine clinical pharmacokinetic data. *J. Pharmacokinet. Biopharm.,* 8:553–571.

36. Sheiner, L. B., Rosenberg, B., and Marathe, V. V. (1977): Estimation of population characteristics of pharmacokinetic parameters from routine clinical data. *J. Pharmacokinet. Biopharm.,* 5:445–479.

37. Tozer, T. N. (1979): Pharmacokinetic principles relevant to bioavailability studies. In: *Principles and Perspectives in Drug Bioavailability,* edited by J. Blanchard, R. J. Sawchuk, and B. B. Brodie, pp. 120–155, S. Karger, Basel.

38. Tozer, T. N., and Winter, M. E. (1980): Phenytoin. In: *Applied Pharmacokinetics: Principles of Therapeutic Drug Monitoring,* edited by W. E. Evans, J. J. Schentag, and W. J. Jusko, pp. 275–314. Applied Therapeutics, San Francisco.

39. Triggs, E. J., and Nation, R. L. (1975): Pharmacokinetics in the aged: A review. *J. Pharmacokinet. Biopharm.,* 3:387–418.

40. Vestal, R. E. (1978): Drug use in the elderly: A review of problems and special considerations. *Drugs,* 16:358–382.

41. Vestal, R. E., and Wood, A. J. J. (1980): Influence of age and smoking on drug kinetics in man: Studies using model compounds. *Clin. Pharmacokinet.,* 5:309–319.

42. Vozeh, S., Muir, K. T., Sheiner, L. B., and Follath, F. (1981): Predicting individual phenytoin dosage. *J. Pharmacokinet. Biopharm.,* 9:131–146.

43. Wagner, J. G. (1975): Linear compartment models. In: *Fundamentals of Clinical Pharmacokinetics,* edited by J. G. Wagner, pp. 57–126. Drug Intelligence Publications, Hamilton, Illinois.

44. Whiting, B., Kelman, A. W., and Grevel, J. (1986): Population pharmacokinetics: Theory and clinical application. *Clin. Pharmacokinet.,* 11:387–401.

45. Wilkinson, G. R. (1980): Influence of liver disease on pharmacokinetics. In: *Applied Pharmacokinetics: Principles of Therapeutic Drug Monitoring,* edited by W. E. Evans, J. J. Schentag, and W. J. Jusko, pp. 57–75. Applied Therapeutics, San Francisco.

46. Wilkinson, G. R., and Shand, D. G. (1975): A physiological approach to hepatic drug clearance. *Clin. Pharmacol. Ther.,* 18:377–390.

47. Williams, R. L., Blaschke, T. F., Meffin, P. J., Melmon, K. L., and Rowland, M. (1976): The influence of acute viral hepatitis on the disposition and plasma binding of tolbutamide. *Clin. Pharmacokinet.,* 5:528–547.

Antiepileptic Drugs, Third Edition, edited by
R. Levy, R. Mattson, B. Meldrum,
J. K. Penry, and F. E. Dreifuss.
Raven Press, Ltd., New York © 1989.

2

General Principles

Biotransformation

Emilio Perucca and Alan Richens

The term biotransformation is used to indicate the process by which the organism metabolizes an exogenous substrate into one or more structurally different derivatives known as metabolites. Teleologically, this process provides an important means for the elimination of a variety of potentially harmful compounds. In fact, many xenobiotics, including drugs, are too lipid-soluble to be excreted efficiently by the kidney and, after being filtrated at the renal glomeruli, they are readily reabsorbed by diffusion from the tubular epithelium. Biotransformation allows the conversion of these compounds to polar, water-soluble metabolites suitable for renal excretion. Although generally drug metabolism represents a detoxication process, there are important exceptions to this rule and in some cases the metabolic products are biologically active and contribute in full or in part to the pharmacological and/or toxic activity of the parent compound. In either situation, changes in the rate of drug metabolism play a fundamental role in determining the intensity and duration of drug action.

PATHWAYS OF DRUG METABOLISM

There are four fundamental types of drug metabolism: oxidation, reduction, hydrolysis, and conjugation. The first three, which precede conjugation in time, are collectively known as phase I reactions, while conjugations are generally referred to as phase II reactions.

In phase I reactions, functional groups such as -OH, -COOH and -NH_2 are introduced into the drug molecule, resulting in the formation of more polar metabolites which may or may not retain pharmacological activity. In phase II reactions, the functional group is coupled with an endogenous substrate such as glucuronic acid, acetic acid, or inorganic sulfate, resulting in the formation of water-soluble conjugates that are generally, though not invariably, inactive and are readily eliminated in the urine or in the bile. Sometimes the metabolic process may be restricted to phase I or phase II reactions only; in the latter case, functional groups suitable for conjugation must already be present in the original molecule.

Almost invariably, the reactions involved in the biotransformation of drugs involve enzymatic catalysis. The enzymes occur for the most part in the smooth endoplasmic reticulum (microsomes) of the liver cells, although a significant degree of enzymatic activity may be present in the microsomes and the cytosol of other organs such as the kidney, the gut, the adrenals, the lung, the skin, and the brain.

Phase I Reactions

Oxidation

Although drug oxidation may take place outside the endoplasmic reticulum (e.g., metabolism of amines by mitochondrial monoamino oxidases), most of these reactions are catalyzed by a microsomal membrane-bound mixed function oxidase containing a cytochrome known as cytochrome P-450.

The metabolism of substrates by this system is effected through a group of P-450 terminal oxidases with electrons supplied by reduced nicotinamide-adenine dinucleotide phosphate (NADPH) and reduced nicotinamide-adenine dinucleotide (NADH), by way of one or more reductases and either directly or by way of cytochrome b5 (59). A trimolecular complex is formed among substrate, enzyme, and molecular oxygen, and one atom of oxygen is incorporated into the cellular water, the other into various reactive intermediates (13,59).

Apart from drugs and other xenobiotics, numerous lipid-soluble endogenous substrates such as free fatty acids, prostaglandins, leukotrienes, steroid hormones, and vitamins function as substrates for the cytochrome P-450 monooxygenase. However, despite the wide variety of biochemical reactions catalyzed, the system is characterized by a high degree of substrate and product specificity that varies in exacting fashion not only with species, strain, sex, tissue, and subcellular compartment, but also with age, hormonal status, disease, and exposure to drugs and environmental chemicals (13,55,56,59). It is known that this specificity of the system can be ascribed to the marked heterogenicity of the P-450 enzyme system, i.e., to the existence of multiple types of these enzymes (22,104). In fact, it has been shown that P-450 enzymes (isozymes) share a common component (the heme group of the cytochrome) but may differ widely with respect to the sequence of about 500 amino acids which constitute the proteic chains.

If the analogy in amino acid sequence between different isozymes is greater than 36%, these isozymes are said to be codified by the same gene "family." At present, several "families" of P-450 genes have been identified in the living organisms, with at least eight of them being detectable in the human DNA (54,55,56). Within each family, it is usually possible to identify "subfamilies" of genes, codifying isozymes with relatively similar (>70% analogy) amino acid sequence. If one considers that each gene may be further subject to considerable polymorphism, it is easy to understand how the system can interact in different ways with an extremely wide variety of substrates. Interestingly, P-450 enzymes obtained from different families of bacterial and human genes show similar amino acid sequences in the portion of the molecule which is proximal to the heme group, providing further support to the hypothesis that all P-450 genes originate from a common ancestor (Fig. 1).

The majority of currently used antiepileptic drugs are extensively metabolized by the mixed function oxidases. Examples of such reactions include the aromatic hydroxylation of phenytoin, phenobarbital, primidone, and carbamazepine; the alkyl oxidation of valproic acid and ethosuximide; the N-demethylation of chlordiazepoxide and trimethadione; and the $S \rightarrow O$ substitution in the conversion of thiopental to pentobarbital. Some of these reactions occur sequentially in the same molecule. Diazepam, for example, is first demethylated in position 1 to nordiazepam and subsequently hydroxylated in position 3 to yield oxazepam, its final phase I metabolite.

Although in many cases phase I metabolites are relatively stable, unstable oxidized intermediates may be formed that undergo rapid hydrogenation or conjugation

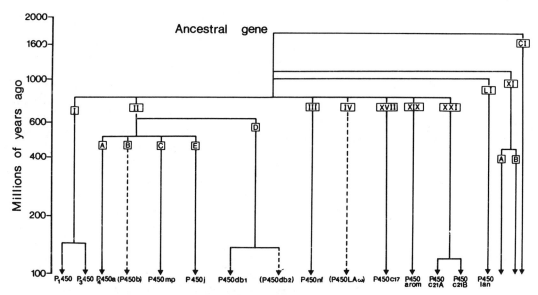

FIG. 1. The evolution of the superfamily of P-450 genes, hypothesized on the basis of the analogies in amino acid sequences of the corresponding enzymes, probably started from a common ancestral gene more than 1,700 million years ago. Gene families I, II, II, IV, XVII, XVII, XIX, and XXI are human or probably human. Enzymes controlled by gene families I, II, III, and IV are predominantly hepatic whereas enzymes codified by gene families XI, XVII, XIX, and XXI are predominantly found in the adrenal cortex and other endocrine organs. Family XI includes mitochondrial genes which are also considered to belong to the human genoma. Family LI is found in vegetals and family CI in bacteria. Based on Nebert and Gonzalez (54,55).

with glutathione, glucuronic acid, or sulfate. The generation of intermediates has considerable practical implications because these compounds, when they are not adequately detoxified, can react with endogenous macromolecules and thereby produce toxic effects such as tissue necrosis, mutagenesis, and carcinogenesis (71). For example, a toxic intermediate, probably the arene oxide (Fig. 2) has been held responsible for phenytoin teratogenicity (19,48), hepatotoxicity (95), and bone marrow toxicity (28). Carbamazepine is also converted to an epoxide intermediate (carbamazepine-10,11-epoxide) which is, however, much more stable than other metabolites and accumulates in serum, possibly contributing to the therapeutic effects of the parent drug. Whether carbamazepine-10,11-epoxide plays any role in mediating serious toxicity, e.g., teratogenic effects, is unclear.

Reduction

Several types of reductive reactions of drugs have been described, the most important examples being the reduction of nitro-compounds (e.g., chloramphenicol) and azocompounds (e.g., Prontosil) to amines and the reduction of ketones (e.g., cortisone) to secondary alcohols (cortisol). The enzymes catalyzing these reactions are predominantly microsomal; certain azo- and nitro-compounds, however, are reduced by gut bacteria and not by mammalian enzymes (16). The role of reductive reactions in the metabolism of antiepileptic drugs is limited, examples being the reduction of nitrazepam to the corresponding amine, the reduction of chloral hydrate to trichloroethanol, and the reduction of nafimidone to its active alcohol metabolite.

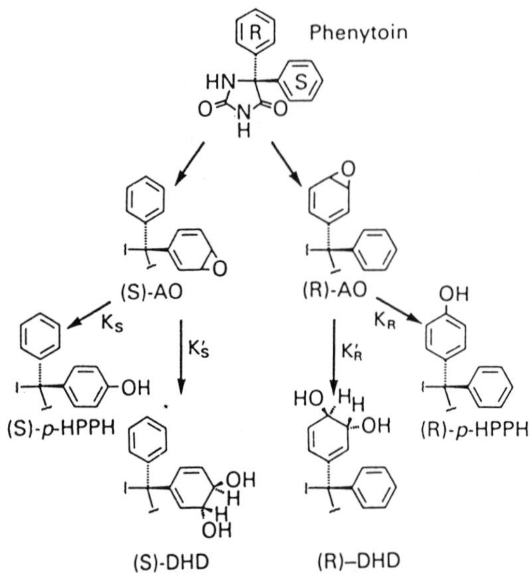

FIG. 2. Stereoselective metabolic pathways of phenytoin to arene oxide (AO), dihydrodiol (DHD) and phenolic (pHPPH) metabolites. From Maguire et al. (46).

Hydrolysis

Hydrolytic reactions are catalyzed by a variety of enzymatic systems that are located not only in the hepatic cells but also in the brain, the blood, and many other tissues. Enzymes such as cholinesterases, carbon anhydrase, and aryl esterases play an important role in phase I metabolism of a number of drugs containing ester groups (110). Another group of hydrolytic enzymes, the epoxide hydrolases, provide a critical protection against tissue damage induced by reactive electrophilic epoxide intermediates.

Phase II Reactions

Phase II reactions can be defined as "a group of synthetic reactions in which a foreign compound or a metabolite thereof is covalently linked with an endogenous molecule or grouping to give a characteristic product known as a conjugate" (18). The

classical conjugation reactions include glucuronidation, glucose conjugation, sulfation, methylation, acetylation, cyanide detoxication, glutathione conjugation, and amino acid conjugation. Several additional types of conjugation with less usual substrates have been described (18). The covalent binding of reactive phase I metabolites to tissue macromolecules can also be considered a form of conjugation.

Most conjugation reactions involve families of specific transferase enzymes, require high-energy nucleotide intermediates, and give rise to more polar, water-soluble metabolites suitable for renal excretion. In some cases, the conjugation product may undergo further metabolism, as in the case of glutathione conjugates ultimately excreted as mercapturic acids. In addition, conjugates may be hydrolyzed by glucuronidases, sulfatases, and amidases. Hydrolysis of enterally secreted glucuronides, for example, may release the lipid-soluble, readily absorbable parent compound thereby providing a crucial step in the enterohepatic circulation of a number of drugs.

Conjugated metabolites are usually pharmacologically inactive, but there are important exceptions to this rule.

Glucuronidation

Conjugation with glucuronic acid, the most common of the synthetic reactions, may occur with compounds containing functions such as the hydroxyl, the carboxyl, the amino, the mercapto, and the dithiocarboxyl groups. The reaction involves the transfer of glucuronic acid from uridine diphosphate (UDP)-glucuronic acid to the aglycone by UDP-glucuronyl transferase, a microsomal enzyme system independent of but functionally related to the mixed function oxidase. Apart from drugs, glucuronide-forming enzymes are actively involved in the metabolism of endogenous substrates such as steroids, bilirubin, and catecholamines. In general, conjugation with glucuronic acid results in drug inactivation, but there are exceptions. The 6-glucuronide of morphine, for example, retains potent analgesic properties, whereas the glucuronic acid and sulfate conjugation of N-hydroxylamines and -amides favors formation of reactive electrophilic ultimate carcinogens (18).

In humans, hepatic UDP-glucuronyl transferases are controlled by genetic and environmental factors and can be drastically reduced in a number of inherited diseases. Patients with Gilbert's syndrome, for example, show a defective conjugation not only of bilirubin but also of a variety of glucuronized drugs.

Examples of glucuronidation reactions involving antiepileptic drugs are plentiful. The majority of phase I metabolites of phenytoin, phenobarbital, primidone, carbamazepine, ethosuximide, valproic acid, and many benzodiazepine drugs are all excreted in urine as glucuronide derivatives. Lamotrigine and lorazepam are examples of drugs whose elimination is primarily dependent upon glucuronidation of the immodified drug molecule.

Acetylation

In acetylation reactions, amino groups situated on the drug molecule or its phase I metabolite(s) react with acetylCoA to form an amide bond. The reaction is catalyzed by nonmicrosomal enzymes, the activity of which may in some cases exhibit marked genetic polymorphism. Not infrequently, N-acetylated metabolites may not be readily excreted and may retain pharmacological activity, thereby contributing to the effects of the parent drug. Examples of drugs yielding acetylated active metabolites include sulfanilamide, procainamide, and acebutolol.

Other Conjugation Reactions

Conjugation with glutathione in its thiol form (GSH) is a crucial reaction in the detoxication of quinones, electrophilic cations, and arene oxides which may result from phase I metabolism of a number of compounds. Several other phase II reactions are known to occur which involve conjugation with glycine, glutamine, cysteine, methyl groups, glucose, sulfate, and many other substrates. The reader is referred elsewhere for detailed information (16,18).

FACTORS INFLUENCING DRUG METABOLISM

It is known that drug metabolism shows remarkable quantitative and, sometimes, qualitative differences not only between different species and between individuals in the same species, but also within the same individual from one time to another. This variability arises as a consequence of different order of factors. Interspecies and interindividual differences in the genes controlling the synthesis and the expression of drug metabolizing enzymes may have a profound influence in determining the mode and rate of biotransformation of a given substrate. Such genetic variation is compounded with the effect of environmental factors that may further modulate the enzymatic profile in different tissues. Some drug metabolizing enzymes, those involved in the metabolism of essential endogenous substrates for example, may be physiologically expressed throughout life whereas others may be synthesized only in certain periods in response to changing hormonal status or exposure to dietary constituents, drugs, and industrial contaminants. Biotransformation may also be influenced by many other factors, e.g., rate of delivery of the drug to the enzyme, pathological changes, and interference by metabolic inhibitors.

The following sections will deal with some of the main sources of variation in hepatic drug metabolism in man. It should be understood, however, that the same factors may also influence the rate of drug metabolism at extrahepatic sites. For certain drugs, e.g., estrogens, the latter may actually be quantitatively more important than metabolism in the liver itself.

Genetic Factors

Since the synthesis of enzymes involved in drug metabolism is controlled by genes, it is not surprising that genetic variation is a main source of differences in drug metabolism among species, sex, and individuals.

Acetylator Phenotype

In a given population, large interindividual differences are observed in the acetylation of drugs such as isoniazid, sulfonamides, hydralazine, amrinone, dapsone, aminogluthetimide and aminonitrazepam, and subjects can be classified as slow or fast metabolizers depending on the rate at which they acetylate these drugs. Slow acetylation is inherited as an autosomal recessive trait, the frequency of the latter being approximately 50% in a Caucasian population. Slow acetylators generally have higher serum levels of the parent drug and, usually, a higher incidence of adverse drug reactions. In some cases, however, the fast acetylator phenotype may also be disadvantageous (82).

Evidence has been accumulating that the acetylator phenotype is not independent of environmental (e.g., nutritional) and developmental factors. The incidence of the slow acetylator status, for example, is much higher in newborns (97) and in the elderly (27) than in nongeriatric adults.

TABLE 1. *Drugs subject to polymorphic oxidation associated with the autosomal recessive trait related to the P-450dbl gene in man*

Antidepressants	Antidysrhythmics
(+)-Amiflamine	Encainide
Amitryptiline	Perhexiline
Chlomipramine	Propaphenone
Desipramine	Propylajmaline
Desmethylchlo-	Sparteine
mipramine	
Nortriptyline	

Beta-blockers	Miscellaneous
Alprenolol	Amphetamine
Bopindolol	Captopril
Bufuraral	Debrisoquine
Metoprolol	Dextrometorphan
Penbutolol	Guanoxan
Propranolol	Indoramin
Timolol	p-Methoxyamphetamine
	Methoxyphenamine
	Phenacetine
	Phenphormin

About 9% of a Caucasian population show defective metabolism of these drugs.

Debrisoquine Hydroxylator Phenotype

About 9% of subjects in a Caucasian population show defective metabolism of debrisoquine, sparteine, and many other drugs (Table 1) (36,39,97). The defect is transmitted as an autosomal recessive trait associated with the P450dbl gene located on chromosome 22 (39,54). The affected cytochrome is a constitutive enzyme not subject to enzyme induction by known inducers in ordinary doses (39). Subjects who are poor metabolizers of debrisoquine show an increased susceptibility to develop adverse reactions to many of the drugs listed in Table 1. On the other hand, these subjects seem to have an advantage compared with the remaining population, since they exhibit a 5- to 40-fold reduction of the risk of developing cancer of the liver and the gastrointestinal tract, probably due to a lower rate of bioactivation of certain dietary constituents such as aflatoxin (39,54). Poor debrisoquine metabolizers also seem less vulnerable to develop lung cancer induced by cigarette smoking.

Mephenytoin Hydroxylator Phenotype

A minority of subjects (approximately 5% of a Caucasian population and 18% of a Japanese population) show a defective capacity to metabolize mephenytoin and mephobarbital (39). The defect is related to polymorphism of the gene P450mp, which belongs to the same family of the P450dbl gene (Fig. 1) and is transmitted as an autosomal recessive trait (105). The implications of the poor mephenytoin hydroxylator status will be discussed in the section dealing with stereoselective metabolism.

Other Genetically Determined Metabolic Defects in Man

Kutt et al. (43) described a genetically transmitted defect in the ability to parahydroxylate phenytoin. Unusually slow hydroxylators of phenytoin have been subsequently described in other studies (68), as have interethnic differences in the rate of phenytoin metabolism (1,39). Although the suggestion has been made that phenytoin metabolism is controlled by the same alleles that regulate debrisoquine hydroxylation (94), a recent study failed to show a correlation between debrisoquine hydroxylator phenotype and metabolism of phenytoin (96).

Other examples of enzymatic defects affecting the metabolism of specific drugs and xenobiotics (e.g., carbocysteine, coumarin, tolbutamide, nifedipine acetophenetidin, benzo(a)pyrene, etc.) have been reported (39,56,75).

Developmental Factors

Age is a well known determinant of the rate of drug metabolism in all species, including man.

Phase I Reactions

In general, although not invariably, phase I reactions are performed at a slower rate in the newborn, especially if premature.

It has been shown that at term, cytochrome P-450, NADPH, and cytochrome c reductase activity approach about one-half the adult value (2). In view of the heterogenicity of the P-450 system, however, the measurement of total P-450 content does not allow a meaningful prediction of the rate at which individual substrates are metabolized. In fact, not only the absolute amount but also the relative proportion of different isozymes may change strikingly during development, thereby providing an explanation for the finding that enzymatic activities involving different substrates are not influenced by gestational age to the same extent and do not follow identical maturational patterns (50,66). The situation *in vivo* is further complicated by the fact that biotransformation rate is affected not only by enzyme activity but also by factors such as hepatic content of the Y anion binding protein, liver blood flow, degree of drug binding to plasma proteins, and presence of endogenous inducers and inhibitors, all of which may be altered in the human neonate (66).

An example of the complexity of the situation is illustrated by the perinatal metabolic pattern of theophylline. Premature newborns are generally unable to demethylate theophylline to 3-methylxanthine (the normal metabolic pathway in infants, children, and adults) but can paradoxically N-methylate the drug to caffeine, a reaction that does not occur in infants and adults (12). Caffeine, in turn, is metabolized at an extremely slow rate in these babies, resulting in accumulation at clinically significant levels. As far as antiepileptic drugs are concerned, their biotransformation is generally reduced in newborns, even though in the case of transplacentally acquired drugs the metabolic rate may be relatively high (compared to nonexposed babies) as a result of enzyme induction occurring during intrauterine life (for review, see Nau et al. [53], Perucca and Richens [76,78] and Perucca [66]).

With most drugs, the biotransformation rate increases gradually over a period of several weeks to several years to peak rates that are often higher than those observed in adults. For some oxidized drugs, the increased metabolic activity is very evident during the period between 2 to 3 months to 2 to 3 years of age, after which the rate of metabolism tends to decline slowly, reaching adult values after puberty. For other oxidized drugs, the maturation of the enzyme system proceeds more slowly and peak values of metabolic rates are reached at a later stage (66). Finally, there are also drugs whose oxidation rate during development never exceeds the level observed in adults.

A typical example of age-dependent changes in metabolic rate is provided by diazepam, the elimination half-life of which varies from 55 ± 35 hr in premature newborns to 31 ± 2 hr in full-term newborns, 10 ± 2 hr in infants, 17 ± 3 hr in children, and 24 ± 12 hr in young adults (49). Phenobarbital shows similar changes, with a serum half-life ranging from 234 ± 43 hr in premature newborns to 146 ± 23 hr in full-term newborns, 58 ± 7 hr in infants, 37–73 hr in children, and 132 ± 18 hr in adults (data from separate studies) (24,49). An increased rate of metabolism in childhood (compared with both neonatal and adult values) has been described also with phenytoin, carbamazepine, ethosuximide, and valproic acid, thereby providing an explanation for the observation that compared to adults, young children (1 to 6 years of age) require larger doses (on a mg/kg basis) of these drugs for therapeutic serum concentrations to be achieved (66).

At the other extreme of life, old age, the rate of metabolism may also be altered. Evidence of a decreased metabolic clearance in the elderly has been provided for a number of oxidized drugs including antipyrine, quinidine, nortriptyline, and verapamil, but for several other drugs oxidation rate shows negligible changes (32,45,90). It has also been reported that the response to enzyme inducers may be decreased in old age (32,90), but evidence for this is conflicting (45). As far as anticonvulsants are concerned, a reduced oxidation rate in the elderly has been reported for various benzodiazepines, including diazepam, chlordiazepoxide, desmethyldiazepam, desalkylflurazepam, alprazolam, and clobazam. A similar effect has been reported also for chlormethiazole, the serum levels of which after an ordinary oral dose are higher in the elderly than in the young (52). Serum phenytoin levels also tend to be higher in the elderly compared with young patients receiving comparable doses (35); in elderly patients with hypoalbuminemia, however, phenytoin clearance may be accelerated, probably because the lower degree of plasma protein binding facilitates drug uptake into the hepatic cell (33). The ability to metabolize valproic acid is also moderately impaired in the elderly, as indicated by a decrease in the clearance of free drug (intrinsic clearance). This results in the elderly having higher free (nonprotein-bound) plasma valproic acid levels compared to young subjects given equivalent doses, even though the total plasma levels of the drug may not differ in the two groups because of the concomitant reduction in valproate plasma protein binding in old age (66). The kinetics of a single dose of carbamazepine are reportedly unaltered in old age (34) but these data may not be necessarily representative for the kinetics of the drug after long-term dosing.

Phase II Reactions

Most phase II reactions take place at a slower rate in the newborn, especially if premature (6,66). The impairment in conjugating capacity affects particularly the glucuronidation pathway, while sulfate conjugation may occur at a relatively efficient rate.

As babies grow older, the enzyme systems responsible for conjugation mature at different rates. Maturation proceeds more slowly for glucuronide conjugation compared with other pathways, even though the development of glucuronizing capacity varies depending on the substrate being investigated due to heterogenicity of UDP-glucuronyl transferases. In any case, adult values of glucuronizing activity are usually reached within 3 years of age (66).

Information on the efficiency of phase II reactions in elderly patients is still limited. Aging, however, seems to affect glucuronide conjugating capacity much less than oxidation capacity (45,90). The glucuronidation of oxazepam, lorazepam, and temazepam is not much different in the elderly compared with the young (32).

Sex, Pregnancy, and Other Factors

Sex

Marked sex-linked differences in rate of drug metabolism are seen in laboratory animals, but in man these differences are usually relatively minor and of little importance. After correction for height and/or body weight, serum phenytoin, primidone, and phenobarbital levels are reported to be higher in males than in females receiving equivalent doses (35,102). Whether these findings reflect differences in metabolizing capacity is unknown.

Sex may also modulate the response to a variety of factors affecting drug metabolism. The decrease in the rate of oxidation of various drugs in the elderly, for example, is much more marked in men than in women (32).

Pregnancy

Several factors may affect the rate of drug metabolism during pregnancy. These in-clude hormonal changes, a physiological rise in body temperature, the contribution of the fetoplacental unit to drug metabolism, alterations in drug binding to plasma proteins, and hemodynamic changes affecting the rate of delivery of the drug to the site of metabolism (66).

Although in rodents pregnancy is usually associated with a decrease in rate of drug metabolism, the situation in humans is much more complex. In a recent review of the literature on drug disposition in pregnant women, Perucca (66) concluded that no univocal pattern of metabolic changes could be characterized from the data surveyed. Although for most drugs metabolic clearance is usually increased during the last trimester of pregnancy, there are examples of compounds whose metabolism is not significantly affected by the pregnant state (e.g., propranolol). Others, notably caffeine and theophylline, may actually exhibit a clear-cut reduction of biotransformation rate as gestation progresses.

As far as anticonvulsants are concerned, evidence has been provided that the biotransformation rate of phenytoin, carbamazepine, and valproic acid frequently increases in pregnant women, leading to a reduction of the levels of these drugs in serum (Fig. 3) (44,66,76). Serum phenobarbital levels also tend to decrease during pregnancy, but the effect may be mediated by an increased renal clearance of the drug and may not necessarily involve increased metabolism. An increased renal and hepatic elimination during pregnancy has also been reported for primidone (66), although a recent study suggests that in some pregnant patients with epilepsy the conversion of primidone to phenobarbital may actually be inhibited (9).

Nutritional Factors, Physical Activity, and Circadian Rhythms

Diet, nutritional status, physical activity, and circadian rhythms may have an appre-

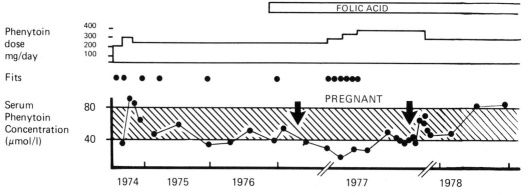

FIG. 3. Serum phenytoin concentrations in an epileptic woman who was followed prospectively throughout pregnancy. Arrows indicate times of conception and delivery. The hatched area corresponds to the commonly quoted optimal serum concentration range. Note the changes in dosage requirements during pregnancy (probably due to increased metabolic clearance) and the worsened seizure control associated with the fall in serum drug levels. From Perucca and Richens (76).

ciable influence on the rate of drug metabolism. The reader is referred elsewhere for detailed information (26,51,84).

Influence of Dosage and Substrate Selectivity

Enzyme Saturation

The biotransformation of most drugs administered in therapeutic doses *in vivo* follows first-order kinetics, i.e., the metabolizing organs remove a constant percentage of the amount of drug delivered to them during a unit of time.

If the amount of drug presented to the metabolism site exceeds a given limit, however, the enzymes will become saturated and the percentage of the substrate metabolized per unit of time will decrease with increasing drug concentration: first-order kinetics no longer apply. A situation of this kind sometimes occurs during the absorption of orally administered drugs when high concentrations of newly absorbed drug molecules reach the liver via the portal vein. This phenomenon has practical implications

for certain drugs undergoing significant "first-pass" metabolism (see Chapter 2) because enzyme saturation results in a higher proportion of the dose escaping presystemic elimination. This explains why the oral availability of certain drugs increases with increasing dosages.

Saturation kinetics occurring during the postabsorptive (elimination) phase is a much less common phenomenon affecting a limited number of drugs, phenytoin being the most prominent example (87). The saturable nature of phenytoin metabolism has two important practical implications:

1. When the phenytoin parahydroxylating enzyme gradually becomes saturated, the percentage of the drug in the body which is metabolized per unit of time decreases with increasing drug concentration. This implies that the rate of elimination of the drug decreases progressively as dosage and serum concentrations are increased. When treatment is discontinued, the elimination phase is not log-linear and the half-life shortens with decreasing concentrations.

2. The relationship between the steady-state serum concentration and the admin-

istered dose is nonlinear; a change in dosage produces a disproportionately large change in serum concentration and, thereby, pharmacological effect. As illustrated in Fig. 4, the limit at which the dose-concentration relationship steepens shows considerable intersubject variability, making the effect of dose increments on the serum concentration poorly predictable in the individual patient.

In the presence of saturable metabolism, the metabolic pattern can be described at best by using the classic equation of enzyme kinetics: the Michaelis-Menten equation. In its original form, this equation states that the velocity of any enzyme-catalyzed reaction (V) is related to the concentration of the substrate (S) by the relationship:

$$V = V_{max} \, S/(K_m + S) \qquad (1)$$

where V_{max} is the maximum rate of metabolism and K_m a proportionality constant for that enzyme, defined as the concentration

of substrate at which $V = \frac{1}{2} V_{max}$. When the system operates under nonsaturable conditions, $S \ll K_m$ and equation (1) reduces to:

$$V = V_{max} \, S/K_m \qquad (2)$$

i.e., the velocity of the reaction is linearly related to the concentration of the substrate (first-order kinetics).

Various rearrangements of the Michaelis-Menten equation have been proposed in order to allow a more or less accurate prediction of the phenytoin dosage adjustments acquired to produce a desired serum concentration (87,107). Although it must be accepted that an experienced clinician can usually tailor satisfactorily phenytoin dosage without resorting to nomograms or mathematical calculations, some of these methods can be useful in particular cases and have a considerable didactical value in allowing a more rapid familiarization with the practical problem posed by saturation kinetics.

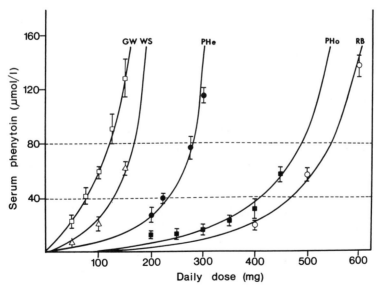

FIG. 4. Relationship between steady-state serum phenytoin concentration and phenytoin dosage in patients studied at different doses. Each point is the mean (± s.d.) of 3 to 8 determinations at each dose level. The horizontal lines represent the limits of the commonly quoted optimal range. Modified from Richens and Dunlop (88).

Feedback Inhibition by Metabolite Formation

Animal experiments have suggested that the dose-dependency of phenytoin metabolism may in fact be caused not by enzyme saturation but by feedback inhibition by the main biotransformation product, 5-p-hydroxphenyl-5-phenylhydantoin (p-HPPH). *In vitro*, the addition of phenytoin at different concentrations to fortified 9,000 × g rat liver supernatants does not affect the rate of hydroxylation of the drug, whereas addition of p-HPPH to the system inhibits hydroxylation in a competitive manner (14,29). *In vivo*, direct administration of p-HPPH to rats (5) and to monkeys (30) also has a dramatic inhibitory effect on phenytoin metabolism.

In order to examine the possibility that product inhibition may also operate in man, we determined the total body clearance of phenytoin during an intravenous infusion of the metabolite and during a control infusion of the solvent in three healthy volunteers (70). Under these conditions, p-HPPH did not produce any consistent change in phenytoin elimination. Together with other lines of evidence (78), these data suggest that feedback inhibition does not occur in man.

Stereoselectivity in Drug Metabolism

A significant proportion of drugs, including many anticonvulsants, exist as enantiomers (optical isomers). The importance of differentiating between individual isomers is becoming increasingly clear to scientists involved in the study of drug action and disposition. In fact, enantiomers of the same drug may differ enormously with respect to both pharmacological properties and pharmacokinetic profile. A case especially relevant to this chapter is where two enantiomers may be differently metabolized, i.e., may be subject to stereoselective metabolism.

One of the first documented examples of stereoselective drug metabolism in man concerned the barbiturate R,S-hexobarbital, a drug which is virtually entirely cleared by oxidation in the hepatic microsomes. Although hexobarbital is normally administered as a racemic mixture, Breimer and Van Rossum (15) have shown that significant central nervous system (CNS) depressant effects can be observed after administration of the S-isomer but not after intake of equivalent doses of the R-isomer. In the same study, the metabolic clearance of S-hexobarbital was found to be about one-third of that of R-hexobarbital. Thus, even though it is likely that the two isomers also differ in intrinsic activity, their potency differences in man could be explained at least in part on the basis of stereoselectivity in hepatic drug oxidation. Metabolic stereoselectivity has been demonstrated recently for another barbiturate, pentobarbital, even though for this compound differences in elimination rate between individual enantiomers are not as marked as with hexobarbital (21). Another important example of a drug undergoing enantioselective metabolism is acenocoumarol. The metabolic inactivation of R-acenocoumarol is only about one-tenth of that of S-acenocoumarol, an observation which explains the much greater anticoagulant activity of the former isomer (31). It should be noted that the stereoselective metabolism is not restricted to differences in metabolic fate of enantiomeric substrates. As pointed out by Testa (99), a wide variety of metabolic reactions result in the creation of new centers of asymmetry that did not exist in the original substrate. Phenytoin is a good example of a nonenantiomeric drug which is converted to enantiomeric metabolites (Fig. 2).

Stereoselective metabolism may be importantly affected by genetic factors, one of the best examples being that of R,S-mephenytoin, an anticonvulsant metabolized by different cytochrome P-450 isozymes. While S-mephenytoin ($t\frac{1}{2} \approx 1$ h) is rapidly parahydroxylated, its R-enantiomer ($t\frac{1}{2}\approx70$ h) is slowly demethylated to the pharmacologically active metabolite 5-ethyl-5-phenylhydantoin (nirvanol) which, in turn, is eliminated very slowly ($t\frac{1}{2}\approx150$ to 200 h) and accumulates in serum. Under normal conditions, therefore, the pharmacological effects of R,S-mephenytoin are entirely dependent on accumulation of the R-isomer and its N-demethylated metabolite.

Approximately 5% of Caucasians, however, have a genetic defect resulting in deficiency of the isozyme responsible for parahydroxylation of the S-isomer. In these subjects, both isomers are cleared slowly but at similar rates by N-demethylation and therefore contribute equally to pharmacological effects. In these poor metabolizers, the N-demethylated active metabolite (nirvanol) is present at concentrations several-fold higher than in extensive metabolizers (106); interestingly, nirvanol is also enantioselectively parahydroxylated and the same defect exists for its S-isomer, proving that a single cytochrome P-450 isozyme catalyzes S-mephenytoin and S-nirvanol hydroxylation (42). A situation similar to that described for mephenytoin has been described for the beta-blocker R,S-metoprolol and for the anticonvulsant R,S-mephobarbital. The genetic defect in the R-metoprolol poor hydroxylators is linked to the debrisoquine phenotype, unlike the defect in poor hydroxylators of R-mephobarbital which seems to be linked to the mephenytoin phenotype. In the case of mephobarbital, stereoselective metabolism has considerable practical implications. In fact, in extensive metabolizers, R-mephobarbital is cleared very rapidly and only S-mephobarbital is available for conversion to phenobarbital, which is responsible for the antiepileptic effect. In poor metabolizers, the clearance of R-mephobarbital is dramatically reduced and this isomer is also converted to phenobarbital, which accumulates at concentrations much higher than those seen in fast hydroxylators.

Drug interactions at metabolic level may also show a high degree of stereoselectivity. For example, sulfinpyrazone has been shown to increase the metabolic clearance of R-warfarin (probably by displacing it from plasma protein binding sites) while inhibiting the metabolism of the more potent S-warfarin (101). This results in a markedly higher concentration of the S-enantiomer, explaining the potentiation of the anticoagulant response. If the plasma levels of racemic warfarin are measured, the opposing effects of the interaction on the R- and S-isomers cancel out reciprocally and no apparent changes in warfarin kinetics are seen. This example emphasizes the important point that blood levels and pharmacokinetic parameters of racemates often do not reflect those of the active enantiomers (3,26,103).

Enzyme Induction

In 1956, Conney and co-workers (20) at the University of Wisconsin first reported that administration of a xenobiotic, 3-methylcholanthrene, causes an increase ("induction") in the activity of certain microsomal enzymes in rat liver. At about the same time, Remmer (85) showed that phenobarbital also induces the hepatic microsomal enzymes. Subsequent studies demonstrated that 3-methylcholanthrene and related polycyclic hydrocarbons are very potent inducers of the intracellular concentration of a specific form of cytochrome P-450, namely the variety that exhibits a spectral absorption of the reduced carbon monoxide complex at 448 nm. Conversely, the cytochrome P-450 induced by phenobarbital exhibits an absorption peak at exactly 450 nm (58).

During the last 30 years, evidence has accumulated that, in addition to phenobarbital and 3-methylcholanthrene, several other pharmacological agents, industrial contaminants, voluctuary substances, and dietary substances possess the ability to stimulate the drug metabolizing enzymes in the liver and/or other organs. Typically, this stimulatory effect affects especially the P-450 microsomal monooxygenases, although induction of other enzymatic pathways (e.g., epoxide hydrolase or glucuronide conjugation) has also been documented. The main features of the induction of the P-450 enzymes have been reviewed recently (58):

1. Enzyme induction is demonstrable only *in vivo*, requires *de novo* synthesis of proteins, and can be demonstrated only with some delay following exposure to the inducing agent. In this respect, the phenomenon of enzyme induction differs from the instantaneous enhancement of reaction velocity caused by metyrapone and a number of other compounds. The latter enhancement occurs also *in vitro*, does not require synthesis of new enzymes, and has been variably ascribed to a selective inhibition of the less active variant of cytochrome P-450 in the constitutive enzyme or to preferential channeling of electrons to a particular enzyme-substrate complex leading to accelerated hydroxylation;

2. Particular inducers induce particular forms of cytochrome P-450 and, therefore, may have strikingly different effects on the metabolism of specific substrates. The two best known prototypes are the phenobarbital and the 3-methylcholanthrene types of induction, but it is now clear that there are other inducers that stimulate the enzyme system with a pattern not completely overlapping those typical of 3-methylcholanthrene or phenobarbital;

3. Morphologically, enzyme induction is associated with a proliferation of the smooth endoplasmic reticulum and, in some species, hepatic hypertrophy.

Further information on the biochemical features and clinical significance of the induction of the P-450 enzymes caused by 3-methylcholanthrene (and related polycyclic hydrocarbons) and phenobarbital are reviewed in the sections below. Induction of conjugating enzymes will also be discussed briefly under a separate heading. Induction of steroid-responsive forms of cytochrome P-450 by steroid hormones will not be reviewed here and the reader is referred elsewhere (89) for detailed information on this topic.

Polycyclic Hydrocarbons Type of Induction

As mentioned above, polycyclic hydrocarbons predominantly cause induction of the P448 variety of the cytochromic enzymes. During treatment with compounds such as benzo(a)pyrene and 3-methylcholanthrene the oxidation of barbiturates and the N-demethylation of ethylmorphine (two reactions markedly accelerated by phenobarbital pretreatment) are not induced, although arylhydrocarbon hydroxylase (AHH) activity increases several-fold. The mechanism responsible for the induction of AHH activity has been elucidated (56) and involves the interaction of the inducing agent with a cytosolic receptor, known as the Ah receptor. The inducer-receptor complex undergoes temperature-dependent translocation into the nucleus, where it causes transcriptional activation of the P_1-450 and P_3-450 genes (Fig. 1) and the synthesis of new enzymes that will metabolize the inducing chemical(s) to innocuous products. In addition, the induced enzymes are responsible for the production of reactive intermediates, leading to tissue necrosis or cancer.

Animal studies have demonstrated that there are genetic differences in the expression of the Ah receptor and, therefore, of the induction process (39). Differences in the expression of the Ah receptor also exist in the human species and are likely to be a major determinant of the individual susceptibility to the carcinogenic effects of environmental or voluctuary contaminants. The practical importance of this is highlighted by the observation that subjects belonging to that proportion of the population with a high AHH inducibility present a 20- to 40-fold increase in the risk of cigarette smoke-induced lung cancer (40).

In addition to 3-methylcholanthrene and benzo(a)pyrene, molecules that interact with the Ah receptor include 2-, 3-, 7-, 8-tetrachlorodibenzo(p)dioxin (TCDD), benzo(a)anthracene, and beta-naphthoflavone.

Since polycyclic hydrocarbons are among the 3,000 chemicals identified so far in cigarette smoke, many investigators have compared the effect of cigarette smoking on drug metabolism with those of Ah-type inducers. In man, cigarette smoke has been reported to induce the oxidation of diazepam, desmethyldiazepam, phenacetin, nicotine, antipyrine, theophylline, propranolol, imipramine, and pentazocine, but not to affect significantly the metabolism of meperidine, nortriptyline, ethanol, phenytoin, phenobarbital, and carbamazepine (10,38,51). It is unlikely, however, that the inducing properties of tobacco smoke are related to an important extent to its content in polycyclic hydrocarbons (86). It has been repeatedly demonstrated, for example, that in experimental animals polycyclic hydrocarbons accelerate markedly the metabolism of benzo(a)pyrene and other substrates both in the liver and in extrahepatic tissues, whereas the inducing effect of cigarette smoke is much more prominent at extrahepatic sites such as the placenta. Differences in tissue reactivity also exist in humans.

Recently, Pelkonen and co-workers (60,61,62) examined AHH, 7-ethoxycoumarin deethylase (ECDE), and 7-ethoxyresorufin O-deethylase (ERDE) activities, three markers of hepatic induction by polycyclic hydrocarbons, in human liver and placental samples obtained from both smokers and nonsmokers. In the placenta all enzyme activities were found to be increased by cigarette smoking, but in the

liver only ERDE activity was enhanced significantly. Evidence was also obtained that the cytochrome P-450 responsible for hepatic AHH and ECDE is different from the cytochromes that are responsible for the induced levels of AHH and ECDE in the placenta. These findings highlight the importance of exploring factors affecting drug metabolism at extrahepatic sites. Inducibility of certain drug-metabolizing enzymes in the placenta intestine, kidney, and lung is probably a primary determinant of the susceptibility to cancer caused by environmental agents in these organs. Depending on the type of carcinogen and type of inducer being considered, enzyme induction may either enhance or reduce the tumorigenic response (86).

Phenobarbital Type of Induction and Induction by Other Drugs

The cytochromic enzymes stimulated by phenobarbital differ from those induced by polycyclic hydrocarbons in the spectral properties of their carbon monoxide complex, and they also differ markedly in respect to their activity toward certain substrates. The cluster of enzymes induced by phenobarbital appears to be codified by genes located on human chromosome 19 (39) and includes those responsible for the hepatic metabolism of a variety of drugs and endogenous compounds such as cortisol, testosterone, and vitamin D_3. Unlike polycyclic hydrocarbons, phenobarbital appears to be devoid of effects stimulating the placental monooxygenases (62).

Although the ability of phenobarbital to stimulate the microsomal drug metabolizing enzymes has been known for about 30 years, the mechanism responsible for this effect has not been fully clarified. It seems that phenobarbital induces a 2 kilobase (kb) mRNA which carries the code for the translation of the induction process. The basic mechanism, in any case, does not appear to require a specific receptor of the type involved in the induction of AHH activity (58).

Many other compounds have been shown to stimulate the hepatic mixed function oxidases with an induction pattern overlapping, at least in part, that observed with barbiturates. The list of such compounds identified in laboratory animals exceeds several hundred but, due to differences in dosage and interspecies variation in response, those causing clinically significant enzyme induction at therapeutic doses in man are much fewer. Examples of the latter include antipyrine, ethanol, glutethimide, aminoglutethimide, medroxyprogesterone, the combination metaqualone-diphenydramine, sulfinpyrazone, rifampicin, and the anticonvulsants phenytoin, carbamazepine, and primidone.

The comparative enzyme-inducing properties of different anticonvulsants in epileptic patients have recently been examined by measuring two indirect indices of induction, the clearance of antipyrine and the urinary excretion of D-glucaric acid (Fig. 5) (69). Compared with drug-free controls, patients receiving chronic treatment with phenytoin, phenobarbital, carbamazepine, and primidone showed a marked increase in both antipyrine metabolism and D-glucaric acid excretion, whereas in valproate-treated patients these parameters were usually within the control range. Within groups receiving a single enzyme inducer, the degree of stimulation of the hepatic microsomal enzymes was positively correlated with the prescribed daily dosage, confirming that enzyme induction is a dose-dependent phenomenon. Although the increase in antipyrine clearance caused by average therapeutic dosages of these anticonvulsants is relatively similar, evidence has been provided that the P-450 isozymes induced by carbamazepine and phenytoin are different from those induced by barbiturates (92).

The clinical consequences of hepatic mi-

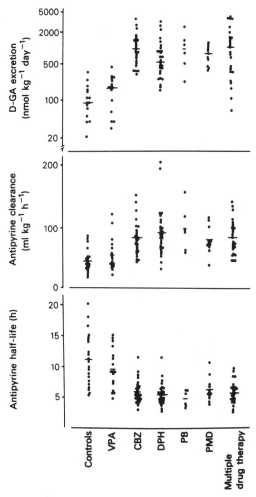

FIG. 5. Antipyrine clearance, antipyrine half-life, and urinary excretion of D-glucaric acid in normal control subjects and in epileptic patients receiving chronic therapy with valproic acid (VPA), carbamazepine (CBZ), phenytoin (DPH), phenobarbital (PB), and primidone (PMD) alone or in combination (Multiple Drug Therapy). Each symbol represents individual subjects. From Perucca et al. (69).

crosomal enzyme induction by antiepileptic drugs are considerable (63,64,65). Self-stimulation of metabolism (autoinduction) is most clearly observed with carbamazepine and is responsible for the progressive decline of the serum concentration and the shortening of the serum half-life of the drug

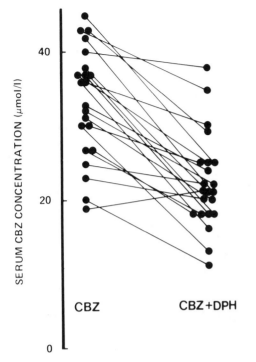

FIG. 6. Steady-state serum carbamazepine levels in 22 pairs of patients receiving long-term treatment with equivalent doses of carbamazepine (CBZ) alone or in combination with phenytoin (DPH). Due to induction of carbamazepine metabolism, serum carbamazepine is lower in patients also taking phenytoin. From Perucca and Richens (72).

TABLE 2. *Drugs whose metabolism may be stimulated by enzyme-inducing anticonvulsants*

Acetanilide	Lidocaine
Acetaminophen	Meperidine
Aminopyrine	Mesoridazine (active
Antipyrine	metabolite of thiori-
Benzodiazepines	dazine)
(many)	Methadone
Carbamazepine	Metronidazole
Chloramphenicol	Methylprednisolone
Chlorimipramine (and	Metyrapone
desmethyl-chlori-	Mexiletine
mipramine)	Mianserin
Chlorpromazine	Misonidazole
Chlorpropamide	Nitroglycerine
Cimetidine	Nomifensine
Cortisol	Nortriptyline
Cyclophosphamide	Phenacetin
Cyclosporin	Phenylbutazone
Dexamethasone	Prednisone (and pred-
Dicoumarol	nisolone)
Digitoxin	Propoxyphene
Disopyramide	Propranolol (and other
Doxycycline	beta-blockers)
Estrogens	Protriptyline
Ethosuximide	Quinine
Felodipine	Quinidine
Flunarizine	Testosterone
Folic acid	Theophylline
Fenoprofen	Thyroxine
Haloperidol	Valproic acid
Hexobarbital	Vitamin D
Imipramine (and des-	Warfarin
methyl-imipramine)	

The list is not exhaustive and not all inducers may share the stimulating effect. Modified from Perucca (65).

a few weeks after initiation of treatment. Stimulation of metabolism of other concurrently administered drugs also occurs and is responsible for a number of interactions which are seen in patients treated with phenytoin, barbiturates, carbamazepine, and other enzyme inducing drugs (Fig. 6 and Table 2). Some of these interactions may have considerable clinical importance, as in the case of the enhanced elimination and consequent reduction of the efficacy of conventional doses of various steroids, antibiotics, oral anticoagulants, antidysrhythmics, and psychotropic drugs. Since the induction profile caused by phenobarbital, primidone, phenytoin, and carbamazepine may not be exactly overlapping, stimulation of the metabolism of all the compounds listed in Table 2 may not necessarily be observed with each of these anticonvulsants.

Perhaps even more important are the clinical consequences of the metabolism of endogenous substrates (see ref. 65 for review). Increased metabolism of vitamin D_3 is probably responsible for the development of anticonvulsant-induced rickets and osteomalacia. Also hypothesized is a possible role of enzyme induction in the development of anticonvulsant-induced folate deficiency and in the pathogenesis of the vitamin K-responsive hemorrhagic disorder in neonates born to drug-treated epileptic mothers, although in the case of these disorders other mechanisms are more likely to be operating. Additional examples of clinical or biochemical abnormalities possibly related to enzyme induction include: altered metabolism of cortisol (with increased production of 6-beta-hydroxycortisol), of other steroid hormones, and of thyroid hormones; increased serum levels of alpha$_1$ acid glycoprotein, sex hormone-binding globulin, gamma-glutamyltransferase, and alkaline phosphatase; precipitation of porphyric attacks in patients with acute intermittent prophyria; and enhancement of insulin-mediated glucose disposal rate (65).

Induction of Conjugating Enzymes

Similar to cytochromes P-450, conjugating enzymes consist of families of isozymes, some of which may be subject to induction. Induction of reduced glutathione (GSH) transferases by phenobarbital has been known for several years and may have considerable biological significance in view of the role played by these enzymes in the detoxication of reactive electrophilic phase I metabolites such as epoxides.

Induction of glucuronizing enzymes also occurs, as exemplified by the elevation in phenol-UDP glucuronyl transferase (UDP-GT) by 3-methylcholanthrene and bilirubin UDP-GT by phenobarbital. The latter phenomenon is responsible for the decrease in serum unconjugated bilirubin in patients receiving enzyme-inducing anticonvulsants (91) and has been exploited therapeutically in the management of neonatal unconjugated hyperbilirubinemia. Animal experiments suggest that different classes of inducers stimulate the synthesis of different types of UDP-GT enzymes: examples include the preferentially increased glucuronidation of chloramphenicol and morphine by phenobarbital, of polar phenols by 3-methylcholanthrene, of bilirubin by clofibrate, and of digitoxigenin-monodigitoxoside by spironolactone (11).

Unlike GSH-transferases and UDP-GTs, sulfotransferases do not appear to be inducible by xenobiotics (100).

Enzyme Inhibition

Inhibition of the drug metabolizing enzymes may be caused by a variety of mechanisms, the most common of which is competition by alternative substrates (58). Similarly to inducers, inhibitors usually interfere with only a limited number of isozymes and may therefore be used as discriminators between different enzymatic forms.

Not surprisingly, many of the best known examples of interactions resulting in inhibition of metabolism *in vivo* involve those drugs which exhibit saturation kinetics at therapeutic dosages, such as phenytoin. The list of drugs reported to more or less consistently inhibit phenytoin metabolism is impressive (64,77) and includes dicoumarol, phencoupromon, disulfiram, sulthiame, pheneturide, methsuximide, imipramine, chlorpromazine, methylphenydate, phenyramidol, chlorphenyramine, propoxyphene, phenylbutazone, chloramphenicol, isoniazid, trimethoprim, various sulphonamides, valproic acid, omeprazole and cimetidine. The clinical implications of these interactions may be considerable: due to the saturable nature of phenytoin metabolism, even a moderate degree of enzyme inhibition can result in a marked rise in the serum phenytoin concentration at steady-state, and clinical intoxication is likely to occur. Usually, the elevation of serum phenytoin after addition of the interfering agent occurs rapidly, but there are exceptions to this rule: in the case of sulthiame, for example, a period of 10 to 20 days may elapse before the interaction becomes manifest (Fig. 9), suggesting that a noncompetitive type of inhibition may be operating.

The metabolism of other antiepileptic drugs is also vulnerable to inhibition. Clinically important examples include the inhibition of phenobarbital metabolism by valproic acid and the inhibition of carbamazepine metabolism by propoxyphene (23) and macrolide antibiotics (7,8). In the case of macrolides, the mechanism of the interaction is known to involve the binding of reactive intermediates to cytochrome P-450-Fe(II) (47).

Interactions involving inhibition of non-oxidative enzymes are also known. An important example is the inhibition of epoxide hydrolase by valpromide, the amide derivative of valproic acid (Figs. 8 and 9) (80,81). If valpromide is added to the therapeutic regimen of patients stabilized on carbamazepine therapy, the resulting inhibition of epoxide hydrolase results in reduced breakdown of the active metabolite carbamazepine-10,11-epoxide, which accumulates at high levels and produces toxicity (80). Valproic acid also shows an elevating effect on carbamazepine-10,11-epoxide lev-

els, but this is less marked than that observed with valpromide (Fig. 7) (80). Since epoxide hydrolases are involved in the detoxication of harmful epoxide intermediates derived from the metabolism of various xenobiotics, inhibition of these enzymes may have implications beyond the interaction with carbamazepine.

Another group of enzymes that is important in inactivation/detoxication is represented by conjugating enzymes. In animal experiments, inhibition of GSH-transferases, UDP-glucuronyl-transferases, and sulfotransferases has been shown to enhance the susceptibility to the toxic effects of reactive intermediates derived from chemicals such as benzo(a)pyrene (17). A clinically important example of inhibition of conjugating enzymes is provided by the inhibition of lamotrigine glucuronide formation by valproic acid.

A particular type of noncompetitive metabolic inhibition exploited in recent years

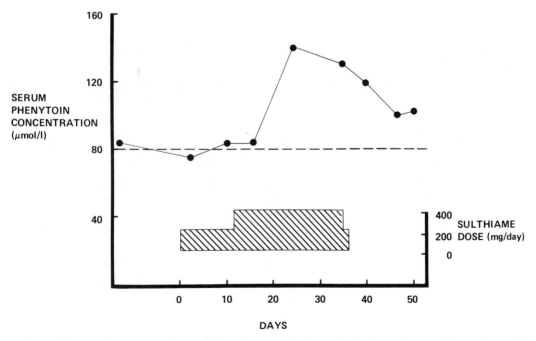

FIG. 7. Changes in serum phenytoin level after addition of sulthiame in a patient stabilized on a constant dose of phenytoin. The horizontal line corresponds to the upper limit of the commonly quoted optimal range. From Perucca and Richens (75).

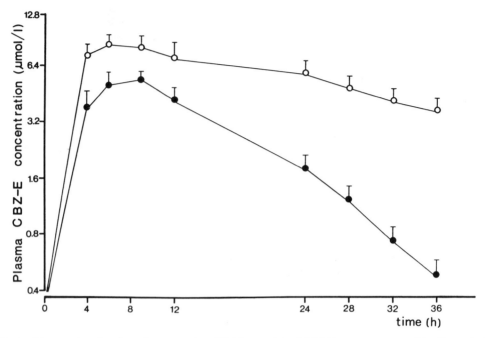

FIG. 8. Plasma levels of carbamazepine-10,11-epoxide (CBZ-E, means, ± s.d.) after administration of a single dose of the metabolite (100 mg) in six subjects in a control session (●) and during coadministration of valpromide (600 mg/day for 8 days) (○). Note the marked inhibitory effect of valpromide on CBZ-E elimination. Data from Pisani et al. (81).

for the development of new pharmacological tools is represented by the irreversible effect of "suicide inhibitors." These compounds are inert *per se*, but are metabolized by a specific enzyme to highly reactive intermediates which bind covalently to the same enzyme and inactivate it. The mode of action of the anticonvulsant vigabatrin is mediated by its capacity to act as an irreversible suicide inhibitor of γ-aminobutyric acid (GABA)-transaminase.

Combined Enzyme Induction and Inhibition

Enzyme induction and inhibition are not mutually excluding phenomena and may occur at the same time. The ability of a given compound to act as an inducer and inhibitor at the same time provides an explanation for the inconsistent and apparently contradictory nature of certain drug interactions. Phenobarbital, for example, may either decrease or increase the serum concentration of phenytoin depending on whether stimulation or inhibition of phenytoin metabolism prevails in an individual patient. In the case of ethanol, inhibition is usually observed after acute ingestion whereas induction prevails in the chronic alcoholic.

Plasma Protein Binding and Blood Flow

The rate at which drugs are biotransformed *in vivo* is determined not only by the activity of the drug metabolizing enzymes but also by the rate of delivery of the individual compounds to the site of metabolism. The degree of drug binding to plasma proteins and the blood flow to the metabolizing organ(s) are important factors to be

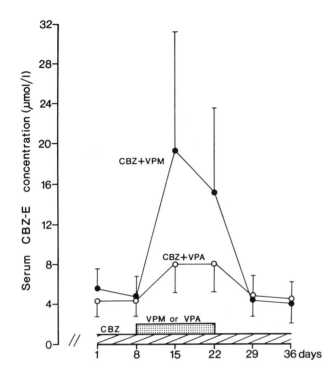

FIG. 9. Changes in serum carbamazepine-10,11-epoxide (CBZ-E) levels after addition of bioequivalent doses of valpromide (VPM) (1,200 mg/day) or sodium valproate (VPA) (1100 mg/day) for 2 weeks to the therapeutic regimen of patients stabilized on a constant dosage of carbamazepine (means ± s.d., n = 6 for each group). Serum carbamazepine (CBZ) levels were not affected by the interaction. The apparent decrease in CBZ-E levels on day 22 in the valpromide group is due to the fact that two patients with very high CBZ-E concentrations required early reduction of valpromide dosage because of side effects. Data from Pisani et al. (80).

considered in this respect. Their role, however, varies depending on the kinetics of the individual compound (74,109).

In the case of drugs taken up avidly by the metabolizing organ, both the free and the protein-bound molecules are extracted during their passage through the organ; under these conditions, an increase in protein binding and/or blood flow may enhance the rate of metabolism by allowing a more efficient delivery of the substrate to the site of metabolism.

The situation is entirely different in the case of drugs poorly extracted by the metabolizing organ (these include most of the major anticonvulsants). In this case, only the free, nonprotein-bound molecules can be taken up and an increase in protein binding actually restricts the amount of drug available for metabolism. The clearance of these drugs will also be independent from blood flow.

A detailed discussion of the effects of protein binding and blood flow on metabolic clearance can be found in Chapter 2 in the sections dealing with restrictive (flow-independent) and nonrestrictive (flow-dependent) elimination.

Disease

Hepatic and Renal Disease

The effect of liver disease on hepatic drug metabolism is complex. On one hand, reduction of drug metabolizing enzyme activity, through hepatocellular damage, and disruption of hepatic vascular architecture, by reducing drug availability at the site of metabolism, tend to decrease the metabolic capacity of the organ. On the other hand, in the case of highly protein-bound drugs characterized by restrictive elimination (Chapter 2), the latter effects may be counterbalanced by a concomitant reduction in the degree of plasma protein binding, which increases the amount of free drug available for metabolism in the liver. Which of these opposing mechanisms will predominate depends on a combination of factors such as the type and the severity of hepatic disease, the degree of hypoalbuminemia, the age of the patient, and the route of drug administration (108). The alteration of the metabolism of individual antiepileptic drugs in hepatic disease has been reviewed by Asconapé and Penry (4).

The metabolic elimination of phenytoin and many other drugs is increased in uremia (4,83). At least for phenytoin, the effect cannot be explained entirely by a reduction in the degree of drug plasma protein binding.

Other Diseases

Apart from hepatic and renal disease, many other pathological conditions may be associated with alterations in drug metabolism (51). An example is provided by the changes in the metabolism of many drugs in patients with thyroid dysfunction (93).

CLINICAL RELEVANCE OF DRUG METABOLISM

Many of the examples presented in this chapter have already highlighted the importance of the biotransformation process in determining drug response. As far as relevance to drug prescribing is concerned, one of the major problems facing the clinician rises from the wide interindividual variability with which these processes occur.

It is well known that in patients with impaired renal function the dosage of drugs which are excreted unchanged in urine must be individualized on the basis of the glomerular filtration rate. For drugs eliminated through biotransformation, dosage also needs to be individualized to take into account the marked interindividual differences in drug metabolism. As a general rule, patients with reduced drug metabolizing capacity are more likely to develop signs of

toxicity when given "standard" doses of a drug and require doses lower than usual for a satisfactory therapeutic effect to be achieved. Most slow metabolizers of phenytoin, for example, will develop marked ataxia when stabilized on an average (300 mg) dose of the drug, whereas fast metabolizers may require doses higher than this. With many drugs (phenytoin is a good example), monitoring of serum drug levels will help to identify the dosage that best suits individual needs.

A particularly complex situation may arise when a drug is converted to active metabolites. In this case, the relative contribution of the metabolite to the overall biological effect will depend on a combination of factors such as the relative potency and the rate of elimination of the metabolite itself, the duration of treatment, and the route of administration of the parent drug. For primidone, for example, there is evidence that much of the antiepileptic efficacy during long-term treatment is in fact mediated by its metabolite phenobarbital. In some of these cases, monitoring serum metabolite levels may prove valuable in individualizing drug dosage. In the future, new techniques (including the use of DNA probes to identify subjects with genetic defects in drug metabolism) are likely to become available to predict accurately the rate of metabolism in individual patients.

A final important aspect that needs to be emphasized at this point is the relevance that biotransformation processes have in fields not strictly related to drug therapy. In view of the role played by the drug metabolizing enzymes in the activation and/or detoxication of many endogenous and exogenous substances, it is not surprising that any factor affecting the function of these enzymes may exert influences which go far beyond an altered responsiveness to a given drug. The study of the relationship between the function of specific isozymes in various tissues and the processes involved in aging, cancerogenesis, teratogenesis, and other disorders represents a fascinating chapter in the history of medicine and is likely to provide in the future additional important clues for the prevention and treatment of disease.

REFERENCES

1. Andoh, B., Idle, J. R., Sloan, T. P., Smith, R. L., and Woolhouse, N. (1980): Inter-ethnic and inter-phenotype differences among Ghanaians and Caucasians in the metabolic hydroxylation of phenytoin. *Brit. J. Clin. Pharmacol.,* 9:282–283P.
2. Aranda, J. V., Louridas, A. T., Vitullo, B. B., Thom, P., Aldridge, A., and Haber, R. (1979): Metabolism of theophylline to caffeine in human fetal liver. *Science,* 206:1319–1321.
3. Ariens, E. J. (1984): Stereochemistry, a basis of sophisticated nonsense in pharmacokinetics and clinical pharmacology. *Eur. J. Clin. Pharmacol.,* 26:663–668.
4. Asconapé, J. J., and Penry, J. K. (1982): Use of antiepileptic drugs in the presence of liver and kidney disease: A review. *Epilepsia,* 23(Suppl. 1):65–80.
5. Ashley, J. J., and Levy, G. (1972): Inhibition of diphenylhydantoin elimination by its major metabolite. *Res. Comm. Chem. Pathol. Pharmacol.,* 4:297–306.
6. Assael, B. M. (1982): Pharmacokinetics and drug distribution during postnatal development. *Pharmacol Ther.,* 18:159–197.
7. Barzaghi, N., Gatti, G., Crema, F., Faja, A., Monteleone, M., Amione, C., Leone, L., and Perucca, E. (1988): Effect of furithromycin, a new macrolide antibiotic, on carbamazepine disposition in normal subjects. *Clin. Pharmacol. Res. (in press).*
8. Barzaghi, N., Gatti, G., Crema, F., Monteleone, M., Amione, C., Leone, L., and Perucca, E. (1987): Inhibition by erythromycin of the conversion of carbamazepine to its active 10,11 epoxide metabolite. *Brit. J. Clin. Pharmacol.,* 24:836–838.
9. Battino, D., Binelli, S., Bossi, L., Como, M. L., Croci, D., Cusi, C., and Avanzini, G. (1984): Changes in primidone/phenobarbitone ratio during pregnancy and the puerperium. *Clinical Pharmacokinetics,* 9:252–260.
10. Benetello, P., Furlanut, M., Pasqui, L., Carmillo, L., Perlotto, N., and Testa, G. (1987): Absence of effect of cigarette smoking on serum concentrations of some anticonvulsants in epileptic patients. *Clinical Pharmacokinetics,* 12:302–304.
11. Bock, K. W., Lilienblum, W., Fischer, G., Schirmer, G., and Bock-Hennig, B. S. (1987): Induction and inhibition of conjugating enzymes with emphasis on UDP-glucuronyltransferases. *Pharmacol. Ther.,* 33:23–27.
12. Bonati, M., Latini, R., Marra, G., Assael, B. M., and Parini, R. (1981): Theophylline metabolism during the first month of life and development. *Ped. Res.,* 15:304–308.
13. Boobis, A., Caldwell, J., De Matteis, F., and Davies, D. (eds.) (1985): *Microsomes and Drug Oxidations.* Taylor and Francis, London.
14. Borondy, P., Chang, T. and Glazko, A. J. (1972): Inhibition of diphenyl-hydantoin hydroxylation by 5-(p-hydroxyphenyl)-5-phenyl-hydantoin. *Fed. Proceed.,* 31:582.
15. Breimer, D. D., and van Rossum, J. M. (1973): Pharmacokinetics of (+)-, (−)-, and (±)-hexobarbitone in man after oral administration. *J Pharm. Pharmacol.,* 25:762–764.
16. Brodie, B. B., and Gillette, J. R. (eds.) (1971): *Concepts in Biochemical Pharmacology,* Vol. 28. Springer-Verlag, Berlin.
17. Burke, M. D., Vadi, H., Jernstrom, B., and Orrenius, S. (1977): Metabolism of benzo(a)pyrene with isolated hepatocytes and the formation and degradation of DNA-binding derivatives. *J. Biol. Chem.,* 252:6424–6431.
18. Caldwell, J. (1982): Conjugation reactions in foreign-compound metabolism: Definition, consequences, and species variations. *Drug Metab. Rev.,* 13:745–777.
19. Clapper, M. L., and Klein, N. W. (1986): Identification of a teratogenic drug-protein complex in sera of phenytoin-treated monkeys. *Epilepsia,* 27:685–696.
20. Conney, A. H., Miller, E. C., and Miller, J. A. (1956): The metabolism of methylated aminoazo dyes. V. Evidence for induction of enzyme synthesis in the rat by 3-methylcholanthrene. *Cancer Res.,* 16:450–459.
21. Cook, C. E., Seltzman, T. B., Tallent, C. R., Lorenzo, B., and Drayer, D. E. (1987): Pharmacokinetics of pentobarbital enantiomers as determined by enantioselective radioimmunoassay after administration of racemate to humans and rabbits. *J. Pharmacol. Exp. Ther.,* 241:779–785.
22. Cresteil, T., Beaune, P., Kremers, P., Celier, C., Guengerich, F. P., and Leroux, J. (1985): Immunoquantification of epoxide hydrolase and cytochrome P-450 isozymes in fetal and adult human liver microsomes. *Eur. J. Biochem.,* 151:345–350.
23. Dam, M., Kristensen, C. B., Hansen, B. S., and Christiansen, J. (1977): Interaction between carbamazepine and propoxyphene in man. *Acta Neurol. Scand.,* 56:633–647.
24. Dodson, W. E. (1984): Antiepileptic drugs utilization in pediatric patients. *Epilepsia,* 25(Suppl. 2):S132–S139.
25. Dossing, M. (1985): Effect of acute and chronic exercise on hepatic drug metabolism. *Clinical Pharmacokinetics,* 10:426–431.
26. Drayer, D. E. (1986): Pharmacodynamic and pharmacokinetic differences between drug enantiomers in humans: An overview. *Clin. Pharmacol. Ther.,* 40:125–133.
27. Gachalyi, B., Vas, A., Hajos, P., and Kaldor, A. (1984): Acetylator phenotypes: Effect of age. *Eur. J. Clin. Pharmacol.,* 26:43.

28. Gerson, W. T., Fine, D. G., Spielberg, S. P., and Sensenbrenner, L. L. (1983): Anticonvulsant-induced aplastic anemia: Increased susceptibility to toxic drug metabolites in vitro. *Blood,* 61:889–893.

29. Glazko, A. J. (1972): Diphenylhydantoin. *Pharmacology,* 8:163–177.

30. Glazko, A. J., Chang, T., Mascewske, E., Hayes, A., and Dill, W. A. (1976): *personal communication.*

31. Godbillon, J., Richard, J., Gerardin, A., Meinertz, T., Kasper, W., and Jahnchen, E. (1981): Pharmacokinetics of the enantiomers of acenocoumarol in man. *Brit. J. Clin. Pharmacol.,* 12:621–629.

32. Greenblatt, D. J., Sellers, E. M., and Shader, R. I. (1983): Drug disposition in old age. *New Engl. J. Med.,* 306:1081–1088.

33. Hayes, M. J. L., Langman, M. J. S., and Short, A. H. (1975): Changes in drug metabolism with increasing age. II. Phenytoin clearance and protein binding. *Brit. J. Clin. Pharmacol.,* 2:73–79.

34. Hockings, N., Pall, A., Moody, J., Davidson, A. V. M., and Davidson, D. L. W. (1986): The effect of age on carbamazepine pharmacokinetics and adverse effects. *Brit. J. Clin. Pharmacol.,* 22:725–728.

35. Houghton, G. W., and Richens, A. (1975): Effect of age, weight and sex on serum phenytoin concentration in epileptic patients. *Brit. J. Clin. Pharmacol.,* 2:251–256.

36. Idle, J. R., and Smith, R. L. (1979): Polymorphism of oxidation at carbon centers of drugs and their clinical significance. *Drug Metab. Rev.,* 9:301–317.

37. Jacqz, E., Hall, S. D., Branch, R. A., and Wilkinson, G. R. (1986): Polymorphic metabolism of mephenytoin in man: Pharmacokinetic interaction with a co-regulated substrate, mephobarbital. *Clin. Pharmacol. Ther.,* 39:646–653.

38. Jusko, W. J. (1978): Role of tobacco smoking in pharmacokinetics. *J. Pharmacokin. Biopharm.,* 6:7–29.

39. Kalow, W. (1987): Genetic variation in the human hepatic cytochrome P-450 system. *Eur. J. Clin. Pharmacol.,* 31:663–641.

40. Kouri, R. E., McKinney, C. E., Slomiany, D. J., Snodgrass, D. R., Wray, T. L., and McLemore, M. P. (1982): Positive correlation between high aryl hydrocarbon hydroxylase activity and primary lung cancer as analyzed in cryopreserved lymphocytes. *Cancer Res.,* 42:5030–5037.

41. Kupfer, A., and Branch, R. A. (1985): Stereoselective mephobarbital hydroxylation cosegregates with mephenytoin hydroxylation. *Clin. Pharmacol. Ther.,* 38:414–418.

42. Kupfer, A., Patwardhan, R., Ward, S., Schenker, S., Preisig, R., and Branch, R. A. (1984): Stereoselective metabolism and pharmacogenetic control of 5-phenyl-5-ethylhydantoin (Nirvanol) in humans. *J. Pharmacol. Exp. Ther.,* 230:28–33.

43. Kutt, H., Wolk, M., Scherman, R., and McDowell, F. (1964): Insufficient para-hydroxyl-

44. Levy, R. H., and Yerby, M. S. (1985): Effects of pregnancy on antiepileptic drug utilization. *Epilepsia,* 26(Suppl. 1): S52–S57.

45. Loi, C.-M., and Vestal, R. E. (1988): Drug metabolism in the elderly. *Pharmacol. Ther.,* 36:131–149.

46. Maguire, J. H., Wettrell, G., and Rane, A. (1987): Apparently normal phenytoin metabolism in a patient with phenytoin-induced rash and lymphadenopathy. *Brit. J. Clin. Pharmacol.,* 24:554–558.

47. Mansuy, D. (1987): Formation of reactive intermediates and metabolites: Effects of macrolide antibiotics on cytochrome P-450. *Pharmacol. Ther.,* 33:41–45.

48. Martz, F., Failinger, C. III, and Blake, D. A. (1977): Phenytoin teratogenesis: Correlation between embryopathic effect and covalent binding of putative arene oxide metabolite in gestational tissue. *J. Pharmacol. Exp. Ther.,* 203:231–239.

49. Morselli, P. L. (1977): Psychotropic drugs. In: *Drug Disposition during Development,* edited by P. L. Morselli, pp. 431–474. Spectrum, New York.

50. Morselli, P. L., Franco-Morselli, R., and Bossi, L. (1980): Clinical pharmacokinetics in newborns and infants. *Clinical Pharmacokinetics,* 5:485–527.

51. Mucklow, J. C. (1988): Environmental factors affecting drug metabolism. *Pharmacol. Ther.,* 36:105–117.

52. Nation, R. L., Vine, J., Triggs, E. J., and Learoyd, B. (1977): Plasma level of chormethiazole and two metabolites after oral administration to young and aged human subjects. *Eur. J. Clin. Pharmacol.,* 12:137–145.

53. Nau, H., Kuhnz, W., Egger, H.-J., Rating, D., and Helge, H. (1982): Anticonvulsants during pregnancy and lactation. Transplacental, maternal and neonatal pharmacokinetics. *Clinical Pharmacokinetics,* 7:508–543.

54. Nebert, D. W., and Gonzalez, F. J. (1985): Cytochrome P-450 gene expression and regulation. *Trends Pharmacol. Sci.,* 6:160–164.

55. Nebert, D. W., and Gonzalez, F. J. (1988): P450 genes: Structure, evaluation and regulation. *Ann. Rev. Biochem. (in press).*

56. Nebert, D. W., and Jaiswal, A. K. (1987): Human drug metabolism polymorphism: Use of recombinant DNA techniques. *Pharmacol. Ther.,* 33:11–17.

57. Netter, K. J. (1980): Inhibition of oxidative drug metabolism in microsomes. *Pharmacol. Ther.,* 10:515–535.

58. Netter, K. J. (1987): Mechanisms of monooxygenase induction and inhibition. *Pharmacol. Ther.,* 33:1–9.

59. Ortiz De Montellano, P. R. (ed) (1986): Cytochrome P-450: *Structure, Mechanism and Biochemistry.* Plenum, New York.

60. Pelkonen, O., Pasanen, M., Kuha, H., Gachalyi, B., Kairaluoma, M., Sotaniemi, E. A., Park, S. S., Friedman, S. K., and Gelboin, H. V. (1986):

ation as a cause of diphenylhydantoin toxicity. *Neurology,* 14:542–548.

The effect of cigarette smoking on 7-ethoxyre-sorufin O-deethylase and other monooxygenase activities in human liver: Analysis with monoclonal antibodies. *Brit. J. Clin. Pharmacol.,* 22:125–134.

61. Pelkonen, O., and Sotaniemi, E. A. (1987): Environmental factors of enzyme induction and inhibition. *Pharmacol. Ther.,* 13:115–120.

62. Pelkonen, O., Vahakangas, K., Karki, N. T., and Sotaniemi, E. A. (1984): Genetic and environmental regulation of aryl hydrocarbon hydroxylase in man: Studies with liver, lung, placenta and lymphocytes. *Toxicol. Pathol.,* 12:256–260.

63. Perucca, E. (1978): Clinical consequences of microsomal enzyme induction by antiepileptic drugs. *Pharmacol. Ther.,* 2:285–314.

64. Perucca, E. (1982): Pharmacokinetic interactions with antiepileptic drugs. *Clinical Pharmacokinetics,* 7:57–84.

65. Perucca, E. (1987) Clinical implications of hepatic microsomal enzyme induction by antiepileptic drugs. *Pharmacol. Ther.,* 33:139–144.

66. Perucca E. (1987): Drug metabolism in pregnancy, infancy and childhood. *Pharmacol. Ther.,* 34:129–143.

67. Perucca, E., Grimaldi, R., Gatti, G., Pirracchio, S., Crema, F., and Frigo, G. M. (1984): Pharmacokinetics of valproic acid in the elderly. *Brit. J. Clin. Pharmacol.,* 17:665–669.

68. Perucca, E., Hebdige, S., Gatti, G., Lecchini, S., Frigo, G. M., and Crema, A. (1980): Interaction between phenytoin and valproic acid: Plasma protein binding and metabolic effects. *Clin. Pharmacol. Ther.,* 28:779–789.

69. Perucca, E., Hedges, A., Makki, K. A., Ruprah, M., Wilson, J. F., and Richens, A. (1984): A comparative study of the enzyme inducing properties of anticonvulsant drugs in epileptic patients. *Brit. J. Clin. Pharmacol.,* 18:401–410.

70. Perucca, E., Makki, K., and Richens, A. (1978): Is phenytoin metabolism dose-dependent by enzyme-saturation or by feed-back inhibition? *Clin. Pharmacol. Ther.,* 24:46–51.

71. Perucca, E., and Manzo, L. (1988): Metabolic activation of neurotoxicants. In: *Recent Advances in Nervous System Toxicology,* edited by C. L. Galli, L. Manzo, and P. S. Spencer. pp. 67–86. Plenum Press, New York.

72. Perucca, E., and Richens, A. (1980): Reversal by phenytoin of carbamazepine-induced water intoxication: A pharmacokinetic interaction. *J. Neurol. Neurosurg. Psych.,* 43:540–545.

73. Perucca, E., Richens, A. (1981): Drug interactions with phenytoin. *Drugs,* 21:120–137.

74. Perucca, E., and Richens, A. (1981): Interpretation of serum drug levels: Relevance of protein binding. In: *Drug Concentrations in Neuropsychiatry,* Ciba Foundation Symposium 74, pp. 51–58. Excerpta Medica, Amsterdam.

75. Perucca, E., and Richens, A. (1981): The pathophysiological basis of drug toxicity. In: *Current Topics in Pathology,* Vol. 69, edited by E. Grundmann, pp. 17–68, Springer-Verlag, Berlin.

76. Perucca, E., and Richens, A. (1983): Antiepilep-

tic drugs, pregnancy and the newborn. In: *Clinical Pharmacology in Obstetrics,* edited by P. Lewis, pp. 264–287. Wright PSG, Bristol.

77. Perucca, E., and Richens, A. (1985): Antiepileptic drug interactions. In: *Antiepileptic Drugs, Handbook of Experimental Pharmacology,* Vol. 74, edited by D. Janz, and H. H. Frey, pp. 661–723, Springer-Verlag, Berlin.

78. Perucca, E., and Richens, A. (1985): Clinical pharmacokinetics of antiepileptic drugs. In: *Antiepileptic Drugs, Handbook of Experimental Pharmacology,* Vol. 74, edited by D. Janz, and H. H. Frey, pp. 661–723. Springer-Verlag, Berlin.

79. Perucca, E., and Richens, A. (1985): Regulation and monitoring of drug therapy. In: *Biochemistry in Clinical Practice, Scientific Foundations of Clinical Biochemistry,* Vol. 2, edited by D. L. Williams, and V. Marks, pp. 379–399. W. Heinemann Medical Books Ltd., London.

80. Pisani, F., Fazio, A., Oteri, G., Ruello, C., Gitto, C., Russo, F., and Perucca, E. (1986): Sodium valproate and valpromide: Differential interactions with carbamazepine in epileptic patients. *Epilepsia,* 27:548–552.

81. Pisani, F., Fazio, A., Oteri, G., Spina, E., Perucca, E., and Bertilsson, L. (1988): Effect of valpromide on the pharmacokinetics of carbamazepine-10,11-epoxide. *Br. J. Clin. Pharmacol.* 25:611–613.

82. Price-Evans, E. (1984): Survey of the human acetylator polymorphism in spontaneous disorders. *J. Med. Genetics,* 21:243–252.

83. Reidenberg, M. M. (1977): The biotransformation of drugs in liver failure. *Am. J. Med.,* 62:482–485.

84. Reinberg, A., and Smolensky, M. H. (1982): Circadian changes of drug disposition in man. *Clinical Pharmacokinetics,* 7:401–420.

85. Remmer, H. (1959): Der beschleunigte Abbau von Pharmaka an den Lebermikrosomen unter dem Einfluss von Luminal. *Naunyn Schmiedeberg's Arch. Exp. Path. Pharmak.,* 235:279–290.

86. Remmer, H. (1987): Induction and its influence on human cancer. *Pharmacol. Ther.,* 33:89–94.

87. Richens, A. (1979): Clinical pharmacokinetics of phenytoin. *Clinical Pharmacokinetics,* 4:153–169.

88. Richens, A., and Dunlop, A. (1975): Serum phenytoin levels in the management of epilepsy. *Lancet,* 2:247–248.

89. Ringold, G. M. (1985): Steroid hormone regulation of gene expression. *Ann. Rev. Pharmacol. Toxicol.,* 25:529–566.

90. Schmucker, D. L. (1985): Aging and drug disposition: An update. *Pharmacol. Rev.,* 37:133–148.

91. Scott, A. K., Jeffers, T. A., Petrie, J. C., and Gilbert, J. C. (1979): Serum bilirubin and enzyme induction. *Brit. Med. J.,* 2:310.

92. Shaw, P. N., Houston, J. B., Rowland, M., Hopkins, K., Thiercelin, J. F., and Morselli, P. L. (1985): Antipyrine metabolite kinetics in healthy human volunteers during multiple dosing of phen-

ytoin and carbamazepine. *Brit. J. Clin. Pharmacol.,* 20:611–618.

93. Shenfield, G. M. (1981): Influence of thyroid dysfunction on drug pharmacokinetics. *Clinical Pharmacokinetics,* 6:275–297.

94. Sloan, R. G., Idle, J. R., and Smith, R. L. (1981): Influence of D^H/D^L-alleles regulating debrisoquine oxidation and phenytoin metabolism. *Clin. Pharmacol. Ther.,* 29:493–497.

95. Spielberg, S. P., Gordon, G. B., Blake, D. A., Goldstein, D. A., and Herlong, H. F. (1981): Predisposition to phenytoin hepatotoxicity assessed in vitro. *New Engl. J. Med.,* 305:722–727.

96. Steiner, E. S., Alvan, G., Garle, M., Maguire, J. H., Lind, M., Nilsson, S-O., Tomson, T., McClanahan, J. S., and Sjoqvist, F. (1987): The debrisoquine hydroxylation phenotype does not predict the metabolism of phenytoin. *Clin. Pharmacol. Ther. (in press).*

97. Szorady, I., Santa, A. (1987): Drug hydroxylator phenotype in Hungary. *Eur. J. Clin. Pharmacol.,* 32:325.

98. Szorady, I., Santa, A., and Veress, I. (1987): Drug acetylator phenotypes in newborn infants. *Biol. Res. Pregn.,* 8:23–25.

99. Testa, B. (1986): Chiral aspects of drug metabolism. *Trends Pharmacol. Sci.,* 7:60–64.

100. Thompson, T. N., Watkins, J. B., Gregus, Z., and Klaassen, C. D. (1982): Effect of microsomal enzyme inducers on the soluble enzymes of hepatic phase II biotransformation. *Toxicol. Appl. Pharmacol.,* 66:400–408.

101. Toon, S., Low, L. K., Gibaldi, M., Trager, W. F., O'Reilly, R. A., Motley, C. H., and Goulart, D. A. (1986): The warfarin-sulfinpyrazone interaction: Stereochemical considerations. *Clin. Pharmacol. Ther.,* 39:16–24.

102. Travers, R., Reynolds, E. H., and Gallagher, B. (1972): Variation in response to anticonvulsants in a group of epileptic patients. *Arch. Neurol.,* 27:29–33.

103. Walle, T., and Walle, U. K. (1986): Pharmacokinetic parameters obtained with racemates. *Trends Pharmacol. Sci.,* 7:155–158.

104. Wang, P. P., Beaune, P., Kaminsky, L. S., Dannan, G. A., Kadlubar, F. F., Larrey, D., and Guengerich, F. P. (1983): Purification and characterisation of six cytochromes P-450 isozymes from human liver microsomes. *Biochemistry,* 22:5375–5383.

105. Ward, S. A., Goto, F., Nakamura, K., Jacqz, E., Wilkinson, G. R., and Branch, R. A. (1987): S-mephenytoin hydroxylation is inherited as an autosomal recessive trait in Japanese families. *Clin. Pharmacol. Ther.,* 42:96–99.

106. Wedlund, P. J., Aslanian, W. S., Jacqz, E., McAllister, C. B., Branch, R. A., and Wilkinson, G. R. (1985): Phenotypic differences in mephenytoin pharmacokinetics in normal subjects. *J. Pharmacol. Exp. Ther.,* 234:662–669.

107. Welty, T. E., Robinson, F. C., and Meyer, P. R. (1986): A comparison of phenytoin dosing methods in private seizure patients. *Epilepsia,* 27:76–80.

108. Wilkinson, G. R., and Schenker, S. (1975): Drug disposition and liver disease. *Drug. Metab. Rev.,* 4:139–175.

109. Wilkinson, G. R., and Shand, D. G. (1975): A physiological approach to hepatic drug clearance. *Clin. Pharmacol. Ther.,* 18:377–390.

110. Williams, F. M. (1985): Clinical significance of esterases in man. *Clinical Pharmacokinetics,* 10:392–403.

Antiepileptic Drugs, Third Edition, edited by
R. Levy, R. Mattson, B. Meldrum,
J. K. Penry, and F. E. Dreifuss.
Raven Press, Ltd., New York © 1989.

3

General Principles

Toxicology

Gabriel L. Plaa

The fact that chemicals can induce toxic reactions in biological systems, particularly in humans, has been known for a long time. Actually, the mechanisms involved in some of these reactions were discovered before modern pharmacology was established. It is said that Claude Bernard's lectures in 1856 on the toxic effects of noxious gases and curare constituted a course in pharmacology (9). The therapeutic effects of many drugs constitute a response that, if exaggerated, can lead to toxic reactions. The problem has been to determine the balance necessary so that chemical interactions with the biological system can be more beneficial than harmful.

CLASSIFICATION OF TOXIC REACTIONS

Drug toxicity usually refers to those properties of a drug that are harmful to the organism or are so undesirable that they greatly limit the therapeutic usefulness of the drug in question. A classification scheme for drug-induced toxic effects is summarized in Table 1. The scheme is partially based on one presented by Rosenheim (21), but deals more completely with underlying mechanisms. Although the scheme is self-explanatory, some comments are in order. Under the category "Primary Toxic Effects," there are two major subdivisions. The first is related to the therapeutic pharmacological properties of the drug; the second concerns adverse effects that are unrelated to pharmacological action. Respiratory depression after phenobarbital overdose serves as an example of the first subdivision, whereas gingival hyperplasia, megaloblastic anemia, and osteomalacia seen with phenytoin, as well as the liver injury associated with valproic acid, would fall in the second subdivision. Liver and renal injury would not be considered an "exaggerated pharmacological effect." Hypokalemia associated with thiazide diuretic therapy would be an "indirect consequence of primary drug action," a subcategory of "exaggerated pharmacological effect," since the benzothiadiazides enhance potassium excretion by the kidney.

In the second category, "Undesirable Side Effects," one includes pharmacological effects other than those used for therapeutic purposes. Dryness of mouth or increased ocular pressure present with anticholinergic drugs, constipation accompanying codeine analgesia, and sedation or somnolence observed with antihistaminics are examples of such side effects. The term side effect implies that the reaction may not be severe. With the scheme in Table 1, one would not classify drug-induced liver or kidney injury, as well as bone marrow depres-

TABLE 1. *Classification of drug-induced toxic reactions*

I. Primary toxic effects
  A. Exaggerated pharmacological effect
    1. Occurs with drug overdosage
    2. Occurs with therapeutic doses if individual is hyperreactive (hypersusceptible, intolerant) to drug
    3. Indirect consequence of primary drug action
  B. Adverse effect unrelated to pharmacological therapeutic effect
    1. Occurs with drug overdosage
    2. Occurs with therapeutic doses
    3. Occurs with therapeutic doses if individual is hyperreactive (hypersusceptible, intolerant) to drug
II. Undesirable side effects
  A. Undesirable pharmacological effect that accompanies the primary drug action
    1. Occurs with therapeutic doses
III. Allergic reactions
  A. Effect based on immunologic reaction (antigen-antibody reaction)
    1. Occurs in sensitized individual
    2. Occurs with therapeutic or subtherapeutic doses
IV. Idiosyncratic reactions
  A. Unexpected or unpredictable reaction, dissimilar from known pharmacological or adverse effects attributable to the drug and is not immunologic in origin
    1. Depends on the personal characteristics of the individual
    2. Occurs in a small number of individuals
    3. May be attributable to the genetic status of the individual
V. Physical dependence
  A. Altered physiological state resulting in abstinence syndrome when drug is discontinued

sion, as "Undesirable Side Effects"; these reactions are examples of "Primary Toxic Effects."

Unfortunately, the fourth category, "Idiosyncratic Reactions," can be confusing. These reactions may be regarded by some authors merely in terms of a low incidence regardless of the underlying mechanism. Others view it as a low-incidence response occurring through an entirely unknown mechanism. Goldstein et al. (9) prefer to restrict the use of the term to describe drug reactions involving a genetically determined abnormal reactivity on the part

of the subject. Most toxicologists would agree that mere frequency of reaction should not be the basis of the definition, but some have reservations about restricting the term "drug idiosyncrasy" to genetically based reactions. Such a restriction does not allow for the truly unexplained reaction. For this reason, the scheme in Table 1 includes genetically based reactions as one type of "Idiosyncratic Reaction," but does not limit the category to only this kind of reaction. The matter is still unresolved, but the reader should be aware that "drug idiosyncrasy" means different things to different authors.

Zbinden (23) classified toxic reactions in three categories of change: functional, biochemical, and structural. He views functional toxicity as "due to the pharmacological effects which are not necessary for the desired action, although they may for another patient and under different circumstances constitute an important therapeutic effect." This corresponds to "Undesirable Side Effects" in Table 1. Table 2 summarizes the major categories of "functional side-effects" as described by Zbinden. The term "functional" activity represents a change in function of an organ system. Each of these major classes can be subdivided into many subcategories. These undesirable side effects are usually reversible on discontinuation of the drug.

Included in Zbinden's second classification, "biochemical toxicity," are reactions that do not produce gross evidence of organ damage but can effect changes in biochemical reactions associated with various organs. By Zbinden's definition, these biochemical changes are not accompanied by marked anatomical changes. Shifts in hormonal balance and changes in acid-base balance, serum electrolytes, and blood coagulation are examples of this type of drug-related toxic change. Again, these changes are usually reversible on discontinuation of the drug. Depending on the underlying mechanisms, the drugs would be included

TABLE 2. *Functional side effects associated with drug therapy*

1. Changes in wakefulness, general well-being, emotions, and personality
   Aggressiveness, agitation, anxiety, depression, insomnia, psychosis, sedation, etc.
2. Central and peripheral nervous system
   Convulsions, ataxia, extrapyramidal reaction, paresthesia, etc.
3. Sensory organs
   Blurred vision, metallic taste, transient myopia, etc.
4. Skin
   Hot flushes, perspiration, etc.
5. Musculoskeletal system
   Cramps, fasciculations, etc.
6. Cardiovascular and respiratory system
   Angina, bradycardia, fibrillation, dyspnea, hypertension, nasal congestion, etc.
7. Gastrointestinal system, including salivary glands, pancreas, and liver
   Constipation, dry mouth, emesis, nausea, salivation, etc.
8. Urinary system
   Nocturia, voiding difficulty, etc.
9. Genital system, including mammary glands
   Amenorrhea, breast engorgement, decrease of libido, impotence, etc.
10. Local drug effects
    Burning in esophagus, pain on injection, etc.
11. Changes involving the whole body
    Fever, hypothermia, weight gain, etc.

From Zbinden (23).

as "Primary Toxic Effects" or as "Undesirable Side Effects" in the scheme in Table 1.

Zbinden's third category, "structural toxicity," involves an actual change in the structure of the organ or the tissue involved. Obviously, these structural changes can also bring about biochemical and functional changes (for example, drug-induced liver injury, kidney injury, and cataracts). These would be classified as "Primary Toxic Effects" in the scheme in Table 1.

PRESENCE OF ADVERSE DRUG REACTIONS

In 1963, the results of a retrospective survey on the frequency of biochemical and structural drug toxicity in humans following the use of drugs were published (23). All reports involving drug overdosage or the treatment of very serious diseases were specifically excluded. In the reports retained, over 20,000 patients were included, and more than 100 different drugs were involved. Of these patients, 7.3% exhibited structural or biochemical changes related to drug action. Toxic effects on the hematopoietic system were the most frequent, followed by the liver, skin, sensory organs, myocardium, fetal development, bone and joints, gastrointestinal tract, and kidney.

In the last 15 years, considerable interest in adverse drug reactions has been generated (3,13,15). Many of the published reports give inadequate information for determination of cause-and-effect relationships. In most, there is a notable lack of data concerning appropriate control groups. Therefore, quantitative assessment of incidences of 6% to 15%, 1% to 6%, 1% to 28%, and 10% to 20% have been reported (3,13,15); the precise incidence is still unknown.

It is of interest to determine whether these adverse drug reactions represent known properties of drugs involved, or if they represent aberrant, undetectable types of responses. Such data are also imprecise. Estimates (3,15) indicate that about 80% of the reactions responsible for patient hospitalization are considered to be traceable to known pharmacological or toxicological mechanisms, less than 10% are immunologic (allergic) in character, and less than 5% are attributable to idiosyncratic and other unknown mechanisms. The data, although imprecise, lead to the conclusion that 70% to 80% of the adverse drug reactions are at least understandable and predictable.

Karsh and Lasagna (13) defined an adverse drug reaction as one that is noxious and unintended, occurring at dosages of drugs used appropriately in humans for prophylaxis, diagnosis, or therapy, excluding therapeutic failures. They developed a clas-

TABLE 3. *Cause-and-effect relationships for reporting adverse drug reactions*

Definite	A reaction that follows a reasonable temporal sequence from administration of the drug or in which the drug level has been established in body fluids or tissues, that follows a known response pattern to the suspected drug, and that is confirmed by improvement on stopping the drug (dechallenge) and reappearance of the reaction on repeated exposure (rechallenge).
Probable	A reaction that follows a reasonable temporal sequence from administration of the drug, that follows a known response pattern to the suspected drug, that is confirmed by dechallenge, and that could not be reasonably explained by the known characteristics of the patient's clinical state.
Possible	A reaction that follows a reasonable temporal sequence from administration of the drug, that follows a known response to the suspected drug, but that could have been produced by the patient's clinical state or other modes of therapy administered to the patient.
Conditional	A reaction that follows a reasonable temporal sequence from administration of the drug, that does not follow a known response pattern to the suspected drug, but that could not be reasonably explained by the known characteristics of the patient's clinical state.
Doubtful	Any reaction that does not meet the criteria above.

From Karsh and Lasagna (13).

TABLE 4. *Routine animal toxicologic tests*

Acute tests with single dose
1. Median lethal dose (LD_{50} or equivalent) in rodents
2. Pyramiding single-dose studies in dogs
3. Local effects on rabbit skin (for agents to be used topically)

Prolonged tests with daily doses
1. Subchronic, up to 3 months, using rats and dogs, three dose levels
2. Chronic, 6 months to 2 years, using rats and dogs, two to three dose levels

Special tests
1. For effects on fertility and reproduction
2. For teratogenicity
3. For carcinogenicity and mutagenicity
4. For effects on behavior
5. For interactions with other chemical agents

reporting of the reaction as defined in Table 3. In most studies, there is a notable lack of data concerning controls. Relatively minor symptoms thought to be drug-related can occur frequently in patients who are not taking medication (20).

DETECTION OF DRUG TOXICITY

Tests in Laboratory Animals

Table 4 summarizes various toxicologic procedures that are routinely employed in the preclinical testing of new potential drugs in laboratory animals. Four types of studies are carried out: (a) acute toxicity, (b) subchronic toxicity, (c) chronic toxicity, and (d) special tests. In the subchronic and chronic studies, the highest dose level selected is one that is sufficiently high to produce signs of toxicity in that species. In these phases, hematologic and organ function tests are done routinely; also autopsies and histologic examination of organs are performed.

In acute toxicity studies, one purpose is to determine the toxic signs that occur when the drug is given only once and in high dosages. A second purpose is to obtain some idea of the quantitative relationships involved (toxic dosage versus probable ther-

sification scheme to establish cause-and-effect relationships for adverse drug reactions. This scheme is summarized in Table 3. Unfortunately, many of the reports in the medical literature suffer from inadequate descriptions of cause-and-effect relationships. The physician interested in establishing whether an untoward reaction is attributable to a specific drug should verify the adequacy of the methods employed in the apeutic dosage). In addition, close observation and physical examination of the animals can yield some insight into the mechanisms involved.

Since most drugs are given to humans for a prolonged period, one must determine the toxicological profile of a new drug under these circumstances. This is the purpose of the subchronic and chronic studies. These are designed to uncover biochemical and morphologic abnormalities that might occur after repetitive exposures. Again, quantitative comparisons of the dosages involved are made to establish the relative safety of the drug.

A battery of special tests is designed to detect toxic manifestations that are not likely to be encountered in routine acute, subchronic, and chronic studies. Such studies include those used for measuring teratogenesis, effects on reproduction, mutagenesis, and carcinogenesis. Quantitative comparisons of the dosages involved are essential for establishing relative safety.

Interest in teratogenicity arose because of the thalidomide tragedy. Since then, suitable methods have been devised for detection of possible teratogens in laboratory animals. Tests using nonplacental species such as the developing chicken embryo were among the first to be utilized. However, such tests are open to considerable criticism; since many factors influence the results, little confidence can be placed in them. Rats and rabbits are the test animals most frequently used. The range of dosages should be such that maternal toxicity itself does not influence the outcome. Live and dead fetuses are counted, the uterus is examined for resorptions, and all fetuses are systematically examined for evidence of malformations.

There are three components to the tests for assessing reproduction: (a) effects on fertility (both males and females), (b) effects on gestation (fetal development, teratogenicity, mutagenicity, intrauterine mortality), and (c) effects on the progeny (maternal lactation and acceptance of the offspring; growth, development, and sexual maturity of the offspring).

Testing for possible carcinogenic properties has become a major preoccupation of toxicologists involved in the safety evaluation process. It is an extremely complex problem that has created emotional reactions because of the possible impact on society. Carcinogenicity testing is usually performed in rodents maintained over their entire life span. The chemical is given by the intended route of exposure in humans, and at least two dosage levels are used. It is common to describe the chemicals that produce any type of tumor as "tumorigenic agents" and those that produce malignant tumors as "carcinogenic agents." However, a controversy still exists since the ultimate fate of benign tumors in animals has not been resolved. A potentially carcinogenic chemical may produce the following in animals: (a) the occurrence of a type of tumor not seen in normal control animals, (b) an increased incidence of normally occurring spontaneous tumors, and (c) a combination of these two events. Furthermore, qualitative differences exist between types of carcinogenic agents. Some chemicals are strongly carcinogenic (small doses produce the effect, a small number of animals is needed to demonstrate the response, and the time needed to produce the tumors is relatively short), whereas others are weak carcinogens (near-toxic dosages have to be employed, a large number of animals are required to show the effect, and near-lifetime exposures are needed). All of these elements must be considered when making a reasoned judgement on the possible carcinogenic properties of a chemical.

There is considerable interest in the testing for mutagenicity. Both mammalian and nonmammalian (bacteria, yeast, plants, insects) systems have been devised. The latter have one serious disadvantage in that they lack the physiological and biotransformation components known to affect toxicity in mammals. Attempts have been made to overcome the biotransformation aspect by the addition of mammalian metabolizing systems to some of the test systems. Both *in vitro* and *in vivo* assays are utilized; this field is evolving very rapidly. There is considerable controversy, however, about the extrapolation of such data to possible toxic manifestations in humans. A battery of mutagenicity tests is employed, since no single method is adequate for determining the possible risk to humans. The various procedures vary considerably in terms of sensitivity, specificity, and applicability. Furthermore, the distinctively artificial nature of the test systems make interpretations regarding safety rather tenuous; unfortunately, quantitative interpretations needed for safety evaluation are extremely limited.

Untoward Effects in Humans

It is now quite apparent that regardless of extensive toxicologic testing carried out under the present regulations of government agencies, significant toxic effects can sometimes be discovered only when a drug has been introduced into the market and administered to a great number of patients. There are several explanations why certain toxic reactions may not be uncovered in preclinical testing: (a) the toxic response is a rare event, (b) the toxic effect appears only after prolonged drug administration, (c) the toxic effect is not reproducible under laboratory conditions used for preclinical testing in animals, or (d) the toxic response occurs only in humans.

The rarity of a toxic event is certainly a reasonable explanation. If the toxic effect occurs only about once in 1,000 or 10,000 cases, it is highly unlikely that the reaction will be uncovered in preclinical testing. Only when the substance is used extensively will it be possible to establish a cause-and-effect relationship. An example of this

type of toxic event is the aplastic anemia associated with the antibiotic chloramphenicol. It took several years of clinical experience before the association was made. Drug toxicities based on genetic abnormalities are also examples of this type of event.

Reactions that are not readily observable in laboratory animals include headache, nausea, insomnia, and psychotic disturbances. With liver injury, some drugs are associated with cholestatic reactions in humans but do not produce the same effects in laboratory animals, although signs of hepatobiliary dysfunction are observed. This situation creates problems, because it is difficult to determine experimentally whether it is the species that is responding differently or whether multiple factors involved in the toxic reaction are not reproduced in all species. Toxic reactions involving metabolic transformations (e.g., of the drugs) can cause this type of aberrant response in different species. Halothane-induced liver damage, a toxic event well characterized in humans, is produced only with difficulty in rats; in this species, one must stimulate hepatic enzymes involved in the biotransformation of halothane and develop a tissue state of relative hypoxia in order to produce a liver lesion resembling that seen in humans.

DOSE-RESPONSE RELATIONSHIPS

The concept of a dose-response relationship is extremely important in toxicologic evaluations. Generally, as one increases the dose of a chemical, the appearance of toxic signs and their severity increases; furthermore, the number of subjects affected increases with the dose. When lethality is the endpoint being measured, it is obvious that there can only be an all-or-none response. Therefore, if one uses a population of animals given a range of dosages, one calculates the percentage of animals at each dosage level that show the lethal response. It is possible to calculate (7) the dosage that kills 50% of the population, the median lethal dosage (LD_{50}). Dose-response relationships can be determined for responses other than lethality. In these cases, the median effective dosage (ED_{50}) is calculated (7). If quantal (all-or-none) data (e.g., percentage of subjects affected) are desired, the measured responses are merely converted into all-or-none units after establishing an appropriate cutoff value between "no effect" and "effect."

Dose-response curves can be used to compare quantitatively the differences in toxic potencies observed in a series of different drugs. Furthermore, for a single compound one can derive a quantitative estimate of its relative potency for producing several different toxic effects. Dose-response relationships are also used to estimate the "no adverse effect level" in the safety evaluation process of drugs. This is the dosage that results in no detectable injurious effect and is used to establish safety factors for the safe use of chemicals (14).

Some untoward drug reactions in humans are uncovered only after widespread use in large patient populations because the toxic reaction may be a rare event. These are known as low-incidence toxic reactions. Frequencies of 0.1%, 0.01%, and 0.001% are examples of such reactions. Toxicologists tend to deemphasize abnormal responses in laboratory animals if a clear dose-response relationship is not observed, particularly when the abnormal response is seen in a low-dosage group but not at higher dosages. One normally assumes that the laboratory animal sampling selected for test purposes represents a homogeneous population. However, subpopulations can exist within a supposedly homogeneous population; such an occurrence was demontrated in rats for sodium chloride-induced hypertension (2). Thus, a low-incidence toxic reaction in a test population may be the reflection of the presence of a susceptible

subpopulation that is diluted out by a larger subpopulation of nonrespondents. One can calculate how many subjects would be required to uncover such a situation in a test population (24). If the incidence of the reaction is 1% (1:100), one would have to test 299 subjects in order to have a 95% probability of detecting at least one respondent. If the incidence is 0.1% (1:1000), 2,995 subjects would have to be tested. With incidences of 0.01% (1:10,000) and 0.001% (1:100,000), the required number of test subjects increases to 29,956 and 299,572, respectively, to detect at least one respondent. These calculations show why it is virtually impossible to expect to detect low-incidence toxic reactions in animal studies if a classic dose-response relationship cannot be demonstrated.

DRUG INTERACTIONS

The use of multiple drugs in current medical practice has created the problem of drug interaction and its sequelae of undesirable or even toxic reactions. The clinical implications of such interactions are now reasonably well known, and appropriate references for specific drug interactions mentioned below can be rapidly obtained (12,22). The fact that two or more drugs are administered to a patient does not mean that a drug interaction will necessarily occur. Whether or not an interaction will be seen depends entirely on the particular drugs involved. Also, the fact that an interaction can occur does not mean that it will always occur; patient variability is the most evident feature of drug interactions. If an interaction does occur, it need not always result in a toxic response. Furthermore, among those that do result in toxic effects, fortunately only a few are life threatening. Some dangerous drug interactions are those that involve the combination of different drugs that affect the pharmacokinetics of coumarin-type anticoagulants, oral hypoglycemic agents, and agents acting on the myo-cardium. The interaction between the tricyclic antidepressants and guanethidine-type antihypertensive drugs is also danger-ous and is due to an interaction at the site of action.

Drug interactions can occur at many lev-els. However, many of them are due to al-terations in pharmacokinetics because of modifications in absorption, distribution, biotransformation, or excretion. Those drugs whose pharmacologic actions are particularly affected by modifications in plasma concentrations are more prone to re-sult in interactions. Furthermore, when the difference between the therapeutic and the toxic plasma concentrations is small, it is more likely that the interaction may result in a toxic effect. However, the interaction can lead to a loss of therapeutic effect if the combined administration of the drugs causes the plasma concentrations of the af-fected agent to drop below its therapeutic level.

Decreased absorption can obviously lower plasma concentrations. Such events have been observed when tetracyclines are coadministered with calcium, aluminum, or ferrous salts. Poorly soluble complexes be-tween the tetracycline and the ions are formed, resulting in poor absorption of these broad-spectrum antibiotics.

Diminished drug binding to plasma pro-teins can lead to an increase in circulating free drug and an increase in tissue distri-bution. The problem of sulfonamides and kernicterus in the premature infant (17) due to displacement of bilirubin from plasma protein binding sites is one example. Drugs can also displace each other. Displacement of anticoagulants by phenylbutazone ana-logs has led to serious bleeding episodes. Methotrexate can be displaced by salicy-lates and may result in hepatotoxicity.

By far the greatest interest in drug inter-action has been at the level of biotransfor-mation. The induction of mixed-function oxidases in the liver by a multitude of drugs

increases the possibilities of such drug in-teractions. The classic example is the in-ductive effect of phenobarbital on dicou-marol biotransformation in patients on anticoagulant therapy (1). Plaa et al. (19) showed that combined used of phenobar-bital and primidone in epileptics could re-sult in toxicity due to enhanced conversion of primidone to phenobarbital. Adverse ef-fects of phenobarbital on corticosteroids in asthmatics are believed to be due to induc-tion of corticosteroid metabolism. Inhibi-tion of drug metabolism also can lead to drug interactions. Treatment with disulfi-ram results in discomforting symptoms when ethanol is ingested (10). This is sup-posedly due to the accumulation of acetal-dehyde caused by an interference of its me-tabolism by disulfiram. Dicoumarol and chloramphenicol can decrease tolbutamide biotransformation. Phenytoin metabolism can be inhibited by several drugs (dicou-marol, chloramphenicol, isoniazid, disulfi-ram, sulfamethizole) and may result in phenytoin toxicity. Carbamazepine metab-olism can be inhibited by erythromycin, isoniazid, and propoxyphene. Valproic acid can inhibit the metabolism of phenobar-bital.

Interactions at sites of elimination are also known. Both in the kidney and in the liver, transport systems for acidic and basic substances have been demonstrated. In the kidney use has been made of this phenom-enon to increase blood levels of penicillin by the coadministration of probenecid. The uricosuric effects of sulfinpyrazone are sig-nificantly reduced by the concurrent ad-ministration of salicylates. It is now be-lieved that it is the nonionic moiety that is involved in back diffusion in the tubules. Therefore, alkalinization has been em-ployed to enhance the excretion of barbi-turates and salicylates in drug intoxications. In the liver, much less is known about pos-sible drug interactions. However, it was ob-served that administration of radiocontrast material can affect the subsequent excretion of Bromosulphalein (BSP), thus resulting in a false abnormal liver function profile. In rats, diazepam and BSP inhibit the biliary excretion of each other (11,18), and diazepam modifies the biliary excretion of phenytoin and certain cardiac glycosides (4–6). Since the importance of the enterohepatic circulation in determining drug action is yet to be determined, the clinical implications of possible drug interactions at the level of biliary excretion are unknown. However, it is known that cholestyramine can lower serum levels of digitoxin through binding of digitoxin in the gut and thereby interrupting the enterohepatic circulation; digitoxin intoxication has been treated successfully by this procedure. Cholestyramine can bind thyroid hormone as well.

Another type of interaction has been observed with the monoamine oxidase inhibitors of the hydrazide type. These substances interfere with normal degradation of certain endogenous biogenic amines. Tyramine metabolism, in particular, is affected by these inhibitors. Individuals treated with these inhibitors may show exaggerated hypertensive, even fatal, effects if they simultaneously ingest foodstuffs such as cheese that contain high levels of tyramine.

The tricyclic antidepressants can antagonize the antihypertensive effect of guanethidine. This interaction has been shown to occur in every patient studied. Guanethidine uptake into the adrenergic neuron (its site of antihypertensive action) is inhibited by the tricyclic antidepressants.

In addition to these types of drug interactions, others occur that are not well understood. These are associated primarily with agents that act on the central nervous system and result in enhanced responses when given in combination. Everyone is aware that ethanol ingestion with barbiturates and other sedatives can result in enhanced depression. This is a particular problem in our society since drug ingestion and the use of ethanol are quite prevalent;

this situation is a serious problem as far as motor vehicle operation is concerned. There are reports that claim that the effects are merely additive, whereas others claim synergy. Gebhardt et al. (8) carried out a study in animals with ethanol, phenobarbital, chlorpromazine, and chlordiazepoxide. It was concluded that additive and synergistic effects can be shown by the combination of ethanol with any of the substances studied but that the effect depended on the level of central nervous system depression being measured. They were able to show that with a mild degree of depression that resulted in the inability of the animals to remain on an inclined screen, the interaction with ethanol usually resulted in additive effects. However, if a more severe index of depression was employed, such as loss of the righting reflex, the interaction usually indicated a synergistic (supra-additive) action.

In laboratory animals, another type of drug interaction can occur with substances acting on the central nervous system. Mice treated with sodium bromide are much more responsive to the subsequent effects of chlorpromazine than are control animals. It was established (16) that bromides enhanced the loss of the righting reflex induced by chlorpromazine. The interaction is dose and time dependent on both the dose of sodium bromide and the dose of chlorpromazine. There is a definite relationship between the plasma bromide concentration and the enhanced effect seen with chlorpromazine; the critical bromide concentration in mice is about 650 μg/ml. This particular effect of sodium bromide is quite interesting because it seems to be a relatively specific effect on central nervous system-depressing properties of chlorpromazine in that the hypothermic response to chlorpromazine is not enhanced by bromide pretreatment. This kind of interaction is thought to occur in humans (16). The mechanism of the interaction is unknown. However, the doses of sodium bromide employed in animals are well below those causing loss of the righting reflex by itself, and the lowest dose of sodium bromide employed to cause this potentiation is remarkably low, less than one-fourth that required to protect against convulsions induced by electroshock and pentylenetetrazol.

SUMMARY

This chapter discusses the various methods of classifying undesirable or toxic effects of therapeutic agents and describes the use and limitations of animal studies for the detection of these effects. It illustrates the concept of the dose-response relationship and tells how such data can be utilized to describe toxic effects. Finally, it discusses the problem of drug interaction and how it can lead to unexpected and even undesirable side effects.

REFERENCES

1. Cucinell, S. A., Conney, A. H., Sansur, M., and Burns, J. J. (1965): Drug interactions in man. I. Lowering effect of phenobarbital on plasma levels of bishydroxycoumarin (Dicoumarol) and diphenylhydantoin (Dilantin). *Clin. Pharmacol. Ther.*, 6:420–429.
2. Dahl, L. K., Heine, M., and Tassinari, L. (1962): Effects of chronic excess salt ingestion: Evidence that genetic factors play an important role in susceptibility in experimental hypertension. *J. Exp. Med.*, 115:1173–1190.
3. Davies, D. M. (1981): *Textbook of Adverse Drug Reactions*, Second Edition. Oxford University Press, Oxford.
4. El-hawari, A. M., and Plaa, G. L. (1976): Effects of diazepam on the biliary excretion of cardiac glycosides. *Pharmacologist*, 18:199.
5. El-hawari, A. M., and Plaa, G. L. (1977): Effects of diazepam on the biliary excretion of diphenylhydantoin in the rat. *J. Pharmacol. Exp. Ther.*, 201:14–25.
6. El-hawari, A. M., and Plaa, G. L. (1978): Role of the enterohepatic circulation in the elimination of phenytoin in the rat. *Drug Metab. Disposit.*, 6:59–69.
7. Gad, S. C., and Weil, C. S. (1982): Statistics for toxicologists, In: *Principles and Methods of Toxicology*, edited by A. W. Hayes, pp. 273–320. Raven Press, New York.
8. Gebhardt, G. F., Plaa, G. L., and Mitchell, C. L. (1969): Effects of ethanol alone and in combination with phenobarbital, chlorpromazine, or chlordiazepoxide. *Toxicol. Appl. Pharmacol.*, 15:405–414.
9. Goldstein, A., Aronow, L., and Kalman, S. M. (1974): *Principles of Drug Action: The Basis of Phamacology*, Second Edition. John Wiley & Sons, New York.
10. Hald, J., and Jacobsen, E. (1948): The formation of acetaldehyde in the organism after ingestion of Antabuse (tetraethylthiuramdisulphide) and alcohol. *Acta Pharmacol. Toxicol. (Kbh.)*, 4:305–310.
11. Hanasono, G. K., deRepentigny, L., Priestly, B. G., and Plaa, G. L. (1976): The effects of oral diazepam pretreatment on the biliary excretion of sulfobromophthalein in rats. *Can. J. Physiol. Pharmacol.*, 54:603–612.
12. Hansten, P. D. (1985): *Drug Interactions*, Fifth Edition. Lea & Febiger, Philadelphia.
13. Karsh, F. E., and Lasagna, L. (1975): Adverse drug reactions. A critical review. *J. Am. Med. Assoc.*, 234:1236–1241.
14. Lu, F. C. (1985): *Basic Toxicology*. Hemisphere, Washington.
15. Melmon, K. L., and Morrelli, H. F. (1978): *Clinical Pharmacology—Basic Principles in Therapeutics*, Second Edition. Macmillan, New York.
16. Norden, L. G., and Plaa, G. L. (1963): Interaction between sodium bromide and chlorpromazine. *Toxicol. Appl. Pharmacol.*, 5:437–444.
17. Nyhan, W. L. (1961): Toxicity of drugs in the neonatal period. *J. Pediatr.*, 59:437–444.
18. Plaa, G. L., Besner, J.-G., and Caillé, G. (1975): Effect of diazepam on sulfobromophthalein excretion. In: *Clinical Pharmacology of Psychoactive Drugs*, edited by E. M. Sellers, pp. 203–218. Addiction Research Foundation, Toronto.
19. Plaa, G. L., Fujimoto, J. M., and Hine, C. H. (1958): Intoxication from primidone due to its biotransformation to phenobarbital. *J. Am. Med. Assoc.*, 168:1769–1770.
20. Reidenberg, M. M., and Lowenthal, D. T. (1968): Adverse nondrug reactions. *N. Engl. J. Med.*, 279:678–679.
21. Rosenheim, M. L. (1962): Symposium on drug sensitization. General introduction. *Proc. Roy. Soc. Med.*, 55:7–8.
22. Shinn, A. F., and Shrewsbury, R. P. (1985): *Evaluations of Drug Interactions*, Third Edition. C. V. Mosby, St. Louis.
23. Zbinden, G. (1963): Experimental and clinical aspects of drug toxicity. In: *Advances in Pharmacology, Vol. 2*, edited by S. Garattini and P. A. Shore, pp. 1–112. Academic Press, New York.
24. Zbinden, G. (1973): *Progress in Toxicology, Vol. 1*. Springer-Verlag, New York.

Antiepileptic Drugs, Third Edition, edited by
R. Levy, R. Mattson, B. Meldrum,
J. K. Penry, and F. E. Dreifuss.
Raven Press, Ltd., New York © 1989.

4

General Principles

Principles of Antiepileptic Drug Action

Robert L. Macdonald and Brian S. Meldrum

What is an antiepileptic drug? In common usage, it is a drug that, when administered over a prolonged period, will decrease the incidence or severity of spontaneous seizures occurring in patients with epilepsy. Any drug that on single-dose administration leads to long-term abolition of seizures would also, no doubt, be accepted as an antiepileptic drug. Specific antidotes for symptomatic seizures are not, in general, considered antiepileptic drugs. Antipyretic or antibiotic drugs may prevent febrile convulsions when promptly administered to a child at the onset of a febrile illness. Many drug intoxications are associated with seizures, and there may be specific remedies such as atropine for convulsions associated with organophosphorus insecticide poisoning. There are, however, many borderline cases of intoxications or metabolic disturbances in which seizures occur and in which conventional antiepileptic drugs may provide appropriate treatment. These include withdrawal of barbiturates or other antiepileptic drugs, and alcohol.

The established antiepileptic drugs that provide the subject matter for most of this volume belong to about eight classes of chemical compound. Curiously, four or five of these classes appear to have certain features of the molecular structure in common (Fig. 1).

There is little evidence for a common pharmacological effect of this supposed "pharmacophore"; the strongest candidate site of action appears to be the sodium channel (see below). It might be proposed that the common structural features arise because of the limited imagination of synthetic chemists, given that the original "lead" compound was phenobarbital and secondarily phenytoin. However, this is not a satisfying explanation, as over the last 50 years it has been standard practice in a large number of pharmaceutical companies to screen every compound with signs of central nervous system activity for anticonvulsant activity. Thus, if there were a wider range of structures with such activity, we would likely know about them. It is possible, however, that the range of chemical compounds that we consider antiepileptic has been artificially restricted by the type of screening tests employed. Virtually all screening tests depend on suppression of chemically or electrically induced seizures by the single-dose administration of the test drug. Thus, drugs with a direct action on nerve membranes or synaptic function are preferentially selected. Drugs that might suppress seizures by inducing slow changes in ionic distribution or in endocrine and metabolic function would not be identified. In particular, trophic agents that might alter the pattern of connectivity in damaged nerve systems or agents that might act on gene

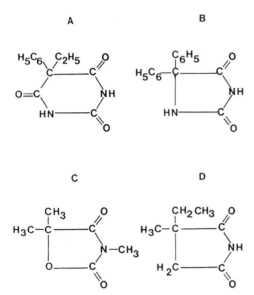

FIG. 1. Several structural features are common to four classes of antiepileptic drugs: **A**, phenobarbital; **B**, phenytoin; **C**, trimethadione; **D**, ethosuximide. (From Porter, ref. 120, with permission.)

expression to modify the specific receptor densities in critical brain areas would not be detected. Thus, we may have failed to identify major types of antiepileptic agents.

Even if we confine our attempts at understanding mechanisms of action of antiepileptic drugs to those mechanisms that lead to acute suppression of convulsions in animals and to chronic elevation of seizure threshold in patients with epilepsy, we still need to consider how many different types of action we seek. It has long been agreed that there must be at least two major functional types of antiepileptic drug. Screening tests separate two classes of drug—those, such as phenytoin and carbamazepine, that are most active against tonic extension in the maximal electroshock test, and those, such as clonazepam and the succinimides, that are more potent in the threshold pentylenetetrazol test (65,117). Similarly, in the clinic there is a clear differentiation between drugs that are effective only in absence-type seizures (ethosuximide, trime-

thadione), those that are effective in myoclonic seizures (benzodiazepines, barbiturates, sodium valproate), those that are effective in focal and secondarily generalized seizures (phenytoin, carbamazepine), and those that are active in all of these seizures (e.g. sodium valproate) (Table 1). This implies two or three mechanisms of action. It is possible, however, that any one compound may have multiple mechanisms of action. Indeed, one compound could produce numerous actions on membrane conductances and synaptic function, some of which are anticonvulsant and some proconvulsant, with such effects interacting to produce different outcomes in different types of seizures. These possibilities can be explored only in specialized test systems which may, of course, introduce particular biases into interpretation of mechanisms of action.

When discussing antiepileptic drugs' mechanisms of action, there is a strong tendency to think only of direct pharmacological actions. This tendency is facilitated both by the acute procedures that are used to identify novel antiepileptic drugs and by the *in vitro* methods used for their assessment. That a similar correlation between plasma antiepileptic drug levels and therapeutic effect is found both in single-dose animal models and in patients receiving prolonged therapy, supports the importance of direct pharmacological actions as opposed to long-term processes of neuronal regulation or growth. For sodium valproate, however, correlations of effect with plasma concentration are sometimes poor, and delayed therapeutic effects have been reported in both man and animal models (54,69).

TEST SYSTEMS

Test systems for studying the mechanisms of action of antiepileptic drugs must be differentiated from test systems intended to identify novel antiepileptic drugs. The

TABLE 1. *Clinical classification of some antiepileptic drugs*

Drug	Generalized tonic-clonic and partial seizures	Myoclonic seizures	Generalized absence seizures
Phenytoin	+ +	−	−
Carbamazepine	+ +	−	−
Sodium valproate	+ +	+ +	+ +
Phenobarbital	+	+	−
Clonazepam	+	+ +	+
Ethosuximide	−	−	+ +

+ +, efficacy against the seizure type at nontoxic serum concentrations.
+, efficacy against the seizure type at toxic serum concentrations.
−, no efficacy.

latter are discussed by Meldrum (94) and Löscher and Schmidt (73) and in Chapter 5. Epilepsy can be studied definitively only *in vivo*. However, analysis of the mechanisms of action of antiepileptic drugs requires *in vitro* test systems. These have the advantage that drug concentrations can be precisely controlled, and complications introduced by drug metabolism or secondary metabolic changes can be largely avoided. Studies of antiepileptic drug actions on ionic conductances have been conducted principally in dispersed neuronal cultures. The use of the patch-clamp technique now allows the study of the effects of antiepileptic drugs on the kinetic properties of single ion channels.

Membrane responses to neurotransmitters and their modification by antiepileptic drugs can be studied in cell culture, either in dispersed neuronal or organotypic cultures. They can also be studied in tissue slices in which specific pathways can be stimulated electrically. In such systems presynaptic effects can be separated from postsynaptic effects and the interaction of effects on inhibitory and excitatory mechanisms can be studied. Epileptiform activity of various kinds can be induced in hippocampal or cortical brain slices (23,154). The properties of such epileptiform activity may depend in part on the circumstances required to initiate it. Possible epileptogenic alterations include decreasing the extracellular concentration of Ca^{++} or

Mg^{++} or raising that of K^+, or the introduction of a variety of convulsant agents (4-aminopyridine, penicillin, bicuculline, picrotoxin, kainate, *N*-methyl-*D*-aspartate) (60,113,118,124,136). Remarkably consistent effects of antiepileptic agents are observed when comparing suppression of burst discharges evoked in slices by diverse procedures. It is also possible to study hippocampal slices from animals made epileptic by kindling or focal injection of long-term epileptogens (e.g., tetanus toxin).

In vivo studies in which the antiepileptic drug is administered systemically commonly pose problems in defining the drug's site of action. This can sometimes be aided by making specific lesions in the brain, or by focal electrical or chemical stimulation to trigger seizure activity. An alternative is to use focal microinjections of antiepileptic agents (although in this case it is often difficult to know the locally effective drug concentration).

SEIZURE INITIATION AND SPREAD

It is possible that different antiepileptic mechanisms contribute to the prevention of initiation of epileptic activity and to the prevention of its spread. Thus, initiation of burst discharges at the cellular level may be seen as a question of stability of membrane potential, whereas the synchronization of bursting within an aggregate may be an ionic or synaptic mechanism and the propagation to distant aggregates is most probably synaptic.

Since the study of Ayala et al. (8), paroxysmal events have been differentiated into "ictal" and "interictal" on the basis of certain electrophysiological features. An interictal event is usually a spike, polyspike, or spike and wave on the EEG, correlating with (in microelectrode records) a brief burst of neuronal firing and a paroxysmal depolarization shift (PDS) of membrane potential followed by an afterhyperpolarization. An ictal event provides a more sustained burst of fast activity or spikes on the EEG associated with (at cellular level) sustained spikes and depolarization, not usually interrupted or followed by an inhibitory hyperpolarization. However, such electrophysiologically defined ictal and interictal events are not necessarily consistent. Interictal events are associated with surround inhibition and remote inhibition, but may, if repetitive, propagate as interictal or ictal events. Ictal events more readily propagate as epileptiform activity. Recruitment and propagation are facilitated by repetition of interictal or ictal events. This process has been studied in hippocampal slices in which afferent tetanization reveals latent excitatory pathways capable of transmitting interictal bursts (100).

Antiepileptic drug effects may be selective in that they can preferentially suppress either interictal or ictal events. The mechanisms by which they do this are discussed below.

PATHWAYS OF SEIZURE PROPAGATION

Seizure activity initiated focally in the neocortex propagates to other cortical areas and to various subcortical nuclei (e.g., thalamus and basal ganglia) and to the brain stem and spinal cord before clinical seizures are manifest (20,55,95). Limbic seizures

also depend on multiple relays in limbic and basal ganglia pathways before being fully expressed clinically. The site of initiation of "primary" generalized seizures is harder to define (see Gloor, 45). Generalized seizures induced in rats by systemic pentylenetetrazol apparently involve an ascending pathway from rostral medulla, via the mamillary bodies and anterior thalamus (102).

Drugs can therefore act at many different sites to provide suppression of clinical seizures. Evidence of this can be provided by the focal injection of drugs at critical relay sites. Thus, in rodent models of epilepsy, seizure manifestations can be suppressed by the focal injection of GABAergic agents (e.g., muscimol or γ-vinyl-GABA) or excitatory amino acid antagonists (e.g., 2-amino-7-phosphonoheptanoate [2-APH]) into a variety of sites depending on the model tested. Sound-induced seizures in the genetically epilepsy prone rat can be suppressed by the focal injection of these agents in the inferior colliculus (101). Pilocarpine-induced limbic seizures can be suppressed by the focal injection of 2-APH or muscimol into the entopeduncular nucleus, the substantia nigra, the lateral habenula, the mediodorsal nucleus of the thalamus, or the prepyriform cortex (114,115). All these regions provide potential sites for antiepileptic drug action.

CELLULAR MECHANISMS LEADING TO BURST FIRING

Study of the mechanisms underlying abnormal paroxysmal activity in the nervous system has been performed primarily on animal models of partial seizures. There is less known of the mechanisms underlying generalized seizures. The two major preparations that have been used to study the cellular mechanisms underlying interictal and ictal events in partial seizures have been the hippocampus and the neocortex *in vivo* and in slice. In the hippocampus several phenomena are important in producing interictal spikes. When a convulsant agent such as penicillin, bicuculline, or picrotoxin is applied to the hippocampus, spontaneous interictal spikes can be recorded with extracellular electrodes. During the interictal spike, intracellular recordings from individual hippocampal pyramidal neurons contain spontaneous firing of bursts consisting of a membrane depolarization, which evokes a train of action potentials followed by a membrane hyperpolarization (33). The occurrence of synchronous burst firing during a spontaneous interictal spike has been termed a PDS (84,121). It is the PDS which is the intracellular correlate of an interictal spike.

Substantial investigation has been directed toward understanding the cellular mechanisms underlying the development of burst firing and the PDS. There appear to be three essential elements (141).

First, hippocampal pyramidal and neocortical neurons have intrinsic burst mechanisms (128,153). As mentioned above, hippocampal pyramidal cells have appropriate conductances on their somatic and dendritic membranes to produce bursts (152). A typical pyramidal cell burst consists of an initial series of sodium-dependent action potentials riding upon a depolarizing potential which is calcium-dependent (151). With sustained and continued depolarization, high-threshold, voltage-dependent calcium channels are activated producing a series of one or more calcium-dependent action potentials. The burst of action potentials is followed by a potassium-dependent afterhyperpolarization (AHP) (5,129). The AHP has at least two slow components: a slow potassium-dependent inhibitory postsynaptic potential (4,104,140) and a slow calcium-dependent potassium potential (5). The AHP also has at least one fast component, a transient calcium-dependent potassium potential (6).

Second, disinhibition is important. Although individual pyramidal neurons can produce a burst when directly stimulated, orthodromic (synaptic) stimulation does not evoke bursts. Reduction of GABAergic inhibition is required to produce synaptically evoked synchronous burst discharges in populations of hippocampal neurons and thus to produce PDS (151). In the hippocampus there is both feed-forward and feedback GABAergic inhibition which is activated when afferents are stimulated. For example, when the Schaffer collateral system is stimulated to activate CA_1 hippocampal pyramidal neurons, the collaterals contact inhibitory interneurons which then inhibit the CA_1 pyramidal cells. Furthermore, when the CA_1 pyramidal neurons fire, pyramidal neuron axon collaterals contact interneurons which feed back to produce inhibition. Thus, there is feed-forward and feed-back inhibition. The GABAergic inhibition limits the ability of these neurons to produce burst firing on synaptic stimulation. In the presence of an antagonist of GABA receptors, feed-back and feed-forward inhibition are blocked, allowing trains of action potentials to be produced that can be transmitted in a forward, or orthodromic, fashion to other hippocampal pyramidal neurons.

Third, feed-forward excitation has been shown to be important. In the CA_3 and CA_2 regions of hippocampus, there are feed-forward excitatory connections among hippocampal pyramidal neurons (79,99). Apparently, in CA_1 there are many fewer excitatory connections among pyramidal cells. The feed-forward synaptic connections among pyramidal cells allow them to fire synchronously. The synaptically induced firing of bursts is due, in part, to the presence of *N*-methyl-*D*-aspartate (NMDA) receptors on these pyramidal cells (34). The NMDA receptor channel has a voltage-dependency conferred upon it by the blocking action of magnesium ions (87,108). At negative membrane potentials, magnesium ions reside in NMDA receptor channels and prevent glutamate activation of current flow through their channels. However, following membrane depolarization, magnesium ions dissociate from the NMDA receptor channel, and glutamate produces large membrane depolarizations. In the presence of disinhibition and feed-forward excitatory connections, excitatory synaptic input produces larger and more sustained depolarization. The sustained depolarization produces high frequency trains of action potentials that evoke further depolarizations in connected cells. When sufficient numbers of neurons are recruited synchronously, simultaneous burst discharges and an interictal spike are produced.

Although it is important that neurons possess intrinsic burst mechanisms and that excitatory interconnections and disinhibition are present, a number of additional mechanisms are required for propagation of burst discharges to other brain regions. In the hippocampus, burst-generating mechanisms are present in CA_3 or CA_2 pyramidal cells (128). Action potentials are generated in the CA_3 and CA_2 pyramidal cells and are transmitted to CA_1 pyramidal cells by Schaffer collaterals to drive the CA_1 cells to burst synchronously (74,153). Thus, the excitatory effects seen in CA_3 and CA_2 can be propagated to another neuronal region, the CA_1 hippocampal pyramidal cell region. In the neocortex, bursts may originate in layers IV and V (22). It is thought that similar mechanisms may underlie the propagation of abnormal electrical excitability from one region to another in the nervous system, and therefore, to produce partial seizures.

All three of these essential features are subject to regulation by antiepileptic drugs (Table 2). First, drugs that block the ability of cells to fire at high frequency, and therefore to disrupt the bursts and feed-forward excitation, would be effective antiepileptic drugs. Second, drugs that enhance inhibition and therefore reduce pathologically produced disinhibition would be effective antiepileptic drugs. Third, drugs that modify synaptic excitation, specifically, that

block NMDA-induced depolarization, would be effective antiepileptic drugs. These three mechanisms are discussed in the following sections.

EFFECTS OF ANTIEPILEPTIC DRUGS ON SODIUM CHANNELS

All antiepileptic drugs have been shown to alter some membrane property of neurons and axons (39,56,77,122). However, to be potential antiepileptic drug mechanisms, the membrane effects must be produced at concentrations achieved in the cerebrospinal fluid (CSF) and in plasma free of protein binding in ambulatory patients. A direct membrane effect produced only at toxic free plasma levels is unlikely to be a relevant antiepileptic drug mechanism. Phenytoin, carbamazepine, sodium valproate, anticonvulsant benzodiazepines (diazepam, clonazepam, and lorazepam), phenobarbital, and primidone block sustained high-frequency repetitive firing (SRF) of action potentials in vertebrate cortical and spinal cord neurons in cell culture (77,88). However, only phenytoin, carbamazepine, and sodium valproate reduce SRF (Fig. 2) at therapeutic free plasma concentrations. The antiepileptic drug-induced block of SRF has several important properties.

First, the block is voltage-dependent. When neurons are held at large negative potentials, membrane depolarization can produce SRF. However, following membrane depolarization, SRF is limited to a few action potentials. Second, the effect of the antiepileptic drugs is use-dependent. Under normal circumstances, neurons fire a train of action potentials with varying degrees of spike frequency adaptation after membrane depolarization. In the presence of an antiepileptic drug, there is a progressive alteration of action potentials within the train. The initial action potential is unaffected but each subsequent action potential has a smaller amplitude and a lower rate of rise.

TABLE 2. *Antiepileptic drug patterns of action against different channel types*

Drug	Sodium channels	GABA receptor channels	T calcium channels
Phenytoin	+ +	−	−
Carbamazepine	+ +	−	?
Sodium valproate	+ +	+ (?)	−
Phenobarbital	+	+	−
Clonazepam	+	+ +	?
Ethosuximide	−	−	+

This pattern of efficacy may correlate with the drugs' actions against generalized tonic-clonic and partial seizures, myoclonic seizures, and generalized absence seizures (see text for details).

Eventually, firing of action potentials fails during the depolarization. Third, the effect of the antiepileptic drugs is time-dependent. Under normal circumstances a train of action potentials can be elicited in neurons, and following membrane repolarization, a depolarization can evoke an action potential which is unaffected. However, in the presence of antiepileptic drug, a train can be evoked with limitation of repetitive firing. Following membrane repolarization for several hundred msec, an evoked action po-

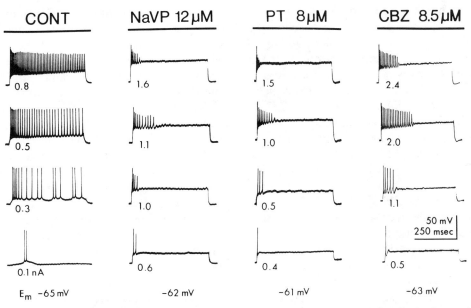

FIG. 2. Sodium valproate (NaVP), phenytoin (PT), and carbamazepine (CBZ) limited sustained high frequency repetitive firing (SRF) of action potentials. Intracellular recordings were made from spinal cord neurons in cell culture and increasing depolarizing current pulses were applied. Magnitude of the current pulses (in namoamps, nA) is shown below each of the traces. The membrane potentials (in mV) from which the depolarizing pulses were applied are shown below each column. In control medium (CONT) SRF was obtained throughout all ranges of depolarization. In the presence of NaVP, PT, and CBZ, limitation of SRF was seen at each of the membrane potentials. (From McLean and Macdonald, ref. 88–90.)

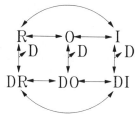

FIG. 3. Voltage-activated sodium channels have three main states. Sodium channels are at rest (R), open (O), or inactivated (I). The distribution of channels among these states in a given neuron is a function of membrane potential and time. When a local anesthetic or antiepileptic drug (D) binds to the channel (DR, DO, DI), the distribution of channels among states may change and the transition rates between states may change. See text for further discussion.

tential will still be of reduced amplitude and rate of rise; i.e., once the effect of the antiepileptic drug has been produced it takes several hundred msec to be removed.

Phenytoin and carbamazepine reduce the amplitude of sodium-dependent action potentials by increasing the voltage-dependency of steady-state inactivation and by reducing the rate of recovery from inactivation of sodium channels (26,83,88, 89,148). Phenytoin, carbamazepine, phenobarbital, and diazepam all inhibit the binding of [H³]batrachotoxin A 20-α-benzoate (BTX-B), a toxin which binds to sodium channels at a site related to activation of sodium channel ion flux (147), and reduce batrachotoxin-stimulated ^{22}Na influx in brain synaptic terminals (149).

The effects of the antiepileptic drugs on sodium channels are similar to those of local anesthetic drugs (25,57,64,137). The action of these drugs has been interpreted using the modulated receptor hypothesis (26,57). The sodium channel exists in three main conformations: a resting (R) or activatable state, an open (O) or conducting state, and an inactive (I) or nonactivatable state (Fig. 3). Under normal circumstances when membrane potential is large and negative,

most of the sodium channels are in the activatable state. With membrane depolarization, a large number of the sodium channels open depending upon the level of the membrane depolarization. With progressive depolarization, some channels are converted to the inactive state and membrane depolarization now will produce opening of fewer channels. If the membrane is held at a very depolarized potential, all channels may be in the inactive state and no channels will open. To remove channel inactivation, the membrane must be again hyperpolarized to a large negative voltage. In the modulated receptor hypothesis, it has been postulated that drugs bind to the different forms of these channels with different affinity. In the case of the antiepileptic drugs, it is likely that they bind to the inactive form of the channel. Therefore, when a neuron has a large negative membrane potential, all of the channels are in the closed conformation and are not bound with high affinity by the antiepileptic drugs. In contrast, when the cell is depolarized, a fraction of the channels are in an inactive state allowing equilibrium to shift toward the bound, inactive conformation of the channel. In such a model, antiepileptic drugs can produce time-, voltage- and use-dependent block of sodium-dependent action potentials because the fraction of inactive channels is increased by membrane depolarization and by repetitive firing. Since the drug which is bound to the inactive channels takes time to dissociate, there is time-dependence of the block. Therefore, it is likely that antiepileptic drugs block SRF of sodium action potentials by selectively binding to the inactive form of the sodium channel.

Although the apparent mechanism of action of sodium valproate is similar to that of phenytoin and carbamazepine, sodium valproate has not been shown to bind to the BTX-B binding site on sodium channels (147) or to block batrachotoxin-stimulated ^{22}Na influx in brain synaptic terminals (149). Thus, it is possible that sodium valproate may bind to a different site on sodium channels than phenytoin and carbamazepine.

Barbiturates, primidone, and benzodiazepines also block SRF, but only at supratherapeutic concentrations (77,91). However, barbiturates and benzodiazepines block SRF at concentrations that are achieved in the treatment of generalized tonic-clonic status epilepticus. Thus, it is likely that phenobarbital and diazepam both block SRF at concentrations achieved in the treatment of generalized tonic-clonic status epilepticus and that this effect may contribute to their anticonvulsant action in this clinical situation.

In contrast, the antiabsence drugs ethosuximide and trimethadione do not block SRF (77,90), BTX-B binding (147), or batrachotoxin-stimulated ^{22}Na influx in brain synaptic terminals (149). Thus, it is likely that blockade of SRF may be responsible, at least in part, for preventing generalized tonic-clonic and partial seizures, but not for generalized absence seizures.

EFFECTS OF ANTIEPILEPTIC DRUGS ON CALCIUM CHANNELS

In addition to effects on sodium channels, the clinically used antiepileptic drugs have been demonstrated to have effects on calcium channels (77). Calcium entry into neurons has been shown to be through three different voltage-dependent calcium channels (109). These channels have been called the L channel, the N channel, and the T channel (Fig. 4). These calcium channels differ in their voltage-dependency for activation and inactivation, the rate of inactivation, and the individual channel conductance. In addition, they have a different agonist and antagonist pharmacology. L channel conductance is large, and L current is long-lasting and slowly inactivating. T channel conductance is small, and T currents are transient and inactivate rapidly. N

channel conductance is intermediate in magnitude, and N current inactivates at a rate between that of the T and L currents. Phenytoin, barbiturates, and benzodiazepines have been demonstrated to reduce calcium influx into synaptic terminals (10,43,67,112) and to block presynaptic release of neurotransmitter (63,103,123, 135,156) at supratherapeutic concentrations. Barbiturates block both L and N currents without affecting T current at anesthetic but not free serum antiepileptic drug concentrations (48,49) (Fig. 4). Similarly, phenytoin (88) and diazepam (134) have been demonstrated to block calcium current at supratherapeutic concentrations.

In contrast, ethosuximide and the trimethadione metabolite dimethadione have recently been demonstrated to affect T current in thalamic neurons (24) and in primary afferent neurons (48) at therapeutically relevant concentrations (Fig. 5). It has been proposed that T calcium currents are important pacemaker currents in thalamic neurons and that these currents may be responsible, in part, for the 3 Hz rhythm seen in the electroencephalogram of patients with generalized absence seizures (24). Blockade of T calcium current by ethosuximide or trimethadione, then, would disrupt the slow rhythmic firing of thalamic neurons and disrupt the spike-and-wave discharge. However, sodium valproate and clonazepam did not alter T calcium currents in primary afferent neurons (48). Thus, it is possible that this effect on T calcium current may underlie the effect of ethosuximide and trimethadione on generalized absence seizures, but not the effect of sodium valproate and the benzodiazepines.

EFFECTS OF ANTIEPILEPTIC DRUGS ON INHIBITORY MECHANISMS

Synaptic inhibition is an important mechanism for regulation of central nervous system excitability. Enhancement of inhibi-

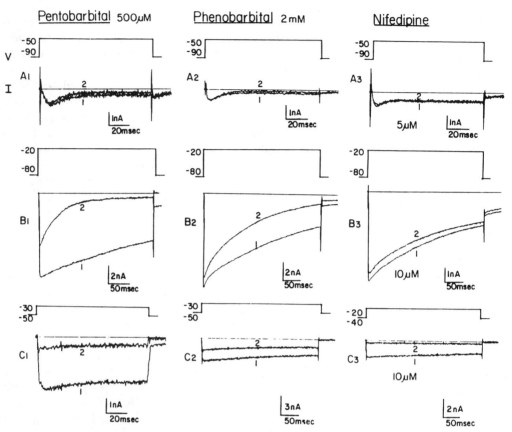

FIG. 4. Pentobarbital and phenobarbital reduced N and L but not T calcium currents, while nifedipine selectively reduced L calcium current. T-, L-, and N/L-currents were evoked using different membrane holding potentials and depolarizing commands. A control current was obtained (**1**) and the effect of pentobarbital (**A₁, B₁, C₁**), phenobarbital (**A₂, B₂, C₂**) and nifedipine (**A₃, B₃, C₃**) were determined by applying the drugs locally to the neuron from a glass micropipette. The current was then evoked again (**2**) and superimposed on the control current. **A,** None of the drugs altered T calcium current. **B,** pentobarbital and phenobarbital, but not nifedipine, increased the rate of inactivation of primarily the N component of the N/L calcium current. **C,** pentobarbital, phenobarbital, and nifedipine decreased L-calcium current. Recordings were made from mouse dorsal root ganglion neurons grown in cell culture. (From Gross and Macdonald, ref. 50, with permission.)

tion, therefore, would be an effective means for decreasing abnormal excitability. Inhibition in the nervous system is mediated by a number of neurotransmitters and their corresponding receptors. Rapid inhibition is mediated primarily by amino acid neurotransmitters including γ-aminobutyric acid (GABA) and glycine acting on postsynaptic GABA$_A$ receptors and glycine receptors, respectively. Additional postsynaptic inhi-

bition which has a slower time course may be mediated by GABA acting at GABA$_B$ receptors (12,105), norepinephrine acting at α_2 receptors (146), and opioid peptides acting at μ- and δ-opioid receptors (107). Inhibition can also be produced presynaptically by reducing the release of neurotransmitter. It is likely that a number of amino acid and neuropeptide transmitters interact with presynaptic receptors to

CONTROL   ETHOSUXIMIDE 1 mM

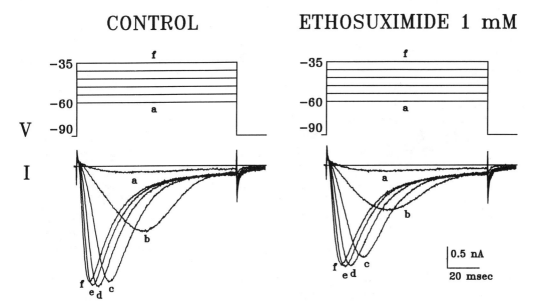

FIG. 5. Ethosuximide reduced T calcium current. Voltage clamp recordings were obtained from acutely dissociated rat nodose ganglion neurons using the whole cell recording technique. The neurons were held at −90 mV and depolarizing commands in 5 mV increments were applied to −60 to −35 mV. Under control conditions this voltage clamp sequence evoked a series of T calcium currents. In the presence of ethosuximide, currents at each command were reduced in amplitude. (From Gross and Macdonald, *unpublished data*).

reduce calcium entry and therefore, to block synaptic transmitter release (38). These neurotransmitters include GABA (37), adenosine (80), neuropeptide Y (40), dynorphin A (17,145), and norepinephrine (38). Rapid forms of inhibition mediated by glycine and GABA_A receptors are produced by activation of neurotransmitter receptors where the proteins forming the receptor also form the channel (47,126). The slower forms of inhibition and the presynaptic regulation of calcium entry are likely mediated by receptors that bind transmitter and then bind guanosine triphosphate (GTP) binding proteins (G-proteins). The G-proteins are heterotrimers that, on interaction with a neurotransmitter-bound receptor, dissociate into a GTP-bound α-subunit and a β-γ dimer (44). It is likely that the α-subunit of the G-protein interacts with calcium channels to reduce presynaptic calcium entry (40,58,130). It has also been demon-

strated that the postsynaptic GABA_B (7), α_2 adrenergic (3) and μ-opioid (3) receptors are coupled to potassium channels via G-proteins.

Of these many forms of inhibition, the only form that has been shown clearly to be regulated by antiepileptic drugs is the GABA_A receptor. The GABA_A receptor has been shown to be an oligomeric complex consisting of at least two binding sites for GABA, allosteric regulatory binding sites for benzodiazepines and β-carbolines, picrotoxin-like convulsant drugs and barbiturates, and a chloride channel (111,119,139). The receptor appears to be formed from four peptide subunits, two α chains and two β chains with a stoichiometry of $\alpha_2\beta_2$ (126), and there are at least three different forms of α chains (68). The GABA binding site is on the β chain and the benzodiazepine binding site is on the α chain. Each peptide chain spans the membrane at least four times, having four membrane or M regions. The juxtaposition of the 16 M units are thought to form the chloride ion channel which is opened by GABA binding. There are series of positive charges around the extracellular portion of the M proteins which presumably are involved in regulating negatively charged chloride ion entry and repelling positively charged cations.

Barbiturates and benzodiazepines bind to specific allosteric regulatory binding sites on the GABA_A receptor. Benzodiazepines have been shown to enhance the binding of GABA to its receptor (93,134) and to enhance GABA receptor current (18,75) (Fig. 6A). Phenobarbital, however, has been demonstrated not to enhance the binding of GABA to its receptor (110); rather, it enhances GABA receptor current (76) (Fig. 6B). The benzodiazepines, diazepam, clonazepam, and nitrazepam, have all been shown to enhance GABA chloride current at low nanomolar concentrations that are achieved in CSF and in plasma, unbound to plasma proteins (132). Similarly, phenobar-

bital has been demonstrated to enhance GABA receptor current at a concentration achieved in ambulatory patients in CSF and in plasma unbound to plasma proteins (127).

Both benzodiazepines and barbiturates enhance GABA receptor current, but they do so by different mechanisms (138,142) (Fig. 7). When GABA binds to its receptor and gates open the chloride ion channel, the channel opens and closes rapidly, forming bursts of openings interrupted by brief closures (53,79) (Fig. 7A, B). This bursting behavior of GABA receptor currents appears to be a general property of neurotransmitter-gated receptor channels (21). Benzodiazepines have been demonstrated to increase the frequency of occurrence of these bursting GABA receptor currents (11,142) (Fig. 7C). Barbiturates, however, do not modify the frequency of occurrence of bursting GABA receptor currents, but instead appear to modify the stability of individual openings (78,142) (Fig. 7D). The GABA receptor bursts are still present but the openings within the bursts are prolonged and there is more current flow per

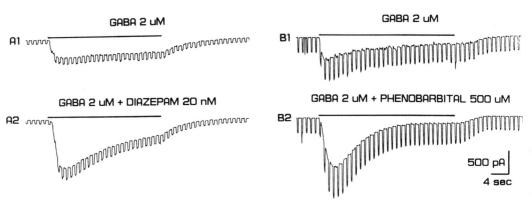

FIG. 6. GABA receptor chloride currents were enhanced by diazepam (DZP) and phenobarbital (PB). Mouse spinal cord neurons were voltage clamped at −75 mV using the whole cell recording technique. GABA (2μM) was applied by pressure ejection from blunt tipped micropipettes positioned adjacent to the neuron. a) GABA receptor current (**A1**) was enhanced when DZP (20 nM was applied with GABA (**A2**). b) GABA receptor current (**B1**) was also enhanced when applied with the PB (500 μM) (**B2**). The equilibrium potential for chloride ions was 0 mV and therefore the GABA receptor currents were inward (downgoing). (From Twyman et al., ref. 142.)

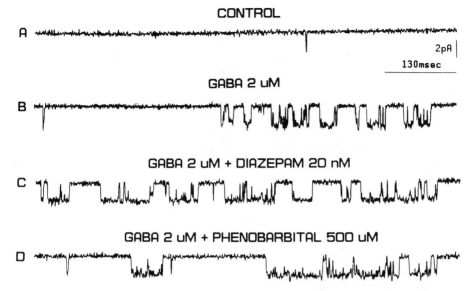

FIG. 7. Single-channel GABA receptor currents were enhanced by diazepam and phenobarbital. Patches of mouse spinal cord neurons were removed using the "outside-out" configuration for patch clamp recording. GABA was applied to the excised patches by local pressure ejection. a) Prior to application of GABA, only rare, brief spontaneous currents were recorded. When channel opening occurred, it produced a downward deflection of the current recording. b) Following application of GABA (2µM), single-channel currents increased in frequency and occurred as single individual openings or in bursts of openings. c) In the presence of DZP (20nM), GABA evoked increased single-channel activity. d) In the presence of PB (500 µM), GABA again increased GABA receptor channel activity. Membrane patches were voltage clamped at −75 mV, and chloride equilibrium potential was 0 mV. It can be seen that DZP increased the frequency of channel opening without altering the basic duration of openings, and PB did not increase the frequency of channel openings but prolonged individual openings. (From Twyman et al., ref. 142.)

burst. Thus, benzodiazepines and barbiturates enhance GABA receptor currents by binding to different binding sites and by regulating different properties of the GABA receptor channel (Fig. 8).

In addition to enhancement of postsynaptic GABA receptor channel properties, drugs that enhance the release of or impair the reuptake of GABA are likely to have anticonvulsant properties (see below).

EFFECTS OF ANTIEPILEPTIC DRUGS ON EXCITATORY MECHANISMS

Excitation in the nervous system is produced primarily by the acidic amino acid glutamate and possibly by aspartate and small dipeptide acidic amino acid (86). Glutamate binds to three different receptors which have been named for agonists that are selective for those receptors, the NMDA receptor, the quisqualate receptor, and the kainate receptor (31,61,92,143). These three receptors are most probably different proteins with different physiological and pharmacological properties. The NMDA receptor operates a channel permeable to Na^+ and Ca^{++} but showing a voltage-dependent block by Mg^{++}.

Of the conventionally used antiepileptic drugs, none of them appear to affect glutamate receptors at therapeutic concentrations (77). The only exception to this is

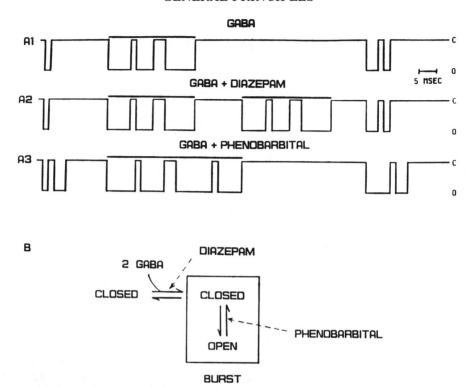

FIG. 8. Barbiturates and benzodiazepines had different sites of action to enhance GABA receptor current. a) GABA (**A₁**) invoked frequent channel openings in isolation or in bursts. Prolonged bursts are overscored. In the presence of DZP (**A₂**), bursts with stable long openings were of the same duration but were more frequent. This resulted in more GABA receptor current. In the presence of PB (**A₃**), bursts were prolonged and consisted of longer single-channel openings. b) In a simplified burst kinetic model for the GABA receptor channel complex, two molecules of GABA bind to the receptor to gate open the chloride channel into bursts. DZP enhanced GABA binding affinity to increased burst frequency without altering individual GABA receptor bursts. PB altered the GABA receptor bursts by prolonging the time spent in the open state. This site of action may be at or near the channel to modify the properties of channel gating. (From Twyman et al., ref. 142.)

phenobarbital which has been shown to block glutamate responses in high magnesium solution, an effect probably at the quisqualate receptor (76,106). Barbiturates do not, however, modify the binding of quisqualate to its receptor at therapeutic plasma concentrations (59). Despite the absence of an action of clinically used antiepileptic drugs on glutamate receptors, there are a number of experimental drugs which have been demonstrated to have anticonvulsant action in experimental animals. Initially it was shown that competitive NMDA receptor antagonists such as 2-APH and 2-amino-5-phosphonovalerate (27,96,97) are potent antiepileptic drugs in rodent and primate models of epilepsy. Similarly, the NMDA channel antagonist MK-801 (150) has been shown to be an effective antiepileptic drug in experimental animals. Whether these antiepileptic drugs will be of clinical use depends on their effects on NMDA receptors involved in the normal functioning of the brain. NMDA receptors are involved in synaptic plasticity and learning; thus, it is possible that NMDA antagonists will have significant cognitive side effects. Whether these antiepileptic drugs will be of clinical use remains an open question.

PRESYNAPTIC ACTIONS OF ANTIEPILEPTIC DRUGS

Presynaptic terminals release one or more neurotransmitters. These include the amino acids acting as fast excitatory neurotransmitters (glutamate, aspartate, and possibly homocysteate) and those acting as inhibitory neurotransmitters (GABA and glycine), and various monoamines whose inhibitory or excitatory effects can vary according to the subtype of receptor present postsynaptically and the nature of ongoing inhibitory or excitatory activity. There is also a very wide range of neuropeptides, some of which are co-released either with amino acids or with monoamines. Synaptic vesicles also contain and apparently release ATP and various cations (including Zn^{++} and Ca^{++}). The effects of co-released neurotransmitters and neuropeptides are not necessarily synergistic but may be in opposition. Thus, GABA and glycine are apparently co-released in the cerebellum, GABA having a direct postsynaptic inhibitory action and glycine having an indirect action via a receptor on the NMDA receptor to enhance the excitatory action of glutamate.

Synaptic release of neurotransmitter substances is primarily determined by the depolarization of the membrane due to the arrival of action potentials. This leads to the entry of Ca^{++} through voltage-sensitive Ca^{++} channels. As already noted, there are three types of voltage-sensitive Ca^{++} channels with different pharmacological characteristics (109). Phenytoin, phenobarbital, and carbamazepine can block voltage-dependent calcium entry into synaptosomes (43). The increase in cytosolic $[Ca^{++}]$ causes synaptic vesicles to fuse with the membrane and release their contents into the synaptic cleft. This process is subject to control or modification by a wide variety of receptors and ionic channels in the presynaptic membrane. So-called "autoreceptors" respond to the released neurotransmitter (e.g., the dopamine and noradrenaline autoreceptors). Other types of presynaptic receptors include those responding to adenosine and those responding to GABA. The latter include the $GABA_B$ receptors which are bicuculline-insensitive and respond to baclofen. There are possibly also $GABA_A$ receptors responding to GABA and benzodiazepines acting presynaptically.

Compounds acting presynaptically can act through various second messenger systems to influence enzymic and membrane functions. These systems include phosphatidylinositol hydrolysis yielding diacylglycerol, which can have the effect of liberating intracellular calcium from the endoplasmic reticulum. The increase in intracellular free $[Ca^{++}]$, besides influencing neurotransmitter release directly, influences the activity in various calcium-calmodulin–dependent enzymes including Ca^{++} calmodulin-dependent ATPases and various protein kinases. Test systems in which the effects of antiepileptic drugs have been evaluated include various *in vitro* preparations (brain slices, synaptosomes, etc.) in which release of excitatory and inhibitory neurotransmitters can be measured, and systems in which the Ca^{++}-calmodulin–dependent phosphorylation of proteins is measured. Phenytoin, carbamazepine, and diazepam inhibit calmodulin kinase II activity (at concentrations higher than their therapeutic CSF levels) (32).

THE ADENOSINE SYSTEM AS A SITE OF ANTIEPILEPTIC DRUG ACTION

Several types of interaction between adenosine systems and antiepileptic drugs have been described (see 36). Inhibition of adenosine uptake is produced by benzodiazepines and some other antiepileptic drugs (116). Inhibition of the binding of adenosine analogs to brain membranes has been shown for carbamazepine and barbiturates (70,144). In rats, long-term carbamazepine administration increases brain adenosine receptors (82). Proof that the antiepileptic drugs act as adenosine-like agents either pre- or postsynaptically is, however, lacking.

EFFECTS OF ANTIEPILEPTIC DRUGS ON NEUROTRANSMITTER METABOLISM, RELEASE, AND UPTAKE

Actions on receptor sites and their associated ion-channels tend to provide the most direct and specific mechanism for modifying inhibitory and excitatory transmission. Significant effects on seizures can also be produced by drugs that either modify the synthesis or further metabolism of neurotransmitters or alter their release or reuptake. The most powerful and general effects concern compounds acting on GABA-mediated inhibition. Effects on excitatory transmission mediated by glutamate, aspartate, or related compounds are also potentially important. Many actions on monoaminergic systems have also been described; their overall importance is uncertain.

GABA Metabolism: Synthesis

The principal pathways of GABA metabolism are shown in Fig. 9. GABA is synthesized directly from glutamate by glutamate decarboxylase (GAD), a cytosolic enzyme that is specifically localized in GABAergic neurons. Glutamate decarboxylase requires pyridoxal phosphate as a coenzyme. Correction of a dietary deficiency of pyridoxine in infants prevents seizures by restoring GABA synthesis to normal. In the normal brain it is probably not possible to enhance GABA synthesis either by precursor loading or by any procedure intended to enhance GAD activity. An enhancement of GAD activity has been described after sodium valproate treatment (71). Other studies, however, indicate a reduced rate of GABA synthesis after sodium valproate administration (16).

GABA Metabolism: Degradation

The further metabolism of GABA to succinate is provided by two mitochondrial enzymes, GABA-transaminase (4-aminobutyrate:2-oxoglutarate aminotransferase, GABA-T) and succinic semialdehyde dehydrogenase (succinate-semialdehyde: NAD(P)oxidoreductase, SSADH). These enzymes occur in neurons and glia, and complete the GABA shunt pathway between the two tricarboxylic acid cycle intermediates, 2-oxoglutarate and succinate. Inhibition of these enzymes can lead to accumulation of GABA in the brain. If this accumulation is presynaptic, it may lead to enhanced inhibitory function through augmented synaptic release of GABA.

Some compounds that act as irreversible or catalytic inhibitors of GABA-T have been shown to be potent antiepileptic drugs in animal test systems (e.g., ethanolamine-O-sulphate, γ-acetylenic GABA and γ-vinyl GABA) (62,98). The latter (as vigabatrin) has been extensively tested in man (see Chapter 68). Administration of these GABA-T inhibitors to rodents produces a massive increase in brain GABA content (4–10-fold after 6–48 hr) (15,125). Vigabatrin enhances the release of preloaded GABA from synaptosomes (2) and the release of GABA from cultured neurons (46). An increase of the release of GABA into cortical superfusates has been demonstrated following the intraperitoneal administration of γ-vinyl GABA or γ-acetylenic GABA in rats (1). In patients, the concen-

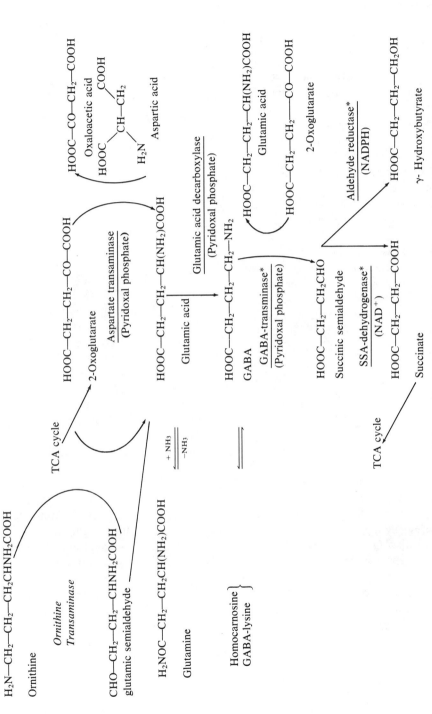

FIG. 9. Metabolic pathways of GABA and glutamate. The route from 2-oxoglutarate to succinate is the "GABA shunt" on the tricarboxylic acid (TCA) cycle. Enzymes inhibited by antiepileptic drugs (sodium valproate, phenobarbital) *in vitro* are marked with an asterisk.

tration of GABA in CSF is increased by therapeutic doses of vigabatrin (51).

GABA Release

Decisive evidence for enhanced release of GABA from presynaptic terminals following antiepileptic drug treatment is largely lacking. The strongest data concerns γ-vinyl-GABA (vigabatrin) where evidence concerning *in vitro* GABA release and *in vivo* GABA increases in cortical superfusates is supplemented by evidence that the concentration of GABA in the CSF of patients treated with vigabatrin rises significantly (52).

Benzodiazepines undoubtedly act postsynaptically to enhance GABA-mediated inhibition, but some physiological experiments suggest that a presynaptic effect is also involved (30). That benzodiazepines enhance the release of GABA is supported by the observation that CSF GABA concentration increases 3–8 min after the intravenous injection of diazepam (72).

GABA Uptake

Synaptically released GABA is inactivated by re-uptake into neurons and glia. Inhibition of this uptake enhances the inhibitory effect of iontophoretically applied GABA (29), and of physiological activation of GABAergic synapses (85). Some compounds inhibiting GABA uptake show selectivity for neuronal versus glial uptake. An anticonvulsant effect of GABA uptake inhibitors has been observed using intracerebroventricular injections in mice with audiogenic seizures (28). Active compounds include such polar molecules as nipecotic acid, *cis*-4-hydroxynipecotic acid, and THPO. Guvacine and nipecotic acid can be made more lipophilic by forming esters (e.g., SKF 100330A and SKF 89976A). Such compounds are anticonvulsant following systemic administration to rodents

(42,66,157). This remains a potential approach to the design of novel antiepileptic drugs. No existing antiepileptic drugs are thought to act by this mechanism, however.

Glutamate and Aspartate Metabolism

Glutamate and aspartate are probably the most important neurotransmitters for fast synaptic excitation in the central nervous system. Sulfonic and sulfinic analogs may play a lesser role as may various di- and tripeptides. The transmission of seizure activity from one neuronal aggregate (e.g., cortical, hippocampal) to another or to subcortical centers involved in the propagation of seizure activity undoubtedly involves activation of glutamatergic synapses. Decreasing the maximal rate of synthesis of glutamate or aspartate could thus suppress the spread of seizure activity. This cannot be achieved by decreasing precursor availability. The main metabolic precursor of cerebral glutamate is glucose. Hypoglycemia, however, increases brain aspartate concentration and facilitates some myoclonic seizure phenomena. Other precursors are glutamine and ornithine (see Fig. 9). Glutamine is of particular interest as it is formed in glial cells from glutamate and is released into the extracellular space where it is taken up by glutamatergic nerve terminals. In the latter site glutamate is reformed by the action of glutaminase. Inhibitors of glutaminase such as azaserine and DON (6-diazo-5-oxo-1-norleucine) have some anticonvulsant activity against sound-induced seizures in rodents (19). Synthesis of glutamate from ornithine requires ornithine aminotransaminase activity which can be inhibited by L-canaline (155). L-Canaline is anticonvulsant when injected focally into the inferior colliculus in rats that show sound-induced seizures (41). Whether any established antiepileptic drugs have primary effects on excitatory amino acid synthesis is not established. Changes in glutamate and aspartate content in the brain are seen acutely after the administration of various antiepileptic drugs. Glutamate is decreased and aspartate increased after phenobarbital or diazepam (13,74), whereas aspartate is decreased and glutamate increased after sodium valproate (16).

Glutamate and Aspartate Release

The synaptic release of glutamate and aspartate can be reduced by acting on a variety of presynaptic receptors, by acting on calcium entry, and by acting on various second messenger systems including the protein kinases that play a role in regulating synaptic release. Adenosine and adenosine analogs can selectively decrease glutamate release (relative to GABA release) (35). The effect of phenytoin, carbamazepine, and benzodiazepines on calmodulin-dependent protein kinases has been described above.

Effects of antiepileptic drugs on stimulated release of endogenous or preloaded acidic amino acids have been demonstrated *in vitro*. Thus, diazepam inhibits the release of preloaded [^{14}C]cysteine sulphate or [^{3}H]glutamate from hippocampal slices (9). Phenytoin and carbamazepine have also been shown to decrease excitatory amino acid release (131).

Whether the reduction in brain aspartate content induced by sodium valproate is associated with reduced synaptic release of aspartate is not certain.

Glutamate and Aspartate Uptake

Impaired re-uptake of glutamate or aspartate could contribute to epileptic phenomena (it occurs during hypoxia or cerebral ischemia and may contribute to the observed facilitation of seizure activity). Drugs enhancing glutamate re-uptake could diminish seizure activity, but evidence for this mechanism of activity is not available.

SUMMARY

The above review suggests that antiepileptic drugs can be divided on a mechanistic basis into at least three classes based on their ability to block SRF by enhancing sodium channel inactivation, to enhance GABAergic inhibition, and to block slow pacemaker-driven repetitive firing by blocking T calcium current. Antiepileptic drugs such as phenytoin and carbamazepine limit SRF but do not modify GABAergic synaptic transmission or T calcium current (Type I drugs). Drugs such as phenobarbital, valproic acid, and the benzodiazepines have dual actions to enhance GABAergic synaptic transmission and to block SRF but do not alter T calcium current (Type II drugs). Ethosuximide and dimethadione, on the other hand, have no effect on either postsynaptic GABA responses or SRF, but block T calcium currents (Type III drugs).

These results further suggest that the ability of a Type I antiepileptic drug to block generalized tonic-clonic seizures and some forms of partial seizures and to block maximal electroshock seizures in experimental animals may correlate with the drug's ability to block SRF. On the other hand, the ability of a Type II antiepileptic drug to enhance GABAergic synaptic transmission may be one mechanism to block myoclonic seizures and pentylenetetrozol-induced seizures in experimental animals. Whether or not generalized absence seizures are blocked by enhancement of GABAergic inhibition is uncertain but remains a possibility. Type III antiepileptic drugs may be effective against generalized absence seizures in humans and pentylenetetrozol-induced seizures in experimental animals due to their effect on T calcium current. This mechanistic classification must remain tentative at the present time since the actions described have not been directly demonstrated to be antiepileptic in experimental animals. Nonetheless, it is likely that cellular mechanisms such as those demonstrated in *in vitro* models are important for antiepileptic efficacy. Further investigation may lead in future to a classification of antiepileptic drugs based on mechanistic rather than empirical bases.

REFERENCES

1. Abdul-Ghani, A. S., Coutinho-Netto, J., and Bradford, H. F. (1980): The action of γ-vinyl-GABA and γ-acetylenic GABA on the resting and stimulated release of GABA *in vivo*. *Brain Res.*, 191:471–481.
2. Abdul-Ghani, A. S., Norris, P. J., Smith, C. C. T., and Bradford, H. F. (1981): Effects of γ-acetylenic GABA and γ-vinyl GABA on synaptosomal release and uptake of GABA. *Biochem. Pharmacol.*, 30:1203–1209.
3. Aghajanian, G. K., and Wang, Y.-Y. (1986): Pertussis toxin blocks the outward currents evoked by opiate and α₂-agonists in locus coeruleus neurons. *Brain Res.*, 371:390–394.
4. Alger, B. E. (1984): Characteristics of a slow hyperpolarizing synaptic potential in rat hippocampal pyramidal cells *in vitro*. *J. Neurophys.*, 52:892–910.
5. Alger, B. E., and Nicoll, R. A. (1980): Epileptiform burst after-hyperpolarization: Calcium-dependent potassium potential in hippocampal CA₁ pyramidal cells. *Science*, 210:1122–1124.
6. Alger, B. E., and Williamson, A. (1988): A transient calcium-dependent potassium component of the epileptiform burst after-hyperpolarization in rat hippocampus. *J. Physiol. (Lond.)*, 399:191–205.
7. Andrade, R., Malenka, R. C., and Nicoll, R. A. (1986): A G protein couples serotonin and GABA_B receptors to the same channels in hippocampus. *Science*, 234:1261–1265.
8. Ayala, G. F., Matsumoto, H., and Gumnit, R. J. (1970): Excitability changes and inhibitory mechanisms in neocortical neurons during seizures. *J. Neurophysiol.*, 33:73–85.
9. Baba, A., Okumura, S., Mizuo, H., and Iwata, H. (1983): Inhibition by diazepam and γ-aminobutyric acid of depolarization-induced release of [4C]cysteine sulfinate and [dH]glutamate in rat hippocampal slices. *J. Neurochem.*, 40:280–284.
10. Blaustein, M. P., and Ector, A. C. (1975): Barbiturate inhibition of calcium uptake by depolarized nerve terminals *in vitro*. *Mol. Pharmacol.*, 11:369–378.
11. Bormann, J. (1988): Electrophysiology of GABA_A and GABA_B receptor subtypes. *TINS*, 11:112–116.
12. Bowery, N. G., Doble, A., Hill, D. R., Hudson, A. L., Middlemiss, D. N., Shaw, J., and Turnball, M. J. (1980): (−)-Baclofen decreases neurotransmitter release in the mammalian CNS by an action at a novel GABA receptor. *Nature*, 283:92–94.
13. Carlsson, C., and Chapman, A. G. (1981): The effect of diazepam on the cerebral metabolic state in rats and its interaction with nitrous oxide. *Anesthesiol.*, 54:488–495.
14. Chapman, A., Keane, P. I., Meldrum, B. S., Simiand, J., and Vernieres, J. C. (1982): Mechanism of anticonvulsant action of valproate. *Prog. Neurobiol.*, 19:315–359.
15. Chapman, A. G., Nordström, C. H., and Siesjö, B. K. (1978): Influence of phenobarbital anesthesia on carbohydrate and amino acid metabolism in rat brain. *Anesthesiol.*, 48:175–182.
16. Chapman, A. G., Riley, K., Evans, M. C., and Meldrum, B. S. (1982): Acute effects of sodium valproate and γ-vinyl GABA on regional amino acid metabolism in the rat brain. *Neurochem. Res.*, 7:1089–1105.
17. Chavkin, C., James, I. F., and Goldstein, A. (1982): Dynorphin is a specific endogenous ligand of the κ opioid receptor. *Science*, 215:413–415.
18. Choi, D. W., Farb, D. H., and Fischbach, G. D. (1977): Chlordiazepoxide selectively augments GABA action in spinal cord cell cultures. *Nature*, 269:342–344.
19. Chung, S. H., and Johnson, M. S. (1984): Studies on sound-induced epilepsy in mice. *Proc. Roy. Soc. B.*, 221:145–168.
20. Collins, R. C. (1989). Prefrontal-limbic systems: Evolving clinical concepts. In: *Advances in Contemporary Neurology Series*, edited by F. Plum. F. A. Davis (*in press*).
21. Colquhoun, D., and Sakmann, B. (1985): Fast events in single-channel currents activated by acetylcholine and its analogues at the frog muscle endplate. *J. Physiol. (Lond.)*, 369:501–557.
22. Connors, B. W. (1984): Initiation of synchronized neuronal bursting in neocortex. *Nature*, 310:685–687.
23. Connors, B. W., and Gutnick, M. J. (1984): Cellular mechanisms of neocortical epileptogenesis in an acute experimental model. In: *Electrophysiology of Epilepsy*, edited by P. A. Schwartzkroin and H. V. Wheal, pp. 79–105. Academic Press, London.
24. Coulter, D. A., Hugenard, J. R., and Prince, D. A. (1989): Specific petit mal anticonvulsants reduce calcium currents in thalamic neurons. *Neurosci. Lett.* (*in press*).
25. Courtney, K. R. (1975): Mechanism of frequency-dependent inhibition of sodium currents in myelinated nerve by the lidocaine derivative GEA 968. *J. Pharmacol. Exp. Ther.*, 195:225–236.
26. Courtney, K. R., and Etter, E. F. (1983): Modulated anticonvulsant block of sodium channels in nerve and muscle. *Eur. J. Pharmacol.*, 88:1–9.
27. Croucher, M. J., Collins, J. F., and Meldrum, B. S. (1982): Anticonvulsant action of excitatory amino acid antagonists. *Science*, 216:899–901.
28. Croucher, M. J., Meldrum, B. S., and Krogsgaard-Larsen, P. (1983). Anticonvulsant activity of GABA uptake inhibitors and their prodrugs following central or systemic administration. *Eur. J. Pharmacol.* 89:217–228.

29. Curtis, D. R., Game, C. J. A., and Lodge, D. (1976): The *in vivo* inactivation of GABA and other inhibitory amino acids in the cat nervous system. *Exp. Brain Res.*, 25:413–428.

30. Curtis, D. R., Lodge, D., Johnson, G. A. R., Brand, S. I. (1976): Central actions of benzodiazepines. *Brain Res.*, 118:344–347.

31. Davies, J. D., Evans, R. H., Francis, A. A., et al. (1982): Conformational aspects of the actions of some piperidine dicarboxylic acids at excitatory amino acid receptors in the mammalian and amphibian spinal cord. *Neurochem Res.*, 7:1119–1133.

32. DeLorenzo, R. J. (1986): A molecular approach to the calcium signal in brain: Relationship to synaptic modulation and seizure discharge. In: *Advances in Neurology, Vol. 44.*, edited by A. V. Delgado-Escueta, A. A. Ward, D. M. Woodbury, and R. J. Porter, pp. 435–464. Raven Press, New York.

33. Dichter, M., and Spencer, W. A. (1969): Penicillin-induced interictal discharges from the cat hippocampus. I. Characteristics and topographical features. *J. Neurophysiol.*, 32:649–662.

34. Dingledine, R., Hynes, M. A., and King, G. L. (1986): Involvement of *N*-methyl-*D*-aspartate receptors in epilepitform bursting in the rat hippocampal slice. *J. Physiol. (Lond.)*, 380:175–189.

35. Dolphin, A. C., and Archer, E. R. (1983): An adenosine agonist inhibits and a cyclic AMP analogue enhances the release of glutamate but not GABA from slices of rat dentate gyrus. *Neurosci. Lett.*, 43:49–54.

36. Dragunow, M. (1988): Purinergic mechanisms in epilepsy. *Progress in Neurobiology*, 31:85–108.

37. Dunlap, K. (1981): Two types of γ-aminobutyric acid receptor on embryonic sensory neurones. *Br. J. Pharmac.*, 74:579–585.

38. Dunlap, K., and Fischbach, G. D. (1978): Neurotransmitters decrease the calcium component of sensory neurone action potentials. *Nature*, 276:837–839.

39. Esplin, D. (1957): Effect of diphenylhydantoin on synaptic transmission in the cat spinal cord and stellate ganglion. *J. Pharmacol. Exp. Ther.*, 120:301–323.

40. Ewald, D. A., Sternweis, P. C., and Miller, R. J. (1988): Guanine nucleotide-binding protein G_o-induced coupling of neuropeptide Y receptors to Ca^{2+} channels in sensory neurons. *Proc. Natl. Acad. Sci. USA*, 85:3633–3637.

41. Faingold, C. L., Copley, C. A., and Boersma, C. A. (1987): Blockade of audiogenic seizures (AGS) in genetically epilepsy-prone rats (GEPR) by the microinjection into inferior colliculus (IC) of blockers of inhibitory and excitant amino acid (EAA) metabolism. *Society for Neuroscience Abstracts*, p. 1158.

42. Falch, E., Meldrum, B. S., and Krogsgaard-Larsen, P. (1987): GABA uptake inhibitors, synthesis and effects on audiogenic seizures of ester prodrugs of nipecotic acid, guvacine and *Cis*-4-hydroxynipecotic acid. *Drug Design and Delivery*, 2:9–21.

43. Ferrendelli, J. A., and Daniels-McQueen, S. (1982): Comparative actions of phenytoin and other antiepileptic drugs on potassium- and veratridine-stimulated calcium uptake in synaptosomes. *J. Pharmacol. Exp. Ther.*, 220:29–34.

44. Gilma, A. G. (1984): Guanine nucleotide-binding regulatory proteins and dual control of adenylate cyclase. *J. Clin. Invest.*, 73:1–4.

45. Gloor, P. (1979): Generalized epilepsy with spike-and-wave discharge: A re-interpretation of its electrographic and clinical manifestations. *Epilepsia*, 20:577–588.

46. Gram, L., Larsson, O. M., Johnsen, A. H., and Schousboe, A. (1988): Effects of valproate, vigabatrin and aminooxyacetic acid on release of endogenous and exogenous GABA from cultured neurons. *Epilepsy Res.*, 2:87–95.

47. Grenningloh, G., Rienitz, A., Schmitt, B., Methfessel, C., Zensen, M., Beyreuther, K., Gundelfinger, E. D., and Betz, H. (1987): The strychnine-binding subunit of the glycine receptor shows homology with nicotinic acetylcholine receptors. *Nature*, 328:215–220.

48. Gross, R. A., Kelly, K. M., and Macdonald, R. L. (1989): Ethosuximide and dimethidione selectively reduce calcium currents in cultured sensory neurons by different mechanisms. *Neurology*, 39(suppl. 1)412.

49. Gross, R. A., and Macdonald, R. L. (1987): Barbiturates and nifedipine have different and selective effects on calcium currents of mouse DRG neurons in culture: A possible basis for differing clinical actions. *Neurology*, 18:443–451.

50. Gross, R. A., and Macdonald, R. L. (1988): Differential actions of pentobarbitone on calcium current components of mouse sensory neurones in culture. *J. Physiol (Lond.)*, 405:187–203.

51. Grove, J., Schechter, P. J., Tell, G., Koch-Weser, J., Sjoerdsma, A., Warter, J. M., Marescaux, C., and Rumbach, L. (1981): Increased γ-aminobutyric acid (GABA), homocarnosine and β-alanine in cerebrospinal fluid of patients treated with γ-vinyl GABA (4-amino-hex-5-enoic acid). *Life Sci.*, 28:2431–2439.

52. Halonen, T., Lehtinen, M., Pitkänen, A., Ylinen, A., and Riekkinen, P. J. (1988): Inhibitory and excitatory amino acids in CSF of patients suffering from complex partial seizures during chronic treatment with γ-vinyl-GABA (vigabatrin). *Epilepsy Res.*, 2:246–252.

53. Hamill, O. P., Bormann, J., and Sakmann, B. (1983): Activation of multiple-conductance state chloride channels in spinal neurones by glycine and GABA. *Nature*, 305:805–808.

54. Harding, G. F. A., Herrick, C. E., and Jeavons, P. M. (1978): A controlled study of the effect of sodium valproate on photosensitive epilepsy and its prognosis. *Epilepsia*, 19:555–565.

55. Hayashi, T. (1952): A physiological study of epileptic seizures following cortical stimulation in animals and its application to human clinics. *Jap. J. Pharmacol.*, 3:46–64.

56. Hershkowitz, N., and Raines, A. (1978): Effects

of carbamazepine on muscle spindle discharges: *J. Pharmacol. Exp. Ther.*, 204:581–591.

57. Hille, B. (1977): Hydrophilic and hydrophobic pathways for the drug-receptor reaction. *J. Gen. Physiol.*, 69:497–515.

58. Holz, G. G., Rane, S. G., and Dunlap, K. (1986): GTP binding proteins mediate transmitter inhibition of voltage-dependent calcium channels. *Nature,* 319:670–672.

59. Honoré, T., Davies, S. N., Drejer, J., Fletcher, E. J., Jacobsen, P., Lodge, D., and Nielsen, F. E. (1988): Quinoxalinediones: Potent competitive non-NMDA glutamate receptor antagonists. *Science,* 241:701–703.

60. Hood, T. W., Siegfried, J., and Haas, H. L. (1983): Analysis of carbamazepine actions in hippocampal slices of the rat. *Cell. and Mol. Neurobiol.*, 3:213–222.

61. Jones, A. W., Smith, D. A. S., and Watkins, J. C. (1984): Structure-activity relations of dipeptide antagonists of excitatory amino acids. *Neuroscience,* 13:573–581.

62. Jung, M. J., Lippert, B., Metcalf, B. W., Böhlen, P., and Schechter, P. J. (1977): γ-Vinyl GABA (4-amino-hex-5-enoic acid), a new selective inhibitor of GABA-T: Effects on brain GABA metabolism in mice. *J. Neurochem.,* 29:797–802.

63. Kalant, H., and Grose, W. (1967): Effects of ethanol and pentobarbital on release of acetylcholine from cerebral cortex slices. *J. Pharmacol. Exp. Ther.*, 158:386–393.

64. Khodorov, B. I. (1981): Sodium inactivation and drug-induced immobilization of the gating charge in nerve membrane. *Prog. Biophys. Mol. Biol.,* 37:49–89.

65. Krall, R. L., Penry, J. K., White, B. G., Kupferberg, H. J., and Swinyard, E. A. (1978): Antiepileptic drug development: II. Anticonvulsant drug screening. *Epilepsia,* 19:409–428.

66. Krogsgaard-Larsen, P., Falch, E., Larsson, O. M., and Schousboe, A. (1987): GABA uptake inhibitors: Relevance to antiepileptic drug research. *Epilepsy Res.,* 1:77–93.

67. Leslie, S. W., Friedman, M. B., and Coleman, R. R. (1980): Effects of chlordiazepoxide on depolarization-induced calcium influx into synaptosomes. *Biochem. Pharmacol.,* 29:2439–2443.

68. Levitan, E. S., Schofield, P. R., Burt, D. R., Rhee, L. M., Wisden, W., Köhler, M., Norihisa, J., Rodriguez, H. F., Stephenson, A., Darlison, M. G., Barnard, E. A., and Seeburg, P. H. (1988): Structural and functional basis for GABA_A receptor heterogeneity. *Nature,* 335:76–79.

69. Lockard, J. S., and Levy, R. H. (1976): Valproic acid: Reversibly acting drug? *Epilepsia,* 17:477–479.

70. Lohse, M. J., Klotz, K.-N., Jakobs, K. H., and Schwabe, U. (1985): Barbiturates are selective antagonists at A₁ adenosine receptors. *J. Neurochem.,* 45:1761–1770.

71. Löscher, W. (1981): Valproate induced changes in GABA metabolism at the subcellular level. *Biochem. Pharmacol.,* 30:1364–1366.

72. Löscher, W., and Schmidt, D. (1987): Diazepam

73. Löscher, W., and Schmidt, D. (1988): Which animal models should be used in the search for new antiepileptic drugs? A proposal based on experimental and clinical considerations. *Epilepsy Res.,* 2:145–181.

74. Lothman, E. W., Collins, R. C., and Ferrendelli, J. A. (1981): Kainic acid-induced limbic seizures: Electrophysiologic studies. *Neurology,* 31:806–812.

75. Macdonald, R. L., and Barker, J. L. (1978): Benzodiazepines specifically modulate GABA-mediated postsynaptic inhibition in cultured mammalian neurones. *Nature,* 271:563–564.

76. Macdonald, R. L., and Barker, J. L. (1978): Different actions of anticonvulsant and anesthetic barbiturates revealed by use of cultured mammalian neurons. *Science,* 200:775–777.

77. Macdonald, R. L., and McLean, M. J. (1986): Anticonvulsant drugs: Mechanisms of action. In: *Advances in Neurology, Vol. 44,* edited by A. V. Delgado-Escueta, A. A. Ward, Jr., D. M. Woodbury, and R. J. Porter, pp. 713–736. Raven Press, New York.

78. Macdonald, R. L., Rogers, C. J., and Twyman, R. E. (1989): Barbiturate regulation of kinetic properties of the main conductance state of the GABA_A receptor channel of mouse spinal cord neurones in culture. *J. Physiol. (Lond.), (in press)*.

79. Macdonald, R. L., Rogers, C. J., and Twyman, R. E. (1989): Kinetic properties of the GABA_A receptor main conductance state of mouse spinal cord neurones in culture. *J. Physiol. (Lond.),* 410:479–499.

80. Macdonald, R. L., Skerritt, J. H., and Werz, M. A. (1986): Adenosine agonists reduce voltage-dependent calcium conductance of mouse sensory neurones in cell culture. *J. Physiol. (Lond.),* 370:75–90.

81. MacVicar, B. A., and Dudek, F. R. (1980): Local synaptic circuits in rat hippocampus: Interactions between pyramidal cells. *Brain Res.,* 184:220–223.

82. Marangos, P. J., Weiss, S. R. B., Montgomery, P., Patel, J., Narang, P. K., Cappabianca, A. M., and Post, R. M. (1985): Chronic carbamazepine treatment increases brain adenosine receptors. *Epilepsia,* 26:493–498.

83. Matsuki, N., Quandt, F. N., Ten Eick, R. E., and Yeh, J. Z. (1984): Characterization of the block of sodium channels by phenytoin in mouse neuroblastoma cells. *J. Pharmacol. Exp. Ther.,* 228:523–530.

84. Matsumoto, H., and Ajmone Marsan, C. (1964): Cortical cellular phenomena in experimental epilepsy: Interictal manifestations. *Exptl. Neurol.,* 9:286–304.

85. Matthews, W. D., McCafferty, G. P., and Setler, P. E. (1981). An electrophysiological model of GABA-mediated neurotransmission. *Neuropharmacol.,* 20:561–565.

86. Mayer, M. L., and Westbrook, G. L. (1987): The

physiology of excitatory amino acids in the vertebrate central nervous system. *Prog. Neurobiol.*, 28:197–276.

87. Mayer, M. L., Westbrook, G. L., and Guthrie, P. B. (1984): Voltage-dependent block by Mg^{2+} of NMDA responses in spinal cord neurones. *Nature*, 309:261–263.

88. McLean, M. J., and Macdonald, R. L. (1983): Multiple actions of phenytoin on mouse spinal cord neurons in cell culture. *J. Pharmacol. Exp. Ther.*, 227:779–789.

89. McLean, M. J., and Macdonald, R. L. (1986): Carbamazepine and 10,11-epoxycarbamazepine produce use- and voltage-dependent limitation of rapidly firing action potentials of mouse central neurons in cell culture. *J. Pharmacol. Exp. Ther.*, 238:727–738.

90. McLean, M. J., and Macdonald, R. L. (1986): Sodium valproate, but not ethosuximide, produces use- and voltage-dependent limitation of high frequency repetitive firing of action potentials of mouse central neurons in cell culture. *J. Pharmacol. Exp. Ther.*, 237:1001–1011.

91. McLean, M. J., and Macdonald, R. L. (1988): Benzodiazepines, but not beta carbolines, limit high frequency repetitive firing of action potentials of spinal cord neurons in cell culture. *J. Pharmacol. Exp. Ther.*, 244:789–795.

92. McLennan, H. (1983): Receptors for excitatory amino acids in the mammalian central nervous system. *Prog. Neurobiol.*, 20:251–271.

93. Meiners, B. A., and Salama, A. I. (1982): Enhancement of benzodiazepine and GABA binding by the novel anxiolytic, tracazolate. *Eur. J. Pharmacol.*, 78:315–322.

94. Meldrum, B. S. (1986): Preclinical test systems for evaluation of novel compounds. In *New Anticonvulsant Drugs*, edited by B. S. Meldrum and R. J. Porter, pp. 31–48. John Libbey, London.

95. Meldrum, B. S. (1988): *In vivo* and *in vitro* models of epilepsy and their relevance to man. In *The Anatomy of Epileptogenesis*, edited by B. S. Meldrum, J. A. Ferrendelli, and H. G. Wieser, pp. 27–42. John Libbey, London.

96. Meldrum, B. S., Croucher, M. J., Badman, G., and Collins, J. F. (1983): Antiepileptic action of excitatory amino acid antagonists in the photosensitive baboon, *Papio papio. Neurosci. Lett.*, 39:101–104.

97. Meldrum, B. S., Croucher, M. J., Czuczwar, S. J., Collins, J. F., Curry, K., Joseph, M., and Stone, T. W. (1983): A comparison of the anticonvulsant potency of (+/−) 2-amino-5-phosphonopentanoic acid and (+/−) 2-amino-7-phosphonoheptanoic acid. *Neuroscience*, 9:925–930.

98. Metcalf, B. W. (1979): Inhibitors of GABA metabolism. *Biochem. Pharmacol.*, 28:5–1712.

99. Miles, R., and Wong, R. K. S. (1983): Single neurones can influence synchronized population discharge in the CA_3 region of the guinea pig hippocampus. *Nature*, 306:371–373.

100. Miles, R., and Wong, R. K. S. (1987): Latent synaptic pathways revealed after tetanic stimulation in the hippocampus. *Nature*, 328:724–726.

101. Millan, M. H. (1988). Sound-induced seizures in rodents. In: *Anatomy of Epileptogenesis*, edited by B. S. Meldrum, J. A. Ferrendelli, and H. G. Wieser, pp. 43–56. John Libbey, London.

102. Miller, J. W., and Ferrendelli, J. A. (1988): Brain stem and diencephalic structures regulating experimental generalised (pentylenetetrazol) seizures in rodents. In: *Anatomy of Epileptogenesis*, edited by B. S. Meldrum, J. A. Ferrendelli, and H. G. Wiese, pp. 57–69. John Libbey, London.

103. Mitchell, P. R., and Martin, I. L. (1978): The effects of benzodiazepines on K^+-stimulated release of GABA. *Neuropharmacology*, 17:317–320.

104. Newberry, N. R., and Nicoll, R. A. (1984): A bicuculline-resistant inhibitory post-synaptic potential in rat hippocampal pyramidal cells *in vitro*. *J. Physiol. (Lond.)*, 348:239–254.

105. Newberry, N. R., and Nicoll, R. A. (1985): Comparison of the action of baclofen with γ-aminobutyric acid on rat hippocampal pyramidal cells *in vitro*. *J. Physiol. (Lond.)*, 265:465–488.

106. Nicoll, R. A. (1975): Pentobarbital: Action on frog motoneurons. *Brain Res.*, 96:119–123.

107. North, R. A. (1986): Receptors on individual neurones. *Neuroscience*, 17:899–907.

108. Nowak, L., Bregostovski, P., Ascher, P., Herbet, A., and Prochiantz, A. (1984): Magnesium gates glutamate-activated channels in mouse central neurones. *Nature*, 307:462–465.

109. Nowycky, M. C., Fox, A. P., and Tsien, R. W. (1985): Three types of neural calcium channels with different calcium agonist sensitivity. *Nature*, 316:440–443.

110. Olsen, R. W., and Snowman, A. M. (1982): Chloride-dependent enhancement by barbiturates of γ-aminobutyric acid receptor binding. *J. Neurosci.*, 2:1812–1823.

111. Olsen, R. W., and Venter, J. C. (eds.) (1986): Benzodiazepine/GABA receptors and chloride channels: Structure and functional properties. In: *Receptor Biochemistry and Methodology, Vol. 5*, pp. 1–351. Alan R. Liss, New York.

112. Ondrusek, M. G., Belknap, J. K., and Leslie, S. W. (1979): Effects of acute and chronic barbiturate administration on synaptosomal calcium accumulation. *Mol. Pharmacol.*, 15:386–395.

113. O'Shaughnessy, C. T., Aram, J. A., and Lodge, D. (1988): A1 adenosine receptor-mediated block of epileptiform activity induced in zero magnesium in rat neocortex *in vitro*. *Epilepsy Res.*, 2:294–301.

114. Patel, S., Millan, M. H., and Meldrum, B. S. (1988): Decrease in excitatory transmission within the lateral habenula and the mediodorsal thalamus protects against limbic seizures in rats. *Exp. Neurol.*, 101:63–74.

115. Patel, S., Millan, M. H., Mello, L. M., and Meldrum, B. S. (1986): 2-Amino-7-phosphonoheptanoic acid (2-APH) infusion into entopeduncular nucleus protects against limbic seizures in rat. *Neurosci. Lett.*, 64:226–230.

116. Phillis, J. W., Wu, P. H., and Bender, A. S. (1981): Inhibition of adenosine uptake into rat

brain synaptosomes by the benzodiazepines. *Gen. Pharmacol.,* 12:67–70.

117. Piredda, S. G., Woodhead, J. H., and Swinyard, E. A. (1985): Effect of stimulus intensity on the profile of anticonvulsant activity of phenytoin, ethosuximide and valproate. *J. Pharmacol. Exptl. Therap.,* 232:741–745.

118. Piredda, S., Yonekawa, W., Whittingham, T. S., and Kupferberg, H. J. (1985): Potassium, pentylenetetrazol, and anticonvulsants in mouse hippocampal slices. *Epilepsia,* 26:167–174.

119. Polc, P., Bonetti, E. P., Schaffner, R., and Haefely, W. (1982): A three-state model of the benzodiazepine receptor explains the interactions between the benzodiazepine antagonist Ro 15-1788, benzodiazepine tranquilizers, β-carbolines, and phenobarbitone. *Naunyn-Schmiedeberg's Arch. Pharmacol.,* 321:260–264.

120. Porter, R. J. (1986): Antiepileptic drugs: Efficacy and inadequacy. In: *New Anticonvulsant Drugs,* edited by B. S. Meldrum and R. J. Porter, pp. 3–15. John Libbey & Co., London.

121. Prince, D. A. (1968): The depolarization shift in "epileptic" neurons. *Exptl. Neurol.,* 21:467–485.

122. Raines, A., and Standaert, F. G. (1966): Pre- and post-junctional effects of DPH at the cat soleus neuromuscular junction. *J. Pharmacol. Exp. Ther.,* 153:361–366.

123. Richter, J. A., and Waller, M. B. (1977): Effects of pentobarbital on the regulation of acetylcholine content and release in different regions of rat brain. *Biochem. Pharmacol.,* 26:609–615.

124. Rose, G. M., Olpe, H.-R., and Haas, H. L. (1986): Testing of prototype antiepileptic drugs in hippocampal slices. *Arch. Pharmacol.,* 332:89–92.

125. Schechter, P. J., Tranier, Y., Jung, M. J., and Böhlen, P. (1977). Audiogenic seizure protection by elevated brain GABA concentration in mice, effects of γ-acetylenic GABA and γ-vinyl GABA, two irreversible GABA-T inhibitors. *Eur. J. Pharmacol.,* 45:319–328.

126. Schofield, P. R., Darlison, M. G., Fujita, N., Burt, D. R., Stephenson, F. A., Rodriguez, H., Rhee, L. M., Ramachandran, J., Reale, V., Glencorse, T. A., Seeburg, P. H., and Barnard, E. A. (1987): Sequence and functional expression of the GABA$_A$ receptor shows a ligand-gated receptor super-family. *Nature,* 328:221–227.

127. Schulz, D. W., and Macdonald, R. L. (1981): Barbiturate enhancement of GABA-mediated inhibition and activation of chloride ion conductance: Correlation with anticonvulsant and anesthetic actions. *Brain Res.,* 209:177–188.

128. Schwartzkroin, P. A., Prince, D. A. (1978): Cellular and field potential properties of epileptogenic hippocampal slices. *Brain Res.,* 147:117–130.

129. Schwartzkroin, P. A., and Stafstrom, C. E. (1980): Effects of EGTA on the calcium-activated afterhyperpolarization in hippocampal CA$_3$ pyramidal cells. *Science,* 210:1125–1126.

130. Scott, R. H., and Dolphin, A. C. (1986): Regulation of calcium currents by a GTP analogue:

Potentiation of baclofen-mediated inhibition. *Neurosci. Lett.,* 69:59–64.

131. Skerritt, J. H., and Johnston, G. A. R. (1984): Modulation of excitant amino acid release by convulsant and anticonvulsant drugs. In: *Neurotransmitters, Seizures and Epilepsy, II,* edited by R. G. Fariello, pp. 215–226. New York, Raven Press.

132. Skerritt, J. H., and Macdonald, R. L. (1984): Benzodiazepine receptor ligand actions on GABA responses. Benzodiazepines, CL 218872, Zopiclone. *Eur. J. Pharmacol.,* 101:127–134.

133. Skerritt, J. H., Werz, M. A., McLean, M. J., and Macdonald, R. L. (1984): Diazepam and its anomalous *p*-chloro-derivative Ro 5-4864: Comparative effects on mouse neurons in cell culture. *Brain Res.,* 310:99–105.

134. Skerritt, J. H., Willow, M., and Johnston, G. A. R. (1982): Diazepam enhancement of low affinity GABA binding to rat brain membranes. *Neurosci. Lett.,* 29:63–66.

135. Somjen, G. G. (1963): Effects of ether and thiopental on spinal presynaptic terminals. *J. Pharmacol. Exp. Ther.,* 140:393–402.

136. Stanton, P. K., Jones, R. S. G., Mody, I., and Heinemann, U. (1987): Epileptiform activity induced by lowering extracellular [Mg^{2+}] in combined hippocampal-entorhinal cortex slices: Modulation by receptors for norepinephrine and *N*-methyl-*D*-aspartate. *Epilepsy Res.,* 1:53–62.

137. Strichartz, G. R. (1973): The inhibition of sodium currents in myelinated nerve by quaternary derivatives of lidocaine. *J. Gen. Physiol.,* 62:37–57.

138. Study, R. E., and Barker, J. L. (1981). Diazepam and (+/−)-pentobarbital: Fluctuation analysis reveals different mechanisms for potentiation of γ-aminobutyric acid responses in cultured central neurons. *Proc. Natl. Acad. Sci. U.S.A.,* 78:7180–7184.

139. Tallman, J., and Gallager, D. (1985): The GABAergic system: A locus of benzodiazepine action. *Annual Rev. Neurosci.,* 8:21–44.

140. Thalmann, R. H. (1984): Reversal properties of an EGTA-resistant late hyperpolarization that follows synaptic stimulation of hippocampal neurons. *Neurosci. Lett.,* 46:103–108.

141. Traub, R. D., and Wong, R. K. S. (1982): Cellular mechanism of neuronal synchronization in epilepsy. *Science,* 216:745–747.

142. Twyman, R. E., Rogers, C. J., and Macdonald, R. L. (1989): Differential regulation of GABA$_A$ receptor channels by diazepam and phenobarbital. *Ann. Neurol.,* 25:213–220.

143. Watkins, J. C., and Evans, R. H. (1981): Excitatory amino acid transmitters. *Ann. Rev. Pharmacol. Toxicol.,* 21:165–204.

144. Weir, R. L., Padgett, W., Daly, J. W., and Anderson, S. M. (1984): Interaction of anticonvulsant drugs with adenosine receptors in the central nervous system. *Epilepsia,* 25:492–498.

145. Werz, M. A., and Macdonald, R. L. (1984): Dynorphin reduces calcium-dependent action potential duration by decreasing voltage-dependent calcium conductance. *Neurosci. Lett.,* 46:185–190.

146. Williams, J. T., Henderson, G., and North, R. A. (1985): Characterization of α_2-adrenoceptors which increase potassium conductance in rat locus coeruleus neurones. *Neuroscience,* 14:95–101.

147. Willow, M., and Catterall, W. A. (1982): Inhibition of binding of [^{3}H]Batrachotoxinin A 20-α-benzoate to sodium channels by the anticonvulsant drugs diphenylhydantoin and carbamazepine. *Mol. Pharmacol.,* 22:627–635.

148. Willow, M., Gonoi, T., and Catterall, W. A. (1985): Voltage clamp analysis of the inhibitory actions of diphenylhydantoin and carbamazepine on voltage-sensitive sodium channels in neuroblastoma cells. *Mol. Pharmacol.,* 27:549–558.

149. Willow, M., Kuenzel, E. A., and Catterall, W. A. (1984): Inhibition of voltage-sensitive sodium channels in neuroblastoma cells and synaptosomes by the anticonvulsant drugs diphenylhydantoin and carbamazepine. *Mol. Pharmacol.,* 25:228–234.

150. Wong, E. H. F., Kemp, J. A., Priestley, T., Knight, A. R., Woodruff, G. N., and Iversen, L. L. (1986): The anticonvulsant MK-801 is a potent *N*-methyl-*D*-aspartate antagonist. *Proc. Natl. Acad. Sci. USA,* 83:7104–7108.

151. Wong, R. K. S., and Prince, D. A. (1979): Dendritic mechanisms underlying penicillin-induced epileptiform activity. *Science,* 204:1228–1231.

152. Wong, R. K. S., Prince, D. A., and Basbaum, A. I. (1979): Intradendritic recordings from hippocampal neurons. *Proc. Natl. Acad. Sci. USA,* 76:986–990.

153. Wong, R. K. S., and Traub, R. D. (1983): Synchronized burst discharge in disinhibited hippocampal slice. I. Initiation in CA2–CA3 region. *J. Neurophysiol.,* 49:442–458.

154. Wong, R. K. S., Traub, R. D., and Miles, R. (1984): Epileptogenic mechanisms as revealed by studies of the hippocampal slice. In: *Electrophysiology of Epilepsy,* edited by P. A. Schwartzkroin and H. V. Wheal, pp. 253–275. Academic Press, London.

155. Wroblewski, J. T., Blaker, W. D., and Meek, J. L. (1985): Ornithine as a precursor of neurotransmitter glutamate: Effect of canaline on ornithine aminotransferase activity and glutamate content in the septum of rat brain. *Brain Res.,* 329:161–168.

156. Yaari, Y., Pincus, J. H., and Argov, Z. (1977): Depression of synaptic transmission by diphenylhydantoin. *Ann. Neurol.,* 1:334–338.

157. Yunger, L. M., Fowler, P. J., Zarevics, P., and Setler, P. E. (1984): Novel inhibitors of γ-aminobutyric acid (GABA) uptake: Anticonvulsant actions in rats and mice. *J. Pharmacol. Exptl. Therap.,* 228:109–115.

Antiepileptic Drugs, Third Edition, edited by
R. Levy, R. Mattson, B. Meldrum,
J. K. Penry, and F. E. Dreifuss.
Raven Press, Ltd., New York © 1989.

5

General Principles

Experimental Selection, Quantification, and Evaluation of Anticonvulsants

Ewart A. Swinyard, Jose H. Woodhead, H. Steve White, and Michael R. Franklin

More than five decades have passed since Putnam and Merritt (16) first demonstrated that drugs effective in epilepsy can be identified from other organic chemicals by testing their ability to suppress experimentally induced convulsions in laboratory animals. Since that time, virtually all species of laboratory animals have been subjected to a wide variety of electrical, chemical, and sensory seizure-evoking techniques in anticipation of finding a model that would be more representative of the clinical disorder. Ideally, such models should duplicate the human clinical condition. Unfortunately, knowledge of the underlying causes of various types of convulsive disorders is still incomplete and the development of laboratory models based on etiology is not yet possible.

Goodman and co-workers (7,23) demonstrated over 35 years ago that the intensity of the convulsive stimulus is of major importance in evaluating the anticonvulsant properties of chemical substances. More recently, Pirreda et al. (14) have re-emphasized the importance of this concept. They demonstrated that the specificity of experimental models of epilepsy is primarily due to the intensity rather than the nature of the stimulus used or the kind of seizure component evoked. Thus, *minimal threshold tests* (clonic response; minimal stimulus intensity) identify substances that raise the seizure threshold (ethosuximide and valproate), whereas *supramaximal tests* (tonic extension of the hind limbs; high stimulus intensity) identify substances that prevent seizure spread (phenytoin, carbamazepine, and valproate). In contrast, *maximal threshold tests* (tonic extension of the hind limbs; minimal stimulus intensity) are non-discriminatory; they may identify anticonvulsant activity but they do not differentiate between substances that increase seizure threshold and those that prevent seizure spread.

The tests described herein were selected for their ability to detect substances with anticonvulsant activity, to determine whether such activity results from the prevention of seizure spread or from the elevation of seizure threshold, and to provide some insight into their mechanisms of action. Since antiepileptic drugs must be taken for prolonged periods and in many instances in combination with other drugs throughout the patient's life, it is also important to assess whether these two factors alter anticonvulsant potency and to determine the mechanism, either pharmacokinetic and/or pharmacodynamic, of any altered response.

The procedures described have evolved from more than 14 years' experience with the Anticonvulsant Drug Development (ADD) Program (9,21). During this time, over 13,000 chemical substances have been screened for anticonvulsant activity and neurotoxicity; more than 2,000 of these have been subjected to anticonvulsant quantification and evaluation; approximately 100 have been subjected to most of the tests described in Table 1; and 14 are in various phases of clinical trial. It is of particular interest that the clinical spectrum of activity of these compounds and the currently available anticonvulsant drugs closely parallel their laboratory spectrum of action.

MATERIALS AND METHODS

Experimental Animals

Adult male CF No. 1 albino mice (18 to 25 g) and adult male Sprague-Dawley albino rats (100 to 150 g) are used as experimental animals. These particular strains are preferred for anticonvulsant studies because they are docile and easy to handle. Moreover, in CF No. 1 mice, maximal electroshock seizures are rarely lethal (24). Animals of the same sex, age, and weight are employed to minimize biological variability (27). The animals are maintained on a 12-hr light/dark cycle and allowed free access to food (Agway Prolab animal diet) and water, except during the short time they are removed from their cages for testing. Animals newly received in the laboratory are allowed 24 hr to compensate for the food and water restriction and stress incurred during transit. This is necessary since starvation increases the severity of maximal electroshock seizures (3). All animals are maintained and handled in a manner consistent with the recommendations in HEW publication (NIH) No. 7423, "Guide for the Care and Use of Laboratory Animals." Animals are used only once and then disposed of in a humane manner. In the rare instance where they are used a second time, at least a one-week interval is allowed for the animal to eliminate the test drug.

Electroshock Apparatus and Convulsant Chemicals

For the test based on maximal electroshock convulsions (Maximal Electroshock Seizure [MES] test), corneal electrodes are used and 60 Hz alternating current is delivered for 0.2 sec by means of an apparatus similar to that originally designed by Dr. L. A. Woodbury (26); the current delivered by this instrument is independent of the external resistance. Supramaximal seizures are elicited with a current intensity five times that necessary to evoke maximal threshold seizures, i.e., 50 mA in mice and 150 mA in rats. Approximately 10% of rats fail to give a full hind limb tonic extension; the incidence of this is higher in older rats. These animals are not used for the MES test.

For tests based on chemically induced convulsions, the convulsant chemical is made up in a concentration that will induce convulsions in more than 97% of animals when injected in mice in a volume of 0.01 ml/g body weight or in rats in a volume of 0.02 ml/10 g body weight. For mice, pentylenetetrazol (Metrazol), picrotoxin, and strychnine are dissolved in 0.9% saline sufficient to make a 0.85%, 0.032%, and 0.012% solution, respectively. For rats, Metrazol is given in a concentration of 3.5%. Bicuculline is dissolved in 1.0 ml of warmed 0.1N hydrochloric acid (HCl) with the aid of a micro-mixer and sufficient 0.9% sodium chloride solution added to make a 0.027% solution. The solution is used within

30 min. All chemical convulsants are administered subcutaneously (sc) into a loose fold of skin in the midline of the neck. Since the doses employed in the above tests induce convulsions in over 97% of mice, it is unnecessary to run control groups simultaneously with the test groups.

Preparation and Injection of Test Drugs

Test drugs soluble in water are administered in 0.9% sodium chloride solution; those insoluble in water are administered as a suspension in 0.5% methylcellulose or in 30% polyethylene glycol 400 (PEG). The test substance is given in a concentration that permits optimal accuracy of dosage without the volume contributing excessively to total body fluid. Thus, the volume employed in mice is 0.01 ml/g body weight; the volume employed in rats is 0.04 ml/10 g body weight. Test drugs are administered either intraperitoneally (I.P.) or orally (P.O.), as indicated in Table 1. The chemical convulsants are administered subcutaneously. No other drugs or chemicals are injected in the same subcutaneous site. The judicious selection of injection sites avoids false positives induced by vasoconstrictor substances retarding the absorption of the convulsant agents.

Anticonvulsant and Differentiation Tests

Five tests are used for the routine identification, quantification, and evaluation of anticonvulsant activity: maximal electroshock seizure test, subcutaneous pentylenetetrazol (Metrazol) seizure threshold test, subcutaneous bicuculline seizure threshold test, subcutaneous picrotoxin seizure threshold test, and subcutaneous strychnine seizure pattern test. The methods employed in these tests have been reported previously (9,15,18,19,20,23). Selected substances are further characterized in special studies. Benzodiazepine and γ-aminobutyric acid (GABA) receptor binding studies and adenosine uptake studies are performed to differentiate possible mechanisms of action. The timed intravenous infusion of Metrazol is used to measure an increase or decrease in seizure threshold. Studies in kindled rats are used to identify substances that may be useful in complex partial seizures.

Maximal Electroshock Seizure (MES) Test

At the previously determined time of peak effect (TPE) of the test substance, a drop of electrolyte solution (local anesthetic in 0.9% sodium chloride solution) is applied to the eyes of each animal, the corneal electrodes are applied, and the electrical stimulus (50 mA in mice; 150 mA in rats; 60 Hz) is delivered for 0.2 sec. The animals are restrained by hand and released immediately following stimulation in order to permit observation of the seizure throughout its entire course. Abolition of the hindleg tonic extensor component after drug treatment is taken as the end point for this test. The tonic component is considered abolished if the hindleg tonic extension does not exceed a 90° angle with the plane of the body; absence of this component indicates that the test substance has the ability to prevent seizure spread.

Subcutaneous Pentylenetetrazol (Metrazol) Seizure Threshold (scMet) Test

The convulsive dose (CD_{97}) of Metrazol (85 mg/kg, mice; 70 mg/kg, rats) is injected into each of the requisite number of animals at the previously determined TPE for the test substance. The animals are placed in isolation cages and observed for the next 30 min for the presence or absence of an episode of clonic spasms persisting for at least five sec. Absence of a clonic seizure indicates that the test substance has the ability to elevate Metrazol seizure threshold.

TABLE 1. *Anticonvulsant drug development*[a]

Phase 1. Anticonvulsant identification
- a. mice I.P.
  - Dose range: 30, 100, and 300 mg/kg
  - Tests: MES, scMet, rotorod, and general behavior
  - Time of test: $\frac{1}{2}$ and 4 hr
- b. rats P.O.
  - Dose: 50 mg/kg
  - Tests: MES or scMet and minimal neurotoxicity
  - Time of test: $\frac{1}{4}$, $\frac{1}{2}$, 1, 2, and 4 hr

Phase 2. Anticonvulsant quantification
- a. mice I.P.
  - TPE: MES, scMet, rotorod
  - ED_{50}: MES, scMet
  - TD_{50}: rotorod
- b. mice P.O.
  - TPE: MES, scMet, rotorod
  - ED_{50}: MES, scMet
  - TD_{50}: rotorod
- c. rats P.O.
  - TPE: MES, scMet, minimal neurotoxicity
  - ED_{50}: MES, scMet
  - TD_{50}: minimal neurotoxicity

Phase 3. Anticonvulsant drug differentiation
- a. mice I.P.
  - ED_{50}: scBic
  - ED_{50}: scPic
  - ED_{50}: scStr
- b. mouse whole brain (*in vitro*)
  - BDZ receptor binding
  - GABA receptor binding
  - Adenosine uptake
- c. mice I.P.
  - Timed i.v. infusion of Metrazol
- d. rats P.O.
  - TPE: EST (kindled)
  - ED_{50}: EST (kindled)

Phase 4. Toxicity profile, mice I.P.
- behavior induced by $1TD_{50}$, $2TD_{50}$s, and $4TD_{50}$s
- TPE: loss of righting reflex
- HD_{50}: loss of righting reflex

Phase 5. Subchronic administration and overt tolerance studies
- a. Subchronic administration: *in vivo* tolerance
  - ED_{50} for 5 days
    - MES or scMet
    - hexobarbital sleep time
- b. Subchronic administration: liver parameters
  - 1) ED_{97} or TD_3 or 100 mg/kg for 7 days
    - weight
    - microsomal
    - protein yield
      - cytochrome P-450 concentration
      - p-nitroanisole 0-demethylase
      - NADPH cytochrome c reductase
      - UDPglucuronosyltransferase (p-nitrophenol)
    - cytosol
      - glutathione S-transferase (1-chloro-2,4 dinitrobenzene)
    - *in vitro*
      - IC_{50} and inhibitory mechanism of p-nitroanisole 0-demethylase

(*continued*)

TABLE 1. (*continued*)

2) significant differences in 1) then all or some additional isozyme selected
    cytochrome P-450 oxidations:
        ethoxyresorufin deethylase activity (c)
        pentoxyresorufin dealkylase activity (b)
        norbenzphetamine MI complex formation (b)
        p-nitrophenol hydroxylase activity (j)
        erythromycin demethylase activity (p)
        troleandomycin MI complex formation
    UDPglucuronosyltransferase of:
      morphine
      1-naphthol
      testosterone
      estrone
    sulfotransferase (cytosol)
      p-nitrophenol
3) significant induction in 1) or 2)
    a) phenytoin ED_{75} MES
    b) phenytoin hydroxylase *in vitro*
4) significant inhibition in 1), acute dose (ED_{16}) on
    a) phenytoin (ED_{25}) MES
    b) phenytoin hydroxylase *in vitro*
    c) hexobarbital sleep time
Phase 6. Pharmacodynamic interactions (with prototype drugs), mice I.P.
    TPE: MES, scMet, rotorod
    ED_{50}: MES, scMet
    TD_{50}: rotorod

[a] The various neurotoxicity, anticonvulsant and liver studies listed above have been integrated into an anticonvulsant drug development procedure designed to identify, quantify, and evaluate the anticonvulsant potential and metabolic interactions of candidate chemical substances.

MES, maximal electroshock seizure test; scMet, subcutaneous pentylenetetrazol (Metrazol) seizure threshold; I.P., intraperitoneally; P.O., *per os* (orally); TPE, time of peak effect; ED_{50}, median effective dose; TD_{50}, median toxic dose; scBic, subcutaneous bicuculline test; scPic, subcutaneous picrotoxin test; scStr, subcutaneous strychnine test

Subcutaneous Bicuculline (scBic), Picrotoxin (scPic), and Strychnine (scStr) Tests

The CD_{97} of bicuculline (2.70 mg/kg), picrotoxin (3.15 mg/kg), or strychnine (1.2 mg/kg) is injected into each of the requisite number of mice at the previously determined TPE for the test substance. The mice are placed in isolation cages and, except for picrotoxin, observed for the next 30 min for the presence or absence of a seizure. Picrotoxin-treated animals are observed for 45 min because of the slower absorption of this convulsant. Absence of a clonic seizure in bicuculline- and picrotoxin-treated animals indicates that the substance has the ability to elevate the respective seizure threshold. In strychnine-treated animals, abolition of the hindleg tonic-extensor component is taken as the end point and indicates that the test substance has the ability to prevent seizure spread.

Receptor Binding Studies

For receptor binding studies, crude synaptic membranes (mouse whole brain) are prepared according to the method of Enna and Snyder (6). [^{3}H]Flunitrazepam receptor binding studies are performed by a slightly modified Braestrup and Squires method (1). GABA receptor binding studies are done by a centrifugation assay as described by Zukin et al., (28) and Enna and Snyder (5). Briefly, membranes are incubated at 0° to 2°C with [^{3}H]flunitrazepam (1 to 10 nM) or [^{3}H]GABA (50 nM), the test substance (0.01 to 100 μM), and sufficient buffer (Tris-HCl or Tris-Citrate, respectively) to make a final volume of 1 ml. The amount of specific [^{3}H]flunitrazepam or [^{3}H]GABA bound is then determined by scintillation counting of the membranes isolated by filtration ([^{3}H]flunitrazepam) or centrifugation ([^{3}H]GABA). Nonspecific binding is determined in the presence of clonazepam (2 μM) or GABA (2 μM). An inhibitory concentration (IC)$_{50}$ of the test substance is calculated by probit analysis and compared with that obtained for prototype benzodiazepines or prototype GABAergic compounds.

Adenosine Uptake Studies

For adenosine uptake studies, the synaptosomes (mouse whole brain) are prepared by differential centrifugation according to Cotman's method (2). [^{3}H]Adenosine uptake is determined by the method of Phillis et al. (13). Briefly, freshly prepared whole brain synaptosomes in phosphate buffered balanced salt solution are incubated at 37°C with [^{3}H]adenosine for 40 sec in the presence of 0.1 to 100 μM test substance. The assay is terminated by filtration through Whatman GF/B filters. Nonspecific binding is determined by incubation of [^{3}H]adenosine with boiled synaptosome membranes.

Timed Intravenous Infusion of Metrazol

This test measures the minimal seizure threshold of each animal (11). The convulsant solution (0.5% Metrazol in 0.9% sodium chloride containing 10 U.S.P. units/ml of heparin sodium) is infused into the tail vein at a constant rate of 0.37 ml/min. The time in seconds from the start of the infusion to the appearance of the first twitch and onset of clonus is recorded for each experimental and control animal. These values

are converted to mg/kg of Metrazol and the mean doses and standard errors (first twitch and clonus) for each group (9 to 11 mice each) are calculated.

Kindled Rats

Seizures evoked in electroshock-kindled rats provide a very sensitive model for the evaluation of drugs that increase minimal seizure threshold. At least 24 hr after the rats have been kindled (2 sec stimulation; 8 mA, 60 Hz, corneal electrodes, twice daily for 5 to 7 days) to stage 4 seizures as described by Racine (17), the test substance is administered orally. At the previously determined TPE, each animal is given the electrical stimulus indicated above and the animals are observed for the presence or absence of forelimb clonus. Abolition of the forelimb clonus is taken as the end point. This indicates that the test substance has the ability to elevate seizure threshold in the kindled animal.

Determination of Acute Toxicity

Abnormal neurological status disclosed by the rotorod test (4) and loss of righting reflex are commonly taken as the end points for minimal neurotoxicity and the hypnotic state, respectively, in mice. Abnormal neurological status disclosed by the positional sense test, or the gait and stance test, is taken as the end point for minimal neurotoxicity in rats. Inability of a rat to perform normally in at least two of these tests indicates that the animal has some neurological deficit. Rats which are to be used for evaluating drug toxicity should be examined by the battery of toxicity tests before the test drug is administered. Individual animals may have peculiarities in gait, equilibrium, muscle tone, and placing response that might erroneously be attributed to the test substance. The names assigned to the above tests are those employed in the authors' laboratory and do not necessarily refer to the specific neurological reflexes involved (18,19).

Rotorod Test

The rotorod test is used exclusively in mice to assess minimal neurotoxicity (TD_{50}). When a normal mouse is placed on a rod that rotates at a speed of 6 rpm, the mouse can maintain its equilibrium for long periods of time. Neurological deficit is indicated by inability of the animal to maintain its equilibrium for 1 min on this rotating rod in each of three trials.

Positional Sense Test

If the hindleg of a normal mouse or rat is gently lowered over the edge of a table, the animal will quickly lift its leg back to a normal position. Neurological deficit is indicated by inability to correct rapidly such an abnormal position of the limb.

Gait and Stance Test

Neurological deficit is indicated by a circular or zigzag gait, ataxia, abnormal spread of the legs, abnormal body posture, tremor, hyperactivity, lack of exploratory behavior, somnolence, stupor, catalepsy, etc.

Muscle Tone Test

Normal animals have a certain amount of skeletal muscle tone which on handling is apparent to the experienced observer. Neurological deficit is indicated by a loss of skeletal muscle tone characterized by hypotonia or flaccidity.

Righting Test

If a mouse or rat is placed on its back, the animal will quickly right itself and as-sume a normal posture. Neurological deficit is indicated by inability to regain a normal body posture within 5 sec. This test is used as a measure of the median hypnotic dose (HD_{50}).

Acute Toxicity Profile

The overt signs and symptoms of acute toxicity induced by each test substance may be determined in intact animals by a modification of the procedure described by Irwin (8). This procedure provides a systematic method for obtaining time-response data on the behavioral and physiologic state of a drug-treated mouse.

Time of Peak Effect

Examination of the Phase 1a results (see Table 2) usually reveals the approximate range of anticonvulsant activity and neurotoxicity. An approximate median effective dose (ED_{50}) or toxic dose (TD_{50}) is then estimated by giving four groups of animals (two animals in each group) a range of four doses between no activity or no toxicity and some activity or some toxicity; these animals are then subjected to the appropriate anticonvulsant or neurotoxicity test(s) at 15 min, 30 min, and 1, 2, and 4 hr. The approximate ED_{50} is then administered to five groups of animals (four animals in each group) and tested at 15 min, 30 min, and 1, 2, and 4 hr, respectively. In the determination of the TPE for toxicity, an approximate TD_{50} is administered to a single group of eight animals; these animals are then subjected to the appropriate toxicity tests for mice or rats at the time intervals indicated above or until peak toxicity has obviously passed. The responses observed are recorded and plotted against time and the TPEs are determined by visual inspection of the graph.

Determination of the Median Effective or Toxic Dose

Quantitative studies (anticonvulsant or toxicity) should be conducted at the TPE of the candidate substance as determined by the specific test procedure (e.g., rotorod test, MES test, scMet test). In the determination of the ED_{50} by the respective anticonvulsant procedure, eight animals are injected with the dose used in the determination of the TPE and subjected to the respective anticonvulsant test at the TPE. The percent of animals protected is plotted against the dose on log-probit paper and another dose level, usually one-half or double the initial dose, is selected. This procedure is repeated until at least three points have been established between the dose level which protects 0% of the animals and the dose level which protects 100% of the animals. These data are then subjected to statistical analysis (see below) and the ED_{50}, 95% confidence interval, and the slope of the regression line are calculated.

In the determination of the TD_{50}, it should be remembered that one point was previously established in the TPE experiment. The percent toxic is plotted against the dose on log-probit paper and another dose, based on the one-half or double rule mentioned above, is selected. This dose is administered to eight animals. The animals are then subjected to the respective toxicity test for mice or rats at the previously determined TPE. This procedure is repeated until three points have been established between the dose level which induces no signs of toxicity in any of the animals and that dose which is toxic to all of the animals. These data are then subjected to statistical analysis (see below) and the results recorded.

The procedures for the determination of the HD_{50} are the same as those described for the TD_{50}. The end point employed is the loss of righting reflex. The data obtained are subjected to statistical analysis as described below.

The various median effective doses (MES, scMet, scBic, scPic, and scStr) and the median toxic doses (TD_{50} and HD_{50}) are calculated by a FORTRAN probit analysis program. This program also provides the 95% confidence intervals, the slopes of the regression lines, and the standard error of the slopes. Reasonable estimates of these values may be determined by the log-probit method of Litchfield and Wilcoxon (10). This statistical treatment provides the kind of data essential to a critical evaluation of anticonvulsant activity and toxicity for structure-activity relations.

Overt Tolerance and Liver Enzyme Studies

Subchronic Administration: Overt Tolerance in Rats

To determine the effect of 5-day subchronic treatment on anticonvulsant activity (MES or scMet test), three groups of eight animals are treated as follows. One group is given the MES (or scMet) ED_{50} of the test drug for 5 days; the second group is given the requisite volume of vehicle for 4 days and a single dose (ED_{50}) of the test drug on day 5; the third group is given the requisite volume of vehicle daily for 5 days. On day 5 at the time of peak effect of the candidate substance (determined from single dose studies), all groups are subjected to the MES (or scMet) test and the number protected is recorded. If the number protected in the treated group is less than that in the single dose control group, it suggests tolerance; conversely, if the number protected in the treated group is more than the number protected in the control group, it suggests potentiation. All three groups of rats are maintained in their home cages for 24 hr and then (day 6) subjected to the hexobarbital sleep time test (100 mg/kg of hexobarbital I.P. and sleep time measured to the nearest minute). If the mean sleep time of the treated group is significantly less than that in the single dose control group, it suggests pharmacokinetic tolerance (induction), whereas an increase suggests potentiation (inhibition).

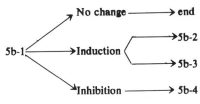

FIG. 1. Flow chart.

Subchronic Administration: Liver Studies

Four animals from each chronically treated and vehicle control group subjected to the hexobarbital sleep time test are continued on their respective treatment regimens 2 more days (days 6 and 7) and 24 hr later subjected to a short screen that determines changes in some hepatic parameters. In addition to these two groups, four rats are given either the MES (or scMet) ED_{97}, the TD_3, or 100 mg/kg for 7 days. The livers are removed and homogenized and subcellular fractions are prepared by differential centrifugation. These subcellular fractions are analyzed as indicated in 5b-1, Table 1, and compared to values from livers of the four vehicle-treated rats (controls). The parameters monitored initially are liver weight, microsomal protein yield, microsomal cytochrome P-450 concentration, p-nitroanisole demethylase, reduced nicotinamide-adenine dinucleotide phosphate (NADPH) cytochrome c reductase, uridine diphospho (UDP)-glucuronosyltransferase (p-nitrophenol), and cytosolic glutathione S-transferase (1-chloro-2,4-dinitrobenzene) activities. All enzyme activities are determined by simple spectrophotometric assays (12). Possible inhibitory influences of the candidate substance on hepatic oxidative drug metabolism are assessed by its ability to extend hexobarbital sleep time *in vivo* and inhibit p-nitroanisole demethylase activity *in vitro*. This is quantitated by the determination of an IC_{50}. If the IC_{50} is low, the mechanism of inhibition (competitive, noncompetitive) is also determined. Further studies are contingent upon the results obtained as shown below in the flow chart

(Fig. 1). Thus, if the short screen (5b-1) does not show significant differences in liver parameters, it will be assumed that further liver studies are unwarranted at this time. If the short screen yields significant differences in liver parameters, more definitive characterization on the same or new livers is undertaken. These include the cytochrome P-450 isozyme-selective oxidations of ethoxyresorufin deethylation (isozyme c), pentoxyresorufin dealkylation (isozyme b), norbenzphetamine metabolic intermediate (MI) complex formation (isozyme b), p-nitrophenol hydroxylation (isozyme j), and erythromcyin demethylation (isozyme p). Changes in the isozymes of UDP-glucuronosyltransferase can be elucidated by using four isozyme selective substrates (morphine, 1-naphthol, testosterone, and estrone) and utilizing high-performance liquid chromatography (HPLC) separation of the glucuronides for quantitation. The uniqueness of any changes in glutathione S-transferase activity in the cytosol can be assessed by monitoring another cytosolic conjugation reaction, sulfotransferase activity toward p-nitrophenol.

Potential drug interactions from inductive and inhibitory effects can be evaluated by some simple tests. If the results suggest induction by the candidate substance, the effect of 7-day prolonged administration (ED_{97} or TD_3 or 100 mg/kg) to (a) decrease phenytoin (ED_{75}) protection against the MES test, (b) decrease hexobarbital sleep time, and (c) increase the *in vitro* metabolism of phenytoin can be examined. If the results suggest potent inhibition by the candidate substance, the ability of an acute dose (ED_{16}) to (a) potentiate phenytoin (ED_{25}) protection against the MES test, (b) increase hexobarbital sleep time, and (c) decrease the *in vitro* metabolism of phenytoin can be investigated.

Pharmacodynamic Interaction

The first step is to establish log-probit regression lines for each of the two component drugs by the same test that is to be used to evaluate the combination. In order to form an isobologram (22,25), these two regression lines must not differ significantly from parallelism. This isobologram is then used to select appropriate doses of the candidate substance and the prototype antiepileptic to be tested in combination. With this procedure, a dose of one drug is selected and added to a calculated amount of a second drug so that the predetermined dose of the combination is expected to produce a 50% response. The formula is as follows: ED_x of drug A + (ED_{50} of drug B − ED_x of drug B) = expected ED_{50} of the combination. Briefly, the TPE of each selected combination is determined for both anticonvulsant activity and minimal neurotoxicity in mice (I.P. or P.O.) and a new TD_{50} and ED_{50} is determined at the TPE. These data are then evaluated with respect to anticonvulsant activity, neurotoxicity, and protective index (PI = TD_{50}/ED_{50}). (For a description of the use of isobolograms and the limitations of combination studies, see refs. 22 and 25.) The primary objective is to show that there is no significant change in the margin of safety (PI) of the combination.

DETECTION AND QUANTIFICATION OF ANTICONVULSANT ACTIVITY

Phase 1

Two tests are used in Phase 1a for the detection of anticonvulsant activity in can-

TABLE 2. *Phase 1a, anticonvulsant identification, mice, I.P.*

		Results[a]		
Test	Time (hr)	30 mg/kg	100 mg/kg	300 mg/kg
MES	½	1/1	3/3	1/1
scMet	½	0/1	0/1	0/1
Toxicity	½	0/4	0/8	4/4
MES	4	0/1	0/3	1/1
scMet	4	0/1	0/1	0/1
Toxicity	4	0/2	0/4	0/2

[a] Number protected or toxic/number tested.

didate substances: the MES pattern test to detect agents that prevent seizure spread and the scMet threshold test to detect agents that elevate minimal seizure threshold. In addition, the rotorod test is used to identify minimal neurotoxicity. Sixteen mice are randomly divided into three groups of four, eight, and four mice each; each group is then given either 30, 100, or 300 mg/kg, respectively, of the test substance intraperitoneally. Thirty min after administration of the test substance, all animals are subjected to the rotorod test; one animal in the 30 and 300 mg/kg group and three animals in the 100 mg/kg group are then subjected to the MES test and one animal in each group to the scMet test. Four hr after drug administration, all remaining animals in each group are subjected to the rotorod test; the animals are then subjected to the MES and scMet test, respectively, as indicated above. Thus, it requires only 16 mice to cover the dose range of 30, 100, and 300 mg/kg and the time periods of one-half and 4 hr.

Typical results obtained with the Phase 1a screening procedure are shown in Table 2, which shows that the test substance is effective in nontoxic doses against the MES test but ineffective by the scMet test; minimal neurotoxicity is >100 mg/kg but <300 mg/kg. Thus, the PI appears to be at least 3 by the MES test. The test substance also appears to have a relatively rapid onset and

TABLE 3. *Phase 1b, anticonvulsant identification, rats, oral[a]*

	Results[b]				
Test	¼ hr	½ hr	1 hr	2 hr	4 hr
MES	1/4	2/4	4/4	4/4	2/4
Toxicity	0/4	0/4	0/4	0/4	0/4
scMet	—	—	—	—	—

[a] Dose: 50 mg/kg
[b] Number protected or toxic/number tested.

short duration of action, since both the anticonvulsant and neurotoxic effects are significantly greater at 30 min than at 4 hr.

Phase 1b provides information relative to whether or not the test substance is active or toxic in a dose of 50 mg/kg after oral administration in rats. It also discloses the time of onset, time of peak effect, and the duration of anticonvulsant activity and/or neurotoxicity, and an estimate of the PI. The results obtained in Phase 1b with the same test substance as used in Phase 1a are shown in Table 3, which shows that some anticonvulsant activity is present within 15 min, the TPE is 1 to 2 hr, the duration of action is about 3½ hr, and, since no neurotoxicity was observed, the PI will most likely be greater than 2. The Phase 1a and b results indicate that further experimental work is justified since the favorable anticonvulsant profile suggests possible clinical usefulness in generalized tonic-clonic and complex partial seizures.

Phase 2

Phase 2a, anticonvulsant quantification, reveals the TPE, the ED_{50}s by the MES and scMet tests, the TD_{50} by the rotorod test, the 95% confidence intervals, slopes of the regression lines, and protective indices. The TPE data provide further insight into the time of onset and the duration of anticonvulsant and toxic activity. Also, the median effective dose information and protec-

tive indices reveal, for the first time, reliable information as to possible clinical usefulness.

Phase 2b provides information similar to that in Phase 2a, except the test substance is given by the oral route of administration. The TPE indicates how rapidly the test substance is absorbed; a comparison of the ED_{50}s and TD_{50} with similar data obtained after intraperitoneal administration (Phase 2a) discloses how adequately the test substance is absorbed after oral administration. All of these factors are important since clinically useful antiepileptic drugs are usually given by the oral route of administration. Consequently, test substances that reach this point and still exhibit satisfactory anticonvulsant activity, margin of safety, and adequate absorption after oral administration usually proceed to Phase 2c.

Phase 2c, anticonvulsant quantification in rats after oral administration, defines the TPE, quantitates the experimental anticonvulsant activity and neurotoxicity in another rodent species, and develops dose information prerequisite to subsequent chronic toxicity studies. More importantly, the Phase 2c data obtained in rats must be carefully reviewed and compared with similar data in mice before it can be determined if the accumulated results are sufficiently promising to warrant moving the candidate substance into costly pharmacokinetic and chronic toxicity studies.

Phase 3

Phases 3a and 3b, anticonvulsant drug differentiation in mice, are designed to delineate more clearly the anticonvulsant profile and possible mechanisms of the candidate substance. Phase 3c and 3d studies are used to evaluate more definitively the effect of the candidate substance on seizure threshold in mice (Phase 3c) and rats (Phase 3d). For Phase 3a studies, the candidate substance is subjected to the scBic, scPic, and scStr tests and the ED_{50}s by these three tests are determined. Each of these convulsants and Metrazol act through a somewhat different neurotransmitter system. For example, Metrazol stimulates neuronal membranes directly; bicuculline blocks GABA receptors and thus interferes with GABA-mediated inhibitory transmission; picrotoxin interferes with chloride channels regulated by GABA receptors; and strychnine blocks postsynaptic inhibition mediated by glycine.

Phase 3b studies are designed to characterize the effect of the candidate substance on [^{3}H]flunitrazepam and [^{3}H]GABA receptor binding and [^{3}H]adenosine uptake. It is generally recognized that benzodiazepine agonists inhibit [^{3}H]flunitrazepam binding, whereas GABA agonists enhance [^{3}H]flunitrazepam binding and inhibit GABA receptor binding. Furthermore, benzodiazepines enhance GABA-mediated neurotransmission; this may be the mechanism whereby benzodiazepines decrease neuronal transmission. Also, some antiepileptic agents inhibit adenosine uptake and thereby decrease neuronal excitability. In these studies, the IC_{50} of the test substance is compared with the IC_{50}s of prototype agents (clonazepam, muscimol, and dipyridamole) in order to identify, at the receptor level, possible sites at which the test substance may act. Thus, Phase 3b contributes significant information with respect to how the test substance obtunds seizures.

Phase 4

Phase 4, toxicity profile, reveals the dose-time relations and the profile of overt toxic manifestations as well as an additional quantitative measure of toxicity (HD_{50}). Six mice are randomly divided into three groups of two mice each, and each group is administered a dose equivalent to either one TD_{50}, two TD_{50}s, or four TD_{50}s of the test substance. A comprehensive assessment of the symptoms of toxicity is made 10, 20, and 30 min and 1, 2, 4, 6, 8, and 24 hr after administration of the test substance. The median hypnotic dose (HD_{50}) is an additional quantitative measure of a higher level of toxicity. Thus, toxicity data obtained in Phases 2a and 4 provide an extensive profile of all levels of toxicity.

EVALUATION OF ANTIEPILEPTIC POTENTIAL

The results obtained with five commonly used antiepileptic drugs subjected to the above procedures are summarized in Tables 4 and 5. The drugs included in these tables were selected for two reasons. First, they are representative of the chemical structures of commonly employed antiepileptic agents: hydantoins (phenytoin), iminostilbenes (carbamazepine), succinimides (ethosuximide), carboxylic acids (valproate), and benzodiazepines (clonazepam). Second, they are the drugs of choice or alternates for either generalized tonic-clonic (grand mal) and complex partial (psychomotor) seizures or generalized absence (petit mal) seizures. Table 4 summarizes the results obtained with Phase 2a, 3a, and 4 procedures after intraperitoneal administration to mice; Table 5 summarizes the results with Phase 2b and 2c procedures after oral administration to mice and rats. These kinds of data correlate well with the clinical use of these agents and provide a basis for the evaluation of the antiepileptic potential of candidate substances. Such an evaluation involves loss of righting reflex doses (HD_{50}s), minimal neurotoxic doses (TD_{50}s), anticonvulsant potencies by the various tests (ED_{50}s), protective indices (PIs), and safety ratios (TD_3/ED_{97}).

The anticonvulsant potential of a candidate substance is usually assessed by comparing the results obtained with well-standardized test procedures with similar

TABLE 4. *Minimal neurotoxicity and profile of anticonvulsant activity of intraperitoneally administered prototype antiepileptic drugs in mice (Phases 2a and 3a)[a]*

Drug	Time of test (hr)	Righting reflex HD$_{50}$ (mg/kg)	Rotorod TD$_{50}$ (mg/kg)	ED$_{50}$s (mg/kg) and PIs[b]				
				MES	scMet	Bicuculline	Picrotoxin	Strychnine
Phenytoin	2	178 (153–195) [14.0]	65.5 (52.5–72.1) [15.2]	9.50 (8.13–10.44) [13.7] PI = 6.89	No protection	No protection	No protection	Max. prot. 50% at 55–100
Carbamazepine	¼	172 (134–198) [5.92]	71.6 (45.9–135) [4.77]	8.81 (5.45–14.1) [3.62] PI = 8.12	Potentiates	Max. prot. 62.5% at 50–130	37.2 (25.3–59.7) [3.86] PI = 1.92	78.8 (39.4–132) [2.85] PI = 0.91
Valproate	¼	886 (821–957) [12.5]	426 (369–450) [20.8]	272 (247–338) [12.8] PI = 1.57	149 (123–177) [11.8] PI = 2.87	360 (294–439) [7.51] PI = 1.18	387 (341–444) [8.35] PI = 1.10	293 (261–323) [11.8] PI = 1.45
Ethosuximide	½	851 (751–918) [16.4]	441 (383–485) [18.4]	>1000 PI = <0.44	130 (111–150) [10.1] PI = 3.38	459 (350–633) [3.21] PI = 0.96	243 (228–255) [26.4] PI = 1.82	Max. prot. 62.5% at 360
Clonazepam	½	>6000	0.18 (0.16–0.23) [14.4]	92.7 (44.9–189) [1.90] PI = 0.002	0.01 (0.005–0.02) [13.9] PI = 20.4	0.01 (0.004–0.02) [1.35] PI = 21.4	0.04 (0.03–0.06) [3.51] PI = 4.28	No protection

[a] The 95% confidence interval is given in parentheses; the slope of the regression line is in brackets.
[b] Protective index (PI) = TD$_{50}$/ED$_{50}$.
HD$_{50}$, median hypnotic dose; TD$_{50}$, median toxic dose; ED$_{50}$, median effective dose; MES, maximal electroshock seizure test; scMet, subcutaneous penylenetetrazol (Metrazol) seizure threshold.

TABLE 5. Neurotoxicity and profile of anticonvulsant activity of orally administered prototype antiepileptic drugs in mice and rats (Phases 2b and 2c)[a]

Drug	Time of test (hr) Mice	Time of test (hr) Rats	Rotorod TD$_{50}$ (mg/kg) Mice	Rotorod TD$_{50}$ (mg/kg) Rats[b]	MES ED$_{50}$ and PI[c] (mg/kg) Mice	MES ED$_{50}$ and PI[c] (mg/kg) Rats	scMet ED$_{50}$ and PI (mg/kg) Mice	scMet ED$_{50}$ and PI (mg/kg) Rats
Phenytoin	2,2,2	½,4,4	86.7 (80.4–96.1) [13.0]	>3000	9.04 (7.39–10.6) [6.28] PI = 9.59	29.8 (21.9–38.9) [2.82] PI = >100	No protection	No protection
Carbamazepine	½,½,½	2,1,1	217 (131–270) [3.47]	813 (489–1234) [6.07]	15.4 (12.4–17.3) [9.07] PI = 14.1	8.50 (3.39–10.5) [4.50] PI = 95.7	48.1 (40.8–57.4) [5.50] PI = 4.52	No protection
Valproate	2,1,1	1,½,½	1264 (800–2250) [4.80]	280 (191–353) [4.63]	665 (605–718) [18.2] PI = 1.90	490 (351–728) [2.90] PI = 0.57	388 (349–439) [8.12] PI = 3.26	180 (147–210) [8.62] PI = 1.56
Ethosuximide	1,½,½	2,2,2	879 (840–934) [30.5]	1012 (902–1109) [15.3]	>1000 PI < 0.88	>1200 PI < 0.84	193 (159–218) [7.39] PI = 4.36	54.0 (45.6–60.9) [9.05] PI = 18.8
Clonazepam	½,½,1	½,1,1	3.39 (1.30–4.51) [2.49]	71.6 (35.7–101) [3.66]	78.35 (55.8–110) [2.30] PI = 0.04	186 (70–500) [1.17] PI = 0.39	0.06 (0.01–0.12) [2.85] PI = 56.5	0.06 (0.02–0.13) [1.17] PI = 1156

[a] The 95% confidence interval is given in parentheses; the slope of the regression line is in brackets.
[b] Minimal neurotoxicity based on ataxia.
[c] Protective index (PI) = TD$_{50}$/ED$_{50}$.
MES, maximal electroshock seizure test; ED$_{50}$, median effective dose; scMet, subcutaneous pentylenetetrazol (Metrazol) seizure threshold.

results obtained with prototype agents (see Tables 4 and 5). The HD_{50}s, TD_{50}s, and ED_{50}s provide important information, but they reveal little when viewed alone. For example, the HD_{50}s of the five prototype agents (see Table 4) range from 172 to >6000 mg/kg and the TD_{50}s range from 0.18 to 441 mg/kg, whereas the ED_{50}s by the MES test range from 8.81 to 272 mg/kg and those by the scMet test range from 0.01 to 149 mg/kg. Considerably more can be learned from a comparison of the ratios between the HD_{50}/TD_{50} and the TD_{50}/ED_{50}. The former provides additional information on the relative safety of the test substance, whereas the latter reveals the protective index (PI = TD_{50}/ED_{50}). The HD_{50}/TD_{50} ratios for phenytoin, carbamazepine, valproate, and ethosuximide range from 1.8 to 2.4. These ratios indicate that prototype antiepileptic drugs exhibit a reasonable spread between minimal and severe toxicity.

PIs are based on the assumption that the slope of the two regression lines (toxicity and anticonvulsant potency) are parallel. If the regression lines are parallel, the calculated PI will be the same at any particular point on the regression lines. If the regression lines are not parallel, the PI is only valid at the D_{50} level. Above or below this median level the PI may be either higher or lower. Therefore, in terms of drug safety, the calculated PI may be misleading. For example, clonazepam has an scBic PI (TD_{50}/ED_{50}) of 21.40; however, the TD_{84}/ED_{84} and TD_{16}/ED_{16} ratios are 4.78 and 104, respectively.

Ideally, an anticonvulsant drug should be capable of suppressing experimental seizures in all animals at dose levels devoid of even minimal toxic effects. Thus, it is more informative to calculate a "safety ratio" (TD_3/ED_{97}) for the candidate substance and to compare this with similar ratios for prototype drugs. The safety ratios for phenytoin, ethosuximide, and valproate in mice are listed (Table 6).

It may be seen that phenytoin can completely suppress MES seizures and ethosuximide can completely suppress scMet seizures in 97% of animals at dose levels devoid of even minimal neurotoxicity. Valproate can provide a similar level of protection by the scMet test after I.P. administration in mice but requires doses in the minimal neurotoxic range to protect 97% of animals by the MES test and after P.O. administration by the scMet test.

Since antiepileptic drugs are generally administered orally, it is important to know how well the candidate drug is absorbed from the gastrointestinal tract. This question can be resolved by comparing the data obtained by a particular test after both oral and intraperitoneal administration of the candidate substance to either mice or rats. For example, it may be seen from Table 5 that the oral TD_{50} and MES and scMet ED_{50}s in mice for valproate are 1,264, 665, and 388 mg/kg, respectively; Table 4 indicates the intraperitoneal TD_{50} and MES and scMet ED_{50}s are 426, 272, and 149 mg/kg,

TABLE 6. *Safety ratios (TD_3/ED_{97}) for i.p. and p.o. administered phenytoin, ethosuximide, or valproate to mice*

	Phenytoin		Ethosuximide		Valproate	
	MES	scMet	MES	scMet	MES	scMet
I.P.	3.5	NA	NA	1.8	0.9*	1.6
P.O.	3.3	NA	NA	2.3	0.6*	0.7*

* Ratios less than 1 indicate that 97% protection is obtained only with some minimal neurotoxicity.

respectively. Thus, the ratios (oral dose/intraperitoneal dose) are 2.97, 2.45, and 2.60 for the TD_{50}, MES ED_{50}, and scMet ED_{50}, respectively. It is generally agreed that the absorption ratio should be equal to or less than 4. Therefore, valproate is well absorbed after oral administration.

Since most antiepileptic medication is taken for prolonged periods and often in combination with other drugs, and because most anticonvulsant drugs undergo significant hepatic metabolism, it becomes important to assess the effect of subchronic therapy and combination therapy on anticonvulsant efficacy and on liver metabolizing enzymes. A special experimental design for such a study has been outlined in Table 1 (see Phases 5a, b, and 6) and is intended to serve primarily as a guide. The Phase 5a studies identify compounds which are significantly less effective after subchronic administration in blocking seizure activity. The Phase 5b procedures reveal whether or not the decreased efficacy results from increased metabolism of the test substance. Likewise, the combination studies outlined in Phase 6 are designed to assess whether a particular combination of a test substance with a prototype antiepileptic is antagonistic, additive, or supra-additive. These investigations become particularly important

as a drug enters clinical testing, since most clinical trials are conducted as "add-on" studies.

The results presented in Tables 4 and 5 provide information relative to clinical use. It may be seen from Table 7 that the three drugs clinically useful in generalized tonic-clonic seizures and complex partial (temporal lobe) seizures (phenytoin, carbamazepine, and valproate) are characterized in the laboratory by ability to prevent seizure spread (anti-MES activity) and may (valproate) or may not (phenytoin and carbamazepine) increase Metrazol seizure threshold. The three drugs effective in generalized absence seizures (ethosuximide, valproate, and clonazepam) are characterized by marked ability to increase Metrazol seizure threshold and may (valproate) or may not (ethosuximide and clonazepam) have an effect on seizure spread (anti-MES activity). The two drugs useful in myoclonic seizures (valproate and clonazepam) are effective in nontoxic doses by all three threshold tests (scMet, scBic, and scPic). Valproate is the only one of the five substances effective by all five tests in nontoxic doses. The broad anticonvulsant profile of valproate correlates well with its wide spectrum of clinical efficacy.

TABLE 7. *Correlation between the profile of anticonvulsant activity in laboratory animals[a] and the clinical use in man*

Antiepileptic drug	Seizure spread		Seizure threshold			Clinical use[b]
	MES	scStr	scMet	scBic	scPic	
Phenytoin	+	±	−	−	−	GTC, CP
Carbamazepine	+	±	−	−	+	GTC, CP
Valproate	+	+	+	+	+	GA, GTC, CP myoclonic
Ethosuximide	−	±	+	±	+	GA
Clonazepam	−	−	+	+	+	GA, myoclonic

[a] Mice; drugs administered I.P.

[b] Clinical spectrum: GTC = generalized tonic-clonic seizures; CP = complex partial seizures; GA = generalized absence seizures.

MES, maximal electroshock seizure test; scStr, subcutaneous strychnine test; scMet, subcutaneous pentylenetetrazol (Metrazol) seizure threshold test; scBic, subcutaneous bicuculline test; scPic, subcutaneous picrotoxin test.

+, effective in nontoxic doses; ±, effective in minimal doses; −, ineffective.

SUMMARY

The technical procedures and statistical analysis of the Anticonvulsant Drug Development Program sponsored by the Epilepsy Branch of the National Institute of Neurological and Communicative Disorders and Stroke are described. Special attention is directed to the order in which these procedures are employed and to factors that may compromise the results. A six-phase anticonvulsant drug development flow chart is presented. The use of these tests in the detection and quantification of anticonvulsant activity and minimal neurotoxicity and in the development of a profile of neurotoxicity is explained. Special attention is directed to the effect of subchronic administration on anticonvulsant activity and various parameters of liver function. Procedures for evaluating the effect of such changes on anticonvulsant potency, pharmacodynamic interactions, and toxicity are described. Data obtained by subjecting five prototype antiepileptic drugs (phenytoin, carbamazepine, ethosuximide, valproate, and clonazepam) to the anticonvulsant identification and quantification procedures are presented. Particular attention is given to the use of anticonvulsant efficacy, acute toxicity, protective indices (TD_{50}/ED_{50}), safety ratio (TD_3/ED_{97}), extent of oral absorption (P.O. ED_{50}/I.P. ED_{50}), results from subchronic and combination therapy, and liver microsomal enzyme data in the evaluation of anticonvulsant potential. Examples are given as to how these procedures are applied in order to assist the inexperienced investigator in the evaluation of candidate substances.

ACKNOWLEDGMENT

This work was supported by a contract (N01-NS-4-2361) from the National Institute of Neurological and Communicative Disorders and Stroke, National Institutes of Health.

REFERENCES

1. Braestrup, C., and Squires, R. F. (1977): Specific benzodiazepine receptors in rat brain characterized by high affinity [^{3}H]diazepam binding. *Proc. Nat. Acad. Sci. U.S.A.*, 74(9):3805–3809.
2. Cotman, C. W. (1974): Isolation of synaptosomal and synaptic plasma fractions. *Methods in Enzymology*, 31A:445–452.
3. Davenport, V. D., and Davenport, H. W. (1948): The relation between starvation, metabolic acidosis and convulsive seizures in rats. *J. Nutr.*, 36:139–152.
4. Dunham, N. W., and Miya, T. A. (1957): A note on a simple apparatus for detecting neurological deficit in rats and mice. *J. Amer. Pharm. Ass. Sci. Ed.*, 46:208–209.
5. Enna, S. J., and Snyder, S. H. (1975): Properties of γ-aminobutyric acid (GABA) receptor binding in rat brain synaptic membrane fractions. *Brain Res.*, 100:81–97.
6. Enna, S. J., and Snyder, S. H. (1977): Influences of ions, enzymes, and detergents on γ-aminobutyric acid receptor binding in synaptic membranes of rat brain. *Mol. Pharmacol.*, 13:442–453.
7. Goodman, L. S., Grewal, M. S., Brown, W. C., and Swinyard, E. A. (1953): Comparison of maximal seizures evoked by pentylenetetrazol (Metrazol) and electroshock in mice, and their modification by anticonvulsants. *J. Pharmacol. Exp. Ther.*, 108:168–176.
8. Irwin, S. (1968): Comprehensive observational assessment: Ia. A systematic, quantitative procedure for assessing the behavioral and physiologic state of the mouse. *Psychopharmacologia* (Berl.), 13:222–257.
9. Krall, R. L., Penry, J. K., White, B. G., Kupferberg, H. J., and Swinyard, E. A. (1978): Antiepileptic drug development: II. Anticonvulsant drug screening. *Epilepsia*, 19:409–428.
10. Litchfield, J. R., Jr., and Wilcoxon, R. (1949): A simplified method of evaluating dose-effect experiments. *J. Pharmacol.*, 96:99–113.
11. Orlof, M. J., Williams, H. L., and Pfeiffer, C. C. (1949): Timed intravenous infusion of Metrazol and strychnine for testing anticonvulsant drugs. *Proc. Soc. Exper. Biol. & Med.*, 70:254–257.
12. Papac, D. I., and Franklin, M. R. (1988): N-benzylimidazole, a high magnitude inducer of rat hepatic cytochrome P-450 exhibiting both polycyclic aromatic hydrocarbon- and phenobarbital-type induction of Phase I and Phase II metabolizing enzymes. *Drug Metab. and Disposition*, 16:259–264.
13. Phillis, J. W., Wu, P. H., and Bender, A. S. (1981): Inhibition of adenosine uptake into rat brain synaptosomes by the benzodiazepines. *General Pharmacol.*, 12:67–70.
14. Pirreda, S. G., Woodhead, J. H., and Swinyard, E. A. (1985): Effect of stimulus intensity on the profile of anticonvulsant activity of phenytoin, ethosuximide, and valproate. *J. Pharmacol. Exp. Ther.*, 222:741–745.
15. Purpura, D. P., Penry, J. K., Tower, D., Woodbury, D. M., and Walter, R., eds. (1972): *Exper-*

imental Models of Epilepsy—A Manual for the Laboratory Worker. Raven Press, New York.

16. Putnam, T. J., and Merritt, H. H. (1937): Experimental determination of the anticonvulsant properties of some phenyl derivatives. *Science*, 85:525–526.

17. Racine, R. J. (1972): Modification of seizure activity by electrical stimulation: II. Motor seizure. *Electroenceph. Clin. Neurophysiol.*, 32:281–294.

18. Swinyard, E. A. (1949): Laboratory assay of clinically effective antiepileptic drugs. *J. Amer. Pharm. Ass.*, 38:201–204.

19. Swinyard, E. A. (1969): Laboratory evaluation of antiepileptic drugs. Review of laboratory methods. *Epilepsia*, 10:107–119.

20. Swinyard, E. A., Brown, W. C., and Goodman, L. S. (1952): Comparative assays of antiepileptic drugs in mice and rats. *J. Pharmacol. Exp. Ther.*, 106:319–330.

21. Swinyard, E. A., and Kupferberg, H. J. (1985): Antiepileptic drugs: Detection, quantification, and evaluation. *Fed. Proc.*, 44:2629–2633.

22. Swinyard, E. A., Woodhead, J. H., and Wolf, H. H. (1988): The use of isobolograms in predicting drug interactions. In: *Antiepileptic Drug Interactions*. Demos Publications, New York (*in press*).

23. Toman, J. E. P., Swinyard, E. A., and Goodman, L. S. (1946): Properties of maximal seizures and their alteration by anticonvulsant drugs and other agents. *J. Neurophysiol.*, 9:231–240.

24. Torchiana, M. L., and Stone, C. A. (1959): Postseizure mortality following electroshock convulsions in certain strains of mice. *Proc. Soc. Exp. Biol. Med.*, 100:290–293.

25. Weaver, L. C., Swinyard, E. A., Woodbury, L. A., and Goodman, L. S. (1955): Studies on anticonvulsant drug combinations: Phenobarbital and diphenylhydantoin. *J.P.E.T.*, 113(3):359–370.

26. Woodbury, L. A., and Davenport, V. D. (1952): Design and use of a new electroshock seizure apparatus, and analysis of factors altering seizure threshold and pattern. *Arch. Int. Pharmacodyn. Ther.*, 92:97–104.

27. Woolley, D. E., Timiras, P. S., Rosenzweig, M. R., Krech, D., and Bennett, E. L. (1961): Sex and strain differences in electroshock convulsions of the rat. *Nature*, 190:515–516.

28. Zukin, S. R., Young, A. B., and Snyder, S. H. (1974): Gamma-aminobutyric acid binding to receptor sites in the rat central nervous system. *Proc. Natl. Acad. Sci. U.S.A.*, 71(12):4802–4807.

Antiepileptic Drugs, Third Edition, edited by
R. Levy, R. Mattson, B. Meldrum,
J. K. Penry, and F. E. Dreifuss.
Raven Press, Ltd., New York © 1989.

6

General Principles

Selection of Antiepileptic Drug Therapy

Richard H. Mattson

The selection of a drug to prevent the recurrence of seizures or to decrease their severity is made on the basis of its efficacy for specific types of seizure and epilepsy. Seizures refer to electroclinical events, whereas epilepsy indicates a tendency for recurrent seizures. Certain epileptic syndromes can be recognized on the basis of a constellation of characteristics, including not only types of seizures but also, for example, age at onset, electroencephalographic findings, etiology and prognosis. Classifications of seizure types (Table 1) and epileptic syndromes (Table 2) have been proposed by the International League Against Epilepsy (9,10) Although admittedly imperfect, these classifications provide our best current understanding and serve as a frame of reference for communication.

Drug selection is often the same for adults and children, but special types of seizures and epilepsies, such as West syndrome, may require quite specific and selective treatments with different expectations of successful outcomes. Some particular problems in seizure treatment, such as status epilepticus, also call for different drug selection. The details of how to initiate and maintain therapy with one drug or combinations of drugs are presented in Chapter 7. Other chapters describe in greater depth the efficacy and toxicity of the various antiepileptic drugs.

GENERALIZED IDIOPATHIC EPILEPSIES

The generalized idiopathic epilepsies most frequently begin in childhood, but some, including juvenile myoclonic epilepsy, may not appear until the teenage years. It is unusual for these epileptic syndromes to begin after the second decade of life, although pre-existing absence or myoclonic seizures may not be medically documented until tonic-clonic seizures occur in adulthood. These generalized epilepsies sometimes remit, but a large number of patients continue to be susceptible to recurrent seizures throughout some or all of their adult life. No specific etiology is known for this group of disorders other than a significant genetic factor. Evidence of other brain dysfunction or disease is not found except coincidentally. The electroencephalographic pattern associated with these epilepsies is that of generalized spike-and-wave or polyspike-and-wave discharges. Associated with these epilepsies are absence, myoclonic, and tonic-clonic seizures.

Valproate (VPA) is usually the drug of choice for the generalized idiopathic

TABLE 1. *International classification of epileptic seizures*

I. Partial (focal, local) seizures
  A. Simple partial seizures
  B. Complex partial seizures
    1. With impairment of consciousness at onset
    2. Simple partial onset followed by impairment of consciousness
  C. Partial seizures evolving to generalized tonic-clonic convulsions (GTC)
    1. Simple evolving to GTC
    2. Complex evolving to GTC (including those with simple partial onset)
II. Generalized seizures (convulsive or nonconvulsive)
  A. 1. Absence
     2. Atypical absence
  B. Myoclonic
  C. Clonic
  D. Tonic
  E. Tonic-clonic
  F. Atonic
III. Unclassified epileptic seizures (includes some neonatal seizures)

Abbreviated from ref. 9.

TABLE 2. *International classification of epilepsies and epileptic syndromes*

1. Localization-related (focal, local, partial) epilepsies and syndromes
  A. Idiopathic with age-related onset
    Benign childhood epilepsy with centrotemporal spikes
    Childhood epilepsy with occipital paroxysms
  B. Symptomatic
2. Generalized epilepsies and syndromes
  A. Idiopathic, with age-related onset, listed in order of age
    Benign neonatal epilepsy
    Childhood absence epilepsy (pyknolepsy)
    Juvenile myoclonic epilepsy (impulsive petit mal)
    Juvenile absence epilepsy
    Epilepsy with grand mal seizures (GTCS) on awakening
  B. Secondary-idiopathic and/or symptomatic
    West syndrome (infantile spasms)
    Lennox-Gastaut syndrome
  C. Symptomatic
    1. Nonspecific etiology
     Early myoclonic encephalopathy
    2. Specific syndromes
     Epileptic seizures which may complicate many diseases, e.g., Ramsay Hunt, Unverricht's, etc.

Modified and abbreviated from ref. 10.

epilepsies. Efficacy is equal to or greater than that of carbamazepine (CBZ) or phenytoin (PHT) for tonic-clonic seizures (4,6,8,11,60) (Table 3) and equal to that of ethosuximide (ESM) for absence seizures (43,54). Valproate is the only drug that can control all seizure types when patients have combinations of tonic-clonic, absence, and/or myoclonic seizures. Low to moderate dosage and blood levels often suffice (4). Because these patients can be treated with modest doses of VPA, very few neurologic or systemic side effects are evident with long-term use (4,21).

Absence Seizures

Absence seizures respond well to both ESM and VPA. Controlled trials indicate that 70%–90% of patients can obtain marked or virtually complete control with use of either of these antiepileptic drugs (4,43,48,54). Although efficacy is comparable between the two drugs, ESM is usually selected for patients with pure childhood absence epilepsy (pyknolepsy) because its side effects are generally fewer or less serious. A trial of VPA is indicated when ESM provides inadequate control after being increased to a dosage causing side effects. For more difficult problems, a combination of the two drugs may provide better control (42). A number of other drugs provide variable success in control of absence seizures and are most often used in patients who are unable to take ESM or VPA because of their adverse effects. Acetazolamide has been reported to be of moderate efficacy, although no controlled trials are available. Side effects are minimal, but evidence of tolerance limits efficacy for long-term use (30). Similarly, the benzodiazepines, including diazepam, clonazepam, and nitrazepam, provide good control but may lose their efficacy after several months of use (5). They usually produce much more

TABLE 3. *Comparative studies of antiepileptic drug efficacy*

Study	Seizure type	Drug monotherapy	N	Treatment period	N (%)	
Shakir et al. (47)	Generalized	Valproate	18	31 months (mean)	15 (83%)	
Wilder et al. (62)	Primary tonic-clonic	Valproate	34	6 months	28 (82%)	
		Phenytoin	17	13 months	13 (76%)	
Loiseau et al. (27)	Partial	Valproate	19	12 months	11 (58%)	
		Carbamazepine	19		8 (42%)	
Callaghan et al. (6)	Generalized	Valproate	37	24 months (median)	22 (59%)	7 (19%)[b]
		Phenytoin	37	18 months (median)	27 (73%)	3 (8%)[b]
		Carbamazepine	28	15 months (median)	11 (44%)	10 (36%)[b]
	Partial	Valproate	27	24 months (median)	12 (44%)	9 (33%)[b]
		Phenytoin	21	24 months (median)	12 (57%)	4 (19%)[b]
		Carbamazepine	31	14 months (median)	11 (34%)	12 (39%)[b]
Turnbull et al. (56, 60)	Tonic-clonic	Valproate	37	2–4 years	27 (73%)[a]	
		Phenytoin	39		22 (56%)[a]	
	Partial	Valproate	33	2–4 years	9 (27%)[a]	
		Phenytoin	31		9 (29%)[a]	

The first two columns under "Patients seizure-free" are Study and Seizure type.

[a] 2-year remission.
[b] >75% reduction in seizure frequency.
(From Chadwick, ref. 8, with permission.)

sedation than ESM or VPA. The oxazolidinediones (trimethadione and paradione) are used infrequently. These compounds have more frequent and serious side effects than currently used medications. The teratogenic risk of trimethadione is especially high, and this drug should be avoided in fertile women (63). The other commonly used antiepileptic drugs have demonstrated little efficacy in the treatment of absence seizures, and there is some evidence that CBZ may increase the frequency of attacks (53).

Myoclonic Seizures

Myoclonic seizures are associated with many epileptic syndromes. Successful control is more often associated with the epileptic syndrome than with the seizure type. Consequently, seizures occurring in generalized idiopathic epilepsy, such as juvenile myoclonic epilepsy, can be fully controlled in 75%–90% of patients (8,11,14). Myoclonic seizures occurring with degen-

erative central nervous system disease or postanoxic encephalopathy may be refractory to any form of therapy. Despite the variable probability of good control with treatment, VPA is the drug of choice in most cases. Ethosuximide is less effective, but methsuximide has been used with some success in patients unresponsive to other drugs. The benzodiazepines are quite effective but, as mentioned above, cause sedative side effects, and in many patients some loss of efficacy is noted after several months of treatment.

Primary Generalized Tonic-Clonic Seizures

Tonic-clonic seizures associated with idiopathic generalized epilepsy occur alone or in association with absence and/or myoclonic seizures. Response to treatment is excellent (Table 3). Approximately 75%–85% of patients can be completely controlled with VPA monotherapy. Some studies did not clearly distinguish between primary and secondarily generalized tonic-clonic seizures, but the response is especially favorable in those patients with generalized idiopathic epilepsy (8). Control was the same or better than obtained with the use of PHT or CBZ (8,62). Half the patients in the study of Bourgeois et al. (4) were not controlled with other antiepileptic drugs including CBZ, phenobarbital (PB), and PHT alone or in combination with other drugs (2). In more refractory patients with generalized idiopathic epilepsy, we were able to obtain complete control with VPA monotherapy in 80% of patients who had not responded to CBZ, PB, PHT, or a combination of these drugs, in addition to ESM or benzodiazepines. This high success rate was achieved only after a lengthy crossover and high doses of VPA initially (32). No entirely satisfactory controlled trial has yet been done to compare all available drugs. Earlier studies suggest PB and primidone (PRM) are as effective as CBZ and PHT for control of tonic-clonic seizures and also could be used as alternative drugs for treatment of this seizure type if VPA is ineffective or not tolerated because of side effects.

SYMPTOMATIC GENERALIZED EPILEPSIES

West Syndrome

West syndrome is characterized by myoclonic seizures (infantile spasms), an hypsarrhythmic electroencephalographic pattern and, in most cases, mental retardation. The seizures begin in the first 2 years of life, but especially between 4 and 6 months of age. Adrenocorticotropic hormone (ACTH) or corticosteroids are usually considered the treatment of choice (1,22,29). Controversy continues as to whether ACTH or corticosteroids have better effect on the long-term outcome than antiepileptic drugs such as VPA. In a recent prospective study of high-dose VPA treatment (associated

with a high mean plasma concentration of 113 µg/ml), 20 of 22 patients achieved total seizure control after 6 months, an outcome comparable to that achieved with ACTH treatment and with less adverse effect (49). This result is somewhat better than that found with nitrazepam or other benzodiazepines (24).

Lennox-Gastaut Syndrome

Lennox-Gastaut syndrome begins in early childhood, and the seizures rarely remit entirely. Seizures are of multiple types with myoclonic, atonic, and atypical absence attacks occurring with great frequency. Tonic-clonic or fragments of these seizures as well as partial attacks may also be seen. These patients have an associated slow spike-and-wave electroencephalographic pattern and some degree of mental retardation. Some variation on these characteristics can be seen in individual patients.

Treatment is very difficult with any single drug or combination of drugs. Seizures often occur many times daily, although occasionally remissions occur for weeks without obvious explanation. Valproate has the greatest spectrum of activity for treatment of the multiple seizure types. The dosage should be increased until side effects appear, and a month or more of therapy should be tried before other medications are added or substituted. Carbamazepine, PHT, and PB may be useful in controlling the tonic-clonic or tonic seizures, and clonazepam or other benzodiazepines are quite effective, at least temporarily, in controlling myoclonic or absence attacks. Ethosuximide is also effective for the treatment of absence attacks, although these atypical, sometimes prolonged, confusional states are much less responsive than those associated with generalized idiopathic epilepsy. Inability to obtain adequate control frequently leads to the use of multiple drug combinations with increased side effects and questionable benefit. Subsequent attempts to withdraw a benzodiazepine or a barbiturate may be difficult due to exacerbation of seizures during withdrawal.

LOCALIZATION-RELATED (FOCAL, PARTIAL) EPILEPSIES

Localization-related (focal, local, partial) epilepsies and associated seizures are responsive to a number of antiepileptic drugs (51). Because more than half of all patients with this type of epilepsy have both partial and secondarily generalized tonic-clonic seizures at some time (35), it is reasonable to select the drugs most likely to provide optimal efficacy against both types of seizures with minimal toxicity. As evidenced by successful long-term adult monotherapy in the Veterans Administration Cooperative Study (VA study) (35), CBZ and PHT in general show the best balance of seizure control with fewer side effects than PB or PRM for treatment of patients with partial epilepsy. Life table analyses demonstrate that patients placed on either of these drugs were most likely to continue to be satisfactorily managed for up to 3 years, the follow-up period (Fig. 1). Valproate may be equally effective and/or have fewer side effects, but insufficient controlled studies have been done to resolve this question (6,8,27,59).

Idiopathic Benign Childhood Epilepsy with Centrotemporal Spikes

Idiopathic benign childhood epilepsy is characterized by partial and secondarily generalized tonic-clonic seizures occurring in early to mid-childhood and usually remitting spontaneously during adolescence or the teenage years (2,28). Despite the focal character of the seizures associated with this syndrome, no evidence by medical history, neurological examination, or diagnostic imaging indicates structural brain disease. Characteristic centrotemporal sharp waves and spikes often occur independently bilaterally and are very prominent during light sleep. This relatively benign condition may be so infrequent and mild that no treatment is required, particularly if the attacks are of the partial type and limited to occurrence in sleep. When treatment is advisable, both CBZ and PHT are quite effective, and complete control is often possible with modest dosage. Dysmorphic side effects and subtle cognitive compromise reported with use of PHT in some individuals, especially in this age group, makes CBZ the drug of choice (15,21,56,58). Phenobarbital and PRM may also prove effective, but behavioral or sedative side effects may make them less desirable (57,61). No comparative trials are available using VPA in this subgroup of patients.

Symptomatic Epilepsies

The symptomatic epilepsies are most common and may begin at any time of life and have multiple etiologies. Among the most frequent causes are head trauma (including birth injury), neoplasms, vascular lesions, and infection. The neurologic examination, brain imaging, and electroencephalogram may indicate areas of abnormal brain function responsible for the seizures. In a considerable number of patients, the etiology or the site of abnormality may escape detection despite all diagnostic efforts.

Secondarily Generalized Tonic-Clonic Seizures

Multiple controlled trials have failed to demonstrate evidence of superiority of any one antiepileptic drug for control of secondarily generalized tonic-clonic seizures. In the VA study of 622 adults with partial epilepsy having tonic-clonic seizures, equal

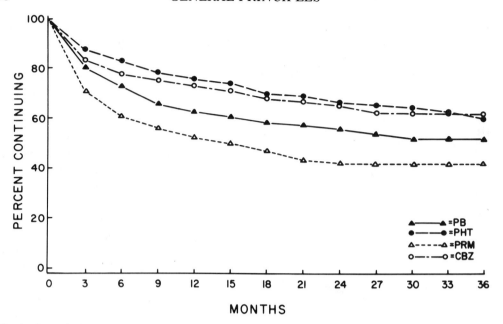

FIG. 1. Cumulative percentage of patients successfully treated with each drug during 36 months of follow-up. PB, phenobarbital; PHT, phenytoin; PRM, primidone; CBZ, carbamazepine. (From Mattson et al. ref. 37, with permission.)

efficacy for CBZ, PB, PHT, and PRM was found after 1, 2, or 3 year follow-up (35). Measures included seizure rate, total number of seizures, seizure severity, seizure-free interval, 100% control, and a special seizure rating scale (12). Few controlled comparative studies are available concerning the efficacy of VPA, but the existing evidence suggests that this drug also is comparable to the others in prevention of secondarily generalized tonic-clonic seizures (6,8,59). Consequently, the choice of treatment is based primarily on differences in side effects among these drugs. Complete control of seizures in patients continuing on a drug can be expected in approximately half of them throughout the first year of follow-up (Table 4).

Partial Seizures

Although the International Classification of Epileptic Seizures (see Table 1) separates partial seizures into simple and complex types with various subgroups included in each category, no studies have shown selective efficacy for one subtype of partial seizure. Indeed, exact determination as to whether partial seizures are of the simple or complex type may be difficult, and many patients have both types at different times. In the VA study, CBZ, PB, PRM, and PHT had similar efficacy in partial seizures. As was true for tonic-clonic seizures, there were no statistically significant differences in seizure number, seizure rate, seizure-free intervals, or seizure rating score. One important difference was found: complete control was more frequently achieved with CBZ than with the barbiturates at 1, 2, and 3 years of follow-up (35). This outcome was found for all patients in the study (i.e., those continuing on a drug with or without those who left the study) (Table 4). There was no statistically significant difference between CBZ and PHT nor between PHT and the barbiturates.

TABLE 4. *Adult patients with partial epilepsy: Percent of patients seizure-free for 12 months*

Drug	Seizure type		
	Tonic-Clonic	Partial	All types
CBZ	58	44	47
PB	45	18	36
PHT	43	32	38
PRM	45	22	35
ALL	45	29	39

Includes all patients randomized to receive a study drug and followed for at least a year, or failing to complete the study because of uncontrolled seizures.
(From Mattson et al. ref. 35, with permission.)

The efficacy of VPA in the treatment of partial seizures is not fully established. The few comparative or controlled studies conducted thus far have shown no statistically significant differences in complete seizure control between CBZ, PHT, and VPA (6,27,61). Overall, the percentage of patients experiencing complete control of partial seizures was low and similar to the results in the VA study (see Tables 3 and 4). More recently, Dean and Penry (13) found that VPA improved seizure control in 73% of patients with partial epilepsy in an open crossover trial involving 30 patients who failed other monotherapy due to side effects, seizures, or both. In all these studies of VPA for treatment of partial seizures, the number of patients and length of the trials have not been sufficient for full comparison of VPA with the other drugs, or the trials have not been controlled to prevent patient or investigator bias.

OTHER SPECIAL EPILEPSY TYPES

Alcoholic Epilepsy

Long-term antiepileptic drug treatment of alcohol withdrawal seizures is not required. The short-term management of these seizures, however, remains controversial (31,40,50). Paraldehyde and the benzodi-azepines show cross-tolerance to alcohol and are highly effective in preventing recurrent seizures. When parenteral drug administration is necessary, use of intravenous benzodiazepines is preferable for reasons of safety. Phenobarbital also shows cross-tolerance to alcohol and has been found to be effective (64), but the drug's long duration of action and sedative effects may complicate diagnosis and management of associated cerebral and systemic disorders. Both PHT and CBZ have been used with inconsistent results. Phenytoin is usually not effective (50). Carbamazepine also has been used, especially in Scandinavia (19), but sufficient comparative controlled trials have not been done to establish its relative efficacy. Treatment with PHT or CBZ is indicated when associated partial epilepsy is suspected to coexist. Valproate has been used successfully, but the concern about hepatic effects in this population and its slow onset of action make it less suitable.

SIDE EFFECTS AND SPECIAL FACTORS INFLUENCING DRUG SELECTION

Certain characteristics such as age, sex, or concomitant medical problems may alter the selection of an antiepileptic drug. These considerations usually concern side effects but may involve pharmacokinetics as well.

Side Effects

Efficacy is often similar among the antiepileptic drugs used for treatment of specific seizure types or epileptic syndromes. Differences in associated side effects may be a major factor in the selection of drugs for each individual patient. The frequency and severity of the side effects vary with the dose, method of administration, co-administration of other drugs, and patient population, but certain side effects are characteristic of each drug. Side effects can be

TABLE 5. *Percent of patients with side effects (n = 247)*

Week	GI distress	Sedation	Dizziness
1	10.2	32.7	9.4
2	6.3	31.7	6.7
4	5.2	27.3	4.1
8	3.6	28.3	1.6
11	3.4	21.4	1.9

Patients received CBZ, PB, PHT, or PRM as monotherapy.
GI, gastrointestinal.
(From Mattson et al. ref. 34, with permission.)

classified according to neurotoxicity or systemic toxicity. In addition, different problems may be noted during initiation of treatment than during prolonged usage.

Initiation of Therapy

Initiation of PRM therapy is difficult because of acute gastrointestinal distress, dizziness, and sedation unless the initial dosage is low and gradually increased (35,46,56). Similar but less severe complaints often accompany the startup of CBZ (7,41). Visual or motor disturbances such as incoordination also may appear. In the VA study (34), PHT and PB were better tolerated than the other drugs at initiation of treatment. Indeed, PB was associated with significantly fewer gastrointestinal and dizziness complaints compared to the other drugs. Phenytoin caused sedation the least frequently but, surprisingly, significant differences among the drugs could not be found. Despite increasing blood levels of the four antiepileptic drugs, the side effects eased spontaneously during subsequent weeks as tolerance developed (Table 5). Similar transient side effects of VPA have been reported (8,20,45,58). Idiosyncratic hypersensitivity reactions can occur with any of these drugs and usually are seen within the first 3 months. They are less commonly reported with VPA therapy. Leukopenia frequently follows initiation of treatment with any of these drugs and is not significantly more common with any one drug. In the VA study (35), 27% of the patients were found to have a white blood cell count of <5,000/mm^3 on at least one occasion in the first year, but none developed a clinically significant granulocytopenia. Valproate can cause dose-related thrombocytopenia or minor platelet dysfunction in some patients (26). Hepatotoxicity constitutes a rare but potentially serious early side effect, specifically in young children (18).

Long-Term Use

Some side effects may be seen with long-term antiepileptic drug therapy, especially in those patients for whom the dosage is raised to produce high blood levels when needed to provide adequate seizure control. Carbamazepine usually produces minimal adverse effects although visual and coordination disturbances are reported as the dosage rises, particularly at times of peak levels (7,41). Phenobarbital often causes sedation in the dosage range needed for treatment (38). Mood and behavior problems, especially in children, are well documented (61) (see also Chapter 23). Uncommon but important connective tissue changes may appear with long-term use of PB or PRM. These include Dupuytren's contracture, frozen shoulder, and generalized aches and pains (36,44). Phenytoin use is associated with significantly more frequent dysmorphic side effects than other drugs (35), and selected neuropsychological testing has revealed some subtle cognitive impairments with long-term use (15,55,57). In long-term use PRM may have fewer cognitive side effects than PB (52), but is associated with significantly more complaints of impotence and decreased libido than CBZ or PHT (35). Ethosuximide causes gastrointestinal symptoms most often.

Valproate therapy is associated with

dose-related tremors and alopecia. Increased appetite and weight gain present both a cosmetic problem and a potential health risk. Like CBZ, cognitive, affective, and behavior effects are uncommon with use of VPA (61).

For any given person, some types of side effects may be important, but for another person the same effects will be of little consequence. For example, the mild acne, hirsutism, and gum hypertrophy sometimes associated with PHT use are likely to be of considerable concern to an adolescent female. These side effects would be of little concern to the adult male. On the other hand, some compromise of potency and libido associated with PRM therapy would be of great importance to the adult male. These examples illustrate the principle that drug selection should be individualized and no single agent can be considered *the* drug of choice for all patients.

Age

Antiepileptic drug treatment always assumes the diagnosis and correction of specific reversible causes of seizures, especially in neonates and infants. Some controversy exists concerning the need for drug therapy for nonconvulsive seizures. It is unclear whether the seizures or the drug constitutes a greater risk for the developing brain (34). When antiepileptic drugs are used in neonates and infants, PB is the drug most frequently used for a variety of seizures. It has the advantage of being available for parenteral administration with predictable absorption from intramuscular or intravenous injection (25). Phenytoin may be as effective, but its absorption from oral administration and its biotransformation are less predictable and pose problems with dosage regulation (16,39). Lack of a parenteral formulation for CBZ limits its usefulness.

For long-term use in children, PB is as-sociated with a high incidence of behavioral problems, sedation, and cognitive dysfunction (see Chapter 23). Carbamazepine is the drug of choice for children with localization-related (partial) epilepsy with tonic-clonic and/or partial seizures. The drug is effective and relatively free of side effects (17). Valproate also is frequently the drug of first choice in this age group, especially because of the common occurrence of generalized idiopathic epilepsies. In addition VPA, like CBZ, is relatively free of long-term sedative, behavioral, or cognitive side effects (62). The use of VPA in infants and children under age 2 carries an increased risk of fatal hepatotoxicity (18). Despite good efficacy PHT is not the drug of first choice in children because of its dysmorphic side effects, as well as subtle compromise of cognitive function (15,21,55,57).

In a comparative study of antiepileptic drug side effects in children, Herranz et al. (21) found that certain side effects were more common with the use of some drugs than others. For example, PB most often caused behavioral problems, VPA was most often associated with digestive complaints, and PHT most often resulted in dysmorphic or motor problems. In keeping with the VA study in adults, CBZ had fewer side effects overall. Interestingly, the side effects were infrequent with long-term PRM use (Fig. 2).

Sex

Special consideration should be given to the use of antiepileptic drugs in women who may become pregnant. A major concern in this population is the risk of teratogenic effects. In epidemiological studies of animals and humans, there is evidence of variable risk to fetal development with the use of all antiepileptic drugs (23,63). Much controversy surrounds the degree of risk from each drug and the relative risk among the various drugs. However, trimethadione has

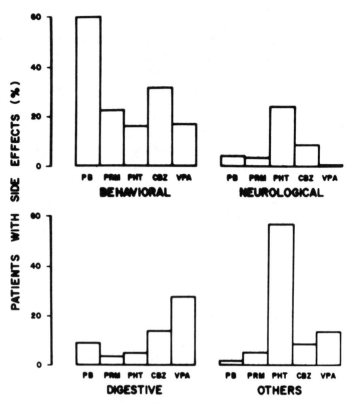

FIG. 2. Percentage of patients treated with phenobarbital (PB, *n* = 99), primidone (PRM, *n* = 85), phenytoin (PHT, *n* = 63), carbamazepine (CBZ, *n* = 35), or valproate (VPA, *n* = 110) with behavioral, neurologic, digestive tract, or other side effects. (From Herranz et al., ref. 21, with permission.)

been associated with a high probability of developmental anomalies and is contraindicated in women who may become pregnant. There is considerable cumulative evidence that PHT, CBZ, PRM, and PB also are capable of causing developmental fetal abnormalities. The relative risk of these drugs is often difficult to ascertain due to the frequent administration of several drugs together. In general, multiple drugs at high doses are associated with a greater frequency of anomalies (23). It is generally thought that the lowest dosage possible should be given as monotherapy to minimize the teratogenic risks regardless of the antiepileptic drug used. Both animal and human studies continue to provide evidence of teratogenic risks from VPA, particularly in failure of midline structures to close (23).

For women of childbearing age who wish to use contraceptive hormones, the choice of antiepileptic drug may be important. Enzyme-inducing antiepileptic drugs (e.g., CBZ, PB, PHT, PRM) may increase hormone clearance and be associated with irregular menses. Likewise, these drugs may cause oral contraceptives to be less dependable in preventing pregnancy. Valproate does not cause enzyme induction and may be optimal for women who elect to use oral contraceptives (37).

PHARMACOKINETIC CONSIDERATIONS

A variety of other circumstances may influence the selection of a specific antiepileptic drug when several of equal efficacy may be available. For example, VPA and PHT are highly protein-bound so that systemic conditions that alter this usual equilibrium may make the management of epilepsy more complicated. Changes in protein concentration or binding characteristics, as in uremia or hepatic disease, may significantly shift the concentration of physiologically active free PHT or VPA. The monitoring of total serum levels becomes less meaningful in guiding treatment. Similarly, the addition of PHT or VPA to CBZ causes increased levels of CBZ epoxide by different mechanisms of interaction. This pharmacologically active metabolite is not usually measured but contributes to CBZ's efficacy and toxicity. The combination of two antiepileptic drugs may alter the pharmacokinetics of either or both (33). Valproate is especially complicated when given with other drugs (see Chapter 43). Enzyme-inducing antiepileptic drugs may have important life-threatening effects by decreasing the drug's plasma levels and efficacy (33) when co-administered with drugs such as coumadin or cyclosporine.

The potential for disturbed drug absorption in patients with significant gastrointestinal disease or frequent elimination may make the use of more slowly absorbed and delayed release capsules or tablets less desirable. On the other hand, epileptic patients with multiple medical illnesses interfering with regular oral ingestion or at times requiring parenteral administration of drugs may be most easily managed with PHT or PB, which have parenteral formulations.

SUMMARY

Specific antiepileptic drugs have some selective efficacy for different types of seizures or epilepsy or are preferable at certain times of life and under specific conditions. Often the selection may be based on expected or observed toxicity, because efficacy differences are often minimal except in absence and myoclonic seizures. Comparative studies may show some superiority of one drug over another in terms of efficacy and freedom from toxicity for large populations, but for a given individual an alternate drug may prove more effective or cause fewer side effects and should be tested if management of the epilepsy is not optimal.

The co-administration of antiepileptic drugs has not yet been proved to provide more antiseizure efficacy than use of one drug without concurrently increasing toxicity. A few combinations have been found to optimize the therapeutic index in experimental models (3), but adequate controlled clinical trials have yet to be done to address this important issue (51) (see also Chapter 7).

ACKNOWLEDGMENTS

This work was supported by the Veterans Administration Medical Research Service and NINCDS Grant No. NS06208-22.

REFERENCES

1. Aicardi, J. (1986): Infantile spasms and related syndromes. In: Aicardi, J., ed. *Epilepsy in Children,* pp. 17–38. edited by Raven Press, New York.
2. Blom, S., and Heijbel, J. (1982): Benign epilepsy of children with centrotemporal EEG foci: A follow-up study in adulthood of patients initially studied as children. *Epilepsia,* 23:629–632.
3. Bourgeois, B. (1989): Antiepileptic and neurologic interactions between antiepileptic drugs. In: *Antiepileptic Drug Interactions,* edited by W. H. Pitlick. Demos Publications, New York.
4. Bourgeois, B., Beaumanoir, A., Blajev, B., de la Cruz, N., Despland, P., Egli, M., Geudelin, B., and Kaspar, W. (1987): Monotherapy with valproate in primary generalized epilepsies. *Epilepsia,* 28 (Suppl. 2):S8–S11.
5. Browne, T. (1976): A review of a new anticonvulsant drug. Clonazepam. *Arch. Neurol.,* 33:326–332.
6. Callaghan, N., Kenny, R. A., O'Neill, B., Crowley, M., and Goggin, T. (1985): A prospective study between carbamazepine, phenytoin and sodium valproate as monotherapy in previously untreated and recently diagnosed patients with epilepsy. *Psychiatry,* 48:639–644.

7. Cereghino, J. J., Brock, J. T., Van Meter, J. C., Penry, J. K., Smith, L. D., and White, B. G. (1974): Carbamazepine for epilepsy: A controlled prospective evaluation. *Neurology*, 24:401–410.

8. Chadwick, D. W. (1987): Valproate monotherapy in the management of generalized and partial seizures. *Epilepsia*, 28 (Suppl. 2):S12–S17.

9. Classification Commission (1981): Proposal for revised clinical and electroencephalographic classification of epileptic seizures. *Epilepsia*, 22:489–501.

10. Classification Commission (1985): Proposal for classification of epilepsies and epileptic syndromes. *Epilepsia*, 26:268–278.

11. Convanis, A., Cupta, A. K., and Jeavons, P. M. (1982): Sodium valproate: Monotherapy and polytherapy. *Epilepsia*, 23:293–320.

12. Cramer, J. A., Smith, D. B., Mattson, R. H., Escueta, A. V. D., Collins, J. F., Browne, T. R., Crill, W. E., and Homan, R. W., Mayersdorf, A., McCutchen, C., McNamara, J., Rosenthal, N. P., Treiman, D., Wilder, J., and Williamson, P. (1983): A method of quantification for the evaluation of antiepileptic drug therapy. *Neurology*, 33 (Suppl. 1):26–37.

13. Dean, J., and Penry, J. (1988): Valproate monotherapy in 30 patients with partial seizures. *Epilepsia*, 29:140–144.

14. Delgado-Escueta, A. V., and Enrile-Bascal, F. (1984): Juvenile myoclonic epilepsy of Janz. *Neurology*, 34:285–294.

15. Dodrill, C. B., and Troupin, A. S. (1977): Psychotropic effects of carbamazepine in epilepsy: A double-blind comparison with phenytoin. *Neurology*, 27:1023–1028.

16. Dodson, W. E. (1980): Phenytoin elimination in childhood: Effect of concentration-dependent kinetics. *Neurology*, 30:196–199.

17. Dodson, W. E. (1987): Carbamazepine efficacy and utilization in children. *Epilepsia*, 28 (Suppl. 2):S17–S24.

18. Dreifuss, F. E., Santilli, N., Langer, D. H., Sweeney, K. P., Moline, K. A., and Menander, K. B. (1987): Valproic acid hepatic fatalities: A retrospective review. *Neurology*, 37:379–385.

19. Flygenring, J., Hansen, J., Holst, B., Peterson, E., and Sorensen, A. (1984): Treatment of alcohol withdrawal symptoms in hospitalized patients. *Acta Psychiatr. Scand.*, 69:398–408.

20. Henricksen, O., and Johannessen, S. I. (1982): Clinical and pharmacokinetic observations on sodium valproate—A 5 year followup study in 100 children with epilepsy. *Acta Neurol. Scand.*, 65:504–523.

21. Herranz, J. L., Armijo, J. A., and Artega, R. (1988): Clinical side effects of phenobarbital, primidone, phenytoin, carbamazepine, and valproate during monotherapy in children. *Epilepsia*, 29:794–804.

22. Hrachory, R. A., Frost, J. D., Kellaway, P., and Zion, T. (1983): Double blind study of ACTH vs. prednisone therapy in infantile spasms. *J. Pediatrics*, 103:641–645.

23. Kaneko, S., Otani, K., Fukushima, Y., Ogawa, Y., Nomura, Y., Ono, T., Nakane, Y., and Teranishi, T. (1988): Teratogenicity of antiepileptic drugs: Analysis of possible risk factors. *Epilepsia*, 29:459–467.

24. Lacy, C. R., and Penry, J. K. (1976): *Infantile Spasms*. Raven Press, New York.

25. Lockman, L. A., Kriel, R., Zaske, D., Thompson, T., and Virnig, N. (1979): Phenobarbital dosage for control of neonatal seizures. *Neurology*, 29:1445–1449.

26. Loiseau, P. (1981): Sodium valproate, platelet dysfunction and bleeding. *Epilepsia*, 22:141–146.

27. Loiseau, P., Cohadon, S., Jogeix, M., Legroux, M., and Artigues, J. (1984): Efficacité du valproate de sodium dans les epilepsies partielles. *Rev. Neurol.*, 140:434–437.

28. Loiseau, P., Duche, B., Cordova, S., Dartigues, J. F., and Cohadon, S. (1988): Prognosis of benign childhood epilepsy with centrotemporal spikes: A follow-up study of 168 patients. *Epilepsia*, 29:229–235.

29. Lombroso, C. T. (1983): A prospective study of infantile spasms: Clinical and therapeutic correlations. *Epilepsia*, 24:135–158.

30. Lombroso, C. T., and Forsythe, I. (1960): A long-term follow up of acetazolamide (Diamox) in the treatment of epilepsy. *Epilepsia*, 1:493–500.

31. Mattson, R. H. (1983): Seizures associated with alcohol use and alcohol withdrawal. In: *Epilepsy: Diagnosis and Management*, edited by T. R. Browne, and R. G. Feldman, pp. 325–333. Little, Brown and Company, Boston.

32. Mattson, R. H., and Cramer, J. A. (1988): Crossover from polytherapy to monotherapy in primary generalized epilepsy. *Am. J. Med.*, 84:23–28.

33. Mattson, R. H., and Cramer, J. A. (1989): Antiepileptic drug interactions in clinical use. In: *Drug Interactions*, edited by W. Pitlick, pp. 75–85. Demos Press, New York.

34. Mattson, R. H., Cramer, J. A., and Collins, J. F. (1986): Early tolerance to antiepileptic drug side effects: A controlled trial of 247 patients. In: *Tolerance to Beneficial and/or Adverse Effects of Antiepileptic Drugs*, edited by W. P. Koella et al. pp. 149–156. Raven Press, New York.

35. Mattson, R. H., Cramer, J. A., Collins, J. F., Smith, D. B., Delgado-Escueta, A. V., Browne, T. R., Williamson, P. D., Treiman, D. M., McNamara, J. O., McCutchen, C. B., Homan, R. W., Crill, W. E., Lubozynski, M. F., Rosenthal, N. P., and Mayersdorf, A. (1985): Comparison of carbamazepine, phenobarbital, phenytoin, and primidone in partial and secondary generalized tonic-clonic seizures. *N. Engl. J. Med.*, 313:145–151.

36. Mattson, R. H., Cramer, J. A., and McCutchen, C. B., the VA Cooperative Study Group. (1989): Barbiturate related connective tissue disorders. *Arch. Int. Med.* 149:911–914.

37. Mattson, R. H., Cramer, J. C., Darney, P. D., and Naftolin, F. (1986): Use of oral contraceptives by women with epilepsy. *J.A.M.A.*, 256:238–240.

38. Mattson, R. H., Williamson, P. D., and Hanahan,

E. (1976): Eterobarb therapy in epilepsy. *Neurology*, 26:1014–1017.

39. Painter, M. J., Pippenger, C. E., Wasterlain, C., Barmada, M., Pitlick, W., Carter, G., and Abern, S. (1981): Phenobarbital and phenytoin in neonatal seizures: Metabolism and tissue distribution. *Neurology*, 31:1107–1112.

40. Porter, R. J., Mattson, R. H., Cramer, J. A., and Diamond, I. (1989): *Alcohol and Seizures.* F. A. Davis & Company, Philadelphia.

41. Rodin, E. A., Rim, C. S., and Rennick, P. M. (1974): The effects of carbamazepine on patients with psychomotor epilepsy: Results of a double-blind study. *Epilepsia*, 15:547–561.

42. Rowan, A. J., Meijer, J. W., de Beer-Pawlikowski, N., Vandergeest, P., and Meinardi, H. (1983): Valproate-ethosuximide combination therapy for refractory absence seizures. *Arch. Neurol.*, 40:797–802.

43. Sato, S., White, B. G., Penry, J. K., Dreifuss, F. E., Sackellares, J. C., and Kupferberg, H. J. (1982): Valproic acid versus ethosuximide in the treatment of absence seizures. *Neurology*, 32:157–163.

44. Schmidt, D. (1983): Connective tissue disorders induced by antiepileptic drugs. In: *Antiepileptic Drug Therapy: Chronic Toxicity of Antiepileptic Drugs*, edited by J. Oxley et al., pp. 115–124. Raven Press, New York.

45. Schmidt, D. (1984): Adverse effects of valproate. *Epilepsia*, 25 (Suppl. 1):544–549.

46. Sciarra, D., Carter, S., Vicale, C. T., and Merritt, H. H. (1954): Clinical evaluation of primidone (Mysoline), a new anticonvulsant drug. *J.A.M.A.*, 154:827–829.

47. Shakir, R. A., Johnson, R. H., Lambie, D. G., Melville, I. D., and Nanda, R. H. (1981): Comparison of sodium valproate and phenytoin as single drug treatment. *Epilepsia*, 22:27–33.

48. Sherwin, A. L., Robb, J. P., and Lechter, M. (1973): Improved control of epilepsy by monitoring plasma ethosuximide. *Arch. Neurol.*, 28:178–181.

49. Siemes, H., Spohr, H. L., Michael, T. H., and Nau, H. (1988): Therapy of infantile spasms with valproate: Results of a prospective study. *Epilepsia*, 29:553–560.

50. Simon, R. (1988): Alcohol and seizures. *N. Engl. J. Med.*, 319:715–716.

51. Smith, D. B., Esuceta, A. V. D., Cramer, J. A., and Mattson, R. H. (1983): Historical perspective on the choice of antiepileptic drugs for the treatment of seizures in adults. *Neurology*, 33 (Suppl. 1):S2–S7.

52. Smith, D. B., Mattson, R. H., Cramer, J. A., Collins, J. F., Novelly, R. A., Craft, B., and VA Cooperative Study Group (1987): Results of a nationwide Veterans Administration Cooperative Study comparing the efficacy and toxicity of carbamazepine, phenobarbital, phenytoin, and primidone. *Epilepsia*, 28 (Suppl. 3):S50–S58.

53. Snead, O. C., and Hosey, L. C. (1985): Exacerbation of seizures in children by carbamazepine. *N. Engl. J. Med.*, 313:916–921.

54. Suzuki, M., Maruyama, H., Ishibashi, Y., Ogawa, S., Seki, T., Hoshino, M., Maekawa, K., and Yogo, T. (1972): A double-blind comparative trial of sodium dipropylacetate and ethosuximide in epilepsy in children with special emphasis on pure petit mal seizures. *Med. Prog.*, 82:470–488.

55. Thompson, P., Huppert, F., and Trimble, M. (1981): Phenytoin and cognitive function: Effects on normal volunteers and implications for epilepsy. *Br. J. Clin. Psychol.*, 20:155–162.

56. Timberlake, W. H., Abbott, J. A., and Schwab, R. S. (1955): An effective anticonvulsant with initial problems of adjustment. *N. Engl. J. Med.*, 7:252–304.

57. Trimble, M. R. (1987): Anticonvulsant drugs and cognitive function: A review of the literature. *Epilepsia*, 28 (Suppl. 3):S37–S45.

58. Turnbull, D. M. (1983): Adverse effects of valproate. *Adv. Drug React. Ac. Pois. Rev.*, 2:191–216.

59. Turnbull, D. M., Rawlins, M. D., Weightman, D., and Chadwick, D. W. (1982): A comparison of phenytoin and valproate in previously untreated adult epileptic patients. *J. Neurol. Neurosurg. Psych.*, 45:55–59.

60. Turnbull, D. M., Rawlins, M. D., Weigtman, D., and Chadwick, D. W. (1983): Long term comparative study of phenytoin and valproate in adult onset epilepsy. *Br. Med. J.*, 290:815–819.

61. Vining, E. P. G., Mellits, E. D., Dorsen, M. M., Cataldo, M., Quaskey, S., Spielberg, S., and Freeman, J. (1987): Psychologic and behavioral effects of antiepileptic drugs in children. A double-blind comparison between phenobarbital and valproic acid. *Pediatrics*, 80:165–174.

62. Wilder, B. J., Ramsay, R. E., Murphy, J. V., Karas, B. J., Marquardt, K., and Hammond, E. J. (1983): Comparison of valproic acid and phenytoin in newly diagnosed tonic-clonic seizures. *Neurology*, 33:1474–1476.

63. Yerby, M. S. (1987): Problems and management of the pregnant woman with epilepsy. *Epilepsia*, 28 (Suppl. 3):S29–S36.

64. Young, G. P., Rores, C., Murphy, C., and Dailey, R. (1987): Intravenous phenobarbital for alcohol withdrawal and convulsions. *Ann. Emerg. Med.*, 16:847–850.

Antiepileptic Drugs, Third Edition, edited by
R. Levy, R. Mattson, B. Meldrum,
J. K. Penry, and F. E. Dreifuss.
Raven Press, Ltd., New York © 1989.

7

General Principles

How to Use Antiepileptic Drugs

Roger J. Porter

The selection of a pharmaceutical regimen appropriate for the patient with epilepsy is followed by the complex process of administering the medication. The second task involves a surprising number of variables, ranging from determining the size of the starting dose to monitoring the saturation kinetics, which are as important to the success of therapy as the initial drug selection. Unfortunately, such factors are often ignored; if the patient does poorly, the drug is often considered a failure. This chapter reviews the important factors in the administration of the primary antiepileptic drugs and establishes a framework to guide the prescribing physician and to allow the patient to obtain the most benefit from the regimen.

DIAGNOSIS

Three levels of diagnosis should be considered in all patients with epilepsy. The first of these is the *etiologic diagnosis*—the cause of the epilepsy. The second is the *seizure diagnosis*—the empirical seizure types suffered by the patient. The third is the *syndrome diagnosis*—the classification of the patient. The suspected etiologic diagnosis is most important in determining which neurologic investigations and interventions, if any, must be performed for the proper evaluation of the cause of the epilepsy. The seizure diagnosis largely determines the type of antiepileptic medication chosen. The syndrome classification gives insight into long-term prognosis and potential for eventual drug discontinuation. Of the three levels, the seizure diagnosis most immediately affects appropriate therapy. Medical therapy can be initiated even though the etiology of the seizures is undetermined or a logical syndrome is unidentified. Without a seizure diagnosis, however, medical therapy is likely to fail.

These levels of diagnosis are predicated on the assumption that the patient does indeed have epilepsy and not some other process that mimics the disorder. The differential diagnosis of epileptic seizures and syndromes and the appropriate choice of antiepileptic medications are considered in Chapter 8.

WHICH PATIENTS TO TREAT

Most patients with epilepsy are started on antiepileptic medication after they have experienced more than one seizure, and the medication is chosen primarily on the basis of the seizure type. The question of whether to prescribe antiepileptic drugs for patients who have had only a single seizure is controversial. Unfortunately, the decision is often based on the erroneous assumption that the epilepsy in all such patients is homogeneous. It is not uncommon, of course, for a patient to present with a single, unprovoked, generalized tonic-clonic seizure, and most clinicians—barring evidence for possible repetitive seizures—would choose not to treat the seizure. On the other hand, what approach should be taken with a single partial seizure? A single partial seizure is much less common than a single generalized tonic-clonic seizure. Is it likely to recur? Do patients ever present with a single absence seizure or a single myoclonic seizure? The interpretation of single seizures is obviously more complex than it appears at first glance.

Most epileptologists hold an important assumption about the presentation of a single seizure. The assumption is that generalized tonic-clonic seizures, even when uncommon in an individual patient, are usually detected, but that virtually all other seizures may quite easily go undetected, especially if they occur infrequently. The first generalized tonic-clonic seizure may properly go untreated; however, when other seizure types are diagnosed, one frequently assumes (very often correctly) that the detected event is not the first occurrence and that multiple seizures have in fact previously occurred. Such seizures are likely to continue to occur and treatment is required. The reason for not treating single generalized tonic-clonic attacks is that a significant percentage of patients (albeit determined by many risk factors) will never have another seizure and have only toxicity to gain from medication.

Neurologic concomitants such as an obvious focal brain lesion or a prominently epileptiform EEG may affect the decision to treat a single seizure. Social factors must also be taken into account. In children and elderly persons, determining factors may be different from those of a working adult.

Discontinuation of antiepileptic drugs is a major consideration in deciding to treat or not to treat seizures, and is the subject of Chapter 10. Furthermore, some patients, after multiple trials of appropriate medications, do not reasonably respond to the prescribed drugs, even though ingestion is documented by adequate blood drug levels and occasional mild, dose-related toxicity. Some patients may be better off without treatment. In many patients, withdrawal of the drugs should be considered after two seizure-free years (3).

HOW TO INITIATE THERAPY

It is the obligation of the prescribing physician to choose the correct medication, explain the choice to the patient (or patient's parent/guardian), warn of unusual, but sometimes life-threatening idiosyncratic adverse effects, describe the dose-related side effects, and consider the next step, especially if the first medication is unsuccessful. Whether to start an antiepileptic drug with vigor and haste or to begin slowly depends on both the drug and the clinical situation. If seizures, especially generalized tonic-clonic seizures, are expected to occur frequently, some drugs can be given in loading doses to attain a rapid antiepileptic effect. Certain drugs, on the other hand, have side effects that limit the ability of the patient to tolerate high initial doses. Each drug needs to be considered separately.

Phenytoin can be given in loading doses either orally or intravenously. In nonacute situations, it can be started at the expected oral maintenance dose. The usual dose of 300 mg/day will achieve steady-state levels in 7 to 10 days and provide only a low therapeutic level in most patients (28). Once-a-day dosing is possible only with the older, slow-release formulations.

Carbamazepine is only available in oral form. Attempts to start the drug at maintenance doses often result in toxic side effects (Fig. 1). In both children and adults, therefore, one should start slowly and grad-

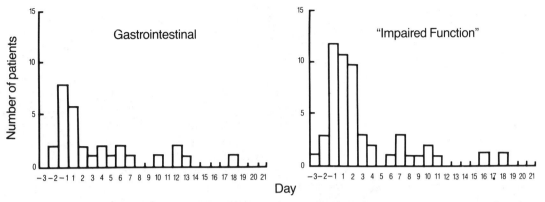

FIG. 1. In an early study in the United States, 45 patients were given carbamazepine (in addition to concomitant antiepileptic drugs) in rapidly increasing doses: 400 mg on the first day, 800 mg on the second day, and 1,200 mg on the third day. Although the dose was divided during the day, both gastrointestinal disturbance and "impaired function" were early complaints. The side effects gradually disappeared, usually without cessation of the drug. Modified from Cereghino et al., 1974 (4).

ually increase the dose over days or weeks (26).

Phenobarbital can be given by any route, but loading doses are highly sedating. Gradually increasing doses are usually required to reach a satisfactory plasma drug level. Phenobarbital can usually be given once a day.

Primidone can only be given orally. Sedation, gastrointestinal distress, and dizziness are most prominent with initiation; increasing the dose very gradually is almost always necessary. Primidone is usually given in divided doses throughout the day.

Ethosuximide may cause nausea, especially at the onset of therapy and with higher doses. Gradually increasing doses are required. Ethosuximide is usually given in divided doses.

Valproic acid, like ethosuximide, is limited by initial dose-related nausea. The drug is usually started slowly and given in divided doses.

Timing of Drug Administration

The optimal timing of the medication intake reflects both pharmacokinetic and toxicity considerations. In general, multiple daily doses are important for drugs with short half-lives and/or gastrointestinal toxicity. For a drug with a short half-life, frequent administration during the day will reduce peaks and troughs in the plasma drug level. If the drug is administered after meals, the absorption rate will be retarded, and the smoothing effect on the plasma drug level will be enhanced. When mixed with food, the drug gradually enters the bloodstream, avoiding a peak plasma drug level, which can cause toxicity. In addition, patients usually tolerate bedtime doses quite well unless they get up after retiring for the night (25).

The administration of drugs after meals and at bedtime is especially effective for patients requiring maximal doses for seizure control. Taking the drug after meals also ameliorates gastric irritation, regardless of whether the drug has a short half-life (e.g., valproate) or a long half-life (e.g., ethosuximide). For example, many patients who routinely omit breakfast have gastric distress from the morning dose. This local effect may be important for patients who have sensitive gastrointestinal tracts even though they require only a moderate amount of drug for seizure control (25).

Some antiepileptic drugs can be administered infrequently and with little attention to the time of day or relation to meals. The most well known is phenytoin, of which once-a-day administration has become popular. Some patients find such a regimen convenient and entirely satisfactory, but others are bothered by toxic effects and find that twice-a-day administration eliminates unpleasant side effects. More importantly, some generic phenytoin preparations are more rapidly absorbed than proprietary formulations. The rapidly absorbed preparations (called "prompt release") are even more likely to cause toxicity on a once-a-day regimen, and package inserts may specifically contraindicate a single daily dose (7).

Timing of Drug Intake Intervals

From a purely pharmacokinetic standpoint, the optional spacing of drug administration throughout the day can be scientifically determined. It makes no difference whether long half-life drugs are given frequently or infrequently. If maximum therapeutic effectiveness of the short half-life drugs is desired, however, they must be delivered frequently—often four times a day. The rule is simple: give short half-life drugs frequently. If the importance of this regimen is carefully explained, most patients will adhere to it (25).

The principle behind this recommendation is that short half-life drugs are cleared from the body faster than long half-life drugs. Indeed, the time a drug takes to decline to half its previous (arbitrary) level in the blood is defined as its half-life. For example, a drug that has a plasma level of 20 μg/ml at noon and a level of 10 μg/ml at 6 P.M. (assuming no drug intake during the interval) has a half-life of 6 hours, which is a rather short half-life for an antiepileptic drug (25).

Valproate and carbamazepine have short half-lives. When valproate is given only every 12 hours, its plasma drug level fluctuates widely (Fig. 2). Similar observations have been made with carbamazepine and have been correlated with adverse drug effects (44). It is most important, therefore, to space out the administration of these drugs during the day, especially in patients whose seizures are not completely controlled and who require maximum therapeutic effectiveness. The same recommendation applies to a lesser extent to primidone, whose action is complicated by its metabolite, phenobarbital, which has a long half-life (25).

Timing of Changes in Drug Dose

Sooner or later a drug reaches a steady state, a more or less constant level, that is achieved by the particular daily dose administered. When a total daily dose is changed, the pharmacokinetic rule is simple: after every dose change it takes five half-lives to reach 97% of a new steady-state plasma drug level. Only after the new steady-state level is reached can drug efficacy be evaluated. For example, accurate evaluation of the efficacy of phenobarbital a few days after a dose change is not possible. The half-life of phenobarbital may be 96 hours or more, and 3 weeks will often be required to reach a new steady-state level. With carbamazepine or valproate, however, a new steady state will be achieved within a few days, and the efficacy of the drug can be more rapidly determined. Of the antiepileptic drugs most commonly used, only carbamazepine and valproate, and to some extent primidone, have short half-lives which allow relatively rapid achievement of a steady-state level after a dose change (Table 1).

The need to wait for the achievement of the steady-state plasma drug level prior to evaluation of the drug's efficacy at the new

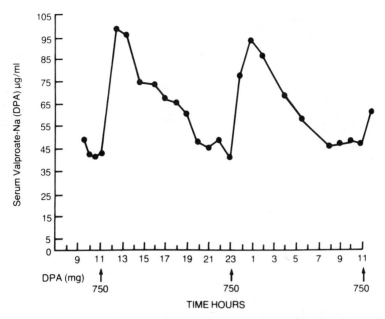

FIG. 2. Serum valproate fluctuations in a 12-hr dosing schedule. Modified from Rowan et al., 1979 (37).

level is important. The same caveat also applies to dose-related toxicity, which, like efficacy, cannot be fully evaluated until the new steady-state level is achieved. Because a patient tolerates a 400 mg daily dose of phenytoin for the first 3 days of administration does not mean that toxicity will not occur after 1 week or more at that dose (25).

TABLE 1. *Plasma half-life of six antiepileptic drugs*

Drug	Half-life[c]	Time to reach steady state
Carbamazepine	12 hr	3 days
Valproate	12 hr	3 days
Primidone[a]	12 hr	3 days
Phenytoin	1 day	5 days[b]
Ethosuximide	2 days	10 days
Phenobarbital	4 days	3 weeks

[a] Primidone is converted rapidly to phenobarbital.
[b] Phenytoin obeys saturation kinetics.
[c] Half-life is usually shorter when coadministered with enzyme inducing drugs.
From Porter, 1984 (25). Modified from Penry and Newmark, 1979 (21).

Occasionally, toxicity occurs before a steady-state level is reached, and a dosage decrease is indicated. Seizure control theoretically could be assessed before a steady-state level is attained, allowing for a lower dosage, but efficacy is best evaluated after steady state is achieved.

Seizure frequency will also affect the time required for efficacy evaluation. If a patient is having five seizures a day, a drug's efficacy can be determined quickly. If the patient is having only two seizures a year, a long time will be required to see whether the regimen is satisfactory (25).

Reaching Steady State

Whether the daily dose of an antiepileptic drug is increased by 15 mg or 150 mg, the time necessary to achieve a new steady-state level is the same. Although this assumption is based on linear kinetics, only phenytoin deviates from this model. Explained another way, the eventual height of

TABLE 2. *Effective plasma drug levels of six antiepileptic drugs*

Drug	Effective level (ug/ml)	High effective level[a] (ug/ml)	Toxic level (ug/ml)
Carbamazepine	4–10	7	>8
Primidone	5–15	10	>12
Phenytoin	10–20	18	>20
Phenobarbital	10–40	35	>40
Ethosuximide	50–100	80	>100
Valproate	50–100	80	>100

[a] Level that should be achieved, if possible, in patients with refractory seizures, assuming that the blood samples are drawn before administrtion of the morning medication. Higher levels are often possible—without toxicity—when the drugs are used alone, i.e., as monotherapy.

From Porter, 1984 (25).

the new steady-state plasma drug level is a function of the daily dose of the drug, whereas the time needed to reach this steady-state level is related not to the total dose or the amount of the dose change, but to the drug's half-life. The longer the half-life, the longer the time needed to reach steady state, regardless of the dose or the amount of dose change (25).

One way to avoid the long time needed to reach a steady-state level when using long half-life drugs is to use an initial large loading dose. This procedure is most useful with phenytoin and is least practical, but still possible, with barbiturates or benzodiazepines.

When changing the dose of a drug, especially at higher plasma levels, changes should be made slowly and in small increments. Dose-related toxicity, if it occurs, will thereby be relatively mild (25).

Value of Monitoring Plasma Drug Levels

Many tables of optimal therapeutic plasma drug levels for various antiepileptic drugs have been published; a simplified version is shown in Table 2. The usual therapeutic level of phenytoin is 10 to 20 μg/ml, which suggests that most patients will ex-

perience optimal seizure control with minimal toxicity if their plasma phenytoin level is within this range. There are many exceptions to this guideline, however, and many patients are well controlled at higher or lower levels. For example, some patients tolerate phenytoin levels exceeding 20 μg/ml and require these high levels for seizure control. The concept of seizure control and its relation to plasma phenytoin levels has been reviewed by Kutt (12).

The main considerations in monitoring plasma drug levels are as follows:

1. Antiepileptic drug monitoring is used only as a guide to changes in therapy; it is not a substitute for clinical judgment.

2. Expected therapeutic plasma drug levels are average values; each patient will have an individually optimal value.

3. Monitoring helps achieve maximal effects of each medication. The use of gradually increasing doses to establish the maximally tolerated dose is a valid concept in patients with refractory seizures.

4. Monitoring is invaluable in the presence of toxic side effects, especially in patients taking multiple drugs and when using phenytoin, which has nonlinear kinetics.

5. Noncompliance, malabsorption, and altered metabolism can be identified, but only noncompliance is a common problem.

6. A reliable laboratory is critical to proper interpretation of the results.

7. If the blood samples for determination of plasma drug levels are drawn at various times during the day, the levels may be misleading.

Limited Importance of Free Drug Levels

In research involving determination of free and bound antiepileptic drugs, numerous studies have emphasized that the free fraction (i.e., the portion not bound to plasma proteins) is the only portion of the circulating drug that can diffuse through plasma membranes. Until recently, however, the question of clinical relevance has been largely ignored. The fundamental argument is not whether the free fraction is the fraction that is diffusable, but whether changes in the free fraction are relevant in clinical practice. Clearly, in certain circumstances, such as uremia or hypoalbuminemia, the free fraction may be dramatically reduced with highly bound drugs such as phenytoin (28). The likelihood, however, of a rapid redistribution of drugs (from bound to free) following diffusion into tissues almost certainly negates the clinical relevance of alterations of the free fraction in drugs that are less than 90% bound; carbamazepine is a good example (1).

Only phenytoin and valproate are sufficiently bound to plasma proteins to be of even theoretical clinical importance. A controlled study of phenytoin binding failed to document the utility of routine free level determinations in the outpatient clinic (43). More recently, a study of the utility of measuring free serum valproate levels pointed to a similar conclusion (6): free levels were not better related to either seizure control or liver enzyme activity than were the total valproate levels. Except in special metabolic circumstances, the need for clinical measurement of free levels of antiepileptic drugs remains in doubt (27).

MONOTHERAPY AND MULTIPLE DRUG REGIMENS

A great deal has been written in the past few years regarding the merits of monotherapy, which has been canonized as the only reasonable approach to antiepileptic drug therapy, especially as compared to the evils of polytherapy. The latter, which involves the treatment of a patient with more than one drug at a time, has been declared in a somewhat mindless way unnecessary and inappropriate, without adequate and reasoned consideration that multiple drugs

may, in fact, be useful in some patients. The following statements offer some of the arguments for and against monotherapy, which tends, by itself, to be treatment by slogan rather than by reason. Some of these statements are provocative by design.

1. The best state of health is the medication-free state. Any therapy, including monotherapy, is inferior to a drug-free state when such a state is possible. Some patients with epilepsy prefer to risk an occasional seizure rather than experience drug-induced toxicity. Others benefit so little from therapy that they may be better off without medication. Such patients are uncommon, but clearly monotherapy is second best to the absence of therapy when none is needed or indicated. Finally, and perhaps most important, some patients who once required medical therapy may no longer need it (see Chapter 10).

2. There are advantages to limiting the number or quantity of antiepileptic drugs. Adverse drug-drug interactions are much less likely; they obviously do not even occur with monotherapy. Side effects may be fewer, but this issue is complex (see discussion below). Compliance by the patient may be better, but compliance problems may also relate to inadequate attention by the physician. Cost of therapy may be lower, but it may also be higher if more expensive drugs are chosen. Seizure control is better in some patients, but may be related to increased compliance because of few adverse side effects and not to fundamental alteration in the propensity for seizures. For all of these reasons, patients should first be tried on a single medication. Before being abandoned as ineffective, the drug should be pushed gently to the point of dose-related side effects. Should the first medication fail, a trial of another single agent should probably be attempted before considering a multidrug regimen.

3. Adverse effects are generally less likely with a single medication than with multiple drugs. Adverse effects of antiepileptic drugs can, in a somewhat oversim-

plified way, be divided into four fundamental groups, each of which may be
affected differently by single or multiple
drug therapy.

a. Dose-related adverse effects: The
most important reason for maintaining patients on fewer medications is the difficulty
of dealing with dose-related side effects.
Multiple drug therapy is more likely to
cause such effects for two reasons. First,
the control of reasonable, nontoxic levels is
clearly more difficult with multiple drugs
than with single medications; physicians
vary in their ability to successfully manage
multidrug regimens. Second, some dose-related adverse effects are additive: ataxia
may appear sooner with modest levels of
carbamazepine combined with phenytoin
than with either drug used singly at higher
doses and levels.

b. Idiosyncratic adverse effects: Most
idiosyncratic side effects occur within the
first few months of therapy; some are severe and most require complete cessation
of the medication. Because of greater patient exposure, the risk of such effects is
clearly higher with multiple drugs than with
single medications. However, little evidence exists for more than a simple additive
effect; the idiosyncratic skin rash of phenobarbital, for example, is not more likely to
occur in the presence of ethosuximide,
which may also cause a rash. Unlike dose-
related side effects (e.g., drowsiness or
ataxia) in which the combination of drugs
may cumulatively aggravate the toxicity,
idiosyncratic reactions are usually related
to a single medication. Patients on multiple
drugs who have an idiosyncratic reaction
present the difficult problem of identifying
which drug is the culprit. Because of the
nature of these reactions, however, the likelihood of an idiosyncratic reaction falls dramatically once a patient tolerates a drug for
several months.

c. Drug interactions: The possibility of
drug-drug interactions increases with the
number of medications used. Furthermore,
combinations of antiepileptic drugs may
alter metabolism to produce changes in the
levels of active and/or toxic metabolites; examples include the effect of phenytoin on
carbamazepine and the effect of phenobarbital on valproate.

d. Teratogenicity: Little is known about
the possible cumulative effects of multiple
drugs on the developing fetus. In practice,
most agree that teratogenic effects are, at
least in part, idiosyncratic effects and that
few drugs are better than many drugs. It has
not been proven, however, that high doses
of monotherapy are safer than moderate
doses of multiple drugs. Is a high dose of
phenytoin really safer for the fetus than
moderate doses of phenytoin plus carbamazepine? Answers to such questions are
not available from controlled studies or currently available data. One of the interaction
effects that is most common with polytherapy is the direct effect on plasma levels.
Monotherapy with carbamazepine, for example, may yield well-tolerated plasma levels in the range of 14 to 16 μg/ml. When
phenytoin is added to the regimen, the maximal tolerated carbamazepine levels may be
8 to 10 μ/ml, with some dose reduction required. Likewise, phenytoin levels of 20 to
25 μ/ml or higher may be tolerated with
monotherapy, but lower levels (and doses)
are often necessary when phenytoin is combined with other drugs.

*4. A multidrug regimen may occasion-
ally be superior to monotherapy.* In certain
patients, usually those with severe, difficult-to-control epilepsy, multiple drugs appear to be more effective than single medications. This issue was addressed in the
Veterans Administration study of partial
and generalized tonic-clonic seizures (17).
Of 522 patients participating in this controlled trial, 82 were considered failures on
monotherapy and were placed on a two-
drug regimen. Of these, almost 40% were
judged to be improved, and 11% became
seizure-free. Although only a minority of

patients may respond, the physician should not automatically reject a multidrug regimen as having no potential benefit for the patient.

5. *A nonsedative regimen may be more important than monotherapy.* In the past decade, numerous studies have suggested that certain antiepileptic drugs, notably those with sedative-hypnotic effects, may cause drowsiness and cognitive dysfunction in many patients with epilepsy. If barbiturates and benzodiazepines are, with certain exceptions, considered second-line antiepileptic drugs because of their sedating properties, then the choice is limited, in most cases, to four primary antiepileptic drugs: phenytoin, carbamezepine, valproic acid, and ethosuximide.

Logically, treatment should begin with one of these four drugs; if it fails, a second drug should be tried before a multiple-drug regimen is prescribed. When a multidrug regimen is indicated, combinations of nonsedative medications are preferable to combinations including barbiturates or benzodiazepines. There have been no adequate studies of whether monotherapy with barbiturates or benzodiazepines is worth the effort before embarking on a multidrug regimen. Only scanty data are available to support a regimen of monotherapy with sedative-hypnotic antiepileptic drugs except for (a) certain specific seizure types, such as the myoclonias, which respond to long-term benzodiazepine therapy, and (b) patients who are intolerant of the usual first-line drugs.

COMPLIANCE AND NONCOMPLIANCE

One of the major causes of uncontrolled seizures is the failure of the patient to follow the prescribed regimen (15). Poor compliance with the physician's instructions regarding medication is not a problem unique to epilepsy; it is a difficulty encountered in the therapy of any chronic disease for which daily therapy is indicated. The typical patient with infrequent seizures forgets for a myriad of reasons to take the medications and continues to have seizures. The frustrated doctor prescribes higher and higher doses of drugs, observing neither toxic effects nor seizure control. Then, if the patient suddenly becomes compliant, toxicity occurs swiftly, the doctor is dumbfounded, and the patient disillusioned. It is an even more difficult problem if the patient has intractable seizures or deliberately omits medication. Poor compliance is by no means limited to patients of lower socioeconomic backgrounds. Children from socioeconomically advantaged families may resist compliance in spite of logical explanations and emotional cajoling. Sometimes such forgetfulness can be detected by the pattern of the plasma drug levels (25).

There are several ways to improve compliance (25). Even with complicated regimens, compliance is possible if the patient is capable of learning:

1. For patients who seem apathetic about their problems, emphasize the importance of taking the prescribed doses so that the physician can interpret the results of therapy.

2. Be understanding and forgiving but firm with patients who are capable of good compliance. At the first visit, it may be useful to reach an understanding of the importance of regular drug intake. Compliance is a reasonable price to pay for improved seizure control, and the physician should expect it.

3. Ask frequently about drug compliance. Have the patient (or guardian who manages the pills) recite, at each visit, the number of each tablet taken and when each is taken during the day. The patient will come to expect the question and will therefore learn the daily regimen. Since alternate day regimens (e.g., 300 and 400 mg of phenytoin on alternate days) are unnecessary and a good excuse for getting confused,

they should not be used (instead, for example, give 350 mg/day of phenytoin).

4. An effective technique for improving compliance, and one that the physician should insist on in difficult cases, is the "morning set-up" plan. Insist that the patient (or guardian) count out the entire day's dose of medications on awakening in the morning; place the tablets in a designated place such as a cup or separate pillbox. Draw from this receptable as needed for the day's dose and inspect it at bedtime to be sure the day's dose is entirely consumed. Repeat the procedure each day. Well-educated patients will resist such an elementary procedure; ignore these complaints and insist that it be followed.

WHEN THE PROPER MEDICAL REGIMEN FAILS

As many as 25% of patients fail to respond to the medical regimen prescribed. For some, the drug failure may be related to seizure-inducing factors such as alcohol withdrawal or sleep deprivation; in rare instances, it may have very specific causes, such as intermittent photic stimulation, that require manipulation of the environment. In other patients, especially those in which the diagnosis is not completely secure, a reevaluation of the diagnosis is necessary. Simply put, some patients with refractory seizures do not have epilepsy and therefore would not be expected to respond to antiepileptic drugs.

Such patients have nonepileptic attacks resembling seizures of epileptic origin but not arising from abnormal neuronal discharge. Any paroxysmal dysfunction with apparent alteration of responsiveness and/or motor, sensory, or autonomic dysfunction may mimic epileptic seizures. These nonepileptic attacks include organic seizures which involve other systems, such as the cardiovascular system. Metabolic disorders may also be associated with sei-

zures. Narcolepsy, cataplexy, and other sleep disorders can be confused with epilepsy. An overlap between epileptic and other organic seizures is apparent (5). Nonorganic seizures are those in which no clear anatomic-pathologic change can be correlated with the disorder.

In 84 patients with nonepileptic seizures studied by Mattson (16), the most common attacks were associated with hysterical (psychogenic) causes (34 patients), drug toxicity (15 patients), and cerebral ischemia (10 patients). A surprising 75% of the patients improved after appropriate diagnosis and therapy.

When the data on seizure characteristics are inadequate, the seizure diagnosis will be in doubt, and intensive monitoring is sometimes necessary to establish a seizure diagnosis. If the physician is forced to make a tentative diagnosis with inadequate data, an erroneous decision can result in inappropriate therapy. Even if the seizure diagnosis is correct, multiple medications may be unnecessarily prescribed or plasma drug levels may be inadequate. Intensive monitoring is an extension of the physician's usual skills; it allows more rational diagnostic and therapeutic decisions in the approximately 5% of patients with epilepsy who fail to respond to conventional approaches (22).

In recent years, there has been increased interest in all types of monitoring devices (9). Although monitoring of the vital functions of critically ill patients has been the most dramatic development in this area, advanced techniques for monitoring patients with epilepsy have also emerged. Advances have occurred in EEG monitoring (10,24,30,32) and in video recording of epileptic and nonepileptic seizures (5,20,23). Simultaneous EEG and video recordings have been combined with intensive pharmacologic monitoring in intractable epilepsy (29).

Prolonged monitoring of the EEG is not new. Many clinicians and investigators have advocated a departure from the routine 20 min recording, and good laboratories are as flexible with the amount of recording time as they are with modification of montages. Prolonging a routine EEG recording, however, has the limitations and disadvantages of an artificial environment, confined observation space, prominent artifact if the patient moves about, electrode problems, and excessive accumulation of paper records. In order to collect long-term EEG data for quantification, classification, and localization, two acceptable alternatives have been devised to alleviate these problems. The first is cable telemetry, in which the weak scalp signals are preamplified and then transmitted through a long cable to the EEG machine. The second is radiotelemetry, in which the signal is transmitted by FM radio signal to a receiver and then to the EEG machine. Both systems are effective.

Intensive monitoring with video recording is a more recent advance than EEG monitoring, and it has added an important dimension to our understanding of seizures. There are three basic elements to any video system: cameras, tape recorders, and video monitors. Although integrated systems are available, the best systems are of modular construction, utilizing the best model and manufacturer for each piece of equipment. Adequate technical staff is needed to maintain the equipment in working order. Further discussion of the technical aspects of video recording of seizures is beyond the scope of this chapter.

Simultaneous video and EEG recording has been combined with frequent monitoring of antiepileptic plasma drug levels with encouraging results in patients with intractable seizures (29). Further, in a study of 69 patients followed for 2 years after intensive monitoring, 58% had improved seizure control, 58% had also maintained a reduction in medication toxicity, and 39% had attained improvement in social adjustment (31). In a larger study of 388 intensively monitored patients, severe epilepsy was documented in 267. Improvement in seizure control was effected in 68% of this group; most of the remaining patients had non-epileptic seizures (16). Newer pharmacologic techniques allow appropriate collection of important seizure data during controlled medication withdrawal (36).

Intensive monitoring units have proliferated throughout the world. Although only 29 units were estimated to be in place in the United States in August 1980 (31), such units are now internationally commonplace.

Long-term ambulatory EEG monitoring without video recording is now possible because of advances in miniaturization of various electronic components (39). The wearable cassette EEG recording device can be used to establish the diagnosis as well as to quantify electrographic discharges.

REFER DIFFICULT PATIENTS TO AN EPILEPSY CENTER

Every patient with uncontrolled epilepsy should have the satisfaction of knowing that all measures capable of producing improvement have been exhausted. Although most diagnostic and therapeutic possibilities can be adequately evaluated by the primary care physician or neurologist, specialized investigation and management can occasionally lead to revision of the diagnosis of epilepsy, a better pharmacologic regimen, a trial of an experimental antiepileptic agent (18) or the use of surgical therapy; dramatic improvement may be the result.

There are several kinds of comprehensive epilepsy centers. In the United States, for example, many research centers are funded by the National Institutes of Health (NIH); these programs are not only involved in clinical research, but also have capabilities for extensive inpatient evaluation. All NIH programs offer outpatient opinions as well. The U.S. Veterans Administration Epilepsy Centers treat veterans; some also treat non-veterans. There are other outstanding clinics and university centers in the United States to which appropriate referrals can be made. The best way to be certain of the expertise available in a particular area of this country is to write to the Epilepsy Foundation of America, 4351 Garden City Drive (Suite 406), Landover, Maryland 20785 U.S.A.

The United States, however, is less advanced in the comprehensive care of epilepsy than many other countries in which long-term comprehensive care is available in nationally funded centers. Such centers emphasize not only the need for long-term hospitalization for proper evaluation and treatment of epilepsy, but also the need for eventual deinstitutionalization to the maximum extent possible. In addition to such centers, there are many outstanding clinics and hospitals throughout the world in which patients with refractory seizures can be definitively evaluated. Information on the location of specialized epilepsy centers and clinics can be obtained from the national or local voluntary or professional epilepsy society. The addresses of the local societies around the world are available from the Epilepsy Foundation of America.

SURGICAL INTERVENTION

Surgical therapy should be considered for medically intractable epilepsy, especially patients with partial seizures (2,19). The number of epileptic patients whose attacks remain uncontrolled by current forms of treatment is quite large. The number of patients with uncontrolled partial seizures was estimated in 1983 to be about 360,000 (46). Although many of these patients could benefit from improved medical therapy, including advanced clinical pharmacologic techniques, the majority will not become seizure free (29). These patients deserve consideration for surgical therapy, as the localized nature of the causal lesion makes them prime candidates for such intervention.

Such consideration is important even though many will be eventually rejected on various criteria (see below).

Ward (46) has estimated that at least 15% of the 360,000 patients with uncontrolled partial seizures are candidates for surgery—54,000 candidates, yet the number of operations for epilepsy in the United States is probably less than 1,000 per year. The underutilization of surgical therapy for epilepsy is presumably related to an assumption that medical therapy is more effective than it actually is, to the need for expensive and dedicated teams to evaluate patients and to perform appropriate surgical procedures, and to inadequate education of the primary care physician about the value of surgical therapy (46).

The selection of patients for surgical intervention is constantly being reevaluated. The patient with intractable complex partial seizures and a clear-cut unilateral temporal lobe focus is the ideal candidate for surgical intervention. A series of decisions must be made for each surgical therapy candidate. These decisions are discussed below in the approximate order of their consideration; the approach is basically taken from Rasmussen (34).

1. *Is the patient's epilepsy medically intractable?* The majority of epileptic patients considered for surgical therapy will have partial seizures. The use of maximally tolerated doses of phenytoin and/or carbamazepine is the most reasonable approach to establish whether medical therapy will be adequate. The addition of primidone or other sedative drugs to such a regimen is unlikely to improve seizure control and will add toxicity. Some investigators feel that other such drugs should, nevertheless, be tried for completeness of effort.

   After the patient is receiving a maximally tolerated regimen of antiepileptic drugs, the significance of the seizures and their frequency must be evaluated in terms of the resulting disability. Some patients can easily tolerate brief or nocturnal seizures without noticeable interference in daily activities (34). In others, even brief seizures may jeopardize a job or prevent driving a car. In patients who are on sedative-hypnotic drugs, the incapacity caused by the side effects of the medication must also be considered. The intractability of the seizures should be prolonged, that is, spontaneous improvement of the disorder should clearly be unlikely before surgical therapy is considered.

2. *Does the patient really want the operation?* The patient must be motivated to undergo the testing necessary to establish eligibility for surgical therapy and to localize the lesion, and finally the patient must be willing to cooperate with the surgical procedure itself. The prolonged process and the associated discomfort and risks should be carefully explained to the patient. The motivation should not come primarily from the family or from the physician (34).

3. *How well localized is the epileptogenic lesion?* Many criteria can be applied to localization of the lesion, which must be somewhat discrete and not located in or closely adjacent to vital structures, such as the speech area. Clinical clues come directly from the history of the seizures; auras need to be evaluated, aphasia or other localizing symptoms must be sought, and the onset of the attack should be determined in detail. Neuropsychologic studies will add to the data on localization.

Electroencephalographic data are critical in the effort to localize the lesion. Initial studies are routine, but the addition of more specialized efforts include simultaneous video and EEG recordings, the use of sphenoidal leads, and the intracarotid sodium amytal test (33). The need for invasive studies to obtain electrographic evidence of the seizure focus is controversial and evolving. Some investigators routinely implant depth electrodes to assure maximal information. Others use depth electrodes sparingly and prefer subdural electrodes when scalp recordings do not give definitive results. Direct cortical recording during the operation to confirm and further define the lesion is performed in some centers.

Computed tomography may be of great assistance in localizing the lesion (8). Other specialized brain imaging techniques, especially positron emission tomography (PET) (42) and nuclear magnetic resonance (NMR) (11; 13) have already helped to refine the approach for selecting surgical candidates and to define surgical lesions. Single photon emission computed tomography may also become more important (14). In the future, magnetoencephalography may play an important role in such localization (35,41).

For those patients with temporal lobe lesions who undergo cortical excision, the results are quite promising. In 653 patients with a median follow-up of 11 years, Rasmussen (34) reported that 71% either had become seizure free or had a marked reduction in frequency of attacks. The current morbidity and mortality rates of the excisional procedures are quite low.

Some progress is now being made in surgical approaches to nonlocalized lesions following such failures as the cerebellar stimulator, which was initially received enthusiastically but in a double-blind study (45) was shown to be ineffective. The major approach now is the splitting of the corpus callosum (corpus callosotomy), a procedure which appears to be most effective for secondary generalized tonic-clonic seizures and for atonic seizures. Spencer et al. (40) noted that more than 70% of their patients remained improved after 2 years' follow-up. In some patients, deterioration of motor function or impairment of memory was documented (38). Nevertheless, the procedure improves the quality of life for many patients with the most intractable epilepsies.

SUMMARY

The proper use of antiepileptic drugs is just as important as the appropriate choice of medication. After deciding whether to treat, the physician must combine a detailed understanding of the pharmacologic principles with an in-depth knowledge of the characteristics of the various antiepileptic drugs. For example, knowledge of pharmacokinetic principles must be combined with specific knowledge about the drugs in question. Monitoring drug levels is required for proper therapy. Intensive monitoring of seizures may improve medical therapy. Some patients fail to respond to medication even when the antiepileptic drugs have been carefully chosen and properly utilized; for these patients, surgical intervention may be necessary.

REFERENCES

1. Agbato, O. A., Elyas, A. A., Patsalos, P. N., Brett, E. M., and Lascelles, P. T. (1986): Total and free serum concentrations of carbamazepine and carbamazepine-10,11-epoxide in children with epilepsy. *Arch. Neurol.*, 43:1111–1116.
2. Cahan, L. C., and Engel, J. (1986): Surgery for epilepsy: A review. *Acta Neurol. Scand.*, 73:551–560.
3. Callaghan, N., Garrett, A., and Goggin, T. (1988): Withdrawal of anticonvulsant drugs in patients free of seizures for two years: A prospective study. *N.E.J.M.*, 318:942–946.
4. Cereghino, J. J., Brock, J. T., Van Meter, J. C., Penry, J. K., Smith, L. D., and White, B. G. (1974): Carbamazepine for epilepsy: A controlled prospective evaluation. *Neurology*, 24:401–410.
5. Desai, B. T., Porter, R. J., and Penry, J. K. (1982): Psychogenic seizures: A study of 42 attacks in six patients, with intensive monitoring. *Arch. Neurol.*, 39:202–209.
6. Farrell, K., Abbott, F. S., Orr, J. M., Applegarth, D. A., Jan, J. E., and Wong, P. K. (1986): Free and total serum valproate concentrations: Their relationship to seizure control, liver enzymes and plasma ammonia in children. *Can. J. Neurol. Sci.*, 13:252–255.
7. Food and Drug Administration (1981): New standards for phenytoin products. *FDA Drug Bulletin*, 11:4.
8. Gammel, T. E., Adams, R. J., King, D. W., So, E. L., and Gallagher, B. B. (1987): Modified CT techniques in the evaluation of temporal lobe epilepsy prior to lobectomy. *A.J.N.R.*, 8:131–134.
9. Gotman, J., Ives, J. R., and Gloor, P. (eds.) (1985): *Long-Term Monitoring in Epilepsy*. EEG, Suppl. No. 37. Elsevier, Amsterdam.
10. Ives, J. R., Thompson, C. J., and Gloor, P. (1976): Seizure monitoring: A new tool in electroencephalography. *Electroencephalography and Clinical Neurophysiology*, 41:422–427.
11. Jabbari, B., Gunderson, C. H., Wippold, F., Citrin, C., Sherman, J., Bartoszek, D., Daigh, J. D., and Mitchell, M. H. (1986): Magnetic resonance imaging in partial complex epilepsy. *Arch. Neurol.*, 43:869–872.
12. Kutt, H. (1982): Phenytoin: Relation of plasma concentration to seizure control. In: *Antiepileptic Drugs*, Second Edition, edited by D. M. Woodbury, J. K. Penry, and C. E. Pippenger, pp. 241–246. Raven Press, New York.
13. Kuzniecky, R., de la Sayette, V., Ethier, R., Melanson, D., Andermann, F., Berkovic, S., Robitaille, Y., Olivier, A., Peters, T., and Feindel, W. (1987): Magnetic resonance imaging in temporal lobe epilepsy: Pathological correlations. *Ann. Neurol.*, 22:341–347.
14. Lee, B. I., Markand, O. N., Siddiqui, A. R., Park, H. M., Mock, B., Wellman, H. H., Worth, R. M., and Edwards, M. K. (1986): Single photon emission computed tomography (SPECT) brain imaging. *Neurology*, 36:1471–1477.
15. Leppik, I. (1988): Compliance during the treatment of epilepsy. The Development of Antiepileptic Drugs. *Epilepsia* (Suppl.) (*in press*).
16. Mattson, R. H. (1980): Value of intensive monitoring. In: *Advances in Epileptology: The Xth Epilepsy International Symposium*, edited by J. A. Wada and J. K. Penry, pp. 43–51. Raven Press, New York.
17. Mattison, R. H., Cramer, J. A., Collins, J. F., Smith, D. B., Delgado-Escueta, A. V., Browne, T. R., Williamson, P. D., Treiman, D. M., McNamera, J. O., McCutchen, C. B., Homan, R. W., Crill, W. E., Lubozynski, M. F., Rosenthal, N. P., and Mayersdorf, A. (1985): Comparison of carbamazepine, phenobarbital, phenytoin, and primidone in partial and secondarily generalized tonic-clonic seizures. *New Engl. J. Med.*, 313:145–151.
18. Meldrum, B. S., and Porter, R. J. (eds.) (1986): *New Anticonvulsant Drugs, vol. 4, Current Problems in Epilepsy*. John Libbey, London.
19. Ojemann, G. A. (1987): Surgical therapy for medically intractable epilepsy. *J. Neurosurg.*, 66:489–499.
20. Penry, J. K., and Dreifuss, F. E. (1969): Automatisms associated with the absence of petit mal epilepsy. *Archives of Neurology*, 21:142–149.
21. Penry, J. K., and Newmark, M. E. (1979): The use of antiepileptic drugs. *Annals of Internal Medicine*, 90:207–218.
22. Penry, J. K., and Porter, R. J. (1977): Intensive monitoring of patients with intractable seizures. In: *Epilepsy: The Eighth International Symposium*, edited by J. K. Penry, pp. 95–101. Raven Press, New York.
23. Penry, J. K., Porter, R. J., and Dreifuss, F. E. (1975): Simultaneous recording of absence seizures with video tape and electroencephalography: A study of 374 seizures in 48 patients. *Brain*, 98:427–440.
24. Porter, R. J. (1980): Methodology of continuous monitoring with videotape recording and electroencephalography. In: *Advances in Epileptology: The Xth Epilepsy International Symposium*, edited by J. A. Wada and J. K. Penry, pp. 35–42. Raven Press, New York.

25. Porter, Roger J. (1984): *Epilepsy: 100 Elementary Principles*. Saunders, London.
26. Porter, R. J. (1987): How to Initiate and Maintain Carbamazepine Therapy in Children and Adults. *Epilepsia*, 28(Suppl. 3):S59–63.
27. Porter, R. J. (1988): Therapy of epilepsy. In: *Current Opinion in Neurology and Neurosurgery*, edited by F. C. Rose. Gower Academic Journals, London (*in press*).
28. Porter, R. J., and Layzer, R. B. (1975): Plasma albumin concentration and diphenylhydantoin binding in man. *Archives of Neurology*, 32:298–303.
29. Porter, R. J., Penry, J. K., and Lacy, J. R. (1977): Diagnostic and therapeutic reevaluation of patients with intractable epilepsy. *Neurology*, 27:1006–1011.
30. Porter, R. J., Penry, J. K., and Wolf, A. A., Jr. (1976): Simultaneous documentation of clinical and electroencephalographic manifestations of epileptic seizures. In: *Quantitative Analytic Studies in Epilepsy*, edited by P. Kellaway and I. Petersen, pp. 253–268. Raven Press, New York.
31. Porter, R. J., Theodore, W. H., and Schulman, E. A. (1981): Intensive monitoring of intractable epilepsy: A two-year follow-up. In: *Advances in Epileptology: XIIth Epilepsy International Symposium*, edited by M. Dam, L. Gram, and J. K. Penry, pp. 265–268. Raven Press, New York.
32. Porter, R. J., Wolf, A. A., Jr., and Penry, J. K. (1971): Human electroencephalographic telemetry: A review of systems and their applications and a new receiving system. *American Journal of Electroencephalographic Technology*, 11:145–159.
33. Powell, G. E., Polkey, C. E., and Canavan, A. G. M. (1987): Lateralisation of memory functions in epileptic patients by use of the sodium amytal (Wada) technique. *J. Neurol. Neurosurg. Psychiat.*, 50:665–672.
34. Rasmussen, T. (1975): Surgical treatment of patients with complex partial seizures. In: *Advances in Neurology, Vol. 11: Complex Partial Seizures and Their Treatment*, edited by J. K. Penry and D. D. Daly, pp. 415–449. Raven Press, New York.
35. Rose, D. F., Smith, P. D., and Sato, S. (1987): Magnetoencephalography and epilepsy research. *Science*, 238:329–335.
36. Rosenfeld, W. E., Leppik, I. E., Gates, J. R., and Mireles, R. E. (1987): Valproic acid loading during intensive monitoring. *Arch. Neurol.*, 44:709–710.
37. Rowan, A. J., Binnie, C. D., de Beer-Pawlikowski, N. K. B., Goedhart, D. M., Gutter, T., van der Geest, P., Meinardi, H., and Meijer, J. W. A. (1979): Sodium valproate: Serial monitoring of EEG and serum levels. *Neurology*, 29:1450–1459.
38. Sass, K. J., Spencer, D. D., Spencer, S. S., Novelly, R. A., Williamson, P. D., and Mattson, R. H. (1988): Corpus callosotomy for epilepsy: Neurologic and neuropsychological outcome. *Neurology*, 38:24–28.
39. Sato, S., Penry, J. K., and Dreifuss, F. E. (1976): Electroencephalographic monitoring of generalized spike-wave paroxysms in the hospital and at home. In: *Quantitative Analytic Studies in Epilepsy*, edited by P. Kellaway and I. Petersen, pp. 237–251. Raven Press, New York.
40. Spencer, S. S., Spencer, D. D., Williamson, P. D., Sass, K., Novelly, R. A., and Mattson, R. H. (1988): Corpus callosotomy for epilepsy: Seizure effects. *Neurology*, 38:19–24.
41. Sutherling, W. W., Crandall, P. H., Engel, J., Darcey, T. M., Cahan, L. D., and Barth, D. S. (1987): The magnetic field of complex partial seizures agrees with intracranial localizations. *Ann. Neurol.*, 21:548–558.
42. Theodore, W. H., Dorwart, R., Holmes, M., Porter, R. J., and DiChiro, G. (1987): Neuroimaging in epilepsy: Comparison of positron emission tomography, magnetic resonance imaging, and computed tomography. In: *Advances in Epileptology: The XVIth Epilepsy International Symposium*, edited by P. Wolf, pp. 283–286. Raven Press, New York.
43. Theodore, W. H., Yu, L., Price, B., Yonekawa, W., Porter, R. J., Kapetanovik, I., Moore, H., and Kupferberg, H. J. (1985): The clinical value of free phenytoin levels. *Ann. Neurol.*, 18:90–93.
44. Tomson, T. (1984): Interdosage fluctuations in plasma carbamazepine concentration determine intermittent side effects. *Arch. Neurol.*, 41:830–834.
45. Van Buren, J. M., Wood, J. H., Oakley, J., and Hambrecht, F. (1978): Preliminary evaluation of cerebellar stimulation by double-blind stimulation and biological criteria in the treatment of epilepsy. *Journal of Neurosurgery*, 48:407–416.
46. Ward, A. A., Jr. (1983): Perspectives for surgical therapy of epilepsy. In *Epilepsy*, edited by A. A. Ward, Jr., J. K. Penry, and D. Purpura, pp. 371–375. Raven Press, New York.

Antiepileptic Drugs, Third Edition, edited by
R. Levy, R. Mattson, B. Meldrum,
J. K. Penry, and F. E. Dreifuss.
Raven Press, Ltd., New York © 1989.

8

General Principles

Discontinuation of Antiepileptic Drugs

J. Christine Dean and J. Kiffin Penry

When a patient who is taking antiepileptic drugs has remained seizure-free for several years, the question arises whether the drugs may be withdrawn. The advantages of reducing or discontinuing antiepileptic drugs are evident: a dose reduction means fewer side effects and less risk of teratogenesis and drug withdrawal reactions, removes the stigma of epilepsy, decreases health care costs, and offers greater social freedom. The increasing awareness of subtle toxicity (31,36) and adverse effects of antiepileptic drugs on cognitive function (45) makes urgent the need to study discontinuation of drugs in epileptic patients. A clinician who advises a patient with epilepsy to discontinue antiepileptic drugs lacks adequate information on the prognosis of certain types of epilepsy and does not understand how antiepileptic drugs influence continuing freedom from seizures.

POTENTIAL CANDIDATES FOR DRUG WITHDRAWAL

Although little is known about the true prognosis of patients with epilepsy, there is concrete evidence of remission of seizures in long-term follow-up. The disadvantage of surveying the literature to answer the question of which patients are candidates for drug withdrawal is that populations differ in their potential for seizure control (i.e., intractable patients versus easily controlled patients) and in their heterogeneity. Annegers et al. (2) found that 42% of patients experience remission for at least 5 years within a year of diagnosis. At 20 years after diagnosis, 50% have been seizure-free without antiepileptic drugs for at least 5 years, 20% will have continued to take antiepileptic drugs with freedom from seizures for at least 5 years, and the remaining 30% will have continued to have seizures in spite of medication. Once a long remission has been achieved a relapse is unusual, but the chance of achieving remission falls rapidly if remission is not achieved in the first or second year of treatment (7). The interval between the second and third seizures is shorter than between the first and second seizures, which substantiates the Gowerian ethic that seizures beget seizures. It appears, therefore, that early treatment with antiepileptic drugs alters the natural history of epilepsy and the earlier the treatment, the better the control of seizure activity and the more certain continued remission. A corollary is that if seizures are allowed to continue in the early stages of treatment, subsequent control may become more difficult.

It is generally agreed that the factors influencing successful withdrawal of antiepileptic drugs are the same factors that influence the prognosis of epilepsy (33). No

TABLE 1. *Factors affecting successful withdrawal of antiepileptic drugs in patients seizure-free for 2 to 5 years*

Age at onset of seizures
Duration, severity, and frequency of seizures, including number of years seizure-free with antiepileptic drug therapy and number of years from first seizure to seizure control
Etiology of epilepsy and associated neurological deficits
Type of seizure
Normalization of EEG with antiepileptic drug therapy

Based on literature review (1952–1988) of prospective and retrospective studies of children and adults.

single factor determines the probability of a patient remaining seizure-free, but a combination of factors can help predict the successful withdrawal of drugs.

Factors favoring antiepileptic drug withdrawal in children and adults are shown in Table 1. These factors were identified in a review of studies of the prognosis of epilepsy and prediction of seizure recurrence after withdrawal of antiepileptic drugs (Table 2). These mainly involve hospital-based populations, but also include patients with severe and refractory epilepsy, patients treated in comprehensive epilepsy centers, and community populations of newly diagnosed, newly treated patients. In the retrospective studies (8,10,14,16, 18,24,28), a bias exists for the successful seizure-free patients since these patients were selected on the basis of their continued remission. Although all studies excluded single seizures, febrile seizures, expired patients, and noncompliant patients, none of the authors used all four criteria as a basis for exclusion of patients. Statistical accountability, especially with large studies, was difficult unless survival study statistics were used. Two studies (8,37) surveyed populations of under 100 children and one study surveyed up to 500 adults (24). Relapse rates for children were amazingly similar (22–35%), but this was not the case for adults (8–66%).

Age at Onset of Seizures

Emerson et al. (8) showed that the earlier the disorder manifests itself, the higher the risk of recurrent seizures when medication is withdrawn. Opinions to the contrary are also drawn from the literature (14,16,17, 21,44,46). If the epilepsy begins before 2 years of age and if it is symptomatic of cerebral pathology, the prognosis is poor (13,19). Seizures beginning before age 1 compared with those beginning between age 1 and 10 years also have a poor prognosis (4). One study (17) deals with late onset epilepsy, but the definition of late onset epilepsy is not well established. Benign epilepsy of childhood usually resolves whether treated or untreated, as does 70% to 80% of absence seizures. Early onset of seizures in infancy suggests that perinatal factors may be causative. In 63% (22 of 35) of children exhibiting serious neurological or psychological deficits, seizures began earlier than age 3 (14). The most significant factors predicting recurrence were symptomatic epilepsy and presence of focal neurological abnormality with or without mental retardation. Focal neurological deficit and mental retardation are two factors that are linked because of their similarity. In general, the patient's age at onset of seizures may be of value in predicting the outcome of drug withdrawal, but is likely to be most important in conjunction with the duration, severity, and frequency of epilepsy before treatment, the EEG findings (spikes, spike-and-wave, sharp waves, paroxysmal slowing), and the time required for seizure control (8).

Duration, Severity, and Frequency of Seizures

Greater relapse rates were found in patients with a history of frequent seizures (8), but there was no relation between the frequency of recurrence and the number of years the patient had been seizure-free on medication (14). When patients were seizure-free more than 5 years, continued sei-

TABLE 2. *Studies on withdrawal of antiepileptic drugs in children and adults*

Study	Study type	Patients No.	age (yr)	Seizure-free with treatment (yr)	Follow-up after withdrawal (yr)	Relapse rate
Children						
Holowach-Thurston (14)	Retrospective	148	x = 13	4.0	5–12	36(24%)
Emerson et al. (8)	Retrospective	68	6–22	4.9	0.5–6	18(26%)
Holowach-Thurston (15)	Long-term follow-up	148	x = 23	4.0	15–23	41(28%)
Foerster and Schmidtberger (10)	Retrospective	114	—	4–5	0.5	31(27%)
Todt (44)	Prospective	433	0.5–15	4.0	5–6	157(35%)
Shinnar et al. (37)	Prospective	88	2–24	2–4	0.5–6	22(25%)
Bouma et al. (4)	Prospective	116	—	2.0	5.0	26(22%)
Arts et al. (3)	Prospective	146	—	2.0	1–10	37(25%)
Adults						
Juul-Jensen (17)	Retrospective	200	—	—	4–5	73(37%)
Juul-Jensen (18)	Long-term follow-up	196	—	—	5–6	79(40%)
Janz et al. (16)	Retrospective	253	2	1–69	2	86(34%)
		253	2	1–69	5	136(54%)
Oller-Daurella et al. (26)	Retrospective	356	5	—	5–27	29 (8%)
Oller-Daurella et al. (24)	Retrospective	522	5	—	10–30	82(34%)
Overweg et al. (29)	Retrospective	134	3	18–50	0.75–1.6	29(22%)
Overweg et al. (28)	Prospective	62	3	18–60	0.5–0.75	41(66%)
Callaghan et al. (5)	Prospective	92	2	x = 24	0.5–5	31(24%)

[a] 22 patients not accounted for.
[b] 218 patients not accounted for.

zure freedom was more favorable in some studies (24,25,46) than in others (16–18,29). The relapse risk decreased after a seizure-free period of at least 3 years before drug withdrawal (43,44). The differences in the findings relate to different remission periods before withdrawal and to the heterogeneity of the patient populations. Patients with a higher frequency of seizures whose need for reduced seizure frequency is recognized earlier than in patients who have long intervals between seizures, need to have longer remission periods before withdrawal (8,28,43). The duration of epilepsy in adults did not differ significantly for relapsed and nonrelapsed groups (16), but in children (8) the likelihood of relapse increased if more than 7 years had passed before seizure control. Todt (43,44) saw a

clear correlation between duration of illness and relapse risk. Of 94 children whose length of time after illness before complete control was longer than 2 years, 51 (54%) had relapses in comparison with 106 (31%) of 339 children with a seizure history of less than 2 years. This relationship was not found in children with absence seizures. Patients with a shorter duration of epilepsy carry a better prognosis, as demonstrated by Holowach-Thurston et al. (15), who found a relapse rate in 36 of 48 (24%) children with epilepsy of less than 6 years duration compared with 112 children whose epilepsy was of longer duration (76%).

There is agreement that the severity of epilepsy is judged by the number and frequency of seizures prior to control and is directly related to the likelihood of relapse

(8,16,17,24). Little information is available about the importance of remission duration and the likelihood of subsequent relapse. Oller-Daurella et al. (24) commented that relapse is more likely in patients who have been seizure-free for many years, but the literature does not support this opinion.

Type of Seizure

Relapse in patients with absence seizures is a relatively rare finding (14,15, 16,23,26,47). However, the combination of absence seizures with other types of primary generalized seizures such as tonic-clonic seizures or myoclonic seizures significantly increases the increase of relapse (16,46). A patient with only primary generalized tonic-clonic seizures has a relatively good prognosis with relapse rates between 8% and 33% (16,24), but the relapse rate for all seizure types in adults is 22% to 54% (4,16,18,26,29). Patients with partial seizures are more likely to relapse and those with a combination of simple partial and complex partial seizures carry a particularly high risk of relapse (15,26). Patients with complex partial seizures that are quickly controlled for 2 years with antiepileptic drugs have a good prognosis for drug withdrawal (37).

Electroencephalogram

The electroencephalogram (EEG) as a prognostic aid for successful drug withdrawal is controversial. Holowach-Thurston et al. (14) reported relapse in 16% of children with normal recordings at the time of withdrawal. The rate of relapse was greater in patients whose prewithdrawal record showed paroxysmal activity. Emerson et al. (8) reported similar findings, in which 12% of patients with a normal EEG immediately before drug withdrawal relapsed, compared with 57% of those who had definitely abnormal EEGs. Juul-Jensen

(17) found that a degree of abnormality in the initial EEG did not correlate well with the prognosis following drug withdrawal. However, relapses were associated with 31% of patients with normal EEGs and 38% of patients with slightly abnormal EEGs obtained immediately before withdrawal. The presence of delta wave foci or bilateral paroxysmal activity was associated with a relapse rate of 100% and 75%, respectively. Strobos (38) demonstrated that bilateral paroxysmal discharges that disappeared with antiepileptic drug therapy were less likely to return when therapy was withdrawn. Janz et al. (16) commented on focal EEG abnormalities as being prognostically poor. Overweg et al. (29) found that the EEG, where normal or abnormal to any degree, was not predictive of outcome. Two studies in children (8,15) found that any number of factors in conjunction with a normal EEG resulted in a good prognosis. The duration of epilepsy appeared to be most important, but a history of focal seizures or combined types of seizures and a neurological deficit had an adverse effect on prognosis (15).

About half of the studies reviewed concluded that an EEG was of little prognostic value whether it was recorded before or during withdrawal. Most authors agreed that the EEG in association with other important factors such as age at seizure onset, severity of seizures, and etiology of epilepsy was prognostic of outcome for withdrawal of drugs. Nine of the studies found a relationship between the EEG and clinical improvement after drug treatment, and patients with primary generalized epilepsy (15,38,39) have a definite positive correlation. The presence of focal epileptiform or background abnormalities on pretreatment EEGs in the patients with newly diagnosed epilepsy were not of prognostic value (7). Rowan et al. (35) reported that paroxysmal discharges and background slowing on initial EEGs of mentally subnormal patients were significant indicators of prognosis and that the degree of brain damage is a major determinant of seizure prognosis, as Rodin had written in 1968 (33). The predictive value of the EEG in various types of seizures prior to termination of medication is apparently determined by the nature and degree of associated brain damage. Perhaps the single consistent correlation between EEG abnormality and seizure frequency occurs in absence seizures (30). It is generally agreed that normalization of the EEG after drug treatment represents a favorable prognosis for withdrawal of antiepileptic drugs.

Etiology of Epilepsy

The causes of epilepsy in infancy, early childhood, later childhood, and adult life are many and diverse, but all of these have one aspect in common: epileptogenicity of brain tissue, or simply stated, the brain's propensity to have seizures. Rodin's (33) approach to the etiology of epilepsy emphasized that additional change must take place beyond and independent of the obvious cause. He defined seizure disposition as the process that periodically changes the substrate of the brain to such extent that an epileptic seizure occurs. The approach seems tenable because a presumed cause (e.g., cerebral injury, brain tumor, vascular disease, or anoxia) or its effects are constantly present, yet patients tend to have seizures at specific intervals. A convulsive threshold may be inherited in patients independently of specific brain tissue substrate and perhaps polygenically. The best evidence of predisposition to seizures is the increased risk of seizures among members of a population with a family history of seizures following additional neurological insult compared with those without such a family history. Nevertheless, the extent of inquiry about family history is rarely adequate to classify the seizure type or elicit the etiology. The importance of etiological factors for successful discontinuation of

antiepileptic drugs is this: if the etiology is unknown, the prognosis tends to be more favorable than if the etiology is known.

PRINCIPLES AND PRACTICAL ASPECTS OF DRUG WITHDRAWAL

With the availability of increasingly sophisticated antiepileptic drugs effective in controlling specific types of seizures, the need for precise diagnosis has become acute. Many clinicians emphasize the importance of monotherapy in prescribing treatment for patients with newly diagnosed epilepsy or for patients whose treatment is being reevaluated. In a multicenter Veterans Administration cooperative study, it was shown that 60% of the patients were adequately managed on the first antiepileptic drug for the first 2 years, and more than half of the 40% that did not respond to the first antiepileptic drug derived benefit from two drugs (22). The goals of epilepsy treatment are to reduce the severity and frequency of seizures and improve the patient's quality of life. These goals are well served by the principle of monotherapy. First, it is easier to monitor plasma concentrations of a single antiepileptic drug in order to assess the therapeutic level or to detect noncompliance, a frequent cause of treatment failure in epilepsy. Second, side effects, especially the more subtle cognitive or behavioral effects, are minimized. Finally, medication toxicity is less likely and the incidence of drug reaction is reduced.

Pharmacokinetics is a quantitative study of the combined processes of drug absorption, distribution, biotransformation, and excretion to produce mathematical models that will predict the concentration of the drug in various parts of the body as a function of dosage, route administration, and time after administration (12). Knowledge of the basic pharmacokinetic principles allows the physician to administer, and later remove, antiepileptic drugs more safely and effectively. Important principles include knowledge of first-order and zero-order enzyme processes, definitions of steady-state levels, therapeutic blood drug levels, dosing intervals, and drug interactions, especially protein binding and displacement reactions.

Two questions are important: who is a candidate and how and when to withdraw the drugs? A patient who has remained seizure-free with treatment for 2 to 5 years may become a candidate for withdrawal or dose reduction. Other candidates are patients who are seizure-free while taking two antiepileptic drugs and are willing to be tapered from one of the drugs.

After a seizure-free period of 2 to 5 years on medication, the incidence of relapse varies from 8% to 60% (34) in adults and 20% to 30% (8,14,15) in children over 2 to 4 years after drug withdrawal. The wide variability in the rate for adults reflects variabilities among studies. Drug withdrawal should be offered to candidates whose prognosis for continued remission is judged to be good based on the factors shown in Table 2, and who have complied with treatment. The decision to withdraw drugs is made between patient and physician, taking into account not only the medical factors, but also social and emotional influences on the patient's life during the projected withdrawal period. Although studies indicate that the EEG and various clinical factors may be of prognostic significance, the probability of successful withdrawal from antiepileptic drugs is about 20% in adults and 75% in children. The reason for the disparity in withdrawal rates between children and adults may well relate to the type of seizures occurring in children compared with adult onset seizures. Adults are prognostically more difficult because etiological factors are accumulated over time.

Withdrawal Duration and Withdrawal Seizures

The duration of antiepileptic drug withdrawal depends on the number of drugs taken and their pharmacokinetic properties. Withdrawal time (weeks or months) does not influence the outcome. One study (41) showed no difference in relapse rates between the short taper group (6 weeks) and the long taper group (9 months). The studies reviewed used various durations for tapering the drugs; there was no consensus of specific timing for decreasing the drugs or decreasing the dosage. However, 93% to 98% of all relapses occurred during the reduction period and within the first year thereafter (15,16,18,43,44). Most studies found that 93% of relapses occurred within 2 years after medication withdrawal. Although it is ill-advised to abruptly terminate drug treatment, this may happen when a patient discontinues his own treatment. Recurrent seizures after withdrawal occurred in direct relationship to a decrease in dosage or within the first 3 months after stopping medication (28).

Although not documented, experience shows that if an antiepileptic drug is maintained at a subtherapeutic level over a period of time in a patient who remains seizure-free, withdrawal of the drug by tapering over a short period of time is indicated.

In epilepsy surgery centers, drugs are often tapered rapidly or terminated abruptly for the purpose of localizing the epileptogenic focus. Rapid antiepileptic drug withdrawal can provoke generalized seizures, particularly in the case of barbiturates and benzodiazepines (4,27). Gradual withdrawal of antiepileptic drugs does not influence the EEG spiking rate and the rate does not change before seizures but increases markedly after them, particularly secondarily generalized seizures (11). The vast majority of the studies reviewed did not mention determination of plasma drug levels during withdrawal and at the time of relapse. Although a more recent report (28) specified drug levels in relation to dose, the older studies often did not mention plasma drug levels before tapering. In general, however, modern drug monitoring concepts were not in use until the mid-1970s.

Drug Withdrawal Protocol

Although no standardized protocol for tapering antiepileptic drugs exists, it is suggested that most drugs can be tapered over 5 to 6 weeks by decreasing the dosage 12% to 20% weekly. Certain practical guidelines can be followed during the transition. First, determine or verify the seizure type and the choice of drug for that type. Perform essential laboratory examinations, including liver function and hematological tests. Frequently, acetazolamide and clorazepate dipotassium can be stopped because they are adjunctive antiepileptic drugs highly implicated in developing tolerance. Assess the length or duration of treatment with long-acting drugs such as barbiturates and primidone. These drugs may cause sedation or side effects and can be withdrawn in outpatients over a prolonged period of time (2–6 months) after removing adjunctive drugs. While gradually tapering the sedative-hypnotic drugs from the regimen, maintain either a preexisting drug or a drug appropriate for the seizure type (phenytoin or carbamazepine for partial seizures; phenytoin or valproate for generalized seizures) at optimal plasma levels for the patient's protection. If it is determined that the patient can be completely tapered off drugs or maintained on a single drug and that drug is already present in the regimen, reduce all others slowly, one at a time, until the goal is reached. A preferred drug for the seizure type may alternatively be added at the transition point where other drugs have been discontinued; the drug of choice then should be raised slowly to an optimal level (level at which the patient has complete benefit of the drug without side effects). Monitoring plasma drug levels plays an important role in the transition of adding or discontinuing drugs. Adjunctive drug levels do not need to be monitored since patients are protected on concomitant primary antiepileptic drugs, but these drugs must be tapered. During drug withdrawal, seizure activity should be recorded on a calendar by date and hour, and precipitants should be noted.

Risk-Benefit Ratio

The patient's consent to withdraw antiepileptic drugs must be in concert with family members and significant others, and the risks and advantages must be weighed carefully. For adults, the risks involve the workplace and driving. Patients who have tremor, blurred vision, or heat intolerance are usually enthusiastic about discontinuing the drugs. Patients may have chronic toxic effects (31,32,36) and late side effects are encountered in offspring of women taking antiepileptic drugs (16,40). In males, antiepileptic drugs may cause infertility (6). Idiosyncratic and dose-related drug effects are less likely to be long-term considerations because both are transient, but an idiosyncratic reaction may be fatal. The central nervous system may be involved in long-term treatment with certain drugs, resulting in neuropathies (phenytoin and carbamazepine), behavioral disorders (phenobarbital), or pseudodementia (phenytoin), even in therapeutic doses.

Removal of sedative-hypnotic drugs in outpatients is not difficult providing the patients are well aware of the side effects of withdrawal and have adequate social support. A major risk in drug withdrawal is status epilepticus, which is more likely to occur when drugs are abruptly terminated, especially the sedative-hypnotic types. Theodore and Porter (42) tapered phenobarbital and benzodiazepines in 78 patients with intractable epilepsy (48 outpatients and 30 inpatients) without a single case of status epilepticus. Nonsedative drugs were continued without change. It appears that risk of status epilepticus as the result of antiepileptic drug withdrawal is significantly less dangerous than previously thought. In children, antiepileptic drug withdrawal appears more prognostically sound and less difficult. Children can be safely withdrawn from antiepileptic drugs after complete seizure freedom for 2 to 5 years if they have none of the risk factors for a poor prognosis after seizure cessation.

Table 3 gives profiles of patients who may benefit from antiepileptic drug withdrawal and predicts a 75% chance of successful withdrawal and continued remission for children (3,4,8,10,14,15,37,43) and a 20% chance for adults (5,16,18,24,28,29).

RESEARCH RECOMMENDATIONS

The literature offers guidelines for determining who may be safely and successfully withdrawn from antiepileptic drugs. However, it is difficult to compare the studies because only some of them (3,4,5,37) surveyed adequate populations of patients with well-documented seizure records and a minimum of 2 years of seizure control, using actuarial methods of analysis and prospective designs. These types of studies represent a more standardized approach to the question of candidacy for drug withdrawal. Future studies should document compliance and identify precipitating factors which have been the most neglected in past studies. Many patients are able to identify factors that they believe precipitate seizures. This is especially true in patients with refractory epilepsy. Difficulty studying precipitants lies in the lack of objective measures of these subjective factors. In Aird's study of 500 patients (1), intense emotional reactions were the common inducing factor reported by patients. This specific precipitant can be resolved by stabilization of the patient's social and emotional environment with facilitation by clinical intervention. Sleep deprivation, alcohol use, and specific drugs lower the seizure threshold. Boredom is often an anecdotal precipitant for seizures.

Techniques of drug withdrawal and the importance of plasma level/dose relationships in patients anticipating withdrawal also have been uniformly neglected. Early relapse has been attributed to a decrease in dose that may have long-term effects on relapse up to a year after total drug reduction. This area of study is best approached through understanding level/dose relationships and fluctuations of these relationships in context with seizure events. Prospective studies of a large number of patients with well-documented seizure histories and evidence of compliance and randomization of patients to study groups are needed to clarify the discrepancy seen in adult relapse rates in the current literature.

TABLE 3. *Profiles of potential candidates for withdrawal of antiepileptic drugs*

Patients	Profile	Success rate[a]
Children (≤15 yr)	Single type of primary generalized seizure, seizure onset after 2 years of age, no neurological abnormalities, normal IQ, seizure-free for 2 to 5 years with antiepileptic drug therapy	75%
Adults (>15 yr)	Single type of primary generalized seizure, seizure onset before 30 years of age, prompt seizure diagnosis and control, normal serial EEGs with treatment, seizure-free for 2 to 5 years with antiepileptic drug therapy	20%

Based on 1,113 children and 1,815 adults reported in the literature.
[a] Successful withdrawal and continued remission of seizures.

SUMMARY

An adult or child who has been seizure-free for 2 to 5 years may become a candidate for drug withdrawal. Discrepancies in relapse rates, especially in adults, can be explained by differences in the populations studied, different definitions of epilepsy, retrospective bias, and interstudy variabilities. Prognosis for successful withdrawal of antiepileptic drugs is similar to the prognosis of epilepsy itself. Numerous factors affect the success of drug cessation, but no one factor is predictive of a good outcome. This statement is supported by prospective and retrospective studies of factors influencing drug withdrawal in children and adults. Basic knowledge of the pharmacodynamics and pharmacokinetics of antiepileptic drugs, especially drug interactions, is necessary for safe and optimal withdrawal of the drugs. The practical aspects of drug withdrawal (e.g., duration of taper, order of drugs tapered) are a matter of personal judgment.

The decision to discontinue medications must be made on a case-by-case basis. Previous studies offer guidelines, but do not answer the questions of who is a candidate for withdrawal and when is the discontinuation process initiated. Nevertheless, the reports are extremely encouraging with respect to the number of patients who have been successfully withdrawn from antiepileptic drugs and remain seizure-free.

REFERENCES

1. Aird, R. B. (1983): The importance of seizure-inducing factors in the control of refractory forms of epilepsy. *Epilepsia*, 24:567–583.
2. Annegers, J. F., Hauser, W. A., and Elveback, L. R. (1979): Remission of seizures and relapse in patients with epilepsy. *Epilepsia*, 20:729–737.
3. Arts, W. F. M., Visser, L. H., Loonen, M. C. B., Tjiam, A. T., Stroink, H., Stuurman, P. M., and Poortvliet, D. C. J. (1988): Follow-up of 146 children with epilepsy after withdrawal of antiepileptic therapy. *Epilepsia*, 29:244–250.
4. Bouma, P. A. D., Peters, A. C. B., Arts, R. J. H. M., Stijnen, T., and Van Rossum, J. (1987): Discontinuation of antiepileptic therapy: A prospective study in children. *J. Neurol. Neurosurg. Psychiatry*, 50:1579–1583.
5. Callaghan, N., Garrett, A., and Goggin, T. (1988): Withdrawal of anticonvulsant drugs in patients free of seizures for two years. *N. Engl. J. Med.*, 318:942–946.
6. Christiansen, P., and Lund, M. (1977): Sexual potency, testicular function and excretion of sexual hormones in male epileptics. In: *Epileptology: Proceedings of the Seventh International Symposium on Epilepsy, Berlin (West)*, edited by D. Janz, pp. 190–191. Thieme, Stuttgart.
7. Elwes, R. D. C., Johnson, A. L., Shorvon, S. D., and Reynolds, E. H. (1984): The prognosis for seizure control in newly diagnosed epilepsy. *N. Engl. J. Med.*, 311:944–947.
8. Emerson, R., D'Souza, B. J., Vining, E. P., Holden, K. R., Mellit, E. D., and Freeman, J. M. (1981): Stopping medication in children with epilepsy. *N. Engl. J. Med.*, 304:1125–1129.
9. Essig, C. F., and Fraser, H. F. (1958): Electroencephalographic changes in man during use and withdrawal of barbiturates in moderate dosage. *Electroencephalogr. Clin. Neurophysiol.*, 10:649–656.
10. Foerster, C., and Schmidtberger, G. (1982): Prognosis in childhood epilepsy after discontinuation of therapy. *Monatschr. Kinderheilk.*, 130:225–228.
11. Gotman, J., and Marciani, M. G. (1985): Electroencephalographic spiking activity, drug levels, and seizure occurrence in epileptic patients. *Ann. Neurol.*, 17:597–603.
12. Greenblatt, D. J., and Koch-Weser, J. (1975): Clinical pharmacokinetics. *N. Engl. J. Med.*, 293:702–964.
13. Hedenstroem, I., and Schorsch, G. (1963): Ueber therapierresistente epileptiker. *Arch. Psychiat. Nervenkr.*, 204:579.
14. Holowach-Thurston, D. L., and O'Leary, J. (1972): Prognosis in childhood epilepsy. *N. Engl. J. Med.*, 286:69–74.
15. Holowach-Thurston, J., Thurston, D. L., Hixon, B. B., and Keller, A. J. (1982): Prognosis in childhood epilepsy. Additional follow-up. *N. Engl. J. Med.*, 306:831–836.
16. Janz, D., and Sommer-Burkhardt, E. M. (1976): Discontinuation of antiepileptic drugs in patients with epilepsy who have been seizure-free for more than two years. In: *Epileptology: Proceedings of the Seventh International Symposium on Epilepsy, Berlin (West)*, edited by D. Janz, pp. 228–234. Thieme, Stuttgart.
17. Juul-Jensen, P. (1964): Frequency of recurrence after discontinuance of anticonvulsant therapy in patients with epileptic seizures. *Epilepsia*, 5:352–363.
18. Juul-Jensen, P. (1968): Frequency of recurrence after discontinuance of anticonvulsant therapy in patients with epileptic seizures. A new follow-up after 5 years. *Epilepsia*, 9:11–16.
19. Kiorboe, E. (1961): The prognosis of epilepsy. *Acta Psychiatr. Scand. Suppl.*, 150:166–178.

20. Lindhout, D., and Meinardi, H. (1984): Gebruik van valproinezuur gedurende de zwangerschap: een indicatie voor prenataal onderzoek op spina bifida. *Ned. Tijdschr. Geneeskd.,* 128:2438–2440.
21. Loiseau, D., Henry, P., and Prissard, A. (1972): Considerations sur l'arret des traitements anti-epileptiques. *Bordeau Med.,* 19:2613–2640.
22. Mattson, R. H., Cramer, J. A., and Collins, J. F. (1985): Comparison of carbamazepine, phenobarbital, phenytoin, and primidone in partial and secondary generalized tonic-clonic seizures. *N. Engl. J. Med.,* 313:145–151.
23. Merritt, H. H. (1958): Medical treatment in epilepsy. *Br. Med. J.,* 1:666–669.
24. Oller-Daurella, L., Oller, F. V. L., and Pamies, R. (1977): Clinical, therapeutic and social status of epileptic patients without seizures for more than five years. In: *Epilepsy. Eighth International Symposium,* edited by J. K. Penry, pp. 69–75. Raven Press, New York.
25. Oller-Daurella, L., Pamies, R., and Oller, F. V. (1975): Reduction or discontinuance of antiepileptic drugs in patients seizure-free for more than 5 years. In: *Epileptology: Proceedings of the Seventh International Symposium on Epilepsy, Berlin (West),* edited by D. Janz, pp. 218–227. Thieme, Stutgart.
26. Oller-Daurella, L., Pamies, R., and Oller, F. V. (1976): Reduction or discontinuance of antiepileptic drugs in patients seizure-free for more than 5 years. In: *Epileptology,* edited by D. Janz, pp. 218–227. Publishing Sciences Group, Littleton, Mass.
27. Overweg, J., and Binnie, C. D. (1983): Benzodiazepines in neurological disorders. In: Costa E. (Ed). *The Benzodiazepines: From Molecular Biology to Clinical Practice,* edited by E. Costa, pp. 339–347. New York, Raven Press.
28. Overweg, J., Binnie, C. D., Oosting, J., and Rowan, A. J. (1987): Clinical and EEG prediction of seizure recurrence following antiepileptic drug withdrawal. *Epilepsy Res.,* 1:272–283.
29. Overweg, J., Rowan, A. J., Binnie, C. D., Oosting, J., and Nagelkerke, N. J. D. (1981): Prediction of seizure recurrence after withdrawal of antiepileptic drugs. In: *Advances in Epileptology: XIIth Epilepsy International Symposium,* edited by M. Dam, L. Gram, and J. K. Penry, pp. 503–508. Raven Press, New York.
30. Penry, J. K., Porter, R. J., and Dreifuss, F. E. (1975): Simultaneous recording of absence seizures with video tape and electroencephalography: A study of 374 seizures in 48 patients. *Brain,* 98:427–440.
31. Reynolds, E. H. (1975): Chronic antiepileptic toxicity: A review. *Epilepsia,* 16:319–352.
32. Reynolds, E. H. (1983): How to avoid chronic toxicity. In: *Chronic Toxicity of Antiepileptic Drugs,* edited by Oxley, J., Janz, D., and Meinardi, H., pp. 300–XXX. Raven Press, New York.

33. Rodin, E. A. (1968): *The Prognosis of Patients with Epilepsy.* Charles C Thomas, Springfield, Illinois.
34. Rodin, E. A., and John, G. (1980): Withdrawal of anticonvulsant medication in successfully treated patients with epilepsy. In: *Advances in Epileptology, Epilepsy International Symposium.* edited by J. A. Wada, and J. K. Penry, pp. 183–186. Raven Press, New York.
35. Rowan, A. J., Overweg, J., Sadikoglu, S., Binnie, C. D., Nagelkerke, N. J. D., and Huenteler, E. (1980): Seizure prognosis in long-stay mentally subnormal epileptic patients: Interrater EEG and clinical studies. *Epilepsia,* 21:219–225.
36. Schmidt, D. (1982): *Adverse Effects of Antiepileptic Drugs.* Raven Press, New York.
37. Shinnar, S., Vining, E. P. G., Mellits, E. D., D'Souza, B. N., Holden, K., Baumgardneu, R. A., and Freeman, J. M. (1985): Discontinuing anti-epileptic medication in children with epilepsy after two years without seizures. *N. Engl. J. Med.,* 313:976–980.
38. Strobos, R. R. J. (1959): Prognosis in convulsive disorders. *Arch. Neurol.,* 1:216–225.
39. Strobos, R. J. (1968): Changes in repeat electroencephalograms in epileptics. *Neurology,* 18:622.
40. Swaab, D. F. (1985): Influence of fetal and neonatal environment on physical, psychological, and intellectual development: Workshop summary. In: *Behavioral Teratology, Proceedings World Congr UNAPEI Prevention of physical and mental congenital defects, part B: Epidemiology, early detection and therapy, and environmental factors,* edited by Marois, M., pp. 463–467. Alan R. Liss, New York.
41. Tennison, M. B., Greenwood, R. S., and Lewis, D. V. (1987): Role of taper for antiepileptic drugs. Abstract. *Epilepsia,* 27:640.
42. Theodore, W. H., and Porter, R. J. (1983): Removal of sedative-hypnotic antiepileptic drugs from the regimens of patients with intractable epilepsy. *Ann. Neurol.,* 13:320–324.
43. Todt, H. (1981): Zur spatprognose kindlicher epilepsien—Ergebnisse einer prospektiven langsschnitt studie. *Dt. Gesundh.-Wesen,* 30, Heft 48:2012–2016.
44. Todt, H. (1984): The late prognosis of epilepsy in childhood: Results of a prospective follow-up study. *Epilepsia,* 25:137–144.
45. Trimble, M. (1979): The effects of anticonvulsant drugs on cognitive abilities. *Pharmacol. and Ther.,* 4:677–685.
46. Van Hey Cop Ten Ham, M. W. (1980): Complete recovery from epilepsy? *Huisants en Wetenshap,* 23:309–311.
47. Yahr, M. D., Sciarra, D., Carter, S., and Merritt, H. H. (1952): Evaluation of standard anticonvulsant therapy in three hundred nineteen patients. *J.A.M.A.,* 150:663–667.

Antiepileptic Drugs, Third Edition, edited by
R. Levy, R. Mattson, B. Meldrum,
J. K. Penry, and F. E. Dreifuss.
Raven Press, Ltd., New York © 1989.

9

Phenytoin

Mechanisms of Action

Robert J. De Lorenzo

Phenytoin (diphenylhydantoin, Dilantin®) was synthesized in 1908 by Biltz (5) and was first introduced for the treatment of epilepsy in 1938 by Merritt and Putnam (58). The success of phenytoin as an anticonvulsant was one of the major pharmacological advances in treating neurological diseases and had a major impact on altering the lives of many epileptics worldwide. Phenytoin is still one of the most widely used anticonvulsants, since it can produce effective anticonvulsant action without significant sedation. Phenytoin is also one of the most effective and widely used compounds for treating generalized tonic-clonic seizures.

Phenytoin was the premier drug demonstrating that an anticonvulsant did not need to be hypnotic (62,63). Thus, phenytoin had a major impact on patient care. Overdoses of phenytoin in man and animals were initially limited to excitatory rather than depressant effects (74). Because of its clinical importance, phenytoin has been extensively evaluated in clinical as well as laboratory investigations. Phenytoin has also been a useful compound for neuroscientists studying basic mechanisms in the pathophysiology of epilepsy. Woodbury and his co-workers (79–85) have contributed extensively to our understanding of some of the effects of phenytoin on nervous tissue and have written several reviews concerning the history, clinical uses, and mechanisms of action of this compound. Many of these and other studies on phenytoin clearly document the historical development of molecular neuropharmacology and neurobiology as it applies to phenytoin's mechanisms of action.

Although a complete review of the mechanisms of action of this widely studied compound goes beyond the scope of a single chapter, the major actions of this drug on neuronal tissue are summarized. Despite the fact that research has focused on understanding the basic mechanisms of phenytoin in producing its anticonvulsant effect, the precise molecular mechanisms by which phenytoin regulates seizure discharge have not been completely elucidated. There is still important research that needs to be done to determine exactly how this useful anticonvulsant regulates cellular function.

MULTIPLE ACTIONS OF PHENYTOIN

Early Phenytoin Research

Early research on phenytoin was directed at characterizing the metabolism, toxic side effects, and clinical efficacy of phenytoin. This research is relevant to the basic mechanism of action of phenytoin since numerous aspects of this drug's effect on the body indicated at an early stage that it probably had multiple sites of action on physiological function.

Following absorption from the gastrointestinal tract or intravenous administration, phenytoin is widely distributed in the body with high plasma protein binding giving maximum plasma solubility at 37 C of approximately 75 ug/ml (44). Phenytoin is not given by intramuscular injection, since it would precipitate at the site of injection and only be absorbed slowly. Phenytoin can only be maintained in aqueous fluids as the sodium salt. If the pH of the carrying vehicle is adjusted significantly below 7.8, phenytoin precipitates out of solution. Thus, the high local concentration of the drug in a neutral pH environment around the injection site causes the drug to precipitate out of solution. For this reason, phenytoin is usually administered orally or intravenously.

For many years it was felt that adequate phenytoin levels could only be obtained after several days of phenytoin loading to saturate all the fat and other body stores for phenytoin. Intravenous loading with appropriate doses of phenytoin can produce adequate serum concentrations within 10 to 20 min. This allows phenytoin to be administered acutely for the treatment of status epilepticus and other acute seizure problems. It also provides the laboratory investigator with the ability to administer this drug quickly in high concentrations to various animal models. The wide distribution of phenytoin in the brain and other body tissues has been studied extensively (60,85). Phenytoin clearly has dramatic effects on the skin, gastrointestinal system, and other major organ systems. The classic phenytoin facies has been well documented and demonstrates that the drug is affecting other organ systems besides the central nervous system.

The toxic side effects of phenytoin are numerous and have been extensively characterized. Fortunately, phenytoin has a very high therapeutic index and patients can be maintained on therapeutic levels without significant side effects. As a result, clinical overdoses of phenytoin are usually not severe and are easily recognized. Phenytoin can produce nystagmus, ataxia, and gait instability at lower levels of toxicity. At higher levels, dysarthria, incoordination, and significant unsteadiness are often seen. At very toxic levels exceeding 30 ug/ml, phenytoin can produce drowsiness, lethargy, and coma. Phenytoin in high toxic levels can also produce diplopia, hypotension, cardiac suppression, and even death. An important early finding of the toxic effects of phenytoin on the nervous system indicated that phenytoin can also produce hyperexcitability. Phenytoin can produce irritability, hallucinations, and even psychotic reactions. These early clinical observations contributed significantly to our understanding of the basic actions of this drug by indicating that it must be working on multiple regulatory systems in the nervous system. Under certain conditions, phenytoin can clearly act as an anticonvulsant and neuronal stabilizing compound. However, in other circumstances, this compound can be excitable and even cause psychotic phenomena.

Another hallmark of the multiple effects of phenytoin on the body are clearly seen in the use of this compound in children. Gingival hypertrophy is a major side effect of phenytoin in persons younger than 21 years of age. This effect has significantly limited the use of phenytoin in the pediatric population. In adults, however, phenytoin does not produce significant gingival hypertrophy. The developmental relationship of this side effect to the action of phenytoin and the specific cellular mechanisms by which this drug produces this effect has not been clearly understood and could have important ramifications for developmental neurobiology. Phenytoin also causes hirsutism to a mild degree in 75% of the patients taking phenytoin. Phenytoin also has a significant effect on the hematopoietic system and can produce, under more rare situations, megaloblastic anemia. Phenytoin also has been shown to produce lupus erythematosus as a rare complication and is well known to exacerbate this condition.

These early clinical investigations documented the fact that phenytoin affected many organ systems and clearly suggested that it affected many physiological and biochemical processes in the body. Much of the research directed at understanding the mechanisms of action of phenytoin was initiated to explain the many effects of this compound in clinical and laboratory settings.

Major Sites of Action

Phenytoin is probably the most studied anticonvulsant. The numerous effects of phenytoin on electrophysiological and biochemical systems in brain and other tissues have been extensively reviewed by Woodbury and others (79–85). Phenytoin has been demonstrated to regulate numerous parameters of nerve function, including effects on ion conductances, sodium-potassium adenosine triphosphate (ATP)ase activity, various enzyme systems, synaptic transmission, posttetanic potentiation, neurotransmitter release, cyclic nucleotide metabolism, and numerous other events. This extensive research has lead many investigators to suggest that this drug has many sites of action in the central nervous system. Thus, phenytoin most likely interacts with numerous biochemical processes that regulate neuronal function.

A point of view different from this original theory is that phenytoin may interact with a few important major regulatory systems in the nervous system that could then regulate numerous other cellular processes controlled by these regulators (19–24). Phenytoin has been shown to regulate Na^--K^+-ATPase, and sodium ion channels. This could have widespread regulatory effects on numerous excitatory and inhibitory systems. Phenytoin has also been shown to regulate calcium-calmodulin-dependent enzyme systems, which may also provide insight into the multiple effects of phenytoin by regulating calcium systems. The effects of phenytoin on cyclic nucleotide metabolism levels could also provide a focal point for multiple effects on cell function. Thus, the effects of phenytoin on several second messenger systems such as the cyclic nucleotides and calcium systems could possibly explain the widespread action of this compound on numerous cells and physiological functions. However, it is still clear that no single action of phenytoin is likely to explain all of its diverse effects on the nervous system.

Whether phenytoin has few or numerous sites of action is still clearly a matter of debate. Furthermore, the precise anticonvulsant effect or effects of this compound on neuronal tissue still need to be elucidated. The following sections summarize the major studies exploring the mechanisms of action of phenytoin. The topics selected for review represent those areas of research that scientists generally agree have some importance in the action of phenytoin.

EFFECTS OF PHENYTOIN ON NEURONAL EXCITABILITY

The hallmark of phenytoin is that it can limit the development of maximal seizure activity and is effective in reducing the spread of seizure discharge from a seizure focus. Both of these experimental observations are pertinent to the clinical effects of phenytoin in treating generalized tonic-clonic seizures and focal epilepsy in man. A major anticonvulsant effect of phenytoin is believed to be its ability to block the epileptic focus from recruiting surrounding neurons, which results in the spread of seizure discharge.

In contrast to phenobarbital, phenytoin does not significantly elevate the threshold for seizures that are induced by electrical stimulation with 60-Hz alternating current or by pentylenetetrazol, strychnine, or picrotoxin. Furthermore, phenytoin can actually potentiate the convulsant effect of pentylenetetrazol and picrotoxin. Thus, studies currently indicate that, although there are some similarities between anticonvulsant drugs, there are important differences in their mechanisms of action and the ways they control seizure activity.

Despite its inability to elevate the seizure threshold for electrical stimulation of the brain with 60-Hz alternating current, phenytoin does have a slight effect on elevating the seizure threshold against seizures induced by 6/sec stimulation of the brain. This effect on low-frequency-induced seizures by electrical stimulation is not as dramatic as the effect of phenobarbital in this system, but is clearly distinct from the effects of phenytoin on high-frequency stimulation. Recent studies on the effects of phenytoin on use-dependent inhibition of sodium channel function (see below) might be related to this interesting physiological effect.

A distinguishing characteristic of the effect of phenytoin on seizures is its ability to modify the pattern of maximal tonic-clonic electroshock seizures induced in animals by supramaximal current. Phenytoin characteristically blocks the tonic phase of tonic-clonic seizures. Thus, the animal treated with phenytoin will have a purely clonic seizure following electric convulsive treatment (4,37,77). This effect of phenytoin in animals has also been documented in humans undergoing electroconvulsive therapy (76). Phenytoin has also been observed to block the tonic phase of seizures induced by picrotoxin, pentylenetetrazol, and fluorothyl. Esplin (36,37) has also observed the effects of phenytoin on the tonic phase of maximal seizures in the spinal cord preparation. Massive stimulation of the spinal cord produces motor events in animals similar to those observed in maximal electric shock tonic-clonic seizures. Phenytoin abolishes the tonic aspect of these seizures in the spinal preparation. However, this effect of phenytoin requires higher doses than those able to block the tonic phase of seizures in the cerebral cortex.

Phenytoin has also been observed to affect peripheral excitability in the nervous system. Phenytoin reduces the prolonged increase in excitability and independent repetitive firing that occurs in the peripheral nerve following supramaximal rapid stimulation (74). The hyperexcitability of peripheral nerve that is induced by low calcium or a combination of low calcium and magnesium in the bathing media is also reduced by phenytoin (49,66). These effects in the peripheral nerve suggest that phenytoin has an overall stabilizing effect on the neuronal membrane that may in some way be related to the effects of calcium or sodium on neuronal excitability.

An intriguing observation is that phenytoin has different levels of effects at different anatomic sites in the central nervous system. Phenytoin has been shown to be effective in preventing the spread of seizure activity in most areas of the central nervous system. However, the effects of phenytoin on seizure threshold are somewhat more directed toward the cerebral cortex. In several species, phenytoin has been shown to elevate the seizure threshold of the cortex, including the threshold of the hippocampus, the amygdala, and the anterior dorsal nucleus of the thalamus (3,14). However, phenytoin does not significantly affect the threshold in the reticular activating system and does not influence the sensory relay path to the pyramidal tract (6). Some of these results indicate that phenytoin is most effective in reducing seizure threshold in anatomic regions that contain numerous synaptic connections.

Gangloff and Monnier (42) have shown that phenytoin is able to elevate the seizure threshold of the diencephalon. However,

Morrell et al. (59) did not find an effect of phenytoin on the diencephalon. This effect was in contradiction to the effects of phenobarbital and trimethadione on this region of the nervous system. Morrell et al. (59) felt that the inability of phenytoin to affect the diencephalon is consistent with some of the clinical observations of this anticonvulsant. Phenytoin can block generalized tonic-clonic seizures but may not block tonic-clonic seizures of cortical origin. Phenytoin does not completely block the sensory or other prodromal signs associated with some partial complex seizures. These authors argue that some of these other effects may result from the fact that phenytoin does not alter the seizure threshold in the diencephalon. However, it is possible that at high concentrations it may have significant effects on this structure and that the reported discrepancies may relate to the concentrations of the drug used in each experimental system.

The studies described above pioneered initial research efforts into the mechanisms of phenytoin action on the central nervous system. Phenytoin clearly produced dramatic and clinically useful suppression of the spread of seizure activity in the cortex and other regions of the brain. This effect was not universal and was somewhat selective for specific types of seizures initiated by maximal electric shock but not by several chemical convulsants. In addition, phenytoin is much more potent in inhibiting the tonic phase of tonic-clonic generalized seizures than the clonic phase.

PHYSIOLOGICAL EFFECTS OF PHENYTOIN

The well-documented effects of phenytoin on seizure discharge and the spread of neuronal excitability set the stage to study the physiological mechanisms underlying the effects of phenytoin on neuronal excitability. The rapid advance of molecular neurobiology with sophisticated intra- and extracellular recording techniques over the last two decades has greatly facilitated this research. Phenytoin has been shown to affect several important physiological processes, including posttetanic potentiation and sustained repetitive firing.

Effects on Posttetanic Potentiation

Posttetanic potentiation (PTP) is a physiological phenomenon that has been implicated in the development of hyperexcitable areas in the brain as a result of recurrent feedback circuits during seizure activity (75). Posttetanic potentiation is also felt to be an important mechanism leading to high-frequency trains of impulses in excitatory brain circuits and to the spread of this activity to adjoining neurons as well as to their propagation to distant neuronal aggregates, resulting in uncontrolled spread of excitation to the whole brain in the maximal tonic seizure discharge (68). Thus, PTP was felt to be an important physiological process that was inherent in normal neuronal circuitry that could be regulating the spread of neuronal excitability. This was thought to account in part for the fact that stimulation of normal brain tissue by focal application of convulsive substances or electrical stimulation can lead to a full-blown tonic-clonic seizure through the spread of this focal excitability throughout the central nervous system.

Posttetanic potentiation specifically refers to the augmentation of the postsynaptic compound action potential elicited by presynaptic stimulation following a repetitive stimulus (tetanus) (64,65,75). Thus, repetitively stimulating a neuronal circuit, stopping the stimulus, and then firing that circuit again produces a more dramatic response from that same circuit. The tetanus or intense stimulation somehow alters the normal resting levels of excitability of the system and produces a hyperexcitable state.

This phenomenon suggests that repetitive use of a neuronal pathway sensitizes that pathway for a given time to further discharge. Thus, the more a pathway is fired, the more likely it is to fire on subsequent stimulation. This type of phenomena could develop a reverberating or building hyperexcitability in the neuronal circuitry and is an attractive model, implicating normal neuronal mechanisms in the development of the spread of the epileptic focus. Although such a model is very appealing, it still remains undocumented whether this is a major mechanism involved in the production of the spread of the seizure focus in man.

Phenytoin is one of the most effective compounds in blocking PTP (64,65). It was thought that the effect of phenytoin on PTP may represent one of its major sites of action in preventing the spread of seizures. Phenytoin has been shown to inhibit PTP in spinal cord preparations as well as in preparations of stellate ganglion in the cat (35,65). In addition, phenytoin has been shown to block PTP at intramedullary terminals and the neuromuscular junction (64). The effect of phenytoin on PTP is also of considerable interest in that not all anticonvulsants are effective in blocking PTP. Phenobarbital has no direct effect on PTP. In addition, trimethadione and valproic acid also have no significant effect on PTP. However, carbamazepine and the anticonvulsant benzodiazepines are effective in blocking PTP.

The mechanism by which phenytoin regulates PTP has not been clearly established. However, it is apparent that both the accumulation of calcium within the nerve terminal during the tetanus and the ability of phenytoin to block sodium channels in a use-dependent fashion may be contributing mechanisms of action for phenytoin in blocking PTP (23,24,67).

Effects on Sustained Repetitive Firing

A growing body of evidence (52–57) is accumulating which indicates that sustained high-frequency repetitive firing (SRF) is an important property of vertebrate and invertebrate neurons and plays a role in regulating the excitability state of the cell. SRF is manifested in several types of central nervous system neurons and may be involved in anticonvulsant drug action and epileptogenesis. Although no direct evidence has demonstrated the link between SRF and epilepsy, information obtained from *in vitro* studies on isolated neurons concerning SRF may have some bearing on altered neuronal excitability and anticonvulsant drug action.

Phenytoin is effective in regulating SRF (53). The correlation of specific anticonvulsant drug activity with actions on SRF has indicated that SRF is a good model for studying drug effects on generalized tonic-clonic and maximal electric shock-induced seizures (52–57). Anticonvulsants effective against generalized absence seizures, such as ethosuximide and trimethadione, are not effective against SRF. Thus, different mechanisms of action are implicated by the effects of drugs on this physiological phenomenon.

The potent effect of phenytoin on SRF is consistent with its clinical action as an effective anticonvulsant against generalized tonic-clonic seizures in man and maximal electric shock seizures induced in animals. The therapeutic efficacy of phenytoin in controlling seizures in animals and humans is similar to its therapeutic efficacy in limiting SRF in isolated cultured neurons. These results indicate that therapeutic cerebrospinal fluid (CSF) levels of phenytoin in man are in a concentration range that could inhibit SRF.

The ability of phenytoin to limit SRF has been shown in a wide variety of neurons maintained in culture and several invertebrate preparations. Although it has not been clearly demonstrated that the effect of phenytoin in limiting SRF mediates its anticonvulsant drug action, this is an attractive hypothesis for some of the neuronal stabilizing effects of this drug. Evidence is now accumulating that some of the effects of phenytoin on SRF may be mediated by the use-dependent blockage of sodium channels produced by phenytoin.

EFFECTS OF PHENYTOIN ON ACTIVE SODIUM-POTASSIUM TRANSPORT

In 1955, Woodbury (79) provided evidence that phenytoin played a major role in altering sodium ion movements across nerve cell membranes. This initial work by Woodbury set the stage for much of the following research over the next 30 years in relation to the effects of phenytoin on ion conductances in neuronal membranes. On the basis of calculated intracellular sodium concentrations, Woodbury (15) suggested that phenytoin might regulate the sodium transport in the brain. It was proposed that one mechanism by which this anticonvulsant could increase active sodium transport was by an effect on the sodium-potassium ATPase.

Sodium-Potassium ATPase

Sodium-potassium ATPase and its regulation by phenytoin have been extensively studied and reviewed (15). Phenytoin has been shown to regulate this enzyme under some conditions but not under others. Phenytoin increases the activity of sodium-potassium ATPase both *in vivo* and *in vitro*. In brain synaptosomes, phenytoin increased sodium-potassium ATPase activity after systemic administration to animals (43,50) and after administration *in vitro* (41,78). Phenytoin also increased the activity of sodium-potassium ATPase in the adrenal medulla (45). Some conflict developed in this field when it was found that under some experimental conditions phenytoin did not affect sodium-potassium ATPase in *in vitro* brain synaptosome experiments. These results have been carefully examined by numerous investigators (15) and it now

appears that the difference in experimental results relates to the ratio of sodium to potassium in the experimental systems.

Deupree (32,33) concluded that under certain conditions, phenytoin does not affect sodium-potassium ATPase and that earlier studies may be explained by the contamination of phenytoin with potassium, which would increase the potassium ratio. However, Delgado-Escueta and Horan (15) reviewed these data and found that the effects of phenytoin on active transport of potassium in synaptosomes occur under conditions in which the potassium content of the cell is lowered and the sodium concentration is increased. This latter condition is felt to be more closely analogous to the environment of the epileptogenic focus.

These initially contradictory results might have important ramifications in explaining why phenytoin might not have significant toxic effects on normal neuronal function, but can have a significant neuronal stabilizing effect during an excitable discharge. It is postulated that under normal conditions phenytoin may not play a role in regulating sodium-potassium ATPase activity. However, in an epileptogenic focus where the ratio of sodium to potassium across the membrane may be altered, phenytoin may then be able to regulate the activity of this important membrane enzyme system. These studies on sodium and the sodium-potassium ATPase initiated by Woodbury represented a major advance in understanding the mechanism of action of anticonvulsant drugs. This research represents one of the first neurochemical insights into the mechanism of action of phenytoin and serves as a model by which this drug has been tested in numerous other biochemical systems.

Effects on Sodium Conductances

Following the initial observations by Woodbury that phenytoin may be regulating neuronal excitability by affecting sodium permeability across the membrane, several relevant investigations developed over the next 30 years as new techniques advanced to the point where they could be applied to the study of the action of phenytoin on neuronal tissue. The membrane "stabilizer" effect of phenytoin and its ability to prevent repetitive electrical activity (10,40,47,49) indicate that phenytoin's action on the sodium conductance might be an important area of further research. Lipicky et al. (51) observed that phenytoin decreased the early sodium current in the voltage clamp squid axon. These studies suggested that phenytoin decreased the number of open channels in the early phase of the action potential. Johnson and Ayala (46) also observed in *Aplysia* that phenytoin decreased sodium influx. Further evidence for an effect of phenytoin on sodium influx was provided by Swanson and Crane (72), who utilized guinea pig cerebral cortex slices, and by Schwartz and Vogel (69) in voltage-clamp experiments on single myelinated neurofibers. These studies also suggested that phenytoin decreased the action potential amplitude and increased the threshold. These results were utilized to hypothesize that phenytoin might reduce the conduction velocity by affecting sodium currents.

More recent observations by DeWeer (34) and Perry et al. (61) on the isolated squid axon provide additional evidence that phenytoin affects sodium influx. These investigators postulated that phenytoin behaved like tetrodotoxin in blocking sodium channels. Their studies also confirmed the observations of Schwartz and Vogel (69) that indicated that phenytoin induced membrane hyperpolarization. Thus, numerous studies have demonstrated that phenytoin has a significant effect on sodium influx in neuronal membrane. It appears that phenytoin blocks sodium channels in a manner similar to that of tetrodotoxin or local anesthetics by blocking the actual channel. These results are consistent with Wood-

bury's original observations and may explain some of the neuronal stabilizing effects of this anticonvulsant.

Use-Dependent Inhibition of Sodium Channels

The ability of phenytoin to inhibit sodium channels is use-dependent. This provides an exciting insight into the ability of this anticonvulsant to regulate some physiological processes under abnormal excitable conditions but not have effects at resting or normal neuronal levels of activity. As a nerve cell is fired, sodium enters the cell. Phenytoin is then able to insert in the membrane in a way to block or inhibit further sodium entry. The initial impulse and resultant entry of sodium is not affected by phenytoin. It is only after this initial impulse that phenytoin has the ability to interact with the membrane following depolarization and block subsequent sodium entry. Thus, there is a use-dependent facilitation of the effect of phenytoin on the ability of this drug to inhibit the sodium channel.

These studies have provided an important molecular neurobiological insight into an important regulatory action of phenytoin that may underlie some of its ability to stabilize neuronal membranes and prevent the spread of seizure discharge by dampening sodium entry that would occur in reverberating hyperexcitable circuits. Although this basic mechanism has not been totally proved to mediate the anticonvulsant effects of phenytoin, it is currently a very attractive model of how phenytoin can regulate abnormal neuronal excitability without significantly affecting normal neuronal activity.

EFFECTS OF PHENYTOIN ON CALCIUM CHANNELS AND CALCIUM SYSTEMS

Phenytoin has been able to inhibit calcium influx in numerous preparations. The mechanism by which phenytoin inhibits calcium influx is not completely understood. However, several studies have provided convincing evidence that this drug regulates the calcium conductances in nerve preparations as well as in other tissues.

Effects on Calcium Channels

Studies by Ferrendelli and co-workers (39,70,71) elegantly demonstrated that phenytoin inhibited depolarization-dependent calcium uptake in a preparation of presynaptic nerve terminals *in vitro*. This work provided the initial evidence that phenytoin inhibits both sodium and calcium influx during depolarization and suggests that these conductances are affected independently of each other. Phenytoin has been shown to block calcium uptake in intact neuromuscular junction preparations and the calcium sequestration by motocondria and presynaptic organelles in this synaptosome preparation (86). Several other studies in relation to the effects of phenytoin on calcium uptake and metabolism have been extensively reviewed (73,81).

Thus, an overwhelming body of evidence further suggests that phenytoin can inhibit calcium influx during depolarization and also the uptake and sequestration of calcium in the nerve terminal following its entry. Consequently, phenytoin has both a depressive effect by blocking calcium uptake and a potentially excitatory effect by blocking the uptake and sequestration of calcium in the nerve terminal. The latter effect could result in prolonged elevated calcium concentrations in the nerve terminal following tetanic stimulation or the spread of repetitive firing. This molecular insight might have some bearing on the clinical observations that phenytoin can be both neuronal stabilizing and anticonvulsive, as well as cause hyperexcitability in the nervous system. Depending on the balance in the system and which effect is more pro-nounced, phenytoin can either suppress neuronal activity by decreasing calcium entry or cause hyperexcitability of the nervous system by elevating the resting intracellular level of calcium in the nerve terminal following repetitive discharge. These results have led several investigators (23,24) to suggest that the effect of phenytoin on calcium metabolism may explain some of its effects on both anticonvulsant activity and hyperexcitability of nervous tissue.

Effects on Calmodulin Target Enzymes

Calmodulin is a major calcium-binding protein that has been implicated in mediating some of the second messenger effects of calcium on cell function (11,48). Calmodulin binds calcium and then this calcium-calmodulin complex can regulate several enzyme systems in the cell. The major enzyme regulated by calcium and calmodulin is specific calcium- and calmodulin-dependent protein kinases. Calmodulin kinase II is a major calcium-dependent protein kinase that has been shown to be regulated by calcium and calmodulin. Phenytoin has been shown to inhibit calcium-calmodulin-regulated protein phosphorylation in neuronal preparations and in preparations of presynaptic nerve terminals (17–31). The ability of phenytoin to regulate this major calcium-dependent enzyme system suggests that phenytoin may modulate many of the second messenger effects of calcium in the nervous system.

This action of phenytoin on the second messenger effects of calcium in the nervous system may provide a major pathway by which phenytoin can regulate many cellular processes. This might explain why phenytoin can influence many neuronal and nonneuronal biochemical processes. Calcium has been implicated in regulating many physiological processes in the brain. If phenytoin can influence some of these processes by blocking calcium entry, by regulating intracellular calcium levels, or by affecting a major calcium-calmodulin-regulated enzyme system, this could account for some of the broad anticonvulsant and toxic effects of phenytoin on the central nervous system. The possible effects of phenytoin on other calmodulin enzyme systems require further investigation. It is also possible that the effect of phenytoin on calmodulin-regulated systems may occur at higher than physiological concentrations and thus may account for some of the toxic effects of phenytoin on neuronal tissue. The precise role of phenytoin inhibition of calcium-calmodulin-regulated enzyme systems is an important area for further investigation.

EFFECTS OF PHENYTOIN ON CHLORIDE PERMEABILITY

Phenytoin has been shown to increase chloride conductants in mammalian cortical neurons as well as in crayfish stretch receptor neurons (2). This chloride conductance is regulated by the inhibitory amino acid, gamma aminobutyric acid (GABA). Evidence suggests that phenytoin manifests this effect in a postsynaptic fashion. This action occurs at nanomolar concentrations of phenytoin. It appears from these results that nanomolar concentrations of phenytoin may modify the gating mechanisms of the chloride channel underlying the inhibitory postsynaptic potential (IPSP), thereby decreasing the rate of closing of the chloride channel. Thus, evidence has been developed that phenytoin can regulate the chloride channel leading to the hyperpolarization of neurons. This effect of phenytoin would be similar to that of the benzodiazepines.

Although this is an attractive model, phenytoin is not effective in inhibiting pentylenetetrazol-induced seizures in animals. These seizures are very sensitive to ben-zodiazepines, which work through the benzodiazepine receptor mechanism and modulation of the chloride channel. Thus, if the benzodiazepine receptor GABA complex and its regulation of the chloride channel is involved with pentylenetetrazol-induced seizures, it is somewhat unlikely that phenytoin has a major anticonvulsant role in this system, since it does not affect pentylenetetrazol-induced seizures in the same way as the benzodiazepines. The effect of phenytoin on chloride channels needs further investigation. Its role in the anticonvulsant action of this compound is still unclear.

EFFECTS OF PHENYTOIN ON BIOCHEMICAL SYSTEMS

Phenytoin has been shown to affect numerous biochemical systems, as excellently reviewed by Woodbury (81–83). In toxic concentrations, phenytoin acts on numerous biochemical processes. A complete discussion of all of these effects goes beyond the scope of this chapter. However, several effects of phenytoin on major second messenger or biochemical systems are worth discussing in some detail, since they may have an important contribution to some of the anticonvulsant or toxic effects of this drug.

Effects on Cyclic Nucleotide Metabolism

Phenytoin has been shown to regulate the metabolism of adenosine $3'5'$-monophosphate (cyclic AMP) and guanosine $3'5'$-monophosphate (cyclic GMP). Both of these cyclic nucleotides have been implicated as major second messengers in cell function. The effects of phenytoin on cyclic nucleotide metabolism have been studied and reviewed by Ferrendelli (38,39). Phenytoin depresses the basal levels of cyclic GMP in the cerebellum *in vivo*. Phenytoin also prevents the elevations of brain cyclic AMP and cyclic GMP levels that result from electric shock convulsions of cerebral cortex. *In vitro* studies indicate that phenytoin inhibits the elevation of brain cyclic nucleotides caused by depolarizing agents that increase sodium influx in synaptosome fractions.

These studies suggest that phenytoin may act directly on nucleotide metabolism or that the action may be secondary to some neuronal stabilizing effects of phenytoin that result in alterations of cyclic nucleotide production or metabolism during neuronal depolarization. The effects of phenytoin on cyclic nucleotide metabolism need further investigation. The possible relationship between these effects and the drug's anticonvulsant action or toxicity remains an important area for further research.

Effects on Neurotransmitter Systems

Phenytoin has been shown to influence neurotransmitter release in metabolism in numerous preparations. This literature has recently been reviewed by Woodbury (81). Phenytoin inhibits the release of norepinephrine and other neurotransmitters from intact nerve terminal preparations *in vitro* and *in vivo*. Phenytoin also inhibits neurotransmitter reuptake. These effects are regulated by the dose of phenytoin, since different effects are attained at different concentrations of the drug. These results suggest that phenytoin may be acting at different sites in regulating transmitter release and transmitter uptake.

It has also been observed that phenytoin decreases the concentration of glutamic acid in the brain and increases the concentration of glutamine and GABA. The effect of phenytoin on GABA systems has been observed in different preparations and in different species. It appears that this anticonvulsant may play a role in regulating the level and metabolism of this major inhibitory neurotransmitter. Phenytoin has also been shown to affect the metabolism and

activity of acetylcholine. These examples indicate that phenytoin may play an important role in regulating numerous neurotransmitter systems in brain by influencing the metabolism, storage, release, or uptake of these compounds. These numerous effects may be regulated by the effects of phenytoin on calcium and cyclic nucleotides second messenger systems.

Effects on Calmodulin Systems

Phenytoin has been shown to inhibit calcium-calmodulin-dependent protein kinase in neuronal preparations (17,24,29). Phenytoin's ability to regulate protein phosphorylation may play an important role in regulating some of the anticonvulsant or side effects of this compound on neuronal and nonneuronal tissue. Since calcium-dependent protein phosphorylation may play a major role in regulating numerous cellular processes, the ability of phenytoin to inhibit this system could account for many of its effects on cell metabolism and, ultimately, on numerous cells in the body. The role of phenytoin in regulating other calmodulin-controlled enzyme systems needs further investigation.

EFFECTS OF PHENYTOIN ON NEUROTRANSMISSION

Phenytoin has long been known to effect synaptic activity. Early studies by Woodbury (79,85) and others have indicated that synaptic transmission is depressed by phenytoin. Over the last 10 years, studies employing new techniques in electrophysiology have allowed these effects of phenytoin to be studied in more detail. It appears that phenytoin can inhibit the depolarization-dependent synaptic transmission but can facilitate many endplate potentials at rest in the synapse. These mechanisms provide an insight into the ability of phenytoin to be both excitatory and inhibitory in the nervous system.

It has been shown that in *in vitro* synaptosome preparations, phenytoin inhibits norepinephrine and acetylcholine release (20–22). Phenytoin has been shown in several intact experiments monitored by electrophysiological studies to inhibit synaptic transmission. Studies of the frog neuromuscular synapse have shown that phenytoin has two major effects: (a) phenytoin reduces the quinal content or the number of packets of transmitter released by a nerve impulse, and (b) phenytoin increases the frequency of motor endplate potentials (MEPP), which represent individual packets of transmitter that are released spontaneously while the nerve is at rest. Both of these effects clearly document that phenytoin can have both excitatory and inhibitory effects at the synapse, as it has on other electrophysiological activities.

Studies (20–24) have shown that phenytoin can inhibit neurotransmitter release from synaptasomes both by blocking calcium entry during depolarization and by directly inhibiting intracellular synaptosomal biochemical processes such as protein phosphorylation and other calmodulin regulated events. Under conditions where calcium enters the synaptosomes through an iontophore, phenytoin could still inhibit neurotransmitter release. These studies provide the first evidence that at least two mechanisms exist for explaining the effects of phenytoin on synaptic transmitter release. Phenytoin most likely blocks transmitter release during an action potential by minimizing or limiting calcium entry and by having a specific effect on other molecular processes within the nerve terminal that modulate transmitter release. The effect of phenytoin on many MEEPs have been postulated to be the result of increased intracellular calcium concentrations induced by phenytoin. Phenytoin not only inhibits calcium uptake into synaptosomes but also can block calcium uptake into mitochondria.

The mitochondria serve as an important intracellular calcium buffering system to keep the calcium concentration in the nerve terminal at a low level. By inhibiting this process, phenytoin can effectively slightly increase intrasynaptosomal calcium, causing a slight hyperexcitability with a significant increase in many endplate potentials.

Phenytoin clearly has direct effects on synaptic transmission. However, these effects would occur both during a seizure and during the interictal phase. Thus, the specific effect of phenytoin on reducing seizures but not having a significant effect on mental processing is not easily explained by this mechanism. Perhaps some of the behavioral effects seen by phenytoin on normal functioning may be related to its effect on dampening synaptic transmission.

PHENYTOIN RECEPTOR MOLECULES

Receptor neuropharmacology has played a major role in the development of many drugs over the last 20 years. Specific receptors for the benzodiazepines, steroids, catecholamines, and other neuroleptic compounds have provided important mechanisms of action for several of these neuropharmacological agents. Currently, however, except for the nanomolar benzodiazepine receptor (9), there is no evidence for a specific anticonvulsant binding site. Recent evidence (7,8) has identified a novel class of benzodiazepine-binding proteins that bind benzodiazepines with a potency series and a therapeutic concentration range that are consistent with the effects of the benzodiazepines on SRF and on maximal electric shock-induced seizures in animals. Recent studies have indicated that phenytoin effectively displaces in therapeutic concentrations the benzodiazepines from this receptor. These results suggest that this novel benzodiazepine receptor also binds phenytoin in therapeutic concentrations and provide evidence of a specific phenytoin-binding protein in the central nervous system. Further investigations must be conducted to determine the significance and relevance of this protein to the action of phenytoin in stabilizing neuronal membranes. It is clear that research directed at identifying anticonvulsant receptors would have important implications in developing new therapeutic agents to regulate seizures and in understanding mechanisms of action of anticonvulsant drugs. This is an area that needs significant future research.

UNIFYING MECHANISMS OF ACTION: SUMMARY

This chapter highlights some of the important advances in our understanding of phenytoin's basic mechanisms of action in regulating neuronal excitability. It is clear that there is no single action of phenytoin that can account for its numerous effects on neuronal and nonneuronal tissue. Although each of the numerous effects of phenytoin could account for different mechanisms of action, the preponderance of evidence suggests that this important clinical compound may produce its numerous effects by regulating several important aspects of cellular function. Phenytoin's ability to regulate sodium transport across neuronal membranes is a major mechanism of action that almost certainly underlies some of the drug's clinical effects on neuronal tissue. The use-dependent inhibition of sodium channels characteristic of phenytoin provides an important potential mechanism allowing phenytoin to regulate excitability under abnormal circumstances during seizure discharge while not significantly affecting normal neuronal activity in the interictal period. Further research on the effect of phenytoin on sodium channels will potentially elucidate how this molecular effect of phenytoin might underlie specific clinical effects. The ability of phenytoin to modu-

late sustained repetitive firing may underlie the ability of this compound to inhibit the tonic phase of generalized tonic-clonic seizures. There is growing evidence that phenytoin may regulate sustained repetitive firing by the use-dependent inhibition of sodium channels.

The ability of phenytoin to regulate calmodulin and cyclic nucleotide second messenger systems could account for some of the widespread effects of phenytoin on numerous cellular processes. It is difficult to find a biochemical or physiological process that is not in some way regulated by cyclic nucleotides or calcium. Thus, effects of phenytoin on these second messenger systems would be dramatically amplified in terms of the diverse clinical and toxic side effects that might result from this compound. These effects may account for the wide diversity of phenytoin's actions. The ability of phenytoin to regulate and inhibit the voltage-dependent neurotransmitter release at the synapse may also play an important role in the anticonvulsant action of this compound. Although the precise mechanisms of this effect are not known, it is clear that phenytoin's inhibition of calcium channels and calcium sequestration within the nerve terminals play an important role in the excitatory and inhibitory actions of this anticonvulsant. The effect of phenytoin on posttetanic potentiation also may underlie some of the important anticonvulsant properties of this drug. It appears that some of the effects of phenytoin on posttetanic potentiation may be mediated at the molecular level by the effect of this compound on calcium and sodium systems.

The advances in molecular neurobiology and neuroscience have clearly pushed back our frontiers in understanding the mechanisms of action of phenytoin. Major advances described in this chapter clearly shed light on how this compound may be mediating neuronal stabilizing and excitatory phenomenon. There is great promise that the more specific correlation between biochemical mechanisms and clear clinical and electrophysiological effects will be elucidated in the next decade.

REFERENCES

1. Ayala, G. F., and Johnston, D. (1977): The influences of phenytoin on the fundamental electrical properties of simple neural systems. *Epilepsia*, 18:299–307.

2. Ayala, G. F., Lin, S., and Johnston, D. (1977): The mechanism of action of diphenylhydantoin on invertebrate neurons. I. Effects on basic membrane properties. *Brain Res.*, 121:245–258.

3. Aston, R., and Domino, E. F. (1961): Differential effects of phenobarbital, pentobarbital and diphenylhydantoin on motor cortical and reticular thresholds in the rhesus monkey. *Psychopharmacologia*, 2:304–317.

4. Barany, E. H., and Stein-Jensen, E. (1946): The mode of action of anticonvulsant drugs on electrically-induced convulsions in the rabbit. *Arch. Int. Pharmacodyn. Ther.*, 73:1–47.

5. Biltz, H. (1908): Uber die Konstitution der Einwirkungsprodukte von substituierten Harnstoffen auf Benzil und uber einige neue Methoden zur Darstellung der 5,5 Diphenylhydantoin. *Berl. Dtsch. Chem. Ges.*, 41:1379.

6. Blum, B. (1964): A differential action of diphenylhydantoin on the motor cortex of the cat. *Arch. Int. Pharmacodyn. Ther.*, 149:45–55.

7. Bowling, A. C., and DeLorenzo, R. J. (1982): Micromolar benzodiazepine receptors: Identification and characterization in central nervous system. *Science*, 216:1247–1250.

8. Bowling, A. C., and DeLorenzo, R. J. (1987): Photoaffinity labeling of a novel benzodiazepine binding protein in rat brain. *Eur. J. Pharmacol.*, 135:97–100.

9. Braestrup, C., and Squires, R. F. (1978): Pharmacological characterization of benzodiazepine receptors. *Eur. J. Pharmacol.*, 48:263–270.

10. Carnay, L., and Grundfest, S. (1974): Excitable membrane stabilization by diphenylhydantoin and calcium. *Neuropharmacol.*, 13:1097–1108.

11. Cheung, W. Y. (1970): Cyclic 3′,5′-nucleotide phosphodiesterase: Demonstration of an activator. *Biochem. Biophys. Res. Commun.*, 38:533–538.

12. Cheung, W. Y. (1980): Calmodulin role in cellular regulation. *Science*, 207:19–27.

13. Czuczwar, S., Frey, H., and Loscher, W. (1986): N-methyl-d, L-Aspartic acid-induced convulsions in mice and their blockade by antiepileptic drugs and other agents. In: *Neurotransmitters, Seizures and Epilepsy III*, edited by G. Nistico, P. Morselli, K. Lloyd, R. Fariello, and J. Engle, pp. 235–246. Raven Press, New York.

14. Delgado, J. M. R., and Mihailovic, L. (1956): Use of intracerebral electrodes to evaluate drugs that act on the central nervous system. *Ann. N.Y. Acad. Sci.*, 64:644–666.

15. Delgado-Escueta, A. V., and Horan, M. P. (1980): Phenytoin: Biochemical membrane studies. *Adv. Neurol.*, 27:377–398.

16. Delgado-Escueta, A. V., Ward, A. A., Woodbury, D. M., and Porter, R. J. (eds.) (1986): *Advances in Neurology*, pp. 3–55. Raven Press, New York.

17. DeLorenzo, R. J. (1976): Antagonistic action of diphenylhydantoin and calcium on the endogenous phosphorylation of specific brain proteins. *Neurology*, 26:386.

18. DeLorenzo, R. J. (1977): Antagonistic action of diphenylhydantoin and calcium on the level of phosphorylation of particular rat and human brain proteins. *Brain Res.*, 134:125–138.

19. DeLorenzo, R. J. (1980): Phenytoin: Calcium- and calmodulin-dependent protein phosphorylation and neurotransmitter release. *Antiepileptic Drugs: Mechanisms of Action*, edited by G. H. Glaser, J. K. Penry, and D. M. Woodbury. Raven Press, New York.

20. DeLorenzo, R. J. (1980): Role of calmodulin in neurotransmitter release and synaptic function. *Ann. N.Y. Acad. Sci.*, 356:92–109.

21. DeLorenzo, R. J. (1981): The calmodulin hypothesis of neurotransmission. *Cell Calcium*, 2:365–385.

22. DeLorenzo, R. J. (1982): Calmodulin in neurotransmitter release and synaptic function. *Fed. Proc.*, 41:2275.

23. DeLorenzo, R. J. (1983): Calcium-calmodulin protein phosphorylation in neuronal transmission: A molecular approach to neuronal excitability and anticonvulsant drug action. In: *Advances in Neurology, Vol. 34, Status Epilepticus*, edited by A. V. Delgado-Escueta, C. G. Wasterlain, D. M. Treiman, and R. J. Porter, pp. 325–338. Raven Press, New York.

24. DeLorenzo, R. J. (1986): A molecular approach to the calcium signal in brain: Relationship to synaptic modulation and seizure discharge. *Advances in Neurology*; Vol. 44, pp. 325–338. Raven Press, New York.

25. DeLorenzo, R. J., and Dashefsky, L. (1985): Anticonvulsants. *Handbook of Neurochemistry*. Vol. 9:363–403.

26. DeLorenzo, R. J., Emple, G. P., and Glaser, G. H. (1976): Regulation of the level of endogenous phosphorylation of specific brain proteins by diphenylhydantoin. *J. Neurochem.*, 28:21–30.

27. DeLorenzo, R. J., and Freedman, S. D. (1977): Possible role of calcium-dependent protein phosphorylation in mediating neurotransmitter release and anticonvulsant action. *Epilepsia*, 18:357–365.

28. DeLorenzo, R. J., Freedman, S. D., Yohe, W. B., and Maurer, S. C. (1979): Stimulation of Ca^{2+}-dependent neurotransmitter release and presynaptic nerve terminal protein phosphorylation by calmodulin and a calmodulin-like protein isolated form synaptic vesicles. *Proc. Natl. Acad. Sci. USA*, 76:1838–1842.

29. DeLorenzo, R. J., and Glaser, G. H. (1976): Effect of diphenylhydantoin on the endogenous phosphorylation of brain protein. *Brain Res.*, 105:381–386.

30. DeLorenzo, R. J., and Taft, W. C. (1984): Regulation of depolarization-induced calcium uptake. In: *Advances in Epileptology: XVth Epilepsy International Symposium*, edited by R. J. Porter et al., pp. 37–42. Raven Press, New York.

31. DeLorenzo, R. J., Taft, W. C., and Andrews, W. T. (1985): Regulation of voltage-sensitive calcium channels in brain by n = micromolar affinity benzodiazepine receptors. In: *Calcium, Neuronal Function and Neurotransmitter Release*, edited by B. Katz, and R. Rahamimoff, pp. 375–934. Martinus Nijhoff, Boston.

32. Deupree, J. D. (1976): Evidence that diphenylhydantoin does not affect adenosine triphosphatase from brain. *Neuropharmacol.*, 15:187–195.

33. Deupree, J. D. (1977): The role or non-role of ATPase activation by phenytoin in the stabilization of excitable membranes. *Epilepsia*, 18:309–315.

34. De Weer, P. (1980): Phenytoin: Blockage of resting sodium channels. *Adv. Neurol.*, 27:353–361.

35. Esplin, D. W. (1957): Effects of diphenylhydantoin on synaptic transmission in cat spinal cord and stellate ganglion. *J. Pharmacol. Exp. Ther.*, 120:301–323.

36. Esplin, D. W., and Freston, J. W. (1960): Physiological and pharmacological analysis of spinal cord convulsions. *J. Pharmacol. Exp. Ther.*, 130:68–80.

37. Esplin, D. W., and Laffan, R. J. (1957): Determinants of flexor and extensor components of maximal seizures in cats. *Arch. Int. Pharmacodyn. Ther.*, 113:189–202.

38. Ferrendelli, J. A. (1980): Phenytoin: Cyclic nucleotide regulation in the brain. *Adv. Neurol.*, 27:429–433.

39. Ferrendelli, J. A., and Kinscherf, D. A. (1977): Phenytoin: Effects on calcium flux and cyclic nucleotides. *Epilepsia*, 18(3):331–348.

40. Fertziger, A. P., Liuzzi, S. E., and Dunham, P. B. (1971): Diphenylhydantoin (Dilantin): Stimulation of potassium influx in lobster axons. *Brain Res.*, 33:592–596.

41. Festoff, B. W., and Appel, S. H. (1968): Effect of diphenylhydantoin on synaptosome sodium-potassium ATPase. *J. Clin. Invest.*, 47:2752–2758.

42. Gangloff, H., and Monnier, M. (1957): The action of anticonvulsant drugs tested by electrical stimulation of the rabbit cortex, diencephalon and rhinencephalon in the unanesthetized rabbit. *Electroencephalogr. Clin. Neurophysiol.*, 9:43–58.

43. Gibbs, M. K., and Kim, T. Ng (1976): Diphenylhydantoin facilitation of labile protein-independent memory. *Brain Res. Bull.*, 1:203–208.

44. Glazko, A. J. (1972): Diphenylhydantoin: Chemistry and methods of determination. In: *Antiepileptic Drugs*, edited by D. M. Woodbury, J. K. Penry, and R. P. Schmidt, pp. 103–112. Raven Press, New York.

45. Gutman, Y., and Boonyaviroj, P. (1977): Mechanism of inhibition of catecholamine release form adrenal medulla by diphenylhydantoin and by low concentration of ouabain (10^{-10} M). *Naunyn-Schmiedeberg's Arch. Pharmacol.*, 296:293–296.

46. Johnston, D., and Ayala, G. F. (1975): Diphenyl-hydantoin: The action of a common anticonvulsant on bursting pacemaker cells in *Aplysia*. *Science*, 189:1009–1011.

47. Julien, R. M., and Halpern, L. M. (1972): Effects of diphenylhydantoin and other antiepileptic drugs on epileptiform activity and Purkinje cell discharge rates. *Epilepsia*, 13:387–400.

48. Klee, C. B., Crouch, T. H., and Richmand, P. G. (1980): Calmodulin. *Annu. Rev. Biochem.*, 49:489–515.

49. Korey, S. R. (1951): Effect of Dilantin and Mesantoin on the giant axon of the squid. *Proc. Soc. Exp. Biol. Med.*, 79:297–299.

50. Lewin, E., and Bleck, V. (1971): The effect of diphenylhydantoin administration on cortex potassium-activated phosphatase. *Neurology*, 21:417–418.

51. Lipicky, R. J., Gilbert, D. L., and Stillman, I. M. (1972): Diphenylhydantoin inhibition of sodium conductance in squid giant axon. *Proc. Natl. Acad. Sci.*, 69:1758–1760.

52. Macdonald, R. L., and McLean, M. J. (1982): Cellular bases of barbiturate and phenytoin anticonvulsant drug action. *Epilepsia*, 23:S7–18.

53. Macdonald, R. L., and McLean, M. J. (1986): Anticonvulsant drugs: Mechanisms of action. *Advances in Neurology*.

54. McLean, M. J., and Macdonald, R. L. (1983): Multiple actions of phenytoin on mouse spinal cord neurons in cell culture. *J. Pharmacol. Exp. Ther.*, 227:779–789.

55. McLean, M. J., and Macdonald, R. L. (1984): Limitation of high frequency repetitive firing of cultured mouse neurons by anticonvulsant drugs. *Neurology*, 34(suppl. 1):288.

56. McLean, M. J., and Macdonald, R. L. (1986): Sodium valproate, but not ethosuximide, produces use- and voltage-dependent limitation of high frequency repetitive firing of action potential of mouse central neurons in cell culture. *J. Pharmacol. Exp. Ther.*, June 237(3):1001–1011 (b).

57. McLean, M. J., and Macdonald, R. L. (1986): Carbamazepine and 10,11-epoxycarbamazepine produce use- and voltage-dependent limitation of rapidly firing action potentials of mouse central neurons in cell culture. *J. Pharmacol. Exp. Ther.*, August 238(2):727–738 (a).

58. Merritt, H. H., and Putnam, T. J. (1938): A new series of anticonvulsant drugs tested by experiments on animals. *Arch. Neurol. Psychiatr.*, 39:1003–1015.

59. Morell, F., Bradley, W., and Ptashne, M. (1958): Effect of diphenylhydantoin on peripheral nerve. *Neurology*, 8:140–144.

60. Noach, E. L., Woodbury, D. M., and Goodman, L. S. (1958): Studies on the absorption, distribution, fate and excretion of 4-^{14}C-labeled diphenylhydantoin. *J. Pharmacol. Exp. Ther.*, 122:301–314.

61. Perry, J. G., McKinney, L., and DeWeer, P. (1978): The cellular mode of action of antiepileptic drug 5,5-diphenylhydantoin. *Nature*, 272:271–273.

62. Putnam, T. J., and Merritt, H. H. (1937): Exper-

imental determination of anticonvulsant properties of some phenyl derivatives. *Science*, 85:525–526.

63. Putnam, T. J., and Merritt, H. H. (1941): Chemistry of anticonvulsant drugs. *Arch. Neurol.*, 45:505–516.

64. Raines, A., and Standaert, F. G. (1966): Pre- and post-junctional effects of diphenylhydantoin at the soleus neuromuscular junction. *J. Pharmacol. Exp. Ther.*, 153:361–366.

65. Raines, A., and Standaert, F. G. (1967): An effect of diphenylhydantoin on post-tetanic hyperpolarization of intramedullary nerve terminals. *J. Pharmacol. Exp. Ther.*, 156:591–597.

66. Rosenberg, P., and Bartels, E. (1967): Drug effects on the spontaneous electrical activity of the squid giant axon. *J. Pharmacol.*, 155:532–544.

67. Rosenthal, J. (1969): Post-tetanic potentiation at the neuromuscular junction of the frog. *J. Physiol (Lond.)*, 203:121–133.

68. Schmidt, R. P., and Wilder, J. (1968): *Epilepsy: Contemporary Neurology Series*. Davis, Philadelphia.

69. Schwarz, J. R., and Vogel, W. (1977): Diphenylhydantoin: Excitability reducing action in single myelinated nerve fibers. *Europ. J. Pharmacol.*, 44:241–249.

70. Sohn, R. S., and Ferrendelli, J. A. (1973): Inhibition of Ca^{++} transport into rat brain synaptosomes by diphenylhydantoin (DPH). *J. Pharmacol. Exp. Ther.*, 185:272–275.

71. Sohn, R. S., and Ferrendelli, J. A. (1976): Anticonvulsant drug mechanisms. *Arch. Neurol.*, 33:626–629.

72. Swanson, P. D., and Crane, P. O. (1972): Diphenylhydantoin and movement of radioactive sodium into electrically stimulated cerebral slices. *Biochem. Pharmacol.*, 21:2899–2905.

73. Taft, W. C., and DeLorenzo, R. J. (1987): Regulation of calcium channels in brain: Implications for the Clinical neurosciences. *Yale Jrnl. of Biology and Medicine*, 60:99–106.

74. Toman, J. E. P. (1952): Neuropharmacology of peripheral nerve. *Pharmacol. Rev.*, 4:168–218.

75. Toman, J. E. P. (1969): In: *Basic Mechanisms of the Epilepsies*, edited by H. H. Jasper, A. A. Ward, and A. Pope, pp. 682–688. Little, Brown, Boston.

76. Toman, J. E. P., Loewe, S., and Goodman, L. S. (1947): Physiology and therapy of convulsive disorders. I. Effect of anticonvulsant drugs on electroshock seizures in man. *Arch. Neurol.*, 58:312–324.

77. Toman, J. E. P., Swinyard, E. A., and Goodman, L. S. (1946): Properties of maximal seizures and their alterations by anticonvulsant drugs and other agents. *J. Neurophysiol.*, 9:231–240.

78. Wilensky, A. J., and Lowden, J. A. (1972): The inhibitor effect of diphenylhydantoin and microsomal ATPases. *Life Sci.*, 11:319–327.

79. Woodbury, D. M. (1955): Effect of diphenylhydantoin on electrolytes and on sodium turnover in brain and other tissues of normal, hypernatremic and postictal rats. *J. Pharmacol. Exp. Ther.*, 115:74–95.

80. Woodbury, D. M. (1969): Mechanisms of action of anticonvulsants. In: *Basic Mechanisms of the Epilepsies*, edited by H. H. Jasper, A. A. Ward, Jr., and A. Pope, pp. 647–681. Little, Brown, Boston.

81. Woodbury, D. M. (1980): Phenytoin: Proposed mechanisms of anticonvulsant action. *Adv. Neurol.*, 27:447–471.

82. Woodbury, D. M. (1982): Phenytoin: Mechanisms of action. In: *Antiepileptic Drugs*, Second Edition, edited by D. M. Woodbury, J. K. Penry, and C. E. Pippenger, pp. 269–282. Raven Press, New York.

83. Woodbury, D. M., and Esplin, D. W. (1959): Neuropharmacology and neurochemistry of anticonvulsant drugs. *Res. Publ. Assoc. Res. Nerv. Ment. Dis.*, 37:24–56.

84. Woodbury, D. M., and Kemp, J. W. (1971): Pharmacology and mechanisms of action of diphenylhydantoin. *Psychiatr. Neurol. Neurochir.*, 74:91–117.

85. Woodbury, D. M., and Swinyard, E. A. (1972): Diphenylhydantoin-Absorption, distribution and excretion. In: *Antiepileptic Drugs*, edited by D. M. Woodbury, J. D. Penry, and R. P. Schmidt, pp. 113–123. Raven Press, New York.

86. Yaari, Y., Pincus, J. H., and Argov, Z. (1977): Depression of synaptic transmission by diphenylhydantoin. *Ann. Neurol.*, 1:334–338.

Antiepileptic Drugs, Third Edition, edited by
R. Levy, R. Mattson, B. Meldrum,
J. K. Penry, and F. E. Dreifuss.
Raven Press, Ltd., New York © 1989.

10

Phenytoin

Chemistry and Methods of Determination

Anthony J. Glazko

Phenytoin is the generic name for 5,5-diphenylhydantoin (acid form). The *Chemical Abstracts* name is 5,5-diphenyl-2,4-imidazolidinedione. It has the chemical structure shown in Fig. 1. The free acid has a molecular weight of 252.26; the sodium salt has a molecular weight of 274.25, equivalent to acid content of 91.98%. The acid form is used in formulations of aqueous suspensions (Pediatric Dilantin-30 Suspension and Dilantin-125 Suspension) containing 30 mg or 125 mg of phenytoin acid per 5 ml. The free acid is also used in formulating chewable tablets (Dilantin Infatabs) containing 50 mg phenytoin acid per tablet. However, other products are formulated with the sodium salt of phenytoin (phenytoin sodium; acid equivalents = 91.98%). With these preparations, the drug content is expressed in terms of the sodium salt rather than the free acid. Thus, the gelatine capsules (Dilantin Sodium Kapseals) are formulated to contain either 30 mg or 100 mg of phenytoin sodium (= 27.6 mg or 92.0 mg of phenytoin acid equivalents) per capsule. This 8% difference in drug content should be taken into account when changing from one product to another. The sodium salt is also used in parenteral formulations (Parenteral Dilantin = phenytoin sodium injection). The drug content is given in terms of the sodium salt.

To eliminate any confusion in terminology, phenytoin assays are expressed in terms of free acid equivalents. Concentrations are usually reported as micrograms of phenytoin per milliliter of biological fluid (μg/ml = mg/liter), but there has been an international trend toward expressing concentrations on a molar basis (e.g., micromoles of phenytoin per liter).

Phenytoin is a weak organic acid that is poorly soluble in water. The apparent dissociation constant (pK_a'), representing the pH at which half the drug is ionized, was found to be in the range of 8.3 to 9.2 by nonaqueous titration in earlier work (3,39). Experiments by Schwartz et al. (78) based on solubility measurements indicated a true pK_a' of 8.06 in water. The acid was essentially nonionized at pH 5.4 (solubility about 19.4 μg/g at 25.4°C), whereas the data at pH 7.4 (about 80% nonionized) indicated a water solubility of 20.5 μg/g (25.2°C). Higher concentrations of phenytoin required strongly alkaline solutions, with solubility measurements of 165 μg/ml at pH 9.1 (borate buffer), and 1,520 μg/ml at pH 10 (sodium hydroxide) (38). Parenteral phenytoin sodium is made up in an aqueous vehicle containing propylene glycol, ethanol, and sodium hydroxide. It contains 50 mg phenytoin sodium per ml (= 46 mg phenytoin acid per ml). The solubility of phenytoin in blood plasma is about 75 μg/ml (37°C), at least in part because of binding of the drug on the plasma proteins (38).

Phenytoin sodium is not recommended as an analytical standard because of its vari-

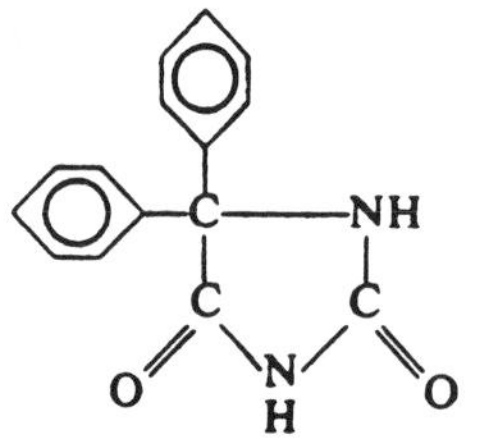

FIG. 1. Structure of phenytoin.

able water content and partial conversion to the free acid on exposure to carbon dioxide (38). Ishiguro et al. (49) measured the vapor pressure of hydrated forms of the sodium salt at different temperatures and concluded that the mono-, tetra-, hepta-, octa-, and hendecahydrates were present. The tetra- and heptahydrates appeared to be most stable under conditions of high humidity, with a moisture content of 20.8% and 31.5%, respectively. This group also reported that the absorption of CO_2 by phenytoin sodium increased with the degree of hydration, forming sodium bicarbonate and phenytoin acid (48).

ASSAY OF PHENYTOIN

The high degree of clinical interest in accurate phenytoin assays is reflected in the large number of papers on this subject that have appeared since our last reviews (38,38a). This period has been marked by rapid expansion in high-performance liquid chromatography (HPLC), enzyme immunoassay (EMIT), fluorescence polarization immunoassays (FPIA), substrate-labeled fluorescence immunoassay (SLFIA), and radioimmunoassay (RIA) techniques. At the same time, many improvements have been made in spectrophotometric techniques based on oxidation procedures and in gas-liquid chromatography (GLC) techniques. Both HPLC and GLC continue to be especially valuable for the rapid detec-

tion and measurement of multiple anticonvulsant and/or metabolite drug concentrations in single plasma specimens.

We have also witnessed the development of new analytical techniques, including the apoenzyme reactive immunoassay system (ARIS) and enzyme immunochromatography (ACCULEVEL), which allow accurate quantitation of anticonvulsant drugs in the physician's office. The next decade will certainly see the development of techniques for routine anticonvulsant quantitation of all drugs at the patient's bedside or in the physician's office.

Spectrophotometric Methods

The colorimetric procedure for phenytoin originally described by Dill et al. (27) has been compared with GLC assays by Berlin et al. (9) using a modification of the procedure described by MacGee (59). Samples included those of patients taking phenobarbital and other drugs as well as those from patients taking phenytoin alone. The two procedures gave essentially the same results, but the standard deviation for single estimates was 0.2 μg/ml for the GLC procedure and 0.6 μg/ml for the colorimetric procedure. At low concentrations of phenytoin, the GLC procedure could be used down to 0.2 μg/ml with 200 μl of plasma, whereas the corresponding limit for the colorimetric procedure was 2 μg/ml with 3-ml plasma samples.

Similar comparisons have been made by Janz and Schmidt (50), between the GLC method of Kupferberg (56) and the ultraviolet absorbance procedure of Svensmark and Kristensen (87). Samples were taken from patients receiving only phenytoin. Assays on the same plasma samples were significantly higher by spectrophotometric assay (mean ± SD = 17.4 ± 11.3 μg/ml) than by GLC assay (11.7 ± 9.2 μg/ml).

Oxidation Procedures

A major step forward in spectrophotometric methods came with the introduction of oxidative procedures by Wallace et al. (95) in which phenytoin was converted to benzophenone. Bromine was first used to effect this conversion, later being replaced by alkaline permanganate (94). The beauty of this procedure is that phenobarbital and most other drugs do not interfere with the assay. However, the original Wallace procedure required large volumes of plasma (5–10 ml), involved extraction with chloroform, which interfered with the assay, and required specialized glassware for refluxing and distillation steps. As a result, numerous modifications of the Wallace procedure were introduced to make the procedure suitable for clinical use (10,25,35,62,65,75,85,89,93,96).

A major breakthrough in 1972 by Dill and Glazko (26) involved the development of a simple fluorometric assay procedure for benzophenone, resulting in greater sensitivity of the assay. In a more recent modification of the fluorometric procedure, Dill et al. (28) ran the permanganate oxidation directly on 0.2 ml of plasma, eliminating the need for preliminary extraction with organic solvents. Ordinary test tubes were used for the oxidation step, the benzophenone was extracted by vortexing with heptane, and fluorescence was developed by vortexing the heptane extract with concentrated sulfuric acid. There were no significant differences in plasma levels of phenytoin in 154 clinical specimens assayed by on-column methylation techniques (GLC) and by the fluorometric assay procedure. One operator can handle 40 to 60 samples per day, and the unit cost per sample is remarkably low. Although this procedure is cost-effective for the quantitation of phenytoin in patients receiving monotherapy, HPLC or GLC techniques would be more appropriate for patients receiving polytherapy, since multiple drugs can be quantitated in the serum specimen.

Gas-Liquid Chromatography

By far the largest number of publications on assay methods for phenytoin deal with gas-liquid chromatography (GLC) procedures. The early phases of development in this area have been covered thoroughly in the first and second editions of *Antiepileptic Drugs* (38,38a). MacGee's on-column methylation procedure with tetramethylammonium hydroxide (TMAH) (59) and Kupferberg's procedure with trimethylanilinium hydroxide (trimethylphenylammonium hydroxide) (TMPAH) (56) are still used today, as is 5-(4-methylphenyl)-5-phenylhydantoin (MPPH), the internal standard originally introduced by Chang and Glazko (16,17). Dudley (32) discussed the desirable features of this internal standard, recommending it for use in GLC assays of multiple antiepileptic drugs. However, problems may arise because of differences in the chemical reactivity or thermal stability of certain drugs, particularly barbiturates, making the use of multiple internal standards desirable.

Current trends are toward multidrug determinations, with more emphasis on derivative than nonderivative techniques. Derivative formation is to be preferred because of more symmetrical peaks and better separation, better thermal stability, and shorter retention times. Also, the added time factor for on-column methylation techniques is negligible. Solow et al. (83,84) used a temperature-programmed version of MacGee's on-column methylation procedure (59) to quantitate numerous hydantoins, succinimides, and barbiturates. A typical run is shown in Fig. 2. Perchalski et al. (67,68) combined the best features of the MacGee (59) and Kupferberg (56) procedures and ran simultaneous assays for phenytoin, phenobarbital, and primidone. Cremers and Verheesen (23) extended the range of as-

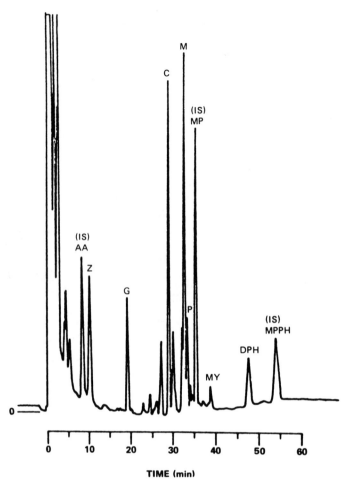

FIG. 2. Chromatograms showing peaks from antiepileptic drug analyses. On-column methylation procedure with tetramethylammonium hydroxide and 5% OV-17 on Gas Chrom Q (100/120 mesh) at 230°C. Z = Zarontin (ethosuximide); G = Gemonil (metharbital); C = desmethyl Celontin (desmethylmethsuximide); M = Milontin (phensuximide); P = phenobarbital; MY = Mysoline (primidone); DPH = diphenylhydantoin; AA = α,α-dimethyl-β-methylsuccinimide; MP = 5-ethyl-5-tolylbarbituric acid; MPPH = 5-(p-methylphenyl)-5-phenylhydantoin. From Solow et al., (ref. 84), with permission of authors and Preston Publications, Inc.

says, using flash methylation for some components, with GLC being run on one column at three different temperatures. More recent multidrug assay procedures with on-column methylation include those of Dorrity and Linnoila (29), Abraham and Joslin (1), and Hill and Latham (44). Different methylation conditions have been examined by Estas and Dumont (33) and by Serfontein and de Villiers (80). Other alkylating agents have also been employed, including flash ethylation with triethylammonium hydroxide (36) and hexylation with tetrahexylammonium hydroxide (37). These may be of value in distinguishing N-demethylated metabolites from the parent compounds but offer no real advantages in the assay of phenytoin.

The GLC assay of phenytoin and other anticonvulsant drugs without derivatization has also been explored in depth (57,60,61,70–74,76,88,92). Pippenger and Gillen (70) used 1% HIEFF-8BP columns for the separation of a series of drugs without forming derivatives, but a plot of peak heights versus amount of drug did not produce a straight line passing through the origin (56). Sampson et al. (76) used a cleanup step to remove lipids as a possible source of interference. The precipitation of cholesterol as the digitonide was used by Driessen and Emonds (30) to reduce plasma blanks. Ritz and Warren (72) reported that a relatively polar liquid phase (3% OV-225) produced chromatograms comparable to those obtained with derivatization techniques. Brien and Inaba (12) used SE-30 columns with good results. Thoma et al. (88) acidified 0.25 to 0.5 ml plasma with 0.5 ml 1.5 M ammonium sulfate plus 3 drops 3 N-HCl and extracted by shaking with 5 ml methylene chloride, resulting in a remarkably clean extract; GLC assays were carried out for underivatized phenobarbital, carbamazepine, primidone, phenytoin, and appropriate internal standards using a newly developed column (2% SP 2110 + 1% SP2510-DA; Supelco, Inc., Bellefonte, Pennsylvania). Toseland et al. (91) reported the use of nitrogen-selective detectors (Hewlett-Packard Model 1516A Nitrogen Detector) with nonderivatized anticonvulsant drugs. Because of the simplicity of these procedures and their applicability to the detection and measurement of many different anticonvulsant drugs, they may find a useful place in the clinical laboratory. However, to the analytical chemist and for reasons already discussed, it is clear that on-column methylation techniques are preferable for most clinical applications.

Mass Spectrometry

Although the mass spectrometer is too highly specialized an instrument to be considered for general use, it can be used as a rather expensive detector for GLC analyses, extending the range of sensitivity five- to 10-fold or more. It plays a more appropriate role as a tool for the structural identification of various derivatives and metabolites of drug products. MacGee (59) showed that the product of on-column methylation of phenytoin was the *N,N*-dimethyl derivative. This was confirmed by Estas and Dumont (33), who also identified the methylated derivative of the major metabolite of phenytoin (*p*-HPPH) as 1,3-dimethyl-5-(*p*-methoxyphenyl)-5-phenylhydantoin. Earlier work by Grimmer et al. (40) indicated that the methylation of phenytoin with diazomethane gave the *N*-3 monomethyl substituent, whereas similar treatment of *p*-HPPH produced the *N*-3 methyl, *p*-methoxyphenyl (dimethylated) derivative.

Rane et al. (71) used mass fragmentography and multiple ion detection to achieve a sensitivity of 0.01 μg phenytoin per ml. They were able to follow the transplacental passage of drug from mother to fetus using 100 μl of plasma for analysis. Hoppel et al. (45) also described the mass fragmentography of phenytoin and *p*-HPPH after extractive alkylation, using 10 to 100 μl of plasma. Baty and Robinson (8) used single and multiple ion detection to study the metabolic profile of subjects who had reached steady-state levels of phenytoin. Horning et al. (46) used chemical ionization techniques and selective ion detection to correlate plasma and breast milk levels after single 100-mg doses of phenytoin. Diazomethane was used as the alkylating agent prior to the introduction of the sample into the mass spectrometer. Lehrer and Karmen (58) also used chemical ionization techniques for the detection and rapid assay of a variety of drugs in serum, including phenytoin (with MPPH internal standard), barbiturates, carbamazepine, nicotine, and caffeine. Assay time in the mass spectrometer was 2 min per sample with direct probe insertion of samples.

Mass spectroscopy is a powerful research tool that can be used to study metabolic patterns, identify metabolic structures, and carry out sophisticated pharmacokinetic studies utilizing stable isotopes in individual patients. However, the expense and time involved in gas chromatography–mass spectrometry assays have prevented its application in routine therapeutic drug monitoring.

High-Performance Liquid Chromatography

The use of HPLC has expanded rapidly in the past few years, with simplified instrumentation and more versatile detection systems readily available. Procedures are rapid, and derivative formation is not usually required. Solvent extraction steps can be eliminated by resorting to protein precipitation with acetonitrile, with assays being run directly on the supernatant. The HPLC technique is amenable to quantitation of multiple drugs and drug metabolites in a single run. High-performance liquid chromatography has displaced GLC as the method of choice for routine monitoring of multiple anticonvulsants in the same specimen.

Anders and Latorre (5) reported the separation of phenytoin and p-HPPH by HPLC on an ion-exchange column, using only standard samples of drug. Evans (34) achieved better separation on silica gel columns and applied the technique to phenytoin and phenobarbital assays on 100-μl serum samples. This was preceded by ether extraction, and the time requirements were about the same as in the usual GLC procedures. Atwell et al. (7) used a silicic acid column but developed a better extraction procedure with methylene dichloride and used an internal standard. Inaba and Brien (47) worked with silica gel columns, but their methodology was directed primarily toward the assay of p-HPPH. Similarly, Albert et al. (4) assayed HPPH but reverted

to the use of ion-exchange columns. Adams and Vandemark (2) separated a number of anticonvulsant drugs from serum by absorption on charcoal and elution with acetonitrile:water (17:83), the same solvent system used later for chromatography on a reversed-phase column. Phenacetin was used as the internal standard, and the phenytoin assay sensitivity was 0.1 μg/ml with 0.5-ml serum samples.

Kabra et al. (51) used MPPH as a more appropriate internal standard for phenytoin assays. Initial separation procedures included solvent extraction of drugs followed by HPLC on silicic acid columns. Later (53), the conditions were altered by eliminating the extraction step, using 2.5 volumes of acetonitrile to precipitate the proteins from 200-μl samples of plasma or serum. The supernatant was then injected onto a reversed-phase μBondapak-C_{18} column (Waters Associates, Inc., Milford, Massachusetts) and developed with a mobile phase consisting of acetonitrile:pH 4.4 phosphate buffer (19:81). Soldin and Hill (82) employed a similar technique with acetonitrile and reversed-phase column chromatography, using a more alkaline solvent. Slonek et al. (81) used essentially the same technique with a more acidic solvent system. Pesh-Imam et al. (69) also used a reversed-phase column with 5-μm Spherisorb-ODS particles (Altex, Inc., Berkeley, California) and a mobile phase consisting of acetonitrile, water, and 1.75 M phosphoric acid (27:72.8:0.2). The method compared favorably with EMIT assays for phenobarbital, primidone, phenytoin, and carbamazepine.

Chamberlain et al. (15) compared their HPLC procedure (extraction with dichloromethane and chromatography on a Partisil-10 column [Whatman, Clifton, New Jersey] using MPPH as an internal standard) with the on-column methylation procedure of MacGee (59) and found no statistically significant differences. The HPLC procedure had the lowest day-to-day variation (CV = 4.0%), cost factors were considerably lower than with the GLC procedure, and assay times were about the same. Helmsing et al. (42) and Schweizer (79) used Extrelut columns (E. Merck, Darmstadt) for preliminary separation of drugs from plasma and other biological fluids, subsequently concentrating the ether eluate with good recovery of drug prior to HPLC or GLC.

Immunoassay Methods

Radioimmunoassay

Radioimmunoassay (RIA) procedures are based on the binding of a radioisotope $I^{125}H^3$ labeled drug to an antibody that specifically recognizes the drug. The key characteristics for antibodies used in RIA (or any immunoassay) are specificity and high affinity. In an RIA for phenytoin, the phenytoin present in a sample at an unknown concentration is allowed to compete with a constant amount of radio-labeled (^3H, ^{125}I) phenytoin for a limited number of antibody-binding sites. At equilibrium both the labeled and unlabeled phenytoin exist either bound to the antibody or "free" (not bound to the antibody). Since the binding is competitive, the amount of labeled phenytoin bound to the antibody is inversely proportional to the amount of unlabeled phenytoin. Drug concentrations in a serum sample can therefore be determined after separation of the bound and free fractions by comparing the amount of radioactivity in either fraction with that obtained from phenytoin standards. A separation step is essential since antibody binding has no effect on radioactive decay, thus it is impossible to determine radio-label distribution between the bound and free forms without separation of the two forms. Radioimmunoassays require a separation step. Immunoassays that require a separation step are referred to as heterogeneous.

Tigelaar et al. (90) prepared an antigen by coupling *p*-HPPH with chicken γ-globulin and produced an antiserum in rabbits. The RIA with ^{14}C-labeled phenytoin (4.65 mCi/mole) had adequate sensitivity to detect 0.03 μg phenytoin in 0.1 ml of sample, but there was strong crossreactivity with the metabolite *p*-HPPH. Similar products are marketed by Wien Laboratories, Inc., Succasunna, New Jersey, and by Clinical Assays, Inc., Cambridge, Massachusetts. Cook et al. (22) attached phenytoin to bovine serum albumin through a 5-carbon side chain in the *N*-3 position of the hydantoin ring and produced an antiserum with high specific activity for phenytoin and virtually no crossreactivity with *p*-HPPH. Orme et al. (66) compared the RIA procedure of Cook et al. (22) with the GLC procedure of Berlin et al. (9), and found excellent correlation.

Although RIA offers the advantage of sensitivity and low cost per test, its disadvantages include the inconvenience associated with radio-labels, short shelf lives of the radio-labeled reagents, special licensing requirements, radioactive waste disposal, and extensive recordkeeping. Since RIA procedures are heterogeneous, it is difficult to completely automate the assays. For these reasons, routine RIA assays for multiple anticonvulsants were never developed. Today, phenytoin RIA assays are utilized primarily in research situations rather than in routine therapeutic drug monitoring.

Enzyme Immunoassay

The enzyme multiplied immunoassay technique (EMIT) and the enzyme-linked immunosorbent assay (ELISA) are the two predominant forms of enzyme immunoassay technique utilized in therapeutic drug monitoring.

ELISA techniques are heterogeneous assays based on the same principles as the RIA methods. The major distinction is the use of an enzyme rather than a radioisotope as the label in ELISA assays. The separated bound or free phase must be treated with a substrate for the labeling enzyme in the ELISA technique. As the enzyme converts the substrate to its product, a spectrophotometric change is monitored and converted to analyte concentration. ELISA assays for digoxin, theophylline, and various endogenous compounds are currently available.

The EMIT methods for monitoring phenytoin and/or phenobarbital in serum were pioneered as the first plasma homogeneous immunoassay (Syva Corp., Palo Alto, California). By definition, a homogeneous assay does not require the separation of bound and free antibody during analysis. The amount of enzyme activity elicited by the bound and free forms of the conjugate are substantially different, so that the activities are easily distinguished from one another. When antibody binds to the drug-enzyme conjugate, the antibody either sterically prevents access of substrate to the active site of the enzyme or causes a conformational change in the enzyme, which alters its activity. Therefore the activity of the bound forms of the conjugate is suppressed and easily distinguished from that of the free forms.

The EMIT system eliminated the use of radioactivity as a measure of substrate release from the antibody. The drug is conjugated with a bacterial enzyme (glucose-6-phosphate dehydrogenase) that has no activity when bound to a drug-specific antibody. Thus, an antibody containing a fixed number of binding sites will equilibrate with free drug to reduce the number of available binding sites. Addition of the drug-enzyme complex will result in less binding to the antibody. This is illustrated schematically in Fig. 3. The decrease in enzyme activity provides a measure of drug concentration present in the EMIT system. The enzyme activity is measured by the rate of reaction with glucose-6-phosphate in the presence of the coenzyme factor NAD (nicotinamide adenine dinucleotide). This in turn is reduced to NADH and measured by its absorbance at 340 nm.

The basic instrumentation used in conjunction with EMIT assays is a pipettor and a spectrophotometer. The EMIT procedure is readily adaptable to any automated chemistry analyzer, which is available in any hospital laboratory. The conversion of NAD to NADPH to the final reaction in the EMIT procedure can also be read fluorometrically. The EMIT assays are convenient to perform, rapid, cost-effective, and provide a broad range of assays which can be performed in a semiautomated or completely automated mode.

Booker and Darcey (11) compared EMIT with their own GLC procedure (chloroform extraction, residue dissolved in carbon disulfide, and GLC on 3% OV-17 with MPPH internal standard) and found good correlation. Spiehler et al. (86) compared phenytoin assays obtained with a commercially available RIA procedure (Wein Laboratories, Inc.), the EMIT system (Syva Corp.) and the GLC procedure of Perchalski et al. (67). A phenytoin level of 10 μg/ml by GLC corresponded with an average value of 12.7 $\pm$ 2.2 μg/ml (RIA), or 11.5 $\pm$ 1.0 μg/ml (EMIT). Castro et al. (14) also compared different assay procedures, including RIA (Wein) and EMIT (Syva), and concluded that the EMIT and HLPC procedures (2) were promising alternatives to the GLC and spectrophotometric methods. The same group (60) automated the EMIT system and found generally good correlation with other methods. Kampa et al. (54) compared the EMIT system with the RIA procedures of Wein Laboratories and Clinical Assays, Inc., and found good correlation among all three procedures.

Substrate-Labeled Fluorescent Immunoassay

The substrate-labeled fluorescent immunoassay (SLFIA) is a homogeneous assay

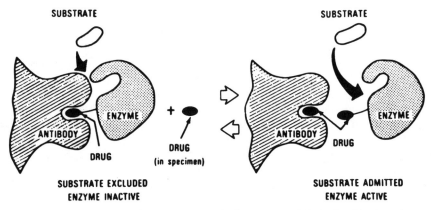

FIG. 3. Homogeneous enzyme immunoassay. **Left:** enzyme labeled with drug bound to the antibody (enzyme inactive). **Right:** drug in patient's serum bound to the antibody, thus preventing binding of the drug-labeled enzyme (enzyme active). From Schottelius (ref. 77), with permission of author and publisher.

developed by the Ames Division of Miles Laboratories, Elkhart, Indiana. The analyte is covalently attached to a fluorogenic enzyme substrate, galactosyl umbelliferone. The substrate-labeled drug is not fluorescent until it reacts with the enzyme, β-galactosidase, to produce a fluorescent product. Wong et al. (98) published a substrate-labeled fluorescent immunoassay (SLFIA) procedure using a single fluorometric reading rather than measurement of enzyme reaction rates. Galactosyl umbelliferone is coupled to a derivative of phenytoin and then bound to a specific antibody. In this form, the substrate is nonfluorescent in the presence of bacterial β-galactosidase. When phenytoin is added to this system, the drug-substrate conjugate is displaced in proportion to the concentration of phenytoin, and enzymatic hydrolysis takes place with the appearance of a fluorescent product. The assay procedure is highly sensitive, with assays possible on 2 μl of undiluted serum or 100 μl of 50-fold diluted serum. There is a 20 min equilibration period, and up to 40 assays can be set up in this time. No interference was encountered from other commonly used drugs. The metabolite p-HPPH at concentrations of 10- to

100-fold greater than normally encountered showed slight interference (10% error at concentrations greater than 35 μg/ml). A side-by-side comparison of clinical serum assays with the SLFIA procedure, the EMIT system, and a GLC assay showed good correlation for all three methods.

When β-galactosidase is added, the fluorescence produced is proportional to the phenytoin concentration in the specimen.

Since the free and antibody-bound forms of the label possess different activities, SLFIA requires no separation steps and is homogeneous. These assays can be performed manually, in a semiautomated or fully automated mode on any clinical analyzer with a fluorescence detector. These systems offer the same advantages as EMIT. The lack of appropriate fully automated clinical analyzers has prohibited the application of SLFIA assays to routine therapeutic drug monitoring.

Fluorescence Polarization Immunoassay

The fluorescence polarization immunoassay (FPIA) is a homogeneous assay developed by Abbott Diagnostics, North Chicago, Illinois. The principles of FPIA are presented schematically in Fig. 4. The phenytoin is covalently bound to a fluorophore derived from fluorescein. The fluorophore-labeled phenytoin conjugate, when excited by polarized light, produces a polarized fluorescence emission. The degree of polarization of a fluorescent solution is correlated to the fluorophore's rotational Brownian movement. Fluorescence polarization is sensitive to changes in the fluorophore's molecular size. The fluorophore-phenytoin is relatively small and has a very rapid rotational Brownian movement which results in fluorescence that is substantially depolarized. When the fluorophore-phenytoin conjugate binds to a phenytoin-specific antibody, the complex has a much greater mass. Thus, the fluorophore-phenytoin bound to antibody has a decreased Brownian rotational motion which is manifested by an increased fluorescence polarization. In competitive binding assays the ratio of free and antibody-bound fluorophore-phenytoin conjugate is governed by the level of analyte in the specimen. As the specimen concentration of phenytoin increases, the amount of antibody-bound phenytoin decreases, resulting in a decreased level of fluorescence polarization.

Fluorescence polarization immunoassay requires an instrument capable of determining the polarization of fluorescence signals. An automated FPIA instrument capable of performing therapeutic drug assays, the Abbott TDX, is capable of determining fluorescence polarization. This system offers a high degree of automation and all the advantages of the EMIT system. FPIA reagents are expensive, but the operational simplicity and speed of the Abbott TDX has made it the most widely used system currently available.

Apoenzyme Reactive Immunoassay

A major technological breakthrough in analytical technology was achieved by the Ames Company with the introduction of their Apoenzyme Reactive Immunoassay System (ARIS). ARIS was the first example of dry-phase immunology (99). The antibody and enzyme necessary for a quantitative immunoassay are impregnated on paper strips. Patient serum is added directly to the strip, and the antibody drug interaction takes place followed by a peroxidase reaction to produce a blue color. The color intensity is proportional to the drug concentration. Quantitative analysis is achieved by measuring the reflectance of light from the strip in a reflectometer (Ames Seralyzer).

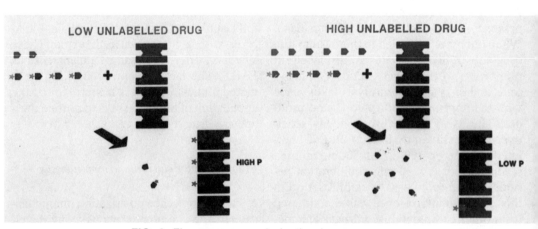

FIG. 4. Fluorescence polarization immunoassay.

At the present time, theophylline, phenytoin, and phenobarbital can be quantitatively determined with the same accuracy and precision as the methods described above. The clear advantage of the system is its rapid, accurate quantitation. The instrument is portable and simple to operate. Thus drug concentrations can be easily measured in the physician's office or at the patient's bedside.

Enzyme Immunochromatography

Recently a method for routine therapeutic drug monitoring which utilizes 100 µl of whole blood and requires no instrumentation has been described (100). This method is based on the principle that plasma can be separated from red blood cells chromatographically followed by an immunoassay to quantitate drug concentrations. The method, enzyme immunochromatography, uses capillary migration to distribute a mixture of patient sample and enzyme-labeled drug on a chromatographic paper strip which has covalently bound monoclonal antibody to the drug of interest.

The test (ACCULEVEL, Syntex Medical Diagnostics, Palo Alto, California) has three main components: a chromatographic paper strip coated with monoclonal antibodies, an enzyme reagent containing horseradish peroxidase-labeled drug and glucose oxidase, and a color developing reagent containing glucose and 4-chloro-1-napthol. The principles of the ACCULEVEL technique are presented schematically in Fig. 5.

The paper strip, contained in a plastic cassette, is placed in a mixture of the patient's whole blood and the enzyme reagent. As the solution migrates up the paper strip by capillary action, drug from the patient sample and peroxidase-labeled drug bind to the immobilized phenytoin antibody sites. The number of occupied antibody sites depends on the concentration of drug components in the solution. Since the concentration of the labeled drug is always the same, the drug concentration in the patient sample determines how far the two components travel up the chromatographic paper.

When the paper strip is immersed in the developing reagent, an insoluble blue product forms on the portions of the chromatographic paper to which enzyme-labeled drug is bound. The color reaction results from coupled enzyme reactions involving glucose oxidase and horseradish peroxidase-drug conjugate (bound to the paper via specific drug antibodies) and their substrates glucose and 4-chloro-1-napthol in the developer reagent.

The height of the color bar is measured in millimeters and converted to a phenytoin concentration using a results table. Although the assay uses whole blood, the table gives assay results in terms of a plasma concentration. This assay provides results consistent with most guidelines for adjusting drug dosages, which are based on serum or plasma concentrations. Since there is a difference between whole blood and plasma concentrations of most therapeutic drugs, the table incorporates a blood-to-plasma ratio factor. This factor is determined in clinical experiments prior to manufacturing ACCULEVEL kits. The blood-to-plasma ratio factor agrees with values reported by other scientists for the specific drug of interest.

With the ACCULEVEL immunochromatographic test system, the manufacturer, rather than the user, has provided the overall quality control needed for the assurance of quality results by establishing a stable calibration curve and a novel use of the control. This new approach to therapeutic drug monitoring represents a step toward immediate laboratory information for better patient care. The ACCULEVEL technique represents a mechanism for routine antiepileptic drug monitoring in the physician's office. It has been demonstrated to actively

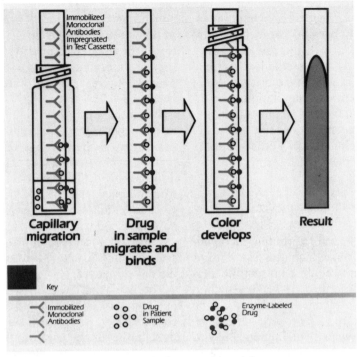

FIG. 5. Phenytoin immunochemistry assay.

and accurately quantitate antiepileptic drug concentrations. Clearly the safeguards built into the assay allow its performance by any person (physician, nurse, office technician) who has been trained in its use. ACCU-LEVEL assays are available for phenytoin, phenobarbital, and carbamazepine.

Differential Pulse Polarography

Brooks et al. (13) applied the principle of controlled nitration to the assay of phenytoin and phenobarbital by differential pulse polarography, with a sensitivity of 1 to 2 μg/ml of blood. Practical difficulties in sample preparation and in the separation of phenobarbital from phenytoin prohibit its application to routine assays, but the technique is of interest from a research standpoint.

METABOLITES OF PHENYTOIN

The major metabolite of phenytoin in human subjects is 5-(4-hydroxyphenyl)-5-

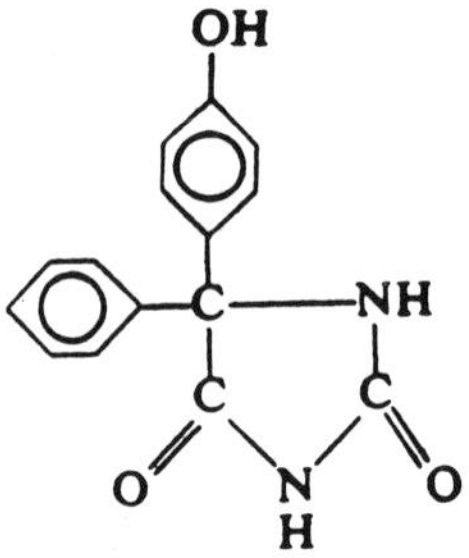

FIG. 6. Structure of 5-(4-hydroxyphenyl)-5-phenylhydantoin (*p*-HPPH).

phenylhydantoin, commonly known as *p*-HPPH. The *Chemical Abstracts* name is 5-(4-hydroxyphenyl)-5-phenyl-2,4-imidazolidinedione. It has the chemical structure shown in Fig. 6. Its molecular weight is 268.26, and phenytoin acid equivalents are 94.04%.

This metabolite is excreted in the urine as a conjugate of the phenolic group with glucuronic acid, yielding a highly water-soluble product. In order to extract the *p*-HPPH with an organic solvent, the conjugate must first be hydrolyzed by heating with hydrochloric acid or by treatment with an enzyme preparation containing β-glucuronidase, such as Glusulase (Endo Laboratories, Inc., Garden City, New York). Dog urine contains large amounts of *meta*-hydroxylated phenytoin (*m*-HPPH) as well as *p*-HPPH (6), but only traces of *m*-HPPH are found in human urine. Most of the analytical methods that have been reported for phenytoin metabolites are directed toward *p*-HPPH because of clinical interest in this product. At the present time there are no well-established assay procedures for the dihydrodiol metabolite or for a number of minor catechol derivatives, although all have been characterized by GLC procedures (18–20).

Early reports indicated that derivatives of phenytoin and *p*-HPPH could be separated by GLC procedures and assayed. Chang and Glazko (16,17) used trimethylsilyl (TMS) derivatives and two internal standards (S_1 = MPPH: S_2 = *m*-HPPH). Grimmer et al. (40) published a GLC assay procedure for *p*-HPPH using diazomethane for methylation and benz(*a*)anthracene as an internal standard. Hammer et al. (41) used flash methylation with trimethylanilinium hydroxide to assay *p*-HPPH. During this period (1968–1971), Dill et al. (24) developed a solvent extraction procedure that effected nearly complete separation of phenytoin and *p*-HPPH, so that separate colorimetric assays could be run on these compounds. The benzophenone procedure does not work with *p*-HPPH, and colorimetric methods lack the sensitivity for quantitating plasma *p*-HPPH concentrations. With single 250-mg intravenous doses of phenytoin in adult subjects, the total *p*-HPPH levels in blood plasma after β-glucuronidase hydrolysis were all below 1 μg/ml. Glazko et al. (39), using a GLC assay procedure, reported total *p*-HPPH plasma levels after 300-mg doses of phenytoin once daily for 15

days to range from 1 to 3 μg/ml for subjects with short phenytoin half-lives and < 1 μg/ml for subjects with long phenytoin half-lives.

Other work on GLC procedures includes the use of flash methylation by Estas and Dumont (33) with MPPH as the internal standard and a 3% OV-17 column. Karlen et al. (55) also used flash methylation techniques. Urine was preextracted with isoamyl alcohol to remove the dihydrodiol metabolite which could interfere with the assay (20). Midah et al. (63) used enzymatic hydrolysis with β-glucuronidase, ether extraction, and flash methylation. Witkin et al. (97) used on-column methylation for GLC determination of *p*-HPPH, using a newly developed internal standard, 5-(*p*-hydroxyphenyl)-5-(*p*-methylphenyl) hydantoin. Acid-treated urine gave *p*-HPPH assays that were not significantly different from those obtained with β-glucuronidase–treated urine.

Driessen and Emonds (31) used short semicapillary columns packed with a mixture of 2.6% OV-17 and 0.4% OV-225 at 260°C to run extracts of underivatized *p*-HPPH after enzymatic hydrolysis. The chemical identity of the *p*-HPPH peak was confirmed by mass spectroscopy. Hoppel et al. (45) used an extractive alkylation procedure with methyl iodide and mass fragmentography for the determination of unconjugated and total *p*-HPPH in 50 μl of plasma. Baty and Robinson (8) used a TMS derivative for mass fragmentography of *p*-HPPH. Deuterated internal standards were used in both of the mass spectrometry methods.

High-precision liquid chromatography assay methods for *p*-HPPH were introduced by Anders and Latorre (5) using an ion-exchange column, but they did not apply this to biological specimens. Inaba and Brien (47) used small-particle silica gel columns following acid hydrolysis of urine and extraction with ethyl acetate. Albert et al. (4) injected plasma samples directly into

DEAE–cellulose anion-exchange columns before and after enzymatic hydrolysis. More recent work has gone in the direction of reversed-phase columns. Kabra and Marton (52) used μBondapak-C_{18} with 27% ethanol in pH 3.2 acetate buffer (0.1 M). Slonek et al. (81) also used μBondapak-C_{18} columns with acetonitrile:water (37:63) as the mobile phase and MPPH as the internal standard. Urine samples were acid hydrolyzed and extracted with ethyl acetate:dichloroethane (1:2). Hermansson and Karlen (43) were able to determine conjugated *p*-HPPH in urine by preliminary extraction with isoamyl alcohol to remove interfering substances, acid hydrolysis of the aqueous residue at 100° for 150 min, subsequent extraction at pH 7.5 with diethyl ether, and return to 0.1 M sodium hydroxide. The HPLC was carried out without derivatization on μBondapak-C_{18} with 27% ethanol in pH 3.2 acetate buffer (0.1 M). Slonek et al. (81) also used μBondapak-C_{18} columns with a mobile phase consisting of acetonitrile:water (30:70), acidified with phosphoric acid to pH 2.65 to 2.69. Deproteinization of spiked plasma specimens with acetonitrile resulted in the recovery of 100% phenytoin and 96% *p*-HPPH.

SUMMARY

The monitoring of phenytoin in plasma or serum has become routine. The methods of choice for routine therapeutic drug monitoring are FPIA and EMIT in the clinical chemistry laboratory. For physician's office testing, ACCULEVEL and ARIS are accurate and simple to use. HPLC has become the optimal technique for monitoring phenytoin and its metabolites. GC and GC-MS analyses are limited to research applications.

CONVERSION

Conversion factor:

$$CF = \frac{1000}{mol.\ wt.} = \frac{1000}{252.3} = 3.96$$

Conversion:

$$(\mu g/ml) \times 3.96 = (\mu moles/liter)$$

$$(\mu moles/liter) \div 3.96 = (\mu g/ml)$$

REFERENCES

1. Abraham, C. V., Joslin, H. D. (1976): Simultaneous gas-chromatographic analysis for phenobarbital, diphenylhydantoin, carbamazepine, and primidone in serum. *Clin. Chem.*, 22:769–771.
2. Adams, R. F., Vandemark, F. L. (1976): Simultaneous high-pressure liquid-chromatographic determination of some anticonvulsants in serum. *Clin. Chem.*, 22:25–31.
3. Agarwal, S. P., and Blake, M. I. (1968): Determination of the pK_a' value for 5,5-diphenyl-hydantoin. *J. Pharm. Sci.*, 57:1434–1435.
4. Albert, K. S., Hallmark, M. R., Carroll, M. E., and Wagner, J. G. (1973): Quantitative separation of diphenylhydantoin and its parahydroxylated metabolites by high-performance liquid chromatography. *Res. Commun. Chem. Pathol. Pharmacol.*, 6:845–854.
5. Anders, M. W., and Latorre, J. P. (1970): High-speed ion exchange chromatography of barbiturates, diphenylhydantoin, and their hydroxylated metabolites. *Anal. Chem.*, 42:1430–1432.
6. Atkinson, A. J., MacGee, J., Strong, J., Garteiz, D., and Gaffney, T. E. (1970): Identification of 5-metahydroxyphenyl-5-phenylhydantoin as a metabolite of diphenyl-hydantoin. *Biochem. Pharmacol.*, 19:2483–2491.
7. Atwell, S. H., Green, V. A., and Haney, W. G. (1975): Development and evaluation of method for simultaneous determination of phenobarbital and diphenylhydantoin in plasma by high-pressure liquid chromatography. *J. Pharm. Sci.*, 64:806–809.
8. Baty, J. D., and Robinson, P. R. (1977): Single and multiple ion recording techniques for the analysis of diphenylhydantoin and its major metabolite in plasma. *Biomed. Mass Spectrom.*, 4:36–41.
9. Berlin, A., Agurell, S., Borga, O., Lund, L., and Sjoqvist, F. (1972): Micromethod for the determination of diphenylhydantoin in plasma and cerebrospinal fluid—A comparison between a gas chromatographic and a spectrophotometric method. *Scand. J. Clin. Lab. Invest.*, 29:281–287.
10. Bock, G. W., and Sherwin, A. L. (1971): The rapid quantitative determination of diphenylhydantoin in plasma, serum, and whole blood of patients with epilepsy. *Clin. Chim. Acta*, 34:97–103.
11. Booker, H. E., and Darcey, B. A. (1975): Enzymatic immunoassay vs. gas/liquid chromatography for determination of phenobarbital and diphenylhydantoin in serum. *Clin. Chem.*, 21:1766–1768.
12. Brien, J. E., and Inaba, T. (1974): Determination of low levels of 5,5-diphenylhydantoin in serum by gas-liquid chromatography. *J. Chromatogr.*, 88:265–270.
13. Brooks, M. A., de Silva, J. A. F., and Hackman,

M. R. (1973): The determination of phenobarbital and diphenylhydantoin in blood by differential pulse polarography. *Anal. Chim. Acta*, 64:165–175.

14. Castro, A., Ibanez, J., DiCesare, J. L., Adams, R. E., and Malkus, H. (1978): Comparative determination of phenytoin by spectrophotometry, gas chromatography, liquid chromatography, enzyme immunoassay, and radioimmunoassay. *Clin. Chem.*, 24:710–713.

15. Chamberlain, R. T., Stafford, D. T., Maijub, A. G., and McNatt, B. C. (1977): High-pressure liquid chromatography and enzyme immunoassay compared with gas chromatography for determining phenytoin. *Clin. Chem.*, 23:1764–1766.

16. Chang, T., and Glazko, A. J. (1968): Quantitative assay of 5,5-diphenylhydantoin (DPH) and 5-(p-hydroxyphenyl)-5-phenylhydantoin (HPPH) in plasma and urine of human subjects. *Clin. Res.*, 16:339.

17. Chang, T., and Glazko, A. J. (1970): Quantitative assay of 5,5-diphenylhydantoin (Dilantin) and 5-(p-hydroxyphenyl)-5-phenylhydantoin by gas-liquid chromatography. *J. Lab. Clin. Med.*, 75:145–155.

18. Chang, T., Okerholm, R. A., and Glazko, A. J. (1972): A 3-0-methylated metabolite of diphenylhydantoin (Dilantin) in rat urine. *Res. Commun. Chem. Pathol. Pharmacol.*, 4:13–23.

19. Chang, T., Okerholm, R. A., and Glazko, A. J. (1972): Identification of 5-(3,4-dihydroxy-phenyl)-5-phenylhydantoin: A metabolite of 5,5-diphenylhydantoin (Dilantin) in rat urine. *Anal. Lett.*, 195–202.

20. Chang, T., Savory, A., and Glazko, A. J. (1970): A new metabolite of 5,5-diphenylhydantoin (Dilantin). *Biochem. Biophys. Res. Commun.*, 38:444–449.

21. Cook, C. E. (1978): Radioimmunoassay. In: *Antiepileptic Drugs: Quantitative Analysis and Interpretation,* edited by C. E. Pippenger, J. K. Penry, and H. Kutt, pp. 163–173. Raven Press, New York.

22. Cook, C. E., Kepler, J. A., and Christensen, H. D. (1973): Antiserum to diphenylhydantoin: Preparation and characterization. *Res. Commun. Chem. Pathol. Pharmacol.*, 5:767–774.

23. Cremers, H. M. H. G., and Verheesen, P. E. (1973): A rapid method for the estimation of antiepileptic drugs in blood serum by gas-liquid chromatography. *Clin. Chim. Acta*, 48:413–420.

24. Dill, W. A., Baukema, J., Chang, T., and Glazko, A. J. (1971): Colorimetric assay of 5,5-diphenylhydantoin (Dilantin) and 5-(p-hydroxyphenyl)-5-phenylhydantoin. *Proc. Soc. Exp. Biol. Med.*, 137:674–679.

25. Dill, W. A., Chucot, L., Chang, T., and Glazko, A. J. (1971): Simplified benzophenone procedure for determination of diphenylhydantoin in plasma. *Clin. Chem.*, 17:1200–1201.

26. Dill, W. A., and Glazko, A. J. (1972): Fluorometric assay of diphenylhydantoin in plasma or whole blood. *Clin. Chem.*, 18:675–676.

27. Dill, W. A., Kazenko, A., Wolf, L. M., and Glazko, A. J. (1956): Studies on 5,5-diphenylhy-

dantoin (Dilantin) in animals and man. *J. Pharmacol. Exp. Ther.*, 118:270–279.

28. Dill, W. A., Leung, A., Kinkel, A., and Glazko, A. J. (1976): Simplified fluorometric assay for diphenylhydantoin in plasma. *Clin. Chem.*, 22:908–911.

29. Dorrity, F., Jr., and Linnoila, M. (1976): Rapid gas-chromatographic measurement of anticonvulsant drugs in serum. *Clin. Chem.*, 22:860–862.

30. Driessen, O., and Emonds, A. (1974): Simultaneous determination of anti-epileptic drugs in small samples of blood plasma by gas chromatography, column technology and extraction procedure. *Proc. Kon. Med. Acad. von Wetenschr.*, C77:171–181.

31. Driessen, O., and Emonds, A. Routine analysis of 5-(p-hydroxyphenyl)-5-phenyl-hydantoin in plasma. *Proc. Kon. Med. Acad. von Wetenschr.*, C78:449–460.

32. Dudley, K. H. (1978): Internal standards in gas-liquid chromatographic determination of antiepileptic drugs. In: *Antiepileptic Drugs: Quantitative Analysis and Interpretation,* edited by C. E. Pippenger, J. K. Penry, and H. Kutt, pp. 19–34. Raven Press, New York.

33. Estas, A., and Dumont, P. A. Simultaneous determination of 5,5-diphenylhydantoin and 5-(-hydroxyphenyl)-5-phenylhydantoin in serum, urine and tissues by gas-liquid chromatography after flash-heater methylation. *J. Chromatogr.*, 82:307–314.

34. Evans, J. E. (1973): Simultaneous measurement of diphenylhydantoin and phenobarbital in serum by high performance liquid chromatography. *Anal. Chem.*, 45:2428–2429.

35. Fellenberg, A. J., Magarey, A., and Pollard, A. C. (1975): An improved benzophenone procedure for the micro-determination of 5,5-diphenylhydantoin in blood. *Clin. Chim. Acta*, 59:155–160.

36. Friel, P., and Troupin, A. S. Flash-heater ethylation of some antiepileptic drugs. *Clin. Chem.*, 21:751–754.

37. Giovanniello, T. J., and Pecci, J. Simultaneous isothermal determination of diphenylhydantoin and phenobarbital serum levels by gas-liquid chromatography following flash-heater hexylation. *Clin. Chim. Acta*, 67:7–13.

38. Glazko, A. J. (1972): Diphenylhydantoin: Chemistry and methods of determination. *Antiepileptic Drugs*, 1st edition, edited by D. M. Woodbury, J. K. Penry, and R. P. Schmidt, pp. 103–112. Raven Press, New York.

38a. Glazko, A. J. (1982): Diphenylhydantoin: Chemistry and methods of determination. *Antiepileptic Drugs*. 2nd edition, edited by D. M. Woodbury, J. K. Penry, and C. E. Pippenger, pp. 177–189. Raven Press, New York.

39. Glazko, A. J., Peterson, F. E., Smith, T. C., Dill, W. A., and Chang, T. (1980): Phenytoin metabolism in human subjects with short and long plasma half-lives. *Fed. Proc.*, 39:1099.

40. Grimmer, G., Jacob, J., and Schafer, H. (1969): Die gaschromatographische Bestimmung von 5,5-diphenylhydantoin und 5-(p-Hydroxyphenyl)-5-

phenylhydantoin im *Blut. Arzneim. Forsch.*, 19:1287–1290.

41. Hammer, R. H., Wilder, B. J., Streiff, R. R., and Mayersdorf, A. (1971): Flash methylation and GLC of diphenylhydantoin and 5-(*p*-hydroxyphenyl)-5-phenylhydantoin. *J. Pharm. Sci.*, 60:327–329.

42. Helmsing, P. J., Van Der Woude, J., Van Eupen, O. M. (1978): A micromethod for simultaneous estimation of blood levels of some commonly used antiepileptic drugs. *Clin. Chim. Acta*, 89:301–309.

43. Hermansson, J., and Karlen, B. (1977): Assay of the major (4-hydroxylated) metabolite of diphenylhydantoin in human urine by reversed-phase high-performance liquid chromatography. *J. Chromatogr.*, 130:422–425.

44. Hill, R. E., and Latham, A. N. (1977): Simultaneous determination of anticonvulsant drugs by gas-liquid chromatography. *J. Chromatogr.*, 131:341–346.

45. Hoppel, C., Garle, M., and Elander, M. (1976): Mass fragmentographic determination of diphenylhydantoin and its main metabolite, 5-(4-hydroxylphenyl)-5-phenylhydantoin, in human plasma. *J. Chromatogr.*, 116:53–61.

46. Horning, M. G., Lertratanangkoon, K., Nowlin, J., Stillwell, W. G., Stillwell, R. N., Zion, T. E., Kellaway, P., and Hill, R. M. Anticonvulsant drug monitoring by GC-MS-COM techniques. *J. Chromatogr. Sci.*, 12:630–635.

47. Inaba, T., and Brien, J. F. (1973): Determination of the major urinary metabolite of diphenylhydantoin by high-performance liquid chromatography. *J. Chromatogr.*, 80:161–165.

48. Ishiguro, T., Kozatani, J., and Otsuka, A. (1955): Absorption of carbon dioxide on diphenylhydantoin sodium hydrates. *J. Pharm. Soc. Jpn.*, 75:1556–1559.

49. Ishiguro, T., Kozatani, J., and Shibata, K. (1958): Physico-chemical studies of sodium salts of diphenylhydantoin hydrates VI. Hydroscopic behavior and dissociation pressure of diphenylhydantoin sodium hydrates. *J. Pharm. Soc. Jpn.*, 391–394.

50. Janz, D., and Schmidt, D. (1974): Comparison of spectrophotometric and gas-liquid chromatographic measurements of serum diphenylhydantoin concentrations in epileptic out-patients. *J. Neurol.*, 207:109–116.

51. Kabra, P. M., Gotelli, G., Stanfill, R., and Marton, L. J. (1976): Simultaneous measurement of phenobarbital, diphenylhydantoin, and primidone in blood by high-pressure liquid chromatography. *Clin. Chem.*, 22:824–827.

52. Kabra, P. M., and Marton, L. J. (1976): High-pressure liquid-chromatographic determination of 5-(4-hydroxyphenyl)-5-phenylhydantoin in human urine. *Clin. Chem.*, 22:1672–1674.

53. Kabra, P. M., Stafford, B. E., and Marton, L. J. (1977): Simultaneous measurement of phenobarbital, phenytoin, primidone, ethosuximide and carbamazepine in serum by high-pressure liquid chromatography. *Clin. Chem.*, 23:1284–1288.

54. Kampa, I. S., Jarzabek, J., and Hundertmark, J. M. (1978): A comparison of the "EMIT" assay with two iodinated radioimmunoassays for diphenylhydantoin. *Clin. Biochem.*, 11:167–168.

55. Karlen, B., Garle, M., Rane, A., Gutova, M., and Lindborg, B. (1975): Assay of the major (4-hydroxylated) metabolites of diphenylhydantoin in human urine. *Eur. J. Clin. Pharmacol.*, 8:359–366.

56. Kupferberg, H. J. (1970): Quantitative estimation of diphenylhydantoin, primidone and phenobarbital in plasma by gas-liquid chromatography. *Clin. Chim. Acta*, 29:283–288.

57. Latham, A. N., and Varlow, G. (1976): Simultaneous quantitative gas-chromatographic analysis of ethosuximide, phenobarbitone, primidone and diphenylhydantoin. *Br. J. Clin. Pharmacol.*, 3:145–150.

58. Lehrer, M., and Karmen, A. (1976): Chemical ionization mass spectrometry for rapid assay of drugs in serum. *J. Chromatogr.*, 126:615–623.

59. MacGee, J. (1970): Rapid determination of diphenylhydantoin in blood plasma by gas-liquid chromatography. *Anal. Chem.*, 42:421–422.

60. Malkus, H., DiCesare, J. L., Meola, J. M., Pippenger, C. E., Ibanez, J., and Castro, A. (1978): Evaluation of EMIT methods for the determination of the five major antiepileptic drugs in an automated kinetic analyzer. *Clin. Biochem.*, 11:139–142.

61. Meijer, J. W. A. (1971): Simultaneous quantitative determination of anti-epileptic drugs, including carbamazepine, in body fluids. *Epilepsia*, 12:341–352.

62. Meulenhoff, J. S., Lojenga, J. C. K. (1972): Details of the Wallace method for the determination of phenytoin in blood, plasma and serum. *Pharm. Weekbl.*, 107:737–744.

63. Midah, K. K., McGilveray, I. J., and Wilson, D. L. (1976): Sensitive GLC procedure for simultaneous determination of phenytoin and its major metabolite from plasma following single doses of phenytoin. *J. Pharm. Sci.*, 65:1240–1243.

64. Morrison, L. D., O'Donnell, C. M. (1974): Determination of diphenylhydantoin by phosphorescence spectrometry. *Anal. Chem.*, 46:1119–1120.

65. Morselli, P. L. (1970): An improved technique for routine determinations of diphenylhydantoin in plasma and tissues. *Clin. Chim. Acta*, 28:37–40.

66. Orme, M. l'E., Borga, O., Cooke, C. E., and Sjoqvist, F. (1976): Measurement of diphenylhydantoin in 0.1-ml plasma samples: Gas chromatography and radioimmunoassay compared. *Clin. Chem.*, 22:246–249.

67. Perchalski, R. J., Scott, K. N., Wilder, R. J., and Hammer, R. H. (1973): Rapid, simultaneous GLC determination of phenobarbital, primidone and diphenylhydantoin. *J. Pharm. Sci.*, 62:1735–1736.

68. Perchalski, R. J., and Wilder, B. J. (1974): GLC microdetermination of plasma anticonvulsant levels. *J. Pharm. Sci.*, 63:806–807.

69. Pesh-Imam, M., Fretthold, D. W., Sunshine, I., Kumar, S., Terrentine, S., and Willis, C. E. (1979): High-pressure liquid chromatography for simul-

taneous analysis of anticonvulsants: Comparison with EMIT system. *Ther. Drug Monit.,* 1:289–299.

70. Pippenger, C. E., and Gillen, H. W. (1969): Gas chromatographic analysis for anticonvulsant drugs in biological fluids. *Clin. Chem.,* 15:582–590.

71. Rane, A., Garle, M., Borga, O., and Sjoqvist, F. (1974): Plasma disappearance of transplacentally transferred diphenylhydantoin in the newborn studied by mass fragmentography. *Clin. Pharmacol. Ther.,* 15:39–45.

72. Ritz, D. P., and Warren, C. G. (1975): Single extraction GLC analysis of six commonly prescribed antiepileptic drugs. *Clin. Toxicol.,* 8:311–324.

73. Rutherford, D. M., and Flanagan, R. J. (1978): Rapid micro-method for the measurement of phenobarbitone, primidone and phenytoin in blood plasma or serum by gas-liquid chromatography. *J. Chromatogr.,* 157:311–320.

74. Sabih, K., and Sabih, K. (1969): Gas chromatographic method for determination of diphenylhydantoin blood level. *Anal. Chem.,* 41:1452–1454.

75. Saitoh, Y., Nishigara, K., Nakagawa, F., and Suzuki, T. (1973): Improved microdetermination for diphenylhydantoin in blood by UV spectrophotometry. *J. Pharm. Sci.,* 62:206–210.

76. Sampson, D., Harasymiv, I., and Hensley, W. J. (1971): Gas chromatographic assay of underivatized 5,5-diphenylhydantoin (Dilantin) in plasma extracts. *Clin. Chem.,* 17:382–385.

77. Schottelius, D. D. (1978): Homogeneous immunoassay system (EMIT) for quantitation of antiepileptic drugs in biological fluids. In: *Antiepileptic Drugs: Quantitative Analysis and Interpretation,* edited by C. E. Pippenger, J. K. Penry, and H. Kutt, pp. 95–108. Raven Press, New York.

78. Schwartz, P. A., Rhodes, C. T., and Cooper, J. W., Jr. (1977): Solubility and ionization characteristics of phenytoin. *J. Pharm. Sci.,* 66:994–997.

79. Schweizer, K., Wick, H., and Brechbuhler, T. (1978): An improved method for preparation of samples for the simultaneous assay of some antiepileptic drugs by gas-liquid chromatography. *Clin. Chim. Acta,* 90:203–208.

80. Serfontein, W. J., de Villiers, L. S. (1977): Quantitative gas chromatographic analysis of barbiturates and hydantoins with quaternary ammonium hydroxides. *J. Chromatogr.,* 130:342–345.

81. Slonek, J. E., Peng, G. W., and Chiou, W. L. (1978): Rapid and micro high-pressure liquid chromatographic determination of plasma phenytoin levels. *J. Pharm. Sci.,* 67:1462–1464.

82. Soldin, S. J., and Hill, J. G. (1976): Rapid micromethod for measuring anticonvulsant drugs in serum by high-performance liquid chromatography. *Clin. Chem.,* 22:856–859.

83. Solow, E. B., and Green, J. B. (1972): The simultaneous determination of multiple anticonvulsant drug levels by gas-liquid chromatography. *Neurology (Minneap.),* 22:540–550.

84. Solow, E. B., Metaxas, J. M., and Summers, T. R. (1974): Antiepileptic drugs: A current assessment of simultaneous determination of multiple drug therapy by gas liquid chromatography on-col-umn methylation. *J. Chromatogr. Sci.,* 12:256–260.

85. Soo Ik Lee, and Bass, N. H. (1970): Microassay of diphenylhydantoin. Blood and regional brain concentrations in rats during acute intoxication. *Neurology (Minneap.),* 20:115–124.

86. Spiehler, V., Sun, L., Miyada, D. S., Sarandis, S., and Jessen, B. (1976): Radioimmunoassay, enzyme immunoassay, spectrophotometry, and gas-liquid chromatography compared for determination of phenobarbital and diphenylhydantoin. *Clin. Chem.,* 22:749–753.

87. Svensmark, O., and Kristensen, P. (1963): Determination of diphenylhydantoin and phenobarbital in small amounts of serum. *J. Lab. Clin. Med.,* 61:501–507.

88. Thoma, J. J., Ewald, T., and McCoy, M. (1978): Simultaneous analysis of underivatized phenobarbital carbamazepine, primidone, and phenytoin by isothermal gas-liquid chromatography. *J. Anal. Toxicol.,* 2:219–225.

89. Thurkow, I., Wesseling, H., and Meijer, D. K. F. (1972): Estimation of phenytoin in body fluids in the presence of sulfonyl urea compounds. *Clin. Chim. Acta,* 37:509–513.

90. Tigelaar, R. E., Rapport, R. L., Inman, J. K., and Kupferberg, H. J. (1973): A radioimmunoassay for diphenylhydantoin. *Clin. Chim. Acta,* 43:231–241.

91. Toseland, P. A., Albani, M., and Gauchel, F. D. (1975): Organic nitrogen-selective detector used in gas-chromatographic determination of some anticonvulsant and barbiturate drugs in plasma and tissues. *Clin. Chem.,* 21:98–103.

92. Van Meter, J. C., Buckmaster, H. S., and Shelley, L. L. (1970): Concurrent assay of phenobarbital and diphenylhydantoin in plasma by vapor-phase chromatography. *Clin. Chem.,* 16:135–138.

93. Vessman, J., Hartvig, P., and Stromberg, S. (1970): Gas chromatography and electron capture detection of benzophenone formed by chromic acid oxidation. Part 3. Applications in the determination of gem-diphenyl–substituted compounds. *Acta Pharm. Suec.,* 7:373–388.

94. Wallace, J. E. (1966): Spectrophotometric determination of diphenylhydantoin. *J. Forensic Sci.,* 11:552–559.

95. Wallace, J., Biggs, J., and Dahl, E. V. (1965): Determination of diphenylhydantoin by ultraviolet spectrophotometry. *Anal. Chem.,* 37:410–413.

96. Wallace, J. E., and Hamilton, H. E. (1974): Diphenylhydantoin microdetermination in serum and plasma by UV spectrophotometry. *J. Pharm. Sci.,* 63:1795–1798.

97. Witkin, K. M., Bius, D. L., Teague, B. L., Wiese, L. S., Boyles, L. W., and Dudley, K. H. (1979): Determination of 5-(*p*-hydroxyphenyl)-5-phenylhydantoin and studies relating to the disposition of phenytoin in man. *Ther. Drug Monitor.,* 1:11–34.

98. Wong, R. C., Burd, J. E., Carrico, R. J., Buckler, R. T., Thoma, J., and Boguslaski, R. C. (1979): Substrate-labeled fluorescent immunoassay for phenytoin in human serum. *Clin. Chem.,* 25:686–691.

99. Leppick, I. E., Oles, K. S., Sheehan, M. L., Penry, J. K., Parker, D. R., Gallagher, T. K., Caron, G. P., Rosenfeld, F. W., and Salomon, J. J. (1989): Phenytoin and phenobarbital concentration in serum: A comparison of Ames Seralyzer with GLC, TDX, and EMIT. *Ther. Drug Monitor.*, 11:73–78.

100. Cramer, J., Mattson, R., Gallagher, B., King, B. W., Wannamaker, B., Denio, L., Shellenberger, M. K., Haibukewych, D., Splane, M. L., Vasos, B., and Searcy, J. (1986): Whole blood/plasma ratio and clinical performance of a non-instituted assay for phenytoin. *Neurol.*, 36: (Suppl. 1)84.

Antiepileptic Drugs, Third Edition, edited by
R. Levy, R. Mattson, B. Meldrum,
J. K. Penry, and F. E. Dreifuss.
Raven Press, Ltd., New York © 1989.

11

Phenytoin

Absorption, Distribution, and Excretion

Dixon M. Woodbury

The many sites at which phenytoin (PHT) acts, its receptors, must be reached before its action can take place. This involves movement of PHT from the site of entrance into the body into the blood stream (absorption), distribution in blood and extracellular fluids to the cell boundaries, and passage across the cell membranes into cells and across subcellular membranes into subcellular organelles. The amount of PHT that reaches the receptor and its duration of stay there depend on its rate of biotransformation and excretion from the body. The absorption, distribution, and excretion of PHT in the body and the factors that affect these processes are of obvious clinical importance, for therapy with the drug is useless if sufficient drug does not reach its site of action. Knowledge and proper use of this information will often change a therapeutic failure into a success.

ABSORPTION

The absorption of PHT from its site of entrance into the body (e.g., oral or intramuscular), as is the case with other drugs, depends on the following factors: its pK_a and lipid solubility, the pH of the medium in which PHT is dissolved, its solubility in the medium, and its concentration. These factors are frequently altered by the pres-

ence of certain foods or drugs in the intestinal tract and by the formulations employed. The latter is of particular importance, since aqueous liquids of the pure chemical are commonly employed in the laboratory, whereas more complex formulations of liquids, capsules, and tablets are employed clinically. As is well known, the chemical form employed, the particle size, the filler and masking agents used in the clinical formulation, and the tablet hardness, all of which can affect dissolution rate, have a marked effect on the absorption of PHT from the gastrointestinal tract.

In the stomach, little absorption of PHT occurs because it is insoluble at the pH of gastric juice (about 2.0). Thus, despite the fact that at the reported pK_a of 8.31 (20, see also 61) PHT exists predominantly in the un-ionized form and should be absorbed readily by passive diffusion, it achieves only a very low concentration in the gastric juice and consequently is only poorly and slowly absorbed (20). The simultaneous administration of PHT and an antacid decreases the absorption of PHT and thereby decreases the plasma drug level below the value it would normally attain.

On passage into the duodenum where the pH is approximately 7 to 7.5, more of the drug exists in the ionized form and hence is considerably more soluble in the intestinal fluid. The bile salts also increase the solu-

TABLE 1. *Absorption of PHT[a] from isolated segments of rat gastrointestinal tract*

Segment injected	Plasma PHT level (μg/ml)
Stomach	0.6
Upper small intestine	3.8
Lower small intestine	1.5
Caecum	0.9
Large intestine	0.7

[a] 100 mg placed in each section; plasma PHT levels determined 4 hr after dosage.
After Dill et al. (20), with permission.

bility of the drug. In addition, the surface area for absorption is much larger in the duodenum and vascularity and blood flow are higher. Thus, absorption can take place rapidly, and it is at this site that the maximum absorption of PHT occurs. Absorption from the jejunum and ileum is slower than from the duodenum and is poor from the colon (70,91). Rectal absorption does not occur (70). The distal portion of the duodenum is also the site of maximum reabsorption of PHT after its intravenous injection (76). As shown in Table 1, 4 hr after 100 mg of PHT was injected into the isolated stomach, Dill et al. (20) demonstrated that the plasma contained 0.6 μg/ml of PHT, whereas with the drug in the upper and lower small intestine, the plasma levels were 3.8 and 1.5 μg/ml, respectively. Lesser amounts, 0.9 and 0.7 μg/ml, appeared in the plasma when the same dose was placed in the caecum and large intestine, respectively. These observations support the fact that PHT is relatively insoluble at the pH of the gastric juice and that significant absorption does not take place until the drug reaches the upper part of the small intestine. However, PHT can rapidly cross the intestinal wall in both directions in all portions of the intestinal tract (76).

Even at the higher pH of the intestinal fluid, PHT is relatively insoluble, and its rate of absorption depends mainly on the rate at which it can enter the blood stream, as discussed below. At pH 7.8 and 37°C,

PHT is soluble in intestinal fluid to the extent of about 100 μg/ml. In man, the usual single oral dose is 100 mg, and this is distributed only in a maximum of 1,000 ml of intestinal fluid even if complete mixing occurs. Since it is soluble to the extent of only 100 μg/ml, and the amount of fluid in which it is actually dissolved is much less than 1,000 ml, some is left undissolved. This remaining portion can be solubilized only after that already in solution is absorbed, a process that is limited by the fact the solubility of PHT in plasma is only 75 μg/ml at 37°C. Thus, absorption can occur only at the rate at which PHT is removed from the blood stream by storage in fat, binding to plasma and tissue constituents, biotransformation by liver, and excretion into bile or urine. Since most of the PHT in solution is in the un-ionized form and is relatively lipid soluble (log octanol/water partition coefficient, 2.23), it is readily absorbed across the lipid membranes of the mucosal cells of the intestinal tract; hence, passage across these cells is not a limiting factor. Dissolution in the gastrointestinal fluids is the rate-limiting process in the absorption of PHT.

The results of experiments in rats and mice (117) show that there is a linear relationship between the percent of PHT absorbed and the dose of drug placed in isolated intestinal loops. Absorption was virtually 100% complete within 90 min in both species when the concentration of PHT was 100 μg/ml. With solutions of 500 μg/ml and above, there was a linear relationship between the log dose placed in the loops and the percent absorbed. Thus, it would appear that the rate of absorption in the two species is the same.

After oral doses of 5 to 250 mg/kg of PHT were given to rats and mice, the plasma drug levels in the rats were always considerably lower than those of the mice. A dose-effect relationship between plasma drug levels of PHT and oral dosage was noted for mice but not for rats, where the levels reached a plateau with dosages above 66 mg/kg. It is likely that this plateau represents a dose range at which PHT is saturating the intestinal fluids and has reached the limit of solubility. Thus, the plateau represents an equilibration between the stabilizing of the PHT in the gastrointestinal tract and absorption into the plasma at a rate determined by the factors mentioned above, of which metabolism by the liver and protein binding are probably most important, since the former is faster and the latter larger in the rat than in the mouse. These differences between rats and mice can explain the greater LD_{50} (median lethal dose) and TD_{50} (median toxic dose) in rats than in mice.

Thus, any factor that interferes with the dissolution of PHT or its solubility in intestinal fluids will delay its absorption. For example, the formulation of PHT preparations for oral use is important, as documented by Glazko and Chang (35). They compared in dogs the absorption of different size particles of PHT. The dissolution rate of the large particles was slower than the small ones; hence, the plasma levels were correspondingly different. That these factors are important in humans was demonstrated by reports from Australia (25,86,106) that a large number of patients showed toxicity with usual doses of PHT given to epileptics because the formulation of the PHT in the capsules given the patients had been changed. The usual capsules contained PHT with an excipient of calcium sulfate, whereas the capsules that produced toxicity in the same dose had lactose as an excipient. Changing back to the usual preparation restored normal plasma drug levels, and the toxic manifestations disappeared. Obviously, the excipient blocked the absorption of the drug by an as yet unknown mechanism. However, in another study (84) in which different brands of PHT were compared in epileptic patients, no significant differences in serum levels were found. Although earlier studies (1,64) had shown that phenytoin sodium in capsules was better absorbed and produced higher plasma drug levels than did phenytoin acid tablets, subsequent reports (49,103) have shown that equivalent oral doses of either phenytoin acid or phenytoin sodium produce equivalent plasma concentrations, providing that high-quality formulations were administered. High quality formulations generally have a proper size and form of phenytoin crystals that are optimum for absorption, since these factors appears to be of major importance for bioavailability of this drug. Thus, Glazko (34) showed that phenytoin acid in microcrystalline suspension was completely absorbed after oral dosage, whereas the amorphous form is generally poorly and erratically absorbed. Thus, bioavailability of the drug is variable, and it is advisable when using this drug that the physician not change preparations once the dose and steady-state plasma level have been established. It is evident, therefore, that in humans the rate of absorption (rate constant, k_a) of PHT is somewhat irregular, not first order, and prolonged (50).

Studies on the bioavailability of PHT have shown that the drug is absorbed nonlinearly and, therefore, that bioavailability must be measured by methods that employ nonlinear pharmacokinetics as described by Martis and Levy (68) and applied to PHT by Jusko and colleagues (50,51).

Utilizing the data of Lund et al. (65) from patients in whom serum concentrations of PHT were compared on intravenous and oral administration of 4.6 mg/kg of this drug, Jusko and colleagues (50,51) showed that absorption of PHT was not uniform and that the data could be fitted by nonlinear kinetics. Thus, on oral administration there was an initial absorption peak at 4 to 7 hr and a secondary peak of 8 to 15 hr after injection of PHT. Thereafter, the absorption continued for a prolonged period of about 2 days. The decline was much flatter with the orally administered drug than with the intravenous administered drug. In intoxicated patients, gastrointestinal absorption of PHT continued for as long as 60 hr after ingestion (110). The secondary absorption peak was assumed to result from dissolution of an appreciable fraction of the residual dosage form when food was ingested. Estimation of the bioavailability of PHT by linear (comparative areas under the plasma concentration-versus-time curves after intravenous and oral administration) and nonlinear calculations showed that the linear method yielded a mean bioavailability estimate of 0.87, whereas the nonlinear method generated a mean value of 0.98 (50,51). Thus, the direct use of area ratios underestimates the essentially complete absorption of PHT from oral capsules. This is explained by the fact that the intravenous route produces an initially higher serum concentration because of the saturation kinetics of these drugs, and this causes a more prolonged retention of phenytoin in the body and produces a slightly larger area value for the intravenous dose.

Therefore, linear (area values) kinetics for bioavailability studies with PHT preparations can be applied only when the study is carried out at relatively low dosages where such kinetics are present. This value for PHT in normal subjects represents an absorption half-life of about 8 hr, but studies are difficult to carry out because the K_m of PHT is small and highly variable (3.4 mg/kg), as discussed below. However, Gugler et al. (41) found that the $T\frac{1}{2}$ for absorption was 1.62 hr.

Kutt et al. (55) reported one case of a defect in gastrointestinal absorption of PHT. In this patient, plasma levels of PHT remained below 1 μg/ml on daily administration of 300 mg given orally; the urinary excretion of the major metabolite of PHT, 5-(p-hydrophenyl)-5-phenylhydantoin (HPPH), was also low (14% of ingested dose). Intravenous injection produced a rise in the plasma level after 5 days to 42 μg/ml, and excretion of HPPH increased to over 60% of the injected dose. During oral administration, large amounts of PHT were recovered from feces. Absorption of other drugs such as salicylates, sulfonamides, and tetracyclines was not impaired, and there was no evidence of malabsorption of fat and carbohydrate. The mechanism of this defect has not been elucidated.

In humans, after oral administration of a single dose, peak blood drug levels are generally reached between 4 and 8 hr after administration, although the peak may be reached as early as 3 hr and as late as 12 hr after ingestion of the drug (20,80). The time of peak effect appears to be independent of the dose. The levels may remain at the peak values for 24 hr.

In newborns and in younger infants (up to 3 months of age), PHT appears to be absorbed very slowly and incompletely after both oral and intramuscular administration (48). In older infants and children, in contrast, the drug is absorbed very efficiently by the oral route, with peak plasma levels usually attained 2 to 6 hr after dosing (11,108).

The absorption of PHT from the gut can be delayed and reduced by concurrent administration of phenobarbital (74,104). Phenytoin is absorbed more slowly when injected intramuscularly than when it is given orally (18,111,112). This is because of its poor water solubility which makes it act as a repository preparation because of deposition of PHT crystals in the muscle. This causes hemorrhagic areas around the crystals (112). It is absorbed only as the free drug is cleared from the plasma by binding to plasma proteins, distribution and binding in tissues, storage in fat, biotransformation in liver, and excretion. If PHT must be given parenterally, it should be administered intravenously rather than intramuscularly. However, brief periods of intramuscular administration after the steady-state has been reached can be used without alterations in serum levels (13,111) because over a 5-day period, complete absorption of the precipitated drug in the muscle does take place (54). The plasma concentration attained after intramuscular administration fits a pharmacokinetic model derived from precipitation and redissolution of PHT at the intramuscular injection site (see 50 for discussion).

DISTRIBUTION

Plasma Binding

On entering the circulatory system, PHT is rapidly and reversibly bound to proteins. The percent bound to protein for different species is shown in Table 2. In man, the average is about 90% (69% to 96%) at 37°C (44,66). The percent bound varies little with plasma concentration, but in the clinically occurring plasma concentration range (5 to 50 μg/ml), there is a small increase in the unbound fraction of PHT with increasing total concentration (19,66). Newborn infants exhibit significantly lower protein binding of PHT than do adults (26,89), as do newborn kittens (28). Binding is even less in fetuses (26). The percent bound decreases (percent unbound increases) with age in normal individuals (90.1% at 17 years and 87.3% bound at 53 years) (44). Binding in males (89.4%) does not differ from binding in females (89%). Binding is directly correlated with plasma albumin and total bilirubin (44). There is probably competition between PHT and endogenous bilirubin for binding sites on the albumin molecule. A Scatchard plot of PHT binding indicates that PHT is bound to several sites on the plasma proteins. At therapeutic concentrations of PHT (<20 μg/ml), one or several sites seem to be involved (66).

Previous studies in neonatal animals had suggested a reciprocal relationship between the unbound fraction of PHT and the albumin level in plasma (89) and indicated that PHT was bound to serum albumin. However, proof of this was not forthcoming

until the studies of Lightfoot and Christian (62). They identified by radioimmunoelectrophoresis of human serum that PHT is bound to albumin and two α-globulin proteins that are identical to those to which thyroxine is bound (see also 73,78). However, unlike thyroxine, PHT is not bound to prealbumin. The observed affinity of both PHT and thyroxine for albumin and the two α-globulins is direct confirmation of previous studies (27,63,81–83,100,113) reporting competition among thyroxine, triiodothyronine, and PHT for binding proteins. The failure of PHT to bind to prealbumin probably accounts for the ability of this drug to displace thyroxine from the thyroxine-binding globulin onto prealbumin (82,100,113); it also displaces thyroxine onto albumin. Fichsel and Knopfle (27) showed that long-term therapy with PHT in epileptic children produced considerable alterations in the thyroidal hormonal state. These consisted of dose-dependent decreases in protein-bound iodine, thyroxine, free thyroxine, triiodothyronine, and also a slight decrease in plasma thyrotropin (TSH). These were a result of displacement of thyroxine and triiodothyronine from their plasma protein binding sites as well as a more rapid conversion and metabolism of thyroxine and triiodothyronine induced by PHT. The decreased TSH was also partly a result of PHT-induced inhibition of TRH release from the hypothalamus. Carbon dioxide decreases the binding power of the α-globulins and presumably therefore decreases the ability of both thyroxine and PHT to bind to them (83).

In addition to thyroxine and triiodothyronine, other drugs bind to these same proteins and compete for the binding sites. Thus, valproic acid, salicylic acid, phenylbutazone, sulfafurazol, and acetazolamide, in concentrations that may be obtained clinically, compete with PHT for these sites and displace it (66,73). Also, endogenous compounds such as fatty acids and bilirubin in the neonate displace PHT from plasma pro-

TABLE 2. Plasma and brain binding, CSF/plasma, brain/plasma and brain/CSF ratios, apparent volume of distribution (V_D), plasma half-life, K_m and V_{max} values of PHT in various species

Species	Protein binding Plasma (%)	Brain (%)	CSF to plasma	Brain to plasma	Brain to CSF	T_1 (hr)	V_D (liter/kg)	K_m (mg/liter)	V_{max} (mg/kg per day)	References
Humans	86 (73–93)		0.17							30,116,117
(4.4 → 6.5 → 13.6 mg/kg orally)						22 → 40 → 59	0.36–0.43			see 117
Normal adults								5.46	6.13	50
								6.77	6.07	33
								4.20	4.76	31
	88							14.40	16.3	4
	90.3		0.12	0.63	5.29	15.4[a]	0.775			38
	(86.9– 91.9)						0.724	11.54	10.3	67
Nonseizure adults (autopsy)										
Gyrus from temporal lobe				1.35						
Gyrus from parietal lobe				1.40						
Gyrus from frontal lobe				1.20						
Gyrus from frontal lobe (gray)				2.25						
Gyrus from frontal lobe (white)				1.37						
Cerebellar hemisphere				1.85						95
Midbrain				1.7						
Thoracic spinal cord				1.0						
Sciatic nerve				0.95						
Median nerve										
Epileptic adults (16.0 mg/kg i.v.)	88		0.12	0.75 (temporal lobe)	6.25	51	0.78			15
										107
	88		0.12	1.13	9.4					98
				gray 1.33	11.1					
				white			0.829	3.34	9.93	50
								14.5	10.9	4

										Ref.
Frontal lobe										
(gray)				1.0						
(white)				0.83						
Parietal lobe										
(gray)				0.90						98
(white)				1.51						
Temporal lobe										
(gray)				1.39						95
(white)				1.73						
Gyrus from temporal lobe				1.55						
lobe				1.73						
Gyrus from frontal lobe										
(gray)				1.73						
Gyrus from frontal lobe										
(white)				2.73						
Normal child				1.72		$6–8^a$	0.783	3.06	6.37	31 / see 117
Monkey, fetal				1.78						35
Dog	64		0.36	1.89	7.09					19
(20 → 50 mg/kg i.v.)	65		0.27 / 0.30	3.50	11.70	2.2 → 6.4	1.04			75 / 87
Cat										
Adult (15 mg/kg i.v.)	76.1	90.3	0.25	2.17	8.76	~72	1.49			28
Newborn (15 mg/kg i.v.)	69.3	84.3	0.32	1.82	5.78	>96	1.32			20
Rat (33 mg/kg i.p.)	80	86		1.35		3.4	1.30	~13		77
				1.50						69
				0.95						33 / 53
Mouse			0.16	1.42						69

^{a} Calculated from formula $T_1 \text{ (min)} = \dfrac{0.693 K_m}{V_{max}}$.

teins and are a potential source of drug interactions (29,40). When these substances (e.g., salicylates) are given, the level of free PHT in the blood increases and, conversely, when PHT is given, the plasma drug levels of free salicylate and thyroxine increase. The unbound fraction of PHT has been reported to increase between 16% and 200% in the presence of salicylate (66), an effect that takes place only with high doses of salicylate and is not clinically important (59). The increased free level increases the anticonvulsant effect of the drug which depends on the unbound drug concentration and not the total plasma concentration (97); it also allows more of the PHT to reach the liver per unit time, and increased biotransformation results, with a consequent more rapid decline in the level of the drug in the plasma. However, this is true only if the enzyme system in the liver that metabolizes PHT is not saturated. If the enzyme is saturated, as is often the case, the plasma half-life increases in the presence of these other drugs. Phenytoin binding is decreased in uremia (e.g., 84.2%) and in hepatic disease (e.g., 84.1%) (6,44,45,78,96) mainly because of the decrease in plasma proteins. It is not altered by oral contraceptives (44) but is decreased in late pregnancy (93). Shavit et al. (94) found that in women with seizures that were more frequent at the time of menstruation, their plasma phenytoin concentrations were also lower during this period then at the midcycle ovulatory phase. This was especially true in patients with high phenytoin concentrations consistent with a greater degree of saturation. This indicates that the female sex steroids compete with phenytoin for biotransformation by the liver microsomal enzymes. A review of PHT binding has been provided by Porter and Layzer (85).

Half-Life

The plasma half-life of PHT in the body is defined as the time it takes for the concentration of the drug in plasma, at the time of its peak level after multiple doses, to decline by 50%. This value is a measure of the rate of metabolism and excretion of the drug and varies quantitatively from species to species, as shown in Table 2. In humans, the half-life after oral administration of doses that result in therapeutic levels averages about 22 hr, with a range of 7.0 to 42.0 hr (3,20); the half-life after intravenous administration is shorter and ranges from 10 to 15 hr (36,101). This difference undoubtedly results from the slow rate of absorption of PHT from the gut, as discussed previously, which maintains the plasma concentration at a high level for a longer period of time.

However, since the half-life increases with dose and exhibits large individual variations, an average value is meaningless. For example, Cranford et al. (15) showed that after intravenous infusion of 15 to 18 mg/kg of PHT, the half-lives varied from 10 to 160 hr, with most values ranging from 20 to 70 hr. The distribution was bimodal, and the long half-lives probably occurred in patients with insufficient parahydroxylation, as originally described by Kutt et al. (57). Drugs that interfere with the metabolism of PHT by the liver (e.g., sulthiame, bishydroxycoumarin, sulfaphenazole, disulfiram, and phenyramidol, and simultaneous administration of p-aminosalicylate and isoniazid) increase its plasma half-life (42,43,56,79,99). Conversely, drugs that accelerate its metabolism by enzyme induction, e.g., phenobarbital (16), shorten its half-life under certain conditions as discussed in chapter 20. For example, sulthiame increased the half-life of a patient on PHT from 12 to 32 hr (42). Genetic factors such as inability of the liver to p-hydroxylate PHT also lengthen its half-life and increase blood levels (57). Although an earlier report (11) presents some evidence that children may metabolize PHT at a slower rate than do adults and that the half-life is longer, subsequent reports (see 74, also

9,14,17,21,22,23,24,31) clearly indicate that PHT is disposed at a faster rate in infants and children than in adults. The $T\frac{1}{2}$ in infants and childen is 1.2 to 16.1 hr at low doses but 11.6 to 31.5 hr at higher doses when plasma levels are between 10 and 20 $\mu g/ml$ (22). Thus, nonlinear (saturation) kinetics are present in newborns, infants, and children as well as adults. For example, in the first week of life, the apparent $T\frac{1}{2}$ of phenytoin ranges from 7 to 140 hr (see 24 for review). Younger children (<5–6 years of age) require larger doses per kilogram than do adults to reach therapeutic levels. Therefore, they have a lower plasma concentration-dose ratio than adults (8,88).

It is evident that an important determinant of PHT plasma half-life is the dose of the drug. In man (3), dog (42), and mouse (32), increasing the dose of PHT increases the plasma half-life (see Table 2). The dose dependency is best explained by saturation of a rate-limiting enzyme reaction in the metabolism of the drug. Saturation of the biotransformation enzymes can also explain the observed fact (3) that the PHT plasma fall-off curves at high doses are not first-order processes (linear on semilogarithmic paper), whereas they are at low doses before saturation occurs. At saturating doses, the curves are characteristic of a zero-order process (linear with time on rectangular paper). Arnold and Gerber (3) have shown that there is a wide variation in the rate of plasma decline of PHT in the population. This variation is probably caused by differences in liver drug-metabolizing activity, variation in the degree of dose dependency among individuals, differences in the plasma concentration of PHT at which enzyme induction may occur, or differences in the level at which rate limiting, drug-metabolizing enzyme reactions become saturated. Since the variability in the half-life of PHT is much less in identical twins than in fraternal twins, the individual variability has been attributed to genetic factors (2). The marked variation in plasma half-life of

PHT in individual patients emphasizes the importance of tailoring the dose of the drug to each patient and of monitoring the patient by measurement of plasma PHT levels.

The dose-dependent kinetics of PHT have been expressed in quantitative terms by using a nonlinear pharmacokinetic model (4,31,33,50,67). Such a model is able to predict plasma levels of the drug based on the dose given and the K_m, V_{max}, and V_D as obtained from experimental subjects. The equation used is based on Michaelis-Menten kinetics and is as follows:

$$[PHT] = \frac{K_m R}{(V_{max} - R)}$$

where R is the dosing rate in mg/kg per day, V_{max} is the maximum rate of metabolism of PHT in mg/kg per day, and K_m is the Michaelis-Menten constant equal to the plasma concentration in mg/liter at which the metabolic rate is one-half maximum. Values of K_m range around 6 to 12 mg/liter. Above these values, zero-order kinetics are more pronounced, and below them, first-order kinetics become more pronounced. The K_m values are usually lower and V_{max} values higher in children than in adults. The nonlinear elimination kinetics for phenytoin make it difficult to regulate the dose in 28% of children. This becomes worse when the K_m is below 2.5 $\mu g/ml$ which makes the dose versus concentration relationship through the therapeutic range very steep (14,22,23,24). However, pharmacogenetic and drug-interaction factors are more important in regulating phenytoin therapy than are age-related kinetic changes. It is evident from these pharmacokinetic data that a very small dosage increment of only 50 to 100 mg can produce an increase in steady-state plasma concentrations over a twofold to threefold range. Prediction of the adjustments needed to obtain proper therapeutic blood drug levels can be made from these equations. Nomograms to aid in calculation of dosage changes have been developed by Richens and Dunlop (92) and Martin et al. (67).

As already mentioned, induction of PHT drug-metabolizing enzyme activity by other drugs or by self-induction appears to occur and results in a decreased plasma half-life. However, this generally takes place only after long-term administration of doses large enough to exceed the saturation concentration of the enzymes; at low doses, PHT does not cause self-induction (12). Febrile illnesses can also alter phenytoin plasma half-life by enhancing biotransformation of the drug (10,39,60). This may result in a marked decrease in phenytoin concentration in serum.

On intravenous administration of PHT to humans (or animals), two components are observed in the plasma decay curve (101). The first component is very rapid and has a half-life of about 6 min and a volume of distribution (based on the free level of PHT in plasma) of 0.79 liters/kg (79%). This probably represents rapid distribution of PHT into extracellular space, cell water, and slight binding to subcellular constituents. The second component is slow and has a half-life of 9 hr. Its volume of distribution is 1.75 liters/kg (175%) and undoubtedly represents further binding to the endoplasmic reticulum in cells, since the binding to tissue fractions is greater than to plasma proteins. Distributions into the gastrointestinal tract via biliary excretion of the metabolites from the liver probably also accounts in part for the large volume of distribution of this component.

Volume of Distribution

Following absorption, PHT distributes freely in the body because at the pH of plasma (7.4) it exists predominantly in the un-ionized form, which allows rapid movement across cell membranes by the process of nonionic diffusion. Much of the drug that enters cells binds to subcellular fractions (see below). Within 15 min, the drug has reached its maximum volume of distribution. Values for V_D based on the total level in the plasma are shown in Table 2 and average about 0.78 liter/kg in humans. Since the free level is 10% of the total, the V_D based on the free level is 10 times higher. Thus, the drug is present in higher concentration in cells than in the extracellular fluid. This is due to avid binding in cells, storage in fat, and binding to plasma proteins. It can be seen in Table 2 that the binding of PHT to brain constituents of adult cats is 90% and 76% to plasma proteins. From the data presented in Fig. 1, it is evident that in rats PHT is present in brain, liver, muscle, and fat at a higher concentration than in plasma. This is also the case for the same tissues in mice and cats and in humans (47,71,98). The accumulation of PHT in tissues occurs mainly by binding, since the concentration of free PHT in all tissues of the body is the same as that in plasma, as shown for the cerebrospinal fluid (CSF) in Table 2.

Phenytoin also distributes into all transcellular fluids as the free form. These fluids include CSF (Table 2), saliva, semen, milk, gastrointestinal fluids, and bile (20,52,76, 77,102,105). Excretion in milk appears to follow saturation kinetics. Phenytoin also freely crosses the human placental barrier and reaches equilibrium between mother and fetus (5,71). The levels of the drug were found to be the same in mother's plasma, cord blood, and in the infant's serum at the time of delivery. Phenytoin also crosses the placenta in monkeys and in rats (109).

Bile contains mainly the metabolites of PHT which are formed in the liver and excreted in the bile. Most of the injected dose is excreted in the bile as metabolites, then enters the intestinal fluid and is subsequently reabsorbed into the blood and excreted in the urine (77). G. Ringham and D. M. Woodbury (*unpublished data*) demon-

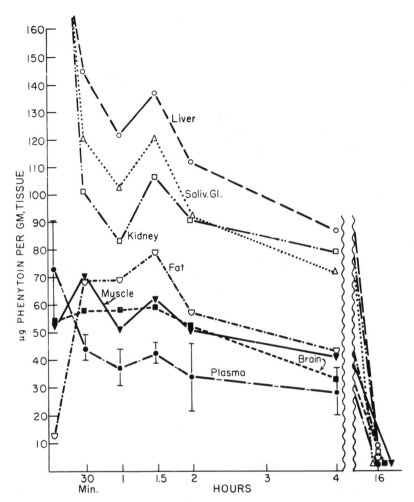

FIG. 1. Distribution of radioactive PHT in various tissues after intravenous administration of 22 mg of PHT labeled with 2-^{14}C-PHT. The ordinate is μg/g tissue, and the abscissa is time (hr) after administration. (From Noach et al., ref. 77, with permission.)

strated that in normal rats 60% of an injected dose of ^{14}C-PHT was excreted from the body in a 48-hr period; of this total, 46% was excreted in urine, and 14% excreted in feces. However, when the bile duct of the rat was cannulated and the bile collected over a 48-hr period, the total excretion (bile, urine, and feces) was 66% to 72%; the bile contained 43% of the injected radioactivity, whereas urine contained only 28%, and feces only 0.6%. Thus, the bile constitutes

a major route of initial excretion of the drug and its metabolites, although ultimately it is mainly excreted from the body in the urine after reabsorption from the intestinal tract.

The amount of PHT that appears in the bile, mainly as HPPH, is influenced by the levels of other drugs. For example, in rats, phenobarbital given acutely appears to compete with the hepatic enzymes and hydroxylates PHT and thereby reduces the rate at which HPPH enters the bile (114).

There is indirect evidence that this also occurs in humans.

Brain and CSF Distribution

The phenomenon of redistribution of PHT occurs after a single dose of the drug. This is analogous to the redistribution of thiopental to muscle and fat following a single dose. On intravenous injection in humans or intraperitoneal administration in rats (see Fig. 2), PHT, because of its high lipid solubility, rapidly enters the brain of either species and reaches a peak level in less than 15 min. However, the concentration immediately falls thereafter as the plasma level declines as a result of redistribution of the drug to binding, storage, or depot sites in other tissues (muscle, liver, fat, or lung). Consequently, the neurophysiological effects of the drug rapidly disappear. This redistribution phenomenon is important to recognize in the treatment of status epilepticus with intravenous PHT, as the seizures may recur unless additional drug is given after the initial dose. On continued administration of the drug, these sites are saturated, and the brain concentration again increases, paralleling the increase in the plasma level; within 4 to 5 days it reaches a steady-state level. This is why it takes several days for a therapeutic plasma drug level of PHT to be reached when therapy is first initiated. However, the steady-state level can be reached rap-

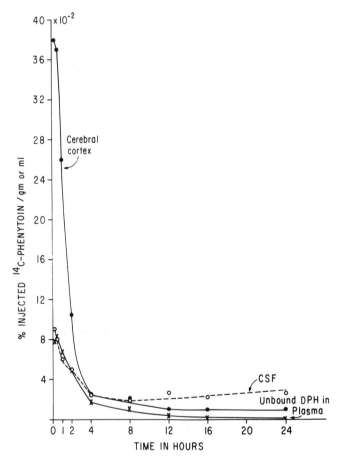

FIG. 2. Distribution of ^{14}C-PHT in plasma, cerebral cortex, and CSF as a function of time in rats. Ordinate is percent of injected dose of ^{14}C-PHT/g wet brain tissue or ml of plasma and CSF, and abscissa is time (hr). The values for plasma represent the free levels of the drug and not the total amount. (From Woodbury and Swinyard, ref. 117, with permission.)

idly by initial administration of loading doses.

The concentration of PHT in brain is about one to three times the concentration of total drug in the plasma and about six to 10 times the concentration of the free drug in plasma (20,28,53,75,77,109). This is a result of binding to various subcellular fractions of brain cells (53, see 115 for review of this aspect).

Preferential accumulation of PHT in the superior and inferior colliculus, amygdala, and hippocampus, compared with 16 other areas of the brain, was observed in dogs and cats receiving PHT at an oral dose of 10 mg/kg for 14 to 16 months (75). The functional significance of this differential distribution in brain is not yet clear. The simultaneous uptake of PHT into the CSF and brain of dogs has been evaluated (87). Two components of uptake into the brain are present. The first has a half-life of 2.1 min and a V_D of 1.9; it represents uptake into the extracellular fluid and cells. The second component has a half-life of 13 min and a V_D of 1.6; it represents penetration into and binding by subcellular fractions of the brain; uptake into the brain is faster than into the CSF ($T\frac{1}{2}$, 7 min) across the choroid plexus (see 116 for discussion).

The levels of PHT in the brain of humans have been tested in patients who have died from overdosage of the drug and in epileptic patients undergoing brain surgery (47,58,95,107). In these cases, the concentration in brain is about one to two times the plasma levels, as is the case for experimental animals. Hence, at least at the levels attainable in humans, the binding to brain substituents are not altered by the dose level in the plasma. This is also the case in mice. In man (95,98,107), rats (69,95), and mice (69), there is a significant correlation between brain and plasma PHT concentrations. In humans, the brain/plasma ratio for PHT averages about 1.52, but white matter (2.73) contains approximately twice as much PHT as gray matter

(1.73). In brain tissues obtained from an autopsy of an individual patient (95), PHT concentrations in cortical gyri containing mostly gray matter averaged 1.3 times the plasma concentration, values close to those observed in tissues obtained from patients in surgery. White matter tissues averaged twice the values in plasma. Cerebellum had the same levels as the cerebrum. Peripheral nerves (sciatic and median) had values equal to those in the plasma. In rats (20,69,77), the brain/plasma ratio ranges from 0.95 to 1.5, and in mice is 1.42 (69) (see Table 2).

In another study, Vajda et al. (107) found that the brain/plasma ratio of PHT was 0.75 in epileptic patients undergoing temporal lobectomy, and the CSF/plasma ratio was 0.12. Thus, the brain/CSF ratio (equivalent to brain/free plasma concentration ratio) is 6.25. There was a significant correlation between brain and plasma levels. Sironi et al. (98) also found that brain, CSF, and plasma levels were correlated. In addition, they found that PHT was slightly higher in white matter than in gray matter in different areas of brain removed surgically from epileptic patients and in normal and scar tissue. The brain/plasma ratio was 1.13 in gray matter and 1.33 in white matter. Phenytoin concentration in the temporal lobes was twice as high as in the frontal lobes, and that in the parietal lobe was also higher than that in the frontal area. These patients were medically resistant and had therapeutic or higher molar levels of PHT in the brain. Thus, despite adequate levels, the drugs were pharmacologically ineffective. The mechanism of this is not known, but the observations of Rapport et al. (90) that PHT concentration in the areas of maximum epileptogenic activity and astrogliosis in patients with epilepsy was much lower than its concentration in normal brain of four controls suggest that the lack of activity may result from failure to bind the drug in the area of the focus. Some evidence suggests that binding may be involved in the action of this drug (see 37,115 for review). However, the lower concentration in the focal area may be due to the astrogliosis since it has been reported that glia concentrate PHT to a lesser extent than do neurons.

The higher levels of PHT in white matter are in part undoubtedly a result of the high lipid content of this tissue, which is 2.5 times greater than in gray matter of cerebral cortex. This can be explained by the observations of Goldberg and colleagues (37,38) and others (see 37,115 for review) that PHT accumulates in brain by avidly binding to brain proteins and phospholipids. The binding to phospholipids depends on the partition coefficient (PC) which is high for PHT (log PC = 2.23) and is altered by the Ca^{2+} concentration (37). Brain levels in humans were four to 10 times higher than the free PHT as measured in the CSF.

The binding in the brain may, however, be influenced by pH, since CO_2 administration increases the level of PHT in brain and lowers the plasma level (114). It is likely that this effect is not related to the pH change increasing the amount of nonionized drug in the plasma. The percentage change in un-ionized drug is much too small to account for the change, and it is more likely that binding to plasma or brain proteins is altered by the pH shift induced by CO_2. In this connection it is of interest that CO_2 does decrease α-globulin binding sites in plasma, as described above.

Since the level of free PHT in plasma is the same as in CSF, it distributes passively between these two fluids (see 116 for review), and the CSF concentration can be used to determine the free level in the plasma and the percentage bound to plasma proteins.

EXCRETION

Phenytoin is excreted in urine and feces mainly as their metabolites. Less than 5% of the total drug is excreted as the unmetabolized form in the urine in experimental animals and humans; only a very small amount is excreted in this form in the feces. In rats, about 70% of PHT is ultimately secreted as HPPH, mainly as HPPH glucuronide (only 1% of unconjugated HPPH is excreted in urine), and about 25% as other metabolites (77). In humans, the amount excreted as HPPH is dose dependent. On oral administration, at a dose of 100 mg, only 50% is excreted as HPPH. However, in clinical doses the excretion of HPPH varies little with dose; about 63% is excreted as this compound. Values as high as 80% to 90% have been reported, but these are probably high. In the first 24 hr after single oral administration of 100 to 150 mg to humans, less than 1% is excreted as PHT, and 27% to 34% as HPPH; after intravenous injection of 50 to 250 mg, 50% to 61% is excreted as HPPH. The dihydrodiol, as well as the catechol and 3-0-methyl catechol derivatives of PHT are formed by rat liver and excreted in urine. However, they have been detected only in small quantities in human urine and are not major excretory products.

Phenytoin must be in the ionized form to be adequately excreted, a process efficiently carried out by the liver to produce HPPH, the dihydroxylated derivative, and the dihydrodiol. The ionized metabolites are excreted by active tubular secretion, as are most organic anions and cations. Thus, Bochner et al. (7) demonstrated that the clearance of PHT (3 to 23 ml/min, depending on urine flow rate) was considerably less than expected for inulin; therefore, it undergoes net resorption in its passage through the kidney. The HPPH glucuronide clearance (76 to 420 ml/min, depending on urine flow rate) exceeded expected inulin clearance if urine flow rates were sufficiently high; thus, this metabolite exhibits net secretion by the renal tubules. However, Hoppel et al. (46) suggest that both HPPH and its glucuronide are mainly filtered in the glomeruli in proportion to creatinine clearance. This is probably true at low urine flow rates, but at high rates, net secretion appears to occur. Alkalinization of the urine enhances the excretion of PHT because the higher pH allows more of the drug to exist in the ionized form; consequently, more leaves by way of tubular secretion and less is reabsorbed, because this occurs by passive diffusion of the un-ionized, lipid-soluble form. The rate of excretion depends on the extent of binding in the plasma, and, since this is high for PHT (80% to 90%), excretion is slow. In rats about 48 to 60 hr are required for complete excretion of an orally or intravenously administered dose; in humans, excretion requires 72 to 120 hr after oral ingestion and about the same time after intravenous administration (36,101).

The excretion of phenytoin in milk, semen, and saliva has implications for its effects on sperm, on nursing infants, and on teeth and gums, especially if toxic doses are attained. Some evidence suggests that viability of sperm may be affected (102). The effects on the child of long-term PHT in milk have not been evaluated, and there is evidence that the level of PHT in saliva is unrelated to the degree of gum hyperplasia produced. The levels in these fluids are about the same as the free levels in the plasma.

SUMMARY

Phenytoin is rapidly and passively absorbed across the intestinal mucosa in the un-ionized form, but absorption is limited by its extremely low solubility in gastrointestinal fluids. Absorption is a nonlinear saturation process that occurs only as the drug is cleared from the plasma and as it goes into solution in the intestinal fluids. After entering the blood, PHT is bound avidly to plasma proteins, but the free form rapidly enters all tissues where it is bound (at least in liver, brain, and muscle) to proteins and phospholipids. Thus, total concentrations in these tissues are higher than in extracellular fluid, but the free levels are the same. Storage in fat also occurs. Concentrations of PHT in transcellular fluids such as CSF, gastrointestinal fluids, bile, saliva, semen, milk, and plasma are the same as the free levels in the blood.

Binding to plasma proteins can be inhibited by drugs such as salicylates, thyroxine, phenylbutazone, and others that compete for the binding sites of the protein. The plasma half-life of the drug in humans is dose dependent and obeys saturation (Michaelis-Menten) kinetics. This can be altered by drugs that compete for binding or inhibit or accelerate biotransformation of the drug in the liver. Large doses of the drug that saturate the enzyme that biotransforms PHT in the liver also increase the plasma half-life.

Phenytoin is handled in the urine by glomerular filtration and tubular resorption, whereas its chief metabolite, HPPH, which represents about 70% of the total excretion of PHT in the urine, is excreted by glomerular filtration and tubular secretion and obeys saturation kinetics in its elimination.

Most of the drug is excreted in the bile as metabolites which are then reabsorbed from the intestinal tract and excreted in the urine; very little drug is lost in the feces.

Saturation of body binding and storage sites is essential before stable plasma and brain levels can be attained.

ACKNOWLEDGMENTS

The author is a Research Career Awardee (5-KO6-NS-13838) of the National Institute of Neurological and Communicative Disorders and Stroke, National Institutes of Health.

REFERENCES

1. Alvan, G., Butler, A., Eeg-Olfsson, O., Karlss E., Sjoqvist, F., and Tomson, G. (1975): Bj

ical availability—A comparison of three phenytoin preparations. *La Kartidningen* 72:2621–2623.

2. Andreasen, P. B., Froland, A., Skovsted, L., Andersen, S. A., and Hauge, M. (1972): Diphenylhydantoin half-life in man and its inhibition by phenylbutazone: The role of genetic factors. *Acta. Med. Scand.*, 193:561–564.

3. Arnold, K., and Gerber, N. (1970): The rate of decline of diphenylhydantoin in human plasma. *Clin. Pharmacol. Ther.*, 11:121–134.

4. Atkinson, A. J., and Shaw, J. M. (1973): Pharmacokinetic study of a patient with diphenylhydantoin toxicity. *Clin. Pharmacol. Ther.*, 14:521–528.

5. Baughman, F. A., Jr., and Randinitis, E. J. (1970): Passage of diphenylhydantoin across the placenta. *J.A.M.A.*, 213:466.

6. Blum, M. R., Riegelman, S., and Becker, C. E. (1972): Altered protein binding of diphenylhydantoin in uremic plasma. *N. Engl. J. Med.* 286:109.

7. Bochner, F., Hooper, W. O., Sutherland, J. M., Eadie, J. J., and Tyrer, J. H. (1973): The renal handling of diphenylhydantoin and 5-(p-hydroxyphenyl)-5-phenylhydantoin. *Clin. Pharmacol. Therap.*, 14:791–796.

8. Borofsky, L. G., Louis, S., Kutt, H., and Roginsky, M. (1972): Diphenylhydantoin: Efficacy, toxicity and dose-serum level relationships in children. *J. Pediatr.*, 81:995–1002.

9. Bourgeois, B. F., and Dodson, W. E. (1983): Phenytoin elimination in newborns. *Neurology*, 23:173–178.

10. Braun, C. W., and Goldstone, J. M. (1980): Increased clearance of phenytoin as the presenting feature of infectious mononucleosis. *Ther. Drug Monogr.*, 26:629–634.

11. Buchanan, R. A., Heffelfinger, J. C., and Weiss, C. F. (1969): The effect of phenobarbital on diphenylhydantoin metabolism in children. *Pediatrics*, 43:114–116.

12. Buchanan, R. A., Kinkel, A. W., Goulet, J. R., and Smith, T. C. (1972): The metabolism of diphenylhydantoin (Dilantin®) following once daily administration. *Neurology* (Minneap.), 22:325–336.

13. Cantu, R. C., Schwab, R. S., and Timberlake, W. H. (1968): Comparison of blood levels with oral and intramuscular diphenylhydantoin. *Neurology* (Minneap.), 18:782–784.

14. Chiba, K., Ishizaki, T., Miura, H. M., and Minagawa, K. (1980): Michaelis-Menton pharmacokinetics of diphenylhydantoin and application in the pediatric age patient. *J. Pediatr.*, 96:479–484.

15. Cranford, R. E., Leppik, I. E., Patrick, B., Anderson, C. B., and Kostick, B. (1978): Intravenous phenytoin: Clinical and pharmacokinetic aspects. *Neurology* (Minneap.), 28:874–880.

16. Cucinelli, A. A., Koster, R., Conney, A. H., and Burns, J. J. (1963): Stimulatory effect of phenobarbital on the metabolism of diphenylhydantoin. *J. Pharmacol. Exp. Ther.*, 141:157–160.

17. Curless, R. G., and Watson, P. D. (1975): Rapid diphenylhydantoin metabolism in infants. *Pediatr. Res.*, 9:282.

18. Dam, M., and Olesen, V. (1966): Intramuscular administration of phenytoin. *Neurology* (Minneap.), 16:288–292.

19. Dayton, P. G., Cucinell, S. A., Weiss, M., and Perel, J. M. (1967): Dose-dependence of drug plasma level decline in dogs. *J. Pharmacol. Exp. Ther.*, 158:305–316.

20. Dill, W. A., Kazenko, A., Wolff, L. M., and Glazko, A. J. (1956): Studies on 5,5-diphenylhydantoin (Dilantin) in animals and man. *J. Pharmacol. Exp. Ther.*, 118:270–279.

21. Dodson, W. E. (1980): Phenytoin elimination in childhood: Effect of concentration dependent kinetics. *Neurology* (Minneap.), 30:196–199.

22. Dodson, W. E. (1980): Phenytoin kinetics in children. *Clin. Pharmacol. Ther.*, 27:704–707.

23. Dodson, W. E. (1982): Nonlinear kinetics of phenytoin in children. *Neurology*, 32:42–48.

24. Dodson, W. E. (1987): Special pharmacokinetic considerations in children. *Epilepsia* 28(suppl 1): 556–570.

25. Eadie, M. J., Sutherland, J. M., and Tyrer, D. H. (1968): Dilantin overdosage. *Med. J. Aust.*, 2:515.

26. Ehrnebo, M., Agurell, S., Jalling, B., and Boreus, L. O. (1971): Age differences in drug binding by plasma proteins: Studies on human fetuses, neonates and adults. *Eur. J. Clin. Pharmacol.*, 3:189–193.

27. Fichsel, H., and Knopfle, G. (1978): Effects of anticonvulsant drugs on thyroid hormones in epileptic children. *Epilepsia*, 19:323–336.

28. Firemark, H., Barlow, C. F., and Roth, L. J. (1963): The entry accumulation and binding of diphenylhydantoin-2-C^{14} in brain. Studies on adult, immature and hypercapnic cats. *Int. J. Neuropharmacol.*, 2:25–38.

29. Fredholm, B. B., Rane, A., and Persson, B. (1975): Diphenylhydantoin binding to proteins in plasma and its dependence on free fatty acid and bilirubin concentration in dogs and newborn infants. *Pediatr. Res.*, 9:26–30.

30. Ganshorn, A., and Kurz, H. (1968): Uterschiede zwischen der Protein bindung Neugeborener and Erwachsener und ihre Bedeutung fur die pharmakologische Wirkung. *Naunyn Schmiedebergs Arch. Pharmacol.*, 260:117–118.

31. Garrettson, L. K., and Jusko, W. J. (1975): Diphenylhydantoin elimination kinetics in overdosed children. *Clin. Pharmacol. Ther.*, 17: 481–491.

32. Gerber, N., and Arnold, K. (1969): Studies on the metabolism of diphenylhydantoin (DPH) in mice. *J. Pharmacol. Exp. Ther.*, 167:77–90.

33. Gerber, N., and Wagner, J. G. (1972): Explanation of dose-dependent decline of diphenylhydantoin plasma levels by fitting to the integrated form of the Michaelis-Menten equation. *Res. Commun. Chem. Pathol. Pharmacol.*, 3:455–466.

34. Glazko, A. J. (1972): Diphenylhydantoin. In: *Proceedings of the Conference on Bioavailability of*

Drugs, edited by B. B. Brodie, and W. M. Haller, pp. 163–177. Karger, Basel.

35. Glazko, A. J., and Chang, T. (1972); 12-Diphenylhydantoin: Absorption, distribution, and excretion (continued). In: *Antiepileptic Drugs*, edited by D. M. Woodbury, J. Kiffin Penry, and R. P. Schmidt, pp. 127–136. Raven Press, New York.

36. Glazko, A. J., Chang, T., Baukema, J., Bill, W. A., Goulet, J. R., and Buchanan, R. A. (1969): Metabolic disposition of diphenylhydantoin in normal human subjects following intravenous administration. *Clin. Pharmacol. Ther.*, 10:498–504.

37. Goldberg, M. A. (1980): Phenytoin: Binding. *Adv. Neurol.*, 27:323–337.

38. Goldberg, M. A., and Crandall, P. H. (1978): Human binding of phenytoin. *Neurology* (Minneap.), 28:881–885.

39. Goulden, K. J., Camfield, P. R., and Camfield, C. S. (1986): Changes in serum anticonvulsant levels with febrile illness in childhood epilepsy. *Ann. Neurol.*, 20:388.

40. Gugler, R., Shoeman, D. W., and Azarnoff, D. L. (1974): Effect of *in vivo* elevation of free fatty acids on protein binding of drugs. *Pharmacology*, 12:160–165.

41. Gugler, R., Mannion, C. V., and Azarnoff, D. L. (1976): Phenytoin: Pharmacokinetics and bioavailability. *Clin. Pharmacol. Ther.*, 19:135–142.

42. Hansen, J. M., Kristensen, M., and Skovsted, L. (1966): Sulthiame (Ospolot®) as inhibitor of diphenylhydantoin metabolism. *Epilepsia*, 9:17–22.

43. Hansen, J. M., Kristensen, M., Skovsted, L., and Christensen, L. K. (1966): Dicoumarol induced diphenylhydantoin intoxication. *Lancet*, 2:265–266.

44. Hooper, W. D., Bochner, F., Eadie, M. J., and Tyrer, J. H. (1973): Plasma protein binding of diphenylhydantoin. Effects of sex hormones, renal and hepatic disease. *Clin. Pharmacol. Ther.*, 15:276–282.

45. Hooper, W. D., Sutherland, J. M., Bochner, F., Tyrer, J. H., and Eadie, M. J. (1973): The effect of certain drugs on the plasma protein binding of phenytoin. *Aust. N.Z. J. Med.*, 3:377–381.

46. Hoppel, C., Garle, M., Rane, A., and Sjoquist, F. (1977): Plasma concentrations of 5-(4-hydroxyphenyl)-5-phenylhydantoin in phenytoin-treated patients. *Clin. Pharmacol. Ther.*, 21:294–300.

47. Houghton, G. W., Richens, A., Toselund, P. A., Davidson, S., and Falconer, M. A. (1975): Brain concentrations of phenytoin, phenobarbitone and primidone in epileptic patients. *Eur. J. Clin. Pharmacol.*, 9:73–78.

48. Jalling, B., Boreus, L. O., Rane, A., and Sjoquist, F. (1970): Plasma concentrations of diphenylhydantoin in young infants. *Pharmacol. Clin.* (Berl.), 2:200–202.

49. Johannessen, S. J., and Strandjord, R. E. (1975): Absorption and protein binding in serum of several antiepileptic drugs. In: *Clinical Pharmacology of Antiepileptic Drugs*, edited by H. Schneider, D. Janz, C. Gardner-Thorpe, H. Meinardi,

and A. L. Sherwin, pp. 262–273. Springer, Berlin, Heidelberg, New York.

50. Jusko, W. J. (1976): Bioavailability and disposition kinetics of phenytoin in man. In: *Quantitative Analytic Studies in Epilepsy*, edited by P. Kellaway and I. Petersen, pp. 115–136. Raven Press, New York.

51. Jusko, W. J., Koup, J. R., and Alvan, G. (1976): Non-linear assessment of phenytoin bioavailability. *J. Pharmacokinet. Biopharm.*, 4:327–336.

52. Kaneko, S., Sato, T., and Suzuki, K. (1979): The levels of anticonvulsants in breast milk. *Brit. J. Clin. Pharmacol.*, 7:624–627.

53. Kemp, J. W., and Woodbury, D. M. (1971): Subcellular distribution of 4-^{14}C-diphenylhydantoin in rat brain. *J. Pharmacol. Exp. Ther.*, 177:342–349.

54. Kostenbauder, H. B., Rapp, R. P., McGoveen, J. P., Foster, T. S., Perrier, D. G., Blacker, H. M., Huylon, W. C., and Kinkel, A. W. (1975): Bioavailability and single dose pharmacokinetics of intramuscular diphenylhydantoin. *Clin. Pharmacol. Ther.*, 18:449–456.

55. Kutt, H., Haynes, J., and McDowell, F. (1966): Some causes of ineffectiveness of diphenylhydantoin. *Arch. Neurol.*, 14:489–492.

56. Kutt, H., Winters, W., and McDowell, F. (1966): Depression of parahydroxylation of diphenylhydantoin by antituberculosis chemotherapy. *Neurology* (Minneap.), 16:594–602.

57. Kutt, H., Wolk, M., Scherman, R., and McDowell, F. (1964): Insufficient parahydroxylation as a cause of diphenylhydantoin toxicity. *Neurology* (Minneap.), 14:542–548.

58. Laubscher, F. (1966): Fetal diphenylhydantoin poisoning. *J.A.M.A.*, 198:1120–1121.

59. Leonard, R. F., Knott, P. J., Rankin, G. O., Robinson, D. S., and Melnick, D. E. (1981): Phenytoin-salicylate interaction. *Clin. Pharmacol. Ther.*, 29:56–60.

60. Leppik, I. E., Fisher, J., Kreil, R., and Sawchuck, R. J. (1986): Altered phenytoin clearance with febrile illness. *Neurology*, 36:1367–1370.

61. Levy, R. H. (1980): Phenytoin: Biopharmacology. *Adv. Neurol.*, 27:315–321.

62. Lightfoot, R. W., Jr., and Christian, C. L. (1966): Serum protein binding of throxine and diphenylhydantoin. *J. Clin. Endocrinol. Metab.*, 16:305–308.

63. Loeser, E. H., Jr. (1961): Studies on the metabolism of diphenylhydantoin (Dilantin®). *Neurology*, (Minneap.), 11:424–429.

64. Lund, L. (1974): Clinical significance of generic inequivalence of three different pharmaceutical preparations of phenytoin. *Eur. J. Clin. Pharmacol.*, 7:119–124.

65. Lund, L., Alvan, G., Berlin, A., and Alexanderson, B. (1974): Pharmacokinetics of single and multiple oral doses of phenytoin in man. *Eur. J. Clin. Pharmacol.*, 7:81–86.

66. Lunde, P. K. M., Anders, R., Yaffe, S. J., Lund, L., and Sjoqvist, F. (1970): Plasma protein binding of diphenylhydantoin in man. Interaction with other drugs and the effect of temperature

and plasma dilution. *Clin. Pharmacol. Ther.*, 11:846–855.

67. Martin, E., Tozer, T. N., Scheiner, L. B., and Riegelman, S. (1977): The clinical pharmacokinetics of phenytoin. *J. Pharmacokinet. Biopharm.*, 5:579–596.

68. Martis, L., and Levy, R. H. (1973): Bioavailability calculations for drugs showing simultaneous first order and capacity-limited elimination kinetics. *J. Pharmacokinet. Biopharm.*, 1:283–294.

69. Masuda, Y., Utsui, Y., Shiraishi, Y., Karasawa, T., Yoshida, K., and Shimizu, M. (1979): Relationships between plasma concentrations of diphenylhydantoin, phenobarbital, carbamazepine, and 3-sulfamoylmethyl-1,2-benzisozazole (AD-810), a new anticonvulsant agent and their anticonvulsant or neurotoxic effects in experimental animals. *Epilepsia*, 20:623–633.

70. Meinardi, H., Kleijn, E. van der, Meijer, J. W. A., and Rees, H. van (1975): Absorption and distribution of antiepileptic drugs. *Epilepsia*, 16:353–365.

71. Mirkin, B. L. (1971): Diphenylhydantoin: Placental transport, fetal localization, neonatal metabolism, and possible teratogenic effects. *J. Pediatr.*, 79:329–337.

72. Mirkin, B. L. (1971): Placental transfer and neonatal elimination of diphenylhydantoin. *Am. J. Obstet. Gynecol.*, 109:930–933.

73. Monks, A., Boobis, S., Wadsworth, J., and Richens, A. (1978): Plasma protein binding interaction between phenytoin and valproic acid in vitro. *Br. J. Clin. Pharmacol.*, 6:487–492.

74. Morselli, P. L. (1977): Pharmacokinetics of antiepileptic drugs during development. In: *Antiepileptic Drug Monitoring*, edited by C. Gardner-Thorpe, D. Janz, H. Meinardi, and C. E. Pippinger, pp. 57–72. Pitman Medical, Kent.

75. Nakamura, K., Masuda, U., Nakatsuji, K., and Kiroka, T. (1966): Comparative studies on the distribution and metabolic fate of diphenylhydantoin and 3-ethylcarbonyldiphenylhydantoin (P-6127) after chronic administration to dogs and cats. *Naunyn Schmiedebergs Arch., Pharmacol.*, 254:406–417.

76. Noach, E. L., and van Rees, H. (1964): Intestinal distribution of intravenously administered diphenylhydantoin in the rat. *Arch. Int. Pharmacodyn. Ther.*, 150:52–61.

77. Noach, E. L., Woodbury, D. M., and Goodman, L. S. (1958): Studies on absorption, distribution, fate and excretion of 4-C^{14} labeled diphenylhydantoin. *J. Pharmacol. Exp. Ther.*, 122:301–314.

78. Odar-Cedarlof, I., and Borga, O. (1976): Impaired protein binding of phenytoin in uremia and displacement effects of salicytic acid. *Clin. Pharmacol. Ther.*, 20:36–47.

79. Olesen, O. V. (1966): Disulfiramum (Antabuse®) as inhibitor of phenytoin metabolism. *Acta Pharmacol. Toxicol.* (Kbh.), 24:317–322.

80. O'Malley, W. E., Denckla, M. A., and O'Doherty, D. S. (1969): Oral absorption of diphenylhydantoin as measured by gas liquid chromatography. *Trans. Am. Neurol. Assoc.*, 94:318–319.

81. Oppenheimer, J. H., Fisher, L. W., Nelson, K. M., and Jailer, J. W. (1961): Depression of the serum protein-bound iodine level by diphenylhydantoin. *J. Clin. Endocrinol.*, 21:252–262.

82. Oppenheimer, J. H., and Tavernetti, R. R. (1962): Studies on the thyroxine-diphenylhydantoin interaction: Effect of 5,5'-diphenylhydantoin on the displacement of L-thyroxine from thyroxine-binding globulin (TBG). *Endocrinology*, 71:496–504.

83. Osorio, C., Jackson, D. J., Gartside, J. M., and Goolden, A. W. G. (1962): Effect of carbon dioxide and diphenylhydantoin on the partition of triiodothyronine labelled with iodine-131 between the red cells and the plasma proteins. *Nature*, 196:275–276.

84. Partington, M. W., Reilly, D. M., Steward, J. H., and Vickery, S. K. (1973): Serum diphenylhydantoin levels following a change in drug brand. *Can. J. Pharm. Sci.*, 91:31–32.

85. Porter, R. J., and Layzer, R. B. (1975): Plasma albumin concentration and diphenylhydantoin in man. *Arch. Neurol.*, 32:298–303.

86. Rail, L. (1968): Dilantin overdosage. *Med. J. Aust.*, 2:339.

87. Ramsay, R. E., Hammond, E. J., Perchalski, R. J., and Wilder, B. J. (1979): Brain uptake of phenytoin, phenobarbital, and diazepam. *Arch Neurol.*, 36:535–539.

88. Rane, A., Lunde, P. K. M., Jalling, B., Yaffee, S. J., and Sjoqvist, F. (1971): Plasma protein binding of diphenylhydantoin in normal and hyperbilirubinemic infants. *Pedr. Pharmacol. Ther.*, 78:877–882.

89. Rane, A., and Wilson, J. T. (1976): Clinical pharmacokinetics in infants and children. *Clin. Pharmacokinet.*, 1:2–24.

90. Rapport, R. L. II, Harris, A. B., Friel, P. N., and Ojemann, G. A. (1975): Human epileptic brain. Na, K, ATPase activity and phenytoin concentrations. *Arch. Neurol.*, 32:549–554.

91. Rees, H. van, and Noach, E. L. (1973): The intestinal absorption of diphenylhydantoin from a suspension in rats. *Arch. Int. Pharmacodyn. Ther.*, 206:76–83.

92. Richens, A., and Dunlop, A. (1975): Serum phenytoin levels in management of epilepsy. *Lancet*, 2:247–248.

93. Ruprah, M., Perrucca, E., and Richens, A. (1980): Decreased serum protein binding of phenytoin in late pregnancy (letter). *Lancet*, 2:316–317.

94. Shavit, G., Lermon, P., Korczyn, A. D., Kivity, S., Bechar, M., and Gitter, S. (1984): Phenytoin pharmacokinetics in catamenial epilepsy. *Neurology*, 34:959–961.

95. Sherwin, A. L., Eisen, A. A., and Sokolowski, C. D. (1973): Anticonvulsant drugs in human epileptogenic brain. Correlation of phenobarbital and diphenylhydantoin levels with plasma. *Arch. Neurol.*, 29:73–77.

96. Shoeman, D. W., and Azarnoff, D. L. (1972): The alteration of plasma proteins in uremia as reflected in their ability to bind digitoxin and diphenylhydantoin. *Pharmacology*, 7:169–177.

97. Shoeman, E. W., and Azarnoff, D. L. (1975): Diphenylhydantoin potency and plasma protein binding. *J. Pharmacol. Exp. Ther.*, 195:83–86.

98. Sironi, V. A., Cabrini, G., Porro, M. G., Ravagnati, L., and Marossero, F. (1980): Antiepileptic drug distribution in cerebral cortex, Ammon's horn, and amygdala in man. *J. Neurosurg.*, 52:686–692.

99. Solomon, H. M., and Schrogie, J. J. (1967): The effect of phenyramidol on the metabolism of diphenylhydantoin. *Clin. Pharmacol. Ther.*, 8:554–556.

100. Squef, R., Martinez, M., and Oppenheimer, J. H. (1963): Use of thyroxine displacing drugs in identifying serum thyroxine-binding proteins separated by starch gel electrophoresis. *Proc. Soc. Exp. Biol. Med.*, 113:837–840.

101. Suzuki, T., Saitoh, Y., and Nishihara, K. (1970): Kinetics of diphenylhydantoin disposition in man. *Chem. Pharm. Bull.* (Tokyo), 18:405–411.

102. Swanson, B. N., Leger, R. M., Gordon, W. P., Lynn, R. K., and Gerber, N. (1978): Excretion of phenytoin into semen of rabbits and man. Comparison with plasma levels. *Drug Metab. Dispos.*, 6:70–74.

103. Tammisto, P., Kauko, K., and Viukari, M. (1976): Bioavailability of phenytoin. *Lancet*, 1:254–255.

104. Tramposch, A. (1977): The effect of simultaneous administration of phenytoin and phenobarbital on their individual absorption from rat ileum *in situ*. M.S. Thesis. St. John's University, New York.

105. Troupin, A. S., and Friel, P. (1975): Anticonvulsant level in saliva, serum, and cerebrospinal fluid. *Epilepsia*, 16:223–227.

106. Tyrer, J. H., Eadie, M. J., Sutherland, J. M., and Hooper, W. D. (1970): Outbreak of anticonvulsant intoxication in an Australian city. *Br. Med. J.*, 4:271–273.

107. Vajda, F., Williams, F. M., Davidson, S., Falconer, M. A., and Breckenridge, A. (1974): Human brain, cerebrospinal fluid, and plasma concentration of diphenylhydantoin and phenobarbital. *Clin. Pharmacol. Ther.*, 15:597–603.

108. Weiss, C. F., Heffelfinger, J. C., and Buchanan, R. A. (1969): Serial Dilantin® levels in mentally retarded children. *Am. J. Ment. Defic.*, 73: 826–830.

109. Westmoreland, B., and Bass, N. H. (1971): Diphenylhydantoin intoxication during pregnancy: A chemical study of drug distribution in the albino rat. *Arch. Neurol.*, 24:158–164.

110. Wilder, B. J., Buchanan, R. A., and Serrono, E. E. (1973): Correlation of acute diphenylhydantoin intoxication with plasma levels and metabolite excretion. *Neurology* (Minneap.), 23:1329–1332.

111. Wilder, B. J., and Ramsay, R. E. (1976): Oral and intramuscular phenytoin. *Clin. Pharmacol. Ther.*, 19:360–364.

112. Wilensky, A. J., and Lowden, J. A. (1973): Inadequate serum levels after intramuscular administration of diphenylhydantoin. *Neurology*, (Minneap.), 23:318–324.

113. Wolff, J., Standaert, M. E., and Rall, J. E. (1961): Thyroxine displacement from serum proteins and depression of serum protein-bound iodine by certain drugs. *J. Clin. Invest.*, 40:1373–1379.

114. Woodbury, D. M. (1969): Role of pharmacological factors in the evaluation of anticonvulsant drugs. *Epilepsia*, 10:121–124.

115. Woodbury, D. M. (1980): Phenytoin: Proposed mechanisms of anticonvulsant action. *Adv. Neurol.* 27:447–471.

116. Woodbury, D. M. (1983): Pharmacology of anticonvulsant drugs in CSF. In: *Neurobiology of Cerebrospinal Fluid 2*, edited by J. H. Woods, Chapter 38, pp. 615–628. Plenum Press, New York.

117. Woodbury, D. M., and Swinyard, E. A. (1972): Diphenylhydantoin: Absorption, distribution, and excretion. In: *Antiepileptic Drugs*, edited by D. M. Woodbury, J. K. Penry, and R. P. Schmidt, pp. 113–123. Raven Press, New York.

Antiepileptic Drugs, Third Edition, edited by
R. Levy, R. Mattson, B. Meldrum,
J. K. Penry, and F. E. Dreifuss.
Raven Press, Ltd., New York © 1989.

12

Phenytoin

Biotransformation

Thomas R. Browne and Tsun Chang

Phenytoin (5,5-diphenylhydantoin; Dilantin) is eliminated almost entirely by metabolic transformation prior to excretion in the form of metabolites. Less than 5% of an administered dose is excreted unchanged in the urine (30,43,66,70). The principal metabolic pathway of phenytoin in man is the 5-(4-hydroxyphenyl)-5-phenylhydantoin (*p*-HPPH) and dihydrodiol pathway, accounting for 70% to 90% of administered phenytoin (Fig. 1). The first step of this pathway (involving the enzyme arene oxidase) exhibits nonlinear enzyme kinetics, which has significant effects on phenytoin's clinical pharmacokinetics. Several minor metabolic pathways for phenytoin also have been described (Fig. 1). Species differences in the biotransformation of phenytoin have been reported.

MAJOR METABOLIC PATHWAYS

The metabolites, *p*-HPPH and dihydrodiol, account for 67% to 88% and 7% to 11%, respectively, of human urinary metabolites of phenytoin (20,29). The first step in the principal metabolic pathway of phenytoin is the formation of an arene oxide intermediate via the cytochrome oxidase system enzyme arene oxidase. Arene oxide is converted spontaneously to *p*-HPPH and is converted by the enzyme epoxide hydrolase to dihydrodiol (Fig. 1).

Arene Oxide

The arene oxide of phenytoin has never been isolated from serum or urine, presumably because it is rapidly converted to further metabolic products. Early kinetic experiments by Tomaszewski et al. (84) suggested the presence of an arene oxide intermediate in the formation of *p*-HPPH. The existence of an arene oxide intermediate in the formation of *p*-HPPH was established using the "N.I.H. shift" technique by Claesen et al. (27) and was confirmed by later studies also using the same technique (68).

The National Institutes of Health (N.I.H.) shift technique depends on the observation that arene oxides spontaneously break down to form a hydroxylated metabolite. When this happens, the hydrogen molecule at the site of the hydroxyl group is lost 50% of the time and is shifted ("N.I.H. shift") to the adjacent carbon where the oxygen molecule had been attached 50% of the time (Fig. 2). In the N.I.H. shift experiment of Claesen et al., (27), racemic 5-(4-deuteriophenyl)-5-phenylhydantoin (*p*-^{2}H-DPH) was administered to four volunteers, and urine was collected.

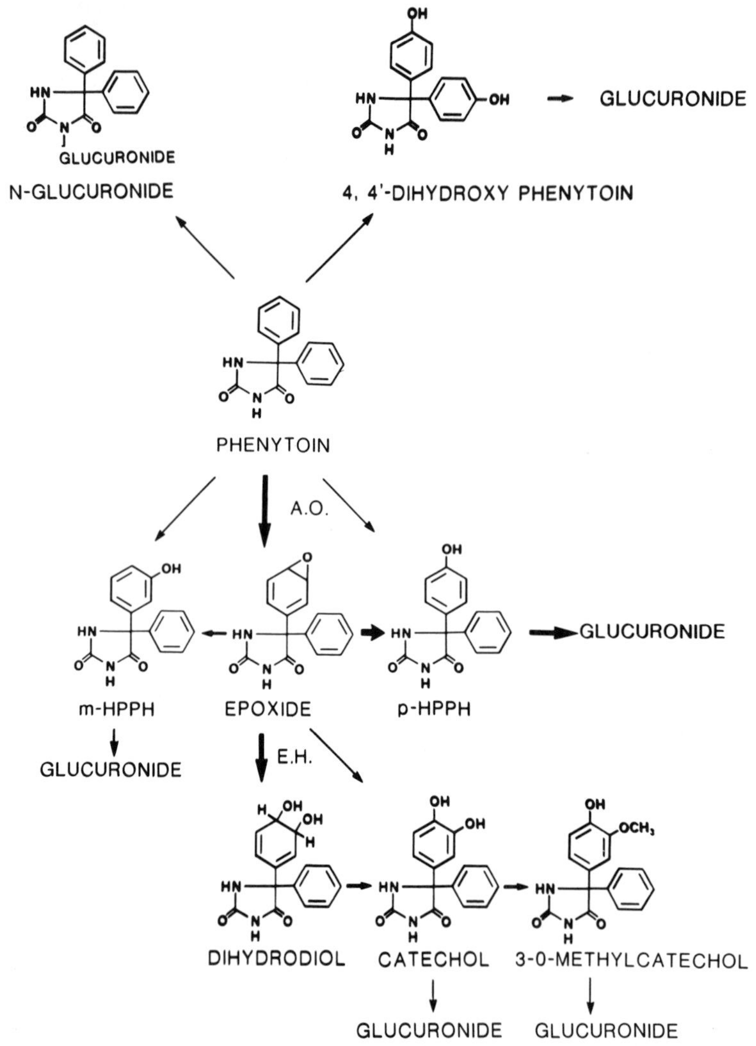

FIG. 1. Pathways of phenytoin metabolism. A. O., arene oxidale; E. H., epoxide hydorldie.

After enzymatic hydrolysis of the urine, deuterium retention by p-HPPH metabolites was determined. The expected percentage of deuterium retention by p-HPPH in the presence of an arene oxide–N.I.H. shift pathway was 75%, and the measured values were 65% to 75%.

Phenytoin is known to exhibit nonlinear pharmacokinetics in man (see below), which implies that substrate saturation occurs in one or more of the metabolizing enzymes. The arene oxidase enzyme appears to be the site of substrate saturation because the rate of urinary excretion of p-HPPH varies inversely with serum phenytoin concentration in man (r = −0.640, p < 0.005) (10), and the rate of formation of p-HPPH from rat hepatocytes and rat hepatic microsomes varies inversely with phenytoin concentration in the medium (85). Phenytoin is the probable substance causing competitive inhibition of the arene oxidase enzyme.

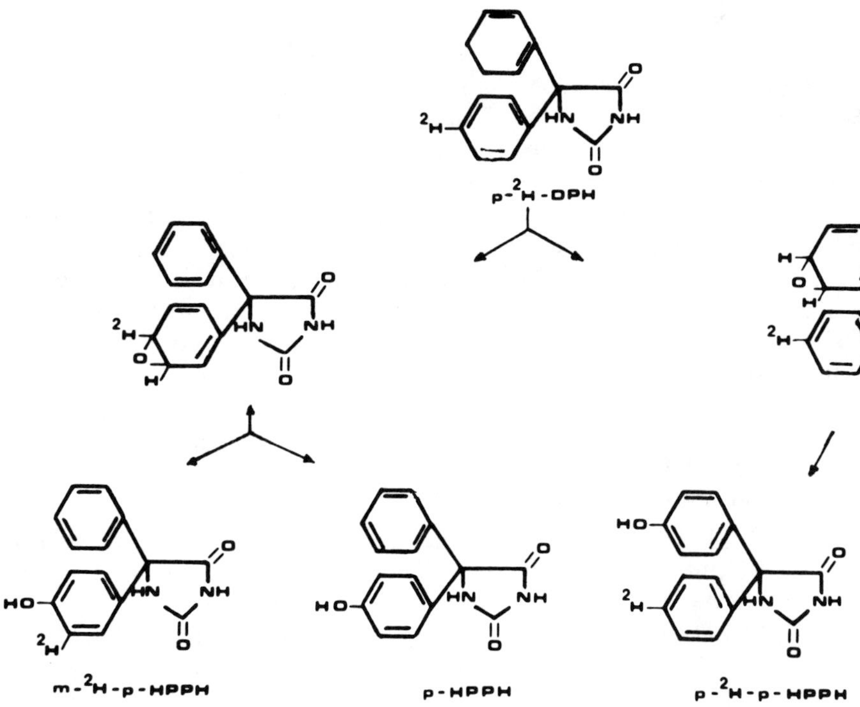

FIG. 2. Arene oxide–N.I.H. shift pathway for *para*-hydroxylation of phenytoin. (From Claesen et al., ref. 27, with permission.)

There is some evidence that p-HPPH competitively inhibits hydroxylation of phenytoin in animals, but this phenomenon has not been demonstrated in man (20).

The arene oxidase enzyme system appears to undergo relatively little or no enzyme induction during phenytoin monotherapy (10), and the addition of phenobarbital or carbamazepine to the regimen does not appear to induce arene oxidase activity (13,15). Carbamazepine competitively inhibits phenytoin metabolism by the arene oxidase enzyme in man (15).

Arene oxides have attracted considerable attention because of their reactivity and possible role in mechanisms of toxicity (8,28,42,71). The teratogenic effect of phenytoin (64) suggests that an arene oxide intermediate may be involved. This possibility was investigated by Martz et al. (63).

Arene oxide is metabolized to a stable dihydrodiol metabolite by the enzyme epoxide hydrolase (see below). When Swiss mice (day 11 of gestation) were given teratogenic doses of phenytoin (50 and 100 mg/kg) together with 1,2-epoxy-3,3,3-trichloropropane (TCPO, 100 mg/kg, an epoxide hydrolase inhibitor), the incidence of cleft lip and cleft palate increased significantly over the phenytoin control group, and the embryo-lethality doubled. Covalent binding of ^{14}C radioactivity in the fetus and placenta 4 hr after administration of [^{14}C]phenytoin plus TCPO was twofold greater than with [^{14}C]phenytoin alone. The TCPO had no marked effect on maternal plasma phenytoin concentration. The authors concluded that the teratogenesis was caused by arene oxide formation and covalent binding to constituents of the gestational tissue.

Para-HPPH and Meta-HPPH

In 1957, Butler (16) isolated and identified p-HPPH as the principal urinary metabolite in man and dog. Fifty percent to 60% of the administered dose was recovered in urine as an acid-labile conjugate of p-HPPH, but only traces of free p-HPPH were detected. Using [^{14}C]phenytoin, Noach et al. (70) demonstrated that 95% of the dose appeared as metabolites in rat urine and that p-HPPH accounted for 60% to 70% of the total metabolites present. Maynert (66) clearly established that the conjugate was a glucuronide from which p-HPPH could be released by incubation with β-glucuronidase. Direct evidence for the structure of p-HPPH glucuronide was provided by Thompson et al. (83) using permethylation and a gas chromatography-mass spectrometry (GC-MS) technique. The possible existence of a sulfate conjugate of p-HPPH in rat and human urine was considered by several investigators (19,66) and rejected when treatment with phenol sulfatase failed to liberate p-HPPH from its conjugate. However, Hassell et al. (47) documented the presence of p-HPPH sulfate conjugate in cat urine after long-term oral administration of phenytoin.

In the early phenytoin metabolic investigations, para-hydroxylation was regarded as the major pathway for phenytoin metabolism in man and laboratory animals. In 1970, Atkinson et al. (1) reported that meta-HPPH (m-HPPH) was the major metabolite in dog, with lesser, variable amounts of p-HPPH also detected. Small amounts of m-HPPH in human urine were also found after acid hydrolysis of the glucuronides. The detection of m-HPPH in human urine was initially thought to be an artifact, arising from degradation of the dihydrodiol metabolite during acid hydrolysis. However, subsequent work (17,44) showed that traces of m-HPPH, much less than the amount reported by Atkinson et al. (1), could be found in

human urine after treatment with β-glucuronidase. According to Butler et al. (17), the ratio of total m-HPPH to p-HPPH in two patients was approximately 1:400.

N.I.H. shift experiments indicate that the majority of p-HPPH in man is produced via an arene oxide intermediate (see above). However, minor differences exist between expected and observed values for deuterium retention by p-HPPH in these experiments. The majority of p-HPPH and dihydrodiol is excreted as (S) enantiomers in man, suggesting a common origin from an (S) arene oxide precursor (see below). However, finite amounts of (R)-p-HPPH and (R)-dihydrodiol are found in human urine, and the (S)-to-(R) ratios of p-HPPH and dihydrodiol are different in human urine (61). These observations suggest that the majority of p-HPPH in man is formed through an (S) stereospecific arene oxide step. However, the formation of relatively small amounts of (S)- or (R)-p-HPPH, or both, via independent pathways cannot be excluded (Fig. 3).

A minority of patients are slow metabolizers of phenytoin (20,44,55,87) and develop toxic serum phenytoin concentrations at average dosing rates. This trait runs in families (55,87) and is genetically determined in animals (20). Glazko et al. (44) reported that the elimination half-life of p-HPPH averaged 30% greater than the phenytoin half-life in normal controls and 50% or more in slow metabolizers. Under comparable conditions, the mean serum concentration of p-HPPH was 1.9 μg/ml and 0.7 μg/ml, respectively. Urinary excretion of total p-HPPH accounted for 65% to 94% of the dose in controls and 52% to 72% of the dose in the metabolically slow group. The preponderance of evidence indicates that slow metabolizers of phenytoin have a genetically determined slower than normal rate of formation of p-HPPH from phenytoin.

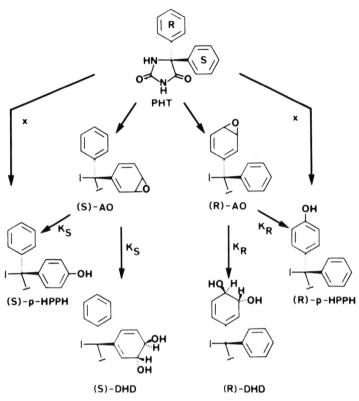

FIG. 3. Scheme depicting stereoselective metabolic pathways involved in the production of *p*-HPPH and dihydrodiol (DHD). Possible stereoselective direct hydroxylation pathways are indicated with an "X". (From Maguire and McClanahan, ref. 61, with permission.)

Dihydrodiol

In 1970, Chang et al. (23) isolated a dihydrodiol metabolite from rat and monkey urine and identified the structure as 5-(3,4-dihydroxy-1,5-cyclohexadien-1-yl)-5-phenylhydantoin. This involved conversion of a phenyl ring to the cyclohexadiene diol with loss of aromaticity. When an acidic solution of the dihydrodiol or the dry powder was heated, approximately equal amounts of *m*-HPPH and *p*-HPPH were formed (23). Preliminary evidence suggested that two hydroxyl groups of the dihydrodiol were oriented in the *trans* configuration (19). The structure of the dihydrodiol was confirmed by Horning et al. (50) using the GC-MS technique. The metabolite was detected in the urine of newborn infants and subsequently in urine of rats (41), mice (80), and humans (37,48).

Phenytoin dihydrodiol is believed to be formed from phenytoin arene oxide via the enzyme epoxide hydrolase (see Figs. 1 and 3). This belief is supported by several lines of evidence. First, the usual metabolic pathway leading to formation of dihydrodiols is conversion of an epoxide intermediate to a dihydrodiol by the enzyme epoxide hydrolase (20,46,53,71). Second, administration of an epoxide hydrolase inhibitor (1,2-epoxy-,3,3,3,-trichloropropane) to pregnant Swiss mice reduced the incidence of phenytoin-related teratogenesis and the covalent binding of ^{14}C radioactivity in the fetus after administration of ^{14}C-labeled phenytoin, whereas the maternal serum phenytoin concentration remained unchanged (63). This implies that the initial step of phenytoin metabolism (presumably arene oxide formation) is unaffected by epoxide hydrolase inhibition and that a metabolic intermediate with teratogenic and covalent binding properties (presumably arene oxide) accumulates in greater than usual amounts when epoxide hydrolase is inhibited. Finally, incubation of phenytoin with human liver fractions known to contain epoxide hydrolase results in the formation of phenytoin dihydrodiol (75). There is evidence that long-term administration of phenytoin may induce epoxide hydrolase activity in man (10,75). The addition of phenobarbital or carbamazepine to phenytoin monotherapy does not appear to induce epoxide hydrolase activity in man (13,15).

Stereoselective Formation of HPPH and Dihydrodiol

Phenytoin is a prochiral compound. Introduction of a hydroxyl group in one of the phenyl rings leads to the creation of a chiral center and results in the formation of enantiomeric phenolic metabolites (see Fig. 3). Butler et al. (17) investigated the stereochemistry of phenytoin hydroxylation in man and the dog. The metabolites (*m*-HPPH or *p*-HPPH) were purified from β-glucuronidase–treated urine using solvent partitioning without crystallization. The results revealed a profound difference in stereoselectivity of phenytoin hydroxylation in the two species. The *m*-HPPH from dog urine was dextrorotatory ($[\alpha]_D = +8.3°$ and $+8.0°$ for two dogs) and was entirely in the form of a pure optical isomer. The *p*-HPPH from dog and human urine consisted of a 2:1 and 10:1 mixture, respectively, of levo- and dextrorotatory isomers. This value for man was later confirmed by others (33,61).

The amount of *m*-HPPH in human urine was too low to permit isolation and measurement of optical rotation.

Maguire et al. (60–62) determined the absolute configuration of the dihydrodiol metabolite in rat, dog, and human urine. As with HPPH, the majority of dihydrodiol in human and rat urine was in the (*S*) configuration [3:1 ratio of (*S*):(*R*) in man], and the dog produced a 2:1 ratio of the (*R*) and (*S*) diastereoisomers. Although an arene oxide of phenytoin has not been directly isolated and characterized, a large body of evidence has accumulated in support of the existence of (*S*) and (*R*) arene oxide intermediates (see above). The proposed pathway is shown in Fig. 3. It is not known whether there are separate (*R*)- and (*S*)-specific arene oxidase enzymes or only one arene oxidase enzyme with incomplete substrate specificity.

NONLINEAR PHARMACOKINETIC PROPERTIES OF PHENYTOIN

The rate of change of serum concentration (C) of a drug by an enzyme system can be expressed by the Michaelis-Menten equation:

$$\frac{dC}{dt} = \frac{V_{max}}{K_m + C} \times C \qquad (1)$$

where t is time, V_{max} is the maximum velocity of the enzyme system, and K_m is the Michaelis constant of the enzyme system (serum concentration at which half of the maximum velocity of the enzyme system is attained). Drug mean steady-state serum concentration (C_{ss}) can be expressed as:

$$C_{ss} = \frac{R \times K_m}{V_{max} - R} \qquad (2)$$

where R is dosing rate. When C is similar to or greater than K_m, dC/dt will vary in a nonlinear fashion with C; when R is equal to or greater than $0.1 \times V_{max}$, C_{ss} will vary in a nonlinear fashion with V_{max}. These observations are the basis of nonlinear pharmacokinetics.

The mean apparent value for phenytoin K_m in adults is 6.2 µg/ml, with a range of 1.5 to 30.7 µg/ml based upon 55 reported determinations; the mean apparent value for phenytoin V_{max} in adults is 0.45 µg/ml/hr with a range of 0.14 to 1.36 µg/ml/hr based upon 54 reported determinations (2,11,32,35,37,40,48,65,74). These values appear to be determined principally by arene oxidase enzyme system K_m and V_{max} values, although the other pathways shown in Fig. 1 presumably have modifying effects on the apparent values of K_m and V_{max} for phenytoin in man. Note that the apparent K_m values computed for man are based upon total (protein-bound and nonprotein-bound) serum phenytoin concentration. Since only nonprotein-bound phenytoin can be acted upon by the metabolizing enzyme system and the nonprotein-bound fraction for phenytoin is approximately 10% in man (89), the K_m of the enzyme responsible for *para*-hydroxylation of phenytoin should actually be approximately 0.6 µg/ml. This prediction has been verified in rat liver microsomes (85).

Eadie et al. (30) performed the largest comprehensive comparison of phenytoin K_m and V_{max} values in children and adults. The K_m values for 21 adults (mean = 5.8 µg/ml) and 15 children (mean, 5.3 µg/ml) were not significantly different. The V_{max} values for 21 adults (mean, 0.48 µg/ml/hr assuming a phenytoin volume of distribution of 0.7 liter/kg) were significantly less than the V_{max} values for 15 children (mean, 0.74 µg/ml/hr assuming a phenytoin volume of distribution of 0.7 liter/kg) ($p < 0.025$). These observations predict that the clearance ($V_{max}/(K_m + C)$) of phenytoin should be greater in children than in adults. This prediction is confirmed by the observations that the elimination half-life of phenytoin is shorter in children than in adults and that the average daily dosing rate of phenytoin (in mg/kg) required to achieve a given serum concentration is greater in children than in adults (9,31,55).

Phenytoin exhibits nonlinear pharmacokinetic properties in the majority of patients because the usual therapeutic serum concentrations (10 to 20 µg/ml, see Chapter 14) exceed the usual K_m value (6.2 µg/ml), and the usual dosing rate (0.15 to 0.45 µg/ml/hr) is greater than $0.1 \times$ the usual value of V_{max} (0.45 µg/ml/hr). The consequences of nonlinear pharmacokinetics are discussed below.

Steady-State Serum Concentration

The steady-state serum phenytoin concentration increases faster than the dosing rate when the rate is increased and decreases faster than the dosing rate when the rate is decreased (equation 2) (Fig. 4) (14,58,76). Thus, the steady-state serum concentration of a drug with nonlinear pharmacokinetic properties at one dosing rate does not directly predict the steady-state serum concentration of the drug at another dosing rate.

If the clinician attempts to increase or decrease the steady-state serum phenytoin concentration by simple linear extrapolation from a known serum concentration versus the dosing rate, the result is often an unexpectedly high or low serum concentration when the new steady-state value is attained (see Fig. 4). Numerous mathematical and tabular methods have been devised to predict the phenytoin dosing rate necessary to produce a given steady state-serum concentration from a single steady-state serum concentration versus time point; these methods have been critically reviewed elsewhere (11,69,74,77,78). A useful rule of thumb for increasing the phenytoin dosage in adults is to increase the dosing rate in increments of 100 mg/day at monthly intervals (see below) until a steady-state serum phenytoin concentration of 5 to 10 µg/ml (a value approximately equal to K_m) is at-

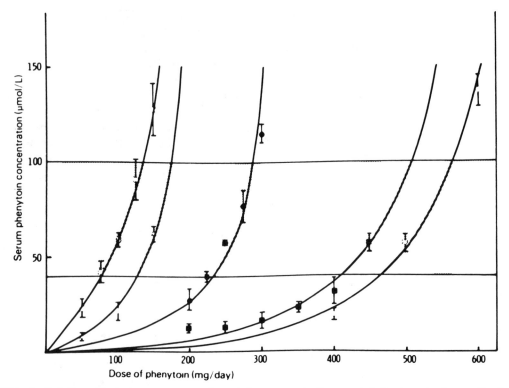

FIG. 4. Relationship between serum phenytoin concentration and daily dose in five patients. Each point represents the mean ($\pm$ S.D.) of three to eight measurements of serum phenytoin concentration at steady state. The curves were fitted by computer using the Michaelis-Menten equation. (From Richens and Dunlop, ref. 76, with permission.)

tained; later increases should not exceed 50 mg/day at monthly intervals.

Nonlinear pharmacokinetics complicate the issue of generic equivalence of phenytoin products. The weighted mean value for absolute bioavailability of brand name phenytoin (Dilantin Kapseals, 100 mg, Parke-Davis) was 86% in three studies (10). Less than complete absorption of Dilantin is at least in part a consequence of the use of a sustained release preparation (see Chapter 11). Different generic preparations of phenytoin thus have the potential to differ in absolute bioavailability from the brand name preparation by approximately 14% or more. Because of phenytoin's nonlinear pharmacokinetics, a 14% difference

in bioavailability would result in a greater than 14% increase or decrease in steady-state serum concentration. A national epidemic of phenytoin intoxication occurred in Australia when a more bioavailable formulation was substituted for an older formulation (73,86).

Clearance and Elimination Half-Life

Drug clearance is equal to $V_{max}/(K_m + C)$. Drug elimination half-life is equal to 0.693 $\times$ volume of distribution/clearance. Thus, phenytoin clearance will vary inversely with serum concentration, and phenytoin elimination half-life will vary directly with serum concentration (Fig. 5) (10,12,14). Browne et al. (12,14) described and validated a method for calculating the phenytoin elimination half-life at any given serum phenytoin concentration if the patient's K_m and V_{max} values for phenytoin are known. The results were as follows for a group of 6 men on phenytoin monotherapy (mean calculated elimination half-life at different serum concentrations): 12.8 hr at 1 µg/ml, 25.8 hr at 10 µg/ml, 40.2 hr at 20 µg/ml, and 69.1 hr at 40 µg/ml. Note that the often-quoted elimination half-life of 24 hr for phenytoin applies principally to serum concentrations in the low therapeutic range (10 µg/ml) and that the elimination half-life is often longer at higher serum concentrations (see also Fig. 5). The range of elimination half-life values at a serum phenytoin concentration of 40 µg/ml was 37.1 to 96.8 hr. Because of phenytoin's long and vari-

able elimination half-life at toxic serum concentrations, one cannot predict the time required for the serum phenytoin concentration to return to the therapeutic level in a given individual. In such circumstances, withhold phenytoin and monitor the serum concentration daily until it returns to the therapeutic range.

Time to Reach Steady-State Serum Concentration

As the serum phenytoin concentration rises, phenytoin clearance decreases (see above). This results in a further rise in serum phenytoin concentration and a further decrease in phenytoin clearance. This self-propagating cycle can require a long period of time to go to completion. The time

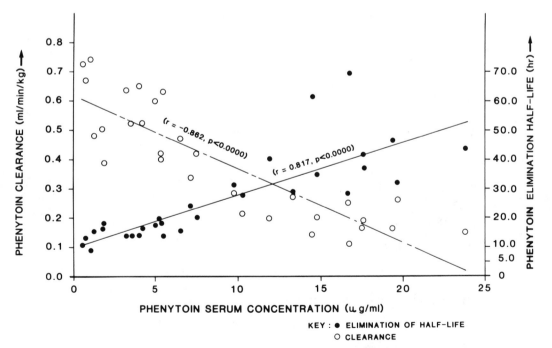

FIG. 5. Phenytoin clearance and elimination half-life values determined by stable isotope tracer techniques at 30 different serum concentration values in 18 adult males on phenytoin monotherapy. (Based in part on data from Browne et al., refs. 10, 13, and 15, with permission.)

(t) required to attain a given serum concentration can be computed by the equation:

$$t = \frac{V_d\,(C_{s,t} - C_{s,0})}{(R - V_{max})} - \frac{V_d\,K_m\,V_{max}}{(R - V_{max})^2}$$
$$\times \ln\left[\frac{(R - V_{max})\,C_{s,t} + RK_m}{(R - V_{max})\,C_{s,O} + RK_m}\right] \quad (3)$$

where V_d = volume of distribution, $C_{s,t}$ = serum concentration at time t, and $C_{s,0}$ = serum concentration at time 0 (57). Assuming average values for K_m and V_{max}, it is possible to compute an accumulation half-life ($t\frac{1}{2}_A$) for phenytoin as follows:

$$t_{1/2A} = 0.270 \times C_{ss} \quad (4)$$

where $t\frac{1}{2}_A$ is expressed in days, and C_{ss} is expressed in μg/ml (88). Equations 3 and 4 predict, and empirical data confirm, that (a) the time to reach steady-state serum concentration will vary nonlinearly with the dosing rate, (b) the time to reach steady-state serum concentration will vary linearly with the serum concentration, and (c) the time required to attain a new steady-state serum concentration after starting phenytoin therapy or increasing or decreasing the phenytoin dosing rate may be as long as 28 days (Figs. 6 and 7) (11,14,57,81,88). Therefore, a serum phenytoin concentration measured less than 28 days after a change in the phenytoin dosing rate may not be an accurate indication of the ultimate new steady-state serum concentration.

Effect of Long-Term Administration

With the initiation of phenytoin monotherapy, the serum phenytoin concentration progressively rises while the rate of formation of p-HPPH decreases, clearance decreases, and the elimination half-life increases (Fig. 5). Table 1 shows typical values for these changes in a group of six patients started on phenytoin monotherapy.

MINOR METABOLIC PATHWAYS

The minor metabolites of phenytoin include those discussed below, as well as some not yet identified (18–20).

Catechol and 3-0-Methyl Catechol Metabolites

Using radioisotopes and GC-MS, Chang et al. (22) identified a 3,4-catechol metabolite, 5-(3,4-dihydroxyphenyl)-5-phenylhydantoin, in rat urine following administration of phenytoin in the diet for 2 weeks (Fig. 1). Borga et al. (7) also detected the same metabolite in rat urine and human urine. Further work by Chang et al. (21) resulted in the identification of a 3-0-methylcatechol metabolite in rat urine as 5-(4-hydroxy-3-methoxyphenyl)-5-phenylhydantoin (Fig. 1). The catechol and the 3-0-methylcatechol represented approximately 2% and 10%, respectively, of the total phenytoin metabolites in rat urine. Later, Midha et al. (67) reported positive identification of the catechol and 3-0-methylcatechol in human, monkey, and dog urine. The same metabolites were also identified as glucuronides in the bile from isolated perfused rat liver (38).

The catechol could be formed via dehydrogenation of the dihydrodiol metabolite by a mechanism similar to that described by Ayengar et al. (4). In a preliminary experiment, ^{14}C-labeled dihydrodiol metabolite isolated from rat urine was administered orally to rats. It did not result in the appearance of the catechol metabolite in urine (22). The catechol metabolite could be formed by further hydroxylation of m-HPPH or p-HPPH. Gerber and Thompson (39) identified small amounts of the catechol and 3-0-methylcatechol in rat bile by GC-MS techniques following administration of m-HPPH or p-HPPH to rats or by addition of these compounds to an isolated perfused rat liver preparation. More recently, Bill-

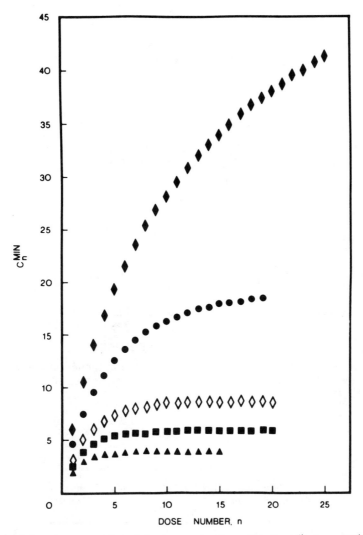

FIG. 6. Plot of minimum serum phenytoin concentration after the Nth dose, C^{min}, versus dose number n. Symbols and dosing rates (g/day) are: (◆) 0.50, (●) 0.40, (◇) 0.30, (■) 0.25, and (▲) 0.20. (From Wagner et al., ref. 88, with permission.)

ings (5), Billings and Fischer (6), Chow, et al. (25), and Chow and Fischer (26) provided evidence that the catechol metabolite of phenytoin was formed from both dihydrodiol and p-HPPH in rats and mice. However, the predominant route was via p-HPPH (26).

In rat urine, the concentration of the 3-0-methylcatechol metabolite was approximately fivefold greater than that of the ca-

techol, indicating extensive 0-methylation in this species (22). Evidence obtained by Chang et al. (21) indicates that the 3-0-methylcatechol metabolite of phenytoin is formed from the catechol. Administration of the synthetic 3,4-dihydroxycatechol to rats resulted in the prompt appearance of 3-0-methylcatechol in the urine (22). It is reasonable to assume that the enzyme catechol-0-methyltransferase is involved in

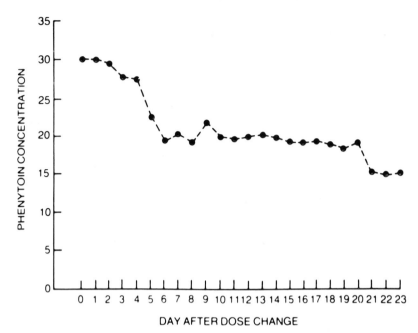

FIG. 7. Changes in serum phenytoin concentration after reduction in phenytoin dosing rate from 250 mg/day to 200 mg/day. Serum phenytoin concentration stabilized after day 23. (From Theodore et al., ref. 81, with permission.)

TABLE 1. *Phenytoin biotransformation and pharmacokinetic values for six patients at three times during monotherapy determined with 150 mg tracer doses of stable isotope-labeled phenytoin*

Week 0[a]	Week 4[b]	Week 12[c]	Significance[d] ($p <$)
Rate of formation of *p*-HPPH (mg labeled *p*-HPPH excreted per 48 hr)			
98.5 ± 31.4[e]	82.2 ± 20.1	69.2 ± 31.9	0.01
Clearance (ml/min/kg)[f]			
0.587 ± 0.149	0.456 ± 0.147	0.387 ± 0.187	0.05
Elimination half-life (hr)[f]			
13.2 ± 3.6	18.4 ± 5.0	25.9 ± 9.7	0.01

[a] Week 0, value from single-dose (150 mg) study performed prior to starting monotherapy.
[b] Week 4, value after 4 weeks on monotherapy (300 mg/day).
[c] Week 12, value after 12 weeks on monotherapy (300–500 mg/day).
[d] Difference among values for weeks 0, 4, and 12 by analysis of variance for one group with repeated measures.
[e] Mean ± standard deviation.
[f] Value for tracer dose of phenytoin.
From Browne et al., ref. 10, with permission.

the formation of this metabolite, since it is known to methylate other catechols, including catecholamines (3).

4,4'-Dihydroxy Metabolite and *N*-Glucuronide of Phenytoin

Two minor metabolites of phenytoin, the 5,5-*bis*(4-hydroxyphenyl) hydantoin (82) and an *N*-glucuronide of phenytoin (79), were identified in rats and humans (Fig. 1). The 4,4'-dihydroxy metabolite was excreted as a glucuronide and accounted for about 1% of the total hydroxylated metabolites. The pathway that leads to the formation of this metabolite is not known. When *p*-HPPH was added to the perfusate of an isolated rat liver preparation, there was no evidence of the formation of the 4,4'-dihydroxy metabolite (82). However, addition of the synthetic 4,4'-dihydroxy compound to the same *in vitro* preparation (82) resulted in the formation of a monoglucuronide, a trihydroxyphenytoin glucuronide, and a dihydroxymethoxyphenytoin glucuronide, indicating further hydroxylation of the dihydroxy metabolite. Whether the trihydroxylated product represents normal phenytoin metabolites in intact animals is not yet known.

The glucuronide of phenytoin was isolated from a patient receiving phenytoin and characterized by GM-MS as the *N*-3 glucuronide. The same metabolite was also present in the bile of an isolated perfused rat liver preparation. The structure assignment was based on the mass spectra of various permethylated derivatives and a comparison of the reaction of the metabolite and 5,5-diphenyl-3-methylhydantoin with diazomethane (79). Subsequently, Hassell et al. (47) reported that phenytoin *N*-glucuronide was the major metabolite in cat urine.

SPECIES DIFFERENCES IN METABOLISM

With the exception of the dog and cat, the major metabolic product of phenytoin in all species, including man, is a glucuronide conjugate of *p*-HPPH (20,22,24,29,36,39, 44). Significant amounts of free *p*-HPPH were observed in the urine of mice and rats (20,30,39). The dihydrodiol metabolite was found in higher concentrations in urine of the rat and monkey than in the mouse, dog, or cat. The catechol and 3-*0*-methylcatechol metabolites were detected in rat urine following repeated administration of phenytoin in the diet and accounted for 2% and 20%, respectively, of the total metabolites present (21). In dog urine, the major metabolite was the glucuronide conjugate of *m*-HPPH, and phenytoin *N*-glucuronide was the major urinary product of cats.

The distribution patterns of metabolites in human urine were reported by Chang and Glazko (20,22,24): 68% to 81% *p*-HPPH, 7% to 11% dihydrodiol, 2.5% 3-*0*-methylcatechol, 1% unchanged phenytoin, and about 1% catechol. Metabolites in human feces (percent of fecal radioactivity) were identified as *p*-HPPH (50% to 80%), dihydrodiol (15% to 35%), and catechol (5% to 10%). Later studies have confirmed these values (29).

Species differences in the formation of glucuronide conjugates of *m*-HPPH or *p*-HPPH in rat or dog liver supernatant were reported by Gabler (34). Conjugation of *m*-HPPH was greater than that of *p*-HPPH in the dog liver, whereas the opposite effect was found with rat liver supernatant.

ACKNOWLEDGMENT

This work was supported in part by the Veterans Administration.

REFERENCES

1. Atkinson, A. J., Jr., MacGee, J., Strong, J., Garteiz, D., and Gaffney, T. E. (1970): Identification

of 5-metahydroxyphenyl-5-phenylhydantoin as a metabolite of diphenylhydantoin. *Biochem. Pharmacol.,* 19:2483–2491.

2. Atkinson, A. J., and Shaw, J. M. (1973): Pharmacokinetic study of a patient with diphenylhydantoin toxicity. *Clin. Pharmacol. Ther.,* 14:521–528.

3. Axelrod, J., and Tomachick, R. (1950): Enzymatic *O*-methylation of epinephrine and other catechols. *J. Biol. Chem.,* 233:702–705.

4. Ayengar, J., and Tomchick, R. (1958): Enzymatic *O*-methylation of epinephrine and other catechols. *J. Biol. Chem.,* 233:702–705.

5. Billings, R. E. (1983): Sex differences in rats in the metabolism of phenytoin to 5-(3,4-dihydroxyphenyl)-5-phenylhydantoin. *J. Pharm. Exper. Therap.,* 225:630–636.

6. Billings, R. E., and Fischer, L. J. (1985): Oxygen-18 incorporation studies of the metabolism of phenytoin to the catechol. *Drug Metab. Dispos.,* 13:312–317.

7. Borga, O., Garle, M., and Gutova, M. (1972): Identification of 5-(3,4-dihydroxyphenyl)-5-phenylhydantoin as a metabolite of 5,5-diphenylhydantoin (phenytoin) in rats and man. *Pharmacology,* 7:129–137.

8. Brodie, B. B., Reid, W. D., Cho, A. K., Sipes, G., Krishna, G., and Gillette, J. R. (1971): Possible mechanism of liver necrosis caused by aromatic organic compounds. *Proc. Natl. Acad. Sci. USA,* 68:160–164.

9. Browne, T. R. (1979): Clinical pharmacology of antiepileptic drugs. *Drug Ther. Rev.,* 2:469–503.

10. Browne, T. R., Evans, J. E., Szabo, G. K., Evans, B. A., Greenblatt, D. J., and Schumacher, G. E. (1985): Studies with stable isotopes I: Changes in phenytoin pharmacokinetics and biotransformation during monotherapy. *J. Clin. Pharmacol.,* 25:43–50.

11. Browne, T. R., Greenblatt, D. J., Evans, J. E., Evans, B. A., Szabo, G. K., and Schumacher, G. E. (1987): Determination of the *in vivo* K_m and V_{max} of a drug with tracer studies. *J. Clin. Pharmacol.,* 27:321–324.

12. Browne, T. R., Greenblatt, D. J., Evans, J. E., Evans, B. A., Szabo, G. K., and Schumacher, G. E. (1987): Estimation of a drug's elimination half-life at any serum concentration when the drug's K_m and V_{max} are known: Calculation and validation with phenytoin. *J. Clin. Pharmacol.,* 27:318–320.

13. Browne, T. R., Szabo, G. K., Evans, J. E., Evans, B. A., Greenblatt, D. J., and Mikati, M. A. (1988): Phenobarbital does not alter phenytoin steady-state serum concentration or pharmacokinetics. *Neurology,* 38:639–642.

14. Browne, T. R., Szabo, G. K., Evans, G. E., Evans, B. A., Greenblatt, D. J., and Schumacher, G. E. (*in press*): Studies of non-linear pharmacokinetics with stable isotope labeled phenytoin. In: *Proceedings of the Third International Symposium on the Synthesis and Applications of Isotopically Labeled Compounds,* edited by T. A. Baillie and J. P. Jones. Amsterdam, Elsevier.

15. Browne, T. R., Szabo, G. K., Evans, J. E., Greenblatt, D. J., and Mikati, M. A. (1988): Carbamazepine increases phenytoin serum concentration and reduces phenytoin clearance. *Neurology,* 38:1146–1150.

16. Butler, T. C. (1957): The metabolic conversion of 5,5-diphenylhydantoin to 5-(*p*-hydroxyphenyl)-5-phenylhydantoin. *J. Pharmacol. Exp. Ther.,* 199:1–11.

17. Butler, T. C., Dudley, K. H., Johnson, D., and Roberts, S. B. (1976): Studies of the metabolism of 5,5-diphenylhydantoin relating principally to the stereoselectivity of the hydroxylation reactions in man and the dog. *J. Pharmacol. Exp. Ther.,* 199:82–92.

18. Chace, D. H., and Abramson, P. P. (*in press*): Selective detection of stable isotope-labeled drugs and metabolites using capillary gas chromatography-reactive interface/mass spectrometry. In: *Proceedings of the Third International Symposium on the Applications of Isotopically Labeled Compounds,* edited by T. A. Baillie and J. P. Jones. Amsterdam, Elsevier.

19. Chang, T., and Glazko, A. J. (1972): Diphenylhydantoin: Biotransformation. In: *Antiepileptic Drugs,* 1st edition, edited by D. M. Woodbury, J. K. Penry, and R. P. Schmidt, pp. 149–162. Raven Press, New York.

20. Chang, T., and Glazko, A. J. (1982): Phenytoin: Biotransformation. In: *Antiepileptic Drugs,* 2nd edition, edited by D. M. Woodbury, J. K. Penry, and C. E. Pippenger, pp. 204–226. Raven Press, New York.

21. Chang, T., Okerholm, R. A., and Glazko, A. J. (1972): A 3-*O*-methylated catechol metabolite of diphenylhydantoin (Dilantin) in rat urine. *Res Commun. Chem. Pathol. Pharmacol.,* 4:13–23.

22. Chang, T., Okerholm, R. A., and Glazko, A. J. (1972): Identification of 5-(3,4-dihydroxyphenyl)-5-phenylhydantoin: A metabolite of 5,5-diphenylhydantoin (Dilantin) in rat urine. *Anal. Lett.,* 5:195–202.

23. Chang, T., Savory, A., and Glazko, A. J. (1970): A new metabolite of 5,5-diphenylhydantoin (Dilantin). *Biochem. Biophys. Res. Commun.,* 38:449–555.

24. Chang, T., Young, R., Maschewske, E., Croskey, L., Smith, T. C., Buchanan, R. A., and Glazko, A. J. (1977): Metabolite studies with ^{13}C-^{14}C doubly labeled phenytoin in human subjects. *Epilepsia,* 18:191.

25. Chow, S. A., Charkowski, D. M., and Fischer, L. J. (1980): Separation of phenytoin and its metabolites by high performance liquid chromatography. *Life Sci.,* 27:2477–2482.

26. Chow, S. A., and Fischer, L. J. (1982): Phenytoin metabolism in mice. *Drug Metab. Dispos.,* 10:156–160.

27. Claesen, M., Moustafa, M. A. A., Adline, J., Vandervorst, D., and Poupaert, J. H. (1982): Evidence for an arene oxide-NIH shift pathway in the metabolic conversion of phenytoin to 5-(4-hydroxyphenyl)-5-phenylhydantoin in the rat and in man. *Drug Metab. Dispos.,* 10:667–671.

28. Daly, J. W., Jerina, D. M., and Witkop, B. (1972): Oxides and the NIH shift: The metabolism, toxicity, and carcinogenicity of aromatic compounds. *Experientia,* 28:1129–1264.

29. Dickinson, R. G., Hooper, W. D., Patterson, M., Eadie, M. J., and Maguire, B. (1985): Extent of urinary excretion of *p*-hydroxyphenytoin in healthy subjects given phenytoin. *Ther. Drug Monit.,* 7:283–289.

30. Dill, W. A., Kazenko, A., Wold, L. M., and Glazko, A. J. (1956): Studies on 5,5-diphenylhydantoin (Dilantin) in animals and man. *J. Pharmacol. Exp. Ther.,* 118:270–279.

31. Dodson, W. E. (1980): Phenytoin elimination in childhood: Effect of concentration-dependent kinetics. *Neurology,* 30:196–199.

32. Eadie, M. J., Tyrer, J. H., Bochner, F., Hooper, W. D. (1976): The elimination of phenytoin in man. *Clin. Exp. Pharmacol. Physiol.,* 3:217–224.

33. Fritz, S., Lindner, W., Roots, I., Frey, B. M., and Kupfer, A. (1987): Stereochemistry of aromatic phenytoin hydroxylation in humans. *J. Pharm. Exper. Ther.,* 241:615–622.

34. Gabler, W. L. (1974): A method for assaying conjugation of diphenylhydantoin metabolites. *Fed. Proc.,* 33:525.

35. Garrettson, L. K., and Jusko, W. J. (1975): Diphenylhydantoin elimination kinetics in overdosed children. *Clin. Pharmacol. Ther.,* 17:481–491.

36. Gerber, N., and Arnold, K. (1969): Studies on the metabolism of diphenylhydantoin in mice. *J. Pharm. Exp. Ther.,* 167:77–90.

37. Gerber, N., Lynn, R., and Oates, J. (1972): Acute intoxication with 5,5-diphenylhydantoin (Dilantin) associated with impairment of biotransformation: Plasma levels and urinary metabolites; and studies in healthy volunteers. *Ann. Intern. Med.,* 77:756–771.

38. Gerber, N., Seibert, R. A., and Thompson, R. M. (1973): Identification of a catechol glucuronide metabolite of 5,5-diphenylhydantoin (DPH) in rat bile by gas chromatography (GC) and mass spectrometry (MS). *Res. Commun. Chem. Pathol. Pharmcol.,* 6:499–511.

39. Gerber, N., and Thompson, R. M. (1974): Identification of catechol glucuronide metabolites of hydroxydiphenylhydantoins (*m*-HPPH, *p*-HPPH) in rat bile. *Fed. Proc.,* 33:525.25.

40. Gerber, N., and Wagner, J. G. (1972): Explanation of dose-dependent decline of diphenylhydantoin levels by fitting to the integrated form of the Michaelis-Menten equation. *Res. Commun. Chem. Pathol. Pharmcol.,* 3:455–466.

41. Gerber, N., Weller, W. L., Lynn, R., Rangno, R. E., Sweetman, B. J., and Bush, M. T. (1971): Study of dose dependent metabolism of 5,5-diphenylhydantoin in the rat using new methodology for isolation and quantitation of metabolites *in vivo* and *in vitro. J. Pharmacol. Exp. Ther.,* 178:567–579.

42. Gillette, J. R. (1974): A perspective on the role of chemically reactive metabolites of foreign compounds in toxicity. I. Correlation of changes in covalent binding of reactive metabolites with changes in the incidence and severity of toxicity. *Biochem. Pharmcol.,* 23:2785–2794.

43. Glazko, A. J., Chang, T., Baukema, J., Dill, W. A., Goulet, J. R., and Buchanan, R. A. (1969): Metabolic disposition of diphenylhydantoin in normal human subjects following intravenous administration. *Clin. Pharmacol. Ther.,* 10:498–504.

44. Glazko, A. J., Peterson, F. E., Smith, T. C., Dill, W. A., and Chang, T. (1982): Phenytoin metabolism in subjects with long and short plasma half-lives. *Ther. Drug Monit.,* 4:281–292.

45. Gorvin, J. H., and Brownlee, G. (1957): Metabolism of 5,5-diphenylhydantoin in the rabbit. *Nature,* 179:1248.

46. Grover, P. L., Hewer, A., and Sims, P. (1971): Epoxides as microsomal metabolites of polycyclic hydrocarbons. *F.E.B.S. Lett.,* 18:76–80.

47. Hassell, T. M., Maguire, J. H., Cooper, C. G., and Johnson, P. T. (1984): Phenytoin administered in the cat after long-term administration. *Epilepsia,* 25:556–563.

48. Holcomb, R., Lynn, R., Harvey, B., Sweetman, B. J., and Gerber, N. (1972): Intoxication with 5,5-diphenylhydantoin (Dilantin): Clinical features, blood levels, urinary metabolites and metabolic changes in a child. *J. Pediatr.,* 80:627–632.

49. Horning, M. G., and Lertratanangkoon, K. (1977): Effect of chronic administration on urinary profiles of phenytoin metabolites. *Fed. Proc.,* 36:966.

50. Horning, M. G., Stratton, C., Wilson, A., Horning, E. C., and Hill, R. M. (1971): Detection of 5-(3,4 - di - *p* - hydroxy - 1,5 - cyclohexadien - 1 - yl) - 5 -phenyl-hydantoin as a major metabolite of 5,5-diphenylhydantoin (Dilantin) in newborn human. *Anal. Lett.,* 4:537–545.

51. Jerina, D. M., and Daly, J. W. (1974): Arene oxides: A new aspect of drug metabolism. *Science,* 185:573–582.

52. Jerina, D., Daly, J., Witkop, B., Zaltmen-Nirenberg, P., and Undenfriend, S. (1968): Role of the oxide-oxepin system in the metabolism of aromatic substrates. 1. *In vitro* conversion of benzene oxide to a permercapturic and dihydrodiol. *Arch. Biochem. Biophys.,* 128:176–183.

53. Jerina, D. M., Daly, J. W., Witkop, B., Zaltzman-Nirenburg, P., and Undenfriend, S. (1970): 1,2-Naphthalene oxide as an intermediate in the microsomal hydroxylation of napthalene. *Biochemistry,* 9:147–155.

54. Jusko, W. J. (1976): Bioavailability and disposition kinetics of phenytoin in man. In: *Quantitative Analytic Studies in Epilepsy,* edited by P. Kellaway and I. Petersen, pp. 115–136. Raven Press, New York.

55. Kutt, H. (1982): Phenytoin: Relation of plasma concentration to seizure control. In: *Antiepileptic Drugs,* 2nd edition, edited by D. M. Woodbury, J. K. Penry, and C. E. Pippenger, pp. 241–246. Raven Press, New York.

56. Kutt, H., Wolk, M., Scherman, R., and McDonald, F. (1964): Insufficient parahydroxylation as a cause of diphenylhydantoin toxicity. *Neurology,* 14:542–548.

57. Lam, G., and Chiou, W. L. (1979): Integrated

equation to evaluate accumulation profiles of drugs eliminated by Michaelis-Menten kinetics. *J. Pharmacokinet. Biopharm,* 7:227–232.

58. Levy, R. H. (1982): General principles: Drug absorption, distribution, and elimination. In: *Antileptic Drugs,* 2nd edition, edited by D. M. Woodbury, J. K. Penry, and C. E. Pippenger, pp. 11–24. Raven Press, New York.

59. Maguire, J. H., Butler, T. C., and Dudley, K. H. (1978): Absolute configuration of (+)-5-(3-hydroxypheny)—5-phenylhydantoin, the major metabolite of 5,5-diphenylhydantoin in the dog. *J. Med. Chem.,* 21:1194–1297.

60. Maguire, J. H., Butler, T. C., and Dudley, K. H. (1980): Absolute configurations of the dihydrodiol metabolites of 5,5-diphenylhydantoin (phenytoin) from rat, dog, and human urine. *Drug Metab. Dispos.,* 8:325–331.

61. Maguire, J. H., and McClanahan, J. S. (1986): Evidence for stereoselective production of phenytoin (5,5-diphenylhydantoin) arene oxides in man.

62. Maguire, J. H., and Wilson, D. C. (1985): Urinary dihydrodiol metabolites of phenytoin: High performance liquid chromatography assay of diastereometric composition. *J. Chromatog.,* 342:323–332.

63. Martz, F., Failinger, C., III, and Blake, D. (1977): Phenytoin teratogenesis: Correlation between embryopathic effect and covalent binding of putative arene oxide metabolite in gestational tissue. *J. Pharcol. Exp. Ther.,* 203:231–239.

64. Massey, K. M. (1966): Teratogenic effect of diphenylhydantoin sodium. *J. Oral. Ther. Pharmacol.,* 2:380–385.

65. Mawer, G. E., Mullen, P. W., Rodgers, M., Robins, A. J., and Lucas, S. B. (1974): Phenytoin dose adjustment in epileptic patients. *Br. J. Clin. Pharmacol.,* 1:163–168.

66. Maynert, E. W. (1960): The metabolic fate of diphenylhydantoin in the dog, rat, and man. *J. Pharmacol. Exp. Ther.,* 130:275–284. In: *Biological Reactive Intermediates III,* edited by J. J. Kocsis, D. J. Jollow, C. M. Witmer, J. O. Nelson, and R. Snyder, pp. 897–902. Plenum, New York.

67. Midha, K. K., Hindmarsh, K. W., McGilvray, I. J., and Cooper, J. K. (1977): Identification of urinary catechol and methylated catechol metabolites of phenytoin in human, monkeys, and dogs by GLC and GLC-mass spectrometry. *J. Pharm. Sci.,* 66:1596–1602.

68. Moustafa, M. A. A., Claesen, M., Adline, J., Vandervorst, D., and Poupaert, J. H. (1983): Evidence for an arene-3,4-oxide as metabolic intermediate in the *meta-* and *para-*hydroxylation of phenytoin in the dog. *Drug Metab. Dispos.,* 11:574–580.

69. Mullen, P. W., and Foster, R. W. (1979): Comparative evaluation of six techniques for determining the Michaelis-Menten parameters relating phenytoin dose and steady state serum concentrations. *J. Pharm. Pharmacol.,* 31:100–104.

70. Noach, E. L., Woodbury, D. M., and Goodman, L. S. (1958): Studies on the absorption, distribution, fate and excretion of 4-^{14}C-labeled diphenylhydantoin. *J. Pharmacol. Exp. Ther.,* 122:301–314.

71. Oesch, F., Kaubisch, N., Jerina, D. M., and Daly, J. W. (1971): Hepatic epoxide hydrase. Structure activity relationships for substrates and inhibitors. *Biochemistry,* 10:4858–4866.

72. Poupaert, J. H., Cavalier, R., Claesen, M. H., and Dumont, P. A. (1975): Absolute configuration of the major metabolite of 5,5-diphenylhydantoin, 5-(4′-hydroxypheny)-5-phenylhydantoin. *J. Med. Chem.,* 18:1268–1271.

73. Rail, L. (1968): Dilantin overdosage. *Med. J. Aust.,* 2:339.

74. Rambeck, B., Boenigk, H. E., Dunlop, A., Mullen, P. W., Wadsworth, J., and Richens, A. (1979): Predicting phenytoin dose: A revised monogram. *Ther. Drug Monit.,* 1:325–333.

75. Rane, A., and Peug, D. (1985): Phenytoin enhances epoxide metabolism in human fetal liver cultures. *Drug Metabol. Dispo.,* 13:382–385.

76. Richens, A., and Dunlop, A. (1975): Serum phenytoin levels in the management of epilepsy. *Lancet,* 2:247–248.

77. Schumacher, G. E. (1980): Using pharmacokinetics in drug therapy: VI. Comparing methods for dealing with nonlinear drugs like phenytoin. *Am. J. Hosp. Pharm.,* 37:128–132.

78. Sheiner, L. B., and Beal, S. L. (1980): Evaluation of population methods for estimating pharmacokinetic parameters: I. Michaelis-Menten model: Routine pharmacokinetic data. *J. Pharmacokinet. Biopharm.,* 8:553–571.

79. Smith, R. G., Daves, G. D., Jr., Lynn, R. K., and Gerber, N. (1977): Hydantoin ring glucuronidation: Characterization of a new metabolite of 5,5-diphenylhydantoin in man and the rat. *Biomed. Mass Spectrom.,* 4:275–279.

80. Sweetman, B. J., Lynn, R., Weller, W. L., Gerber, N., and Bush, M. T. (1977): The urinary metabolite pattern of 5,5-diphenylhydantoin (DPH) in control mice and mice pretreated with DPH. *Pharmacologist,* 13:22.

81. Theodore, W. H., Qu, P., Tsay, J. Y., Pitlick, W., and Porter, R. J. (1984): Phenytoin: The pseudo-steady-state phenomenon. *Clin. Pharmacol. Ther.,* 25:822–825.

82. Thompson, R. M., Beghin, J., Fife, W. K., and Gerber, N. (1976): 5,5-Bis(4-hydroxyphenyl) hydantoin, a minor metabolite of diphenylhydantoin (Dilantin) in the rat and human. *Drug Metab. Dispos.,* 4:349–356.

83. Thompson, R. M., Gerber, N., Seibert, R. A., and Desiderio, D. M. (1973): A rapid method for the mass spectrometric identification of glucuronides and other polar drug metabolites in permethylated rat bile. *Drug Metab. Dispos.,* 1:489–505.

84. Tomaszewski, J. E., Jerina, D. M., and Daly, J. W. (1975): Deuterium isotope effect during formation of phenoes by hepatic monooxygenases. Evidence for an alternative to the arene oxide pathway. *Biochemistry,* 14:2024–2031.

85. Tsuru, M., Erickerson, R. R., and Holtzman, J. L. (1982): The metabolism of phenytoin by isolated

hepatocytes and hepatic microsomes from male rats. *J. Pharm. Exp. Ther.*, 222:658–661.

86. Tyrer, J. H., Eadie, M. J., Sutherland, J. M. (1970): Outbreak of anticonvulsant intoxication in an Australian city. *Br. Med. J.*, 4:271–273.

87. Vasko, M. R., Bell, R. D., Daly, D. D., and Pippenger, C. E. (1979): Inheritance of phenytoin hypometabolism: A kinetic study in one family. *Clin. Pharmacol. Ther.*, 27:96–103.

88. Wagner, J. G. Time to reach steady state and prediction of steady-state concentration for drugs obeying Michaelis-Menten elimination kinetics. *J. Pharmacokinet. Biopharm.*, 6:209–225.

89. Woodbury, D. M. (1982): Phenytoin: Absorption, distribution, and excretion. In: *Antiepileptic Drugs,* 2nd edition, edited by D. M. Woodbury, J. K. Penry, and C. E. Pippenger, pp. 191–207. Raven Press, New York.

Antiepileptic Drugs, Third Edition, edited by
R. Levy, R. Mattson, B. Meldrum,
J. K. Penry, and F. E. Dreifuss.
Raven Press, Ltd., New York © 1989.

13

Phenytoin

Interactions with Other Drugs

Henn Kutt

INTRODUCTION

The majority of interactions between phenytoin and other drugs manifest in changes of the pharmacokinetic parameters of phenytoin or the other drug. Interactions involving pharmacodynamic parameters have been assumed to take place with some drug combinations, but documentation of those is still limited.

Pharmacokinetic interactions become clinically evident by the appearance of signs of intoxication or lack of effectiveness. Monitoring the drug concentrations shows that the plasma concentration has risen or fallen depending on the mechanism of the interaction. Further studies reveal changes in clearance (Cl), elimination half-life ($T_{1/2}$), and area under the curve (AUC) of serial concentrations with or without changes of the volume of distribution (V_d) and protein binding.

It is important to realize that the same drug in combination with phenytoin may not have the same effect in all patients. First, the extent of the interaction-related change in the drug concentration may vary among individuals. Second, the direction of the change may be up in some and down in other patients. The reasons for the variability among individuals in the magnitude or direction of the interaction are only partially understood. The nonlinear kinetics of

phenytoin and the individual's preexisting kinetic parameters (e.g., V_{max}, K_m) play a role. Genetic factors are important; a patient who is a slow metabolizer of phenytoin or the interacting drug is more likely to have a severe interaction. The magnitude of inducibility of hepatic drug-metabolizing enzymes appears to be a factor and is also genetically controlled to some extent. Environmental factors such as previous drug exposure can influence the extent and direction of an interaction, as does the dual effect of some drugs that cause induction of drug-metabolizing enzyme production but inhibit its action. Variable individual susceptibility is a practical phrase to use in this context.

The clinical significance of an interaction depends on whether or not it leads to a need to adjust the drug dosages and whether or not it is likely to occur in the majority of patients. In addition to these criteria is the need for consideration of the end result in an individual patient: a modest or even marked elevation of a low phenytoin level caused by an interaction may merely improve seizure control, a small elevation of a nearly toxic level may cause intoxication, and a marked elevation in an unusually susceptible individual with a combination of drugs that causes little change in the majority of patients is obviously significant.

The early reports about interactions

sometimes warned not to use the "reported" drug in combination with phenytoin. Empirically, it has now become clear that with monitoring plasma drug levels and adjusting dosages, virtually no drug combination is totally incompatible with phenytoin. The critical period with most potentially interacting drug combinations is usually the first few weeks or months. Close clinical and laboratory monitoring in that period is prudent.

MECHANISMS OF PHARMACOKINETIC INTERACTIONS

Pharmaceutical Interaction

Although not an interaction in the conventional sense, the pharmaceutical formulation has an effect on phenytoin bioavailability and on the rate of its absorption. The factors influencing the absorption rate are the granule size, nature of the filler, and whether the free acid or the sodium salt of phenytoin is the active ingredient. Numerous studies (14) have shown that phenytoin products from different manufacturers vary in the absorption rate and differ in the time to reach maximum concentration, even if the area under the curve is adequate to pass the Food and Drug Administration requirements. Therefore the United States Pharmacopeia lists "Phenytoin Prompt" (rapid maximum blood level peak) and "Phenytoin Extended" (delayed maximum blood level peak). This alters the diurnal pattern of plasma phenytoin levels. It is best to prescribe phenytoin from the same manufacturer to maintain stability.

Some calcium-containing fillers can reduce the amount of phenytoin absorbed. An example is the Australian experience of intoxication in patients whose phenytoin levels rose when the filler was changed from calcium sulfate to lactose (7).

A pharmaceutical interaction is to be considered precipitation of parenteral phenytoin in a large-volume, glucose-containing fluid.

Absorption

Absorption interactions can alter the absorption rate or the total amount absorbed or both. The mechanisms involved include changes of gastric pH and emptying time, and the motility of the gastrointestinal tract in general.

Antacids are the agents of concern in this respect and their effects are complex. The magnesium-containing antacids primarily increase the gastric pH that enhances the solubility of weak acids and reduces the absorption rate from the stomach as it increases the ionization of the drug. Aluminum-containing antacids, in addition, prolong gastric emptying time which under these circumstances further slows the rate of absorption (52). The increased gastric motility and diarrhea may add another factor. Chelation or adsorption of phenytoin into the calcium-containing preparations has been suspected. In clinical studies using low doses of antacid (10 ml every 6 hr), little or no effect was seen (64). Higher doses (15 to 45 ml), however, were found to reduce phenytoin bioavailability (14,19). The effect is usually more noticeable if the antacid is given at the same or near time of phenytoin ingestion; therefore, it is practical to stagger the ingestion times in patients whose plasma phenytoin level is on the low side relative to the dose.

Food has been found to have variable but modest, usually enhancing, effects on phenytoin absorption (14). The mechanisms by which food could affect phenytoin absorption include saturation of the first-pass mechanisms, increased phenytoin dissolution in the stomach, and increased splanchnic flow (56). Lipid meals were found to increase phenytoin bioavailability somewhat (84). A protein-rich diet had the same effect on phenytoin acid but not on the sodium salt

(41). A steady relationship in time between food intake and ingestion of phenytoin is recommended (41,56).

Activated charcoal delays and reduces absorption of phenytoin; therefore, it is beneficial to give large doses of charcoal in the early phases of massive phenytoin overdose (102).

There is limited evidence that phenytoin interferes with the absorption of other drugs. Phenytoin reduces the plasma metyrapone level when metyrapone is given orally, but not when it is given intravenously. Decreased effectiveness and low levels of furosemide have been observed to be caused by phenytoin and ascribed in part to a reduction of furosemide absorption (105). The *Physician's Desk Reference* points out that molindone contains calcium, which might influence phenytoin absorption; no clinical reports have appeared so far.

Protein Binding

About 90% of the total phenytoin in the plasma is protein bound; less binding occurs in the very young and in subjects with renal or hepatic diseases. Other strongly binding drugs, such as tolbutamide (103), salicylates (25), valproate (60), and phenylbutazone (86), among others, can displace phenytoin from the binding sites. This effects an increase in the unbound fraction of phenytoin that often leads to increased clearance as the free drug reaches the liver. The result is some lowering of the total plasma concentration of phenytoin. Yet, loss of effectiveness may not occur since at the new lower steady-state level, the percent of free phenytoin is greater than it was before the displacing drug was added, and the actual concentration of the free phenytoin may remain relatively unchanged. However, if the displacing drug also happens to be an inhibitor of the phenytoin-metabolizing system and/or this system was nearly saturated already, the displacing drug may lead to elevation of the total plasma phenytoin level.

Biotransformation

Induction

Phenytoin is metabolized by the hepatic microsomal mixed-function oxidase system, hydroxylation followed by glucuronidation being the major pathway. The production of these enzymes is induced by inducer drugs. As evidence of induction of phenytoin metabolism, traditional plasma phenytoin half-life studies with fixed test doses have been carried out before and after or during the administration of the inducing drug. Shortening of the half-life of a test dose seems to indicate the trend but does not always correlate with the extent of induction during long-term drug administration. This is because phenytoin half-life is complex and concentration dependent. More recent techniques using stable isotope-labeled phenytoin as substrate during steady state are expected to help to characterize the presence of induction (12).

On the other hand, phenytoin can also act as an inducer of the metabolism of various other drugs in animals and humans, notably carbamazepine and anticoagulants. Induction of its own metabolism occurs only to a limited extent (22).

Inhibition

Inhibition of metabolism is the other major mechanism by which interactions between phenytoin and other drugs occur. The binding of phenytoin (a type I substrate) with the enzyme is somewhat unstable, as the magnitude of the phenytoin-induced difference spectra in microsomal preparations is easily reduced by a variety of drugs and chemicals (44). It has been shown that some drugs such as phenobarbital (44,68) and sulthiame (68) are competitive, and others such as disulfiram (47) and isoniazid (44) are noncompetitive inhibitors of phenytoin metabolism. The distinction has some theoretical as well as practical relevance: a noncompetitive inhibitor may cause marked accumulation of phenytoin, whereas a competitive inhibitor would only raise the level to a higher plateau at which phenytoin is again able to compete successfully if the entire system is not yet saturated. The extent of inhibition of phenytoin metabolism *in vitro* is related to the inhibitor's concentration. *In vivo*, increasing accumulation of phenytoin has been observed after an increase of sulthiame dose. With drugs given in conventional fixed doses such as isoniazid, the plasma concentration depends on the genetically determined acetylator phenotype: slow acetylators have a higher plasma concentration of isoniazid than fast acetylators, and they also develop higher phenytoin accumulations.

Induction–Inhibition

The induction and inhibition of phenytoin metabolism can take place at the same time if a drug induces the enzyme production but inhibits its action, as is the case with phenobarbital and probably with pheneturide and ethanol. The net result is no change if both effects are equal, or a rise or fall of the plasma phenytoin level if one dominates. The alterations of phenytoin level in this context may also change with time. If the inducer-inhibitor was just started, the inhibition may dominate first, leading to an early rise of the phenytoin level. Induction takes some time to develop but may then become dominant and cause a later fall of phenytoin level. Other factors that influence the net result of these opposing effects are the state of induction from previous drug contacts and probably the genetic makeup. The extent of inducibility has been shown to be genetically determined (100); a

"good" inducer is likely to have a fall, whereas a "poor" inducer would show no change or a rise of the phenytoin level following inducing-inhibiting drug addition.

ALTERATION OF PHENYTOIN KINETICS BY OTHER DRUGS

Analgesics and Antipyretics

Salicylates can displace phenytoin from the plasma protein binding sites *in vitro* and *in vivo*. In clinical studies, an increase of the unbound fraction of phenytoin from the usual 10% to near 16% and an increase of phenytoin clearance by acetylsalicylic acid were demonstrated (25). These changes were to some degree proportional to the acetylsalicylic acid dose, which ranged from 900 mg to 3,600 mg per day. In epileptic patients, high repeated doses of acetylsalicylic acid are expected to cause a small decline of total plasma phenytoin level but a slight increase in the relative percent of free phenytoin (69). Thus, in terms of effectiveness of phenytoin, no change is expected under these circumstances, and a need for dosage adjustment may not arise.

A small increase of plasma phenytoin level in five patients was observed by Dam et al. (20) after the patients received 65 mg of *propoxyphene* three times daily for 6 days. In another patient who took large amounts (650 mg per day) of propoxyphene for several days (45), phenytoin accumulated to the toxic range. In laboratory studies using rat liver microsomal preparations, propoxyphene has been shown to inhibit phenytoin metabolism (47). In clinical practice, however, with the conventional use of propoxyphene, significant elevations of plasma phenytoin levels are not expected.

Phenylbutazone (100 mg three times daily) has a variable effect on the total phenytoin level, but increases the concentration of unbound phenytoin. Marked prolongation of phenytoin half-life is also caused by phenylbutazone. Phenytoin intoxication has occurred in some epileptic patients taking phenylbutazone (86). The major factor in this interaction is displacement of phenytoin from plasma binding sites associated with some inhibition of phenytoin metabolism. A need to adjust phenytoin dosage may occur in some patients (70).

Doses of 600 mg of ibuprofen four times daily for 5 days did not alter the kinetics of 900 mg test doses of phenytoin in volunteers. Clinically significant interactions are unlikely to occur with this drug combination (96).

Anticoagulants

Bishydroxycoumarin (86) and, to a lesser extent, *phenprocoumon* have been reported to cause elevation of plasma phenytoin levels in some patients. *Warfarin* and *phenindione* have caused no change of plasma phenytoin levels (87). The general experience has been that patients taking phenytoin and anticoagulants together tolerate common doses of phenytoin well.

Antimicrobial Agents

Chloramphenicol has caused modest elevation of plasma phenytoin levels in some patients and marked elevations in others (42,70). The need to reduce the phenytoin dose has varied. It is likely that besides individual disposition, the duration of chloramphenicol administration is a determining factor.

Isoniazid inhibits phenytoin metabolism (Fig. 1) *in vitro* and *in vivo* (44,107). The inhibition is noncompetitive, and the mechanism by which it comes about has not yet been clarified. Noticeable *in vitro* inhibition of phenytoin metabolism occurs with isoniazid concentrations (5 µg/ml) (47) that have been measured in the plasma of patients taking isoniazid, particularly in those who are slow acetylators of isoniazid (44).

In patients taking phenytoin and isoniazid together, the clinical consequences vary and depend on the patient's acetylator phenotype (10,44). The polymorphism in acetylation is controlled by two autosomal alleles on a single gene locus: R and r. This allows three combinations, RR, Rr, and rr, and agrees with the fact that three modes can be distinguished clinically. The fast acetylators generally do not maintain high enough isoniazid concentration to inhibit phenytoin metabolism noticeably. In the intermediate group, a modest elevation of phenytoin level may occur, whereas in the very slow acetylators in whom isoniazid levels are high enough, there may be considerable phenytoin accumulation (44) (Fig. 2.) In patients taking phenytoin and isoniazid together, significant phenytoin accumulation and intoxication have been reported to occur in 10% to 15% of the subjects (10,21,107) who, in some studies, were identified as very slow acetylators (10).

Clinical management of this interaction is handled best by frequent monitoring of plasma phenytoin levels after the onset of combined therapy with conventional doses. If the plasma phenytoin level continues to rise, as is likely in a slow acetylator, the phenytoin dose is reduced. Prophylactic reduction of phenytoin dose is not practical unless the patient is a known very slow acetylator.

The isoniazid-phenytoin interaction is an example of a situation in which the genetic phenotype with regard to one drug determines the extent of its interaction with another and defines one reason for the individual susceptibility.

Rifampin can lower phenytoin levels and increase its clearance by a factor of two. Furthermore, the rifampin comedication minimizes the inhibitory effect of isoniazid even in the slow isoniazid acetylators (40).

A number of bacteriostatic *sulfonamides*, including sulfadiazine, sulfamethizole, sulfamethoxazole, and sulfaphenazole, can re-

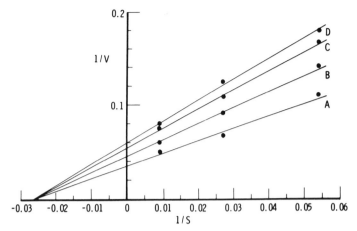

FIG. 1. Noncompetitive inhibition of phenytoin metabolism by isoniazid in rat liver microsomal (9,000 × *g* supernatant) fraction. **Curve A,** control; **curves B, C, and D,** isoniazid added in concentrations of 3.6×10^{-5} M; $1,1 \times 10^{-4}$ M; and 5.4×10^{-4} M, respectively. (From Kutt, ref. 44, with permission.)

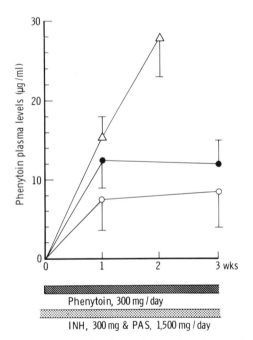

FIG. 2. Plasma levels of phenytoin of patients taking phenytoin and isoniazid together. **Open circles**, fast acetylators; **closed circles**, intermediate slow acetylators; **open triangles**, very slow acetylators. Based on data of Brennan et al. (10).

duce phenytoin clearance and prolong its half-life (59). In some patients, clinically evident phenytoin intoxication has occurred during sulfonamide therapy. The mechanism appears to be inhibition of phenytoin metabolism, and sulfaphenazole is the strongest inhibitor (59). Adjustment of phenytoin dosage may become necessary during sulfonamide therapy.

Metronidazole caused minor variable changes of phenytoin clearance and half-life in five volunteers, although the drug is a structural analog of cimetidine (35).

Antifungal Agents

Miconazole in combination with flucytosine caused elevation of phenytoin levels (78).

Antineoplastic Agents

Low phenytoin levels have been observed in several patients undergoing antineoplastic therapy with *vinblastine*, *cisplatinum*, and/or *bleomycin* (8,93). The reason for this manifestation may be multifactorial. Reduced absorption is likely to play a role and concomitant administration of steroids and antacids may contribute.

Antiulcer Agents

Antacids such as aluminum and magnesium hydroxides and calcium carbonate have been found to reduce or maintain low blood phenytoin levels in some patients but not in others. The complex effects of antacids on drug bioavailability influence drug dissolution, ionization, and gastrointestinal tract motility, in addition to chelation; therefore, variations in their effects in different individuals would be expected. It appears that the total dose of antacid and the time of administration are the determining factors. Empirically, it has been proved that if unexpectedly low phenytoin concentrations occur in patients who take antacids close to the time of phenytoin ingestion, a staggering of the intake times by 1 to 2 hr may result in an increase of phenytoin levels (14,19,45; see also "Absorption," this chapter).

Cimetidine has been found to increase phenytoin concentrations (50,72). In one study (72), 300 mg of cimetidine given four times a day caused elevation of blood phenytoin levels in a few days in five of nine subjects. The elevations were more marked in patients in whom the phenytoin levels were higher before cimetidine administration. In another study (81), phenytoin levels increased in six patients, causing intoxication in two, after addition of cimetidine; no change or slight decline was seen in the remaining three patients. The mechanism of this interaction is inhibition of phenytoin metabolism, as cimetidine has been shown to be an inhibitor of hepatic mixed-function oxidase systems. Phenytoin dosage adjustments with this drug combination may be necessary and are best guided by frequent monitoring of phenytoin levels during cimetidine administration.

Ranitidine has little or no effect on phenytoin metabolism and blood phenytoin levels (58).

Antihistaminics

Phenyramidol caused some elevation of phenytoin levels in several patients, but dosage adjustment was not necessary (90). A modest elevation of plasma phenytoin levels has occurred in some patients after the addition of *chlorpheniramine*, but without the need to change dosages (74).

Cardiac Drugs

Amiodarone, a investigational antiarrhythmic drug, caused two- to threefold increases of plasma phenytoin levels in three patients. Inhibition of phenytoin metabolism was suspected (55). *Diazoxide* reduced the protein binding of phenytoin, with a consequent increase in the free fraction and a slight decrease in the total plasma phenytoin concentration; the clinical consequences are likely to vary (77).

Other Antiepileptic Drugs

Phenobarbital induces the production of the enzymes involved in phenytoin biotransformation (44), but being a competitive inhibitor it also competes as a substrate with phenytoin for that enzyme (see Fig. 3) (44,68). This dual effect leads to variable results in patients taking phenytoin and phenobarbital together. The opposing effects may cancel each other or lead to a rise or fall of the plasma phenytoin level if one dominates. What to expect in an individual patient depends on the individual disposition, i.e., the state of induction by previous drug intake, the doses of phenytoin and phenobarbital, and the genetic background of the patient.

Comparison of groups of patients taking

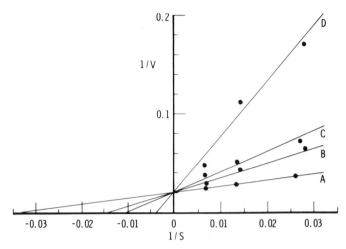

FIG. 3. Competitive inhibition of phenytoin metabolism by phenobarbital in rat liver micro-somal (9,000 × *g* supernatant) fraction. **Curve A,** control; **curves B, C, and D,** phenobarbital added in concentrations of 5.9 × 10^{-4} M; 1.1 × 10^{-3} M and 2.3 × 10^{-3} M, respectively. (From Kutt, ref. 44, with permission.)

phenytoin alone and phenytoin together with phenobarbital reveals, in general, that inductions predominate to some extent, as the phenytoin levels in the combined-therapy groups are usually somewhat lower than in monotherapy groups (46,61). In some patients taking phenytoin, the addition of phenobarbital may cause no change or may lead to a decline or an elevation of the plasma phenytoin level (9,46,61). The changes are rarely large, and seldom lead to a need for dosage adjustments.

The effect of *carbamazepine* on the plasma phenytoin level varies among patients. Several authors have reported a lowering effect (106), whereas others have found no significant changes, and still others have found that, if anything, there is some upward trend (109). Prolongation of phenytoin half-life by carbamazepine was also seen in several but not all patients using a stable isotope-labeled phenytoin test dose (11). What to expect in an individual patient is largely unpredictable.

The effect of *valproate* on the plasma phenytoin level varies among patients and may vary in the same patient during the course of therapy. Thus, a transient fall (13,60) or rise (106) within days after the addition of valproate occurs in some patients, with a return to previous values after days or weeks. In other patients, the recovery may take longer and may not quite reach the starting value (13). In general, marked changes are less frequent than smaller changes, and in many patients no significant change in the plasma phenytoin level occurs after the addition of valproate. A lowering effect is probably more frequent than an elevation (13,106). Clinically, the need to adjust the phenytoin dose is not frequent.

The mechanism for this interaction includes changes in binding to plasma proteins (60). Both drugs are bound to a high degree to plasma proteins and compete for binding sites. There is evidence that valproate in higher concentrations (near 100 μg/ml) reduces phenytoin binding from the usual near 90% to 85% or less. The increase in the free fraction of phenytoin in a patient with unsaturated clearing capacity would result then in a somewhat lower total steady-state phenytoin level (60). Since the valproate level fluctuates considerably during the 24-hr cycle, however, the effective displacement periods are not long, and the increased clearing of phenytoin is not extensive (76). Elevation of the plasma phenytoin level might occur in patients whose phenytoin-clearing system is almost saturated, particularly in view of the fact that valproate inhibits phenytoin metabolism *in vitro* (68).

Clonazepam lowers the plasma phenytoin level in some patients concomitant with an increase of conjugated 5-(4-hydroxyphenyl)-5-phenylhydantoin (*p*-HPPH). In one patient, the phenytoin level fell from 25 to 15 μg/ml after the addition of clonazepam (79). In other studies, clonazepam has been observed to cause a rise of the phenytoin level (106), but more often than not, no significant changes were found (36). This suggests that in the majority of patients, alterations of plasma phenytoin levels by clonazepam are not of great clinical concern.

The effect of *diazepam* on the plasma phenytoin level varies among patients. In some studies, elevations of phenytoin levels in some patients have been reported (99), whereas in other studies and other patients the opposite has occurred (32). In the majority of patients, the commonly used diazepam doses do not seem to cause significant changes in the plasma phenytoin level.

Chlordiazepoxide has caused phenytoin accumulation in some patients (45,99), but this occurs as a rare exception rather than a rule.

Sulthiame has caused elevations of plasma phenytoin levels ranging from modest to considerable and becoming obvious within days or weeks after the addition of sulthiame to phenytoin (28). Comparison with patients taking phenytoin without sulthiame indicated that plasma phenytoin levels were higher in patients taking both drugs, as was the incidence of clinical phenytoin intoxication. Reduction of the phenytoin dose may become necessary if its

plasma concentration reaches the toxic range and continuation of sulthiame seems to be indicated (70).

In groups of patients taking phenytoin with or without *pheneturide*, the plasma phenytoin levels were somewhat higher in the combined-therapy group (32). The addition of pheneturide to the medication of patients stabilized on phenytoin resulted in elevation of the phenytoin levels. These elevations were higher in the early phase of combined therapy and declined in later weeks, which indicates that both inhibition and induction are involved in this interaction. Inhibition can start almost immediately, whereas induction takes time to develop. In the long run, inhibition dominates slightly. The changes were generally not large with this drug combination (32,70).

Comedication of epileptic patients with phenytoin and *methsuximide* caused elevation of plasma phenytoin levels in varying degrees (75).

New and/or Experimental Antiepileptic Drugs

Felbamate increased phenytoin levels in the majority of patients during comedication, and reduction of the phenytoin dose was necessary in some patients (31). In several studies, the addition of *flunarizine* caused little if any changes in phenytoin levels (5). Single doses of *lamotrigine* did not alter phenytoin kinetics significantly (6). Similar lack of interaction has been observed with repeated doses. *Milacemide* was not found to cause marked changes in blood phenytoin levels during comedication (33). *Nafimidone* was demonstrated to be a mixed type inhibitor of phenytoin metabolism *in vitro* (38). In clinical studies, nafimidone caused phenytoin accumulation, and the phenytoin dose had to be reduced in some patients because of intoxication (97).

Progabide given as add-on medication caused elevation of blood phenytoin levels to varying extents in the majority of patients. The phenytoin dose was frequently reduced, particularly to maintain the original phenytoin concentrations, as required in the study protocol (4). *Stiripentol* reduced the clearance of phenytoin in a dose-dependent manner up to 40% (51). The effect of *zonisamide* on blood phenytoin levels was modest and variable, and there was no need to adjust the phenytoin dose because of the interaction (80).

Psychotropic Drugs

The *phenothiazines* chlorpromazine, prochlorperazine, and thioridazine may cause phenytoin accumulation and intoxication (45,101) or have a lowering effect (29). In general, phenothiazine drugs do not cause significant alterations of plasma phenytoin levels in the majority of patients (82). The effect of *methylphenidate* on the plasma phenytoin level varies among patients. A rise has been observed in a few patients, but no change occurred in probably the majority (45).

Imipramine caused an increase in phenytoin levels in some studies but in other studies no significant alteration of phenytoin kinetics was seen. It appears that the tricyclic antidepressants rarely necessitate phenytoin dosage adjustments (70). The phenytoin level increased from 17 to 46 μg/ml in a patient within a few weeks after trazodone administration (23). Clinical intoxication occurred and the phenytoin dose had to be reduced.

Miscellaneous Agents

Disulfiram, an enzyme inhibitor, inhibits phenytoin metabolism and causes accumulation of phenytoin and intoxication in the majority of patients taking it together with phenytoin (66). After disulfiram is discontinued, the plasma phenytoin level slowly declines, probably reflecting the slow elimination of disulfiram. A study by Svendsen et al. (92) with normal volunteers demonstrated that disulfiram reduced phenytoin clearance from approximately 50 to 34 ml/min. Dosage adjustment of phenytoin is necessary if these two drugs are administered together.

Prolonged use of *ethanol* can reduce the plasma phenytoin level (39), perhaps through induction. Elevation of the plasma phenytoin level, on the other hand, has been observed during occasional moderate or heavy intake of ethanol (45). Thus, a dual action is likely; long-term ethanol intake may have an inducing effect on phenytoin and acute intake may have an inhibiting effect. The need for dosage adjustments in this interaction is variable.

Tolbutamide was found to displace phenytoin from the binding sites and to lower plasma phenytoin levels in patients (103). Adding 1,000 mg of tolbutamide daily to the regimen of 17 patients with stable phenytoin levels caused a 10% decline of the total plasma phenytoin level in the majority. The percent of unbound phenytoin increased considerably at first and then declined but remained elevated. The clinical effects of this interaction are likely to be minor in the majority of patients.

Several studies indicate lowering of the phenytoin level by *folic acid*. The mechanism of this interaction is complex, but apparently is related to biotransformation. A recent study in folate-deficient subjects is of interest in this respect. Giving 1 mg of folate daily caused up to a 45% decrease in phenytoin levels, which were greatest in subjects with lowest K_m for phenytoin (3). Dosage adjustments may be needed sometimes.

ALTERATION BY PHENYTOIN OF KINETICS OF OTHER DRUGS OR SUBSTANCES

Analgesics–Antipyretics

Meperidine half-life declined from 6.4 to 4.3 hr and the area under the curve of the primary metabolite of meperidine increased after the addition of phenytoin (73). The clinical implication is that patients given phenytoin may need higher doses of meperidine. The area under the curve of blood *methadone* levels diminished by 50% in five methadone maintenance patients who had received phenytoin for 3 weeks (95). Several of these patients started to have withdrawal signs and symptoms while on the previously adequate methadone maintenance dose. Induction of methadone metabolism by phenytoin was thought to have occurred. Elimination of *acetaminophen* is facilitated to some extent by phenytoin, perhaps through acceleration of its biotransformation (70). *Antipyrine* undergoes a similar fate.

Antiasthma Agents

Daily doses of 300 to 400 mg of phenytoin, producing blood levels of 10 to 20 µg/ml, reduced the half-life of intravenously administered *theophylline* by 40% and increased its clearance in 10 volunteers. It was suggested that patients receiving phenytoin may need higher and/or more frequent doses of theophylline (37,85).

Antibiotics

Phenytoin was found to reduce *chloramphenicol* levels in patients (43). Higher doses of chloramphenicol may be needed during comedication. The elimination rate of *doxycycline* was increased in patients receiving phenytoin (63).

Anticoagulants

Phenytoin can reduce the blood level of *dicoumarol*, leading to a need for increased dosage of that anticoagulant (27). As the anticoagulant doses are usually adjusted on the basis of prothrombin time, clinical management problems from this interaction are alleviated. The effect of phenytoin on *warfarin* is variable, and in some patients phenytoin has even increased the anticoagulant effect (62).

Antidiuretics

Frusemide efficacy is reduced by phenytoin to some degree. There is evidence that phenytoin reduces frusemide absorption, but interference with frusemide action in the kidney may occur as well (1,70,105).

Cardiac Drugs

Phenytoin has been found to reduce the half-life of *quinidine* by 50% and make it necessary to require rather large doses of quinidine in order to maintain effective plasma quinidine levels. The potential danger in this situation is that if phenytoin is discontinued, the quinidine dose may become excessive. Induction of quinidine metabolism is the likely mechanism (70). In some patients receiving phenytoin, *digitoxin* levels were reduced to a modest extent (89). Phenytoin can accelerate the rate of metabolism of *disopyramide*. As the dealkylated metabolite is also pharmacologically active, a loss of effectiveness may not occur. (2).

Immunosuppressants

Phenytoin reduced the maximal concentration, area under the curve, and the half-life of *cyclosporin*, while it increased the clearance; the clinical efficacy was reduced (26).

Other Antiepileptic Drugs

Phenytoin is a potent inducer of *carbamazepine* biotransformation. In numerous studies, the plasma concentrations of carbamazepine are usually higher in those patients taking carbamazepine alone than in

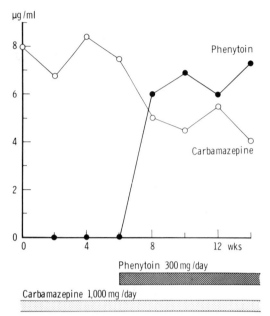

FIG. 4. Decline of plasma carbamazepine level following addition of phenytoin. (Kutt, *unpublished data.*)

those taking phenytoin as well (17). In individual patients taking carbamazepine, addition of phenytoin often causes the carbamazepine level to fall as much as one-half of the original value (see Fig. 4). Lander et al. (48) calculated that in their patients, daily phenytoin doses of 1 mg/kg caused a fall of about 0.5 μg/ml in the plasma carbamazepine level. The plasma concentration of 10,11-carbamazepine epoxide, which usually equals 10% to 30% of the parent compound in patients on monotherapy, may remain unchanged after the addition of phenytoin or may undergo a small rise or fall. In most cases, the ratio of metabolite over the parent compound increases to a variable degree. Since the plasma carbamazepine level tends to decline through autoinduction in the early phase of carbamazepine therapy, it may be difficult to discern the effect of phenytoin if the latter is added soon. Whether the mechanism of this interaction is an increased conversion to the 10,11-epoxide metabolite or acceleration of some other biotransformation step has not yet been fully clarified. The clinical effects of this interaction vary: the decline of the parent compound may be compensated by an increase of the active metabolite.

Phenytoin induces *primidone* biotransformation. The ratio of primidone-derived phenobarbital to primidone in the plasma of patients taking primidone alone usually ranges from 1.5 to 2.5; if phenytoin is added to the medication, this ratio may increase to 4 or higher (24,83). The extent of increase of this ratio varies among individual patients. This phenomenon is not of great clinical concern, since it rarely leads to a need for dosage adjustments.

Phenytoin has been reported to cause an elevation of plasma *phenobarbital* levels in some patients (61,106). Also, in some patients stabilized on combination therapy, a decrease in the plasma phenobarbital level was noted after phenytoin was discontinued (61). In the majority of patients, however, phenytoin has not caused significant changes in plasma phenobarbital levels, and the need to adjust dosages because of this interaction is expected to be quite infrequent. The mechanism is likely to be competitive inhibition.

An analysis of data from 259 epileptic patients indicated that *valproate* levels were lower in those patients who received polytherapy. In particular, phenytoin was shown to be the strongest reducer (up to 50%) of plasma valproate levels (54). Phenytoin was found to increase the levels of the pharmacologically active metabolite (*N*-desmethylmethsuximide) of *methsuximide* during combined treatment in epileptic patients (75).

New and/or Experimental Antiepileptic Drugs

Flunarizine levels were somewhat lower in patients receiving combined medication, including phenytoin (5). With *lamotrigine* therapy, patients who had been receiving phenytoin had shorter elimination half-lives, indicating induction (6). The kinetics of *milacemide* were not significantly altered by phenytoin (33). Patients receiving phenytoin as comedication had lower *zonisamide* levels than those whose comedication was carbamazepine. It was thought that phenytoin is a more effective inducer of zonisamide metabolism than carbamazepine (65).

Steroids

Failure of *oral contraceptives* has been reported in some epileptic patients taking antiepileptic drugs, including phenytoin (30). This has led to the hypothesis that the metabolism of synthetic steroids may be induced by phenytoin (30,67). If breakthrough bleeding occurs, higher-dose contraceptive pills may need to be given during antiepileptic therapy (53).

Phenytoin induces the metabolism of *dexamethasone* considerably. The elimination half-life of 3.5 hr was reduced to 1.8 hr after the addition of phenytoin (15). In six patients, dexamethasone levels dropped by 50% with phenytoin comedication (108). Failure of the low-dose dexamethasone test in patients receiving phenytoin has been reported. Similarly, failure of the metyrapone test has occurred by the same mechanism. Effectiveness of prednisone and prednisolone is reduced in some patients taking antiepileptic drugs, including phenytoin (70).

Endogenous Substances

Phenytoin is known to accelerate cortisol metabolism, but this usually does not lead to clinical consequences, as a homeostatic mechanism compensates with increased synthesis of cortisol (16).

Vitamins

Osteomalacia in some patients taking phenytoin is thought to be related in part to acceleration of the *cholecalciferol* biotransformation pathway (34). If antiepileptic drug-induced bone disease is present, giving cholecalciferol products is indicated, but prophylactic treatment with vitamin D is generally not recommended (94).

Folic acid levels have been found to be reduced in patients taking phenytoin, sometimes leading to macrocytic anemia. The mechanism of this manifestation is complex: altered absorption, utilization, and biotransformation all seem to play a role. Manifest drug-induced folate deficiency is treated with 1 to 2 mg folic acid daily (70).

Vitamin K-dependent coagulation factors may become reduced by phenytoin, occasionally leading to bleeding in neonates born to mothers taking phenytoin (70,88).

Miscellaneous

Phenytoin has been found to reduce the half-life of *misonidazole* and accelerate its demethylation. This may diminish the toxicity of misonidazole while not reducing its effectiveness as an enhancer in radiotherapy (104). Reduction of the blood *psoralen* levels in patients taking phenytoin was accompanied by a reduction in the effectiveness of psoralen as an intensifier of ultraviolet therapy for psoriasis (91).

PHARMACODYNAMIC INTERACTIONS BETWEEN PHENYTOIN AND OTHER DRUGS

Since most interactions between phenytoin and other drugs involve some pharmacokinetic changes, it is extremely difficult to rule in or out the simultaneous presence of alterations of pharmacodynamic parameters. Is the improved seizure control after adding a second drug to phenytoin simply additive or is there potentiation? Measurements of brain phenytoin and phenobarbital concentrations and comparison of the antiepileptic effect in animals by Leppik and Sherwin (49) indicated that the effect was additive under their experimental conditions. Tunnicliff et al. (98) found that phenytoin competes with diazepam for binding sites at rat cortex synaptosomal membranes.

Cohan et al. (18) postulated that suppression of afferent discharges from muscle spindles by phenytoin would potentiate the effectiveness of chlorpromazine in diminishing the extensor tone of decerebrate rigidity in cats. Mendez et al. (57) found that phenytoin may inhibit the uptake or utilization of dopamine by basal ganglia. Ahmad (1) suggested that renal sensitivity to furosemide is reduced by antiepileptic drugs, including phenytoin.

CONCLUSION

Numerous interactions between phenytoin and other drugs have been reported. The majority of these are pharmacokinetic and involve induction or inhibition of biotransformation or alteration of plasma protein binding. The result is a rise or decline in the plasma level of phenytoin or of the other drug.

With many of the reported drug combinations with phenytoin, small changes of plasma levels are not infrequent, but marked changes occur only rarely in apparently unusually susceptible individuals. The plasma level changes may be in opposite directions in different individuals with the same drug combination, particularly if the interacting drug induces enzyme production but inhibits its action.

Interactions with a predictable potential to necessitate adjusted dosages occur only with a few drugs in combination with phenytoin. Cimetidine, chloramphenicol, disulfiram, sulthiame, and isoniazid (in very

slow acetylators) cause elevations of plasma phenytoin levels in the majority of patients. Antacids may reduce phenytoin absorption if taken near the time of phenytoin ingestion. Conversely, phenytoin often causes a decline of the plasma carbamazepine level. A need to adjust dosages depends on the magnitude of these changes.

REFERENCES

1. Ahmad, S. (1974): Renal insensitivity to furosemide caused by chronic anticonvulsant therapy. *Br. Med. J.*, 3:657–659.
2. Aitio, M. L., Mansbury, L., Tala, E., Haataja, M., and Aitio, A. (1981): The effect of enzyme induction on the metabolism of disopyramide in man. *Br. J. Clin. Pharmacol.*, 11:279–286.
3. Berg, M. J., Fischer, L. J., Rivey, M. P., Vern, B. A., and Schottelius, D. D. (1983): Phenytoin and folic acid interaction: A preliminary report. *Ther. Drug Monit.*, 5:389–394.
4. Bianchetti, G., Padovani, P., Thenot, J. P., Thiercelin, J. F., and Morselli, P. L. (1987): Pharmacokinetic interactions of progabide with other antiepileptic drugs. *Epilepsia*, 28:68–73.
5. Binnie, C. D., de Beukelaar, F., Meijer, J. W. A., Meinardi, H., Overweg, J., Wauquier, A., and van Wieringen, A. (1985): Open dose-ranging trial of flunarizine as add-on therapy in epilepsy. *Epilepsia*, 26:424–428.
6. Binnie, C. D., van Emde Boas, W., Kasteleijn-Nolste-Trenite, D. G. A., Meijer, J. W. A., Meinardi, H., Miller, A. A., Overweg, J., Peck, A. W., van Wieringen, A., and Yuen, W. C. (1986): Acute effects of lamotrigine (BW 430C) in persons with epilepsy. *Epilepsia*, 27:248–254.
7. Bochner, F., Hooper, W. D., Tyrer, J. H., and Eadie, M. J. (1972): Factors involved in an outbreak of phenytoin intoxication. *J. Neurol. Sci.*, 16:481–487.
8. Bollini, P., Riva, R., Albani, F., Nicola, I., Cacciari, L., Bollini, C., and Baruzzi, A. (1983): Decreased phenytoin level during antineoplastic therapy: A case report. *Epilepsia*, 24:75–78.
9. Booker, H. E., Tormey, A., and Toussaint, J. (1971): Concurrent administration of phenobarbital and diphenylhydantoin: Lack of an interference effect. *Neurology (Minneap.)*, 21:383–385.
10. Brennan, R. W., Deheija, H., Kutt, H., Verebely, K., and McDowell, F. (1970): Diphenylhydantoin intoxication attendant to slow inactivation of isoniazid. *Neurology (Minneap.)*, 20:687–693.
11. Browne, T. R., Evans, J. E., Szabo, G. K., Evans, B. A., and Greenblatt, D. J. (1985): Effect of carbamazepine on phenytoin pharmacokinetics determined by stable isotope technique. *Neurology*, 35(suppl. I):284.
12. Browne, T. R., Evans, J. E., Szabo, G. K.,

Evans, B. A., Greenblatt, D. J., and Schumacher, G. E. (1985): Studies with stable isotopes I: Changes of phenytoin pharmacokinetics and biotransformation during monotherapy. *J. Clin. Pharmacol.*, 25:43–50.

13. Bruni, J., Wilder, B. J., Willmore, L. J., and Barbour, B. (1979): Valproic acid and plasma levels of phenytoin. *Neurology (Minneap.)*, 29:904–905.

14. Cacek, A. J. (1986): Review of alterations in oral phenytoin bioavailability associated with formulation, antacids and food. *Ther. Drug Monit.*, 8:166–171.

15. Chalk, J. B., Ridgeway, K., Brophy, T., Yelland, J. D. N., and Eadie, M. J. (1984): Phenytoin impairs the bioavailability of dexamethasone in neurological and neurosurgical patients. *J. Neurol. Neurosurg. Psychiatry*, 47:1087–1090.

16. Choi, Y., Thrasher, K., Werk, E., Sholiton, L. J., and Olinger, C. (1971): Effect of diphenylhydantoin on cortisol kinetics in humans. *J. Pharmacol. Exp. Ther.*, 176:27–34.

17. Christiansen, J., and Dam, M (1973): Influence of phenobarbital and diphenylhydantoin on plasma carbamazepine levels in patients with epilepsy. *Acta Neurol. Scand.*, 49:543–546.

18. Cohan, S. L., Anderson, R. J., and Raines, A. (1976): Diphenylhydantoin and chlorpromazine in the treatment of spasticity. *Neurology (Minneap.)*, 26:367.

19. D'Arcy, P. F., and McElnay, J. C. (1987): Drug-antacid interactions of clinical importance. *Drug Intel. Clin. Pharm.*, 21:607–617.

20. Dam, M., Christensen, J. M., Brandt, J., Hansen, B. S., Hvidberg, E. F., Angelo, H., and Lous, P. (1980): Antiepileptic drugs: Interaction with dextropropoxyphene. In: *Antiepileptic Therapy: Advances in Drug Monitoring*, edited by S. I. Johannessen, P. L. Morselli, C. E. Pippenger, A. Richens, D. Schmidt, and H. Meinardi, pp. 299–304. Raven Press, New York.

21. de Wolff, F., Vermeij, P., Ferrari, M. D., Buruma, O. J. S., and Breimer, D. D. (1983): Impairment of phenytoin parahydroxylation as a cause of severe intoxication. *Ther. Drug Monit.*, 5:213–215.

22. Dickinson, R. G., Hooper, W. D., Patterson, M., Eadie, M. J., and Maguire, B. (1985): Extent of urinary excretion of p-hydroxyphenytoin in healthy subjects given phenytoin. *Ther. Drug Monit.*, 7:283–289.

23. Dorn, J. M. (1986): A case of phenytoin toxicity possibly precipitated by trazodone. *J. Clin. Psychiatry*, 47:89–90.

24. Fincham, R. W., Schottelius, D. D., and Sahs, A. L. (1974): The influence of diphenylhydantoin on primidone metabolism. *Arch. Neurol.*, 30:259–262.

25. Fraser, D. G., Ludden, T. M., Evens, R. P., and Sutherland, E. W. (1980): Displacement of phenytoin from plasma binding sites by salicylate. *Clin. Pharmacol. Ther.*, 27:165–169.

26. Freeman, D. J., Laupacis, A., Keown, A., Stiller, C. R., and Carruthers, S. G. (1984): Evaluation of cyclosporin-phenytoin interaction with observations on cyclosporin metabolites. *Br. J. Clin. Pharmacol.*, 18:887–893.

27. Hansen, J. J. M., Siersbaek-Nielsen, K., Kristensen, M., Skovsted, L., and Christensen, L. K. (1971): Effect of diphenylhydantoin on the metabolism of dicoumarol in man. *Acta Med. Scand.*, 189:15–19.

28. Hansen, J. M., Kristensen, M., and Skovsted, L. (1968): Sulthiame (Ospolot) as inhibitor of diphenylhydantoin metabolism. *Epilepsia*, 9:17–22.

29. Haydukewyck, D., and Rodin, E. A. (1985): Effects of phenothiazines on serum antiepileptic drug concentrations in psychiatric patients with seizure disorders. *Ther. Drug Monit.*, 7:401–405.

30. Hempel, E., and Klinger, W. (1976): Drug stimulated biotransformation of hormonal steroid contraceptives: Clinical implications. *Drugs*, 12:442–448.

31. Holmes, G. B., Graves, N. M., Leppik, I. E., and Fuerst, R. H. (1987): Felbamate: Bidirectional effects on phenytoin and carbamazepine serum concentrations. *Epilepsia*, 28:578–579.

32. Houghton, G. W., and Richens, A. (1974): The effect of benzodiazepines and pheneturide on phenytoin metabolism in man. *Br J. Clin. Pharmacol.*, 1:344–345.

33. Houtkooper, M. A., van Oorschot, C. A. E. H., Rentmeester, T. W., Hoppener, P. J. E. A., and Onkelinx, C. (1986): Double-blind study of milacemide in hospitalized therapy resistant patients with epilepsy. *Epilepsia*, 27:255–262.

34. Hunter, J. (1976): Effects of enzyme induction on vitamin D3 metabolism in man. In: *Anticonvulsant Drugs and Enzyme Induction*, edited by A. Richens and F. P. Woodford, pp. 77–84. Elsevier Excerpta Medica North Holland, Amsterdam.

35. Jensen, J. C., and Gugler, R. (1985): Interaction between metronidazole and drugs eliminated by oxidative metabolism. *Clin. Pharmacol. Ther.*, 37:407–410.

36. Johannessen, S. I., Strandjord, R. E., and Munthekaas, A. W. (1977): Lack of effect of clonazepam on serum levels of diphenylhydantoin, phenobarbital and carbamazepine. *Acta Neurol. Scand.*, 55:506–512.

37. Jonkman, J. H. G., and Upton, R. A. (1984): Pharmacokinetic drug interactions with theophylline. *Clin. Pharmacokinet.*, 9:309–334.

38. Kapetanovic, M., and Kupferberg, H. J. (1984): Nafimidone, an imidazole anticonvulsant and its metabolite as potent inhibitor of microsomal metabolism of phenytoin and carbamazepine. *Drug Metab. Dispos.*, 12:560–564.

39. Kater, R. M. H., Roggin, G., Tobon, F., Zieve, P., and Iber, F. L. (1969): Increased rate of clearance of drugs from circulation of alcoholics. *Am. J. Med. Sci.*, 258:35–39.

40. Kay, L., Kampmann, J. P., Svendsen, T. L., Vergman, B., Molholm-Hansen, J. E., Skovsted, L., and Kristensen, M. (1985): Influence of rifampin and isoniazid on the kinetics of phenytoin. *Br. J. Clin. Pharmacol.*, 20:323–326.

41. Kennedy, M. C., and Wade, D. N. (1982): The

effect of food on the absorption of phenytoin. *Aust. NZ. J. Med.*, 12:258–261.

42. Koup, J. R. (1978): Interaction of chloramphenicol with phenytoin and phenobarbital. A case report. *Clin. Pharmacol. Ther.*, 24:571–575.

43. Krasinski, K., Kusmiesz, M., and Nelson, J. D. (1982): Pharmacologic interactions among chloramphenicol, phenytoin and phenobarbital. *Pediatr. Infect. Dis.*, 1:232–235.

44. Kutt, H. (1974): Interactions with antiepileptic drugs involving multiple mechanisms. In: *Drug Interactions*, edited by P. L. Morselli, S. Garattini, and S. N. Cohen, pp. 211–222. Raven Press, New York.

45. Kutt, H. (1984): Interactions between anticonvulsants and other commonly prescribed drugs. *Epilepsia*, 25(Suppl 2):S118–S131.

46. Kutt, H., Haynes, J., Verebely, K., and McDowell, F. (1969): The effect of phenobarbital on plasma diphenylhydantoin level and metabolism in man and in rat liver microsomes. *Neurology (Minneap.)*, 19:611–616.

47. Kutt, H., and Verebely, K. (1970): Metabolism of diphenylhydantoin by rat liver microsomes. I. Characteristics of the reaction. *Biochem. Pharmacol.*, 19:675–686.

48. Lander, C. M., Eadie, M. J., and Tyrer, J. H. (1975): Interactions between anticonvulsants. *Proc. Aust. Assoc. Neurol.*, 12:111–116.

49. Leppik, I. E., and Sherwin, A. (1977): Anticonvulsant activity of phenobarbital and phenytoin in combination. *J. Pharmacol. Exp. Ther.*, 200:570–575.

50. Levine, M., Jones, M. W., and Sheppard, I. (1985): Differential effect of cimetidine on serum concentrations of carbamazepine and phenytoin. *Neurology*, 35:562–565.

51. Levy, R. H., Loisseau, P., Guyot, M., Blehaut, H. M., Tor, J., and Moreland, T. A. (1984): Stiripentol kinetics in epileptic patients: Nonlinearity and interactions. *Epilepsia*, 23:657.

52. Marano, A. R., Caride, V. J., Prokop, E. K., Tronacale, F. J., and McCallum, R. W. (1985): Effect of sucralfate and an aluminum hydroxide gel on gastric emptying of solids and liquids. *Clin. Pharmacol. Ther.*, 37:629–632.

53. Mattson, R. H., and Cramer, J. A. (1985): Epilepsy, sex hormones and antiepileptic drugs. *Epilepsia*, 26(suppl. 1):S40–S55.

54. May, T., and Rambeck, B. (1985): Serum concentrations of valproic acid: Influence of dose and co-medication. *Ther. Drug Monit.*, 7:387–390.

55. McGovern, B., Geer, V. R., Laraia, P. J., Garan, H., and Ruskin, J. N. (1984): Possible interaction between amiodarone and phenytoin. *Ann. Int. Med.*, 101:650–651.

56. Melander, A., Brante, G., Johansson, O., Lindberg, T., and Wallin-Boll, E. (1979): Influence of food on the absorption of phenytoin in man. *Eur. J. Clin. Pharmacol.*, 15:269–274.

57. Mendez, J. S., Cotzias, G. C., Mena, I., and Papavasiliou, P. S. (1975): Diphenylhydantoin. Blocking of levodopa effects. *Arch. Neurol.*, 32:44–46.

58. Mitchard, M., Harris, A., and Mullinger, B. M. (1987): Ranitidine drug interaction. A literature review. *Pharmacol. Ther.*, 32:293–325.

59. Molholm Hansen, J., Kampmann, J. P., Siersbaek-Nielsen, K., Lumholtz, I. B., Arroe, M., Abilgaard, U., and Skovsted, L. (1979): The effect of different sulfonamides on phenytoin metabolism in man. *Acta Med. Scand. (Suppl.)*, 624:106–110.

60. Monks, A., and Richens, A. (1980): Effects of single doses of sodium valproate on serum phenytoin levels and protein binding in epileptic patients. *Clin. Pharmacol. Ther.*, 27:89–95.

61. Morselli, P. L., Rizzo, M., and Garattini, S. (1971): Interaction between phenobarbital and diphenylhydantoin in animals and in epileptic patients. *Ann. N.Y. Acad. Sci.*, 179:88–107.

62. Nappi, J. (1979): Warfarin and phenytoin interaction. *Ann. Int. Med.*, 90:852.

63. Neuvonen, P. J., Penttila, O., Lehtovaara, R., and Aho, K. (1975): Effects of antiepileptic drugs on the elimination of various tetracycline derivatives. *Eur. J. Clin. Pharmacol.*, 9:147–154.

64. O'Brien, L. S. (1978): Failure of antacids to alter pharmacokinetics of phenytoin. *Br. J. Pharmacol.*, 6:176–177.

65. Ojeman, L. M., Shastri, R. A., Wilenski, A. J., Friel, P. N., Leux, R. H., McLean, J. R., and Buchanan, R. A. (1986): Comparative pharmacokinetics of zonisamide (CI-912) in epileptic patients on carbamazepine or phenytoin monotherapy. *Ther. Drug Monit.*, 8:293–296.

66. Olesen, O. V. (1967): The influence of disulfiram and calcium carbimide on the serum diphenylhydantoin. *Arch. Neurol.*, 16:642–644.

67. Orme, M. L. E. (1982): Clinical pharmacology of oral contraceptive steroids. *Br. J. Clin. Pharmacol.*, 14:31–42.

68. Patsalos, P. M., and Lascelles, P. T. (1977): *In vitro* hydroxylation of diphenylhydantoin and its inhibition by other commonly used anticonvulsant drugs. *Biochem. Pharmacol.*, 266:1929–1933.

69. Paxton, J. W. (1980): Effects of aspirin on serum phenytoin kinetics in healthy subjects. *Clin. Pharmacol. Ther.*, 27:170–178.

70. Perucca, E. (1982): Pharmacokinetic interactions with antiepileptic drugs. *Clin. Pharmacokinetics*, 7:57–84.

71. Perucca, E. (1987): Clinical implications of hepatic microsomal enzyme induction by antiepileptic drugs. *Pharmacol. Ther.*, 33:139–144.

72. Phillips, P., and Hansky, J. (1984): Phenytoin toxicity secondary to cimetidine administration. *Med. J. Aust.*, 141:602.

73. Pond, S. M., and Kretschzmar, K. M. (1981): Effect of phenytoin on meperidine clearance and nor-meperidine formation. *Clin. Pharmacol. Ther.*, 30:680–686.

74. Pugh, R. N. H., Geddes, A. M., and Yeoman, W. B. (1975): Interaction of phenytoin and chlorpheniramine. *Br. J. Clin. Pharmacol.*, 2:173–174.

75. Rambeck, B. (1979): Pharmacological interactions of methsuximide with phenobarbital and

phenytoin in hospitalized epileptic patients. *Epilepsia*, 20:147–156.

76. Riva, R., Albani, F., Contin, M., Perucca, E., Ambrosetto, G., Gobbi, G., Santucci, M., Procaccianti, G., and Baruzzi, A. (1985): Time-dependent interaction between phenytoin and valproic acid. *Neurology*, 35:510–515.

77. Roe, T. F., Podosin, R. L., and Blaskovics, M. E. (1975): Drug interaction: Diazoxide and diphenylhydantoin. *J. Pediatr.*, 87:480–484.

78. Rolan, P. E., Somogy, A. A., Drew, M. R., Cobain, W. G., South, D., and Bochner, F. (1983): Phenytoin intoxication during treatment with parenteral miconazole. *Br. Med. J.*, 287:1760.

79. Saavedra, I. N., Aguilera, L. I., and Galdames, D. G. (1985): Phenytoin/clonazepam interaction. *Ther. Drug Monit.*, 7:481–484.

80. Sackellares, J. G., Donofrio, P. D., Wagner, J., Abou-Khalil, B., Berent, S., and Aasved-Hoyt, I. K. (1985): Pilot study of zonisamide (1,2-benzisoxazole-3-methanesulfonamide) in patients with refractory partial seizures. *Epilepsia*, 26:206–211.

81. Salem, R. B., Breland, B. D., Mishra, S. K., and Jordan, G. E. (1983): Effect of cimetidine on phenytoin serum level. *Epilepsia*, 24:284–288.

82. Sands, C. D., Robinson, J. D., Salem, R. B., Stewart, R. B., and Muniz, C. (1987): Effect of thioridazine on phenytoin serum concentration. A retrospective study. *Drug Intell. Clin. Pharm.*, 21:267–272.

83. Schottelius, D. D., and Fincham, R. W. (1977): Clinical application of serum primidone levels. In: *Antiepileptic Drugs: Quantitative Analysis and Interpretation*, edited by C. E. Pippenger, J. K. Penry, and H. Kutt, pp. 273–282. Raven Press, New York.

84. Sekikawa, H., Nakano, M., Takada, M., and Arita, T. (1980): Influence of dietary components on the bioavailability of phenytoin. *Chem. Pharm. Bull.*, 22:2443–2449.

85. Sklar, S. J., and Wagner, J. C. (1985): Enhanced theophylline clearance secondary to phenytoin therapy. *Drug Intell. Clin. Pharm.*, 19:34–36.

86. Skovsted, L., Hansen, J. M., Kristensen, M., and Christensen, L. K. (1974): Inhibition of drug metabolism in man. In: *Drug Interactions*, edited by P. L. Morselli, S. Garattini, and S. N. Cohen, pp. 81–90. Raven Press, New York.

87. Skovsted, L., Kristensen, M., Molholm Hansen, J., and Siersbaek-Nielsen, K. (1976): The effect of different oral anticoagulants on diphenylhydantoin (DPH) and tolbutamide metabolism. *Acta Med. Scand.*, 199:513–515.

88. Solomon, G. E., Hilgartner, M. W., and Kutt, H. (1972): Coagulation defects caused by diphenylhydantoin. *Neurology (Minneap.)*, 22:1165–1171.

89. Solomon, H. M., Reich, S., Spirt, N., and Abrams, W. B. (1971): Interaction between digitoxin and other drugs *in vitro* and *in vivo*. *Ann. N.Y. Acad. Sci.*, 79:362–369.

90. Solomon, H. M., and Shrogie, J. J. (1967): The effect of phenyramidol on the metabolism of digitoxin and other drugs — digitoxin is a phenylhydantoin. *Clin. Pharmacol. Ther.*, 8:554–556.

91. Starberg, B., and Hueg, B. (1985): Interaction between 8-methoxpsoralen and phenytoin. Consequences for PUVA therapy. *Acta Derm. Venereol. (Stockholm)*, 65:553–555.

92. Svendsen, T. L., Kristensen, M., Hansen, J. M., and Skovsted, L. (1976): The influence of disulfiram on the half-life and metabolic clearance rate of diphenylhydantoin and tolbutamide in man. *Eur. J. Clin. Pharmacol.*, 9:439–441.

93. Sylvester, R. K., Lewis, F. B., Caldwell, K. C., Lobell, M., Perri, R., and Sawchuk, R. A. (1984): Impaired phenytoin bioavailability secondary to cisplatinum, vinblastin and bleomycine. *Ther. Drug Monit.*, 6:302–305.

94. Tjellesen, L., Gotfredsen, A., and Christiansen, C. (1985): Different actions of vitamin D_2 and D_3 on bone metabolism in patients treated with phenobarbitone/phenytoin. *Calcif. Tissue Int.*, 37:218–222.

95. Tong, T. G., Pond, S. M., Kreek, M. J., Jaffry, N. F., and Benowitz, N. L. (1981): Phenytoin-induced methadone withdrawal. *Ann. Int. Med.*, 94:349–351.

96. Townsend, R. J., Fraser, D. G., Scavone, J. M., and Cox, S. R. (1985): The effects of ibuprofen on phenytoin pharmacokinetics. *Drug Intell. Clin. Pharm.*, 19:447–448.

97. Treiman, D. M., and Ben-Menachem, E. (1987): Inhibition of carbamazepine and phenytoin metabolism by nafimidone, a new antiepileptic drug. *Epilepsia*, 28:699–705.

98. Tunnicliff, G., Smith, J. A., and Ngo, T. T. (1979): Competition from diazepam receptor binding by diphenylhydantoin and its enhancement by gamma-aminobutyric acid. *Biochem. Biophys. Res. Commun.*, 91:1018–1024.

99. Vaijda, F. J. E., Prineas, R. J., and Lowell, R. R. H. (1971): Interaction between phenytoin and the benzodiazepines. *Br. Med. J.*, 1:346.

100. Vesell, E. S., and Page, J. G. (1969): Genetic control of the phenobarbital-induced shortening of plasma antipyrine half-lives in man. *J. Clin. Invest.*, 48:2202–2209.

101. Vincent, F. M. (1980): Phenothiazine-induced phenytoin intoxication. *Ann. Int. Med.*, 93:56–57.

102. Welling, P. G. (1984): Interactions affecting drug absorption. *Clin. Pharmacokinet.*, 9:404–434.

103. Wesseling, H., and Molsthurkow, I. (1975): Interaction of diphenylhydantoin (DPH) and tolbutamide in man. *Eur. J. Clin. Pharmacol.*, 8:75–78.

104. Williams, K., Begg, E., Wade, D., and O'Shea, K. (1983): Effects of phenytoin, phenobarbital and ascorbic acid on misonidazole elimination. *Clin. Pharmacol. Ther.*, 33:314–321.

105. Williamson, H. E. (1986): Interaction of furosemide and phenytoin in the rat. *Proc. Soc. Exp. Biol. Med.*, 182:322–324.

106. Windorfer, A., Jr., and Sauer, W. (1977): Drug interactions during anticonvulsant therapy in childhood: Diphenylhydantoin, primidone, phe-

nobarbitone, clonazepam, nitrazepam, carbamazepine, and dipropylacetate. *Neuropaediatrie*,
8:29–41.

107. Witmer, D. R., and Ritschel, W. A. 91984): Phen-
ytoin-isoniazid interaction: A kinetic approach to
management. *Drug Intell. Clin. Pharm.*, 18:483–
486.

108. Wong, D. D., Longenecker, R. G., Liepman, M.,

Baker, S., and La Vergne, M. (1985): Phenytoin-
dexamethasone: A possible drug-drug interaction. *J.A.M.A.* 254(15):2062–2063.

109. Zielinski, J., Haydukewych, D., and Leheta,
B. J. (1985): Carbamazepine-phenytoin interaction: Elevation of plasma phenytoin concentrations due to carbamazepine co-medication. *Ther.
Drug Monit.*, 7:51–53.

Antiepileptic Drugs, Third Edition, edited by
R. Levy, R. Mattson, B. Meldrum,
J. K. Penry, and F. E. Dreifuss.
Raven Press, Ltd., New York © 1989.

14

Phenytoin

Clinical Use

B. J. Wilder and Rogelio J. Rangel

In 1937, Putnam and Merritt (18) launched scientific drug testing by using graded electrical stimulation of the brains of cats to produce seizures. They tested a series of drugs containing phenyl groups. Phenytoin demonstrated marked antiseizure activity against seizures induced by maximal electroshock without producing the hypnotic side effects commonly seen with phenobarbital (14). Clinical testing soon demonstrated the efficacy of phenytoin, and in 1938 Merritt and Putnam (15) reported on its use in the treatment of epileptic patients.

EFFICACY IN PARTIAL AND GENERALIZED TONIC-CLONIC SEIZURES

Merritt and Putnam (14) described phenytoin as the most effective drug they had ever used, and later studies (16,17) confirmed its efficacy. Weinberg and Goldstein (25) treated refractory patients with phenytoin and reported seizure cessation in 40% of them. Johnson (9), in a study of the new drug in institutionalized patients, reported the best results in cases of grand mal, phenytoin being more than twice as effective as phenobarbital. Merritt and Putnam (17) reported that phenytoin was effective in 227 of 267 patients who had not responded to other forms of therapy.

Since the introduction of phenytoin, 19 drugs have been licensed in the United States for the treatment of epilepsy. Sixteen of these are recommended for the treatment of partial and tonic-clonic seizures. During the past 12 years, controlled, randomized clinical trials and double-blind studies comparing new antiepileptic drugs with phenytoin have shown that it remains one of the most effective drugs for the treatment of partial and generalized tonic-clonic seizures.

In 1977, Ramsay et al. (20) compared phenytoin and carbamazepine in 87 patients, 19 with partial seizures and secondary generalized tonic-clonic seizures, 37 with partial seizures only, and 31 with generalized tonic-clonic seizures. Phenytoin and carbamazepine were equally efficacious and had equal potential for major side effects (Table 1). Trough plasma levels of carbamazepine and phenytoin in the patients who had a good-to-excellent response ranged from 9.1 to 11.0 μg/ml and 4.7 to 6.5 μg/ml, respectively. In the treatment failure group, mean plasma phenytoin and carbamazepine levels were 14.3 μg/ml and 9.8 μg/ml, respectively.

Wilder et al. (31) compared phenytoin and valproic acid in patients with newly diagnosed generalized tonic-clonic seizures.

TABLE 1. Comparison of carbamazepine and phenytoin in patients with epilepsy

	Carbamazepine	Phenytoin
Patients (60 men, 27 women, aged 18–77 yr)		
Entered study	42	45
Withdrawn from study	7	10
Completed study	27	27
Major side effects	8 (22.9%)	8 (22.9%)
Rash	4	1
Exfoliative dermatitis	1	0
Pruritis	0	1
Impotence	1	2
Dizziness	1	1
Headaches	0	1
Nausea and vomiting	1	0
Impaired cognition	0	1
Elevated liver enzymes	0	1
Minor side effects[a]		
Nausea	14	17
Gingival hyperplasia	0	5
Headaches	10	14
Cognitive impairment	14	7
Nystagmus	22	18
Sedation	14	7
Fine tremor	8	13
Seizures		
Controlled	22 (62.9%)	23 (65.7%)
Uncontrolled	5 (14.2%)	4 (11.4%)

.[a] Mild and transient, did not interfere with daily functioning.

TABLE 2. Comparison of valproic acid and phenytoin in patients with epilepsy

	Valproic acid	Phenytoin
Patients		
Entered study	40	21
Completed study	34	17
Lost to follow-up or noncompliant	6	4
Response		
Excellent (no seizure recurrence)	25[a] (73%)	8 (47%)
Good	3 (9%)	5 (29%)
Poor to fair	6 (19%)	4 (24%)
Side effects		
Tremor	9	1
Nystagmus	1	1
Impotence	0	1
Lethargy	4	6
Irritability	1	0
Gastrointestinal upset, nausea, and/or vomiting	5	2
Alopecia	1	0
Ataxia	1	1
Drug-induced hepatitis	0	1

[a] Four patients had no further generalized tonic-clonic seizures, but subsequently experienced complex partial seizures, which required the addition of another drug.

The response to valproic acid was slightly better than to phenytoin (Table 2), but the difference was not significant. Mean steady-state trough plasma levels were 57 μg/ml (range, 33 to 88 μg/ml) for valproic acid and 12.6 μg/ml (range, 8.3 to 16.9 μg/ml) for phenytoin.

Turnbull et al. (24) randomized 140 patients with untreated tonic-clonic or partial seizures to receive either phenytoin or valproic acid. The drugs were equally efficacious. The only prognostic factor that influenced the achievement of a 2-year remission of seizures was the seizure type. Patients with tonic-clonic seizures did sig-nificantly better than those with a history of partial seizures.

Callaghan et al. (3) compared valproate, phenytoin, and carbamazepine in 181 patients with untreated epilepsy and reported on a 14- to 24-month follow-up. All drugs were highly effective in the control of generalized tonic-clonic seizures, but less effective for partial seizures. Patients with generalized tonic-clonic seizures had an excellent response (i.e., became seizure-free) to phenytoin, which was superior to the other drugs and significantly so to carbamazepine ($p < 0.01$; chi-squared test). In patients with partial seizures with or without secondarily generalized tonic-clonic seizures, phenytoin was superior to valproate and carbamazepine but the difference was not significant (57% had an excellent response to phenytoin, 44% to valproate, and 33% to carbamazepine). A poor response to phenytoin, carbamazepine, and valproate (less than 50% reduction in seizures) was obtained in 24%, 26%, and 22% of the patients, respectively. Excellent or good responses (greater than 50% reduction in seizures) occurred in the nontoxic therapeutic range of plasma drug levels with valproate (300–700 μmol/liter) and carbamazepine (15–40 μmol/liter) and in the subtherapeutic range with phenytoin (40–80 μmol/liter).

The most comprehensive double-blind, controlled study reported to date has been that of the VA Cooperative Group. Mattson et al. (13) compared the efficacy and toxicity of phenytoin, phenobarbital, primidone, and carbamazepine in 622 patients with newly diagnosed partial and secondarily generalized tonic-clonic seizures. Rating scales of seizure frequency, systemic toxicity, and neurotoxicity were completed at each patient's visit for a minimum of 1 year and extended for 6 years. Each patient was given a combined composite score reflecting the clinical response: good (0–20), satisfactory (21–35), fair to poor (36–50), and unacceptable (>50). Mean composite scores for seizure frequency and toxicity at 12, 24, and 36 months, ranked from lowest to highest, indicated that phenytoin was the most efficacious and least toxic, followed by carbamazepine, phenobarbital, and primidone. The scores at 12, 24, and 36 months were 21, 24, and 29 for phenytoin and 22, 27, and 31 for carbamazepine. Phenytoin and carbamazepine were significantly better than phenobarbital and primidone at 12 and 24 months ($p < 0.01$) and at 36 months ($p < 0.25$).

A different picture was revealed by the evaluation of seizure frequency only in patients who were not dropped because of drug failure, toxicity, or loss to follow-up. In controlling generalized tonic-clonic seizures, phenytoin was less efficacious than the other three drugs. In controlling partial seizures, phenytoin was significantly less effective than carbamazepine ($p < 0.05$) and

more effective than the other two drugs. However, the combined results of the study (with assessment of all factors) indicated that phenytoin and carbamazepine are most likely to be successful as initial single-drug therapy in adults with partial or secondarily generalized seizures. One of these two drugs is recommended for the initial treatment of adolescents and adults with these seizure types.

Phenytoin is not efficacious in absence and myoclonic seizures and is not recommended for the treatment of infantile spasms, Lennox-Gastaut syndrome, and the epileptic syndromes of older childhood and adolescence when absence and myoclonus are present.

INITIATION AND MAINTENANCE OF THERAPY

Phenytoin is well tolerated by most patients, and therapy can be initiated in a manner consistent with the clinical situation. In patients in whom epilepsy has recently been diagnosed and seizures are infrequent, 5 to 7 mg/kg of phenytoin can be administered as a single or twice daily dose (30). In patients in whom therapeutic plasma phenytoin levels are more urgent, oral loading can be achieved by giving 15 mg/kg orally in three divided doses over a 2-hr period. Therapeutic plasma levels are achieved within 8 to 10 hr (29). In acute seizures, phenytoin can be loaded intravenously (15 mg/kg) over 20 to 60 min. The drug is soluble in normal saline and can be given by intravenous drip or infusion pump (21,22). Intravenous or oral loading rarely produces adverse reactions. Transient vertigo and nausea may occur.

There may be wide interpatient variations in dosing. Callaghan et al. (3) found that a dose of 4.9 ± 1.70 mg/kg (mean ± SD) produced mean serum phenytoin levels of 26.9 ± 10.8 μmol/liter in patients with an excellent response to phenytoin. Children, because of more rapid metabolism, require a 25% to 50% greater dose (in mg/kg) to achieve therapeutic levels than do postadolescents. Phenytoin monotherapy does not result in autoinduction of metabolism. Ramsay et al. (20) followed patients serially for 6 months after initiation of phenytoin therapy and found no significant changes in the relationship of dose to serum phenytoin level. Wilder (26) surveyed 120 stable adult patients and found the average daily dose of phenytoin to be 342 mg.

The accepted therapeutic serum phenytoin level ranges from 10 to 20 μg/ml (40–80 μmol/liter). However, this range should only be used as a guide; proper management depends on the clinical response (28). Patients with partial seizures require a higher dose and higher serum phenytoin levels to achieve seizure control than do patients with generalized tonic-clonic seizures (23).

STATUS EPILEPTICUS AND ACUTE SEIZURES

Phenytoin is considered by most epileptologists in the United States to be the drug of choice in the treatment of status epilepticus, acute, and serial seizures (5,11,27,32). Phenytoin is ideal for the treatment of status epilepticus or other acute seizures because it is available in an easily administered intravenous solution, rapidly penetrates the blood-brain barrier to achieve therapeutic concentrations at the site of action, effects seizure control in all cases, possesses a time span of action that permits calculated dosing to maintain a therapeutic response, does not cause respiratory or cardiac depression, produces no changes in the neurological examination, and does not potentiate central nervous system depression produced by previously administered agents (e.g., diazepam, barbiturates).

Phenytoin is available in a parenteral formulation that is readily soluble in normal saline (22). Concentrations of 5 to 20 mg of phenytoin per milliliter of normal saline can be administered at a rate of 50 mg/min without producing significant adverse clinical effects (21). Care must be taken to prevent extravasation from the vein, as a severe local reaction may occur. A mild decrease in blood pressure or slowing of the pulse occasionally occurs, but can be controlled by decreasing the rate of administration (11,32). An infusion rate exceeding 50 mg/min may produce a significant decrease in blood pressure and slowing of the pulse rate (4). In personal practice of 15 years, respiratory depression has not been observed in patients receiving intravenous loading doses of 10 to 20 mg/kg of phenytoin. Asystole may occur following bolus intravenous injection. Subjective side effects of intravenous loading are rare, but mainly involve vertigo and nausea. Except for nystagmus, the neurological examination is unchanged.

Phenytoin rapidly penetrates the brain during intravenous infusion (19,32) and is concentrated by brain phospholipids (6,7). One hour after intravenous infusion, the brain-to-plasma ratio is greater than 1.5 in both experimental animals and humans (19,32).

Patients with status epilepticus involving chronic or acute epileptic seizures, alcohol or drug withdrawal seizures, or seizures of undetermined origin respond promptly to intravenous phenytoin. Leppik et al. (11) and Wilder et al. (27,32) reported that 60% to 80% of patients responded within 20 min after the initiation of phenytoin infusion. Wilder et al. (27) reported plasma phenytoin levels of 10 μg/ml or more 12 hr following a mean intravenous dose of 13 mg/kg in 8 of 14 patients, and Leppik et al. (11) found higher levels after higher intravenous doses.

In personal experience with intravenous administration of phenytoin to patients with status epilepticus or serial seizures, potentiation of the effects of previously administered benzodiazepines or barbiturates has not been observed. In contrast, potentiation of respiratory depression secondary to diazepam or a barbiturate when the other is parenterally administered is a common emergency room occurrence and sometimes is the cause of respiratory arrest, ventricular fibrillation, and death.

CLINICALLY RELEVANT PHARMACOKINETICS AND DRUG INTERACTION

Phenytoin in slow release formulation (Dilantin, 30 and 100 mg capsules) is slowly absorbed, reaching peak plasma levels after 8 to 12 hr. In normal persons absorption approaches 95%. The drug is 80% to 95% bound to plasma protein (30). Protein binding is not concentration-dependent, as it is with valproic acid. Phenytoin is metabolized to a single inactive metabolite by hydroxylation, conjugated to glucuronic acid, and excreted in the urine. Only a small amount of free phenytoin (less than 1%) is excreted. Because of high protein binding and a high pK_a, phenytoin is relatively undialyzable. The metabolism of phenytoin is rate limited and metabolizing enzyme saturation usually begins in the low therapeutic range. When dose changes are made, plasma phenytoin levels should be carefully monitored. It is personal practice to use the 30-mg capsules for dose changes when the serum levels range from 8 to 25 µg/ml.

Phenytoin is a potent inducer of the microsomal P450 system. Phenytoin markedly induces the metabolism of valproic acid, carbamazepine, and primidone, and increases by 50% to 100% the dose of carbamazepine or valproic acid needed to achieve therapeutic serum level (26). Phenytoin does not significantly induce the metabolism of the benzodiazepines or succinimides.

The metabolism of phenytoin may be inhibited when the drug is used in combination with carbamazepine (1). The metabolic interaction between phenytoin and phenobarbital is variable (10). At high therapeutic serum levels, phenytoin metabolism is inhibited by phenobarbital and at low levels, phenytoin may be induced. Valproic acid mildly inhibits phenytoin metabolism and may significantly displace phenytoin from protein binding sites, with resulting transient toxicity associated with the higher unbound or free serum levels (2).

Phenytoin interacts with numerous kinds of other drugs (see Chapter 13).

TOXICITY

Phenytoin produces no, or relatively minor, dose-related central nervous system toxicity with serum levels in the low and middle therapeutic range. Impairment of cerebellovestibular integration of motor activity (e.g., nystagmus, ataxia, incoordination, and disintegration of skilled motor activity) begins in most patients when the levels exceed 20 µg/ml. Impairment of cognitive function and behavioral changes may begin to be observed with levels in the high therapeutic range and in most patients when levels exceed 30 µg/ml. Other aspects of phenytoin toxicity are addressed in Chapter 15.

SUMMARY

Phenytoin has been the drug of choice for the treatment of partial and generalized tonic-clonic seizures for more than half a century, and for the past 15 years it has been the major drug used in the management of status epilepticus. Phenytoin possesses several unique characteristics that make it desirable for the long-term management of epileptic patients. The slow release form of the drug (Dilantin capsules) coupled with a relatively long half-life permits once-a-day dosing in most patients. Phenytoin is hydroxylated to a single inactive metabolite, permitting easy correlation of clinical response with serum drug levels. A parenteral preparation is available for the management of emergency seizure situations. Unfortunately, phenytoin follows saturation kinetics so that when the therapeutic range is reached small changes in the daily dose sometimes result in large alterations in serum phenytoin levels and clinical effect.

REFERENCES

1. Browne, T. R., Szabo, G. K., Evans, J. E., Evans, B. A., Greenblatt, D. J., and Mikati, M. A. (1988): Carbamazepine increases phenytoin serum concentrations and reduces phenytoin clearance. *Neurology*, 38:1146–1150.
2. Bruni, J., Gallo, J. M., Lee, C. S., Perchalski, R. J., and Wilder, B. J. (1980): Interactions of valproic acid with phenytoin. *Neurology*, 30:1233–1236.
3. Callaghan, N., Kenny, R. A., O'Neill, B., Crowley, M., and Goggin, T. (1985): A prospective study between carbamazepine, phenytoin, and sodium valproate as monotherapy in previously untreated and recently diagnosed patients with epilepsy. *Journal of Neurology, Neurosurgery, and Psychiatry*, 48:639–644.
4. Cranford, R. E., Patrick B., Anderson, C. B., and Kostick, B. (1978): Intravenous phenytoin: Clinical and pharmacokinetic aspects. *Neurology*, 28:874–880.
5. Delgado-Escueta, A. V., Wasterlain, C., Treiman, D. M., and Porter, R. J. (1982): Management of status epilepticus. *N. Eng. J. Med.*, 306:1337–1340.
6. Goldberg, M. A., and Crandall, P. H. (1978): Human brain binding of phenytoin. *Neurology*, 28:881–885.
7. Goldberg, M. A., and Todoroff, T. (1976): Diphenylhydantoin binding to brain lipids and phospholipids. *Biochem. Pharm.*, 25:2079–2083.
8. Hauptman, A. (1912): Luminal bei epilepsie. *Munch. Med. Wochenschr.*, 59:1907–1909.
9. Johnson, H. K. (1940): The response of various types of epilepsy to Dilantin therapy. *Psychiatry Q.*, 14:612–618.
10. Kutt, H. (1975): Interactions of antiepileptic drugs. *Epilepsia*, 16:393–402.
11. Leppik, I., Patrick, B. K., and Cranford, R. E. (1983): Treatment of acute seizures and status epilepticus with intravenous phenytoin. In: *Advances in Neurology, Vol. 34, Status Epilepticus*, edited by A. V. Delgado-Escueta, C. G. Wasterlain, D. M. Treiman, and R. J. Porter, pp. 447–451. Raven Press, New York.
12. Locock, C. H. (1857): Discussion of paper by Sieve King, analysis of 52 cases of epilepsy observed by author. *Lancet*, 1:527.
13. Mattson, R. H., Cramer, J. A., Collins, J. F., Smith, D. B., Delgado-Escueta, A. V., Browne, T. R., Williamson, P. D., Treiman, D. M.,

McNamara, J. O., McCutchen, C. B., Homan, R. W., Crill, W. E., Lubozynski, M. F., Rosenthal, N. P., and Mayersdorf, A. (1985): Comparison of carbamazepine, phenobarbital, phenytoin, and primidone in partial and secondarily generalized tonic-clonic seizures. *N. Eng. J. Med.*, 313:145–151.
14. Merritt, H. H., and Putnam, T. J. (1938a): A new series of anticonvulsant drugs tested by experiments on animals. *Arch. Neurol. Psychiatry*, 39:1003–1015.
15. Merritt, H. H., and Putnam, T. J. (1938b): Sodium diphenylhydantoinate in the treatment of convulsive disorders. *J.A.M.A.*, 111:1068–1073.
16. Merritt, H. H., and Putnam, T. J. (1939): Sodium diphenylhydantoinate in the treatment of convulsive disorders—Toxic symptoms and their prevention. *Arch. Neurol. Psychiatry*, 42:1053–1058.
17. Merritt, H. H., and Putnam, T. J. (1940): Further experiences with the use of sodium diphenylhydantoinate in the treatment of convulsive disorders. *Am. J. Psychiatry*, 96:1023–1027.
18. Putnam, T. J., and Merritt, H. H. (1937): Experimental determination of the anticonvulsant properties of some phenyl derivatives. *Science*, 85:525–526.
19. Ramsay, R. E., Hammond, E. J., Perchalski, R. J., and Wilder, B. J. (1979): Brain uptake of phenytoin, phenobarbital, and diazepam. *Arch. Neurol.*, 36:535–539.
20. Ramsay, R. E., Wilder, B. J., Berger, J. R., and Bruni, J. (1983): A double-blind study comparing carbamazepine with phenytoin as initial seizure therapy in adults. *Neurology*, 33:904–910.
21. Salem, R. B., Wilder, B. J., Yost, R. L., Doering, P. L., and Lee, C. H. (1981): Rapid infusion of phenytoin sodium loading doses. *Amer. J. Hosp. Pharm.*, 38:354–357.
22. Salem, R. B., Yost, R. L., Torosian, G., Davis, F. T., and Wilder, B. J. (1980): Investigation of the crystallization of phenytoin in normal saline. *Drug Intelligence and Clinical Pharmacy*, 14:605–608.
23. Schmidt, D., Einicke, I., and Haenel, F. (1986): The influence of seizure type on the efficacy of plasma concentrations of phenytoin, phenobarbital, and carbamazepine. *Arch. Neurol.*, 43:263–265.
24. Turnbull, D. M., Howel, D., Rawlins, M. D., and Chadwick, D. W. (1985): Which drug for the adult epileptic patient: Phenytoin or valproate. *Br. Med. J.*, 290:815–819.
25. Weinberg, J., and Goldstein, H. H. (1940): A comparative study of the effectiveness of dilantin sodium and phenobarbital in a group of epileptic patients. *Am. J. Psychiatry*, 96:1029–1034.
26. Wilder, B. J. (*unpublished data*).
27. Wilder, B. J. (1983): Efficacy of phenytoin in treatment of status epilepticus. In: *Advances in Neurology, Vol. 34: Status Epilepticus*, edited by A. V. Delgado-Escueta, C. G. Wasterlain, D. M. Treiman, and R. J. Porter, pp. 441–446. Raven Press, New York.
28. Wilder, B. J., and Bruni, J. (1981): Medical management of seizure disorders. In: *Seizure Disor-*

ders: A Pharmacological Approach to Treatment, pp. 35–39. Raven Press, New York.

29. Wilder, B. J., Serrano, E. E., and Ramsay, R. E. (1973): Plasma diphenylhydantoin levels after loading and maintenance doses. *Clin. Pharmacol. Ther.,* 14:798–801.

30. Wilder, B. J., Streiff, R. R., and Hammer, R. H. (1972): Diphenylhydantoin: Absorption, distribution and excretion. In: *Antiepileptic Drugs,* 1st edition, edited by D. Woodbury, J. K. Penry, and R. P. Schmidt, pp. 137–148. Raven Press, New York.

31. Wilder, B. J., Ramsay, R. E., Murphy, J. V., Karas, B. J., Marquardt, K., and Hammond, E. J. (1983): Comparison of valproic acid and phenytoin in newly diagnosed tonic-clonic seizures. *Neurology,* 33:1474–1476.

32. Wilder, B. J., Ramsay, R. E., Willmore, L. J., Feussner, G. F., Perchalski, R. J., and Schumate, J. B. (1977): Efficacy of intravenous phenytoin in the treatment of status epilepticus: Kinetics of central nervous system penetration. *Ann. Neurol.,* 1:511–518.

Antiepileptic Drugs, Third Edition, edited by
R. Levy, R. Mattson, B. Meldrum,
J. K. Penry, and F. E. Dreifuss.
Raven Press, Ltd., New York © 1989.

15

Phenytoin

Toxicity

E. H. Reynolds

INTRODUCTION

More than 50 years have passed since phenytoin was introduced into clinical practice in 1938. As it remains an economical and effective drug for the treatment of several types of seizure disorders, it has been, like phenobarbital, one of the most widely consumed drugs in the world. It has, therefore, many lessons to teach us about drug toxicity in general. Although the vestibule-ocular cerebellar syndrome of acute toxicity was immediately recognized, it took until the era of blood drug level monitoring in the late 1960s and early 1970s to reveal other acute and subacute toxic effects of the drug. These effects had remained undetected in the absence of classic signs such as nystagmus, especially in the mentally handicapped. In addition, gum hypertrophy and hirsutism were soon described as toxic effects of long-term phenytoin use. There then followed a remarkable delay of some 30 years before many of the chronic toxic effects of phenytoin, with which we are familiar today, were first recognized (78). Drug level monitoring played a part in this detection process, but so did other technological advances, such as vitamin and hormone assays, and other metabolic screening tests. Furthermore, the most common and important of all the chronic toxic effects of phenytoin (as well as other

antiepileptic drugs) that is, subtle effects on cognitive function and behavior, has only received widespread recognition and investigation in the last decade (81,102,103). After 50 years there is, of course, an enormous literature on phenytoin toxicity. This updated picture is based on several reviews in the previous editions of this book (20,30,72,77), as well as reviews from other sources (9,69,73,78,88). Almost every toxic effect of phenytoin has had one or more reviews devoted to it.

ACUTE TOXICITY

Cerebellar Syndrome

The vestibulo-ocular cerebellar syndrome of acute phenytoin toxicity has been described so often (30,73,88) and is generally so well known that detailed description is not required here. Much has been learned about terelationship of the various clinical features to blood drug levels, but the reported step-wise correlation between nystagmus, ataxia, and mental symptoms and increasing phenytoin levels is not always as evident in clinical practice as suggested by Kutt et al (49). There is much individual variation so that one or more of the clinical features (e.g., nystagmus or diplopia) may be absent, especially in the brain damaged or mentally handicapped, in whom toxicity may be overlooked (102). Furthermore, the blood level at which various aspects of the syndrome appear will be influenced by the presence of concomitant antiepileptic medication: indeed, the syndrome appears most often in the context of polytherapy.

The presence of ataxia in an epileptic patient on phenytoin should always lead to the suspicion of drug toxicity until proved otherwise. Much unnecessary investigation for brain tumors and the like has occurred in the past, especially if, for example, the toxicity also results in headache and vomiting (71). One important reason for early accurate diagnosis is that the syndrome is not always so readily reversible as has been thought. Several examples of residual persistent ataxia have been described in patients with prolonged acute toxicity that was not initially recognized for what it was (78). The effect of frequent or prolonged seizures on cerebellar function and pathology may also render some patients more vulnerable to this persisting ataxic syndrome (20). Iivanainen et al. (41) pneumoencephalographically studied 131 mentally retarded epileptic patients treated with phenytoin, only 21 of whom were on this drug alone: 73 were intoxicated with phenytoin, 18 of whom developed persistent "loss of locomotion" after a 22 month mean duration of intoxication. Cerebellar and brain stem atrophy was found in 28% of this series but was not higher than in a control series of patients treated with drugs other than phenytoin. However, the degree of the atrophy was most severe in the 18 patients with persistent phenytoin intoxication. The authors emphasized that brain damaged and mentally retarded patients are particularly vulnerable to this complication of phenytoin, as well as to mental deterioration (55,84,102). Munoz-Garcia et al. (66) compared 28 epileptic patients exhibiting truncal ataxia with 67 patients from the same clinic without ataxia. They found that the distinction between acute and reversible,

and chronic and irreversible, ataxia was not clear-cut. The ataxia appeared after several years of treatment, often without any change in the drug schedule. However, the ataxia tended to fluctuate in degree and to improve, but seldom to disappear, on reducing the medication. The ataxic group had a longer history of epilepsy, were taking a greater number of drugs (only two on single-drug therapy), and had higher serum levels of both phenytoin and phenobarbital.

Involuntary Movements

Another reason for the occasional failure to recognize phenytoin toxicity may be the absence of ataxia or the presence of unusual or atypical clinical features. Among the latter, involuntary movements have received the most attention (12,25,58). In adults and children, phenytoin may produce reversible dyskinesias involving the face, limbs, and trunk, which are clinically indistinguishable from those produced by neuroleptics. However, in the great majority of cases, the patients have been on polytherapy. In many the movements appeared soon after the introduction of phenytoin, after an increase in the dose of phenytoin, or with the addition of another drug. Some, but not all, such patients were found to have high phenytoin levels, and some had other evidence of phenytoin intoxication such as drowsiness or dysarthria, but rarely the classic ataxic syndrome. The dyskinesias may last for hours, days, weeks, or months, may occasionally disappear spontaneously, and are usually reversed by reducing or stopping the phenytoin. They have been reversed with intravenous or oral diazepam. Most authors have emphasized the occurrence of previous brain damage or "encephalopathy" in the majority of patients, but it is clear that the syndrome can occur occasionally in otherwise normal persons. A few case reports have emphasized preexisting radiological or pathological lesions in the basal ganglia (25).

Exacerbation of Epilepsy

Another less well known but potentially very important occasional feature of acute phenytoin toxicity is exacerbation of the epilepsy. There are a few reports that toxic serum concentrations of phenytoin may increase seizure frequency and even precipitate status epilepticus (50,52,76,104). In one study of 18 patients in whom toxic serum levels of the drug were reduced, seizure frequency fell by 50% or more in nine patients in the ensuing 6 months (76).

Mental Symptoms

The mental symptoms of acute phenytoin toxicity, variously described as "delirium," "psychosis," or "encephalopathy," may proceed to severe drowsiness and even coma. In the presence of nystagmus and ataxia, there is no difficulty in recognizing the true nature of this syndrome. With the advent of blood level monitoring, it became clear that there also existed a more insidious toxic encephalopathy (30,76,102). In this syndrome, reversible impairment of intellectual function and memory evolve subacutely or chronically, usually in association with a toxic blood level, but in the absence of nystagmus or ataxia. Occasionally, unusual neurological signs such as dyskinesias have been noted, as already discussed. There may be a modest rise in cerebrospinal fluid (CSF) protein and an excess of slow activity on the EEG. This encephalopathy can occur in adults but has been noted particularly in children, especially those with pre-existing mental retardation or brain damage. In these patients, further deterioration in intellectual function, in the absence of more classic signs of toxicity, may be overlooked or mistakenly regarded as part of an underlying progressive neurological disease (55).

CHRONIC TOXICITY

The distinction between acute and chronic toxicity of phenytoin is not always so clear-cut, as has already been observed above with respect to mental symptoms, involuntary movements, and even ataxia. Nevertheless, the last 20 years have seen a remarkable growth of our awareness and understanding of many subtle chronic effects of phenytoin and other antiepileptic drugs on most tissues of the body. The classification of chronic effects in this present review is a minor modification of a review of this subject in 1975 (78).

Cognitive and Behavioral Effects

The cognitive and behavioral effects of phenytoin have been reviewed by Reynolds (81) and Trimble and Reynolds (103). Although impaired mental function with toxic blood phenytoin levels has long been recognized, more recently it has become apparent that subtle changes in cognitive function and behavior may occur with more modest or "therapeutic" levels.

In a study of 57 epileptic outpatients, Reynolds and Travers (84) found that patients with intellectual deterioration, psychiatric illness, personality change, or psychomotor slowing had significantly higher concentrations of phenytoin or phenobarbital than those without such changes, after exclusion of those with overt drug toxicity, gross cerebral lesions, or mental illness preceding the onset of epilepsy. Furthermore, the mean blood concentrations of the two drugs in the patients with mental changes were within the optimum or therapeutic range. These observations were not simply the reflection of higher anticonvulsant prescribing for more severe epilepsy, because similar differences were noted in those patients with infrequent seizures. Similar findings were reported by Trimble et al. (101) in a study of 312 epileptic children in a residential hospital school. Those children with a fall in IQ of between 10 and 40 points in at least 1 year had significantly higher levels of phenytoin and primidone, and a similar trend was found for phenobarbital. Again, the mean blood drug concentrations were within the optimal range.

Psychometric studies have been undertaken in normal volunteers (40,96), epileptic patients (24,97,98), and newly diagnosed epileptic patients well controlled on monotherapy (4). A fairly consistent picture emerges suggesting that phenytoin may impair memory, concentration, mental and motor speed, and processing, and that these impairments are related to the blood drug levels. Reynolds (81) has discussed various mechanisms by which phenytoin and other antiepileptic drugs may influence mental function. These include effects on folate, monoamine, and hormone metabolism, and possibly central neuropathological damage, as is known to occur in the peripheral nervous system.

Peripheral Neuropathy

There have been widely varying reports on the incidence of clinical or electrical evidence of peripheral neuropathy in selected groups of treated patients (56,91). This subject has been reviewed by Shorvon (89) and Trimble and Reynolds (103). Clinical features, which have been described in up to one-third of patients, have consisted usually of absent lower limb reflexes and impaired vibration sense at the ankles. Distal sensory symptoms and motor weakness are very rare. Electrophysiological abnormalities have been found more often than clinical manifestations and have consisted of a slight reduction in motor or sensory conduction and reduced or absent sensory action potentials. All authors have attributed the neuropathy to phenytoin, but Shorvon and Reynolds (91) found evidence that long-term barbiturate therapy may also lead to clinical or electrical abnormalities of peripheral nerve function.

Several problems in interpreting the published studies have arisen: first, the selected nature of the chronic patients, most of whom were on polytherapy; second, the failure to distinguish acute reversible anticonvulsant-induced electrophysiological changes from chronic irreversible abnormalities; and third, the failure to relate the findings to the duration of the treatment and to clinical and metabolic variables, such as drug toxicity, serum anticonvulsant concentrations, and folate levels. In newly diagnosed epileptic patients followed prospectively on carefully monitored single-drug treatment with either phenytoin or carbamazepine for up to 5 years, Shorvon and Reynolds (91) found no evidence of clinical neuropathy. Slight electrophysiological abnormalities were found in 18% of those on phenytoin but in none of those on carbamazepine. The presence of electrophysiological abnormalities in the phenytoin group was significantly related to previous exposure to high serum phenytoin and low serum folate concentrations, or both. In nonepileptic subjects with megaloblastic anemia due to folate deficiency, clinical evidence of neuropathy was found in 18% (90).

It seems, therefore, that phenytoin and barbiturates can contribute to anticonvulsant neuropathy, but there is no evidence incriminating carbamazepine or sodium valproate. Much of the previously reported clinical and electrical neuropathy has been associated with polytherapy, and perhaps especially with prolonged or repeated exposure to toxic concentrations of phenytoin or phenobarbital and/or prolonged folate deficiency.

Folic Acid Deficiency

This has been reviewed by Reynolds (77,79) and Pisciotta (72). The rare occurrence of megaloblastic anemia, first recognized by Mannheimer et al. in 1952 (61), was followed in the late 1960s and early 1970s by many reports of the high incidence of abnormal serum folate levels. This in turn led to a growing literature on the relationship between folic acid and both epileptic and antiepileptic mechanisms, and between deficiency of the vitamin and neuropsychiatric complications.

Megaloblastic Anemia

Megaloblastic anemia has been reported in 0.15% to 0.75% of drug-treated epileptic patients. It is usually associated with phenytoin, administered either alone or with other drugs (usually barbiturates), but it has been observed rarely in association with phenobarbital or primidone alone. It can occur at any age and after any duration of therapy. Poor diet and pregnancy may sometimes be additional precipitating factors. The anemia is due to folic acid deficiency, confirmed by low serum and red cell folate levels, and always responds to treatment with the vitamin. Serum vitamin B_{12} levels are usually normal or low normal, but occasionally subnormal due to transient malabsorption of the vitamin B_{12} secondary to the folate deficiency.

Macrocytosis, Folic Acid, and Vitamin B_{12} Levels

Mild macrocytosis without anemia has been reported in 8% to 53% of patients, subnormal serum folate levels in 27% to 91% (usually over 50%), and serum vitamin B_{12} in 0% to 11%, the latter usually a secondary phenomenon. Several studies have also shown that low serum folate levels are usually accompanied by corresponding falls in red blood cell and CSF folate. More recent studies of patients on monotherapy with phenytoin and other drugs have shown a lower incidence of folate deficiency than in the older investigations (18,22). The fall in serum, red blood cell, and CSF folate is usually better correlated with the concentration of phenytoin than the duration of treatment (22,83).

Mechanism of Phenytoin-Induced Folate Deficiency

The way in which phenytoin induces folate deficiency is still not clarified. Two of the most favored hypotheses are malabsorption of folic acid or induction of enzymes involved in folate metabolism. Other possibilities include competitive interaction between phenytoin and folate coenzymes, or increased demand for folic acid either for phenytoin hydroxylation or for other hepatic enzymes induced by the drug. Evidence for and against these various hypotheses has been discussed by Chanarin (13), Coggin et al. (18), and Carl et al. (11).

Folic Acid, Seizures and Antiepileptic Mechanisms

There have been several reports of exacerbation of seizures in patients treated with folic acid, giving rise to the suggestion that there may be a relationship between antifolate and antiepileptic mechanisms (74). Although evidence that the vitamin consistently exacerbates epilepsy is lacking, these clinical reports have stimulated considerable experimental research that has shown unequivocally that various folate derivatives have potent excitatory properties in different species (38,39). Furthermore, folic acid enhances electrical kindling and can even kindle seizures on its own in the rat (63,67). It has been demonstrated that there is an active transport and effective blood-brain barrier mechanism for folate. Thus, when the blood-brain barrier is damaged or circumvented, the excitatory properties of folic acid are most apparent (5). Phenytoin, phenobarbital, and possibly valproate have been shown to interfere with folate transport in the nervous system (92). There is also recent experimental evidence that folic acid blocks presynaptic GABA inhibition (105). Finally at least one new antiepileptic drug, lamotrigine (Chapter 69) has been developed from the antifolate-antiepileptic hypothesis. The antifolate drug pyrimethimine was selected for study and its molecule modified such that although it has antiepileptic efficacy, it now has weak or no antifolate action.

Folic Acid and Neuropsychiatric Disorders

There is considerable evidence now that in addition to its excitatory properties, folic acid is involved in many important metabolic pathways in the nervous system, especially methylation reactions, and neurotransmitter and nucleoprotein metabolism, and is implicated in a variety of neuropsychiatric disorders (10,82,90). These disorders include depression and cognitive impairment most commonly, but also, like vitamin B_{12} deficiency, peripheral neuropathy, and rare instances of subacute combined degeneration. Such complications have been described in epileptic patients with drug-induced folate deficiency (75,78). Although there have been some early negative studies of the effect of folic acid on the mental state of epileptic patients (78), more recently the association of drug-induced folate deficiency and mental symptoms has been confirmed in a community study (26) and in children (101). Furthermore, in a double-blind, placebo-controlled study in a nonepileptic folate-deficient psychiatric population, methylfolate treatment for 6 months significantly enhanced psychological and social recovery (31).

Neonatal Coagulation Defects

Clinical bleeding due to coagulation defects has occasionally been reported in infants born to mothers on treatment with phenytoin or phenobarbital (45,93). Bleyer and Skinner (8) reviewed 21 cases. The clinical features differ slightly from other forms of hemorrhagic disease of the newborn in that bleeding tends to occur earlier, usually within the first 24 hrs, and also in unusual sites such as abdominal and pleural cavities. The bleeding is due to depression of vitamin K-dependent coagulation factors (II, VII, IX, and X). Mountain et al. (65) found this coagulation defect in eight of 16 neonates born to 16 unselected epileptic mothers. In seven the defect was severe and in two it led to bleeding. Battino et al. (6) also found slight reductions, but within the normal range, of prothrombin time, partial prothrombin time, and prothrombin activity. Bleeding occurred in only one of 49 neonates.

This coagulation disorder, which has been produced experimentally with phenytoin in cats and kittens (93), may be prevented or corrected by vitamin K. Intramuscular vitamin K up to 10 mg shortly before birth has been recommended for prevention. The neonate may also be treated by intramuscular injections of vitamin K in doses varying from 1 mg to 1 mg/kg daily (65,93,107). Walte et al. (107) also discuss the use of fresh-frozen plasma or concentrates of the missing factors.

Metabolic Bone Disease

Following the reports of Schmid (86) and Kruse (48), rickets in children and osteomalacia in adults have been recognized as occasional complications of phenytoin and other antiepileptic drug therapy, especially polytherapy. This in turn has led to many studies revealing radiological or biochemical evidence of metabolic bone disease in as many as one-third of epileptic patients, most of whom are clinically asymptomatic (34,78,88). In the more florid clinical syndrome, the main features are aches, pains, and weakness. The often vague and indefinite symptomatology of osteomalacia may easily be overlooked, especially in patients who are mentally and physically slowed by their severe epilepsy and polytherapy (23). Fractures, which are not uncommon, especially in institutionalized patients, (3) should always lead to a search for predisposing metabolic bone disease. Postural, growth, or dental abnormalities should also alert the physician. A frank myopathy may occur, as with any osteomalacia (62).

Studies of predominantly asymptomatic epileptic populations have revealed bone disease by X-ray examination, but also by measurements of bone density, bone mass, and bone mineral content (15,47,53,64). The biochemical findings include a slight lowering of serum calcium, elevation of serum alkaline phosphatase of both bone and liver origin, and a lowering of 25-hydroxycholecalciferol. Again such findings are more common in patients on prolonged polytherapy, and precise relationships between the dose and duration of therapy of individual drugs are not easy to establish. Some authors have emphasized the relative importance of phenytoin (44), although florid disease due to phenytoin alone is rare. Gough et al. (33) studied biochemical parameters related to vitamin D metabolism in patients on different monotherapy regimens and found similar changes with all the major enzyme inducing antiepileptic drugs, including phenytoin. Very minor biochemical changes are seen during the first 2 years of monotherapy with phenytoin (22).

There has been considerable interest in and an extensive literature on the possible mechanisms involved (7,34,68,78,88) and in some respects the mechanisms remain uncertain. The most widely favored view is that phenytoin and other enzyme-inducing antiepileptic drugs increase the metabolism of vitamin D and also divert it along pathways that result in more polar and active metabolites. There is some evidence that vitamin D deficiency is aggravated in some patients by relative inactivity and limited exposure to sunlight (33). Another possibility is increased biliary excretion of vitamin D and its metabolites by the drugs. Especially with respect to phenytoin it has been suggested that a defect in the absorp-

tion of calcium may contribute to the hypocalcemia. Finally there is also some evidence of impaired parathormone function, particularly in patients with dental disorders.

Clinically apparent rickets and osteomalacia clearly require treatment, but there is uncertainty as to whether subclinical metabolic bone disease should be treated. In both situations advice has varied about whether to give vitamin D_2 or vitamin D_3, in what doses as initial and as maintenance therapy, and for how long (16,34,46,88). All agree that especially in the subclinical situation, great care should be taken to avoid vitamin D intoxication. It has been asked whether the hypocalcemia of this syndrome aggravates the underlying epilepsy, and if so whether it is reversible by treatment with vitamin D or calcium (17), but these questions have not been clearly answered.

Pituitary-Adrenal Function

As noted above for vitamin D, phenytoin and other enzyme-inducing drugs alter the metabolism of steroids, and this has several other clinical implications (20,78,88). Exogenously administered and endogenous steroids may be more readily catabolized due to enzyme induction. For example, dexamethasone and prednisone, which are widely used in a variety of clinical situations, may be less effective. The low-dose dexamethasone suppression test may give false negative results. The metyrapone test of pituitary-adrenal function may be undermined by phenytoin, both due to the enzyme-inducing action of the drug and by blocking the pituitary release of ACTH. The drug also impairs the immunosuppressive action of corticosteroids. Phenytoin may increase the turnover of cortisol and the excretion of polar conjugated metabolites, especially 6-hydroxycortisol. At autopsy, some epileptic patients have adrenal hyperplasia.

In high doses, phenytoin may interfere with the release of antidiuretic hormone (ADH) in normal subjects and in patients with inappropriate ADH syndrome. Phenytoin has been reported to inhibit the thyroid stimulating hormone (TSH) response to thyroid releasing hormone (TRH) experimentally and in humans (95). It also appears to promote increased secretion of follicle stimulating hormone (FSH) and luteinizing hormone (LH) in epileptic patients (100). Resting levels of prolactin were slightly raised in epileptic patients taking phenytoin (27,100) but dynamic responses to metoclopramide and bromocriptine were unaffected (100). Resting levels of growth hormone were also slightly raised on phenytoin therapy, and paradoxical suppression was seen following bromocriptine (100).

Thyroid Function

The effect of phenytoin on thyroid function has been reviewed by Gharib and Munoz (29), Reynolds (78), and Schmidt (88). Phenytoin depresses protein-bound iodine (PBI), probably due to displacement of thyroxine (T_4) from its binding sites on thyroxine binding globulin (TGB). The drug also lowers concentrations of total thyroxine (T_4) and free thyroxine (FT_4), mainly due to enhanced conversion to triiodothyronine (T_3) (35). However, T_3 and TSH levels usually remain normal and the patient clinically euthyroid. As the lethargy, slowness, and ataxia of phenytoin toxicity can sometimes mimic hypothyroidism, it is important not to be misled by these diagnostically confusing effects of the drug on thyroid function tests. Radioactive iodine tests are not affected by the drug. The determination of thyrotropin concentrations may also be useful to assess thyroid function during phenytoin treatment. Hypothyroidism may occasionally occur in an epileptic patient on phenytoin (1).

The Pancreas and Glucose Metabolism

There have been several case reports of reversible nonketotic hyperglycemia and glycosuria in association with severe phenytoin toxicity (78). The association of drug-induced drowsiness and hyperglycemia gave rise to the mistaken suspicion of diabetic precoma in some of these cases. Experimental studies in animals and man suggest that phenytoin impairs the insulin response to glucose stimulation (19,60). For most epileptic patients this effect is probably of little significance (43), but the drug should obviously be used with caution in diabetics.

Sex Hormones

The effects of antiepileptic drugs on estrogen and progesterone metabolism and on oral contraception have been reviewed by Schmidt (87). The role of drug-induced endocrine changes in the sexual disorders associated with epilepsy has been reviewed by Toone (99). Phenytoin, among other drugs, stimulates the microsomal metabolism of estradiol, estrone, and progesterone in experimental animals and humans. The efficacy of oral contraceptives may be impaired. Breakthrough bleeding and spotting may suggest potential failure of contraceptive action.

Christiansen et al. (14) reported a high incidence of impotence and sperm abnormalities associated with low androgen excretion in men with epilepsy. Phenytoin, among other drugs, was incriminated (57). Phenytoin increases plasma concentrations of sex-hormone–binding globulin and total testosterone (100), but lowers free testosterone (21).

Gum Hypertrophy

Gum hypertrophy was the first recognized and most well known chronic toxic effect of phenytoin. It has been reviewed by Livingstone and Livingstone (54) and Hassell et al. (37). It can occur in up to 50% or more of cases depending on age, dental hygiene, and dose of the drug. It usually appears within 2 or 3 months of commencing therapy and may progress over the following 12 months. A younger age and poor dental hygiene predispose to this complication, which is also more common with high doses and high blood drug levels. The histological picture is of dense collagen tissue with scattered inflammatory cells. The mechanism is still uncertain. On stopping the phenytoin, the gum hypertrophy will regress slowly over 3 to 6 months.

TABLE 1. *Hypersensitivity reactions to phenytoin in 38 patients[a]*

Rashes	28
Licheniform or morbilliform	25
Erythema multiforme	7
Stevens-Johnson syndrome	5
Fever	14
Abnormal liver function tests	11
Lymphoid hyperplasia	9
Eosinophilia	8
Blood dyscrasias	12
Leukopenia	6
Thrombocytopenia	2
Anemia	6
Increased atypical lymphocytes	1
Serum sickness	2
Albuminuria	2
Renal failure	1

[a] From Haruda, ref. 36.

Facial Changes

Enlargement of the lips and nose and coarsening of features due to generalized thickening of subcutaneous tissues of the face and scalp may occur in many patients on prolonged therapy, usually with multiple antiepileptic drugs, especially in institutions and in mentally retarded patients (51,106). There may be associated gum hypertrophy and radiological evidence of calvarial thickening. The addition of acne, pigmentation, and hirsutism may all contribute to a characteristic facial appearance, referred to by Walshe (106) as "family likeness" and illustrated by Falconer and Davidson (28) in two pairs of identical twins, one of each pair suffering from epilepsy.

IDIOSYNCRATIC REACTIONS

The idiosyncratic reactions to phenytoin have been reviewed by Booker (9), Haruda (36) and Schmidt (88). Table 1 shows the type and frequency of hypersensitivity reactions to phenytoin in a series of 38 patients from one center over 14 years. Several of these reactions may occur together. They generally appear within the first few days, weeks, or months of phenytoin ad-

ministration and are more frequent and severe if the initial dose is a high one.

Skin Rashes

The most common skin rashes are itchy maculopapular morbilliform and scarlatiniform exanthemata (Table 2). About half are associated with fever. Exfoliative dermatitis is a more serious but less frequent skin reaction, which may appear within the first 4 weeks of treatment. It may be accompanied by hepatitis, hepatosplenomegaly, jaundice, fever, myalgia, eosinophilia, and lymphadenopathy, which can mimic serum sickness, infectious mononucleosis, or periarteritis nodosa.

The rare erythema exudativum multiforme of Stevens-Johnson syndrome may be associated with conjunctivitis, iritis, keratitis, stomatitis, vulvitis, fever, and arthralgia. Toxic epidermal necrolysis (Lyell syndrome) is also rare but, like the above two conditions, is potentially fatal. It is, therefore, important for the drug to be stopped immediately.

Hemapoietic Reactions

Hemapoietic reactions to phenytoin have been reviewed by Reynolds (77) and Pisciotta (72). Aplastic anemia is extremely rare and most of the reports concern patients who, in addition to phenytoin, have been taking other drugs, some of which are known to cause aplastic anemia.

Phenytoin occasionally causes a mild transient leucopenia in the early months of therapy. A more serious agranulocytosis has been described, but only 11 cases were recorded in the United States by 1982 (72), one of whom died. Thrombocytopenia is even less common than agranulocytosis. A pure red blood cell aplasia has been described in only three patients.

Hepatitis

Phenytoin-induced hepatitis has been reviewed by Parker and Shearer (70) and more recently by Jeavons (42), who summarized 44 cases from the literature, 12 of whom died. Thirty-two patients were on phenytoin alone. In 35 patients the duration of treatment was less than 36 days. The hepatitis was associated with a rash in 86% (exfoliative in 50%). Fever was present in 84%, lymphadenopathy in 66%, and eosinophilia in 77%. Various liver function tests were abnormal in up to 92%; jaundice occurred in 54.4%, and hepatomegaly in 52%. Hepatic pathology, either at autopsy or biopsy, seemed variable, but it is suggested that the pattern of injury is primarily hepatocellular with a prominent inflammatory response. Necrosis is frequently present.

Lymphadenopathy

Lymphadenopathy may be a prominent feature of hypersensitivity reactions to phenytoin. In 89 cases reviewed by Saltzstein and Ackerman (85), the predominantly cervical lymphadenopathy usually appeared within 4 months of starting treatment, often in association with fever and a rash, less commonly with arthritis, conjunctivitis, or hepatosplenomegaly. Patho-logically the nodes show obliteration of the normal architecture, hyperplasia of the reticulum cells, frequent mitoses, and eosinophilic infiltration. There are no Reed-Sternberg cells. Although this is usually a benign condition, it has sometimes been mistaken for reticulum cell sarcoma or Hodgkin's disease. Withdrawal of phenytoin usually leads to regression of the lymphadenopathy within 2 weeks. There are, however, a few reports of an increased incidence of malignant lymphomas occurring after 2 to 28 years of phenytoin therapy and without hypersensitivity phenomena. These are summarized by Schmidt (88), who emphasizes that the nature of this association is not clear. MacKinney and Booker (59) reported a lymphotoxic effect of phenytoin, especially at high serum levels of the drug.

Systemic Lupus Erythematosus

A reversible syndrome indistinguishable from systemic lupus erythematosus (SLE) has rarely been associated with phenytoin or with other antiepileptic drugs (88). As epilepsy may be an early feature of SLE, there remains some uncertainty about the relationship of this syndrome to drug therapy. Some doubt also remains concerning rare reports of an association between antiepileptic drugs and dermatomyositis, scleroderma, or a myasthenic syndrome.

Immunoglobulins and Antibodies

Humeral and cellular immune responses may be impaired during treatment with phenytoin (2,88,94). Several authors have found depression of immunoglobulin A and less often lowering of immunoglobulins M and G. There may be altered cellular immune reactions and delayed hypersensitivity reactions to common antigens, as well as impaired hemagglutinin-induced DNA synthesis. Antinuclear antibodies have been detected in up to 25% or more of epileptic patients, but not necessarily in association with immunoglobulin changes. The significance of the antibodies is unclear.

TERATOGENICITY

The teratogenic effects of phenytoin have been reviewed by Hassell et al. (37) and Schmidt (88). Children of epileptic mothers have malformations 1.25 to 2.24 times as often as the general population. Some malformations such as cardiac abnormalities or cleft palate/hair lip may carry a greater risk. Although animal experiments implicate phenytoin and other drugs, in clinical studies it is more difficult to show correlations with particular drugs. Schmidt (88) criticizes the use of the term "fetal hydantoin syndrome," pointing out that often the incrimination of a particular drug is not adequately supported since many patients are on multiple drugs. He prefers the use of the term "fetal anticonvulsant syndrome," the features of which are summarized in Table 2. The mechanisms of teratogenicity are not well understood but there is interest, for example, in the antifolate effect of some drugs, as this vitamin is important for neural development. Not all malformations are necessarily related to antiepileptic drug therapy.

PREVENTION OF TOXICITY

The prevention of phenytoin toxicity has been reviewed by Reynolds (80). Many factors predispose to the development of chronic toxicity, including recurrent acute toxicity. The old practice of pushing the dose of phenytoin and other drugs up to the point of acute toxicity should and can be avoided by careful monitoring. Treatment should be kept to the minimum dose compatible with seizure control, which for about one-third of newly diagnosed patients

TABLE 2. *Anomalies in the fetal anticonvulsant syndrome[a]*

Growth and performance
  Motor or mental deficiency
  Microcephaly
  Prenatal growth deficiency
  Postnatal growth deficiency
Craniofacial
  Short nose with low nasal bridge
  Hypertelorism
  Epicanthic folds
  Ptosis of eyelid
  Strabismus
  Low-set and/or abnormal ears
  Wide mouth
  Prominent lips
  Cleft palate
  Metopic sutural ridging
  Wide fontanelles
Limb
  Hypoplasia of nails and distal phalanges
  Fingerlike thumb
  Abnormal palmar creases
  Five or more digital arches
Other
  Short or webbed neck, low hairline
  Coarse hair
  Widely spaced, hypoplastic nipples
  Rib, sternal, or spinal anomalies
  Hernias
  Undescended testes

[a] From Schmidt, ref. 88.

is below the so called therapeutic or optimal range. Early age and prolonged therapy increase the risks, but the latter always has to be balanced against the risks of withdrawing therapy. Additional risk factors may include poor diet, pregnancy, intercurrent illness, institutionalization, mental retardation, and genetic predisposition. Greater awareness of the spectrum of toxicity, especially the subtle cognitive and behavioral aspects which may not even be apparent to the patient, is also important. A correct seizure diagnosis and avoidance of unnecessary polytherapy can also help prevent drug-induced toxicity.

REFERENCES

1. Aanderud, S., and Strandjord, E. E., (1980): Hypothyroidism induced by anti-epileptic therapy. *Acta. Neurol. Scand.*, 61:330–332.

2. Aarli, J. A. (1980): Effect of phenytoin on the immune system. In: *Phenytoin-Induced Teratology and Gingival Pathology,* edited by T. M. Hassell, M. C. Johnston, and K. H. Dudley, pp. 25–34. Raven Press, New York.

3. Allen J., and Oxley, J. (1983): Fractures in patients with epilepsy. In: *Chronic Toxicity of Antiepileptic Drugs,* edited by J. Oxley, D. Janz, and H. Meinardi, pp. 205–208. Raven Press, New York.

4. Andrewes, D. G., Bullen, J. G., Tomlinson, L., Elwes, R. D. C., and Reynolds, E. H. (1986): A comparative study of the cognitive effects of phenytoin and carbamazepine in new referrals with epilepsy. *Epilepsia,* 27:128–134.

5. Arends, J., Hommes, O., Doesburg, W., de Boo, T., Kap, J., Schoofs, M., van der Velden, T., and Jansen, M. (1981): Folate activated partial epilepsy: A model for drug study. In: *Advances in Epileptology: XII Epilepsy International Symposium,* edited by M. Dam, L. Gram, and J. K. Penry, pp. 653–669. Raven Press, New York.

6. Battino, D., Bossi, L., Canger, R., Margstkler, E., Molteni, B., Rossi, E., and Spina, S. (1981): Coagulation function in newborns treated *in utero* with antiepileptic drugs. *Epilepsia,* 22:367–368.

7. Bell, R. D., Pak, C. Y. C., Zerwekh, J., Barilla, D. E., and Vasko, M. (1979): Effects of phenytoin on bone and vitamin D metabolism. *Ann. Neurol.,* 5:374–378.

8. Bleyer, W. A., and Skinner, A. L. (1976): Fatal neonatal hemorrhage after maternal anticonvulsant therapy. *J.A.M.A.,* 235:626–627.

9. Booker, H. E., (1975): Idiosyncratic reactions to the antiepileptic drugs. *Epilepsia,* 16:171–181.

10. Botez, M. I., and Reynolds, E. H. (1979): *Folic Acid in Neurology, Psychiatry and Internal Medicine.* Raven Press, New York.

11. Carl, G. F., Gill, M. W., and Schatz, R. A., (1988): Effect of chronic primidone treatment on folate-dependent one carbon metabolism in the rat. *Biochem. Pharmacol.,* 36:2139–2144.

12. Chadwick, D. W., Reynolds, E. H., and Marsden, C. D. (1976): Anticonvulsant-induced dyskinesias—A comparison with dyskinesias induced by neuroleptics. *J. Neurol. Neurosurg. Psychiatr.,* 39:1210–1218.

13. Chanarin, I. (1982): *The Megaloblastic Anaemias.* Blackwell Press, Oxford.

14. Christiansen, P., Deigaard, J., and Lund, M. (1975): Potency, fertility, and sexual hormones in young male epileptics. *Ugeskr. Laeg.,* 137:2402–2405.

15. Christiansen, C., Kristensen, M., and Rodbro, P. (1972): Latent osteomalacia in epileptic patients on anticonvulsants. *Brit. Med. J.,* 3:738–739.

16. Christiansen, C., Rodbro, P., and Lund, M. (1973): Incidence of anticonvulsant osteomalacia and effect of vitamin D: Controlled therapeutic trial. *Br. Med. J.,* 4:695–701.

17. Christiansen, C., Rodbro, P., and Sjo, O. (1974): "Anticonvulsant action" of vitamin D in epileptic patients? A controlled pilot study. *Br. Med. J.,* 2:258–259.

18. Coggin, T., Gough, H., Bissessar, A., Crowley, M., Baker, M., and Callaghan, N. (1987): A comparative study of the relative effects of anticonvulsant drugs and dietary folate on the red cell folate status of patients with epilepsy. *Quart. J. Med.,* 247:911–919.

19. Cudworth, A. G., and Cunningham, J. L. (1974): The effect of diphenylhydantoin on insulin response. *Clin. Sci. Mol. Med.,* 46:131–136.

20. Dam, M. (1982): Phenytoin toxicity. In: *Antiepileptic Drugs,* 2nd edition, edited by D. M. Woodbury, J. K. Penry, and C. E. Pippenger, pp. 247–256. Raven Press, New York.

21. Dana-Haeri, Oxley, J., and Richens, A. (1982): Reduction of free testosterone by antiepileptic drugs. *Br. Med. J.,* 284:85–86.

22. Dellaportas, D. I., Shorvon, S. D., Galbraith, A. W., Laundy, M., Reynolds, E. H., Marshall, W. J., and Chanarin, I. (1982): Chronic toxicity in epileptic patients receiving single-drug treatment. *Br. Med. J.,* 285:409–410.

23. Dent, C. E., Richens, A., Rowe, D. J. F., and Stamp, T. C. B. (1970): Osteomalacia with long-term anticonvulsant therapy in epilepsy. *Br. Med. J.,* 4:69–72.

24. Doddrill, C. B., and Troupin, A. S. (1977): Psychotropic effects of carbamazepine in epilepsy: A double-blind comparison with phenytoin. *Neurology,* 27:1023–1028.

25. Dravet, C., Dalla, B. B., Mesdjian, E., Galland, M. C., and Roger, J. (1983): Phenytoin-induced paroxysmal dyskinesias. In: *Chronic Toxicity of Antiepileptic Drugs,* edited by J. Oxley, D. Janz, and H. Meinardi, pp. 229–235. Raven Press, New York.

26. Edeh, J., and Toone, B. K. (1985): Antiepileptic therapy, folate deficiency and psychiatric morbidity: A general practice survey. *Epilepsia,* 26:434–440.

27. Elwes, R. D. C., Dellaportas, C., Reynolds, E. H., Robinson, W., Butt, W. R., and London, D. R. (1985): Prolactin and growth hormone dynamics in epileptic patients receiving phenytoin. *Clin. Endocrin.,* 23:263–270.

28. Falconer, M. A., and Davidson, S. (1973): Coarse features in epilepsy as a consequence of anticonvulsant therapy. *Lancet,* II:1112–1114.

29. Gharib, H., and Munoz, J. M. (1974): Endocrine manifestations of diphenylhydantoin therapy. *Metabolism,* 23:515–524.

30. Glaser, G. H. (1972): Diphenylhydantoin toxicity. In: *Antiepileptic Drugs,* 1st edition, edited by D. M. Woodbury, J. K. Penry, and R. P. Schmidt, pp. 219–226. Raven Press New York.

31. Godfrey, P., Toone, B. K., Carney, M. W. P., Flynn, T., Bottiglieri, T., Laundy, M. and Reynolds, E. H. (1988): Methyl folate enhances recovery from psychiatric illness. Presentation, British Assoc. for Psychopharmacology (*in press*).

32. Gough, H., Bissesar, A., Goggin, T., Higgins, D., Baker, M., Crowley, M., and Callaghan, N. (1986): Factors associated with the biochemical changes in vitamin D and calcium metabolism in

institutionalized patients with epilepsy. *Ir. J. Med. Sci.,* 155:181–189.

33. Gough, H., Goggin, T., Bissessar, A., Baker, M., Crowley, M., and Callaghan N. (1986): A comparative study of the relative influence of different anticonvulsant drugs, UV exposure and diet on vitamin D and calcium metabolism in out-patients with epilepsy. *Quart. J. Med.,* New Series 59, 230:569–577.

34. Hahn, T. J., (1976): Bone complications of anticonvulsants. *Drugs,* 12:201–211.

35. Haidukewych, D., and Rodin, E. A. (1987): Chronic antiepileptic drug therapy: Classification by medication regimen and incidence of decreases in serum thyroxine and free thyroxine index. *Ther. Drug Mon.,* 9:392–398.

36. Haruda, F. (1979): Phenytoin hypersensitivity: 38 cases. *Neurology,* 29:1480–1485.

37. Hassell, T. M., Johnston, M. C., Dudley, K. H., eds. (1980): *Phenytoin-Induced Teratology and Gingival Pathology.* Raven Press, New York.

38. Hommes, O. R. (1981): Excitatory properties of folate derivatives. In: *Advances in Epileptology: 12th Epilepsy International Symposium,* edited by M. Dam, L. Gram, and J. K. Penry, pp. 641–651. Raven Press, New York.

39. Hommes, O. R., Hollinger, J. L., Jansen, M. J. T., Schoofs, V. D., Wiel, T., and Kok, J. C. N. (1979): Convulsant properties of folate compounds: Some considerations and speculations. In: *Folic Acid in Neurology, Psychiatry, and Internal Medicine,* edited by M. I. Botez and E. H. Reynolds, pp. 285–316. Raven Press, New York.

40. Idestrom, C.-M., Schalling, D., Carlquist, U., and Sjoqvist, F. (1972): Acute effects of diphenylhydantoin in relation to plasma levels. *Psychol. Med.,* 2:111–120.

41. Iivanainen, M., Viukari, M., and Helle, E.-P. (1977): Cerebellar atrophy in phenytoin-treated mentally retarded epileptics. *Epilepsia,* 18:375–386.

42. Jeavons, P. M. (1983): Hepatotoxicity of antiepileptic drugs. In: *Chronic Toxicity of Antiepileptic Drugs,* edited by J. Oxley, D. Janz, and H. Meinardi, pp. 1–45. Raven Press, New York.

43. Karp, M., Lerman, P., Doron, M., and Laron, Z. (1973): Effect of diphenylhdantoin on insulin response in the oral glucose tolerance test in children and adolescents. *Helv. Paediat. Acta,* 28:617–620.

44. Koch, H-U., Kraft, D., Von Herrath, D., and Schaefer, K. (1972): Influence of diphenylhydantoin and phenobarbital on intestinal calcium transport in the rat. *Epilepsia,* 13:829–834.

45. Kohler, H. G. (1966): Haemorrhage in the newborn of epileptic mothers. *Lancet,* 1:267.

46. Krause, K.-H., Berlit, P., and Schmidt-Gayk, H. (1983): Interrelationships between serum 25-hydroxycalciferol and bone mass in adults on long-term antiepileptic drug therapy. In: *Chronic Toxicity of Antiepileptic Drugs,* edited by J. Oxley, D. Janz, and H. Meinardi, pp. 193–200. Raven Press, New York.

47. Krause, K.-H., Prager, P., Schmidt-Gayk, H.,

and Ritz, E. (1977): Diagnostik der Osteopathia antiepileptica in Erwachsenenalter. *Dtsch. Med. Wschr.,* 102:1872–1877.

48. Kruse, R. (1968): Osteopathien bei antiepileptischer Langzeittherapie. *Mschr. Kinderheilk.,* 116:378–380.

49. Kutt, H., Winters, W., Kokenge, R., and McDowell, F. (1964): Diphenylhydantoin metabolism, blood levels, and toxicity. *Arch. Neurol.,* 11:642–648.

50. Lascelles, P. T., Kocen, R. S., and Reynolds, E. H. (1970): The distribution of plasma phenytoin levels in epileptic patients. *J. Neurol. Neurosurg. Psychiat.,* 33:501–505.

51. Lefebvre, E. B., Haining, R. G., and Labbe, R. F. (1972): Coarse facies, calvarial thickening and hyperphosphatasia associated with long-term anticonvulsant therapy. *N. Eng. J. Med.,* 286:1301–1302.

52. Levy, L. L., and Fenichel, G. M. (1965): Diphenylhydantoin activated seizures. *Neurology,* 15:716–722.

53. Linde, J., Hansen, J. M., Siersback-Nilesen, K., and Fuglsang-Fredriksen, V. (1971): Bone density in patients receiving long-term anticonvulsant therapy. *Acta. Neurol. Scand.,* 47:650–651.

54. Livingston, S., and Livingston, H. L. (1969): Diphenylhydantoin gingival hyperplasia. *Amer. J. Dis. Child.,* 117:265–270.

55. Logan, W. J., and Freeman, J. M. (1969): Pseudogenerative disease due to diphenylhydantoin intoxication. *Arch. Neurol.,* 21:631–637.

56. Lovelace, R. E., and Horwitz, S. J. (1968): Peripheral neuropathy in long-term diphenylhydantoin therapy. *Arch. Neurol.,* 18:69–77.

57. Luhdorf, K., Christiansen, P., Hansen, J. M., and Lund, M. (1977): The influence of phenytoin and carbamazepine on endocrine function; preliminary results. In: *Epilepsy, the VIIIth International Symposium,* edited by J. K. Penry. Raven Press, New York.

58. Luhdorf, K., and Lund, M. (1977): Phenytoin-induced hyperkinesia. *Epilepsia,* 18:409–415.

59. MacKinney, A. A., and Booker, H. E. (1972): Diphenylhydantoin effects on human lymphocytes *in vitro* and *in vivo. Arch. Intern. Med.,* 129:988–992.

60. Malherbe, C., Burrill, K. C., Levin, S. R., Karam, J. H., and Forsham, P. H. (1972): Effect of diphenylhydantoin on insulin secretion in man. *N. Engl. J. Med.,* 286:339–342.

61. Mannheimer, E., Pakesch, F., Reimer, E. E., and Vetter, H. (1952): Die hamatologischen Komplikationen der Epilepsiebehandlung mit Hydantoinkorpem. *Med. Klin.,* 47:1397–1401.

62. Marsden, C. D., Reynolds, E. H., Parsons, V., Harris, R., and Duchen, L. (1973): Myopathy associated with anticonvulsant osteomalacia. *Br. Med. J.,* 4:526–527.

63. Miller, A. A., Goff, D., and Webster, R. A. (1979): Predisposition of laboratory animals to epileptogenic activity of folic acid. In: *Folic Acid in Neurology, Psychiatry, and Internal Medicine,*

edited by M. I. Botez, and E. H. Reynolds, pp. 331–334. Raven Press, New York.

64. Mosekilde, L., and Melsen, F. (1976): Anticonvulsant osteomalacia determined by quantitative analysis of bone changes: Population study and possible risk factors. *Acta Med. Scand.,* 199:349–355.

65. Mountain, K. R., Hirsch, J., and Gallus, A. S. (1970): Neonatal coagulation defect due to anticonvulsant drug treatment in pregnancy. *Lancet,* 1:265–268.

66. Munoz-Garcia, D., Del Ser, T., Bermejo, F., and Portera, A. (1982): Truncal ataxia in chronic anticonvulsant treatment. Association with drug-induced folate deficiency. *J. Neurol. Sci.,* 55:305–311.

67. O'Donnell, R. A., Leach, M. J., and Miller, A. A. (1983): Folic acid induced kindling in rats: Changes in brain amino acids. In: *Chemistry and Biology of Pteridines,* edited by J. A. Blair, pp. 801–805. Walter de Gruyter & Co., Berlin.

68. Offermann, G. (1983): Chronic antiepileptic drug treatment and disorders of mineral metabolism. In: *Chronic Toxicity of Antiepileptic Drugs,* edited by J. Oxley, D. Janz, and H. Meinardi, pp. 175–184. Raven Press, New York.

69. Oxley, J., Janz, D., and Meinardi, H., eds. (1983): *Chronic Toxicity of Antiepileptic Drugs.* Raven Press, New York.

70. Parker, W. A., and Shearer, C. A. (1979): Phenytoin hepatoxicity: A case report and review. *Nuerology (Minneap.),* 2:175–178.

71. Patel, H., and Crichton, J. V. (1968): The neurological hazards of diphenylhydantoin in childhood. *J. Pediatr.,* 73:676–684.

72. Pisciotta, A. V. (1982): Phenytoin: Hematological toxicity. In: *Antiepileptic Drugs,* 2nd edition, edited by D. M. Woodbury, J. K. Penry, and C. E. Pippenger, pp. 257–268. Raven Press, New York.

73. Plaa, G. L. (1975): Acute toxicity of antiepileptic drugs. *Epilepsia,* 16:183–191.

74. Reynolds, E. H. (1967): Effects of folic acid on the mental state and fit frequency of drug-treated epileptic patients. *Lancet,* 1:1086–1088.

75. Reynolds, E. H. (1968): Mental effects of anticonvulsants, and folic acid metabolism. *Brain,* 91:197–214.

76. Reynolds, E. H. (1970): Iatrogenic disorders in epilepsy. In: *Modern Trends in Neurology, Vol. 5,* edited by D. Williams, pp. 271–286. Butterworths, London.

77. Reynolds, E. H. (1972): Diphenylhydantoin: Hematologic aspects of toxicity. In: *Antiepileptic Drugs,* 1st edition, edited by D. M. Woodbury, J. K. Penry, and R. P. Schmidt, pp. 247–262. Raven Press, New York.

78. Reynolds, E. H. (1975): Chronic antiepileptic toxicity: A review. *Epilepsia,* 16:319–352.

79. Reynolds, E. H. (1983): Adverse hematological effects of antiepileptic drugs. In: *Chronic Toxicity of Antiepileptic Drugs,* edited by J. Oxley, D. Janz, and H. Meinardi, pp. 91–100. Raven Press, New York.

80. Reynolds, E. H. (1983): How to avoid chronic toxicity. In: *Chronic Toxicity of Antiepileptic Drugs,* edited by J. Oxley, D. Janz, and H. Meinardi, pp. 285–291. Raven Press, New York.

81. Reynolds, E. H. (1983): Mental effects of antiepileptic medication. A review. *Epilepsia,* 24 (Suppl. 2):85–95.

82. Reynolds, E. H. (1985): Folic acid and neuropsychiatry. *Farmaci & Terapia,* 2:163–168.

83. Reynolds, E. H., Mattson, R. H., and Gallagher, B. B. (1972): Relationships between serum and cerebrospinal fluid anticonvulsant drug and folic acid concentrations in epileptic patients. *Neurology (Minneap.),* 22:841–844.

84. Reynolds, E. H., and Travers, R. D. (1974): Serum anticonvulsant concentrations in epileptic patients with mental symptoms. *Br. J. Psychiatr.,* 124:440–445.

85. Saltzstein, S. L., and Ackerman, L. V. (1959): Lymphoadenopathy induced by anticonvulsant drugs and mimicking clinically and pathologically malignant lymphomas. *Cancer,* 12:164–182.

86. Schmid, F. (1967): Osteopathien bei antiepileptischer Damerbehandlung. *Fortschr. Med.,* 9:381–382.

87. Schmidt, D. (1981): Effect of antiepileptic drugs on estrogen and progesterone metabolism and on oral contraception. In: *Advances in Epileptology: XIIth Epilepsy International Symposium,* edited by M. Dam, L. Gram, and J. K. Penry, pp. 423–431. Raven Press, New York.

88. Schmidt, D. (1982): *Adverse Effects of Antiepileptic Drugs.* Raven Press, New York.

89. Shorvon, S. D. (1979): Anticonvulsant therapy and peripheral neuropathy. In: *Folic Acid in Neurology, Psychiatry, and Internal Medicine,* edited by M. I. Botez and E. H. Reynolds, pp. 335–347. Raven Press, New York.

90. Shorvon, S. D., Carney, M. W. P., Chanarin, I., and Reynolds, E. H. (1980): The neuropsychiatry of megaloblastic anaemia. *Br. Med. J.,* 281:1036–1038.

91. Shorvon, S. D., and Reynolds, E. H. (1982): Anticonvulsant peripheral neuropathy: A clinical and electrophysiological study of patients on single drug treatment with phenytoin, carbamazepine or barbiturates. *J. Neurol., Neuros. and Psych.,* 45:620–626.

92. Smith, D. B., and Carl, G. F. (1981): Anticonvulsant-folate interactions. In: *Advances in Epileptology: XIIth Epilepsy International Symposium,* edited by M. Dam, L. Gram, and J. K. Penry, pp. 671–678. Raven Press, New York.

93. Solomon, G. E., Hilgatner, M. W., and Kutt, H. (1972): Coagulation defects caused by diphenylhydantoin. *Neurology (Minneap.),* 22:1165–1171.

94. Sorrell, T. C., and Forbes, I. J. (1975): Depression of immune competence by phenytoin and carbamazepine. *Clin. Exp. Immunol.,* 20:273–285.

95. Surks, M. I., Ordene, K. W., Manu, D. N., and Kumara-Siri, M. H. (1983): Diphenylhydantoin inhibits the thyrotropin response to thyrotropin-

releasing hormone in man and rat. *J. Clin. Endocrinol. Metab.*, 56:940–945.

96. Thompson, P. J., Huppert, F. A., and Trimble, M. R. (1981): Phenytoin and cognitive functions: Effects on normal volunteers and implications for epilepsy. *Br. J. Clin. Psychol.*, 20:155–162.

97. Thompson, P. J., and Trimble, M. R. (1982): Anticonvulsant drugs and cognitive functions. *Epilepsia*, 23:531–544.

98. Thompson, P. J., and Trimble, M. R. (1983): The effect of anticonvulsant drugs on cognitive function: Relation to serum levels. J. Neurol., *Neuros. and Psych.*, 46:227–233.

99. Toone, B. (1986): Sexual disorders in epilepsy. In: *Recent Advances in Epilepsy*, edited by T. A. Pedley and B. S. Meldrum, pp. 233–259. Churchill Livingstone, Edinburgh.

100. Toone, B. K., Wheeler, M., and Fenwick, P. B. C. (1980): Sex hormone changes in male epileptics. *Clin. Endocrin.*, 12:391–395.

101. Trimble, M. R., Corbett, J., and Donaldson, D. (1980): Folic acid and mental symptoms in children with epilepsy. *J. Neurol., Neuros. and Psych.*, 43:1030–1034.

102. Trimble, M. R., and Reynolds, E. H. (1976): Anticonvulsant drugs and mental symptoms: A review. *Psychol. Med.*, 6:169–178.

103. Trimble, M. R., and Reynolds, E. H. (1984): Neuropsychiatric toxicity of anticonvulsant drugs. In: *Recent Advances in Clinical Neurology*, edited by W. B. Matthews and Gilbert H. Glaser, Churchill Livingstone, Edinburgh.

104. Troupin, A. S., and Ojemann, L. M. (1975): Paradoxical intoxication—A complication of anticonvulsant administration. *Epilepsia*, 16:753–758.

105. Van Rijn, C. M., Van der Velden, T. J. A. M., Rodrigues de Miranda, J. F., Feenstra, M. G. P., and Hommes, O. R. (1988): The influence of folic acid on the picrotoxin-sensitive site of the GABA receptor complex. *Epilepsy Res.*, 2:215–218.

106. Walshe, M. M. (1972): Cutaneous drug effects in epilepsy. *Trans. St. John's Hosp. Derm. Soc.*, 58:269–281.

107. Waltl, H., Mitterstieler, G., and Schwingshackl, A. (1974): Hämorrhagische Diathese bei einem Neugeborenen einer Mutter mit antiepileptischler Therapie. *Dtsch. Med. Wschr.*, 99:1315–1317.

Antiepileptic Drugs, Third Edition, edited by
R. Levy, R. Mattson, B. Meldrum,
J. K. Penry, and F. E. Dreifuss.
Raven Press, Ltd., New York © 1989.

16

Other Hydantoins

Mephenytoin and Ethotoin

Harvey J. Kupferberg

The synthesis of 5,5-diphenylhydantoin (phenytoin) preceded Merritt and Putnam's discovery of its anticonvulsant activity by 30 years (44). Since then, a large number of hydantoins have been synthesized and tested for anticonvulsant activity. Many of these compounds are active, but only three have found their way into modern therapy: phenytoin, mephenytoin, and ethotoin. Several hydantoins are no longer used or their efficacy has not been established.

5-Ethyl-5-phenylhydantoin (Nirvanol) was synthesized in 1914 (5) and was used for movement disorders and seizures, but its use declined because of the high frequency of skin rashes and fever. 3-Allyl-5-isobutyl-2-thiohydantoin (albutoin, Co-ord) was evaluated for efficacy in therapy-resistant institutionalized epileptic patients in a randomized blinded comparison with phenytoin and primidone (8). The results showed that albutoin (1,200 mg/day) was not as effective as phenytoin (300 mg/day) or primidone (750 mg/day) in controlling seizures.

5,5-Diphenylimidazolin-4-one (doxenitoine, Glior) has the same structural relationship to phenytoin as primidone has to phenobarbital. It does not, however, appear to be metabolized to phenytoin to any extent in rats (13). Oral doses of doxenitoine (0.8 to 2.4 g) prevented the tonic component of generalized seizures produced by elec-troshock therapy in psychiatric patients (14).

MEPHENYTOIN

Mephenytoin, unlike phenytoin, is effective in both the supramaximal electroshock seizure pattern test (MES) and subcutaneous pentylenetetrazol (sc Met) seizure threshold test in both rats and mice. It is one-sixth as active as phenytoin following intraperitoneal administration to mice (9.5 mg/kg versus 65.5 mg/kg) but has similar activity in rats following oral administration (29.8 mg/kg for phenytoin and 18.1 mg/kg for mephenytoin). Mephenytoin inhibits the clonic seizures induced by subcutaneously administered bicuculline and picrotoxin. The dose of mephenytoin required to inhibit the clonic seizures is, however, near its neurotoxic dose.

Chemistry and Methods of Determination

Physical and Chemical Properties

Mephenytoin (3-methyl-5-ethyl-5-phenylhydantoin) is a white crystalline substance (Fig. 1). Its melting point is 137° to 138°C. It has a molecular weight of 218.25. Commercially available mephenytoin is a ra-

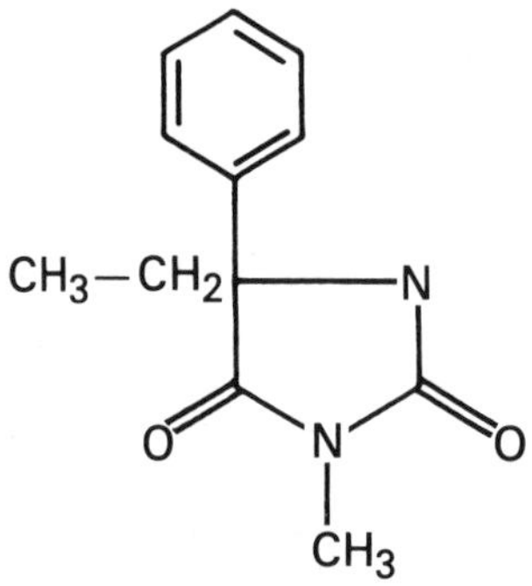

FIG. 1. Structure of mephenytoin (3-methyl-5-ethyl-5-phenylhydantoin).

cemic mixture with its asymmetric carbon in the 5 position of the hydantoin ring. The isomers of mephenytoin can be produced by alkylating the respective isomers of Nirvanol with dimethylsulfate (24). The optical rotations of (R)-$(-)$ mephenytoin are

$[\alpha]\dfrac{125}{D} = -104°$ and $[\alpha]\dfrac{125}{365} = -410°$ and

those of (S)-$(+)$ mephenytoin are $[\alpha]\dfrac{125}{D} =$

$+105°$ and $[\alpha]\dfrac{125}{365} = +416°$.

Nirvanol can be separated into its enantiomers by fractional crystallization of the diastereomeric salts formed with $(-)$-brucine. The rotation of each isomer is 115° with a melting point of 237°C (41). The acidic nature of Nirvanol (pK_a of 8.5) is suppressed by its methylation. Therefore, mephenytoin can be extracted from Nirvanol by organic solvents (e.g., chloroform) from basic solutions.

Methods of Determination

The early methods of analysis of mephenytoin and Nirvanol in plasma and tissue used derivative formation and gas-liquid chromatography, e.g., on-column ethylation (12), trimethylsilyl derivatives (33) propylation (24), ethylation (49), and

capillary column gas chromatography–mass spectrometry (2). A renewed interest in the pharmacogenetic control of mephenytoin metabolism in humans required the development of specific sensitive methods for the determination of mephenytoin and its metabolites in urine and plasma. Kupfer et al. (27) developed high-performance liquid chromatographic analysis (HPLC) using a reversed-phase column to separate mephenytoin, nirvanol, and their metabolites, 3-methyl-5-(4-hydroxyphenyl)-5-ethyl-hydantoin, and 5-(4-hydroxy-phenyl-5-ethyl-hydantoin in urine of patients receiving mephenytoin. 5-Phenyl-5-propyl-hydantoin and 5-(4-bromophenyl)-5-ethylhydantoin were used as internal standards. Complete separation and quantitation of each compound was achieved within 17 min. Meier et al. (37) quantitated the 4-hydroxyphenyl metabolites of mephenytoin and Nirvanol produced from mephenytoin by human microsomes with HPLC using a reversed-phase C-18 column with acetonitrile/methanol/aqueous sodium perchlorate as an eluent. Direct enantiomeric resolution of mephenytoin can be obtained without derivatization using chiral capillary column gas chromatography followed by nitrogen-specific detection (48). The resolution of the enantiomers of Nirvanol requires propylation of the imide nitrogen of the hydantoin ring. Linearity of reproducible standard curves was found between concentrations of 50 ng/ml and 5 μg/ml. Akrawi and Wedlund (1) unexpectedly found that a small amount of Nirvanol was methylated to mephenytoin during the propylation process. The 1-iodopropane used to propylate Nirvanol contained small amounts of iodomethane. Although the contamination was small, methylation of Nirvanol proceeds more rapidly than propylation. Redistillation of the iodopropane decreased the amounts of mephenytoin during the propylation of Nirvanol.

Biotransformation

Mephenytoin is extensively metabolized in humans. The oxidative products of its metabolism have been identified in urine. The major routes of metabolism are de-methylation and *p*-hydroxylation of the phenyl ring (6,17,26,29,34). Other aromatic ring hydroxylated metabolites include the dihydrodiol, catechol, and the 3-methyl ca-techol. Aliphatic hydroxylation of the 5-ethyl side chain and glucuronidation of the imide nitrogen of hydantoin ring also occurs but to a lesser degree (34).

A renewed interest in mephenytoin phar-macokinetics occurred when Kupfer et al. (25) described the stereoselective disposi-tion and metabolism of Nirvanol in the dog. The volume of distribution and protein binding of the two enantiomers of Nirvanol were the same but the levo-form had a longer half-life than the dextro-form (23.3 hr versus 16.3 hr). There appears to be a stereospecific difference in the urinary ex-cretion rate of the isomers of the hydrox-ylated metabolite of Nirvanol. The urinary excretion rate of the dextro-isomer of *p*-hy-droxynirvanol was eight times greater than the levo-form of the metabolite.

Kupfer and Bircher (24) studied the me-tabolism of mephenytoin in dogs and again found stereospecific differences in metab-olism. A dramatic difference in stereoselec-tive metabolism of mephenytoin was ob-served in humans. Kupfer et al. (32), using a novel pseudoracemic mixture of radio-labeled mephenytoin enantiomers, dem-onstrated that the hydroxy metabolite of mephenytoin, 3-methyl-5-(4-hydroxy-phenyl)-5-ethylhydantoin, was derived from the (*S*)-(+) isomer. About 42% of the dose of mephenytoin is recovered in the urine as this metabolite within 24 hr following oral administration. In contrast, the (*R*)-(−) iso-mer of mephenytoin is demethylated slowly to the corresponding isomer of Nirvanol. Nirvanol is not extensively metabolized and

is eliminated by renal excretion. When *R*-Nirvanol was administered to patients for a prolonged period, 86% of the administered dose could be recovered unchanged in the urine. The half-lives ranged from 77 to 176 hr, but the volumes of distribution were similar (4).

Polymorphic Metabolism

Kupfer et al. (28) found a subject who had a defect in the hydroxylation of (*S*)-me-phenytoin. This defect was present in other family members. The urinary recovery of the hydroxy metabolite of mephenytoin represented only 3% of the dose adminis-tered. In the hydroxylation-deficient sub-jects, mephenytoin and Nirvanol accumu-late in the plasma, and both isomers of Nirvanol appear slowly in the urine.

The urinary recovery of the hydroxy me-tabolite of mephenytoin was used to iden-tify the polymorphic frequency in the gen-eral population. Poor metabolizers of mephenytoin excrete approximately 2% of the administered dose as the 4-hydroxy me-tabolite of mephenytoin. The ratio of each enantiomer is close to unity. Extensive me-tabolizers excrete approximately 50% of the dose as the 4-hydroxy metabolite, but the (*S*) configuration is approximately 50 times larger than the (*R*) configuration (47).

The pharmacokinetic parameters of me-phenytoin in the two populations reflect the metabolic specificity for the (*S*)(+) enan-tiomer by the extensive metabolizers (47). The half-life of (*S*)-mephenytoin is 2 hr whereas the (*R*)-enantiomer half-life is approximately 76 hr. The half-life of both enantiomers of mephenytoin in the poor metabolizer's population is equal to the half-life of (*R*)-mephenytoin in extensive metabolizers. Urinary excretion of un-changed mephenytoin and the steady-state volumes of distribution of mephenytoin were the same for the two populations.

Kupfer and Preisig (31) found that approximately 5% of the Swiss subjects studied were poor metabolizers of mephenytoin. A similar frequency of poor metabolizers was found in the Canadian (19) and American Caucasian populations (46). Jurima et al. (22) found a higher frequency of poor metabolizers of mephenytoin in an oriental population living in Canada. A close inspection of the data showed that approximately 23% of the Japanese were hydroxylation deficent, whereas the Chinese population was similar to the Caucasians. Nakamura et al. (40) confirmed this finding in Japanese living in Japan. Another significant finding was that none of the Japanese subjects were poor metabolizers of debrisoquine, another drug used in identifying polymorphism. Family studies among the Japanese indicate that the deficiency in mephenytoin metabolism is an autosomal-recessive trait (18,45).

The metabolism of Nirvanol also appears to be genetically controlled (30). Patients who are poor hydroxylators of mephenytoin also fail to hydroxylate Nirvanol. The recovery of aromatic ring hydroxylated metabolites of Nirvanol from the urine of extensive metabolizers following the administration of (S)-Nirvanol was 20 times greater than from poor metabolizers.

Human liver microsomes have been used to characterize the stereoselectivity of mephenytoin's metabolism. Both the demethylation and hydroxylation are dependent on NADPH and inhibited by carbon monoxide, SKF-525, and metyrapone (16,37). Both reactions appear to be mediated by cytochrome P-450 monooxygenases. The hydroxylation of the aromatic ring followed Michaelis-Menten kinetics whereas the N-demethylation did not show saturation kinetics with steady-state equilibrium constants (K_m) ranging from 59 to 143 μM (23). Meier et al. (35) found an increase in the K_m and a decrease in the maximal velocity for the hydroxylation of (S)-mephenytoin by microsomes obtained from poor metabo-

lizers. A loss of stereospecificity for the hydroxylation of the two enantiomers of mephenytoin was also seen. Gut et al. (15) purified a cytochrome P-450 from human liver which specifically catalyzes the hydroxylation of (S)-mephenytoin. This enzyme was devoid of any demethylation activity. The specific P-450 for mephenytoin hydroxylation, isolated from both populations of metabolizers, were indistinguishable in a variety of immunological and physical properties (38). These data strongly suggest that the hydroxylation deficiency is caused by a minor structural change of the enzyme.

The clinical significance of mephenytoin's polymorphic metabolism is important to the epileptologist. At least 5% of the Caucasian and 20% of the Japanese population treated with mephenytoin will exhibit toxicity because of elevated plasma levels of mephenytoin and Nirvanol. Nakamura et al. (40) found that sleepiness was three times higher in the poor metabolizers.

Clinical Efficacy and Toxicity

The clinical effectiveness of mephenytoin appears to be good in partial and secondarily generalized seizures, although its use remains small compared to phenytoin. Mephenytoin therapy has been associated with idiosyncratic side effects including skin rash, fever, generalized adenopathy, and fatal blood dyscrasias (43). It may be substituted for phenytoin where the peripheral neuropathy, gingival hypertrophy, or hirsutism create problems.

Troupin et al. (43) attempted to relate seizure control to serum mephenytoin and Nirvanol levels. They suggested that the total amount of plasma hydantoin (mephenytoin and Nirvanol) be measured for best seizure control. As most patients metabolize mephenytoin rapidly, the concentration of Nirvanol is most important to seizure control. Levels of 25 to 40 μg/ml usually yield improved seizure control without discomfort.

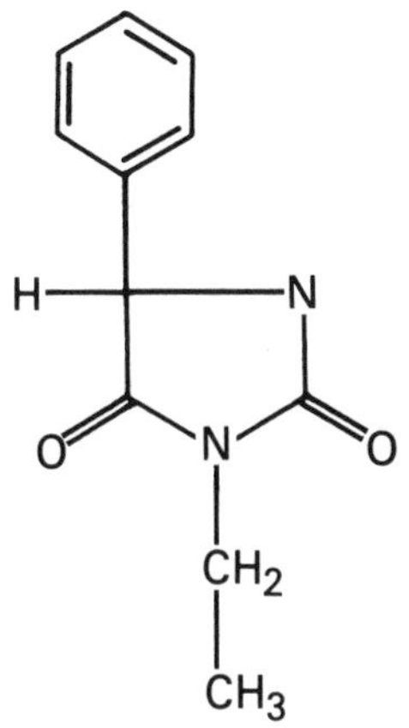

FIG. 2. Structure of ethotoin (3-ethyl-5-phenylhydantoin).

Theodore et al. (42) studied five patients with uncontrolled complex partial seizures. Two patients had reduced seizures during mephenytoin treatment with a dose of 400 mg per day. The average steady-state plasma levels of mephenytoin and Nirvanol were 1.5 µg/ml and 18 µg/ml, respectively. None of the patients had idiosyncratic mephenytoin toxicity.

ETHOTOIN

Ethotoin (Peganone) has been available for over 30 years for the treatment of generalized tonic-clonic seizures. It still remains underused and does not produce the gingival hyperplasia, hirsutism, and ataxia seen with phenytoin therapy. The anticonvulsant profile of ethotoin in experimental animals is similar to that of mephenytoin as it inhibits seizures induced by the MES and sc MET tests in both mice and rats.

Chemistry and Methods of Determination

Physical and Chemical Properties

Ethotoin (3-ethyl-5-phenylhydantoin) is a white crystalline compound (Fig. 2). Its melting point is 94°C. It has a molecular weight of 204.22. Ethotoin has a chiral center at the 5 position of the hydantoin ring and is used as a racemic mixture. The pharmacologic activity of the diastereoisomers of ethotoin has never been reported. Ethotoin is insoluble in water and acidic or basic solutions, but soluble in most organic solvents.

Methods of Determination

Yonekawa et al. (50) developed a gas chromatographic method for ethotoin, but the method did not quantitate 5-phenylhydantoin, an active metabolite of ethotoin. Meyer et al. (36) developed an HPLC method for the pharmacokinetic study of ethotoin in healthy volunteers. Ethotoin was extracted from plasma made basic with trisodium phosphate and extracted with ether. The organic solvent was evaporated to dryness and the residue dissolved in acetonitrile. A C-18 column and a mobile phase of 30% acetonitrile/70% 0.01M sodium phosphate (pH 4.4) was used to separate and quantitate ethotoin. A variable wavelength detector was set at 195 nm. Inotsume et al. (21) quantitated ethotoin by gas chromatography–mass spectrometry. Chloroform extracts of serum were evaporated to dryness and derivatives formed by on-column methylation. Ethotoin was quantitated by selected ion monitoring of the m/z 218 ion. Inotsume and co-workers (20) later separated the enantiomers of ethotoin using chiral stationary phase HPLC.

Absorption, Distribution, and Excretion

The pharmacokinetic parameters of ethotoin were reported by Meyer et al. (36) in five healthy volunteers. Doses of 500, 1,500, and 2,500 mg doses were given to each subject at 7-day intervals. Plasma samples were collected over a 49-hr period. The plasma concentration-time profiles were

analyzed by both one- and two-compartment open models, and with and without
concentration-dependent elimination kinetics. The time to maximal plasma concentration increased with increasing dose, indicating a decrease in absorption rate. The
area under the plasma concentration time
curve (AUC) for each dose, normalized for
body weight, lacked proportionality. The
majority of data sets were best described by
a nonlinear model. Carter et al. (7) characterized the pharmacokinetics of ethotoin
in children and adolescents with uncontrolled seizures. There was no significant
correlation between the dose of ethotoin
and the steady-state serum levels. Five of
17 patients required a change in ethotoin
dose during the study. The steady-state ethotoin plasma levels along with the dose
were used to estimate the maximum metabolic velocity (V_{max}) and K_m for these patients. The V_{max} ranged from 50 to 95 mg/
kg/day and the K_m ranged from 9.3 to 43
mg/liter.

Biotransformation

Ethotoin undergoes ring hydroxylation
similar to that of mephenytoin and phenytoin. Bius et al. (3) found p-hydroxyetho-
toin, m-hydroxyethotoin, o-hydroxyetho-
toin, 3-methoxy-4-hydroxyethotoin, 3,4-
dihydroxyethotoin, and a dihydrodiol,
along with several 5-hydroxy metabolites of
ethotoin and 5-phenylhydantoin. The 5-hy-
droxy-5-phenylhydantoin represented between 17% to 34% of the dose of ethotoin
(39). There was no indication that the
phenyl ring of 5-phenylhydantoin is hydroxylated.

A second pathway of ethotoin metabolism is deethylation. The hydantoin ring of
5-phenylhydantoin is then hydrolyzed by
the enzyme dihydropyrimidinase in a stereospecific manner. (R)-(−)-5-Phenylhy-
dantoin is metabolized to (R)-(−)-2-phen-
ylhydantoic acid. The S(+) isomer of 5-

phenylhydantoin undergoes racemization
before hydrolysis takes place (9). Dihydropyrimidinase is selective for 5-monosubsti-
tuted hydantoins, and therefore the hydan-
toic acids of the 5,5-disubstituted
hydantoins, mephenytoin and phenytoin,
are not produced (10).

Clinical Efficacy and Toxicity

Animal studies have shown that ethotoin
is about one-fourth as active as phenytoin
in inhibiting electrically induced seizures in
mice and rats. The average daily dose
ranges from 0.5 and 1.5 g in children and
2.0 to 3.0 g in adults. The doses are usually
divided and administered four times a day
due to ethotoin's short half-life. In a recent
unblinded study, ethotoin was administered
to 17 children with uncontrolled seizures in
daily doses ranging from 19 to 49 mg/kg (7).
Plasma levels of ethotoin, 2 hr after the
dose, ranged from 14 to 34 μg/ml. Seizures
appeared to be controlled within this range
of plasma levels. Only one of the 17 patients
was not helped by the addition of ethotoin
to the regimen. There were no significant
side effects other than a bitter taste. Ten of
the 17 patients were switched to ethotoin
with improvement in gingival hyperplasia
and hirsutism. Volunteers who received
1,500 mg of ethotoin reported visual disturbances, described as increased brightness
or flashing lights (36). A dose of 2,500 mg
of ethotoin produced both the visual disturbances and ataxia within one hour after
administration.

Teratogenicity may occur with ethotoin
as it does with other anticonvulsants (e.g.,
phenytoin and valproic acid). Fetal-induced
hydantoin syndrome has been associated
with phenytoin and mephenytoin. Finnell
and DiLiberti (11) studied the clinical features of three siblings prenatally exposed to
ethotoin. All children appeared to have features characteristic of this syndrome. Zablen and Brand (51) reported the occurrence

of bilateral cleft lip and cleft palate in a premature infant born to a mother taking ethotoin 2,000 mg/day and mephobarbital 400 mg/day.

CONCLUSIONS

The use of ethotoin and mephenytoin in the treatment of seizure disorders still remains limited. A great deal has been learned about the metabolism and clinical pharmacology of these drugs in the last 10 years. This knowledge can be used to design studies establishing their therapeutic usefulness.

CONVERSION

Mephenytoin

Conversion factor:

$$CF = \frac{1000}{mol.\ wt.} = \frac{1000}{218.25} = 4.58$$

Conversion:

$$(\mu g/ml) \times 4.58 = (\mu moles/liter)$$
$$(\mu moles/liter) \div 4.58 = (\mu g/ml)$$

Ethotoin

Conversion factor:

$$CF = \frac{1000}{mol.\ wt.} = \frac{1000}{204.22} = 4.90$$

Conversion:

$$(\mu g/ml) \times 4.90 = (\mu moles/liter)$$
$$(\mu moles/liter) \div 4.90 = (\mu g/ml)$$

REFERENCES

1. Akrawi, S. H., and Wedlund, P. J. (1986): A problem with quantitation of mephenytoin enantiomers due to chiral interference from its N-demethylated metabolite. *J. Chromatog.*, 381:198–200.
2. Baumann, P., and Jonzier-Perey, M. (1988): GC and GC-MS procedures for simultaneous pheno-typing with dextromethorphan and mephenytoin. *Clin. Chem. Acta,* 171:211–222.
3. Bius, D. L., Yonekawa, W. D., Kupferberg, H. J., Cantor, F., and Dudley, K. H. (1980): Gas chromatographic-mass spectrometric studies on the metabolic fate of ethotoin in man. *Drug Metab. Dispos.,* 8:223–229.
4. Bourgeois, B. F. D., Kupfer, A., Wad, N., and Egli, M. (1986): Pharmacokinetics of R-enantiomeric normephenytoin during chronic administration in epileptic patients. *Epilepsia,* 27:412–418.
5. Burger, A. (1951): Anticonvulsants. In: *Medicinal Chemistry,* pp. 138–151. Academic Press, New York.
6. Butler, T. C. (1952): Metabolic demethylation of 3-methyl-5-ethyl-5-phenyl-hydantoin (Mesantoin). *J. Pharmacol. Exp. Ther.,* 104:299–308.
7. Carter, C. A., Helms, R. A., and Boehm, R. (1984): Ethotoin in seizures of childhood and adolescence. *Neurol.,* 34:791–795.
8. Cereghino, J. J., Brock, J. T., and Penry, J. K. (1972): Other hydantoins, albutin. In: *Antiepileptic Drugs,* 1st edition, edited by D. M. Woodbury, J. K. Penry, and R. P. Schmidt, pp. 283–291. Raven Press, New York.
9. Dudley, K. H., and Bius, D. L. (1976): Buffer catalysis of the racemization reaction of some 5-phenylhydantoins and its relation to *in vivo* metabolism of ethotoin. *Drug Metab. Dispos.,* 4:340–348.
10. Dudley, K. H., Butler, T. C., and Bius, D. L. (1974): The role of dihydropyrimidinase in the metabolism of hydantoin and succinimide drugs. *Drug Metab. Dispos.,* 2:103–112.
11. Finnell, R. H., and DiLiberti, J. H. (1983): Hydantoin-induced teratogenesis: Are arene oxide intermediates really responsible? *Helv. Paediat. Acta,* 38:171–177.
12. Friel, P., and Troupin, A. S. (1975): Flash-heater ethylation of some antiepileptic drugs. *Clin. Chem.,* 21:751–754.
13. Glasson, B., Benakis, A., and Ernst, C. (1963): Metabolisme et excretion comparée de quelques medicaments anti-convulsivants. *Therapie,* 18:1483–1491.
14. Goodman, L. S., Swinyard, E. A., Brown, W. C., and Schiffman, P. O. (1954): Anticonvulsant properties of 5,5-diphenyltetrahydroglyoxalin-4-one (SKF 2599). *J. Pharmacol. Exp. Ther.,* 118:405–410.
15. Gut, J., Meier, U. T., Catin, T., and Meyer, U. A. (1986): Mephenytoin-type polymorphism of drug oxidation: Purification and characterization of a human liver cytochrome P-450 isozyme catalyzing microsomal mephenytoin hydroxylation. *Biochem. et Biophys. Acta,* 886:435–447.
16. Hall, S. D., Guengerich, F. P., Branch, R. A., and Wilkinson, G. R. (1987): Characterization and inhibition of mephenytoin 4-hydroxylase in human liver microsome. *J. Pharmacol. Exp. Ther.,* 240:222.
17. Horning, M. G., Butler, C. M., Lertratanangkoon, K., Hill, R. M., Zion, T. E., and Kellaway, P. (1976): Gas chromatography–mass spectrometry-

computer studies of the metabolism of anticonvulsant drugs. In: *Quantitative Analytic Studies in Epilepsy,* edited by P. Kellaway and I. Petersen, pp. 95–114. Raven Press, New York.

18. Inaba, T., Jurima, M., and Kalow, W. (1986): Family studies of mephenytoin hydroxylation deficiency. *Am. J. Hum. Genet.,* 38:768–772.

19. Inaba, T., Jurima, M., Nakano, M., and Kalow, W. (1984): Mephenytoin and sparteine pharmacogenetics in Canadian caucasians. *Clin. Pharmacol. Ther.,* 36:670–676.

20. Inotsume, N., Fujii, J., Honda, M., Nakano, M., Higashi, A., and Matsuda, I. (1988): Stereoselective analysis of the enantiomers of ethotoin in human serum using chiral stationary phase liquid chromatography and gas chromatography-mass spectrometry. *J. Chromatog.,* 428:402–407.

21. Inotsume, N., Higashi, A., Kinoshita, E., Matsuaoka, T., and Nakano, M. (1986): Rapid and sensitive determination of ethotoin as well as carbamazepine, phenobarbital, phenytoin and primidone in human plasma. *J. Chromatog.,* 383:166–171.

22. Jurima, M., Inaba, T., Kadar, D., and Kalow, W. (1985): Genetic polymorphism of mephenytoin *p*(4')-hydroxylation: Differences between Orientals and Caucasians. *Br. J. Clin. Pharmac.,* 19:483–487.

23. Jurima, M., Tadanobu, I., and Kalow, W. (1985): Mephenytoin metabolism *in vitro* by human liver. *Drug Metab. Dispos.,* 13:151–155.

24. Kupfer, A., and Bircher, J. (1979): Stereoselectivity of differential routes of drug metabolism: The fate of the enantiomers of [¹⁴C] mephenytoin in the dog. *J. Pharmacol. Exp. Ther.,* 209:190–195.

25. Kupfer, A., Bircher, J., and Presig, R. (1977): Stereoselective metabolism, pharmacokinetics and biliary elimination of phenylethylhydantoin (Nirvanol) in the dog. *J. Pharmacol. Exp. Ther.,* 203:493–499.

26. Kupfer, A., Brilis, G. M., Watson, J. T., and Harris, T. M. (1980): A major pathway of mephenytoin metabolism in man. Aromatic hydroxylation to *p*-hydroxymephenytoin. *Drug Metab. Dispos.,* 8:1–4.

27. Kupfer, A., Carr, J. R., and Branch, R. (1982): Analysis of hydroxylated and demethylated metabolites of mephenytoin in man and laboratory animals using gas-liquid chromatography and high performance liquid chromatography. *J. Chromatog.,* 232:93–100.

28. Kupfer, A., Desmond, P., Patwardhan, R., Schenker, S., and Branch, R. A. (1984): Mephenytoin hydroxylation deficiency: Kinetics after repeated doses. *Clin. Pharmacol. Ther.,* 35:30–39.

29. Kupfer, A., Lawson, J., and Branch, R. A. (1984): Stereoselectivity of the arene epoxide pathway of mephenytoin hydroxylation in man. *Epilepsia,* 25:1–7.

30. Kupfer, A., Patwardhan, R., Ward, S., Schenker, S., Preisig, R., and Branch, R. A. (1984): Stereoselective metabolism and pharmacogenetic control of 5-phenyl-5-ethylhydantoin (Nirvanol) in humans. *J. Pharmacol. Exp. Ther.,* 230:28–33.

31. Kupfer, A., and Preisig, R. (1984): Pharmacogenetics of mephenytoin: A new drug hydroxylation polymorphism in man. *Eur. J. Clin. Pharmacol.,* 26:753–759.

32. Kupfer, A., Roberts, R. K., Schenker, S., and Branch, R. A. (1981): Stereoselective metabolism of mephenytoin in man. *J. Pharmacol. Exp. Ther.,* 218:193–199.

33. Kupferberg, H. J., and Yonekawa, W. D. (1975): The metabolism of 3-methyl-5-ethyl-5-phenylhydantoin (mephenytoin) to 5-ethyl-phenyl-hydantoin (Nirvanol) in mice in relation to anticonvulsant activity. *Drug Metab. Dispos.,* 3:26–29.

34. Lynn, R. K., Bauer, J. E., Gordon, W. P., Smith, R. G., Griffin, D., Thompson, R. M., Jenkins, R., and Gerber, N. (1979): Characterization of mephenytoin metabolites in human urine by gas chromatography and mass spectrometry. *Drug Metab. Dispos.,* 7:138–144.

35. Meier, U. T., Dayer, P., Male, P. J., Kronbach, T., and Meyer, U. A. (1985): Mephenytoin hydroxylation polymorphism: Characterization of the enzymatic deficiency in liver microsomes of poor metabolizers phenotyped *in vivo. Clin. Pharmacol. Ther.,* 35:488–494.

36. Meyer, M. C., Holcombe, B. J., Burckart, G. J., Raghow, G., and Yau, M. K. (1983): Nonlinear ethotoin kinetics. *Clin. Pharmacol. Ther.,* 33:329–334.

37. Meier, U. T., Kronbach, T., and Meyer, U. A. (1982): Assay of mephenytoin metabolism in human liver microsomes by high-performance liquid chromatography. *Anal. Biochem.,* 151:286–291.

38. Meier, U. T., and Meyer, U. A. (1987): Genetic polymorphism of human cyctochrome P-450 (*S*)-mephenytoin 4-hydroxylase. Studies with human autoantibodies suggest a functionally altered cytochrome P-450 isoenzyme as a cause of the genetic deficiency. *Biochemistry,* 26:8466–8474.

39. Naestoft, J., and Larsen, N. E. (1977): Mass fragmentographic quantitation of ethotoin and some of its metabolites in human urine. *J. Chromatog.,* 143:161–169.

40. Nakamura, E., Goto, F., Ray, W. A., McAllister, C. B., Jacqz, E., Wilkinson, G. R., and Branch, R. A. (1985): Interethnic differences in genetic polymorphism of debrisoquin and mephenytoin hydroxylation between Japanese and Caucasian populations. *Clin. Pharmacol. Ther.,* 38:402–408.

41. Sobotka, H., Holzman, M. F., and Kahn, J. (1932): Optically active 5,5'-disubstituted hydantoins. *J. Amer. Chem. Soc.,* 55:4697–4702.

42. Theodore, W. H., Newmark, M. E., Desai, B. T., Kupferberg, H. J., Penry, J. K., Porter, R. J., and Yonekawa, W. D. (1984): Disposition of mephenytoin and its metabolite, Nirvanol, in epileptic patients. *Neurology,* 34:1100–1102.

43. Troupin, A. S., Ojemann, L. M., and Dodrill, C. B. (1976): Mephenytoin: A reappraisal. *Epilepsia,* 17:403–414.

44. Vida, J. A., and Gerry, E. H. (1977): Cyclic Ureides. In: *Anticonvulsants,* edited by J. A. Vida, pp. 151–291. Academic Press, New York.

45. Ward, S. A., Goto, F., Nakamura, K., Jacqz, E., Wilkinson, G. R., and Branch, R. A. (1987): *S*-mephenytoin 4-hydroxylase is inherited as an autosomal-recessive trait in Japanese families. *Clin. Pharmacol. Ther.,* 42:96–99.

46. Wedlund, P. J., Aslanian, W. S., McAllister, C. B., Wilkinson, G. R., and Branch, R. A. (1984): Mephenytoin hydroxylation deficiency in Caucasians: Frequency of a new oxidative drug metabolism polymorphism. *Clin. Pharmacol. Ther.,* 36:773–780.

47. Wedlund, P. J., Aslanian, W. S., Jacqz, E., McAllister, C. B., Branch, R. A., and Wilkinson, G. R. (1985): Phenotypic differences in mephenytoin pharmacokinetics in normal subjects. *J. Pharmacol. Exp. Ther.,* 234:662–669.

48. Wedlund, P. J., Sweetman, B. J., McAllister, C. B., Branch, R. A., and Wilkinson, G. R. (1984): Direct enantiomeric resolution of mephenytoin and its *N*-demethylated metabolite in plasma and blood using chiral capillary gas chromatograph. *J. Chromatog.,* 307:121–127.

49. Yonekawa, W. D., and Kupferberg, H. J. (1979): Measurement of mephenytoin (3-methyl-5-ethyl-5-phenylhydantoin) and its demethylated metabolite by selective ion monitoring. *J. Chromatog.,* 163:161–167.

50. Yonekawa, W., Kupferberg, H. J., and Cantor, F. (1975): A gas chromatographic method for the determination of ethotoin (3-ethyl-5-phenyl-hydantoin) in human plasma. In: *Clinical Pharmacology of Antiepileptic Drugs,* edited by H. Schneider, D. Janz, C. Gardner-Thorpe, H. Meinardi, and A. L. Sherwin, pp. 115–121. Springer-Verlag, Berlin.

51. Zablen, M., and Brand, N. (1977): Cleft lip and palate with the anticonvulsant ethotoin. *N. Engl. J. Med.,* 297:1404.

Antiepileptic Drugs, Third Edition, edited by
R. Levy, R. Mattson, B. Meldrum,
J. K. Penry, and F. E. Dreifuss.
Raven Press, Ltd., New York © 1989.

17

Phenobarbital

Mechanisms of Action

James W. Prichard and Bruce R. Ransom

INTRODUCTION

Phenobarbital (PB) is the oldest antiepileptic drug still in use. Although it has been replaced by newer, more selective drugs as the treatment of first choice, it retains an important role as supplementary or alternative therapy, and arguments in favor of its superiority in special applications continue to appear (29). No other antiepileptic drug has been more thoroughly studied. Nevertheless, its basic mechanisms of selective antiepileptic action are not yet fully understood. Much evidence, including studies using new techniques, points toward modulation of the inhibitory postsynaptic actions of γ-aminobutyric acid (GABA) and the excitatory postsynaptic actions of amino acids such as glutamate as key PB-sensitive phenomena relevant to seizure control (see section on "Synaptic Transmission"). However, earlier workers proposed several mechanisms that seemed plausible in light of the data then available, only to see them rendered improbable by the advance of neurobiological knowledge. The history of the subject is a cautionary tale for those who wish to discover the true connection between the overall effect of a drug on the awesomely complex mammalian nervous system and its specific actions at the molecular level. Our current knowledge of epileptic pathophysiology limits

how thoroughly we should expect to understand the fundamental mechanism of any antiepileptic drug action. We know considerably more than the preceding generation did about how seizure discharge involves the major areas of the brain. Available data are numerous and precise enough to support a plausible, carefully reasoned discussion of generalized tonic-clonic and absence seizures in a single theoretical framework that invites refinement by further experimentation (44). We have acquired in the paroxysmal depolarization shift a marker of abnormal cellular behavior apparently fundamental to several kinds of seizures (for references see Gloor [44] and Ayala et al. [6]). Nevertheless, the chain of events from cellular defect to clinical seizure is still too vaguely defined to permit discovery of where along it the critical actions of antiepileptic drugs occur. Much remains to be learned about the vulnerability of the normal brain to epileptogenic stimuli, the properties of permanently abnormal neurons that lead to intermittent entrainment of normal ones to cause a clinical seizure, and, especially, the mechanisms responsible for terminating seizure discharge. These gaps in knowledge, although still important, are not hopelessly large. Experiments designed to fill them can exploit much precise information about the paroxysmal depolarization shift, postactivation potentiation, kindling, synaptic physiology, transmitter metabolism, and energy transfer among and within cells.

Thorough understanding of antiepileptic drug actions also requires detailed knowledge of the neuropharmacological differences among closely related drugs. This is a problem in the study of all antiepileptic drugs, but it is particularly clear for the barbiturates because so many of them have been studied. At present, the only abnormal phenomena that distinguish antiepileptic barbiturates as a group are the seizures used to define antiepileptic potency. It is not yet known in any detail whether the drugs can be sorted the same way by their actions on GABA-mediated synaptic transmission, the paroxysmal depolarization shift, kindling, or other phenomena possibly intermediate between the basic cellular defects of epilepsy and their full expression in clinical seizures. In normal systems, there has been no neuropharmacological action of barbiturates yet demonstrated that is a selective property of the antiepileptic barbiturates. Further work on this problem requires no technological advances and may provide important clues to the intimate mechanisms of the antiepileptic action of PB.

ACTIONS OF PHENOBARBITAL ON ABNORMAL PHENOMENA

Seizures in Humans and Animals

In man, PB is effective against generalized tonic-clonic and partial seizures but not against absence seizures (2,41,65,66, 76,121,158). In these respects, it resembles carbamazepine (CBZ), phenytoin, and primidone. Against partial seizures, however, it is somewhat less effective than CBZ (74), and probably less effective than phenytoin and primidone. This is one of the reasons for suspecting that the antiepileptic potency of primidone is independent of its conversion to PB. Primidone is also metabolized in man to phenylethylmalonamide, and both this compound and unmetabolized primidone have antiepileptic potency in animals (38,39). Thus, any of at least three compounds, or some combination of them, may be responsible for the seizure reduction observed in patients given primidone. At present, it is entirely uncertain whether one or several basic mechanisms of action are involved. Eterobarb (38,148) presents the same problem because of its conversion to PB and monomethoxymethyl PB which may have antiepileptic potency; the unmetabolized drug does not accumulate in detectable quantities. Unmetabolized mephobarbital is antiepileptic in animals (28), but its usefulness in man is probably attributable to its conversion to PB (2,41,66,121; also Chapter 24).

In experimental animals, PB, mephobarbital, and primidone have wide spectra of antiepileptic action (15,28,37,39,45,56, 64,136,139) which are qualitatively similar for particular species, ages, and types of seizure induction (110). All three drugs elevate electroshock seizure threshold and protect against pentylenetetrazol-induced convulsions more effectively than phenytoin does. The limited data available on eterobarb (148) suggest that its spectrum of action in experimental tests resembles that of PB. As noted above, mephobarbital (28) and certain metabolites of primidone (37,39) and eterobarb (38,148) have antiepileptic potency in animals.

The overall picture presented by these data prompts two thoughts. First, the antiepileptic barbiturates must have some property not shared with phenytoin that causes elevation of threshold to electrical and chemical epileptic stimuli. This cannot be a selective effect on abnormal nervous tissue, because elevated thresholds can be demonstrated in normal animals. Second, among the barbiturates and their metabolites, the number of compounds having antiepileptic potency in animals suggests that separate mechanisms of action may be involved. However, it can also be argued that PB alone is responsible for the clinical effectiveness of mephobarbital, primidone, and eterobarb since it accumulates when any of these is given, and that experimental data on the effectiveness of other compounds, although true, are irrelevant.

Focal Epileptic Discharge

There is abundant evidence (4,17,32, 40,48,137,138,146) that subanesthetic concentrations of barbiturates can shorten the duration of and raise the threshold for epileptic after-discharge elicited by electrical stimulation of various brain structures in normal animals. However, this effect is not limited to antiepileptic barbiturates, and quantitative differences among drugs were not defined in most studies. The work of Aston and Domino (4) is a major exception. They determined motor cortical and reticular formation after-discharge thresholds in the monkey and showed that pentobarbital raised both equally, PB raised the cortical threshold more than the reticular one, and phenytoin raised only the cortical threshold. These findings seem quite consistent with the relative antiepileptic and hypnotic potencies of the three drugs. The depression of consciousness, elevation of thresholds for electrical and chemical seizures, and production of EEG fast activity (see below), all of which distinguish PB from phenytoin, could all be related to actions in the reticular formation. Further studies like that of Aston and Domino (4) are necessary to extend their results and move toward a cellular explanation of them.

Studies of drug action on the electrical activity of brain areas made abnormally susceptible to epileptic discharge provide further distinctions that have important implications for mechanisms of antiepileptic action. At present, such epileptic foci define the smallest neuronal populations in which the drug sensitivities of phenomena having a known relationship to behavioral seizures can be studied. Because of this, and the fact that they can be produced in cortical and subcortical structures by several means in common laboratory animals, they offer the best opportunity currently available for bringing the techniques of cellular neurobiology to bear on epileptic events. Notable results of such efforts include definition of the paroxysmal depolarization shift characteristic of many neurons in several kinds of foci (6,44) and detection of certain biochemical differences from nearby normal tissue (49). Pharmacological studies are less advanced. Phenobarbital and other barbiturates suppress the discharge of epileptic foci (21,52,73,79,89,147). Comparison of PB and pentobarbital in the same study showed PB to be more potent against after-discharges in isolated cortex (147) and interictal spikes in hippocampal slices exposed to penicillin (89). The latter study also included phenytoin, which was substantially less potent than PB, and diazepam, which was very slightly more potent; the authors commented on the unexpectedly strong action of PB compared with the other drugs. A study on rabbits with chronic cortical freeze foci (79) provided strong evidence that PB and phenytoin oppose epileptic discharge by different mechanisms. Phenobarbital inhibited spread of abnormal activity from the focus to adjacent cortex and diencephalon and suppressed the firing of the focus itself. Phenytoin was a better inhibitor of cortical spread but had no effect on the focus or on spread to the diencephalon.

Such data suggest that PB exerts an important part of its antiepileptic action on abnormal neurons, in contrast to phenytoin which may act primarily on normal neurons. This is a plausible distinction in modes of antiepileptic action but hardly a proven one. The cellular basis for the difference is unknown. There has been little quantitative comparison of the effects of various barbiturates on epileptic foci. If sedative barbiturates in subsedative concentrations were found to suppress foci as well as anti-epileptic barbiturates, interest in mechanisms of focus suppression would wane; a more selective result (89) would encourage close analysis of them. This is one of several areas in the pharmacology of antiepileptic drugs where useful data not now available could come from fairly simple experiments.

In kindled foci, one can study the development and drug sensitivities of progressively more intense epileptic responses to the same stimulus (148). Phenobarbital retards the kindling process more effectively than other antiepileptic drugs studied so far (3,150,151,156), possibly for the same reasons that it suppresses other kinds of foci. Whether new data support that preeminence or not, experimental kindling seems so likely to proceed by mechanisms relevant to human epilepsy that the cellular basis of the action of PB on it is among the most promising targets for further investigation.

Hyperexcitable Axons

The abnormal firing of frog nerve caused by repetitive stimulation and low Ca was reduced by concentrations of PB below 1 mM (144); similarly, normal action potentials of squid giant axon were blocked only by 100 mM PB, whereas 3 mM were sufficient to block spontaneous firing in low Ca (116). The latter observations suggest that PB is more potent against abnormal than normal forms of excitability. Comparable data are too few to permit a conclusion regarding the possible specificity of this action among barbiturates, but phenytoin had the same effect at lower concentration in the study on squid axon (116). Phenytoin also reduced uptake of sodium by lobster nerves (95) and, after prolonged administration, reduced excitability after repetitive stimulation of rabbit vagus nerve (51); PB also did these things but was less potent. In studies on frog node of Ranvier, phenytoin reduced

sodium permeability and opposed the shift toward increased excitability in low Ca at concentrations less than 5% of those required for PB to exert the same effects (80,125).

ACTIONS OF PHENOBARBITAL ON NORMAL PHENOMENA

Extraneural Tissues

Enzyme induction is the only well-defined barbiturate action outside the nervous system that has received attention as a possible antiepileptic mechanism. Barbiturates caused increased synthesis and concentration of a number of enzymes in a variety of tissues (113,114). Phenobarbital is the most effective inducer among them, but whether this is related to any property also important for its antiepileptic potency is not known. The most thoroughly studied inductions are of hepatic microsomal enzymes, several of which have been implicated in barbiturate toxicity. Reynolds (111) has proposed that some antiepileptic drugs, including PB, act against seizures because they alter folate metabolism; the mechanisms are not completely understood but may involve hepatic enzyme induction. The relevant data as a whole do not provide strong support for this theory (see 113 for references) but do prompt reflection on the possibility that what antiepileptic drugs do in the rest of the body may influence what they do in the brain. At present, however, there is no good evidence that enzyme induction or any other extraneural action of PB is responsible for its antiepileptic potency.

Sleep and Anesthesia

Barbiturates have been used to cause sleep more frequently than for any other purpose. The exact mechanisms of their sedative action are not known, but it is known that the state they produce is not equivalent to physiological sleep. Total time spent in the rapid eye movement phase of sleep is reduced and rebounds after barbiturate use is stopped (54,91). Prolonged use is associated with restlessness in the latter part of the night, ordinarily dominated by rapid eye movement sleep (88). Since all barbiturates and many quite different drugs have similar effects, it seems unlikely that clues to the selective antiepileptic action of PB will be found in the mechanisms by which it can cause sleep. The same is true of barbiturate anesthesia. Behavioral and electrographic measures have provided a detailed description of how barbiturate anesthesia develops (23,117), but the basic mechanisms responsible for it are unknown. It seems probable that they, as well as mechanisms of antiepileptic action, will prove to be related to the cellular actions discussed later in this chapter, but just how is yet unpredictable.

Electroencephalogram and Evoked Potentials

The extensive literature (99) on barbiturates and the electroencephalogram (EEG) offers few clues to the nature of barbiturate antiepileptic action. Most barbiturates appear to exert quite similar actions on the EEGs of man and common experimental animals, although their potencies and durations of action vary greatly. Electroencephalogram power spectrum analysis has revealed some differences among barbiturates (42,120), but these have not been shown to correlate with antiepileptic potency. All barbiturates cause widespread cortical and subcortical 20 to 30 Hz fast activity. This is seen at lower concentrations than any of their other EEG effects; it is commonly present in the EEGs of patients taking PB. Animal experiments show that it results from some action of the drugs on the mesencephalic reticular formation.

Evoked potential studies, like those on EEG, have so far shown no selective effect of antiepileptic barbiturates. In general, barbiturates depress nonspecific and neospinothalamic sensory-evoked potentials at doses that spare or enhance other specific ones (see 99 for references). One study (53) found differences between antiepileptic concentrations of PB and phenytoin at several sites in cat brain, among which the mesencephalic reticular formation was the most sensitive to PB; other barbiturates were not studied.

It is not surprising that the most barbiturate-sensitive brain region detectable by EEG methods should be one known to have powerful influence over the electrical activity of the cerebrum. Nor would it be surprising if the ascending pathways that allow all barbiturates to pace fast activity in large areas of brain were also found to distribute selective effects of the antiepileptic ones. There is no evidence at present that any aspect of barbiturate antiepileptic action depends on the mesencephalic reticular formation, but experiments likely to detect such dependency have not been done.

Synaptic Transmission

The most potent neuropharmacological actions of barbiturates yet demonstrated are on synaptic transmission or phenomena plausibly related to it. Phenobarbital shares this general property of its class. Some of its synaptic actions occur at concentrations as low as 25 μM, which is well within the range of concentrations found in the serum of patients whose seizures are controlled by the drug. These actions therefore deserve close consideration as the possible basis of PB's antiepileptic effectiveness.

The concentration of free PB in serum correlates better with seizure control than does total concentration. About 40% of serum PB is protein-bound. The therapeutic range of free PB concentration is 25 to 100 μM (6–24 μg/ml). In humans, free PB concentrations greater than 100 μM frequently produce sedation, and still higher concentrations produce anesthesia. It is not known whether these clinical effects of high PB concentrations are due to exaggeration of the same mechanisms that are responsible for the drug's antiepileptic action, or to different ones.

Postsynaptic Modulation of Transmitter Action

Phenobarbital shares the general tendency of barbiturates to depress physiological excitations (1,9,10,11,12,68,78,84,86, 102,107,108,112,127,132,140–143,152,153) and enhance inhibitions (8,33,77,82,85, 94,96,122,123,145,157). Many studies that have compared actions of various barbiturates on synaptic transmission have not revealed any selective effect of PB. Direct comparison of PB with pentobarbital showed their actions to be similar and pentobarbital to be at least as potent as PB on frog neuromuscular junction (102,143), sympathetic ganglia of bull frog (84,86) and rat (16), cat dorsal-ventral root preparation (77), rat hippocampus (158), and rat brain slices (75).

Pharmacological studies on mammalian central neurons grown in tissue culture, however, have provided insight into the postsynaptic actions of barbiturates and pointed to important differences between PB and pentobarbital that may account for the relatively selective action of PB as an antiepileptic drug (69,72). Phenobarbital and pentobarbital selectively augmented GABA responses and decreased glutamate responses in frog spinal cord (83) and cultured mouse spinal cord neurons (12,70,107,108,124). Barbiturates block the actions of other excitatory amino acids in the guinea pig hippocampus, especially the responses to quisqualate (119). The mechanism of barbiturate antagonism of glutamate excitation is not clear. GABA re-

sponses may be enhanced by barbiturate enhancement of GABA binding (90,154). Pentobarbital increases the mean channel open time of the chloride ion channel associated with the GABA receptor complex (71), and it is not clear if this represents a distinct interaction with the receptor ionophore or merely the result of enhanced GABA binding. Pentobarbital (100 μM) did not augment inhibitory responses elicited by the GABA B agonist baclofen (81), suggesting that barbiturate modulation of inhibition is limited to responses mediated by the GABA A receptor.

The concentrations of PB that enhance GABA responses and depress glutamate responses are similar and are within the clinically relevant antiepileptic range (25–100 μM). In concentrations of 25 to 500 μM, both pentobarbital and PB suppressed paroxysmal activity induced in cultured mouse neurons by convulsant drugs. Phenobarbital, however, suppressed abnormal neuronal discharge without blocking spontaneous activity, whereas pentobarbital was much less selective (69). These phenomena are illustrated in Fig. 1. We regard selectivity of this kind as the principal clue to better understanding of barbiturate antiepileptic action.

Presynaptic Effects

As little as 40 μM PB inhibited Ca^{++} uptake induced by high K^+ in rabbit neocortical synaptosomes, although the effect continued to increase up to 4 mM PB (131). *In vivo*, such an action might interfere with voltage-dependent transmitter release. Indeed, PB produces a concentration-dependent reduction of Ca^{++}-dependent action potentials in mouse spinal cord neurons (47). These effects on Ca^{++} action potentials, however, occurred at concentrations ranging from 100–500 μM, the same range of barbiturate concentrations that reduced neurotransmitter release from other neuronal preparations (25,30,31,97,115) and re-

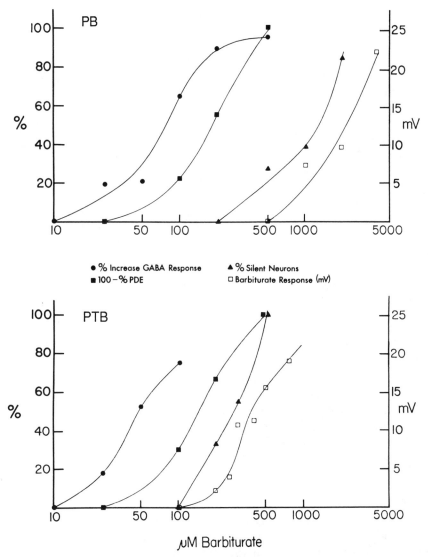

FIG. 1. Dose dependency of phenobarbital (PB) and pentobarbital (PTB) actions. PB antagonized paroxysmal depolarizing events (PDE) induced by the convulsant bicuculline and augmented GABA-mediated responses over a similar concentration range (25–500 μM), but higher concentrations (500–4000 μM) were required to abolish spontaneous activity and to produce direct membrane depolarization. The direct GABA-like action of high concentrations of PB produced a depolarization in the cells, rather than hyperpolarization, because recordings were obtained with KCl-filled micropipettes. In contrast, there was considerable overlap of PTB concentrations at which the same four actions occurred. (Adapted from Schulz and MacDonald, ref. 124 with permission.)

duced Ca uptake by synaptosomes (14). These actions may contribute to the production of anesthesia by reducing presynaptic Ca^{++} entry and resultant neurotransmitter release. As noted above, both PB and pentobarbital cause postsynaptic modulation of neurotransmitter responses at low concentrations, but only pentobarbital also has potent effects on Ca^{++}-dependent action potentials in the same concentration range (47).

Other Effects

Phenobarbital at high concentrations (>500 μM) and pentobarbital at moderate ones (>100 μM) caused direct membrane hyperpolarization of cultured mouse spinal cord neurons (12,47) (see Fig. 1). This effect is antagonized by the GABA A receptor antagonists picrotoxin and bicuculline and is believed to result from direct barbiturate binding to GABA receptors with activation of chloride ion conductance (71,124), that is, at these concentrations, barbiturates act in a manner similar to GABA. This action of PB would not come into play at concentrations that prevent seizures, but a similar action of pentobarbital may be important in the production of anesthesia. It should be emphasized, however, that this may not be a general mechanism of anesthesia, as other general anesthetics cause membrane hyperpolarization and decreased neuronal responsiveness by increasing K^+ conductance, unrelated to GABA receptor activation (87).

The vast majority of experiments concerning PB's actions on synaptic transmission have studied immediate rather than long-term effects. Paucity of information about the latter imposes a limitation of unknown but possibly great importance on efforts to understand mechanisms of antiepileptic action that are exerted during prolonged administration. Long-term PB exposure has been shown to elevate trans-

mitter levels (92), down-regulate GABA binding sites (67), diminish barbiturate depression of stimulated Ca^{++} influx into synaptosomes (34) and alter neuronal survival and morphology (13,126). All of these findings are recent, and any of them might contribute to seizure control. New work is needed to determine which, if any, actually do.

Glia

Glial cells, both oligodendrocytes and astrocytes, exhibit properties that may be influenced by PB (for a general review, see 109). For example, these cells express type A receptors for GABA, and clinically relevant concentrations of PB modulate their Cl^--dependent responses to GABA (7,43). Theories on the pathophysiology of epilepsy have usually not included a role for glial cells, owing to scant understanding of their functions. This area of neurobiology is developing rapidly, and the possibility that direct actions on glia are involved in seizure prevention by antiepileptic drugs may soon become testable.

Action Potentials

Barbiturates affect conduction along excitable membranes only in concentrations substantially above those that affect synapses, and PB is distinguished from other barbiturates and phenytoin mainly by its lower potency. Thus, 0.8 to 2.9 mM PB produced 50% block of compound action potentials in rat nerve, and pentobarbital was equally effective at slightly lower concentrations (135). Both drugs blocked frog sciatic nerve conduction at 1 to 8 mM (62,118,147). In the leech Retzius cell, action potentials were prolonged by six barbiturates; PB was the least potent, being effective only in the low millimolar range (58,59,98,101). Similar phenomena were seen in sensory ganglion (50); the degree of prolongation was characteristic for each type of neuron. Ca^{++} antagonized this action of all the barbiturates tested, including PB. In bursting pacemaker neurons of *Aplysia,* voltage-clamp experiments suggested that PB, 1 to 10 mM, increased, and at higher concentrations suppressed, a slow inward Ca^{++} current responsible for controlling the normal firing pattern (50). An unusually potent action of PB and pentobarbital on limiting repetitive action potential generation in *Aplysia* (155) did not reveal a difference between the drugs. One study (118) on axonal conduction did find a difference: in frog sciatic nerve, the blocking action of pentobarbital appeared to depend on external Ca concentration and adrenergic mechanisms, whereas that of PB did not. At high concentrations (>200 μM), PB limited repetitive action potential discharge in cultured mouse neurons (72), but the relevance of this finding to the drug's antiepileptic action is unclear. Phenytoin and CBZ, on the other hand, may act as antiepileptics primarily by limiting high frequency neuronal discharge (72).

Energy Metabolism

Barbiturates have a variety of effects measurable by chemical methods in nervous tissue. Some of these might be related directly or through the physiological processes discussed above to mechanisms of antiepileptic action. Potentially important effects already mentioned are changes in transmitter metabolism and depression of voltage-dependent Ca^{++} entry into synaptosomes (14,131). Barbiturates can depress cerebral energy metabolism (18,24,26,27,35,36,63,104,129,130), but it is not clear when this is a primary effect and when it is secondary to reduced energy demand, as would occur during periods of decreased electrophysiological activity. Primary depression of energy metabolism could be an important mechanism of anti-epileptic action. A plausible theory of general anesthesia (61) suggests that an early consequence of depressed cerebral respiration would be reduced sequestration of intraneuronal free Ca^{++}, which would accumulate, causing profound effects on transmitter release and membrane excitability. The same reasoning could be extended to antiepileptic mechanisms if depression of energy metabolism by barbiturates was known to occur in the antiepileptic concentration range. Most data support the general assumption that it does not. However, depressed respiration in a small part of the neuronal population might be undetectable by conventional biochemical methods, yet would have consequences as widespread as the physiological influence of the affected neurons on others. Since it is unlikely that respiration in all neurons is affected at the same drug concentration, this interesting possibility has a place in constructive speculation about antiepileptic mechanisms.

Interpretation of data on the metabolic effects of barbiturates is limited in certain ways that obscure the roles some of them may play in clinically useful seizure prevention. First, as in most physiological studies, there are too few directly comparable data on the various barbiturates to reveal any selective action the antiepileptic barbiturates may have. Much progress can be made in this area with currently available techniques. Second, the biochemical systems known to be affected by barbiturates are themselves of uncertain relation to epileptic phenomena. It is useful to know that in low concentrations PB can stimulate, and in higher ones depress, free acetylcholine production in brain slices (75), but the knowledge cannot be translated into understanding of barbiturate antiepileptic action unless one also knows how cholinergic transmission is involved in generation or control of some epileptic event. Progress here depends on better understanding of epileptic pathophysiology. Third, chemical measurements in the nervous system do not yet routinely achieve resolution at the level of the single cell. As such resolution becomes available, correlation of chemical and electrical measurements pertaining to the same identified neurons should provide substantial new insight into mechanisms of antiepileptic drug action.

CONCLUSIONS

Freud is said to have described his method of investigation as "simply staring at the facts until they make sense". Certain defects in the method could be pointed out, but Freud was a doctor, not an epistemologist. We who would understand the mechanisms of antiepileptic drug actions have much the same problem he had. Like him, we contemplate an intricate system and try to squeeze sense from whatever facts are available about it. Like him, we constantly face the seduction of the plausible. If PB is seen to depress some kind of excitation, we say we are on the right track, and so are perplexed when pentobarbital proves to do the same thing better. We next learn that PB strengthens certain inhibitions and are relieved to find such good sense in the facts, only to suffer perplexity again as barbiturates not useful in epilepsy are shown to have the same action. There is nothing wrong with this process. It is, in fact, the basis of empirical science, the means by which simple-minded assumptions about nature are molded toward understanding. It is more advanced for PB than for other antiepileptic drugs. If 2,500 hydantoins had been synthesized, and dozens of them studied in a variety of neurobiological systems, current ideas about how phenytoin prevents seizures might seem quite naive. Because a number of simple explanations for the antiepileptic potency of PB have been eliminated by studies on related drugs, hypotheses for guiding future work can be formulated more precisely than is possible in the case of other antiepileptics.

First of all, unique actions of PB may yet be found, either in preparations already under study (103) or in new ones suggested by better knowledge of epileptic pathophysiology. Phenobarbital is distinguishable from pentobarbital by its more selective actions on motor cortex excitability (55), local electrical seizure thresholds (4), after-discharge of isolated cortex (147), penicillin-induced spikes in hippocampal slices (89), convulsant-induced events in tissue-cultured spinal neurons (124), and enhancement of GABA responses (124). Perhaps when other barbiturates are studied carefully in the same systems, these or related phenomena will indeed prove to be selectively sensitive to PB. If that happens, the mechanisms of action on the distinguishing phenomena will gain high priority as candidates for basic mechanisms of antiepileptic action. However, it may be that even after the appropriate comparisons have been made, there will be no experimental test that segregates barbiturates the way seizures do.

Second, a combination of actions in some critical proportion, rather than a single action, might be what determines the antiepileptic potency of a drug. Phenobarbital, as well as pentobarbital, depressed excitatory postsynaptic potentials in frog neuromuscular junction (102,143) and sympathetic ganglia (84,86), prolonged segmental (33,77) and cuneate (8,96) presynaptic inhibition in cat, prolonged recurrent inhibitions in rat hippocampus (157), prolonged an inhibition possibly mediated by GABA in guinea pig olfactory cortex (122,123), increased action potential duration in leech neurons (57–60,98,101), affected firing thresholds in *Aplysia* neurons (155), and blocked conduction in frog nerve (147). In every case, pentobarbital was of equal or greater potency. That does not necessarily mean that such actions cannot be involved in the antiepileptic action of PB. For the sake of illustration only, suppose that seizure control depends mainly on enhanced inhibition and that loss of consciousness results mainly from direct activation of GABA receptors with consequent hyperpolarization. Suppose further that pentobarbital also exerts both actions but in the same concentration range, and PB is more effective at prolonging inhibition than producing direct hyperpolarization, although weaker than pentobarbital at both. If these things were so, PB would suppress seizures relatively more than consciousness, whereas pentobarbital would simply produce seizure-free anesthesia. This is essentially the argument used by MacDonald et al. (69,72,124) to interpret their experiments with cultured neurons.

Finally, drug distribution in nervous tissue is a possible determinant of antiepileptic potency that has received only occasional attention (99,104,105). Many of the actions already mentioned might suppress seizures if exerted selectively in a part of the nervous system especially important for seizure elaboration. Biochemical (128) and autoradiographic (22) measurements show that PB enters the brain in a manner reflecting blood flow patterns but in the steady state is evenly distributed in gray and white matter. Detection of some barbiturates by immunological methods (133,134) can provide a finer measure of tissue distribution. Immunofluorescent localization of PB in brains of acutely overdosed mice revealed quite uneven distribution among nuclei and among neurons within gray matter (93). The method could be used to learn more about how PB and other barbiturates to which antibodies can be made are distributed in the steady state. Such information combined with other histochemical measurements might offer a great deal of new insight into barbiturate actions.

Abnormal electrical discharge could create local conditions favoring the action of particular barbiturates. One of the most obvious of these is pH change, which bears a complex relation to electrical activity and anatomy in nervous tissue. Activity-dependent alkaline shifts have been observed (19). On the other hand, generalized seizure activity lowers cortical pH (5,20,46); local cortical stimulation for 20 sec can lower local pH 0.15 unit without causing seizure activity (46). It is therefore possible that pH is lower in a chronically discharging epileptic focus than in surrounding tissue. At 7.3, the acid dissociation constant of PB is lower and closer to the physiologic pH range than that of any other common barbiturate; most experiments show that the uncharged form of barbiturates is active, at least for depression of membrane excitability (59,62,125). Local acidosis would shift PB into its active form proportionately more than barbiturates with more alkaline dissociation constants. Thus, PB would tend selectively to suppress firing in regions of vigorous electrical discharge such as seizure foci, while tending to spare regions better able to control hydrogen ion activity. This would be a good arrangement for ensuring that PB act in the right place at the right time. Other local or use-dependent conditions could also be important for other drugs as well as PB. The longer unique actions of antiepileptic drugs elude investigation, the more plausible such explanations will become.

ACKNOWLEDGMENTS

Various phases of the authors' own work were supported by USPHS grants P50-NS06208 and RO1-NS15589 and a grant from the Esther A. and Joseph Klingenstein Fund.

REFERENCES

1. Adams, P. (1976): Drug blockade of open end-plate channels. *J. Physiol. (Lond)*, 260:531–552.
2. Aird, R. B., and Woodbury, D. M. (1974): *The Management of Epilepsy*. Charles C Thomas, Springfield.
3. Albertson, T. E., Peterson, S. L., and Stark, L. G. (1978): Effects of phenobarbital and SC-13504 on partially kindled hippocampal seizures in rats. *Exp. Neurol.*, 61:270–276.
4. Aston, R., and Domino, E. F. (1961): Differential

effects of phenobarbital, pentobarbital, and diphenylhydantoin on motor cortical and reticular thresholds in the rhesus monkey. *Psychopharmacologia*, 2:304–317.

5. Astrup, J., Heuser, D., Lassen, N. A., Nilsson, B., Norberg, K., and Siesjo, B. K. (1978): Evidence against H^+ and K^+ as main factors for the control of cerebral blood flow: A microelectrode study. In: *Ciba Foundation Symposium #56 Cerebrovascular Smooth Muscle and its Control*, edited by K. Elliot and M. O'Connor, pp. 313–332. Elsevier, New York.

6. Ayala, G. F., Dichter, M., Gumnit, R. J., Matsumoto, H., and Spencer, W. A. (1973): Genesis of epileptic interictal spikes. *Brain Res.*, 52:1–17.

7. Backus, K. H., Kettenmann, H., and Schachner, M. (1988): Effect of benzodiazepines and pentobarbital on GABA-induced depolarization in cultured astrocytes. *Glia*, 1:132–140.

8. Banna, N. R., and Jabbur, S. J. (1969): Pharmacological studies on inhibition in the cunneate nucleus of the cat. *Neuropharmacology*, 8:299–307.

9. Barker, J. L. (1975): CNS depressants: Effects on postsynaptic pharmacology. *Brain Res.*, 92:35–56.

10. Barker, J. L. (1975): Inhibitory and excitatory effects of CNS depressants on invertebrate synapses. *Brain Res.*, 93:77–90.

11. Barker, J. L., and Gainer, H. (1973): Pentobarbital: Selective depression of excitatory postsynaptic potentials. *Science*, 182:720–721.

12. Barker, J. L., and Ransom, B. R. (1978): Pentobarbital pharmacology of mammalian central neurons grown in tissue culture. *J. Physiol. (Lond.)*, 280:355–372.

13. Bergey, G. K., Swaiman, K. F., and Schreir, B. K. (1981): Adverse effects of phenobarbital on morphological and biochemical development of fetal mouse spinal cord neurons in culture. *Ann. Neurol.*, 9:584–589.

14. Blaustein, M. P., and Ector, A. (1975): Inhibition of calcium uptake by depolarized nerve *in vitro*. *Mol. Pharmacol.*, 11:369–378.

15. Bogue, J. Y., and Carrington, H. C. (1953): The evaluation of "Mysoline"—A new anticonvulsant drug. *Br. J. Pharmacol. Chemother.*, 8:230–236.

16. Bowery, N. G., and Dray, A. (1976): Barbiturate reversal of amino acid antagonism produced by convulsant agents. *Nature*, 264:276–277.

17. Boyer, P. A. (1966): Anticonvulsant properties of benzodiazepines. *Dis. Nerve Syst.*, 27:35–42.

18. Bunker, J. P., and Vandam, L. D. (1965): Effect of anaesthesia on metabolism and cellular functions. *Pharmacol. Rev.*, 17:182–263.

19. Carlini, W. G., and Ransom, B. R. (1986): Regional variation in stimulated extracellular pH transients in the mammalian CNS. *Neuroscie. Abst.*, 12:452.

20. Caspers, H., and Speckman, E.-J. (1969): DC potential shifts in paroxysmal states. In: *Basic Mechanisms of the Epilepsies*, edited by H. H.

Jasper, A. A. Ward, and A. Pope. pp. 375–388. Little, Brown, Boston.

21. Caspers, H., and Wehmeyer, H. (1957): Die Wirkung von Diphenylhydantoin auf die Krampferregbarkeit der Hirnrinde. *Z. Gesamte. Exp. Med.*, 129:77–86.

22. Cassrano, G. B., Ghetti, B., Gliozzi, E., and Hanson, E. (1967): Autoradiographic distribution study of "short acting" and "long acting" barbiturates: 35S-Thiopentone and 14C-phenobarbitone. *Br. J. Anaesth.*, 39:11–20.

23. Clark, D. L., and Rosner, B. S. (1973): Neurophysiologic effects of general anesthetics: I Electroencephalogram and sensory evoked responses in man. *Anesthesiology*, 38:564–582.

24. Cohen, P. J. (1973): Effect of anesthetics on mitochondrial function. *Anesthesiology*, 39:153–164.

25. Coleman-Riese, D., and Cutler, R. W. P. (1978): Inhibition of gamma-aminobutyric acid release from rat cerebral cortex slices by barbiturate anesthesia. *Neurochem. Res.*, 3:423–429.

26. Corriol, J. H., and Joanny, P. A. (1973): Oxidative and electrolytic metabolism of nervous tissue *in vitro*. In: *Anticonvulsant Drugs*, edited by J. Mercier, pp. 505–532. Pergamon Press, Oxford.

27. Cowger, M. L., and Labbe, R. R. (1967): The inhibition of terminal oxidation by porphyriongenic drugs. *Biochem. Pharmacol.*, 18:2189–2199.

28. Craig, C. R., and Shideman, F. E. (1971): Metabolism and anticonvulsant properties of mephobarbital and phenobarbital in rats. *J. Pharmacol. Exp. Ther.*, 176:35–42.

29. Crawford, T. O., Mitchell, W. G., Fishman, L. S., and Snodgrass, S. R. (1988): Very high dose phenobarbital for refactory status epilepticus in children. *Neurology*, 38:1035–1040.

30. Cutler, R. W. P., Markowitz, D., and Dudzinski, D. S. (1974): The effect of barbiturates on [3H]-GABA transport in rat cerebral cortex slices. *Brain Research*, 81:189–197.

31. Cutler, R. W. P., and Young, J. (1979): Effect of barbiturates on release of endogenous amino acids from rat cortex slices. *Neurochem. Res.*, 4:319–329.

32. Domino, E. F. (1962): Sites of action of some central nervous depressants. *Ann. Rev. Pharmacol.*, 2:215–250.

33. Eccles, J. C., Schmidt, R. F., and Willis, W. D. (1963): Pharmacological studies on presynaptic inhibition. *J. Physiol. (Lond.)*, 168:500–530.

34. Elrod, S. V., and Leslie, S. W. (1979): Acute and chronic effects of barbiturates on depolarization-induced calcium influx into synaptosomes from rat brain regions. *J. Pharmacol. Exp. Ther.*, 212:131–136.

35. Fink, B. R., and Haschke, R. H. (1973): Anesthetic effects on cerebral metabolism. *Anesthesiology*, 39:199–215.

36. Forda, O., and McIlwain, H. (1953): Anticonvulsants and electrically stimulated metabolism of separated mammalian cerebral cortex. *Br. J. Pharmacol.*, 8:225–229.

37. Frey, H. H., and Hahn, I. (1960): Untersuchungen uber die Bedeutung des durch Biotransformation gebildeten Phenobarbital fur die antikonvulsive Wirkung von Primidon. *Arch. Int. Pharmacodyn. Ther.*, 128:281–290.

38. Gallagher, B. B. (1977): Neuropharmacology and treatment of epilepsy. In: *Anticonvulsants*, edited by J. A. Vida, pp. 11–55. Academic Press, New York.

39. Gallagher, B. B., Smith, D. B., and Mattson, R. H. (1970): The relationship of the anticonvulsant properties of primidone to phenobarbital. *Epilepsia*, 11:293–301.

40. Gangloff, H., and Monnier, M. (1957): The action of anticonvulsant drugs tested by electrical stimulation of the rabbit cortex, diencephalon and rhinencephalon in the unanesthetized rabbit. *Electroencephalogr. Clin. Neurophysiol.*, 9:43–58.

41. Gastaut, H., Roger, J., and Lob, H. (1973): Medical treatment of epilepsy. In: *Anticonvulsant Drugs, Vol. 2*, edited by J. Mercier. pp. 535–598. Pergamon Press, Oxford.

42. Gehrmann, J. E., and Killiam, K. F. (1976): Assessment of CNS drug activity in rhesus monkeys by analysis of the EEG. *Fed. Proc.*, 35:2258–2263.

43. Gilbert, P., Kettenmann, H., and Schachner, M. (1984): Gamma-aminobutyric acid directly depolarizes cultured oligodendrocytes. *J. Neurosci.*, 4:561–569.

44. Gloor, P. (1979): Generalized epilepsy with spike-and-wave discharge: A reinterpretation of its electrographic and clinical manifestations. *Epilepsia*, 20:571–588.

45. Goodman, L. S., Swinyard, E. A., Brown, W. C., Schiffman, D. O., Grewal, M. S., and Bliss, E. L. (1953): Anticonvulsant properties of 5-phenyl-5-hexahydropyrimidine-4, 6-dione (Mysoline), a new antiepileptic. *J. Pharmacol. Exp. Ther.*, 108:428–436.

46. Heuser, D. (1978): The significance of H^+, K^+ and Ca^{++} activities for regulation of local cerebral blood flow under conditions of enhanced neuronal activity. In: *Ciba Foundation Symposium #56, Cerebrovascular Smooth Muscle and its Control*, edited by Elliot, K., and O'Connor, M. Elsevier, pp. 339–348. New York.

47. Heyer, E. J., and MacDonald, R. L. (1982): Barbiturate reduction of calcium-dependent action potentials: Correlation with anesthetic action. *Brain Res.*, 236:157–171.

48. Izquierdo, I. (1974): Effect of anticonvulsant drugs on the number of afferent stimuli needed to cause a hippocampal seizure discharge. *Pharmacology*, 11:146–160.

49. Jasper, H. H., Ward, A. A., and Pope, A. (1969): *Basic Mechanisms of the Epilepsies*. Little, Brown, Boston.

50. Johnston, D. (1978): Phenobarbital: Concentration-dependent biphasic effect on Aplysia burst neurons. *J. Pharmacol. Exp. Ther.*, 10:175–180.

51. Julien, R. M., and Halpern, L. M. (1970): Stabilization of excitable membrane by chronic administration of diphenylhydantoin. *J. Pharmacol. Exp. Ther.*, 175:206–213.

52. Julien, R. M., and Halpern, L. M. (1972): Effects of diphenylhydantoin and other antiepileptic drugs on epileptiform activity and Purkinje cell discharge rates. *Epilepsia*, 13:387–400.

53. Kaplan, B. J. (1977): Phenobarbital and phenytoin effects on somatosensory evoked potentials and spontaneous EEG in normal cat brain. *Epilepsia*, 18:397–403.

54. Kay, D. C., Jasinski, D. R., and Eisenstein, R. B. (1972): Quantified human sleep after pentobarbital. *Pharmacol. Ther.*, 13:221–241.

55. Keller, A. D., and Fulton, J. F. (1931): The action of anesthetic drugs on the motor cortex of monkeys. *Am. J. Physiol.*, 47:537.

56. Killam, E. K. (1976): Measurement of anticonvulsant activity in the Papio papio model of epilepsy. *Fed. Proc.*, 35:2265–2269.

57. Kleinhaus, A. L. (1975): Electrophysiological actions of convulsants and anticonvulsants on neurons of the leech subesophageal ganglion. *Comp. Biochem. Physiol.*, 52:27–34.

58. Kleinhaus, A. L., and Prichard, J. W. (1977): A calcium-reversible action of barbiturates on the leech Retzius cell. *J. Pharmacol. Exp. Ther.*, 201:332–339.

59. Kleinhaus, A. L., and Prichard, J. W. (1977): Pentobarbital actions on a leech neuron. *Comp. Biochem. Physiol.*, 581:61–65.

60. Kleinhaus, A. L., and Prichard, J. W. (1979): Interaction of divalent cations and barbiturates on four identified leech neurons. *Comp. Biochem. Physiol.*, [C] 63:351–357.

61. Krnjevic, K. (1975): Is general anesthesia induced by neuronal asphyxia? In: *Molecular Mechanisms of Anesthesia*, edited by B. R. Fink. pp. 92–98. Raven Press, New York.

62. Krupp, P., Bianchi, C. P., and Suarez-Kurtz, G. (1969): On the local anesthetic effect of barbiturates. *J. Pharm. Pharmacol.*, 21:763–768.

63. LaManna, J. C., Cordingly, G., and Rosenthal, M. (1977): Phenobarbital actions *in vivo*: Effects on extracellular potassium activity and oxidative metabolism in cat cerebral cortex. *J. Pharmacol. Exp. Ther.*, 200:560–569.

64. Lembeck, F., and Beubler, E. (1977): Convulsions induced by hyperbaric oxygen: Inhibition by phenobarbital, diazepam and baclofen. *Naunyn. Schmiedebergs Arch. Pharmacol.*, 297:47–52.

65. Lennox, W. G. (1960): *Epilepsy and Related Disorders*. Little, Brown, Boston.

66. Livingston, S. (1963): *Living with Epileptic Seizures*. Charles C Thomas, Springfield.

67. Lloyd, K. G., Thuret, F., and Pilc, A. (1985): Upregulation of gamma-aminobutyric acid (GABA) B binding sites in rat frontal cortex: A common action of repeated administration of different classes of antidepressants and electroshock. *J. Pharmacol. Exp. Ther.*, 235:191–199.

68. Loyning, Y., Oshima, T., and Yokota, T. (1964): Site of action of thiamylal sodium on the mono-

synaptic reflex pathway in cats. *J. Neurophysiol.,* 27:408–428.

69. MacDonald, R. L. (1983): Barbiturate and hydantoin anticonvulsant mechanisms of action. In: *Basic Mechanisms of Neuronal Hyperexcitability,* edited by Jasper, H. H., and van Gelder, N. Alan R. Liss, Inc., pp. 361–387. New York.

70. MacDonald, R. L., and Barker, J. L. (1978): Different actions of anticonvulsant and anesthetic barbiturates resolved by use of cultured mammalian neurons. *Science,* 200:775–777.

71. MacDonald, R. L., and Barker, J. L. (1979): Anticonvulsant and anesthetic barbiturates: Different postsynaptic actions on cultured mammalian neurons. *Neurology,* 29:432–447.

72. MacDonald, R. L., and McLean, M. J. (1986): Anticonvulsant drugs: Mechanisms of action. In: *Advances in Neurology,* edited by A. V. Delgado-Escueta, A. A. Ward, D. M. Woodbury, and R. J. Porter. pp. 713–736. Raven Press, New York.

73. Mares, P., Kolinova, M., and Fischer, J. (1977): The influence of pentobarbital upon cortical epileptogenic focus in rats. *Arch. Int. Pharmacodyn. Ther.,* 226:313–323.

74. Mattson, R. H., Cramer, J. A., Collins, J. F., Smith, D. B., Delgado-Escueta, A. V., Browne, T. R., Williamson, P. D., Treiman, D. M., McNamara, J. O., and McCutchen, C. B. (1985): Comparison of carbamazepine, phenobarbital, phenytoin, and primidone in partial and secondarily generalized tonic-clonic seizures. *N. Engl. J. Med.,* 313:145–151.

75. McLennan, H., and Elliott, K. A. C. (1951): Effect of convulsant and narcotic drugs on acetylcholin synthesis. *J. Pharmacol. Exp. Ther.,* 103:35–43.

76. Millchap, J. G. (1973): Correlations of clinical and laboratory evaluations of anticonvulsant drugs. In: *Anticonvulsant Drugs,* edited by J. Mercier, pp. 189–202. Pergamon Press, Oxford.

77. Miyahara, J. T., Esplin, D. W., and Zablocka, B. (1966): Differential effects of depressant drugs on presynaptic inhibition. *J. Pharmacol., Exp. Ther.,* 154:119–127.

78. Morgan, K. G., and Bryant, S. H. (1977): Pentobarbital presynaptic effect in squid giant synapse. *Experientia,* 33:487–488.

79. Morrell, F., Bradley, W., and Ptashne, M. (1959): Effects of drugs on discharge characteristics of chronic epileptogenic lesions. *Neurology (Minneap.),* 9:492–498.

80. Neuman, R. S., and Frank, G. B. (1977): Effects of diphenylhydantoin and phenobarbital on voltage-clamped myelinated nerve. *Can. J. Physiol. Pharmacol.,* 55:42–47.

81. Newberry, N. R., and Nicoll, R. A. (1984): Comparison of the action of baclofen with gamma-aminobutyric acid on rat hippocampal pyramidal cells. *J. Physiol.,* 360:161–185.

82. Nicoll, R. A. (1972): The effects of anesthetics on synaptic excitation and inhibition in the olfactory bulb. *J. Physiol.,* 223:803–814.

83. Nicoll, R. A. (1975): Pentobarbital: Actions on frog motor neurons. *Brain Res.,* 96:119–123.

84. Nicoll, R. A. (1978): Differential post-synaptic actions on sympathetic ganglion cells. *Science,* 199:451–452.

85. Nicoll, R. A., Eccles, J. C., Oshiwa, T., and Rubia, F. (1975): Prolongation of hippocampal inhibitory postsynaptic potentials by barbiturates. *Nature,* 258:265–267.

86. Nicoll, R. A., and Iwamoto, E. T. (1978): Action of pentobarbital on sympathetic ganglion cells. *J. Neurophysiol.,* 41:977–986.

87. Nicoll, R. A., and Madison, D. V. (1982): General anesthetics hyperpolarize neurons in the vertebrate central nervous system. *Science,* 217:1055–1057.

88. Ogunremi, O. O., Adamson, L., Brezenova, V., Hunter, W., Mclean, A. W., Oswald, I., and Percy-Robb, I. W. (1973): Two antianxiety drugs: A psychoneuroendocrine study. *Br. Med. J.,* 2:202–205.

89. Oliver, A. P., Hoffer, B. J., and Wyatt, R. J. (1977): The hippocampal slice: A system for studying the pharmacology of seizures and for screening anticonvulsant drugs. *Epilepsia,* 18:543–548.

90. Olsen, R. W., and Snowman, A. M. (1982): Chloride-dependent enhancement by barbiturates of gamma-aminobutyric acid receptor binding. *J. Neurosci.,* 2:1812–1823.

91. Oswald, I., and Priest, R. G. (1965): Five weeks to escape the sleeping-pill habit. *Br. Med. J.,* 2:1093–1099.

92. Patsalos, P. N., and Lascelles, P. T. (1981): Changes in regional brain levels of amino acid putative neurotransmitters after prolonged treatment with the anticonvulsant drugs diphenylhydantoin, phenobarbitone, sodium valproate, ethosuximide, and sulthiame in the rat. *J. Neurochem.,* 36:688–695.

93. Pertschuk, L. P., Rainford, E., and Brigati, D. (1976): Localization of phenobarbital in mouse central nervous system by immunofluorescence. *Acta Neurol. Scand.,* 53:325–334.

94. Pickles, H. G., and Simmonds, M. A. (1978): Field potentials, inhibition and the effect of pentobarbitone in the rat olfactory cortex slice. *J. Physiol. (Lond.),* 275:135–148.

95. Pincus, J. H., Grove, I., Marino, B. B., and Glaser, G. H. (1970): Studies on the mechanism of action of diphenylhydantoin. *Arch. Neurol.,* 22:566–571.

96. Polc, P., and Haefely, W. (1976): Effects of two benzodiazepines, phenobarbitone and baclofen, on synaptic transmission in cat cuneate nucleus. *Naunyn Schmiedebergs Arch. Pharmacol.,* 294:121–132.

97. Potashner, S. J., Lake, N., Langlois, E. A., Plouffe, L., and Lecavalier, D. (1980): Pentobarbital: Differential effects on the depolarization-induced release of excitatory and inhibitory amino acids from cerebral cortex slices. *Brain Res. Bull.,* 5:659–664.

98. Prichard, J. W. (1972): Effect of phenobarbital on a leech neuron. *Neuropharmacology,* 11:585–590.

99. Prichard, J. W. (1980): Barbiturates: Physiological effects I. *Adv. Neurol.*, 27:505–522.

100. Prichard, J. W., and Kleinhaus, A. L. (1974): Phenobarbital: Proposed mechanisms of antiepileptic action. *Adv. Neurol.*, 27:553–562.

101. Prichard, J. W., and Kleinhaus, A. L. (1974): Dual action of phenobarbital on leech ganglia. *Comp. Gen. Pharmacol.*, 5:239–250.

102. Proctor, W. R., and Weakly, J. N. (1976): A comparison of the presynaptic and postsynaptic actions of pentobarbitone and phenobarbitone on the neuromuscular junction of the frog. *J. Physiol.*, 258:257–258.

103. Purpura, D. P., Penry, J. K., Tower, D., Woodbury, D. M., and Walter, R. D. (1972): *Experimental Models of Epilepsy*. Raven Press, New York.

104. Quastel, J. H. (1965): Effects of drugs on the metabolism of brain *in vivo. Br. Med. Bull.*, 21:49–56.

105. Raines, A., Blake, G. J., Richardson, B., and Gilbert, M. B. (1979): Differential selectivity of several barbiturates on experimental seizures and neurotoxicity in the mouse. *Epilepsia*, 20:105–113.

106. Raines, A., and Standaert, F. G. (1969): Effects of anticonvulsant drugs on nerve terminals. *Epilepsia*, 10:211–227.

107. Ransom, B. R., and Barker, J. L. (1975): Pentobarbital modulates transmitter effects of mouse spinal neurones grown in tissue culture. *Nature*, 254:703–705.

108. Ransom, B. R., and Barker, J. L. (1976): Pentobarbital selectively enhances GABA-mediated post-synaptic inhibition in tissue cultured mouse spinal neurons. *Brain Res.*, 114:530–535.

109. Ransom, B. R., and Carlini, W. G. (1986): Electrophysiological properties of astrocytes. In: *Astrocytes*, edited by S. Federoff and A. Vernadakis, pp. 1–49. Academic Press, New York.

110. Reinhard, J. F., and Reinhard, J. F. (1977): Experimental evaluation of anticonvulsants. In: pp. 57–111, edited by Academic Press, New York.

111. Reynolds, E. H. (1973): Anticonvulsants, folic acid and epilepsy. *Lancet*, 1:1376–1378.

112. Richards, C. D. (1972): On the mechanisms of barbiturate anaesthesia. *J. Physiol. (Lond.)*, 227:749–768.

113. Richens, A. (1976): *Drug Treatment of Epilepsy*. Kimpton, London.

114. Richens, A., and Woodford, F. P. (1976): *Anticonvulsant Drugs and Enzyme Induction*. Excerpta Medica, Amsterdam.

115. Richter, J. A., and Waller, M. B. (1977): Effects of pentobarbital on the regulation of acetylcholine content and release in different regions of rat brain. *Biochem. Pharmacol.*, 26:609–615.

116. Rosenberg, P., and Bartels, E. (1967): Drug effects on the spontaneous electrical activity of the squid giant axon. *J. Pharmacol. Exp. Ther.*, 155:532–534.

117. Rosner, B. S., and Clark, D. L. (1973): Neurophysiologic effects of general anesthetics II. *Anesthesiology*, 39:59–81.

118. Sabelli, H. C., Diamond, B. I., May, J., and Havdala, H. S. (1977): Differential interactions of phenobarbital and pentobarbital with beta-adrenergic mechanisms *in vitro* and *in vivo*. *Exp. Neurol.*, 54:453–466.

119. Sawada, S., and Yamamoto, C. (1985): Blocking action of pentobarbital on receptors for excitatory amino acids in the guinea pig hippocampus. *Exp. Brain Res.*, 59:226–231.

120. Schallek, W., and Johnson, T. C. (1976): Spectral density analysis of the effects of barbiturates and benzodiazepines on the electrocorticogram of the squirrel monkey. *Arch. Int. Pharmadocyn. Ther.*, 233:301–310.

121. Schmidt, R. P., and Wilder, B. J. (1968): *Epilepsy*. F. A. Davis, Philadelphia.

122. Scholfield, C. N. (1978): A barbiturate induced intensification of the inhibitory potential in slices of guinea pig olfactory cortex. *J. Physiol. (Lond.)*, 275:559–566.

123. Scholfield, C. N., and Harvey, J. A. (1975): Local anesthetics and barbiturates: Effects on evoked potentials in isolated mammalian cortex. *J. Pharmacol. Exp. Ther.*, 195:522–531.

124. Schulz, D. W., and MacDonald, R. L. (1981): Barbiturate enhancement of GABA-mediated inhibition and activation of chloride ion conductance. *Brain Res.*, 209:177–188.

125. Schwarz, J. R. (1979): The mode of action of phenobarbital on the excitable membrane of the node of Ranvier. *Eur. J. Pharmacol.*, 56:51–60.

126. Serrano, E. E., Kunis, D. M., and Ransom, B. R. (1988): Effects of chronic phenobarbital exposure on cultured mouse spinal cord neurons. *Ann. Neurol.* 24:429–438.

127. Seyama, I., and Narahashi, T. (1975): Mechanism of blockade of neuromuscular transmission by pentobarbital. *J. Pharmacol. Exp. Ther.*, 192:95–104.

128. Sherwin, A. L., Harvey, C. D., and Leppik, I. E. (1976): Quantitation of antiepileptic drugs in human brain. In: *Quantitative Analytic Studies in Epilepsy*, edited by P. Kellaway and I. Petersen, pp. 172–182. Raven Press, New York.

129. Siesjo, B. K. (1978): *Brain Energy Metabolism*. John Wiley & Sons, New York.

130. Singh, P., and Huot, J. (1973): Neurochemistry of epilepsy and mechanism of action of antiepileptics. In: *Anticonvulsant Drugs*, edited by J. Mercier, pp. 427–504. Pergamon, Oxford.

131. Sohn, R. S., and Ferrendelli, J. A. (1976): Anticonvulsant drug mechanisms. *Arch. Neurol.*, 33:626–269.

132. Somjen, G. G. (1967): Effects of anesthetics on spinal cord of mammals. *Anesthesiology*, 28:135–143.

133. Spector, S., Berkowitz, B., Flynn, E. J., and Peskar, B. (1973): Antibodies of morphine, barbiturates and serotonin. *Pharmacol. Rev.*, 25:281–292.

134. Spector, S., and Flynn, E. J. (1971): Barbiturates: Radioimmunoassay. *Science*, 174:1036–1038.

135. Staiman, A., and Seeman, P. (1974): The impulse-blocking concentrations of anesthetics, alcohols,

anticonvulsants, barbiturates and narcotics on phrenic and sciatic nerves. *Can. J. Physiol. Pharmacol.*, 52:535–557.

136. Stark, L. G., Killam, K. G., and Killam, E. K. (1970): The anticonvulsant effects of phenobarbital, diphenylhydantoin and two benzodiazapines in the baboon, *Papio papio. J. Pharmacol. Exp. Ther.*, 173:125–133.

137. Straw, R. N., and Mitchell, C. L. (1966): Effect of phenobarbital on cortical after-discharge and overt seizure patterns in the rat. *Int. J. Neuropharmacol.*, 5:323–330.

138. Strobos, R. R. J., and Spudis, E. V. (1960): Effect of anticonvulsant drugs on cortical and subcortical seizure discharges in cats. *Arch. Neurol.*, 2:399–406.

139. Swinyard, E. A., Brown, W. C., and Goodman, L. S. (1952): Comparative assays of antiepileptic drugs in mice and rats. *J. Pharmacol. Exp. Ther.*, 106:47–59.

140. Takeuchi, H. (1968): Modifications par la phenobarbital des pripriétés electriques du neurone à potentiel de membrane stable. *C. R. Soc. Biol.*, (*Paris*), 162:488–490.

141. Takeuchi, M., and Chalazonitis, N. (1968): Effets du phenobarbital sur les neurones autactifs. *C. R. Soc. Biol. (Paris)*, 162:491–493.

142. Thesleff, S. (1956): Effects of anesthetic agents on skeletal muscle membrane. *Acta Physiol. Scand.*, 37:335–349.

143. Thomas, T. D., and Turkanis, S. A. (1973): Barbiturate induced transmitter release at a frog neuromuscular junction. *Br. J. Pharmacol.*, 48:48–58.

144. Toman, J. E. P. (1952): Neuropharmacology of peripheral nerve. *Pharmacol. Rev.*, 4:168–218.

145. Tsuchiya, T., and Fukushima, H. (1978): Effects of benzodiazepines and pentobarbitone on the GABA-ergic recurrent inhibition of hippocampal neurons. *Eur. J. Pharmacol.*, 48:421–424.

146. Vastola, E. F., and Rosen, A. (1960): Suppression by anticonvulsants of focal electrical seizures in the neocortex. *Electroencephalogr. Clin. Neurophysiol.*, 12:237–332.

147. Vazquez, A. J., Diamond, B. I., and Sabelli, H.

C. (1975): Differential effects of phenobarbital and pentobarbital on isolated nervous tissue. *Epilepsia*, 16:601–608.

148. Vida, J. A., and Gerry, E. G. (1977): Cyclic ureides. In: *Anticonvulsants,* edited by J. A. Vida, pp. 152–291. Academic Press, New York.

149. Wada, J. A. (1976): *Kindling.* Raven Press, New York.

150. Wada, J. A. (1977): Pharmacological prophylaxis in the kindling model of epilepsy. *Arch. Neurol.*, 34:389–395.

151. Wauquier, A., Ashton, D., and Melis, W. (1979): Behavioral analysis of amygdaloid kindling in beagle dogs and the effects of clonazepam, diazepam, phenobarbital, diphenylhydantoin and flunarizine on seizure manifestation. *Exp. Neurol.*, 64:579–586.

152. Weakly, J. N. (1969): Effect of barbiturates on quantal synaptic transmission in spinal mononeurones. *J. Physiol. (Lond.)*, 204:63–77.

153. Weakly, J. N., and Proctor, W. R. (1977): Barbiturate induced changes in transmitter release independent of terminal spike configuration in the frog neuromuscular junction. *Neuropharmacology*, 16:507–510.

154. Willow, M., and Johnston, G. A. R. (1981): Enhancement by anesthetic and convulsant barbiturates of GABA binding to rat brain synaptosomal membranes. *J. Neurosci.*, 1:364–367.

155. Wilson, W. A., Zbicz, K. L., and Cote, I. W. (1980): Barbiturates: Inhibition of sustained firing in Aplysia neurons. *Adv. Neurol.*, 27:533–540.

156. Wise, R. A., and Chinerman, J. (1974): Effects of diazepam and phenobarbital on electrically induced amygdaloid seizures and seizure development. *Exp. Neurol.*, 45:355–363.

157. Wolf, P., and Haas, H. L. (1977): Effects of diazepines and barbiturates on hippocampal recurrent inhibition. *Naunyn. Schmiedebergs Arch. Pharmacol.*, 299:211–218.

158. Woodbury, D. M., and Fingl, E. (1975): Drugs effective in the therapy of the epilepsies. In: *The Pharmacological Basis of Therapeutics,* edited by L. S. Goodman and A. Gilman. pp. 201–226. Macmillan, New York.

Antiepileptic Drugs, Third Edition, edited by
R. Levy, R. Mattson, B. Meldrum,
J. K. Penry, and F. E. Dreifuss.
Raven Press, Ltd., New York © 1989.

18

Phenobarbital

Chemistry and Methods of Determination

Svein I. Johannessen

Phenobarbital was introduced into the treatment of epilepsy in 1912. Following barbital, which was introduced in 1903, phenobarbital was the second derivative of barbituric acid marketed for clinical use, and it was the first effective organic antiepileptic agent. Most other antiepileptic drugs were later developed as structural variations of phenobarbital.

PHYSICAL AND CHEMICAL PROPERTIES

Phenobarbital is a 5,5-substituted barbituric acid, 5-ethyl-5-phenylbarbituric acid. The well-known structural formula is shown in Fig. 1. Other barbiturates are formed by various substitutions in the 1 and 5 positions. Phenobarbital is much more potent as an anticonvulsant than as a sedative and is often capable of being used as an antiepileptic drug in nonsedative doses in contrast to other barbiturates. Slight changes in structure may convert barbituric acid derivatives into convulsants. Thus, convulsant properties may appear as hypnotic activity diminishes if the alkyl side chains in the C-5 position are too long. A phenyl group at C-5 or N confers selective anticonvulsant activity on a barbiturate.

Phenobarbital is a white crystalline material with a somewhat bitter taste. The molecular weight is 232.23, and the melting point is 176°C. The free acid is only sparingly soluble in water, whereas the sodium salt is freely soluble. Phenobarbital is soluble in organic solvents such as chloroform, diethyl ether, and ethanol. The partition coefficient between chloroform and water is 4.2 at pH 3.4.

The pK_a is 7.3, and phenobarbital is a considerably stronger acid than other barbiturates. The ionization exponent is lower than that of compounds with only alkyl or alkenyl substituents in the C-5 position. The electron-attracting force of the phenyl group favors the dissociation of a proton from nitrogen. These acidic properties are important in relation to the distribution and excretion of the drug. The effects of a pH change on the distribution of a weak acid across a semipermeable membrane are stronger, the lower the pK_a of the acid. The rate of changes of the urine/plasma concentration with change of urinary pH depends on the pK_a of a weak acid. Thus, the change in the ratio is higher, the lower the pK_a of the acid. The pK_a of phenobarbital is such that a change of extracellular pH without a corresponding change of intracellular pH will cause a shift of the drug from one compartment to the other. Metabolic and respiratory alkalosis and acidosis cause important shifts of phenobarbital between the extracellular and intracellular compart-

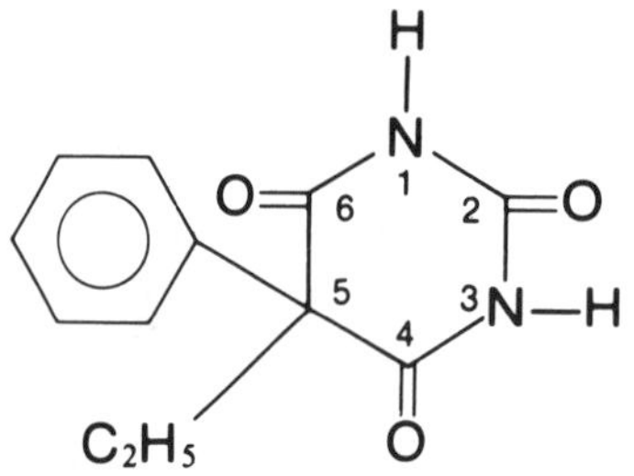

FIG. 1. Structural formula for phenobarbital (5-ethyl-5-phenylbarbituric acid).

ments. The clearance of phenobarbital is much higher when urine is alkaline than when it is acidic, since the pK_a of the drug is such that the renal clearance is largely influenced by change of urinary pH. This is of clinical importance in the treatment of phenobarbital intoxication. The rate of renal excretion of unchanged phenobarbital also varies considerably in patients with uncontrolled water intake and diet.

Phenobarbital and other barbiturates are quite stable in aqueous solutions of low pH. Unlike phenytoin, exposure of phenobarbital to strong aqueous alkali and heating will rupture the barbituric acid ring, mostly at the 1,6 or 3,4 bonds.

The physical properties of a compound are important for separation methods in drug assays. Differences in ionization in aqueous solutions, partition coefficients between organic solvents and aqueous solutions at various pH values, mobility in chromatographic systems, volatility, stability, and absorbance in ultraviolet light all play important roles in an optimal drug assay.

SYNTHESIS

Various reactions described for the chemical synthesis of barbiturates have been reviewed by Vida and Gerry (36). These reactions may take place in acidic, neutral, or alkaline mediums. Some examples are given below.

The barbiturates are commonly synthe-

sized by the condensation of appropriate malonic acid derivatives with urea. Phenobarbital is prepared by ethylating phenylmalonic ester and condensing the product with urea in the presence of sodium alcoholate or, first, preparing phenylbarbituric acid and then ethylating with ethyl bromide and sodium alcoholate. The condensation of malononitrile with urea in alkaline medium also produces barbiturates in good yield. An appropriate malonic acid can be condensed with urea in the presence of phosphorous oxychloride. It is also possible to synthesize 5,5-disubstituted barbituric acids from alkylation of 5-monosubstituted barbiturates with the powerful phenylating agent diphenyliodonium chloride.

METHODS OF DETERMINATION

A variety of techniques have been used for measuring phenobarbital at biological concentration (22,23,26). Early methods were based on gravimetry or the color reaction with cobalt. These methods were abandoned with the introduction of spectrophotometric methods. Different types of chromatography soon followed, first paper and thin-layer chromatography, and later gas-liquid chromatography and high-pressure liquid chromatography. Chromatography has also been combined with mass spectrometry. This technique is known as mass fragmentography or selected ion monitoring. Recently, various immunoassay techniques have also been introduced for routine monitoring of phenobarbital.

Some methods are developed for research purposes, and some are especially designed for routine analysis. Chromatographic techniques allow simultaneous quantitation of several drugs in a single run, whereas immunoassay techniques were developed for specific determination of one drug at a time.

Special precautions are necessary when metabolites or other drugs are present. For determination of phenobarbital, it is, therefore, essential that the drug can be analyzed in the presence of other antiepileptic drugs and other medication, and that interference from the metabolite *p*-hydroxyphenobarbital can be excluded.

Most measurements of phenobarbital concentrations are made on serum, plasma, or whole blood samples. For special investigations, urine, cerebrospinal fluid, saliva, or tears may also be useful. It is beyond the scope of this chapter to discuss the different phenobarbital methods in detail, but some of the general principles will be outlined.

Spectrophotometry

Phenobarbital was initially measured by spectrophotometry (40). Separation from other drugs, especially from phenytoin, was achieved by differential extraction procedures. Even if spectrophotometric methods for determination of phenobarbital can give excellent results in the absence of interfering compounds, these techniques can hardly be recommended today for routine monitoring of patients with epilepsy. Patients are often treated with various drugs, and these are not always reported to the laboratory. Accordingly, there is a great risk of false results, as has been shown in quality control schemes (39).

Thin-Layer Chromatography

To avoid interfering substances and problems with spectrophotometric analysis of phenobarbital, thin-layer chromatographic systems have been useful. This technique also allowed analysis of multiple antiepileptic drugs. Instead of extensive solvent partition extractions, separation was achieved on the chromatographic plate (40). Although many of the thin-layer chromatographic methods are specific and reproducible, they are rather complicated, time

consuming, with low output, and cannot be recommended today.

Gas-Liquid Chromatography

The determination of phenobarbital by gas-liquid chromatography soon followed thin-layer chromatography and has been widely used because of its high selectivity and sensitivity. Most of these methods also include determination of other antiepileptic drugs. In the past years numerous papers on gas chromatographic quantitation of antiepileptic drugs have been published (28). However, a great many of these methods are only modifications of previous techniques, but precise and specific methods for routine application have been developed, taking the best from many of them.

The gas chromatographic determination of phenobarbital depends on various conditions; variables include specific quantitation of phenobarbital alone or multiple drug analysis, simple or complex extraction procedures, choice of internal standards, use of derivatization, type of column, isothermal or programmed temperature, and type of detector.

Early methods were based on a single extraction of the drugs and detection by flame ionization. Even though these methods were handy for routine analysis of several drugs, interfering substances often caused problems, and adsorption of the drug to the column produced peak tailing. For optimal results, a multiple-step extraction scheme able to remove normally occurring serum constituents is preferable. This also gives excellent recoveries of the drugs. Although isothermal separation is possible, a temperature-programmed run tends to give better peak separation (5,26).

Derivatization of phenobarbital produces peaks with little or no tailing and increases the volatility of the drug. On-column or flash-heater methylation is most widely used for derivatization. Both tetramethylammonium hydroxide (TMAH) and trimethylphenylammonium hydroxide (TMPAH) used as the methyl donor produce good results (26).

The controversy over the formation of multiple derivatives with phenobarbital during flash methylation was resolved with the introduction of 5-ethyl-5-(p-methylphenyl)-barbituric acid as an internal standard for phenobarbital. This compound is structurally similar to phenobarbital; it has the same extraction characteristics, and it also undergoes the same decomposition reactions (19,26).

Most gas chromatographic procedures for therapeutic monitoring have involved the use of the flame ionization detector. The sensitivity and selectivity of the nitrogen-phosphorous detector often make it possible to reduce sample size and to eliminate clean-up steps (26,31). However, there are also several problems, usually of chemical origin, in the use of the nitrogen-phosphorous detector, but this detection mode looks promising for routine analysis.

The most precise gas chromatographic method for quantitating phenobarbital is probably comparison of the dimethyl derivative of phenobarbital to a proper internal standard.

Gas chromatographic procedures are also described for determination of p-hydroxyphenobarbital (15,26). Methylation following direct extraction of the free metabolite from urine seems preferable. The conjugated metabolite is determined, following initial acid hydrolysis, to split the conjugation with glucuronic acid.

High-Pressure Liquid Chromatography

Determination of phenobarbital by liquid chromatography is a suitable alternative to gas chromatography (1,3,7,9,14,30,37). Liquid chromatographic separations are based on solubility and not on vapor pressure as in gas chromatography. Various chromatographic conditions may also be used in this method by varying the type and length of column, the type and concentration of the mobile phase solvents and the addition of buffers, the use of isocratic or gradient elution, and the flow rate and temperature (29).

Hence, there are several procedures for determination of phenobarbital based on ion exchange, normal phase, or reverse phase liquid chromatography. Most procedures also include measurements of other antiepileptic drugs and their metabolites. The reverse phase mode is the one most often used, and offers distinct advantages over other modes.

Usually, phenobarbital and other antiepileptic drugs are extracted by simple or complex procedures into an organic solvent that is evaporated to dryness. Alternatively, manual or automatic extractor/concentrator equipment based on resin columns may be used for sample pretreatment. The residue is dissolved in a small volume of solvent and chromatographed by reverse phase. Most often the drugs are detected by an ultraviolet detector at around 200 nm (13).

High-pressure liquid chromatography is the method of choice for simultaneous determination of parent drug and metabolites. However, most often a sample clean-up procedure must be developed first. Recently fully automated pretreatment procedures that include direct injection of serum have been developed, aided by the use of a multicolumn system and a column-switching device, with subsequent analysis of phenobarbital and other antiepileptic drugs and their metabolites (17,21).

Liquid chromatography offers several advantages over gas chromatographic methods, such as lack of derivatization, faster separation, better sample stability, and smaller sample size.

Gas Chromatography-Mass Spectrometry

The quantitation of both phenobarbital and its metabolites using selected ion detection with a gas chromatograph-mass spectrometer-computer system operated in the chemical ionization mode has been reported in several studies (11). Alternatively, phenobarbital can be quantitated using a stable isotope-labeled internal standard and chemical ionization/mass spectrometry without prior chromatographic separation (35). Selected ion monitoring is the most sensitive and specific method for drug analysis. Although this method can be considered a reference procedure, the instrumentation is costly and technically difficult to operate. It is therefore limited to research laboratories.

Immunoassays

Various immunoassays have been widely used in recent years as a technique for analysis of antiepileptic drugs.

Radioimmunoassay

The principle of a radioimmunoassay consists of a radiolabeled ligand that binds to a specific antibody. Added unlabeled ligand competes with the label for binding sites. Measurement of the free or bound label is used for the quantitation of drug present. Specific radioimmunoassays for determination of phenobarbital are not commercially available, but the technique has been described in several reports (40). Generally, radioimmunoassays have the advantage of excellent sensitivity, and it is possible to make the antisera highly specific. Furthermore, a large number of samples can be processed. The disadvantages of this technique are the limited stability of the radioisotope, a separation step that is required to remove the displaced labeled substance from the antibody-bound labeled substance prior to quantitation, and a scintillation counter that is needed.

Homogeneous Enzyme Immunoassay

The development of the homogeneous enzyme immunoassay (EMIT, Syva Company) for phenobarbital and other antiepileptic drugs has been a major advance in the rapid and accurate analysis of microsamples (4,12,26,32,34).

Whereas the label in radioimmunoassays is a radioactive isotope, the homogeneous enzyme immunoassays employ an enzyme as a label. The assay is based on competition between drug in sample and drug labeled with the enzyme glucose-6-phosphate dehydrogenase for antibody binding sites. Enzyme activity decreases upon binding to the antibody, so the drug concentration in the sample can be measured spectrophotometrically in terms of enzyme activity based upon the conversion of oxidized nicotinamide-adenine dinucleotide (NAD^+) to the reduced form of NAD (NADH). No separation step is required in this assay.

The phenobarbital assay is easily run on one of the Syva Lab Systems, including the Syva Advance Fluorescence Immunoassay System. In running phenobarbital EMIT assay on the Advance System, rather than measuring the absorbance of NADH in the turnover of NAD^+ to NADH, the fluorescence emission of NADH is measured. Modified procedures for application on other instrument systems are also available.

Fluorescence Polarization Immunoassay

Another system of therapeutic monitoring of phenobarbital and other drugs is based on fluorescence polarization immunoassay (27). An automated analyzer TDx was introduced for such measurements (Abbott Diagnostics).

This method combines competitive protein binding with fluorescence polarization to give a direct measurement without the need for a separation procedure. All competitive immunoassays for measuring therapeutic drugs are based on competition between the drug in the patient sample and a labeled drug, called tracer. In the TDx system, the label on the tracer drug is the fluorescent dye, fluorescein. The polarization of fluorescent light emitted by fluorescein tracer increases as the tracer is bound to antibody. Polarization is measured using a sophisticated optical detection system. A calibration curve stored in the system memory is used to automatically determine the concentrations of unknown patient samples. Fluorescence polarization is a precise, sensitive measurement technique for rapid analysis of phenobarbital in small sample volumes (20,38).

Substrate-Labeled Fluorescent Immunoassay

This type of test for determination of phenobarbital utilizes a technique in which the drug in the specimen competes with a drug-labeled fluorogenic substrate for binding sites on the antibody (16). The drug is labeled with a derivative of the fluorogenic enzyme substrate umbelliferyl-β-D-galactoside. This fluorogenic drug reagent (FDR) is nonfluorescent under the conditions of the assay. However, hydrolysis catalyzed by β-galactosidase yields a fluorescent product. When antibody to the drug reacts with the FDR, it is virtually inactive as a substrate for the β-galactosidase. Competitive binding reactions are set up with a constant amount of FDR, a limiting amount of antibody to the drug, and the clinical sample containing the drug. The drug in the sample competes with the FDR for antibody binding sites. FDR not bound to antibody is hydrolyzed by β-galactosidase to produce the fluorescent product. Hence, the fluorescence produced is proportional to the drug

concentration in the sample. The intensity of fluorescence is related to the specimen drug concentration by means of a calibrator curve. Each test requires only a small volume of serum or plasma and can be easily run on Ames Fluorescent Chemistry Systems.

Nephelometric Inhibition Immunoassay

Phenobarbital is also measured by a rate nephelometric inhibition immunoassay, which is a homogeneous, competitive binding assay for quantitation of haptens (8). It utilizes a precipitation procedure that does not require the use of fluorescent, radioactive, or enzymatic tracers. The drug in each patient sample competes with a drug-protein conjugate for a fixed amount of antibody that is injected into each test reaction. Since the rate of light scattering results only from the reaction of the antibody with the drug-protein conjugate (and not the reaction with the drug in the patient sample), the nephelometric signal is inversely proportional to the amount of drug present in the test sample. This system has been very convenient for the precise determination of phenobarbital in patient samples (Beckman Immunochemistry Systems).

Radial Partition Immunoassay

A radial partition immunoassay for phenobarbital has also been developed. This assay is an integral part of the Stratus Enzyme Immunoassay System (American Dade) which is a rapid and sensitive procedure for the automated determination of therapeutic phenobarbital levels in serum and plasma, based upon the competitive immunoassay technique (2). The clinical sample is premixed with alkaline phosphatase labeled phenobarbital and spotted onto glass fiber paper containing preimmobilized antiphenobarbital distributed throughout the paper at the analysis site. The two antigens then compete for binding sites on the antibody molecule and any unbound labeled drug is washed out of the field of view of the fluorometric analyzer. A substrate for the enzyme label is incorporated into the wash solution and the enzyme reaction is initiated simultaneously with the wash. The reaction rate of the bound fraction is measured via front surface fluorometry. These rates are inversely proportional to the phenobarbital concentration. This system has proven to be a rapid and sensitive procedure for determination of phenobarbital levels.

Dry-Phase Apoenzyme Reactivation Immunoassay System (ARIS)

The ARIS reagent strip test for determination of phenobarbital is performed on the Seralyzer reflectance photometer (Ames). In the assay, the drug of the sample competes with a flavine adenine dinucleotide (FAD)-drug conjugate for binding to a specific antibody. The unbound conjugate then activates apoglucose oxidase to reconstitute glucose oxidase, whose activity is kinetically monitored by a coupled chromogenic reaction (6).

This homogeneous competitive colorimetric immunoassay is particularly suitable for emergency use, for testing small batches of samples, and wherever prompt results are needed. The dry reagent strip technology is very convenient since all reagents are contained in a ready-to-use cellulose pad fixed to a plastic strip, the color developed on the pad is kinetically monitored by a reflectance photometer, and test results are displayed directly in clinically useful units (6,10).

Enzyme Immunochromatography

A noninstrumented quantitative method for therapeutic monitoring of phenobarbital and other antiepileptic drugs has been developed using a factory-calibrated unit test format and a novel single-level approach to quality control (AccuLevel test, Syntex) (33). This method is based on the principles of immunochromatography, which provides a number of convenient protocol advantages without sacrificing assay performance or quality assurance, mainly because quantification is dependent on enzyme migration rather than enzyme activity. Since migration height is almost solely a function of a highly stable, immobilized, dry antibody reagent, this test is extremely insensitive to environmental factors. The features of stability, factory calibration, and unitized test components make the AccuLevel immunochromatography method amenable to new quality control schemes (24).

The AccuLevel test consists of three main components: a chromatographic paper strip coated with monoclonal antibodies against a specific drug, an enzyme reagent that contains horseradish peroxidase-labeled drug and the enzyme glucose oxidase, and a developing reagent that contains glucose and 4-chloro-1-naphthol. A result can be obtained within 15 min using a simple 2-incubation protocol which requires no sample dilution. Whole blood can be used and no electronic or other instrumentation is required. This new approach to therapeutic drug monitoring represents a step toward immediate laboratory information for better patient care.

COMPARISON OF METHODS

Numerous methods using various instrumental techniques are available for the analysis of phenobarbital. When a new method is established, it is of utmost importance to make sure that results comparable with other techniques are achieved. Several studies are available for comparison of the various techniques used for phenobarbital assays, such as gas chromatography, liquid chromatography, and various immunoassays (2,6,10,12,16,18,20,21,23,25,28,31, 32,33,38,39). Some of the data are summarized in Table 1. In most cases, the comparison data are in good agreement.

The method of choice for determination of phenobarbital depends on the needs of the individual laboratory. Gas chromatography is a suitable method, but highly skilled operators are needed. The choice of proper internal standard, extraction procedure, chromatographic conditions, and derivatization method is essential for optimal results. Liquid chromatography is an alternative method that offers several advantages, including faster separation, absence of need for derivatization, better sample stability, and smaller sample size. Methods involving mass spectrometers are the ultimate methods and serve as a reference source, but are hardly applicable in routine laboratories because of the cost involved.

An immunoassay is the method of choice in many laboratories engaged in therapeutic drug monitoring. These assays have several advantages over other currently used methods and are precise, reproducible, and rapid

TABLE 1. *Phenobarbital analysis: comparison of methods*

Method	N	Serum PB level (μg/ml $\pm$ SD)	Slope	Intercept	r	Reference
EMIT GLC	92	21.2 $\pm$ 10.2 21.9 $\pm$ 9.1	0.840	2.40	0.940	12
EMIT GLC	57	23.3 $\pm$ 10.9 24.7 $\pm$ 12.2	0.860	2.06	0.966	18
EMIT HPLC	50	22.4 $\pm$ 10.6 23.9 $\pm$ 12.3	0.844	2.29	0.976	18
HPLC GLC	140	18.7 $\pm$ 12.0 18.7 $\pm$ 11.5	1.027	−0.50	0.998	18
HPLC EMIT	41	23.1 21.9	1.028	−0.03	0.96	25
GLC-ND HPLC	130	—	0.985	0.43	0.986	31
ARIS SLFIA	50	29.3 29.1	1.013	−0.12	0.992	6
ARIS EMIT	50	28.8 29.2	0.998	0.50	0.994	6
ARIS GLC	31	29.5 28.4	1.019	0.54	0.998	6
HPLC[a] EMIT	80	—	0.997	−0.11	0.976	21
HPLC[a] HPLC	80	—	0.968	0.55	0.989	21
EMIT STRATUS	96	—	0.973	−0.13	0.992	2
SLFIA EMIT	102	—	1.105	−2.71	0.970	16
TDx EMIT	135	—	0.994	0.52	0.982	20
TDx HPLC	46	—	1.070	0.27	0.992	20
AccuLevel TDx	71	—	0.97	−1.34	0.97	33
AccuLevel EMIT	48	—	0.98	−0.73	0.96	33
AccuLevel HPLC	79	—	1.13	−0.77	0.97	33

[a] Automated method, column switching.

methods for determination of phenobarbital in microsamples. However, these methods do not have the same screening potential as chromatographic methods, which also can be used for determination of less common antiepileptic drugs and new drugs. Furthermore, the reagents used in immunoassays are more costly than in chromatographic procedures, but the immunoassays can be performed very rapidly. Thus, it is possible for the physician to know the drug level during examination or when rapid identification, in case of intoxication, is necessary. Small samples are also of considerable importance, both in children and adults, during intensive monitoring. Capillary samples may be used, and a few microliters are sufficient for several determinations of both phenobarbital and other antiepileptic drugs. However, it must be emphasized that the immunoassays are designed for specific determination of a single drug, and therefore simultaneous drug analysis, which is an advantage of certain chromatographic systems, is not possible. No matter which method is chosen, a quality control program is mandatory.

CONVERSION

Conversion factor:

$$CF = \frac{1000}{\text{mol.wt.}} = \frac{1000}{232.2} = 4.31$$

Conversion:

$$(\mu g/ml) \times 4.31 = (\mu moles/liter)$$

$$(\mu moles/liter) \div 4.31 = (\mu g/ml)$$

REFERENCES

1. Adams, R. F., Schmidt, G. J., and Vandemark, F. L. (1978): A microliquid column chromatography procedure for twelve anticonvulsants and some of their metabolites. *J. Chromatogr.,* 145:275–284.
2. American Dade (1983): Package insert for Stratus Phenobarbital Fluorometric Enzyme Immunoassay.
3. Atwell, S. H., Green, V. A., and Haney, W. G. (1975): Development and evaluation of method for simultaneous determination of phenobarbital and diphenylhydantoin in plasma by high pressure liquid chromatography. *J. Pharm. Sci.,* 64:806–809.
4. Booker, H. E., and Darcey, B. A. (1975): Enzymatic immunoassay vs. gas-liquid chromatography for determination of phenobarbital and diphenylhydantoin in serum. *Clin. Chem.,* 21:1766–1768.
5. Bredesen, J. E., and Johannessen, S. I. (1974): Simultaneous determination of some antiepileptic drugs by gas-liquid chromatography. *Epilepsia,* 15:611–617.
6. Croci, D., Nespolo, A., and Tarenghi, G. (1987): Quantitative determination of phenobarbital and phenytoin by dry-phase apoenzyme reactivation immunoassay system (ARIS). *Ther. Drug Monit.,* 9:197–202.
7. Evans, J. E. (1973): Simultaneous measurements of diphenylhydantoin and phenobarbitone in serum by HPLC. *Anal. Chem.,* 45:2428–2429.
8. Finley, P. R., Dye, J. A., Williams, J., and Lichti, D. A. (1981): Rate nephelometric inhibition immunoassay of phenytoin and phenobarbital. *Clin. Chem.,* 27:405–409.
9. Gerson, B., Bell, F., and Chan, S. (1984): Antiepileptic agents—Primidone, phenobarbital, phenytoin, and carbamazepine by reversed-phase liquid chromatography (proposed selected method). *Clin. Chem.,* 30:105–108.
10. Graves, N. M., Holmes, G. B., Leppik, I. E., Galligher, T. K., and Parker, D. R. (1987): Quantitative determination of phenytoin and phenobarbital in capillary blood by Ames Seralyzer. *Epilepsia,* 28:713–716.
11. Horning, M. G., Lertratanangkoon, K., Nowlin, J., Stillwell, W. G., Stillwell, R. N., Zion, T. E., Kellaway, P., and Hill, R. M. (1974): Anticonvulsant drug monitoring by GC-MS-COM techniques. *J. Chromatogr. Sci.,* 12:630–631.
12. Johannessen, S. I. (1977): Evaluation of enzyme multiplied immunoassay technique (EMIT) in routine analysis of antiepileptic drugs. A comparison of methods. In: *Antiepileptic Drug Monitoring,* edited by C. Gardner-Thorpe, D. Janz, H. Meinardi, and C. E. Pippenger, pp. 7–20. Pitman Medical, Kent.
13. Jürgens, U., May T., Hillenkötter, K., and Rambeck, B. (1984): Systematic comparison of three basic methods of sample pretreatment for high-performance liquid chromatographic analysis of antiepileptic drugs using gas chromatography as a reference method. *Ther. Drug Monit.,* 6:334–343.
14. Kabra, P., Nelson, M., and Marton, L. (1983): Simultaneous very fast liquid-chromatographic analysis of ethosuximide, primidone, phenobarbital, phenytoin, and carbamazepine in serum. *Clin. Chem.,* 29:473–476.
15. Kållberg, N., Agurell, S., Ericsson, O., Bucht, E., Jalling, B., and Boréus, L. O. (1975): Quantitation of phenobarbital and its main metabolites in human urine. *Eur. J. Clin. Pharmacol.,* 9:161–168.

16. Krausz, L. M., Hitz, J. B., Buckler, R. T., and Burd, J. F. (1980): Substrate-labeled fluorescent immunoassay for phenobarbital. *Ther. Drug Monit.,* 2:261–272.

17. Kuhnz, W., and Nau, H. (1984): Automated high-pressure liquid chromatographic assay for anti-epileptic drugs and their major metabolites by direct injection of serum samples. *Ther. Drug Monit.,* 6:478–483.

18. Kumps, A., Mardens, Y., and Scharpé, S. (1980): Comparison between HPLC, gas-liquid chromatography, and enzyme-immunoassay for the determination of antiepileptic drugs in serum. In: *Antiepileptic Therapy: Advances in Drug Monitoring,* edited by S. I. Johannessen, P. L. Morselli, C. E. Pippenger, A. Richens, D. Schmidt, and H. Meinardi, pp. 341–347, Raven Press, New York.

19. Kurata, K., Takeuchi, M., and Yoshida, K. (1979): Quantitative flash-methylation analysis of phenobarbital. *J. Pharm. Sci.,* 68:1187–1189.

20. Lu-Steffes, M., Pittluck, G. W., Jolley, M. E., Panas, H. N., Olive, D. L., Wang, C. J., Nystrom, D. D., Keegan, C. L., Davis, T. P., and Stroupe, S. D. (1982): Fluorescence polarization immunoassay IV. Determination of phenytoin and phenobarbital in human serum and plasma. *Clin. Chem.,* 28:2278–2282.

21. Matsumoto, K., Kikuchi, H., Kano, S., Iri, H., Takahashi, H., and Umino, M. (1988): Automated determination of drugs in serum by liquid chromatography with column-switching. I. Separation of antiepileptic drugs and metabolites. *Clin. Chem.,* 34:141–144.

22. Meijer, J. W. A., Meinardi, H., Gardner-Thorpe, C., and van der Kleijn, E. (1973): *Methods of Analysis of Antiepileptic Drugs.* Excerpta Medica, Amsterdam; American Elsevier, New York.

23. Meijer, J. W. A., Rambeck, B., and Riedmann, M. (1983): Antiepileptic drug monitoring by chromatographic methods and immunotechniques—Comparison of analytical performance, practicability, and economy. *Ther. Drug Monit.,* 5:39–53.

24. Opheim, K. E., Statland, B. E., Tillson, S. A., and Litman, D. J. (1987): Calibration, quality control, and stability of a quantitative enzyme immuno-chromatographic method for therapeutic drug monitoring. *Ther. Drug Monit.,* 9:190–196.

25. Pesh-Imam, M., Fretthold, D. W., Sunshine, I., Kumar, S., Terrentine, S., and Willis, C. E. (1979): High pressure liquid chromatography for simultaneous analysis of anticonvulsants: Comparison with EMIT system. *Ther. Drug Monit.,* 1:289–299.

26. Pippenger, C. E., Penry, J. K., and Kutt, H. (1978): *Antiepileptic Drugs: Quantitative Analysis and Interpretation.* Raven Press, New York.

27. Popelka, S. R., Miller, D. M., Holen, J. T., and Kelso, D. M. (1981): Fluorescence polarization immunoassay II: Analyzer for rapid, precise measurement of fluorescence polarization with use of disposable cuvettes. *Clin. Chem.,* 27:1198–1201.

28. Rambeck, B., and Meijer, J. W. A. (1980): Gas chromatographic methods for the determination of antiepileptic drugs: A systematic review. *Ther. Drug Monit.,* 2:385–396.

29. Rambeck, B., Riedmann, M., and Meijer, J. W. A. (1981): Systematic method of development in liquid chromatography applied to the determination of antiepileptic drugs. *Ther. Drug Monit.,* 3:377–395.

30. Riedmann, M., Rambeck, B., and Meijer, J. W. A. (1981): Quantitative simultaneous determination of eight common antiepileptic drugs and metabolites by liquid chromatography. *Ther. Drug Monit.,* 3:397–413.

31. Rovei, V., Sanjuan, M., and Morselli, P. L. (1980): Comparison between HPLC and GLC-ND analytical methods for the determination of AED in plasma and blood of patients. In: *Antiepileptic Therapy: Advances in Drug Monitoring,* edited by S. I. Johannessen, P. L. Morselli, C. E. Pippenger, A. Richens, D. Schmidt, and H. Meinardi, pp. 349–356. Raven Press, New York.

32. Schmidt, D., Goldberg, V., Guelen, P. J. M., Johannessen, S. I., van der Kleijn, E., Meijer, J. W. A., Meinardi, H., Richens, A., Schneider, H., Stein-Lavie, Y., and Symann-Louette, N. (1977): Evaluation of a new immunoassay for determination of phenytoin and phenobarbital. Results of a European collaborative control study. *Epilepsia,* 18:367–374.

33. Syntex (1986): AccuLevel Phenobarbital Test, Clinical Study Summary.

34. Syva (1976): *Antiepileptic Drug Assays, Syva Bulletin 6A164-1.* Syva, Palo Alto, California.

35. Truscott, R. J. W., Burke, D. G., Korth, J., and Halpern, B. (1978): Simultaneous determination of diphenylhydantoin, mephobarbital, carbamazepine, phenobarbital and primidone in serum using direct chemical ionization mass-spectrometry. *Biomed. Mass Spectrom.,* 5:477–482.

36. Vida, J. A., and Gerry, E. H. (1977): Cyclic ureides. In: *Anticonvulsants,* edited by J. A. Vida, pp. 151–291. Academic Press, New York.

37. Wad, N. (1984): Simultaneous determination of eleven antiepileptic compounds in serum by high-performance liquid chromatography. *J. Chromatogr.,* 305:127–133.

38. Wang, S. T., and Peter, F. (1985): The Abbott TDx fluorescence polarization immunoassay and liquid chromatography compared for five anticonvulsant drugs in serum. *Clin. Chem.,* 31:493–494.

39. Wilson, J. F., Marshall, R. W., Williams, J., and Richens, A. (1983): Comparison of assay methods used to measure antiepileptic drugs in plasma. *Ther. Drug Monit.,* 5:449–460.

40. Woodbury, D. M., Penry, J. K., and Pippenger, C. E. (1982): *Antiepileptic Drugs,* 2nd edition. Raven Press, New York.

Antiepileptic Drugs, Third Edition, edited by
R. Levy, R. Mattson, B. Meldrum,
J. K. Penry, and F. E. Dreifuss.
Raven Press, Ltd., New York © 1989.

19

Phenobarbital

Absorption, Distribution, and Excretion

Robert S. Rust and W. Edwin Dodson

Phenobarbital pharmacokinetics have been studied extensively for more than 75 years. They result from the interaction of both drug-related and host-related factors. Important drug-related factors include phenobarbital's relatively low lipid solubility and its ionization constant, which is nearly the same as normal plasma pH. Additional drug-related factors include both the specific formulation of phenobarbital and the characteristics of the drug carrier relative to the specific route of administration. The major host factors include age and gastrointestinal, hepatic, and renal function, which in turn vary due to biological variation, comedication, and the presence of disease.

ABSORPTION

Salts of phenobarbital are more soluble than phenobarbital crystals, which are hygroscopic and have only slight solubility in water and relatively low lipid solubility. Therefore, formulations for intravenous or intramuscular administration are prepared from the sodium salt in slightly alkaline solutions. The sodium salt favors tautomerization of the 2-position carbonyl group from the keto to the enol form, enhancing aqueous solubility. Tablets for oral administration are usually compounded from fine, somewhat polymorphic crystals of the sodium phenobarbital salt.

Most studies of phenobarbital absorption have been based on plasma concentrations of drug after doses of 25 to 200 mg administered orally, intravenously, or intramuscularly to adult volunteers. After oral or intramuscular administration, peak plasma concentrations occur in 2 to 12 hr, and are linearly related to dose within a wide range of doses (100,112,122,129). The average time to peak plasma concentrations is 2 hr after oral dosing (64,93,122), but the peak may be considerably delayed in patients with diminished gastrointestinal motility or poor circulation (73,112). Peak serum concentrations after intramuscular administration to adults and children older than 6 months usually occur within 4 hr (60,112,122,128).

Phenobarbital has high bioavailability in adults after oral or intramuscular administration. Peak levels by these routes are similar (112,122). Studies in dogs and humans based on rates of either drug accumulation or elimination involving doses of 0.59 to 3.2 mg/kg/day and steady-state kinetics assumptions, have shown 80% to 100% absorption of orally administered phenobarbital (21,114). Bioavailability for phenobarbital tablets was 95% and for phenobarbital elixir was 100% in one study (91). Although several investigators have found 12% to 21% greater bioavailability for oral as compared to intramuscularly administered phenobarbital, this difference diminishes if values are corrected for individual variation in drug clearance (112,122,128). Wilensky et al. (128) found equivalent bioavailability for phenobarbital tablets ($100 \pm 11\%$) and intramuscular phenobarbital ($101 \pm 13\%$). Half-time for accumulation of serum phenobarbital to peak was 0.64 ± 0.71 hr for oral and 0.73 ± 0.5 hr for intramuscular administration.

Although older infants (>6 weeks old) and children have similar rates and extent of absorption after either oral or intramuscular administration, newborns (<6 weeks old) are different (70,85,129). Newborns have delayed and incomplete absorption of oral as compared to intramuscular phenobarbital (10,61,124). Jalling (61) found that 90% of the peak plasma concentration of phenobarbital was achieved within 4 hr of intramuscular administration in 8 of 10 neonates. After oral dosing only 3 of 6 newborns had peak concentrations within 4 hr.

When sodium phenobarbital parenteral solutions are administered rectally, the absorption is more rapid than from oral or intramuscular sites in both infants and adults (14,70). On the other hand, phenobarbital suppositories, formulated in lipophilic or hydrophilic solid carriers, are less well absorbed than orally administered standard preparations in dogs (14,71). Only small amounts of barbiturates are absorbed across the buccal mucosa (6).

In the acidic environment of the stomach, phenobarbital is largely un-ionized and diffusable (66). Gastric drug absorption is a function of lipid solubility, concentration of nonionized molecules, and gastric emptying time (106). Thus, phenobarbital is less diffusable across gastric epithelium than highly lipid-soluble barbiturates such as secobarbital (55,107). The bulk of orally administered phenobarbital is absorbed in the small intestine where the un-ionized fraction is smaller, but intraluminal dwell time is longer.

Gastric absorption of sodium phenobarbital is enhanced if it is dissolved prior to administration (18,105,111). Microcrystalline preparations offer the advantage of a large surface area for absorption, but the method of crystal preparation may render certain preparations poorly wettable and resistant to absorption (18,105). The presence of food and neutralizing agents or rapid gastric emptying slows phenobarbital absorption, and the presence of even small amounts of ethanol in the stomach or blood accelerates gastric absorption (54,67).

A majority of orally administered phenobarbital is absorbed in the small intestine because of the extensive surface area and ample time for absorption. This occurs despite the alkaline pH in the small intestine. Interestingly, studies of the rat small intestine indicate that absorption rates are maximal when the pH is between 6.5 and 7.5, an observation that is inconsistent with the Overton-Meyer explanation of absorption as a function of the state of ionization (67, 106). Furthermore, absorption from the small intestine correlates poorly with the lipid/aqueous partition coefficients of several different barbiturates, including phenobarbital. These observations have led to the notion that phenobarbital might bind to a protein on the luminal surface of the small intestine. This has not been substantiated.

The role of enterohepatic circulation in phenobarbital pharmacokinetics is incompletely characterized. Several studies have demonstrated unmetabolized phenobarbital in bile within 1 hr of intravenous administration (25,58,92). Arimori et al. (3) found biliary phenobarbital concentration to be twice the peak serum concentration. Engasser et al. (34) detected rebound elevation of phenobarbital in rat serum 1 hr after intravenous administration, corresponding to the appearance of phenobarbital in bile.

The phenobarbital equilibrium across the gastrointestinal tract can be perturbed by the administration of activated charcoal. Administering charcoal orally reduces the phenobarbital half-life by a factor of 2.4 to 6, and increases total body clearance from 52% to 80% (7,49,92,130). This result is consistent both with diffusion of phenobarbital from serum or tissue to gastrointestinal fluids along a concentration gradient maintained by absorption of the diffusable species to charcoal (7), and with enterohepatic secretion of drug (3,34,92).

DISTRIBUTION

Phenobarbital disseminates into all body tissues. The pK_a of phenobarbital (variously reported as 7.2 to 7.41) (18,21,58,79, 93,123) is nearly the same as the normal pH of plasma. Thus the ratio of neutral to charged species is quite sensitive to changes in pH within the physiologic range.

Lowering serum pH increases the nonionized portion in serum, enhancing diffusion into tissue, whereas higher serum pH has the opposite effect (123). In dogs, acidification of the serum to pH 6.8 by inhalation of CO_2 rapidly decreases serum phenobarbital concentrations while increasing tissue levels. Conversely, alkalinization of serum by the administration of intravenous bicarbonate increases serum and levels and decreases phenobarbital concentrations in tissue. Lowering serum pH increases the nonionized portion in serum enhances diffusion into tissue, whereas raising serum pH has the opposite effect.

Phenobarbital binding to plasma proteins plays a minor role in distribution (48,65). Binding is readily reversible and independent of drug concentration, ionic dissociation, and serum calcium concentration within the physiological range of pH (83,123). However, the extent of phenobarbital binding is dependent on albumin concentration. *In vitro* studies with bovine serum albumin indicate that 46% of phenobarbital is bound at pH 7.6 (123), similar to the magnitude of binding for adult serum

(48,74,93). Since approximately 55% of phenobarbital in serum is unbound, changes in the extent of phenobarbital binding in serum have little effect on the unbound phenobarbital level. For example, reducing phenobarbital binding by 50% leads to only a 33% increase in the unbound concentration.

In newborns and children, the extent of phenobarbital binding to serum proteins is 32% and 51% to 55%, respectively (33,43,118). The lower protein binding of phenobarbital in newborns is most likely due to their relative hypoalbuminemia. Other possible contributors include a lower affinity constant for binding to fetal albumin, competition for binding by bilirubin and free fatty acids, and lower blood pH in the immediate neonatal period (46,84).

Phenobarbital binding in organ homogenates, except for brain and possibly liver, is on the same order as phenobarbital binding to albumin (34,47). In brain, phenobarbital binding correlates with the regional protein concentration except for a slight additional phenobarbital affinity for brain sphingomyelin (48). Brain homogenates have higher fractions of bound phenobarbital than comparable concentrations of albumin. Little if any of this binding can be ascribed to extractable brain lipids.

In immature cats, phenobarbital distribution varies with age (104). In newborn cats, the highest regional brain concentrations occur in unmyelinated white matter. By 4 weeks of age, phenobarbital distributes uniformly throughout white and gray matter. By 8 weeks of age, early phenobarbital concentration is highest in gray matter, just as in mature cats (29,104). In rats, the cerebrospinal fluid (CSF)-to-brain concentration ratio decreases from 0.79 at age 4 weeks to 0.63 at age 18 months (127).

Concentrations of phenobarbital in surgically removed human epileptic brain specimens correlate with plasma concentrations (47,74). However, the reported brain-to-plasma concentration ratios vary widely, ranging from 0.35 to 1.13 (51,57,109,121).

Among 17 newborns who died while taking phenobarbital, brain-to-plasma concentration ratios were 0.71 ± 0.21 (94). The ratio correlated with gestational age with lower brain-to-plasma ratios in premature than in full-term newborns. Gray-to-white matter ratios calculated in three of these infants varied from 0.86 to 1.11. Thus, at equilibrium, phenobarbital concentrations in gray and white matter are similar in human newborns and adults (51,109,121).

Concentrations of phenobarbital in CSF of adults are 43% to 60% of plasma concentrations and correlate well with the unbound phenobarbital concentration in serum (29,74,104,108). The CSF levels in infants are similar, ranging from 48% to 83% of plasma levels (62). In 20 adults, CSF levels correlated with plasma ultrafiltrate levels with a coefficient of variation of 0.53 (74).

The phenobarbital concentration in CSF provides a reliable index of phenobarbital concentration in brain (16,27,126,127). Under nonequilibrium dosing conditions, actions of phenobarbital correlate better with CSF levels than with either dose or the rate of drug administration. For example, the loss of righting reflex in rodents is related to CSF concentration and is independent of either the dose or the rate of administration (126,127).

Phenobarbital concentrations are higher in CSF than saliva, a more acidic but similarly low-protein fluid. Both salivary and sweat phenobarbital concentrations vary with flow rate (87,97,101). The dependence of salivary phenobarbital levels on pH is somewhat controversial. Some investigators have found that salivary phenobarbital concentrations are highly pH dependent (27,31,56,76,93,108,120), whereas others conclude the opposite (39,118). Among children at steady state, the saliva-to-total serum concentration ratios for phenobarbital range from 0.21 to 0.52 (24,56, 59,108,120). Saliva-to-serum phenobarbital ratios have greater interindividual

than intraindividual variation (125) and salivary levels correlate highly with the plasma levels in individual patients (24). However, when equations incorporating phenobarbital's pK_a relative to measured salivary pH are used to adjust the salivary levels, the correlation between salivary and unbound serum phenobarbital concentrations are as high as 0.938 (31,76,93). Since tears have more constant pH than saliva, some investigators suggest that tears may be more reliable than other nonsanguinous fluids for estimating serum phenobarbital concentrations (119).

Phenobarbital readily crosses the placenta and is secreted in breast milk (37,70). Infants born to mothers with steady-state phenobarbital concentrations have equivalent serum concentrations in the immediate postnatal period (12,13,63,82,89,103). Concentrations of phenobarbital in breast milk were $36 \pm 20\%$ and $41 \pm 16\%$ of maternal serum concentration in two studies (69,89).

After intravenous administration, phenobarbital distribution into body organs has two phases. The early phase involves distribution to highly vascular organs including liver, kidney, and heart, but not brain, muscle, or intestine. During the late phase, phenobarbital achieves fairly even distribution throughout the body except for relative exclusion from fat (19,29,34,47,115). During this interval, there is a rapid decline in the plasma concentration with a half-life of 0.13 to 0.7 hr in adults (91,128). This pattern of relatively slow entry into brain and late exclusion from fat is related to phenobarbital's low lipid solubility, as drugs with higher lipophilicity rapidly enter brain (16,80,102).

The relative exclusion of phenobarbital from body fat should be taken into consideration when dosages are based on weight to avoid overdosing obese people (115).

Phenobarbital requires 12 to 60 min for maximal penetrance of adult mammalian brain, as compared to 30 sec for thiopental (34,50,77,78,102,110). The rate of central nervous system penetration is also age-related, with more rapid entry in younger animals (29,35). In mature cats, phenobarbital concentrations rise more rapidly in gray than white matter of brain, probably reflecting the early effect of blood flow, but uniform distribution is achieved after several hours (104,109).

VOLUME OF DISTRIBUTION

Estimates of the apparent volume of distribution for phenobarbital vary nearly fourfold (Table 1). This wide range of values is in part attributable to the different methods that have been employed; most investigators have used a single compartment kinetic model. In dogs, the relative volume of distribution of phenobarbital is 0.75 L/kg after oral administration (20). In adult humans, the relative volume of distribution ranges from 0.36 to 0.67 L/kg after intramuscular doses and from 0.42 to 0.73 L/kg after oral doses (7,112,116). One study after intravenous phenobarbital administration demonstrated a volume of distribution of 0.54 ± 0.03 L/kg in adult volunteers and 0.61 ± 0.05 L/kg in adults with epilepsy (128). A wider range (0.39 to 2.25 L/kg) of volume of distribution values has been reported for newborns than for older children or adults (72,99).

The average volume of distribution for phenobarbital is larger in newborns, averaging appropriately 1.0 L/kg. This is probably the consequence of their relatively larger extracellular fluid volume (10,33,84). The range after intravenous dosing is 0.66 to 1.22 L/kg, and is independent of body weight, dose, or gestational age (30,41,72,96,97,99). These values are stable throughout the neonatal period and are similar in both asphyxiated (0.88 ± 0.08 L/kg) and nonasphyxiated (0.89 ± 0.20 L/kg) newborns (30,41). After oral administration, the range for volume of distribution for newborns has the larger range of 0.56 to

1.54 L/kg, possibly an artifact of slow absorption (53,59). Jalling (59) found a range of 0.59 to 0.84 L/kg after intramuscular but 0.89 ± 1.54 L/kg after oral administration to neonates. Lockman et al. (72) found no significant variation in volume of distribution in neonates for intravenous (0.81 ± 0.19 L/kg) as compared to intramuscular (0.91 ± 0.33 L/kg) administration.

The phenobarbital volume of distribution in older infants and children is similar to adults. One study of 51 children found no age-related variation in volume of distribution between 1 week and 5 years of age (52). In two other studies of children older than 6 months, the volume of distribution was 0.63 ± 0.09 L/kg (range 0.47–0.76) and 0.70 L/kg (15,61).

ELIMINATION

A number of factors contribute to variation in the rate of elimination of phenobarbital. The phenobarbital half-life is the longest among the frequently used antiepileptic drugs. Phenobarbital elimination is slowed when liver metabolism or renal clearance is reduced, or in cases where urine is rendered more acidic (2,38).

Despite the presence of two parallel phenobarbital eliminating mechanisms, phenobarbital clearance rates are very low as compared to other antiepileptic drugs. Phenobarbital is eliminated from the body both by hepatic metabolism and by renal excretion (17,81). In the liver, phenobarbital is parahydroxylated and subsequently conjugated to glucuronic acid. The parahydroxylated metabolite accounts for 0 to 20% of excreted drug in the first few days of life, but up to 50% by day 8 of life (4). The extent of glucuronide formation of phenobarbital varies widely. For example, Kallberg (68) described a 9-year-old whose urinary phenobarbital was 75% unmetabolized. Both unmetabolized and parahydroxylated phenobarbital are excreted

TABLE 1. *Phenobarbital half-lives and relative apparent volume of distribution*

Subjects	n	Route	V_d (L/kg)	$T_{1/2}$ (range) (hours)	Reference
Newborn	18	P		271 ± 238 (77–1060)	60
Newborn	10	P/IM		111 ± 34 (82–199)	11
Newborn	32	IV	0.96		94
Newborn 27–30 wk, prm	26	IV	0.96 ± 0.21		95
Newborn 31–36 wk, prm	10	IV	0.96 ± 0.12		95
Newborn >37 wk	23	IV	0.88 ± 0.16		95
Newborn/Sx	18	IV	0.93 ± 0.15	194 ± 17 (77–404)	96
Newborn	6	IM	0.71 ± 0.10	(59–182)	62
Newborn	5	PO	1.17 ± 0.31	(59–182)	62
Newborn	10	IM/PO		107 ± 33 (69–165)	125
Newborn	15	IM	0.81 ± 0.12	103 ± 49 (43–217)	36
Newborn/Sx	<36	IV	0.81 ± 0.19		72
Newborn/Sx	<36	IM	0.91 ± 0.33		72
Newborn	9	IV	0.89 ± 0.20		42
Asphyxiated newborn	16	IV	0.88 ± 0.08		42
Asphyxiated newborn	10	IV	0.97 ± 0.18	148 ± 55	30
Infant 1–4 wk/Sx	8	IV	0.97 ± 0.15	115	99
Infant 0–4 wk/Sx	14	IV	0.85 ± 0.06	119 ± 16	52
Infant >4 wk	8	IV	0.97 ± 0.15	67	99
Infant 2–3 mo	16	IV	0.86 ± 0.09	63 ± 5	52
Infant 4–12 mo	14	IV	0.57 ± 0.05	63 ± 4	52
Infants >6 mo	33	IM/PO	0.63 ± 0.09	(37–133)	61
Infants 9–26 mo/Sx	7	PO	0.69 ± 0.18	65 ± 31 (46–198)	61
Infants 13–31 mo/Sx	11	IM	0.63 ± 0.09	72 ± 27 (37–119)	61
Children 1–5 yr	7	IV		69 ± 3	52
Children/epilepsy	6	PO		(37–73)	44
Children	39	IM	0.70		15
Normal adult	6	IV	0.54 ± 0.03	99 ± 18 (75–126)	129
Normal adult	6	IM		101 ± 19	129
Normal adult	6	PO		100 ± 17	129
Adult epileptic	6	IV	0.61 ± 0.05	103 ± 21 (77–128)	129
Normal adult	6	IV	0.68 ± 0.04	110 ± 8	7
Normal adult + charcoal	6	IV	0.73 ± 0.06	45 ± 6	7
Adult		PO		110	92
Adult + charcoal		PO		20	92
Adult	11	PO	0.60	87 ± 16 (79–93)	21
Normal adult	5	PO		82 ± 25	122
Normal adult	5	IM		96 ± 21	122
Adult	6	PO		90 ± 18	115

PRM, premature; Sx, seizures; P, transplacental; IM, intramuscular; IV, intravenous; PO, oral.

in urine (1). Enterohepatic circulation and fecal excretion probably are not important contributors to the net phenobarbital disposition under usual circumstances (8,81).

Phenobarbital elimination has first-order kinetics and thus is independent of concentration. From 11% to 50% of phenobarbital is eliminated from the body per day corresponding to a half-life range of 24 to 140 hr. Average half-lives after single doses range from 75 to 126 hr and are not influenced by route of administration (7,22,74,75,86, 98,113,128). However, the rate of urine flow and urinary pH do influence the phenobarbital elimination rate.

Both urinary pH and flow influence phenobarbital reabsorption in the distal nephron (40). Under usual circumstances total renal clearance of phenobarbital ranges from 0.7 to 8.8 ml/kg/hr in adults (17,75,91,112,128). This is much less than the glomerular filtration rate, indicating extensive resorption in the nephron (9,74). Renal clearance is enhanced by diuresis, whether the urine is acidic or alkaline, but clearance is even greater when the urine is alkaline (9,26,73,75,88,123). Diuresis induced by water administration that increases urine flow approximately eightfold (from 0.8–1.2 ml/min to 6.7–9.0 ml/min) increases phenobarbital clearance only three- to fourfold from (2.0–3.0 to 4.3–7.5 ml/min), suggesting that back-diffusion of phenobarbital is restricted in the distal tubule as compared to water (45,80). Thus, the enhancement of renal phenobarbital clearance due to increased water filtration has limits (45). Dopamine- and diamox-induced diuresis also increase the clearance of phenobarbital (26). Probenecid administration does not (123).

Alkalinization of urine increases phenobarbital excretion. Elevation of urinary pH from 6.1 to 8.0 with sodium bicarbonate increased clearance rates up to 29 ml/kg/min in dogs (123). This increase results from trapping of ionized drug in the alkaline tubular urine compartment. At plasma pH 7.4, raising the urinary pH from 6.0 to 7.9 increases the urine-to-plasma phenobarbital ratio from 0.45 to 2.3. (81,123). Alkalinization of urine to pH 8.0 (plasma pH 7.55) increases the fraction of ionized phenobarbital in renal tubular fluid from 69% to 86% (18). Thus, phenobarbital excretion is particularly sensitive to urinary pH. When coupled with diuresis, alkalinization increases renal clearance fourfold.

Other factors that modify phenobarbital elimination include age, nutritional state, and drug interactions (see Chapter 21) but not the duration of phenobarbital administration. Prolonged starvation increases clearance of phenobarbital, possibly due to diminished protein binding, an effect that persists for a considerable period after refeeding (40,127). Phenobarbital elimination is similar among drug-naive adult volunteers, patients treated for less than 2 weeks, or patients treated with phenobarbital for

months to years (20,128). Although valproate retards phenobarbital elimination, other antiepileptic medications, such as phenytoin or carbamazepine, do not significantly alter phenobarbital clearance (32,86,93,128).

The phenobarbital half-life varies with age. It is longest in premature and full-term newborns who have similar values, typically ranging from 59 to 400 hr (53,82,99). These values may also vary considerably from day to day in individual patients (36,53,61,63,82,94,99,124). Newborn infants eliminate maternally derived phenobarbital with a half-life of 77 to 404 hr (63). They also have longer phenobarbital half-lives (111 ± 34 hr, range 82–199 hr) than their mothers (79 ± 23 hr, range 60–128 hr) (11).

Whereas newborns have the longest phenobarbital half-lives, infants (ages 6 weeks to 12 months) have the shortest. Thus, during the first month of life phenobarbital elimination accelerates, often doubling during the first week (52,63,94). Neonatal phenobarbital elimination rates are related to postpartum age but not to gestational age at birth, or to birthweight (63,96,99). Pitlick et al. (99) estimated that the half-life diminishes from an average of 115 hr to 67 hr between birth and 1 month of age. Jalling (60) found half-lives of 37 to 133 hr in 33 infants older than 6 months, after single doses. Other investigators have found serum phenobarbital half-lives to range from 21 to 75 hr in older children, considerably shorter than in adults (44,53,90).

Perinatal asphyxia also retards phenobarbital elimination by newborns. Ten severely asphyxiated infants showed a significant prolongation of serum half-life to 148 ± 55 hr and low clearances 0.08 ± 0.03 ml/kg/min (70). Gal et al. (41,42) measured total clearance of 8.7 ± 3.9 ml/kg/hr in nonasphyxiated versus only 4.1 ± 1.0 ml/kg/hr in asphyxiated newborns. The relative contributions of renal versus hepatic dysfunction to the reduced phenobarbital elimination in perinatal asphyxia is unknown (5,28,42). Both mechanisms are likely.

Intestinal elimination of phenobarbital can be important under certain circumstances. Phenobarbital elimination is increased by oral administration of activated charcoal. Berg et al. (7,8) showed reduction in the serum half-life for a single intravenous dose of phenobarbital from 110.0 ± 8.0 to 45.0 ± 6.0 hr. Total body clearance increased by a factor of 2.8, largely accounted for by the increase in nonrenal clearance from 52% to 80% of total body clearance (7,8). Similar three- to sixfold reductions in the apparent half-life for elimination of phenobarbital have been found by others after single or multiple oral doses of activated charcoal (49,92,130). In rats more than 6% of the dose is exsorbed into the lumen of isolated small intestine after an intravenous dose, with less than 0.54% of the dose distributed into bile even though bile concentrations were twice as high as serum (3).

REFERENCES

1. Algeri, E. J., and McBay, A. J. (1956): Metabolite of phenobarbital in human urine. *Science,* 23:183–184.
2. Alvin, J., McHorse, T., Hoyumpa, A., Bush, M. T., and Schenker, S. (1975): The effect of liver disease in man on the disposition of phenobarbital. *J. Pharmacol. Exp. Ther.,* 192:224–235.
3. Arimori, K., and Nakano, M. (1986): Transport of phenobarbitone into the intestinal lumen and the biliary tract following i.v. administration to rats. *J. Pharm. Pharmacol.,* 38:391–393.
4. Aymard, P., Taburet, A. M., Baudon, J. J., et al. (1980): Kinetics and metabolism of phenobarbital in the neonate. In: *Antiepileptic Therapy: Advances in Drug Monitoring,* edited by S. I. Morselli, P. L. Pippenger, C. E. Richens, A. Schmidt, and D. Meinardi, pp. 1–8. Raven Press, New York.
5. Baumel, I., DeFoe, J. J., and Lal, H. (1970): Effect of acute hypoxia on brain-sensitivity and metabolism of barbiturates in mine. *Psychopharmacologia,* 17:1983–1987.
6. Beckett, A. H., and Moffat, A. C. (1971): The buccal absorption of some barbiturates. *J. Pharm. Pharmacol.,* 23:15–18.
7. Berg, J. M., Berlinger, W. G., Goldberg, M. J.,

Spector, R., and Johnson, G. F. (1982): Acceleration of the body clearance of phenobarbital by oral activated charcoal. *N. Engl. J. Med.,* 307:642–644.
8. Berg, M. J., Rose, J. Q., Wurster, D. E., Rahman, S., Fincham, R. W., and Schottelius, D. D. (1987): Effect of charcoal and sorbitol-charcoal suspension on the elimination of intravenous phenobarbital. *Ther. Drug. Monit.,* 9:41–47.
9. Bloomer, H. A. (1966): A critical evaluation of diuresis in the treatment of barbiturate intoxication. *J. Lab. Clin. Med.,* 67:898–905.
10. Boreus, L. O., Jalling, B., and Kallberg, N. (1975): Clinical pharmacology of phenobarbital in the neonatal period. In: *Basic and Therapeutic Aspects of Perinatal Pharmacology,* edited by P. L. Morselli, S. Garattini, and F. Sereni, pp. 331–340. Raven Press, New York.
11. Boreus, L. O., Jalling, B., and Kallberg, N. (1978): Phenobarbital metabolism in adults and in newborn infants. *Acta Pediatr. Scand.,* 67:193–200.
12. Boreus, L. O., Jalling, B., and Wallin, A. (1978): Plasma concentrations of phenobarbital in mother and child after combined prenatal and postnatal administration for prophylaxis of hyperbilirubinemia. *J. Pediatr.,* 93:695–698.
13. Bossi, L., Battino, D., Caccamo, M. L., De Giambattista, M., Latis, G. O., Oldrini, A., and Spina, S. (1982): Pharmacokinetics and clinical effects of antiepileptic drugs in newborns of chronically treated epileptic mothers. In: *Epilepsy, Pregnancy, and the Child,* edited by D. Janz, M. Dam, A. Richens, L. Bossi, H. Helge, and D. Schmidt, pp. 373–381. Raven Press, New York.
14. Boyd, E. M., and Singh, J. (1967): Acute toxicity following rectal thiopental, phenobarbital and leptazol. *Anesth. Analg. Curr. Res.,* 46:395–400.
15. Brachet-Liermain, A., Gouteres, F., and Aicardi, J. (1975): Absorption of phenobarbital after the intramuscular administration of single doses in infants. *J. Pediat.,* 87:624–626.
16. Brodie, B. B., Kurz, H., and Schanker, L. S. (1960): The importance of dissociation constant and lipid solubility in influencing the passage of drugs into the cerebrospinal fluid. *J. Pharmacol. Exp. Ther.,* 130:20–25.
17. Brodwall, E., and Stoa, K. F. (1956): A study of barbiturate clearance. *Acta Med. Scand.,* 154:139–144.
18. Bush, M. T. (1963): Sedatives and hypnotics: Absorption, fate and excretion. In: *Physiological Pharmacology, Vol. 1,* edited by W. S. Root and F. G. Hofmann, pp. 185–218. Academic Press, New York.
19. Butler, T. C. (1950): The rate of penetration of barbituric acid derivatives into the brain. *J. Pharmacol. Exp. Ther.,* 100:219–226.
20. Butler, T. C. (1952): Quantitative studies on the metabolic fate of mephobarbital (*N*-methylphenobarbital). *J. Pharmacol. Exp. Ther.,* 106:235–245.
21. Butler, T. C. (1954): Metabolic oxidation of

phenobarbital to *p*-hydroxyphenobarbital. *Science*, 120:494.

22. Butler, T. C., Mahaffee, C., Waddell, W. J. (1954): Phenobarbital: Studies of elimination, accumulation, tolerance, and dosage schedules. *J. Pharmacol. Exp. Ther.*, 111:425–435.

23. Butler, T. C., and Waddell, W. J. (1958): *N*-Methylated derivatives of barbituric acid, hydantoin and oxazolidinedione used in the treatment of epilepsy. *Neurology*, 8:106–112.

24. Cook, C. E., Amerson, E., Poole, W. K., Lesser, P., and O'Tuama, L. (1975): Phenytoin and phenobarbital concentrations in saliva and plasma measured by radioimmunoassay. *Clin. Pharmacol. Ther.*, 18:742–747.

25. Cooper, D. Y., Schleyer, H., Levin, S. S., Touchstone, J. C., Eisenhardt, R. H., Vars, H. M., Rosenthal, O., Rastigar H., and Harken, A. (1979): Biliary and urinary excretion of phenobarbital and parahydroxyphenobarbital in rats with bile fistula. In: *The Introduction of Drug Metabolism*, edited by R. W. Estabrook and E. Lindenlaub, pp. 253–256. Symposia Medica Hoechst Verlag, Stuttgart, West Germany.

26. Costello, J. B., and Poklis, A. (1981): Treatment of massive phenobarbital overdose with dopamine diuresis. *Arch. Intern. Med.*, 141:938–940.

27. Danhof, M., and Levy, G. (1984): Kinetics of drug action in disease states. I. Effect of infusion rate on phenobarbital concentrations in serum, brain and cerebrospinal fluid of normal rats at onset of loss of righting reflex. *J. Pharmacol. Exp. Ther.*, 229:44–50.

28. Dauber, I. M., Krauss, A. N., Symchych, P. S., and Auld, P. A. (1976): Renal failure following perinatal anoxia. *J. Pediat.*, 88:851–855.

29. Domek, N. S., Barlow, C. F., and Roth, L. J. (1960): An ontogenetic study of phenobarbital-C^{14} in cat brain. *J. Pharmacol. Exp. Ther.*, 130:285–293.

30. Donn, S. M., Grasela, T. H., and Goldstein, G. W. (1985): Safety of a higher loading dose of phenobarbital in the term newborn. *Pediatrics*, 75:1061–1064.

31. Dvorchick, B. H., and Vessell, E. S. (1977): Pharmacokinetic interpretation of data gathered during therapeutic drug monitoring. *Clin. Chem.*, 22:868–878.

32. Eadie, M. J., Lander, C. M., Hooper, W. D., and Tyrer, J. H. (1977): Factors influencing plasma phenobarbitone levels in epileptic patients. *Br. J. Clin. Pharmacol.*, 4:541–547.

33. Ehrnebo, M., Agurell, S., Jalling, B., and Boreus, L. O. (1971): Age differences in drug binding by plasma proteins: Studies on human foetuses, neonates and adults. *Eur. J. Clin. Pharmacol.*, 3:189.

34. Engasser, J. M., Sarhan, F., Falcoz, C., Minier, M., Letourneur, P., and Siest, G. (1981): Distribution, metabolism, and elimination of phenobarbital in rats: Physiologically based pharmacokinetic model. *J. Pharmaceut. Sci.*, 70:1233–1238.

35. Ferngren, H. (1969): Brain and blood levels of phenobarbital-2-^{14}C during postnatal develop-

ment in the mouse. *Acta Pharm. Suec.*, 6:331–338.

36. Fischer, J. H., Lockman, L. A., Zaske, D., and Kriel, R. (1981): Phenobarbital maintenance dose requirements in treating neonatal seizures. *Neurology*, 31:1042–1044.

37. Fouts, J. R., and Hart, L. G. (1965): Hepatic drug metabolism during the perinatal period. *Ann. N.Y. Acad. Sci.*, 123:245–251.

38. Fowler, G. W. (1978): Effect of dipropylacetate on serum levels of anticonvulsants in children. *Proc. West. Pharmacol. Soc.*, 21:37–40.

39. Friedman, I. M., Litt, I. F., Henson, R., Holtzman, D., and Halverson, D. (1981): Saliva phenobarbital and phenytoin concentrations in epileptic adolescents. *J. Pediatr.*, 98:645–647.

40. Fujimoto, J. M., and Donnelly, R. A. (1968): Effect of feeding and fasting on excretion of phenobarbital in the rabbit. *Clin. Toxicol.*, 1:297–307.

41. Gal, P., Boer, H. R., Toback, J., and Erkan, N. V. (1982): Phenobarbital dosing in neonates and asphyxia. *Neurology*, 32:788–789.

42. Gal, P., Toback, J., Erkan, N. V., Boer, N., and Henry, R. (1984): The influence of asphyxia on phenobarbital dosing requirements in neonates. *Dev. Pharmacol. Ther.*, 7:145–152.

43. Ganshorn, A., and Kurz, H. (1968): Unterschiede zwischen der Proteinbindung Neugeborener und Erwachsener und ihre Bedeutung fur die pharmakologische Wirkung. *Arch. Pharmakol. Exp. Pathol.*, 260:117–118.

44. Garrettson, L. K., and Dayton, P. G. (1970): Disappearance of phenobarbital and diphenylhydantoin from serum of children. *Clin. Pharmacol. Ther.*, 11:674–679.

45. Giotti, A., and Maynert, E. W. (1951): The renal clearance of barbital and the mechanism of its reabsorption. *J. Pharmacol. Exp. Ther.*, 101:296–309.

46. Gitlin, D., and Boesman, M. (1966): Serum fetoprotein, albumin and IgG globulin in the human conceptus. *Clin. Invest.*, 45:1826–1838.

47. Goldbaum, L. R., and Smith, P. K. (1954): The interaction of barbiturates with serum albumin and its possible relation to their disposition and pharmacological actions. *J. Pharmacol. Exp. Ther.*, 111:197–209.

48. Goldberg, M. A. (1980): Antiepileptic drugs. Phenobarbital. In *Antiepileptic Drugs, Mechanisms of Action*, edited by G. H. Glaser, J. K. Penry, and D. M. Woodbury, pp. 501–504. Raven Press, New York.

49. Goldberg, M. J., and Berlinger W. G. (1982): Treatment of phenobarbital overdose with activated charcoal. *J. Am. Med. Assn.*, 247:2400–2401.

50. Goldstein, A., and Aronow, L. (1960): The duration of action of thiopental. *J. Pharmacol. Exp. Ther.*, 128:1.

51. Harvey, C. D., Sherwin, A. L., and Van Der Kleijn, E. (1977): Distribution of anticonvulsant drugs in gray and white matter of human brain. *Can. J. Neurol. Sci.*, 4:89–92.

52. Heimann, G., and Gladtke E. (1977): Pharma-

cokinetics of phenobarbital in childhood. *Eur. J. Clin. Pharmacol.*, 12:305–310.

53. Heinze, E., and Kampffmeyer, H. G. (1971): Biological half-life of phenobarbital in human babies. *Klin. Wochenschr.*, 49:1146–1147.
54. Hogben, C. A. M., Schanker, L. S., Tocco, D. J., and Brodie, B. B. (1957): Absorption of drugs from the stomach. II. The human. *J. Pharmacol. Exp. Ther.*, 120:540.
55. Hogben, C. A. M., Tocco, D. J., Brodie, B. B., and Schanker, L. S. (1959): On the mechanism of intestinal absorption of drugs. *J. Pharmacol. Exp. Ther.*, 125:275.
56. Horning, M. G., Brown, L., Nowlin, J., Lertratananangh, K., Kellaway, P., and Zion, T. E. (1977): Use of saliva for therapeutic drug monitoring. *Clinc. Chem.*, 23:157–164.
57. Houghton, G. W., Richens, A., Toseland, P. A., Davidson, S., and Falconer, M. A. (1975): Brain concentrations of phenytoin, phenobarbital and primidone in epileptic patients. *Eur. J. Clin. Pharmacol.*, 9:73–78.
58. Ioannides, C., and Parke, D. V. (1975): Mechanism of induction of hepatic microsomal drug metabolizing enzymes by a series of barbiturates. *J. Pharm. Pharmacol.*, 27:739.
59. Jalling, B. (1968): Plasma and cerebrospinal fluid concentrations of phenobarbital in infants given single doses. *Dev. Med. Child Neurol.*, 10:626–632.
60. Jalling, B. (1974): Plasma and cerebrospinal fluid concentrations of phenobarbital in infants given single doses. *Dev. Med. Child. Neurol.*, 11:781–793.
61. Jalling, B. (1975): Plasma concentrations of phenobarbital in the treatment of seizures in the newborns. *Acta Paediatr. Scand.*, 64:514–524.
62. Jalling, B. (1976): Plasma and cerebrospinal fluid concentrations of phenobarbital in infants given single doses. *Dev. Med. Child. Neurol.*, 16:781–793.
63. Jalling B., Boreus, L. O., Kallberg, N., and Agurell, S. (1973): Disappearance from the newborn of circulating prenatally administered phenobarbital. *Europ. J. Clin. Pharmacol.*, 6:234–238.
64. Johannessen, S. I., and Strandjord, R. E. (1975): Absorption and protein binding in serum of several anti-epileptic drugs. In: *Clinical Pharmacology of Anti-Epileptic Drugs,* edited by H. Schneider, D. Janz, C. Gardner Thorpe, H. Meinardi, and A. L. Sherwin, pp. 268. Springer-Verlag, New York.
65. Jusko, W., and Gretch, M. (1976): Plasma and tissue binding of drugs in pharmacokinetics. *Drug Metab. Rev.*, 5:43–140.
66. Kakemi, K., Arita, T., Hori, R., and Konishi, R. (1967): Absorption and excretion of drugs. XXX. Absorption of barbituric acid derivatives from rat stomach. *Chem. Pharm. Bull. (Tokyo)*, 15:1534–1539.
67. Kakemi, K., Arita, T., Hori, R., and Konishi, R. (1967): Absorption and excretion of drugs. XXXII. Absorption of barbituric acid derivatives

from rat small intestine. *Chem. Pharm. Bull. (Tokyo)*, 15:1883–1887.
68. Kallberg, N., Agurell, S., Ericsson, O., Bucht, E., Jalling, B., and Boreus, L. O. (1975): Quantitation of phenobarbital and its main metabolites in human urine. *Eur. J. Clin. Pharmacol.*, 9:161–168.
69. Kaneko, S., Suzuki, K., Sato, T., Ogawa, Y., and Nomura, Y. (1982): The problems of antiepileptic medication in the neonatal period: Is breastfeeding advisable? In: *Epilepsy, Pregnancy, and the Child,* edited by D. Janz, M. Dam, A. Richens, L. Bossi, H. Helge, and D. Schmidt, pp. 343–348. Raven Press, New York.
70. Langset, A., Meberg, A., Bredesen, J. E., and Lunde, P. K. M. (1978): Plasma concentrations of diazepam and N-demethyldiazepam in newborn infants after intravenous, intramuscular, rectal and oral administration. *Acta Paed. Scand.*, 67:699–704.
71. Leucuta, S. E., Popa, L., Ariesan, M., Popa, L., Pop, R. D., Kory, M., and Toader, S. (1977): Bioavailability of phenobarbital from different pharmaceutical forms. *Pharm. Acta Helv.*, 52:261–266.
72. Lockman, L. A., Kriel, R., Zaske, D., Thompson, T., and Virnig, N. (1979): Phenobarbital dosage for control of neonatal seizures. *Neurology*, 29:1445–1449.
73. Lous, P. (1954): Barbituric acid concentration in serum from patients with severe acute poisoning. *Acta Pharmacol.*, 10:261.
74. Lous, P. (1954): Blood serum and cerebrospinal fluid levels and renal clearance of phenemal in treated epileptics. *Acta Pharmacol. Toxicol.*, 10:166–177.
75. Lous, P. (1954): Plasma levels and urinary excretion of three barbituric acids after oral administration to man. *Acta Pharmacol. Toxicol.*, 10:147–165.
76. McAuliffe, J. J., Sherwin, A. L., Leppik, I. E., Fayle, S. A., and Pippenger, C. E. (1977): Salivary levels of anticonvulsants: A practical approach to drug monitoring. *Neurology*, 27:409–413.
77. Mark, L. C., Burns, J. J., Brand, L., Campomanes, C. I., Trousef, N., Papper, E. M., and Brodie, B. B. (1958): The passage of thiobarbiturates and their oxygen analogs into brain. *J. Pharmacol. Exptl. Therap.*, 123:70.
78. Mayer, S., Maickel, R. P., and Brodie, B. B. (1959): Kinetics of penetration of drugs and other foreign compounds into cerebrospinal fluid and brain. *J. Pharmacol. Exp. Ther.*, 127:205.
79. Maynert, E. W. (1972): Phenobarbital mephobarbital and metharbital. Absorption, distribution, and excretion. In: *Antiepileptic Drugs,* 1st edition, edited by D. M. Woodbury, J. K. Penry, and R. P. Schmidt, pp. 303–310. Raven Press, New York.
80. Maynert, E. W. (1982): Absorption, distribution, and excretion. In: *Antiepileptic Drugs,* 2nd edition, edited by D. M. Woodbury, J. K. Penry,

and C. E. Pippenger, pp. 309–317. Raven Press, New York.

81. Maynert, E. W., and van Dyke, H. B. (1949): The metabolism of barbiturates. *Pharmacol. Rev.,* 1:217–242.

82. Melchior, J. C., Svensmark, O., and Trolle, D. (1967): Placental transfer of phenobarbitone in epileptic women, and elimination in newborns. *Lancet,* 11:860–861.

83. Melten, J. W., Wittebrood, A. J., Wemer, J., and Faber, D. B. (1986): On the modulating effects of temperature, albumin, pH and calcium on the free fractions of phenobarbitone and phenytoin. *J. Pharm. Pharmacol.,* 38:643–646.

84. Morselli, P. L. (1976): Clinical pharmacokinetics in neonates. *Clin. Pharm.,* 1:81–98.

85. Morselli, P. L. (1983): Development of physiological variables important for drug kinetics. In: *Antiepileptic Drug Therapy in Pediatrics,* edited by P. L. Morselli, C. E. Pippenger, and J. K. Penry, pp. 1–12. Raven Press, New York.

86. Morselli, P. L., Rizzo, M., and Garrattini, S. (1971): Interaction between phenobarbital and diphenylhydantoin in animals and in epileptic patients. *Ann. N.Y. Acad. Sci.,* 179:88–107.

87. Mucklow, J. C., Bending, M. R., Kahn, G. C., and Dollery, C. T. (1978): Drug concentration in saliva. *Clin. Pharmacol. Ther.,* 24:563–570.

88. Myschetzky, A., and Lassen, N. A. (1971): Forced diuresis in treatment of acute barbiturate poisoning. In: *Acute Barbiturate Poisoning,* edited by H. Matthew, pp. 223–232. Amsterdam, Excerpta Medica.

89. Nau, H., Rating, D., Hauser, I., Jager, E., Koch, S., and Helge, H. (1980): Placental transfer and pharmacokinetics of primidone and its metabolites, phenobarbital, PEMA, and hydroxyphenobarbital in neonates and infants of epileptic mothers. *Eur. J. Clin. Pharmacol.,* 18:31–42.

90. Neimann, G., and Gladtke, E. (1977): Pharmacokinetics of phenobarbital in childhood. *Eur. J. Clin. Pharmacol.,* 12:305.

91. Nelson, E., Powell, J. R., Conrad K., et al. (1982): Phenobarbital pharmacokinetics and bioavailability in adults. *J. Clin. Pharmacol.,* 22:141–148.

92. Neuvonen, P. J., and Elonen, E. (1980): Effect of activated charcoal on absorption and elimination of phenobarbitone, carbamazepine and phenylbutazone in man. *Eur. J. Clin. Pharmacol.,* 17:51–57.

93. Nishihara, K., Katsuyoski, U., Saitoh, Y., Honda, Y., Nakagawa, F., and Tamwia, Z. (1979): Estimation of plasma unbound phenobarbital concentration by using mixed saliva. *Epilepsia,* 20:37–45.

94. Painter, M. J., and Pippenger C. E. (1981): Phenobarbital and phenytoin in neonatal seizures: Metabolism and tissue distribution. *Neurology,* 31:1107–1112.

95. Painter, M. J., Pippenger, C. E., MacDonald, H., and Pitlick, W. H. (1977): Phenobarbital and phenytoin blood levels in neonates. *Pediatrics,* 92:315–319.

96. Painter, M. J., Pippenger, C. E., MacDonald, H., and Pitlick, W. (1978): Phenobarbital and diphenylhydantoin levels in neonates with seizures. *J. Pediatr.,* 92:315–319.

97. Parnas, J., Flachs, H., Lennart, G., and Wurtz-Jorgensen, A. (1978): Excretion of antiepileptic drugs in sweat. *Acta Neurol. Scand.,* 58:197–204.

98. Patel, I. H., Levy, R. H., and Cutler, R. E. (1980): Phenobarbital-valproic acid interaction. *Clin. Pharmacol. Ther.,* 27:515–521.

99. Pitlick, W., Painter, M., and Pippenger, C. E. (1978): Phenobarbital pharmacokinetics in neonates. *Clin. Pharmacol. Ther.,* 23:346–350.

100. Plaa, G. L., and Hine, C. H. (1960): Hydantoin and barbiturate blood levels observed in epileptics. *Arch. Int. Pharmacodyn.,* 128:375–382.

101. Porter, R., Penry, J. K., and Kiffin, J. (1980): Phenobarbital: Biopharmacology. In: *Antiepileptic Drugs: Mechanisms of Action,* edited by G. H. Glaser, J. K. Penry, and D. M. Woodbury, pp. 493–500. Raven Press, New York.

102. Ramsay, R. E., Hammond, E. J., Perchalski, R. J., and Wilder, B. J. (1979): Brain uptake of phenytoin, phenobarbital, and diazepam. *Arch. Neurol.,* 36:535–539.

103. Rating, D., Nau, H., Kuhnz, W., Jager-Rom, E., and Helge, H. (1983): Antiepileptika in der neugeborenenperiode. *Monatsschr Kinderheilkd,* 131:6–12.

104. Roth, L. J., and Barlow, C. F., (1961): Drugs in the brain. Autoradiography and radioassay techniques permit analysis of penetration of labeled drugs. *Science,* 132:22–31.

105. Schanker, L. S. (1960): On the mechanism of absorption of drugs from the gastrointestinal tract. *J. Med. Pharm. Chem.,* 2:343.

106. Schanker, L. S. (1961): Mechanisms of drug absorption and distribution. *Ann. Rev. Pharmacol.,* 1:29–44.

107. Schanker, L. S., Shore, P. A., Brodie, B. B., and Hogben, C. A. M. (1957): Absorption of drugs from the stomach. I. The rat. *J. Pharmacol. Exptl. Therap.,* 120:528.

108. Schmidt, D., and Kupferberg, H. J. (1975): Diphenylhydantoin, phenobarbital, and primidone in saliva, plasma, and cerebrospinal fluid. *Epilepsia,* 16:735–741.

109. Sherwin, A. L., Eisen, A. A., and Sagolowski, C. D. (1973): Anticonvulsant drugs in human epileptogenic brain. *Arch. Neurol.,* 29:73.

110. Simon, R. P., Copeland, J. R., Benowitz, N. L., Jacob, P., and Bronstein, J. (1987): Brain phenobarbital uptake during prolonged status epilepticus. *J. Cereb. Blood Flow Metab.,* 7:783–788.

111. Sjogren, J., Solvell, L., and Karlsson, I. (1965): Studies on the absorption rates of barbiturates in man. *Acta Med. Scand.,* 178:553–559.

112. Strandjord, R. E., and Johannessen, S. I. (1977): Serum levels of phenobarbitone in healthy subjects and patients with epilepsy. In: *Antiepileptic Drug Monitoring,* edited by C. Gardner-Thorpe, D. Janz, H. Meinardi, and C. E. Pippenger, pp. 89–103. Pitman Medical, Tunbridge Wells (Kent), England.

113. Sunshine, I., and Hackett, E. R. (1954): Correlation between clinical condition and blood barbiturate levels. *Am. J. Clin. Pathol.*, 24:1133–1138.

114. Svensmark, O., and Buchthal, F. (1963): Accumulation of phenobarbital in man. *Epilepsia*, 4:199–206.

115. Svensmark, O., and Buchthal, F. (1963): Dosage of phenytoin and phenobarbital in children. *Dan. Med. Bull.*, 10:234–235.

116. Svensmark, O., and Buchtal, F. (1964): Diphenylhydantoin and phenobarbital serum levels in children. *Am. J. Dis. Child.*, 108:82–87.

117. Tang, B. K., Inaba, T., and Kalow, W. (1977): *N*-hydroxyphenobarbital—The major metabolite of phenobarbital in man. *Fed. Proc.*, 36:3671.

118. Tokugawa, K., Ueda, K., Fujito, H., and Kurokawa, T. (1986): Correlation between the saliva and free serum concentration of phenobarbital in epileptic children. *Eur. J. Pediatr.*, 145:401–402.

119. Tondi, M., Mutani, R., Mastropaolo, C., and Monaco, F. (1978): Greater reliability of tear versus saliva anticonvulsant levels. *Ann. Neurol.*, 4:154–155.

120. Troupin, A. S., and Friel, P. (1975): Anticonvulsant level in saliva, serum and cerebrospinal fluid. *Epilepsia*, 223–227.

121. Vajda, F., Williams, F. M., Davidson, S., Falconer, M. A., and Breckenridge, A. (1974): Human brain, cerebrospinal fluid, and plasma concentrations of diphenylhydantoin and phenobarbital. *Clin. Pharmacol. Ther.*, 15:597–603.

122. Viswanathan, C. T., Booker, H. E., and Welling, P. G. (1978): Bioavailability of oral and intramuscular phenobarbital. *J. Clin. Pharmacol.*, 18:100–105.

123. Wade, A. (1980): Barbiturates. In: *Pharmaceutical Handbook*. The Pharmaceutical Press, London.

124. Wallin, A., Jalling, B., and Boreus, L. O. (1974): Plasma concentrations of phenobarbital in the neonate during prophylaxis for neonatal hyperbirubinemia. *Journal of Pediatrics*, 85:392–398.

125. Walson, P. D., Mimaki, T., Curless, R., Mayersohn, M., and Perrier, D. (1980): Once daily doses of phenobarbital in children. *Journal of Pediatrics*, 97:303–305.

126. Wanwimolruk, S., and Levy, G. (1987): Effect of age on the pharmacodynamics of phenobarbital and ethanol in rats. *J. Pharmaceutical Sci.*, July (76)7:503.

127. Wanwimolruk, S., and Levy, G. (1987): Kinetics of drug action in disease states. XX. Effects of acute starvation on the pharmacodynamics of phenobarbital, ethanol and pentylenetetrazol in rats and effects of refeddings and diet composition. *J. Pharmacol. Exp. Ther.*, July 242(1):166–172.

128. Wilensky, A. J., Friel, P. N., Levy, R. H., Comfort, C. P., and Kaluzny S. P.: (1982): Kinetics of phenobarbital in normal subjects and epileptic patients. *Eur. J. Clin. Pharmacol.*, 23:87–92.

129. Yaffe, S. J. (1976): Developmental factors influencing interactions of drugs. *Annals of the New York Academy of Sciences*, 281:90–97.

130. Yatzidis, H. (1971): The use of ion exchange resins and charcoal in acute barbiturate poisoning. In: *Acute Barbiturate Poisoning*, edited by H. Matthew, pp. 223–232. Amsterdam, Excerpta Medica.

Antiepileptic Drugs, Third Edition, edited by
R. Levy, R. Mattson, B. Meldrum,
J. K. Penry, and F. E. Dreifuss.
Raven Press, Ltd., New York © 1989.

20

Phenobarbital

Biotransformation

Gail D. Anderson

Even though phenobarbital is one of the oldest and most widely used antiepileptic agents, its fate in man has not been completely elucidated. Evaluation of the mass balance of phenobarbital after a single dose requires complete collection of urine (and possibly feces) for at least 3 weeks to allow for greater than 90% elimination. Therefore quantitative mass balance studies following a single dose have been difficult to carry out. Steady-state experiments after long-term dosing are experimentally less difficult and also more relevant. At steady state, the rate of drug administration during a dosing interval is equal to the rate of drug eliminated during the same time interval. Whyte and Dekaban (41) failed to detect any phenobarbital or any of its metabolites in the feces of four patients on phenobarbital therapy. Therefore, a 24-hr urine collection in patients given prolonged treatment can be used to determine the fraction of the daily dose of phenobarbital eliminated through various pathways.

EXCRETION OF UNCHANGED PHENOBARBITAL

There is considerable intersubject and intrasubject variability in the amount of phenobarbital excreted unchanged in the urine. Single-dose studies in five normal volunteers (36,37) and two patients (30,41) where urine was collected for a minimum of 15 days reported a range of 9% to 33% (average 23%) of the phenobarbital dose as unchanged drug. In a study designed to evaluate the mechanism of the interaction between phenobarbital and valproic acid, Patel et al. (28) administered a single dose of phenobarbital with and without valproic acid to six normal volunteers. They found that the fraction of the dose excreted unchanged in urine (F_e) during the control phase was 22% (range 7%–40%). F_e was determined from the ratio of renal clearance to plasma clearance during two different time intervals (49–96 hr, 216–264 hr) after administration of phenobarbital. Two steady-state studies in epileptic patients given long-term administration of phenobarbital have reported that the percent of the daily phenobarbital dose excreted in a 24-hr urine collection ranged from 11% to 48% (average 24%) in four epileptic patients (22) and from 12% to 55% (average 25%) in eight epileptic patients (41).

There is very little information regarding the disposition of phenobarbital in infants and children. Children under the age of 4 have shorter half-lives (29), which is postulated to be due to a larger clearance. Boréus et al. (8) showed that the 8-day urinary excretion of unchanged phenobarbital after a single dose was similar in four newborn infants (17%) compared to two adult volunteers (16%). This indicates that if there is a larger clearance, it may be due to the non-renal component. However, there are no other data available in children of other age groups.

The renal clearance of phenobarbital is dependent on both urine flow (22,25,40,41) and urine pH (40) due to the lipophilicity and pK$_a$ (7.2) of this drug. This phenomenon may explain some of the intersubject variability found in the fraction of dose excreted unchanged in urine. After a drug is filtered by the glomerulus and possibly actively secreted into the tubule, it may be subject to passive reabsorption. Drug reabsorption takes place primarily in the distal tubule where the tubule membranes favor the transport of lipid-soluble and un-ionized compounds. The efficient reabsorption of water from the proximal tubule and Loop of Henle results in a large concentration gradient between drug in the distal tubule and drug in the plasma. Increasing urine flow decreases this concentration gradient, resulting in a decrease in passive reabsorption. Small changes in urine pH can cause large increases/decreases in the percent of un-ionized weak acid (pK$_l$ 3.0–7.5) like phenobarbital subject to passive reabsorption.

Waddell and Butler (40) first demonstrated the effect of urine flow and urine pH on phenobarbital renal clearance in an anesthetized dog model in which diuresis was induced. The renal clearance of phenobarbital increased linearly with urine flow over an eightfold range of urine flow. Administration of intravenous sodium bicarbonate increased urine pH to 7.8–8.0. At this higher pH, phenobarbital renal clearance increased eightfold at any given urine flow rate. In a study designed to evaluate the mechanism of the phenobarbital and valproic acid interaction, Kapetanovic et al. (22) studied three epileptic patients on prolonged phenobarbital therapy. Twenty-four–hr serial urine samples were collected ($N = 26$). They found a direct linear correlation between urine flow and urinary excretion of unchanged phenobarbital (4 = 0.913) over a fourfold range of urine flow. In a group of 20 epileptic patients Lous (25) demonstrated the same linear correlation between urine flow and phenobarbital renal clearance, but also observed that the phenobarbital renal clearance was independent of phenobarbital concentration in the therapeutic range. The dependence of phenobarbital renal clearance on urine flow and urine pH has provided the basis for the use of urine alkalinization and diuresis in overdose patients (16,40).

In summary, the fraction of dose excreted unchanged accounts for approximately 20% to 25% of the total clearance but there is wide intersubject variability.

MAJOR METABOLIC PATHWAYS

Aromatic Hydroxylation

Butler (10) first reported the formation of p-hydroxyphenobarbital (PBOH) from phenobarbital in the dog and it was later confirmed in man (10,12) that PBOH (Fig. 1A) was a major metabolite. A substantial fraction of the PBOH is then conjugated with glucuronic acid to form PBOH glucuronide. In randomly sampled urine specimens from eight patients on phenobarbital monotherapy, an average of 56% (range 31%–87%) of the PBOH found was excreted as the 0-glucuronide (25). Early reports of possible sulfate conjugate of PBOH have not been substantiated experimentally and may have been due to problems in analytical methodology (26).

There is also a large intersubject variability in the fraction of the phenobarbital dose that is metabolized by aromatic hydroxylation to PBOH. In one patient where urine was collected for 47 days after an oral

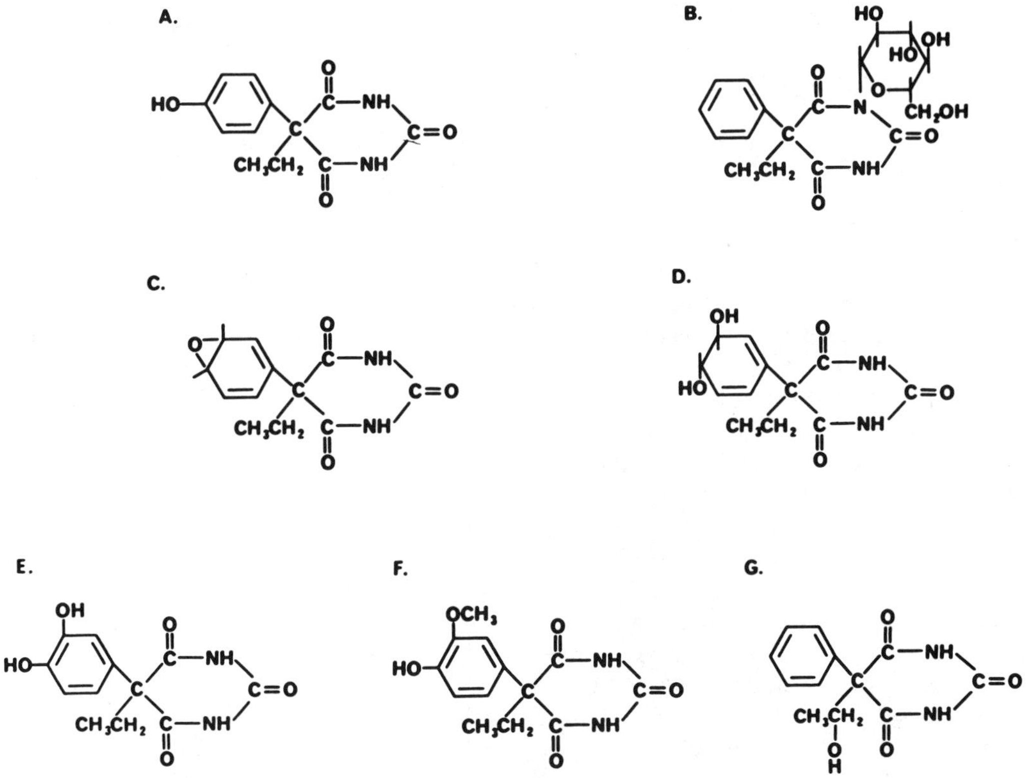

FIG. 1. Chemical structures of some metabolites of phenobarbital: **A,** *p*-hydroxyphenobarbital; **B,** phenobarbital *N*-glucopyranoside; **C,** epoxide; **D,** dihydrodiol; **E,** catechol; **F,** 0-methylcatechol; **G,** 5-(1-hydroxyethyl)-5-phenylbarbituric acid.

dose of phenobarbital, Raven-Jonsen (30) found 34% of the dose as total PBOH (conjugated and unconjugated) in acid-hydrolyzed urine. From the data given by Whyte and Dekaban (41) in a patient where urine was collected 16 days after a single phenobarbital dose, only 8% of the phenobarbital was recovered as total PBOH with approximately 40% of the PBOH found as the glucuronide conjugate in this patient. Tang et al. (36,37) reported an average of 18% of the dose recovered in urine as total PBOH (range 14–22%) in five normal volunteers after a single dose of phenobarbital. Steady-state experiments in eight patients (41) found on the average 20% of the phenobarbital daily dose was total *p*-hydroxyphen-

obarbital (range, 6–24%) with 54% (range, 30–72%) excreted as the glucuronide conjugate. In three patients evaluated in a phenobarbital/valproic acid interaction study, Kapetanovic et al. (22) found that the percent of the phenobarbital daily dose as total PBOH was 24%, 25%, and 34% with 43%, 52%, and 55% as the glucuronide conjugate, respectively.

Boréus (8) found that in four neonates, 15% of the phenobarbital dose was total PBOH with 33% conjugated with glucuronic acid. In two adult volunteers studied concurrently, 25% of the phenobarbital dose was total PBOH with 60% conjugated. These authors concluded that the neonates had a decreased ability to conjugate PBOH.

However, due to the lack of pharmacological activity of PBOH (10,13), this would not be a clinically significant effect.

N-Glucosidation

˙ It has been recently proposed that 1-(β-D-glucopyranosyl) phenobarbital (Fig. 1B) is a quantitatively significant metabolite of phenobarbital. Tang et al. (36) administered a mixture of ^{14}C-labeled and ^{15}N-labeled phenobarbital to two normal volunteers. Thin-layer chromatography of a 16-day urine identified the N-glucoside conjugate of phenobarbital after comparison to a synthetic standard. In five normal volunteers (36,37), phenobarbital N-glucoside accounted for 26% (range, 24–30%) of the phenobarbital dose. Bhargava et al. (7) examined randomly collected urine samples from eight patients treated with phenobarbital monotherapy. Phenobarbital N-glucoside was detected in all but one patient. Bhargava and Garrettson (6) also studied the development of phenobarbital metabolism in four neonates by analyzing serial single daily voided urines. The N-glucosidation pathway was not active at birth and onset occurred after 2 weeks of age. However, by day 20, PNG accounted for 50% of the drug and metabolites in the urine sample. This indicates that glucosidation may be a significant pathway in the disposition of phenobarbital in the neonate.

Glucosidation in plants and insects has been known for many years to be analogous to glucuronidation in mammals (15). 0-Glucoside conjugation of several compounds (i.e., 4-nitrophenol, bilirubin, and isoflavones) have been reported in mammals. Duggan et al. (14) reported the first instance of N-glucosidation as a detoxification mechanism in mammals. A xanthine oxidase inhibitor, 3-(4-pyrimidinyl)-5-(4-pyridyl) 1,2,3-triazole, forms an N-glucoside in dog, rat, and rhesus monkey. In the dog, 60% of the dose was recovered in the bile

as the N-glucoside metabolite. Tang et al. (35) have also documented that amobarbital forms the N-glucoside metabolite in man as one of its major metabolites. However, the fraction of dose metabolized through this pathway has not been established. A set of twins exhibiting a genetic deficiency in the formation of the metabolite now known as amobarbital N-β-D-glucopyranoside has been reported (20). Based on the results of Bhargava and Garrettson (6), a deficiency of this kind may have marked clinical implications in a neonate treated with phenobarbital.

OTHER ROUTES OF METABOLISM

Epoxidation and Subsequent Reactions

The hydroxylation of phenobarbital to PBOH is presumed to be mediated by the cytochrome P-450 system. Cytochrome P-450–mediated aromatic hydroxylation is postulated to occur through epoxide intermediates. Due to the highly unstable nature of epoxides, they can undergo spontaneous rearrangement to phenols primarily in the *para* orientation. Theoretically, *meta* hydroxyphenobarbital could also be formed. Metahydroxyphenobarbital has been identified by gas chromatography-mass spectrometry (GC-MS) analysis as a minor metabolite in rats and guinea pigs (17). Quantitative studies in our laboratory (5) have indicated that less than 2% of the phenobarbital dose is recovered as *m*-hydroxyphenobarbital in the urine of rats. Whyte and Dekaban (41) failed to detect any *m*-hydroxyphenobarbital in the urine of four patients receiving long-term phenobarbital.

The phenobarbital epoxide (Fig. 1C) could also spontaneously or enzymatically yield the corresponding dihydrodiol (Fig. 1D). Harvey et al. (17) were able to obtain GC-MS evidence that the dihydrodiol was present in rat, guinea pig, and human urine in small amounts. Theoretically, oxidation of the dihydrodiol could yield the corresponding catechol (Fig. 1E). This substance has been tentatively identified in rat and human urine by GC-MS analysis (18). Recently, the 4-hydroxy 3-methoxy derivative of phenobarbital (0-methylcatechol) has been isolated from human urine and its structure (Fig. 1F) was confirmed by comparison to synthetic compound. In six normal volunteers who received a single dose of phenobarbital, approximately 1% of the dose was recovered as this metabolite (38).

Aliphatic Hydroxylation

Due to steric hindrance, cytochrome P-450–mediated aliphatic oxidation of the ethyl group of phenobarbital is not a favored reaction. However, small amounts of 5(1-hydroxyethyl)5-phenylbarbituric acid (Fig. 1G) was detected by GC-MS analysis of the urine of rats and guinea pigs (17). This metabolite has not been found in human urine.

Hydrolysis

Phenobarbital in aqueous solution is subject to spontaneous hydrolysis to a greater extent than any of the dialkylbarbiturates (27). The extent to which phenobarbital is subject to hydrolysis in the human body is unknown. Studies with 2-^{14}C phenobarbital in mice (2) and rats (3,11) found only trace amounts of ^{14}C-labeled CO_2 in expired air. However, since there is still a significant part of the phenobarbital dose that is not accounted for by excretion of unchanged phenobarbital and metabolites, this mode of elimination cannot be totally discounted.

IN VITRO MODELS

There are only a few examples of *in vitro* metabolic studies using phenobarbital as a substrate. Due to the low hepatic extraction of phenobarbital, incubation of the drug with rat liver microsomes (4,21) or in an isolated perfused rat liver (4) results in only a marginal disappearance of phenobarbital. Seago and Garrod (32) were able to produce an 8% overall metabolism of ^{14}C-phenobarbital using hamster liver microsomes and a multiple cofactor addition technique. *p*-Hydroxyphenobarbital was the only identifiable metabolite in this system. However, *in vitro* systems have been used very successfully to evaluate the formation of phenobarbital metabolites. Kapetanovic and Kupferberg (21) used a liver microsomal preparation obtained from phenobarbital-induced rats to study the inhibition of PBOH formation by valproic acid. They were also able to document formation of *m*-hydroxyphenobarbital. The formation of PBOH glucuronide from PBOH has also been successfully characterized in the phenobarbital-induced rat liver microsomal preparation (33). In our laboratory (4), the isolated perfused rat liver was used to evaluate the effect of valproic acid on the formation of *p*-hydroxyphenobarbital and its glucuronide conjugate. An advantage of the isolated perfused rat liver is that it maintains the intact architecture of the liver and allows evaluation of the sequential metabolism of phenobarbital. In addition, biliary clearance can also be assessed. The single-pass extraction of phenobarbital to form PBOH was approximately 2%. Approximately 40% of the PBOH was then sequentially conjugated to the glucuronide. Greater than 95% of the PBOH glucuronide formed was eliminated into the bile. In contrast, less than 5% of the unconjugated PBOH and unchanged phenobarbital were eliminated by biliary excretion.

The fecal route has been shown not to be important in phenobarbital elimination in man (41). However, in the rat enterohepatic recirculation is more prominent than in any other species. Levin et al. (24) found approximately 45% to 50% of the ^{14}C-phenobarbital dose eliminated in the bile in Fisher-Vars rats with biliary fistulas. However, with no fistula present, greater than 80% of the phenobarbital dose was excreted in the urine indicating substantial entero-hepatic recycling. Similar results were found by Caldwell et al. (11). Studies in our laboratory (3) with Sprague-Dawley rats showed that after administration of an intravenous bolus of 2-^{14}C-phenobarbital, approximately 16% of the phenobarbital dose was eliminated in the feces. It was determined by isolation and identification of fecal radioactivity that 50% of the radioactivity in feces was PBOH glucuronide, unchanged phenobarbital accounted for 20%, and the remainder was unknown metabolite(s). Approximately 25% of the PBOH formed from phenobarbital was eliminated by fecal elimination. There was not an acid labile conjugate of phenobarbital identified in bile or urine indicating that phenobarbital N-glucosidation appears not to be a major route of biotransformation in the Sprague-Dawley rat.

Tang and Carro-Ciampi (34) reported a method for the study of N-glucosidation of amobarbital *in vitro* using incubations with human liver and UDP-glucose. Preliminary results indicated that this method may be useful for further characterization of this metabolic pathway.

AUTOINDUCTION

Phenobarbital is the classic inducer of hepatic microsomal metabolism. Surprisingly, it appears not to alter its own metabolism in humans. Butler et al. (10) found little difference in the elimination rates of phenobarbital among six patients who had received the drug between several months or years and five normal volunteers who received the drug for 12 days. Browne et al. (9) gave tracer doses of stable isotope-labeled phenobarbital intravenously to six normal volunteers before, at 4 weeks, and 12 weeks after receiving phenobarbital, 90 mg daily. Based on the results of this study,

the authors concluded that phenobarbital does not undergo time-dependent changes in total plasma clearance. An earlier study (39) of three volunteers suggested that the elimination rate may actually decrease after prolonged dosing of phenobarbital. However, the results of this study have been questioned due to problems in analytical methodology and small group size (9).

In contrast to the results in humans, there is evidence in both dog and rat that autoinduction occurs. During prolonged dosing in the dog, the daily elimination rate increases twofold (31). In a study designed to evaluate the effect of age on the pharmacokinetics of phenobarbital, Kapetanovic et al. (23) found that the apparent clearance of phenobarbital was approximately two times higher after a 5-day continuous infusion that following a single intravenous bolus in the Fischer rat. Caldwell et al. (11) used ^{14}C-phenobarbital in Wistar rats to compare the excretion of metabolites after single and repeated doses. The rate of appearance of the isotope in the urine and feces did not change on prolonged dosing. In contrast, in studies in our laboratory (4) comparing 3-day urine and fecal recovery in two groups of Sprague Dawley rats, induced and noninduced, we found a significantly lower recovery of total radioactivity in the induced rats than the noninduced rats. This result would be consistent with the effect of induction on metabolites, in addition to PBOH in the rat resulting in a decreased fraction of the dose metabolized to PBOH or excreted as phenobarbital. The pathway of metabolism involved at this time is unknown as only 40% to 50% of the phenobarbital dose in the rat has been isolated and identified.

SUMMARY

In spite of decades of use and the introduction of other agents, phenobarbital has remained the most widely used antiepileptic drug in the world. Although the main pathways of phenobarbital clearance have been identified, our knowledge of its quantitative disposition is based on a series of observations rather than definitive studies. This is surprising in light of recent advances in analytical and enzymatic techniques. Few studies have been performed in the last few years and today we remain with a large discrepancy between the degree of investigation and the degree of use. For example, phenobarbital is widely used in children but disposition in this population is virtually unknown. Definitive quantitative investigations of phenobarbital metabolism are still warranted.

REFERENCES

1. Algeria, E. J., and McBay, A. J. (1956): Metabolite of phenobarbital in human urine. *Science,* 123:183–184.
2. Aliprandi, B., and Masironi, R. (1958): Research on radioactive barbiturates: Distribution of phenobarbital in the animal organism. *Ric. Sci.,* 28:1611–1615.
3. Anderson, G. D. (1987): The interaction of phenobarbital and valproic acid in the rat. Dissertation, University of Washington, Seattle, Washington.
4. Anderson, G. D., and Levy, R. H. (1985): Phenobarbital/valproic acid interaction in the isolated perfused rat liver (abstract). *APHA Academy of Pharmaceutical Sci.,* 15:158.
5. Anderson, G. D., and Levy, R. H. (1987): Effect of valproic acid on the elimination of phenobarbital and parahydroxyphenobarbital in the rat (abstract). *J. Pharm. Sci.,* 76:S39.
6. Bhargava, V. O., and Garrettson, L. K. (1985): Phenobarbital glucosidation in the human neonate (abstract). *APHA Academy of Pharmaceutical Sci.,* 15:147.
7. Bhargava, V. O., Soine, W. H., and Garrettson, L. K. (1985): High performance liquid chromatographic analysis of 1-(β-D-glucopyranosyl)-phenobarbital in urine. *J. Chromatogr.,* 343:219–223.
8. Boréus, L. O., Jalling, B., and Kållberg, N. (1978): Phenobarbitral metabolism in adults and in newborn infants. *Acta Paediatr. Scand.,* 67:193–200.
9. Browne, T. R., Evans, J. E., Szabo, G. K., Evans, B. A., and Greenblatt, D. J. (1985): Studies with stable isotopes II: Phenobarbital pharmacokinetics during monotherapy. *J. Clin. Pharmacol.,* 25:51–58.
10. Butler, T. C. (1956): The metabolic hydroxylation of phenobarbital. *J. Pharmacol. Exp. Ther.,* 116:326–336.
11. Caldwell, J., Croft, J. E., Smith, R. L., and Snedden, W. (1977): The metabolic fate of [^{14}C]-phenobarbital in the rat and the effect of chronic administration and dose size. *Br. J. Pharmacol.,* 60:295P–296P.
12. Curry, A. S. (1955): A note on a urinary metabolite of phenobarbitone. *J. Pharm. Pharmacol.,* 7:1072–1073.
13. Danhof, M., and Levy, G. (1984): Kinetics of drug action in disease states. I. Effect of infusion rate on phenobarbital concentrations in serum, brain and cerebrospinal fluid of normal rats at onset of loss of righting reflex. *J. Pharmacol. Exp. Ther.,* 229:44–50.
14. Duggan, D. E., Baldwin, J. J., Arison, B. H., and Rhodes, R. E. (1974): N-Glucoside formation as a detoxification mechanism in mammals. *J. Pharmacol. Exp. Ther.,* 190:563–569.
15. Dutton, G. J. (1980): *Glucuronidation of Drugs and other Compounds.* CRC Press Inc., Boca Raton, Florida.
16. Gary, N. E., and Tresznewsky, O. (1983): Barbiturates and a potpourri of other sedatives, hypnotics and tranquilizers. *Heart and Lung,* 12:122–127.
17. Harvey, D. U., Glazner, L., Stratton, G., Nowlin, J., Hill, R. M., and Horning, M. (1972): Detection of a 5-(3,4-dihydroxy-1,5-cyclohexadien-1-yl)-metabolite of phenobarbital and mephobarbital in rat, guinea pig, and human. *Res. Commun. Chem. Pathol. Pharmacol.,* 3:557–565.
18. Horning, E. C., and Horning, M. G. (1971): Metabolic profiles. The study of human metabolites by gas phase analytical methods. *Clin. Chem.,* 17:802–809.
19. Hvidberg, E. F., and Dam, M. (1976): Clinical pharmacokinetics of anticonvulsants. *Clin. Pharmacokinet.,* 1:161–188.
20. Kalow, W., Kadar, D., Inaba, T., and Tang, B. K. (1977): A case of deficiency of N-hydroxylation of amobarbital. *Clin. Pharmacol. Ther.,* 21:530–535.
21. Kapetanovic, I. M., and Kupferberg, H. J. (1981): Inhibition of microsomal phenobarbital metabolism by valproic acid. *Biochem. Pharmacol.,* 30:1361–1363.
22. Kapetanovic, I. M., Kupferberg, H. J., Porter, R. J., Theodore, W., Schulman, E., and Penry, J. K. (1981): Mechanism of valproate-phenobarbital interaction in epileptic patients. *Clin. Pharmacol. Ther.,* 29:480–486.
23. Kapetanovic, I. M., Sweeney, D. J., and Rapoport, S. I. (1982): Phenobarbital pharmacokinetics in rats as a function of age. *Drug Met. Disp.,* 10:586–588.
24. Levin, S. S., Vars, H. M., Schleyer, H., and Cooper, D. Y. (1986): The metabolism and excretion of enzyme-inducing doses of phenobarbital by rats with bile fistulas. *Xenobiotica,* 16:213–224.
25. Lous, P. (1954): Blood serum and cerebrospinal fluid levels and renal clearance of phenemal in treated epileptics. *Acta Pharmacol. Toxicol. (Kbh.),* 10:261–280.
26. Maynert, E. W. (1982): Phenobarbital: Biotransformation. In: *Antiepileptic Drugs,* 2nd edition, edited by D. M. Woodbury, J. K. Penry, and C.

E. Pippenger, pp. 319–327. Raven Press, New York.

27. Maynert, E. W., and van Dyke, H. B. (1949): The metabolism of barbiturates. *Pharmacol. Rev.,* 1:217–242.

28. Patel, I. H., Levy, R. H., and Cutler, R. E. (1980): Phenobarbital-valproic acid interaction. *Clin. Pharmacol. Ther.,* 27:515–521.

29. Rane, A. (1978): Clinical pharmacokinetics of antiepileptic drugs in children. *Pharmacol. Ther.,* 2:251–267.

30. Raven-Jonsen, A., Lundin, M., and Secher, O. (1969): Excretion of phenobarbitone in urine after intake of large doses. *Acta Pharmacol. Toxicolo, (Kbh),* 27:193–201.

31. Remmer, H., and Siegert, M. (1962): Kumulation and elimination von phenobarbital. *Naunyn-Schmiedeberg's Arch. Exp. Path. U. Pharmak.,* 243:479–494.

32. Seago, A., and Garrod, J. W. (1987): The *in vitro* metabolism of [14C] pentobarbitone and [14C] phenobarbital by hamster liver microsomes. *J. Pharm. Pharmacol.,* 39:84–89.

33. Taburet, A. M., and Aymard, P. (1983): Valproate glucuronidation by rat liver microsomes. Interaction with parahydroxyphenobarbital. *Biochem. Pharmacol.,* 32:3859–3861.

34. Tang, B. K., and Carro-Ciampi, G. (1980): A method for the study of N-glucosidation *in vitro*— Amobarbital-N-glucoside formation in incubations with human liver. *Biochem. Pharmacol.,* 29:2085–2088.

35. Tang, B. K., Kalow, W., and Grey, A. A. (1978): Amobarbital metabolism in man: N-glucoside formation. *Res. Commun. Chem. Pathol. Pharmacol.,* 21:45–53.

36. Tang, B. K., Kalow, W., and Grey, A. A. (1979): Metabolic fate of phenobarbital in man. N-glucoside formation. *Drug Metab. Dispos.,* 7:315–318.

37. Tang, B. K., Yilmaz, B., and Kalow, W. (1984): Determination of phenobarbital, p-hydroxyphenobarbital and phenobarbabital-N-glucoside in urine by gas chromatography chemical ionization mass spectrometry. *Biomed. Mass Spectrom.,* 11:462–465.

38. Treston, A. M., Philippides, A., Jacobsen, N. W., Eadie, M. J., and Hooper, W. D. (1987): Identification and synthesis of 0-methylcatechol metabolites of phenobarbital and some n-alkyl derivatives. *J. Pharm. Sci.,* 76:496–501.

39. Viswanathan, C. T., Booker, H. E., and Welling, P. G. (1979): Pharmacokinetics of phenobarbital following single and repeated doses. *J. Clin. Pharmacol.,* 19:282–289.

40. Waddell, W. J., and Butler, T. C. (1957): Distribution and excretion of phenobarbital. *J. Clin. Invest.,* 36:1217–1226.

41. Whyte, M. P., and Dekaban, A. S. (1977): Metabolic fate of phenobarbital. A quantitative study of p-hydroxyphenobarbital elimination in man. *Drug Metab. Disp.,* 5:63–70.

Antiepileptic Drugs, Third Edition, edited by
R. Levy, R. Mattson, B. Meldrum,
J. K. Penry, and F. E. Dreifuss.
Raven Press, Ltd., New York © 1989.

21

Phenobarbital

Interactions with Other Drugs

Henn Kutt

INTRODUCTION

Interactions between phenobarbital and other drugs result in alterations of pharmacokinetic or pharmacodynamic parameters of the involved agents. Information on these interactions is still limited. Observations of alterations of pharmacokinetic parameters, however, are numerous. The majority of these deal with situations in which phenobarbital has caused changes in the kinetics of other drugs. Situations where other drugs alter phenobarbital kinetics are relatively fewer. The kinetic interactions are usually documented from the measurements of plasma concentrations of the drug and expressed as change of maximal blood level (C_{max}), steady-state blood level (C_{ss}), clearance (Cl), elimination half-life ($T_{1/2}$), and volume of distribution (V_d). Area under the curve (AUC) of concentrations measured after a dose is another parameter. Sometimes the biotransformation products are measured as well.

The clinical significance of phenobarbital interactions with other drugs varies. Practically no drug combination with phenobarbital is incompatible. Only a few drugs in combination with phenobarbital cause predictable changes in the majority of patients and lead to the need for adjusted dosages. Furthermore, the same drug combination with phenobarbital may lower the plasma drug concentration in some patients, cause no change in others, and raise the concentration in still others. The variability in response is best understood by accepting the fact that not all patients are genetically alike, nor are the clinical conditions alike with regard to previous drug history and current drug dosages. Thus, it is not necessarily contradictory or conflicting if reported results of different studies disagree or point in opposite directions with the same drug combinations.

MECHANISMS INVOLVED IN PHARMACOKINETIC INTERACTIONS

Changes in Absorption

Phenobarbital is usually almost completely absorbed, and there have been no reports of its absorption being directly altered by other drugs through chelation. It is conceivable that drugs that greatly facilitate intestinal motility and emptying time may reduce the amount of drug absorbed. In particular, activated charcoal reduces phenobarbital absorption, which is relevant in the early treatment of phenobarbital overdose (64,91).

It has been suspected that absorption of griseofulvin (76) is reduced by phenobarbital and phenobarbital may cause a modest reduction of cimetidine absorption (83).

Changes in Protein Binding

Only approximately 50% of phenobarbital is bound to plasma protein. Therefore it is unlikely that it would displace other drugs or be displaced by other drugs to any significant extent. This mechanism has not yet been implicated as a major factor in any of the reported interactions.

Altered Biotransformation

Induction and inhibition of biotransformation are key elements in the majority of the reported interactions between phenobarbital and other drugs, with induction being far more prevalent.

Induction of Drug Metabolism by Phenobarbital

Phenobarbital is the prototype among inducers of the hepatic mixed-function oxidase system which affects the biotransformation of numerous drugs and endogenous substances. The important components of this system affecting electron transport and oxygen transfer include cytochrome P-450 (which may exist in several subforms) and NADPH-cytochrome *c* reductase, contained predominantly in the smooth-membraned endoplastic reticulum of the liver cells. The heme component of membrane-bound cytochrome P-450 is ferroprotoporphyrin IX; the compound requires close association with phospholipid phosphatidylcholine for proper functioning. Several other hepatic enzymes, such as UDP-glucuronyl transferase and those involved in glucuronic acid synthesis, are utilized for conjugation of drug metabolites with glucuronic acid (14,86).

Mechanism of Induction by Phenobarbital

The mode of action by which phenobarbital produces induction is complex and only partially understood. It appears that both an increase of production and a decrease of degradation of enzymes occur (86). Thus, actinomycin D, an inhibitor of DNA-RNA transcription, reduces or prevents induction by phenobarbital (67). There is evidence that phenobarbital stabilizes the messenger RNA, perhaps by inhibiting the ribonuclease activity (24,57). The changes in turnover of microsomal protein caused by phenobarbital are thought to be due to stabilization of lysosomes or inhibition of lysosomal enzymes. The increase of phospholipid concentration is thought to be due to a decrease of phospholipid degradation (31). One of the current concepts is that induction of cytochrome P-450 by phenobarbital is mediated at the level of transcription (71).

There is some evidence that phenobarbital induces its own metabolism in animals to a modest extent (14). There is no clinical or laboratory evidence that autoinduction of phenobarbital metabolism occurs in humans. The recently introduced technique using stable isotope-labeled substrate is helpful in further investigations (9).

Induction in Animals

Treatment of rats with phenobarbital in doses of 50 to 75 mg/kg for 3 to 7 days causes an increase of total liver weight and a proliferation of endoplasmic reticulum demonstrable with electron microscopy. The content of microsomal protein per gram of liver increases as do the concentrations of cytochrome P-450, NADPH-cytochrome *c* reductase, and UDP-glucuronyl transferase, as well as phospholipids. The activity (V_{max}) of various steps involved in drug metabolism, such as hydroxylation and dealkylation of a number of endogenous (such as steroids) and exogenous (drugs) substrates, is increased considerably following phenobarbital treatment, as has been shown *in vitro* with isolated microsomal preparations. Figure 1 shows the increase of phenytoin hydroxylation by rat liver microsomes following phenobarbital treatment. A twofold increase of V_{max} was seen with both the washed microsomes and the 9,000 × *g* supernatant, the latter containing microsomes and the hepatic soluble fraction (43). Other substrates commonly used to demonstrate the induction of microsomal drug metabolism by phenobarbital are hexobarbital, aniline, benzphetamine, and ethylmorphine, among others. The activity with some of these substrates may increase up to sixfold following phenobarbital treatment (14,86).

The substrate-induced difference spectra, Type I and Type II, are both enhanced in the microsomes from phenobarbital-treated animals, although phenobarbital itself is a Type I substrate (45).

The induced changes last for several days following discontinuation of phenobarbital administration and then slowly decline. The extent of inducibility by phenobarbital is to a degree related to its dose but is saturable. Furthermore, there are species differences in the extent of induction as well as differences among strains in the same animal species that are thought to be genetically determined (86,88).

Induction in Man

Changes analogous to those seen in animals have been observed in the hepatic mixed-function oxidase system of humans following treatment with phenobarbital. Lecamwasam et al. (48) gave phenobarbital in a dose of 90 mg daily for 7 days to patients with Hodgkin's disease who were scheduled to undergo laparotomy and liver biopsy. There was an increase of microsomal protein, and the cytochrome P-450 content

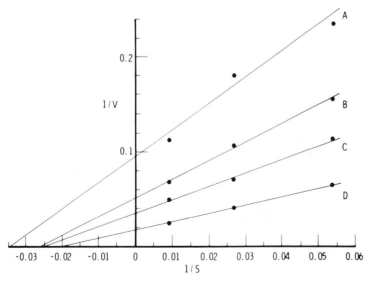

FIG. 1. Increase of phenytoin metabolism by phenobarbital in rat liver microsomal preparations. **A**, activity in washed control microsomes; **B**, activity in control 9,000 × *g* supernatant; **C**, activity in washed microsomes following phenobarbital treatment in animals; **D**, activity in 9,000 × *g* supernatant following phenobarbital treatment in animals. Phenobarbital dose: 75 mg/kg for 7 days. Based on data of Kutt and Fouts (43).

was found in eight patients to be nearly twice that in subjects without phenobarbital treatment. The hexobarbital oxidase activity was doubled, and the urinary excretion of D-glucaric acid increased severalfold. Other investigators have made similar observations regarding P-450 content in liver biopsy material from patients treated sporadically with phenobarbital (72). With higher phenobarbital doses (180 mg daily), an increase of UDP-glucuronyl transferase was also observed (6). In an epileptic patient, needle biopsy of liver revealed an increase of P-450, NADPH-cytochrome c reductase, and drug-oxidizing activity (80). Thus, the biochemical parameters of induction by phenobarbital can be observed in man. Determination of a test-drug half-life before and after phenobarbital treatment, such as antipyrine which undergoes complete hepatic biotransformation, has been utilized as an indicator of induction. Although not an ideal representative of all drugs, the changes of antipyrine half-life seem to provide some clinically useful evidence of induction of microsomal enzymes by phenobarbital (69,78,89).

Effect of Age and Environment on Induction

Induction of the mixed-function oxidase system by phenobarbital in man is influenced to some extent by environmental factors as well as by the age and possibly the sex of the subject. The age may not matter so much directly, but younger subjects may have had less contact with inducing agents than older subjects. There is little evidence that sex has a great influence, but empirically, females are sometimes somewhat better inducers than males (88).

Environmental factors that influence the response of a given patient to the inducing effect of phenobarbital are lifestyle and previous drug history. Chronic consumption of alcohol has some inducing effect per se, but it also causes liver damage that may alter the response to induction by phenobarbital. Other influences are tobacco smoking and probably a variety of environmental and food chemicals, all having an inducing effect to some degree. Previous and/or current contact with other drugs or medications may have some inducing effects and thus possibly reduce the phenobarbital effect (88).

Genetic Influence on Induction in Man

Genetic influence on the extent of induction by phenobarbital has been well documented. It appears that there are individuals with genetically determined high inducing capacity as well as subjects in whom only modest induction takes place. A good example is Vesell and Page's study (90) of pairs of identical and fraternal twins (see Fig. 2). The overall induction of antipyrine metabolism by phenobarbital, evidenced by shortening of antipyrine half-life, varied in this study from 0 to 68% among individual subjects. However, the extent of induction in each of the identical twins within a pair was nearly identical despite different living habits (intrapair difference, 0 to 2.6%). In the fraternal twins, on the other hand, the intrapair differences in inducibility ranged from 8% to 31%. It has not yet been ascertained what genetic structures or mechanisms regulate the inducibility of the mixed-function oxidase system, but it is clear from the results with identical twins that heredity has a strong influence on the extent of inducibility by phenobarbital.

In practical terms, then, the effects of induction by phenobarbital on other drugs in individual patients are largely unpredictable. In subjects with genetically high inducing capacity and little environmental inducer contact, the phenobarbital effect may be noticeable and require adjustment of the induced drug dosage. In others with genetically low inducing capability and consid-

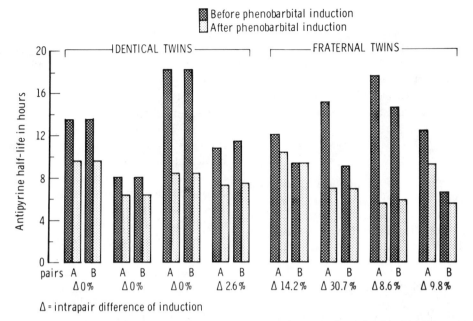

FIG. 2. Genetic influence on induction of drug metabolism by phenobarbital in humans. The intrapair difference in the extent of shortening of antipyrine half-life varied from 0 to 2.6% in identical twins in contrast with 8.6 to 31% variation in fraternal twins. Based on data of Vesell and Page (90).

erable environmental inducer contact, the effect is negligible. Empirically, only a few drug combinations with phenobarbital are predictable candidates for clinically significant interactions based on phenobarbital as an inducer. The effects of the inducer usually become noticeable within days or early weeks of comedication and last a week or two after discontinuation of phenobarbital. Despite being an excellent inducer of drug metabolism in animals, phenobarbital in humans appears to be inferior to phenytoin (a modest inducer in animals) in this respect.

Inhibition of Drug Metabolism by Phenobarbital

Phenobarbital may also inhibit drug metabolism, particularly if it competes with another Type I drug as substrate. Thus, competitive inhibition of phenytoin hydroxylation has been demonstrated *in vitro* (44) and observed clinically in some patients (7,44). Inhibition of phenobarbital metabolism (parahydroxylation) by other drugs also occurs, most notably that caused by valproate (34,35). These events are described in detail below.

CLINICAL INTERACTIONS MANIFESTED IN CHANGES OF PHENOBARBITAL KINETICS BY OTHER DRUGS

Analgesics and Antipyretics

Dam and co-workers (16) reported a study in which four epileptic patients who were stabilized on phenobarbital monotherapy were given *dextropropoxyphene* in a dose of 65 mg three times a day for 6 days. A modest (10–15%) elevation of plasma phenobarbital levels occurred in all patients by the sixth day. As the rise in plasma phenobarbital level was small and dextropropoxyphene is seldom taken regularly in large amounts, it is likely that the need to change phenobarbital dosage with this drug combination would occur only rarely.

Antibiotics

An elevation of phenobarbital level was observed in a patient after *chloramphenicol* was added to the medication regimen. Phenobarbital clearance was reduced by 40% in this patient (40).

Other Antiepileptic Drugs

Accumulation of phenobarbital caused by *valproate* is probably one of the clinically most important interactions in this group since it occurs predictably in the majority of patients taking these two drugs together. The clinical manifestation was increasing somnolence, sometimes resulting in coma, within days or weeks after the initiation of valproate administration, and increased plasma phenobarbital while patients continued taking their usual doses of phenobarbital (10,92). This phenomenon is illustrated in Fig. 3. The rate and magnitude of phenobarbital accumulation vary among individual patients, being negligible in some but reaching double the initial value in others, and phenobarbital dosage reductions have been necessary in up to 80% of patients (19,92). Whether the dosage of phenobarbital needs to be reduced depends on the initial dosage and plasma phenobarbital level and the extent of the rise. The magnitude of the necessary dose reduction is best indicated by the rate of the rise of the plasma phenobarbital level.

In patients taking primidone the plasma level of derived phenobarbital also tends to rise, but not as predictably as in patients taking phenobarbital. The possibility that valproate reduces the conversion of primidone into phenobarbital has been offered as an explanation for the less predictable and sometimes smaller rise of the plasma level of phenobarbital derived from primidone (94).

The mechanism by which valproate causes phenobarbital accumulation is thought to involve inhibition of phenobarbital metabolism. Kapetanovic et al. (34) demonstrated that elimination of *para*-hydroxyphenobarbital in the urine declined by 30% following valproate administration, mainly because of a reduced output of the conjugated fraction of the metabolite, since the excretion of free *p*-hydroxyphenobarbital remained virtually unchanged after addition of valproate. No change in distribution volume accompanied this reduction of total body clearance of phenobarbital, which indicated inhibition of phenobarbital metabolism. Further experiments by the same authors utilizing rat liver microsomal preparations *in vitro* provided direct evidence that valproate inhibits phenobarbital hydroxylation (35). In another study, a decrease of urinary *p*-hydroxyphenobarbital was also noted following addition of valproate (10).

Whether or not this reduction of phenobarbital biotransformation is sufficient alone to explain the accumulation of a drug which is excreted unchanged to a great extent (20–40%) remains to be clarified. Another theoretically possible mechanism is a reduction of renal excretion of phenobarbital by valproate by lowering the pH. Measurements of plasma and urine pH of patients taking valproate, however, have not revealed drastic changes (10,34); thus, the role of pH in the mechanism of this interaction remains uncertain. It is of interest that short-chain fatty acids from another source, such as ketogenic diet, have also caused phenobarbital accumulation (54). Most likely, the valproate-induced phenobarbital accumulation is multifactorial.

In some patients, *phenytoin* has been

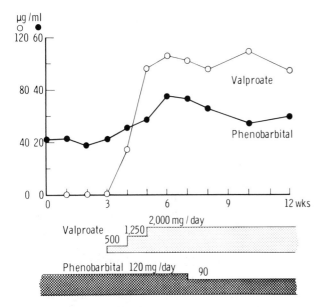

FIG. 3. Increase of plasma phenobarbital levels by valproate (*from author's unpublished case material.*)

noted to raise the plasma phenobarbital level. Also, the phenobarbital level fell in a few patients after phenytoin was discontinued (61,95). Eadie et al. (21) failed to find among 121 patients any significant elevations of plasma phenobarbital levels attributable to phenytoin, which is in accordance with our experience. Thus, elevation of plasma phenobarbital levels by phenytoin is generally an infrequent manifestation occurring, apparently, in susceptible individuals; if it does occur, it is rarely of significant magnitude. The mechanism could be inhibition of phenobarbital biotransformation, as both drugs are hydroxylated by hepatic microsomal enzymes.

It has been shown that *carbamazepine*, *clonazepam*, and *diazepam* usually do not alter plasma phenobarbital levels (42,68). However, *acetazolamide* (36), *phenylethylacetylurea* (68), and *methsuximide* (74), may cause a modest elevation of phenobarbital level.

The new experimental antiepileptic drug *flunarizine* was found to cause little if any change of phenobarbital level during comedication (4,23). Single doses of *lamotri-*

gine has no significant effect on phenobarbital kinetics (5). Only a modest elevation of phenobarbital level in some patients was caused by *progabide* (3). *Stiripentol* was found to reduce phenobarbital clearance somewhat (50). *Zonisamide* effect on phenobarbital kinetics was modest and variable (79).

Psychotropic Drugs

Elevations of phenobarbital levels in three out of five subjects occurred after addition of *thioridazine* (25). Phenothiazines, including *chlorpromazine*, *thioridazine*, or *prochlorperazine*, had a lowering effect on phenobarbital levels in psychiatric patients in another study (28).

CLINICAL INTERACTIONS MANIFESTED IN CHANGES OF KINETICS OF OTHER AGENTS BY PHENOBARBITAL

Analgesics and Antipyretics

Phenobarbital induces the metabolism of *antipyrine* (90) and *amidopyrine* (14) as evidenced by shortening of their half-lives. After addition of phenobarbital the trough and peak levels of *methadone* in a subject declined and allowed withdrawal signs and symptoms to occur with the previously adequate methadone maintenance dose (53). It is thought that phenobarbital induces *acetaminophen* metabolism and increases the production of a toxic product, which could be relevant in cases of acetaminophen overdose (18). *Meperidine* demethylation became accelerated, resulting in increased normeperidine concentration when phenobarbital was added; an increase in toxicity has been suggested to occur as a result of this interaction (85).

Antiasthma Agents

Phenobarbital given 90 mg daily for 4 weeks increased *theophylline* clearance by 33%. In another study a reduction of theophylline elimination half-life by 12% and an increase of clearance by 17% was seen in eight volunteers. The conclusion was that phenobarbital may increase the dosage requirement of theophylline (33).

Antibiotics

Induction of the metabolism of *chloramphenicol* by phenobarbital has been observed (41,93). Phenobarbital was observed to cause an increased elimination rate of *doxicycline* in patients receiving these drugs together (65). Decreased levels of *griseofulvin* have been noted in patients taking phenobarbital. It is thought that this manifestation is caused by interference with griseofulvin absorption, acceleration of its metabolism, or both (2).

Anticoagulants

The anticoagulant effects of *bishydroxycoumarin* and *warfarin* often decline after the start of phenobarbital administration (14,15,56). This leads to appropriate dosage adjustments of anticoagulants guided by prothrombin time determinations. Following discontinuation of phenobarbital, the anticoagulant dose is then readjusted. Because of present-day controlled management routines, which include continuous monitoring of prothrombin time and anticoagulant dosage adjustments, this potentially dangerous interaction seldom leads to grave consequences (38). Although the mechanism of anticoagulant activity reduction by phenobarbital is generally thought to be caused by induction of the anticoagulant metabolism, interference with absorption may also be partly involved. Thus, fecal excretion of bishydroxycoumarin after oral ingestion is doubled by barbiturates but remains unchanged when bishydroxycoumarin is administered intravenously.

Antiulcer Agents

Phenobarbital has been reported to reduce *cimetidine* blood levels, and increase of cimetidine clearance was observed in those patients. Urinary output of cimetidine products was reduced at the same time, suggesting that both induction of metabolism and reduction of absorption had occurred (83).

Immunosuppressants

Phenobarbital markedly reduced the levels and desired clinical effects of *cyclosporine* in a 4-year-old child (11). In animal experiments, cyclosporine nephrotoxicity was reduced by treatment with phenobarbital (81). The mechanism in these interactions was thought to be induction of cyclosporine metabolism.

Other Antiepileptic Drugs

Phenobarbital predictably induces *phenytoin* metabolism in experimental animals, doubling the rate in rats, for example (43). It also acts as a competitive inhibitor with phenytoin as substrate (44) since both drugs undergo parahydroxylation and glucuronidation. It appears that the effects of these interactions in humans often balance out, leading to no change or to only minor changes in the form of decline or elevation of plasma phenytoin levels. Furthermore, humans, unlike naive laboratory animals, are likely to be at least partially induced by previous drug contacts and/or food chemicals.

In clinical studies in which groups of patients taking phenytoin alone or phenytoin combined with phenobarbital were compared, the maintenance plasma phenytoin levels tended to be somewhat lower in the group on combined therapy (7,44,61,84). When individual patients were studied before and after the addition of phenobarbital to phenytoin, the plasma phenytoin levels declined in some, rose in others, and remained unchanged in still others, rarely leading to a need to readjust dosages (7,15,44,61). It is fair to assume that the patients who showed a more marked decline in plasma phenytoin levels are genetically "good inducers" or had less previous contact with inducing agents. The patients in whom a rise occurred, on the other hand, may already have been fully induced and/or had a low saturation point of the hydroxylating system. It also appears that in some patients, higher phenobarbital doses cause more marked changes in plasma phenytoin levels. Similarly, the changes tend to be greater when the starting plasma phenytoin levels are higher.

Phenobarbital may cause a decline of plasma *carbamazepine* levels in some patients. The plasma level of 10,11-carbamazepine epoxide, the pharmacologically active circulating carbamazepine metabolite, may also decline but to a smaller extent. This increases the ratio of metabolite to parent compound in the plasma (17,32,77). The extent of these changes varies from negligible or small in the majority of patients to considerable in some presumably good inducers, and in the latter patients, dosage readjustments may become necessary (47). If groups of patients who are taking carbamazepine alone and carbamazepine together with phenobarbital are compared, the plasma levels of carbamazepine tend to be somewhat higher in the group on monotherapy (12,13,32). It is worth mentioning here that phenytoin is a stronger inducer of carbamazepine metabolism than phenobarbital.

Valproate levels are often lower in patients taking it together with phenobarbital than in patients taking valproate alone (59,70). Valproate dosage adjustments may be necessary.

Induction of valproate metabolism by phenobarbital has potential relevance to hepatotoxicity of valproate. Recent studies (75) have shown that treatment of rats with phenobarbital increased the production of several valproate metabolites including the "4-en" (2-n-propyl-4-pentenoic acid). The latter compound has been shown to damage liver cells under experimental conditions (37,73). It is normally present in low amounts in subjects receiving valproate but was found in quite large amounts in a patient with fatal liver failure (39). The finding of increased 4-en production due to induction by phenobarbital is an important link in understanding the potential mechanism of valproate-induced hepatotoxicity. It is obvious, however, that additional risk factors (possibly genetic and/or environmental) have to be present to produce clinical hepatotoxicity since numerous patients have been and still are treated with phenobarbital and valproate without clinical liver complications.

Nor-methsuximide blood levels were found to be higher in epileptic patients receiving phenobarbital as comedication compared to those taking equivalent doses of methsuximide alone (74). *Flunarizine* levels were somewhat lower in patients who received combined medication including phenobarbital (4,23).

Psychotropic Drugs

Loga et al. (55) studied the effect of phenobarbital on blood *chlorpromazine* levels in a group of schizophrenic patients. After treatment for 2 weeks with 300 mg of chlorpromazine daily, the mean blood levels of chlorpromazine in six patients ranged from 25 to 35 ng/ml. Then, phenobarbital (150 mg daily) was given for 3 weeks. Soon after the onset of phenobarbital administration, blood chlorpromazine levels declined to near 20 ng/ml. Considerable interindividual variation was observed in the extent of decline of blood chlorpromazine levels caused by phenobarbital. Antipyrine half-lives determined before and after phenobarbital administration paralleled the decline of blood chlorpromazine levels. The clinical effectiveness of chlorpromazine evaluated by psychiatric rating scores was not considered to be adversely influenced by phenobarbital in these patients (46).

After addition of phenobarbital to the medication schedule, *thioridazine* levels changed little if any but there was a considerable reduction of active metabolite levels, i.e., mesoridazine (52). There was a marked drop of *haloperidol* levels after addition of phenobarbital with or without loss of psychotropic efficacy (52). Phenobarbital has been reported to cause a decline of plasma *desipramine* levels. In a group of epileptic patients whose medication included phenobarbital or primidone, the steady-state nortriptyline levels were lower than in nonepileptic patients (8). It thus appears that phenobarbital induction can lower the plasma levels of tricyclic antide-

pressant drugs, and it may be necessary to adjust dosages.

Miscellaneous Agents

Osteomalacia related to deficiency of *vitamin D* has occurred in some epileptic patients. Low plasma levels of 25-hydroxycholecalciferol, the active metabolite of vitamin D, are usually seen in these patients. Although the mechanism producing this manifestation appears to be complex and incompletely understood, induction of microsomal enzymes may be involved as well. Studies of the clearance rate of radioactive cholecalciferol indicated that the clearance was faster in induced (epileptic) patients than in normal subjects. Since the rate of synthesis of 25-hydroxycalciferol was the same in both groups, it was concluded that some of the calciferol was metabolized by a different route in the induced patients, producing inactive metabolites (30,69). Similar conclusions have been reached on the basis of animal experiments (27). Other environmental factors such as the amount of sunlight and the content of vitamin D in the diet seem to be the factors determining which patients develop clinical osteomalacia. Treatment of symptomatic patients is usually 4,000 units of vitamin D daily. The mono- and dihydroxy active metabolites of vitamin D have also been effective in experimental treatment programs. In a recent study vitamin D_2 was found primarily to increase the bone mass, and vitamin D_3 increased calcium excretion in patients treated with 4,000 units daily (87). Prophylactic treatment with vitamin D of patients taking phenobarbital is generally not recommended.

Several authors have reported contraceptive failures among epileptic women taking *oral steroid contraceptives* (62,69). Hempel and Klinger (29) reported that breakthrough bleeding occurred in over 50% of 52 subjects taking phenobarbital and was positively correlated with the phenobarbital dose. In the control population, the incidence of breakthrough bleeding was only 4%. Laboratory studies usually show reduced free hormone concentrations and an increase of sex hormone binding protein (SHBP). It is generally recommended that patients taking phenobarbital use medium or high dose steroid preparations (58,66).

Phenobarbital Effect on Endogenous Substances

The elimination of bilirubin is enhanced by phenobarbital. This effect has been utilized clinically to treat Gilbert's disease as well as newborns with hyperbilirubinemia. The need to have exchange transfusions was considerably reduced by phenobarbital treatment in infants (95). The metabolism of endogenous steroids is enhanced to some extent by phenobarbital, manifested by an increase of urinary excretion of 6-β-hydroxycortisol. No clinical problems have been ascribed to this manifestation. Bile salts, cholesterol, and lipids in plasma (51,69) as well as levels of folate (22) can be reduced by phenobarbital.

INDUCTION OF DRUG METABOLISM BY PHENOBARBITAL AS A POTENTIAL CAUSE OF INCREASED DRUG TOXICITY

In most instances the induction of drug metabolism by phenobarbital is expected to result in a reduction of the effects of other drugs. With some drugs, however, increased toxicity may occur, specifically if the induction causes an increased production of a metabolite that has toxic effects (26). Thus, phenobarbital enhances the production of 2-hydroxyphenetidin from acetophenetidin, particularly in patients whose normal metabolic pathways for acetophenetidin are deficient because of their genetic makeup (82). 2-Hydroxyphenetidin is responsible for methemoglobin formation. Similarly, induction increases the hepatotoxicity of acetaminophen by increasing the production of a toxic intermediary metabolite; this is particularly relevant in cases of acetaminophen overdose (18,60). Increase of toxicity from fluroxene in phenobarbital-induced subjects has been observed; the toxic metabolite is trifluoroethanol (63). There is also evidence that induction by phenobarbital increases the toxicity of various laboratory chemicals such as carbon tetrachloride and bromobenzene, the latter via enhanced production of the 3,4-epoxide metabolite (26). A phenobarbital dose-related increase of promotion of liver tumor production by nitrosamines has been demonstrated (20). The increase of potentially toxic valproate metabolites by phenobarbital induction (75) was discussed under valproate.

PHARMACODYNAMIC INTERACTIONS BETWEEN PHENOBARBITAL AND OTHER DRUGS

Little information is available on this subject. It has been suggested that antiepileptic drugs, including phenobarbital, reduce renal sensitivity to the diuretic action of frusemide (1). The earlier notions that phenobarbital might potentiate the effect of phenytoin at the sites of action probably are not true. Animal experiments evaluating the brain concentrations of these two drugs indicate that, if given together, the increase of anticonvulsant effect is additive and proportional to the sum of drug concentrations and does not demonstrate potentiation (49).

REFERENCES

1. Ahmad, S. (1974): Renal insensitivity to frusemide caused by chronic anticonvulsant therapy. *Br. Med. J.*, 2:657–659.

2. Beurey, J., Weber, M., and Vignaud, J. M. (1982): Treatment of tinea capitis: Metabolic interference of griseofulvin with phenobarbital. *Ann. Dermatol. Venereol.*, 109:567–570.

3. Bianchetti, G., Padovani, P., Thenot, J. P., Thiercelin, I. F., and Morselli, P. L. (1987): Pharmacokinetic interactions of progabide with other antiepileptic drugs. *Epilepsia*, 28:68–73.

4. Binnie, C. D., de Beukelaar, E., Meijer, J. W. A., Meinardi, H., Overweg, J., Wauquier, A., van Wieringen, A. (1985): Open dose-ranging trial of flunarizine as add-on therapy in epilepsy. *Epilepsia*, 26:424–428.

5. Binnie, C. D., van Emde Boas, W., Kasteleijn-Noliste-Trenite, D. G. A., de Korte, R. A., Meijer, J. W. A., Meinardi, H., Miller, A. A., Overweg, J., Peck, A. W., van Wieringen, A., and Yuen, W. C. (1986): Acute effects of lamotrigine (BW 430C) in persons with epilepsy. *Epilepsia*, 27:248–254.

6. Black, M., Perret, R. D., and Carter, A. E. (1973): Hepatic bilirubin UDP-glucuronyl transferase activity and cytochrome P-450 content in surgical population and the effect of preoperative drug therapy. *J. Lab. Clin. Med.*, 81:704–712.

7. Booker, H. E., Tormey, A., and Toussaint, J. (1971): Concurrent administration of phenobarbital and diphenylhydantoin: Lack of an interference effect. *Neurology (Minneap.)*, 21:383–385.

8. Braithwaite, R. A., Flanagan, R. A., and Richens, A. (1975): Steady state plasma nortriptyline concentrations in epileptic patients. *Br. J. Clin. Pharmacol.*, 2:469–471.

9. Browne, T. R., Evans, V. E., Szabo, G. K., Evans, B. A., and Greenblatt, D. J. (1985): Studies with stable isotopes II: Phenobarbital pharmacokinetics during monotherapy. *Clin. Pharmacol.*, 25:51–58.

10. Bruni, J., Wilder, B. J., Perchalski, R. J., Hammond, E. J., and Villarreal, H. J. (1980): Valproic acid and plasma levels of phenobarbital. *Neurology (Minneap.)*, 30:94–97.

11. Cartstensen, H., Jacobsen, N., and Dieperink, H. (1986): Interaction between cyclosporin and phenobarbitone. *Br. J. Clin. Pharmacol.*, 21:550–551.

12. Cereghino, J. J., van Meter, J. C., Brock, J. T., Penry, J. K., Smith, L. D., and White, B. G. (1973): Preliminary observations of serum carbamazepine concentration in epileptic patients. *Neurology (Minneap.)*, 23:357–366.

13. Christiansen, J., and Dam, M. (1973): Influence of phenobarbital and diphenylhydantoin on plasma carbamazepine levels in patients with epilepsy. *Acta Neurol. Scand.*, 49:543–546.

14. Conney, A. H. (1967): Pharmacological implications of microsomal enzyme induction. *Pharmacol. Rev.*, 19:317–366.

15. Cucinell, S. A., Conney, A. H., Sansur, M. S., and Burns, J. J. (1965): Drug interactions in man. I. Lowering effect of phenobarbital on plasma levels of bishydroxycoumarin (Dicumarol) and diphenylhydantoin (Dilantin). *Clin. Pharmacol. Ther.*, 6:420–429.

16. Dam, M., Christensen, J. M., Brandt, J., Hansen, B. S., Hvidberg, E. F., Angelo, H., and Lous, P. (1980): Antiepileptic drugs: Interaction with dextropropoxyphene. In: *Antiepileptic Therapy: Advances in Drug Monitoring*, edited by S. I. Johannessen, P. L. Morselli, C. E. Pippenger, A. Richens, D. Schmidt, and H. H. Meinardi, pp. 299–304. Raven Press, New York.

17. Dam, M., Jensen, A., and Christiansen, J. (1975): Plasma levels and effect of carbamazepine in grand mal and psychomotor epilepsy. *Acta Neurol. Scand.* (Suppl.), 60:33–38.

18. Davis, M., Simmons, C., Harrison, N. G., and Williams, R. (1976): Paracetamol overdose in man: Relationship between pattern of urinary metabolites and severity of liver damage. *Q. J. Med.*, 45:181–191.

19. de Gatta, M. R. F., Gonzales, A. C. A., Sanchez, M. J. G., Hurle, A. D. G., Borbujo, J. S., and Corral, L. M. (1986): Effect of sodium valproate on phenobarbital serum levels in children and adults. *Ther. Drug Monit.*, 8:416–420.

20. Driver, H. E., and McLean, A. E. M. (1986): Dose-response relationship of phenobarbitone promotion of liver tumors initiated by single dose dimethylnitrosamine. *Br. J. Exp. Pathol.*, 67:131–139.

21. Eadie, M. J., Lander, C. M., Hooper, W. D., and Tyrer, J. H. (1977): Factors influencing plasma phenobarbitone levels in epileptic patients. *Br. J. Clin. Pharmacol.*, 4:541–547.

22. Eadie, M. J., Lander, C. M., and Tyrer, J. H. (1977): Plasma drug level monitoring in pregnancy. *Clin. Pharmacokinet.*, 2:427–436.

23. Fröscher, W., Bulau, P., Burr, W., Penin, H., Rao, M. L., de Beukelaar, F. (1988): Double-blind placebo-controlled trial with flunarizine in therapy-resistant epileptic patients. *Clin. Neuropharmacol.* 232–240.

24. Fonne, R., and Meyer, U. A. (1987): Mechanism of phenobarbital-type induction of cytochrome P-450 isozymes. *Pharmacol. Ther.*, 33:19–22.

25. Gay, P. E., and Madsen, J. A. (1983): Interaction between phenobarbital and thioridazine. *Neurology*, 33:631–632.

26. Gillette, J. R. (1974): A perspective on the role of chemically reactive metabolites of foreign compounds in toxicity. *Biochem. Pharmacol.*, 28:2927–2938.

27. Hahn, T. J., Birge, S. J., Shapp, C. R., and Avioli, L. V. (1972): Phenobarbital-induced alterations in vitamin D metabolism. *J. Clin. Invest.*, 51:741–748.

28. Haydukewyck, D., and Rodin, E. A. (1985): Effects of phenothiazine on serum antiepileptic drug concentrations in psychiatric patients with seizure disorder. *Ther. Drug Monit.*, 7:401–405.

29. Hempel, E., and Klinger, W. (1976): Drug stimulated biotransformation of hormonal steroid contraceptives: Clinical implications. *Drugs*, 12:442–448.

30. Hunter, J. (1976): Effects of enzyme induction on vitamin D_3 metabolism in man. In: *Anticonvulsant Drugs and Enzyme Induction*, edited by A. Richens and F. P. Woodford, pp. 77–84. Elsevier/Excerpta Medica/North-Holland, New York.

31. Infante, R., Petit, D., Polonovski, J., and Caroli, J. (1971): Microsomal phospholipid biosynthesis after phenobarbital administration. *Experientia*, 27:640–642.

32. Johannessen, S. I., and Strandjord, R. E. (1975): The influence of phenobarbitone and phenytoin on carbamazepine serum levels. In: *Clinical Pharmacology of Antiepileptic Drugs*, edited by H. Schneider, D. Janz, C. Gardner-Thorpe, H. Meinardi, and A. Sherwin, pp. 201–205. Springer-Verlag, Berlin.

33. Jonkman, J. H. G., and Upton, R. A. (1984): Pharmacokinetic drug interactions with theophylline. *Clin. Pharmacokinet.*, 9:309–334.

34. Kapetanovic, I. M., Kupferberg, H. J., Porter, R. J., and Penry, J. K. (1980): Valproic acid-phenobarbital interaction: A systematic study using stable isotopically labeled phenobarbital in an epileptic patient. In: *Antiepileptic Therapy: Advances in Drug Monitoring*, edited by S. I. Johannessen, P. L. Morselli, C. E. Pippenger, A. Richens, D. Schmidt, and H. Meinardi, pp. 373–380. Raven Press, New York.

35. Kapetanovic, I. M., Kupferberg, H. J., Porter, R. J., Theodore, W., Schulman, E., and Penry, J. K. (1981): Mechanism of valproate-phenobarbital interaction in epileptic patients. *Clin. Pharmacol. Ther.*, 29:480–486.

36. Kelly, W. N., Richardson, A. P., Mason, M. F., and Rector, F. C. (1966): Acetazolamide in phenobarbital intoxication. *Arch. Intern. Med.*, 117:64–69.

37. Kesterson, J. W., Granneman, G. R., and Machinist, J. M. (1984): The hepatotoxicity of valproic acid and its metabolites in rats. I. Toxicologic, biochemical and histopathologic studies. *Hepatology (Baltimore)*, 4:1143.

38. Kleinman, P. D., and Griner, P. F. (1970): Studies of the epidemiology of anticoagulant drug interactions. *Arch. Intern. Med.*, 126:522–523.

39. Kochen, W., Schneider, A., and Ritz, A. (1983): Abnormal metabolism of valproic acid in fatal hepatic failure. *Eur. J. Pediatr.*, 141:30–35.

40. Koup, J. R., Gibaldi, M., McNamara, P., Hilligoss, D. M., Coburn, W. A., and Bruck, E. (1978): Interaction of chloramphenicol with phenytoin and phenobarbital. *Clin. Pharmacol. Ther.*, 24:571–575.

41. Krasinski, K., Kusmiesz, H., and Nelson, J. D. (1982): Pharmacologic interactions among chloramphenicol, phenytoin and phenobarbital. *Pediatr. Infect. Dis.*, 1:232–235.

42. Kutt, H. (1984): Interactions between anticonvulsants and other commonly prescribed drugs. *Epilepsia* 25 (Suppl. 2), S118–S131.

43. Kutt, H., and Fouts, J. R. (1971): Diphenylhydantoin metabolism by rat liver microsomes and some of the effects of drug or chemical pretreatment on diphenylhydantoin metabolism by rat liver microsomal preparations. *J. Pharmacol. Exp. Ther.*, 176:11–26.

44. Kutt, H., Haynes, J., Verebely, K., and McDowell, F. (1969): The effect of phenobarbital on plasma diphenylhydantoin level and metabolism in man and rat liver microsomes. *Neurology (Minneap.)*, 19:611–616.

45. Kutt, H., Waters, L., and Fouts, J. R. (1971): The effects of some stimulators (inducers) of hepatic microsomal drug-metabolizing enzyme activity on substrate-induced difference spectra in rat liver microsomes. *J. Pharmacol. Exp. Ther.*, 179:101–113.

46. Lader, M. (1977): Drug interactions and the major tranquilizers. In: *Drug Interactions*, edited by D. G. Grahame-Smith, pp. 159–170. University Park Press, Baltimore.

47. Lander, C. M., Eadie, M. J., and Tyrer, J. H. (1977): Factors influencing plasma carbamazepine concentration. *Clin. Exp. Neurol.*, 14:184–193.

48. Lecamwasam, D. S., Franklin, C., and Turner, P. (1975): Effect of phenobarbitone on hepatic drug-metabolizing enzymes and urinary D-glucaric acid excretion in man. *Br. J. Clin. Pharmacol.*, 2:257–262.

49. Leppik, I. E., and Sherwin, A. (1977): Anticonvulsant activity of phenobarbital and phenytoin in combination. *J. Pharmacol. Exp. Ther.*, 200:570–575.

50. Levy, R. H., Loisseau, P., Guyot, M., Blehaut, H. M., Tor, J., and Moreland, T. A. (1984): Stiripentol kinetics in epileptic patients: Nonlinearity and interactions. *Epilepsia*, 25:657.

51. Linarelli, L. G., Hengstenberg, F. H., and Drash, A. L. (1973): Effect of phenobarbital on hyperlipemia in patients with intrahepatic and extrahepatic cholestasis. *J. Pediatr.*, 83:291–293.

52. Linnoila, M., Viukari, M., Vaisanen, K., and Auvinen, J. (1980): Effect of anticonvulsants on plasma haloperidol and thioridazine levels. *Am. J. Psychiatry*, 137:819–821.

53. Liu, S. J., and Wang, R. I. H. (1984): Case report of barbiturate-induced enhancement of methadone metabolism and withdrawal syndrome. *A. J. Psychiatry*, 141:1287–1288.

54. Livingstone, S. (1972): *Comprehensive Management of Epilepsy in Infancy, Childhood and Adolescence*. Charles C Thomas, Springfield, Illinois.

55. Loga, S., Curry, S., and Lader, M. (1975): Interactions of orphenadrine and phenobarbitone with chlorpromazine: Plasma concentrations and effects in man. *Br. J. Clin. Pharmacol.*, 2:197–208.

56. MacDonald, M. G., and Robinson, D. S. (1968): Clinical observations of possible barbiturate interference with anticoagulation. *J.A.M.A.*, 204:97–100.

57. Matsumura, S., and Omura, T. (1973): The effects of phenobarbital on the turnover of messenger RNA's for microsomal enzymes. *Drug Metab. Dispos.*, 1:248–250.

58. Mattson, R. H., and Cramer, J. A. (1985): Epilepsy, sex hormones and antiepileptic drugs. *Epilepsia*, 26 (suppl. 1):S40–S55.

59. May, T., and Rambeck, B. (1985): Serum concentrations of valproic acid: Influence of dose and comedication. *Ther. Drug Monit.*, 7:387–390.

60. McLean, A. E. M., and Day, P. (1975): The effect of diet on the toxicity of paracetamol. *Biochem. Pharmacol.*, 23:37–42.

61. Morselli, P. L., Rizzo, M., and Garattini, S. (1971): Interaction between phenobarbital and diphenylhydantoin in animals and in epileptic patients. *Ann. N. Y. Acad. Sci.*, 179:88–107.
62. Mumford, J. P. (1974): Drugs affecting oral contraceptives. *Br. Med. J.*, 2:333–334.
63. Munson, E. S., Malagodi, M. H., Shields, R. P., Tham, M. K., Fiserova-Bergerova, V., Holaday, D. A., Perry, J. C., and Embro, W. J. (1975): Fluroxene toxicity induced by phenobarbital. *Clin. Pharmacol. Ther.*, 18:687–699.
64. Neuvonen, P. J., and Elonen, E. (1980): Effect of activated charcoal on absorption and elimination of phenobarbitone, carbamazepine and phenylbutazone in man. *Eur. J. Clin. Pharmacol.*, 17:51–57.
65. Neuvonen, P. J., Penttila, O., Lehtovaara, R., and Aho, K. (1975): Effects of antiepileptic drugs on the elimination of various tetracycline derivatives. *Eur. J. Clin. Pharmacol.*, 9:147–154.
66. Orme, M. L. E. (1982): Clinical pharmacology of oral contraceptive steroids. *Br. J. Clin. Pharmacol.*, 14:31–42.
67. Orrenius, S., Ericson, J. E., and Ernster, L. (1965): Phenobarbital-induced synthesis of the microsomal drug-metabolizing enzyme system and its relationship to the proliferation of endoplasmic membranes. *J. Cell. Biol.*, 25:627–639.
68. Perruca, E. (1982): Pharmacokinetic interactions with antiepileptic drugs. *Clin. Pharmacokinet.*, 7:57–84.
69. Perruca, E. (1987): Clinical implications of hepatic microsomal enzyme induction by antiepileptic drugs. *Pharmacol. Ther.*, 33:139–144.
70. Perucca, E., Gatti, G., Frigo, G. M., Crema, A., Calzetti, S., and Visintini, D. (1978): Disposition of sodium valproate in epileptic patients. *Br. J. Clin. Pharmacol.*, 5:495–499.
71. Pike, S. F., Shephard, E. A., Rabin, B. R., and Phillips, I. R. (1985): Induction of cytochrome P-450 by phenobarbital is mediated at the level of transcription. *Biochem. Pharmacol.*, 34:2489–2494.
72. Pirttiaho, H. I., Sotaniemi, E. A., Ahokas, J. T., and Pitkanen, J. (1978): Liver size and indices of drug metabolism in epileptics. *Br. J. Clin. Pharmacol.*, 6:273–278.
73. Prickett, K. S., and Baillie, T. A. (1986): Metabolism of unsaturated derivatives of valproic acid in rat liver microsomes and destruction of cytochrome P-450. *Drug Metab. Dispos.*, 14:221–229.
74. Rambeck, B. (1979): Pharmacological interactions of mesuximide with phenobarbital and phenytoin in hospitalized epileptic patients. *Epilepsia*, 20:147–156.
75. Rettie, A. E., Rettenmeier, A. W., Howald, W. N., and Baillie, T. A. (1987): Cytochrome P-450-catalyzed formation of delta-four VPA, a toxic metabolite of valproic acid. *Science*, 235:890–893.
76. Riegelman, S., Rowland, M., and Epstein, W. L. (1970): Griseofulvin-phenobarbital interactions in man. *J.A.M.A.*, 213:426–431.
77. Riva, R., Contin, M., Albani, F., Perucca, E., Procaccianti, G., and Baruzzi, A. (1985): Free concentration of carbamazepine and carbamazepine-10-11-epoxide in children and adults. Influence of age and phenobarbitone co-medication. *Clin. Pharmacokinet.*, 10:524–531.
78. Rosalki, S. B. (1976): Plasma enzyme changes and their interpretation in patients receiving anticonvulsant and enzmye-inducing drugs. In: *Anticonvulsant Drugs and Enzyme Induction*, edited by A. Richens and F. P. Woodford, pp. 27–35. Elsevier/Excerpta Medica/North Holland, New York.
79. Sackellares, J. G., Donofrio, P. D., Wagner, J., Abou-Khalil, B., Berent, S., and Aasved-Hoyt, K. (1985): Pilot study of zonisamide (1,2-benzisoxazole-3-methanesulfonamide) in patients with refractory partial seizures. *Epilepsia*, 26:206–211.
80. Schone, B., Fleischmann, R. A., Remmer, H., and von Oldershausen, H. P. (1972): Determination of drug-metabolizing enzymes in needle biopsies of human liver. *Eur. J. Clin. Pharmacol.*, 4:65–73.
81. Schwass, D. E., Sasaki, A. W., Houghton, D. C., Benner, K. E., and Bennett, W. M. (1986): Effects of phenobarbital and cimetidine on experimental cyclosporine nephrotoxicity: Preliminary observations. *Clin. Nephrol.*, 25 (suppl. 1):117–120.
82. Shahidi, N. T. (1968): Acetophenetiden-induced methemoglobinemia. *Ann. N.Y. Acad. Sci.*, 151:822–831.
83. Somogyi, A., and Gugler, R. (1982): Drug interaction with cimetidine. *Clin. Pharmacokinet.*, 7:23–41.
84. Sotaniemi, E., Arvela, P., Hakkarainen, H., and Huhti, E. (1970): The clinical significance of microsomal enzyme induction in the therapy of epileptic patients. *Ann. Clin. Res.*, 2:223–227.
85. Stambaugh, J. E., Hemphill, D. M., Wainer, I. W., and Schwartz, I. (1977): A potentially toxic drug interaction between pethidine (meperidine) and phenobarbital. *Lancet*, 1:398–399.
86. Testa, B., and Jenner, P. (1976): *Drug Metabolism: Chemical and Biochemical Aspects*. Marcel Dekker, New York, Basel.
87. Tjellesen, L., Gotfredsen, A., and Christiansen, C. (1985): Different actions of vitamin D_2 and D_3 on bone metabolism in patients treated with phenobarbitone/phenytoin. *Calcif. Tissue Int.*, 37:218–222.
88. Vesell, E. S. (1977): Genetic and environmental factors affecting drug interactions in man. In: *Drug Interactions*, edited by D. G. Grahame-Smith, pp. 119–143. University Park Press, Baltimore.
89. Vesell, E. S. (1979): The antipyrine test in clinical pharmacology: Conceptions and misconceptions. *Clin. Pharmacol. Ther.*, 26:275–288.
90. Vesell, E. S., and Page, J. G. (1969): Genetic control of the phenobarbital-induced shortening of plasma antipyrine half-lives in man. *J. Clin. Invest.*, 48:2202–2209.
91. Welling, P. G. (1984): Interactions affecting drug absorption. *Clin. Pharmacokinet.*, 9:404–434.
92. Wilder, B. J., Willmore, L. J., Bruni, J., and Villarreal, H. J. (1978): Valproic acid: Interaction with other anticonvulsant drugs. *Neurology (Minneap.)*, 28:892–896.

93. Windorfer, A., Jr., and Pringsheim, W. (1977): Studies on the concentrations of chloramphenicol in the serum and cerebrospinal fluid of neonates, infants and small children. Reciprocal reactions between chloramphenicol, penicillin and phenobarbitone. *Eur. J. Pediatr.*, 124:129–138.

94. Windorfer, A., Jr., and Sauer, W. (1977): Drug interactions during anticonvulsant therapy in childhood: Diphenylhydantoin, primidone, phenobarbitone, clonazepam, nitrazepam, carbamazepine and dipropylacetate. *Neuropediatrie*, 8:29–41.

95. Yeung, C. Y., and Field, C. E. (1969): Phenobarbital therapy in neonatal hyperbilirubinaemia. *Lancet*, 2:135–139.

Antiepileptic Drugs, Third Edition, edited by
R. Levy, R. Mattson, B. Meldrum,
J. K. Penry, and F. E. Dreifuss.
Raven Press, Ltd., New York © 1989.

22

Phenobarbital

Clinical Use

Michael J. Painter

Phenobarbital, discovered in 1912, is the oldest anticonvulsant in common use, and is safe, effective, and inexpensive. However, conflicting reports exist regarding its effects on behavior and its teratogenicity and efficacy. This drug is largely confined to use in generalized tonic, clonic, tonic–clonic, and partial seizures in children or adults and most seizures in neonates. Its pharmacokinetic properties are such that phenobarbital achieves predictable plasma levels that are therapeutically efficacious with oral, intravenous, or intramuscular doses. Despite relatively slow equilibrium between brain and plasma, this drug retains a place in the treatment of status epilepticus. Phenobarbital, however, induces hepatic metabolism and alters the disposition of other drugs administered to patients.

USE IN NEONATAL SEIZURES

Among anticonvulsants used in the treatment of neonatal seizures, phenobarbital is the first drug most frequently chosen (19,28,33,47). The choice of phenobarbital in the treatment of neonatal seizures is not based on its proven superiority as an anticonvulsant agent but on tradition and many years of familiarity with this drug among pediatricians. Until the last decade, the use of phenobarbital for treatment of neonatal

seizures was based on empiric information of clinical response rather than plasma or brain tissue concentrations attained during therapy. The relatively recent knowledge that a significant number of clinically classified neonatal seizures are unaccompanied by electrical seizure patterns and are due to nonictal abnormal neonatal movement renders a discussion of the efficacy of any anticonvulsant, including phenobarbital, incomplete (31). Subcortical gray matter is relatively nonepileptogenic, but clinical and EEG seizure patterns have been described in an atelencephalic infant (8). The proportion of neonatal seizures that may have clinical expression without concomitant cortical electrical seizures is unknown. All studies describing the efficacy of phenobarbital in the treatment of neonatal seizures are based on clinical criteria of diagnosis and efficacy. Studies utilizing video-EEG monitoring for the proper diagnosis and treatment of neonatal seizures will certainly alter our current understanding of phenobarbital's place in their treatment.

It is apparent that the neonate does not metabolize phenobarbital in a manner that might be predicted from data obtained in older children and adults (28,33). All investigators agree that to obtain therapeutically effective but nontoxic concentrations of phenobarbital promptly, loading doses of

the drug should be administered intravenously. The volumes of distribution reported by Donn (12) (0.97 ± .18 l/kg) and
Lockman (28) (0.81 ± .12 l/kg) with loading
doses of 15 to 20 mg/kg indicate that a rather
predictable plasma level is achieved following the administration of loading doses
within these ranges. Both Lockman (17) and
Painter (32) have noted that plasma levels
of phenobarbital can be maintained in the
range of 20 μg/ml with doses of 3 to 4 mg/
kg/day following loading (17). The plasma
concentrations achieved and the calculated
volumes of distribution do not appear to differ significantly in infants of various gestational ages and are followed by a gradual
decrease in plasma levels. In infants subsequently treated with phenobarbital at 5
mg/kg/day orally as a maintenance dosage,
initial accumulation of the drug is noted. In
infants treated with a dosage regimen of 3
to 4 mg/kg/day, accumulation is not seen
and concentrations between 10 and 20 μg/
ml are maintained. The decreasing plasma
concentrations in infants sequentially followed from 7 to 28 days of therapy are reflected in a decreasing half-life of phenobarbital during exposure to this drug over
time. The plasma concentrations of phenobarbital do not bear a constant relationship
with gestational age but correlate well with
duration of phenobarbital therapy. Lockman (28) and Painter (33) noted that a clinical response to phenobarbital therapy is
uncommon below concentrations of 16 μg/
ml. In infants studied immediately following
death, brain-to-plasma ratios were found to
be 0.71 ± 0.21 in 15 neonates (33). Within
this population, there appeared to be a trend
to lower brain-to-plasma ratios with increasing plasma protein concentration. The
brain-to-plasma ratio appeared to be constant during phenobarbital therapy, and
there is no evidence of drug accumulation
in the brain. There is, however, a significant
increase in the brain-to-plasma ratio with
increasing gestational age. Tissue-to-
plasma ratios for liver, heart, and muscle
are significantly higher than those of brain.

TABLE 1. *Phenobarbital efficacy in neonatal seizures*

	Response rate	Loading doses
Lockman (1979)	32%	15–20 mg/kg
Painter (1981)	36%	15–20 mg/kg
Gal (1982)	85%	up to 40 mg/kg
VanOrman (1985)	33%	15–20 mg/kg

Three series show very close agreement
regarding the efficacy of phenobarbital as
the initial agent in the treatment of neonatal
seizures (Table 1). Lockman (28), in a
study of 39 neonates utilizing loading doses
of approximating 20 mg/kg, noted seizure
control in 32% of the infants. VanOrman
(47), in a study of 81 neonates who had received adequate loading doses of phenobarbital at 15 to 20 mg/kg, noted control in
33% of the population. Painter (33), in a
study of 77 neonates, noted that 36% of the
population was controlled following loading
doses of 15 to 20 mg/kg of phenobarbital.
Gal (19), however, reported efficacy of 85%
in 71 neonates in whom phenobarbital was
used as monotherapy, and doses as high as
40 mg/kg were given to achieve or surpass
plasma concentrations of 40 μg/ml. There
are significant differences in the response
of this population compared to the other series. Gal (19) had about a 60% response with
plasma levels achieved by the other authors, an almost twofold difference. In 13
infants with seizures due to hemorrhage,
Gal (19) noted an 85% success rate compared to an 11% success rate noted by
Painter and a 30% response reported by
VanOrman using phenobarbital alone or
phenobarbital and phenytoin in combination. The lack of specific seizure definition,
electrically or clinically, in all of these series makes the interpretations of the differences in data difficult, but there appears to
be a significant clinical difference in Gal's
population.

Although all potential toxicities of phenobarbital are important, two are of immediate

concern in neonates. First, as any change in heart rate in the neonate may not be accompanied by a change in stroke volume to maintain cardiac output, the cardiovascular effects of anticonvulsants are of paramount importance. Second, as the neonate represents a growing organism, the effects of phenobarbital on brain growth are of long-term concern. The potential toxicity of phenobarbital in the neonate has been inadequately addressed. All of the series previously summarized have noted only lethargy and no apparent change in cardiovascular status. In none of these series were sequential heart rates and blood pressures systematically recorded and reported. Svenningson (42) noted an invariable decrease in heart rate below 100 with lack of variability at plasma concentrations of 52 μg/ml. Donn (12) studied pharmacokinetic and cardiovascular parameters in 10 severely asphyxiated term newborns who were given loading doses of 30 mg/kg of phenobarbital intravenously over 15 min. Observations were made immediately before and 30 min after the loading dose. There was a trend to decreasing heart rate, respiratory rate, and increasing blood pressure, but the changes were not statistically significant. Since the time of maximum distribution of phenobarbital to the central nervous system is unknown but possibly as long as 60 min, an observation time of 30 min following the load may not have been sufficient. Observations of cardiovascular effects following phenobarbital administration need to be performed for a longer time following treatment, with preterm infants included.

Kuban et al. (22) evaluated the ventilatory requirements of 127 infants who received phenobarbital for 5 days compared to 111 infants who received placebo. All infants were intubated and weighed less than 1,750 grams at birth. Infants receiving phenobarbital did not require ventilatory assistance for more time than did those receiving placebo, but pneumothorax and pulmonary interstitial emphysema were more likely to develop in infants who had received phenobarbital. The mechanism of this complication is not clear, but infants receiving phenobarbital did not have more severe pulmonary disease.

In an elegant rat pup model controlled for nutrition, Diaz and Schain (9) noted that phenobarbital interferes with brain growth. Yanai et al. (51) also noted neuronal deficits in mice pups exposed to phenobarbital. As the metabolism and distribution of phenobarbital in the rat is significantly different from the human and the velocity of brain growth significantly different between species, the importance of these findings to humans is uncertain, but concerns regarding the effects of phenobarbital on central nervous system development in neonates are justified.

We noted that protein binding was significantly decreased in 11 neonates receiving phenobarbital for the treatment of neonatal seizures (32). Protein binding varied from 6% to 42%, representing a 50% decrease compared to values obtained in older children and adults. The problem appears most acute in the sick preterm infant, and great variability of protein binding among sequential measurements in individual patients and within the entire population was noted. Because autopsy studies in the frontal pole have demonstrated a trend to a higher brain-to-plasma ratio with decreasing plasma protein concentrations, protein binding is an important consideration when evaluating the efficacy and toxicity of phenobarbital in neonates.

USE IN INFANTS AND CHILDREN

Specific indications for use of phenobarbital for seizure types in children are similar to those for adults with a few exceptions. Dosage is different due to changing pharmacokinetics. Although there is a significant overlap among ages, there is a trend

TABLE 2. *Phenobarbital dose to achieve plasma concentrations of 16–25 mg/L relative to age*

Age groups	Loading dose	Maintenance dose
Neonates	20 mg/kg/i.v.	3–4 mg/kg/day p.o. or i.v.
Infants	6–8 mg/kg/d, p.o. for 2 days	3–4 mg/kg/d
Children and adults	10–20 mg/kg/i.v.	1–4 mg/kg/d

to decreasing dosage requirements of phenobarbital with increasing age (10,11,13,37) (Tables 2 and 3). This change is accompanied by a decrease in volume of distribution of phenobarbital with age, with ranges between 0.45 to 0.55 l/kg in adults, approximately half that reported in neonates. In young adults, phenobarbital half-life ranges from 53 to 140 hr, with an average of 96 hr. The range in neonates is wide: from 43 to 217 hr, with a median of 83 hr in 1 study and an average of 114.4 hr in another study. In one study six infants had an average half-life of 47 ± 8 hr by 2 months of age. Among children 1 to 15 years of age, a representative range of half-lives is from 37 to 73 hr. After the age of 15, the half-life and the clearance of phenobarbital remains stable until age 40. Rossi (37) studied the dosage of phenobarbital relative to age in children to achieve concentrations of 10 to 25 μg/ml. Infants from 2 months to 1 year of age require 2.31 ± 0.74 mg/kg, children ages 1 to 3 require 3.5 ± 0.99 mg/kg,

TABLE 3. *Phenobarbital dose to achieve plasma concentrations of 10–25 mg/L in children relative to age*

Age	Dose	Range
2 mos–1 yr	2.3 ± .7 mg/kg/d	4–11 mg/kg/d
1–3 yr	3.5 ± 1 mg/kg/d	3–7 mg/kg/d
3–6.5 yr	4.8 ± 2.3 mg/kg/d	2.2–5 mg/kg/d

Modified from Rossi et al., ref. 37.

and children from 3 to 6.5 years of age require 4.79 ± 1.31 mg/kg in order to achieve these plasma concentrations. There was a significant increase in dosage of phenobarbital per kilogram of body weight with increasing age, which is in accord with half-life values of 64 to 141 hr over 15 years of age, 37 to 73 hr from age 1 to 15, 47 ± 8 hr at 1 to 12 months, and 63 to 98 hr below 1 year of age. There is significant overlap within these populations. Infants from 2 months to 1 year of age required doses of 4 to 11 mg/kg/day, those from 1 to 3 years of age required 3 to 7 mg/kg/day, and those from 3 to 6.5 years of age required 2.2 to 5 mg/kg/day to achieve desired plasma levels.

Although one can anticipate a decreasing dose requirement for phenobarbital with increasing age, the interpatient metabolic variation is such as to require close monitoring of plaama concentrations at the beginning of therapy. Buchthal and Lennox-Buchthal (6) also observed that the elimination rate for phenobarbital in infants and children is much greater than in adults. As a rule, drugs reach their plateau after about 3.5 times their biological half-life, amounting to 3 weeks in the case of phenobarbital. During this interval, changes in dose will cause unpredictable changes in plasma level. In adolescents and adults, doses of approximately 1 to 1.3 mg/kg/day will result in concentrations between 10 and 16 μg/ml, which is in agreement with the linear regression curves calculated by Eadie et al. (13) showing little difference between ages 15 and 40 years. The available half-life data would indicate that only daily administration should provide adequate concentrations with minimal fluctuation in most children. In a study of 12 children aged 1.3 to 8.8 years, Watson (49) demonstrated no significant variation in plasma concentrations of phenobarbital when converting from multiple daily to single dose administrations. Watson (49) also noted that salivary concentrations of phenobarbital could be used to predict serum concentrations reliably.

Febrile Seizures

A major area of interest concerning phenobarbital use is in the prophylaxis of febrile seizures. Although there is controversy today regarding which patients should receive phenobarbital for febrile seizure prophylaxis, there is agreement that phenobarbital cannot be used intermittently with success. Among pediatricians a common practice has been to administer phenobarbital at the time of fever in an attempt to prevent febrile seizures. When phenobarbital is administered at 6 to 8 mg/kg/day orally, it takes approximately 48 hr before a concentration above 15 μg/ml is achieved (15). In the study by Faero et al. (15), concentrations of 16 to 30 μg/ml were required to prevent recurrent febrile seizures, and these concentrations could not be achieved by the time a febrile seizure occurred after fever was recognized. Wolfe (50) also noted that there was no decrease in the incidence of febrile seizures in a pediatric population receiving intermittent phenobarbital therapy. Recurrent febrile seizures, however, are reduced by continuous treatment commencing with oral loading doses of 6 to 8 mg/kg/day for two days followed by a maintenance dose of 3 to 4 mg/kg/day (15).

A consensus panel of the National Institutes of Health (18) concluded that in view of the benign nature and outcome of most febrile seizures, there is no need for medication. Anticonvulsant prophylaxis, however, could be considered in the presence of neurological abnormalities, prolonged (> 15 min) or focal seizures, febrile seizures associated with transient or permanent neurologic deficits, or a family history of nonfebrile seizures.

It is important to remember that even when two of these risk factors are present, only 13% of the children develop epilepsy and 87% of this high risk group do not. If phenobarbital is chosen for prophylaxis in the treatment of febrile seizures, it should not be utilized intermittently, but must be administered daily. Faero et al. (15) compared 59 patients under the age of 3 years with 172 untreated children of the same age. Of 27 children who maintained plasma levels of 16 to 30 μg/ml only one (4%) developed a new febrile seizure compared with seven (22%) of 33 children who maintained plasma levels between 8 and 15 μg/ml. The rate of febrile seizure development in the untreated population was 20%.

Mitchell et al. (30) found equal efficacy of phenobarbital and carbamazepine in partial onset seizures in children followed for 1 year.

Effects on Behavior and Cognition

The effect of phenobarbital on the behavior of children is of great concern. Wolfe and Forsythe (50), in a study of 109 children treated daily with phenobarbital following their first febrile seizure, noted that 42% developed a behavioral disorder, usually hyperactivity. The behavioral disturbance appeared within several months of therapy and was not correlated with plasma phenobarbital concentrations. The behavioral disorder disappeared in 73% and improved in all children when phenobarbital was discontinued. There were no characteristics of the initial or recurrent febrile seizures that predicted the behavior disorder in this population. The children with behavioral disturbances, however, had a lower incidence of family history of seizures, especially febrile seizures, and a higher frequency of abnormalities of pregnancy, labor, delivery, and the neonatal period, as well as delayed milestones, short seizures, normal electroencephalograms, and recurrent febrile seizures. It is important to note that 18% of the children who received no phenobarbital developed a behavior disorder, most often hyperactivity, which subsequently disappeared in 52%. The role of a pre-existing predisposition to behavioral abnormalities that may become manifest with or without phenobarbital therapy is unclear at this time.

In spite of over a half century's experience with phenobarbital, its effect on cognition has been poorly studied. Tchicaloff et al. (43) assessed 20 epileptic patients with psychometric tests and noted a correlation between the dose of phenobarbital administered and impaired performance on subsets of the Wechsler Adult Intelligence Scale (WAIS). Camfield et al. (7), in a double-blind study in which children were given phenobarbital to prevent recurrent febrile seizures, noted no significant differences on a scale of infant development when the children were followed for 8 to 12 months. When serum phenobarbital concentrations were correlated to five Binet subscores, however, they noted a significant negative relationship to memory tasks. The effect was greater in those children taking the drug for 12 months compared to those taking the drug for 8 months. Hutt et al. (21) in a study of four normal adults, noted impairments on various measures of perceptual motor performance in those taking phenobarbital for up to 1 month. Tasks requiring sustained performance were most affected. Key pressing, vigilance, verbal learning, and speech rate were affected, especially at higher levels of the drug. In a study of 66 patients with epilepsy and depression aged 18 to 70 years, Robertson et al. (36) noted that nine patients on phenobarbital as a part of polytherapy were more significantly depressed than those not receiving this agent, as rated on the Beck Depression Inventory. Although these findings may have been a part of epilepsy or polytherapy rather than phenobarbital per se, it is in keeping with anecdotal reports suggesting an association and improvement in depressive symptoms if barbiturates are withdrawn (44).

Anecdotally, mephobarbital has been reported to cause fewer behavioral side effects than phenobarbital. This assertion has never made sense, as the action of mepobarbital is attributed to its hepatic conver-sion to phenobarbital. Young et al. (53) studied eight children with an average age of 9 ± 1 year in a prospective double-blind randomized crossover study of these two anticonvulsants. There was no deterioration of behavior with either phenobarbital or methobarbital regardless of which drug was administered first. The levels of phenobarbital were 23.5 ± 1.8 µg/ml with administration of phenobarbital and 17.6 ± 1.3 µg/ml with mephobarbital. The study by Wolfe and Forsythe (50) noting a high incidence of behavioral side effects was not blinded and used no systematic behavioral inventory, but a double-blind crossover trial of phenobarbital and valproic acid conducted by Vining et al. (48) noted a statistically significant worsening on eight of 48 items utilizing a standardized behavioral questionnaire in children receiving phenobarbital.

Camfield et al. (7) in a double-blind, placebo-controlled study noted that most toddlers do not have major phenobarbital side effects. Mitchell and Chavez (30) also failed to find behavioral impairment in children with partial onset seizures treated with phenobarbital. Neither Camfield et al. (7), Mitchell and Chavez (30), nor Young et al. (53) noted a significant increase in complaints regarding hyperactivity. Although Wolfe and Forsythe (50) did not note a relationship of plasma concentrations of phenobarbital to behavioral effects, Camfield et al. (7) noted behavioral side effects to be dose related in four of 35 children. Certainly the frequency of adverse behavioral effects of phenobarbital are lower in double-blind, placebo-controlled studies than in nonblinded studies. In addition, pre-seizure behavioral status may also be relevant to subsequent development of adverse behavioral effects. Wolfe and Forsythe (50) did note that the frequency of behavioral disorder was 80% in children who had a history of abnormal behavior before the onset of seizures, compared to 20% in controls. In interpreting the effects of phenobarbital on behavior and cognition in populations of patients with seizures, it is important to remember that among patients taking phenobarbital, 65% gain seizure control and 30% experience cognitive improvement (23,24,26). Cognitive improvement is more common than deterioration. Thompson et al. (46) noted that in a group of patients whose IQ dropped a mean of 26 over time, while taking anticonvulsants their episodes of intoxication were more frequent when compared to a control group matched for age at onset of seizures, duration of seizures, and initial IQ. This experience suggests that behavioral and cognitive changes will depend on the presence of a sufficiently large drug-sensitive subgroup within the study, drug levels at the time of testing, and the particular assessment modality used.

USE IN ADULTS

Phenobarbital is widely used in the treatment of simple and complex partial seizures as well as generalized tonic-clonic seizures in all age groups (29,30,38). The therapeutic range of phenobarbital has been reported as 10 to 40 µg/ml (14). In a study of 78 patients with various types of epileptic seizures, Schmidt et al. (38) noted that in 16 patients taking either phenobarbital or primidone, the phenobarbital plasma concentrations necessary to control generalized tonic-clonic seizures was 18 ± 10 µg/ml in 10 patients and 38 ± 6 µg/ml in six patients with simple or complex partial seizures with or without secondary generalization. Complete control of simple or complex partial seizures appears to require significantly higher plasma concentrations of phenobarbital compared to concentrations required for complete control of tonic-clonic seizures alone. These data suggest that uncritical reliance on published therapeutic ranges of plasma phenobarbital concentrations will result in incomplete control in some patients. Feely et al. (16) studied

phenobarbital in previously untreated epilepsy. In 13 new patients with epilepsy (eight adults and five children), they found that complete seizure control was achieved in 11 patients. Doses sufficient to attain a mean steady-state plasma concentration of more than 10 µg/ml were associated with better seizure control than lower doses. As expected from previous reports, doses necessary to achieve these plasma concentrations were 1.0 to 1.5 mg/kg for adult patients and 1.5 to 3 mg/kg for children. One adult tolerated a dose of 2 mg/kg. Their data were similar to those of Schmidt et al. (38) in that eight of nine patients with generalized motor seizures were controlled completely with phenobarbital. One patient incompletely controlled was improved but had poor compliance. Three of four patients with complex partial seizures were seizure-free and one improved. It appears that in previously untreated patients, a success rate of 89% to 95% can be obtained with phenobarbital monotherapy. Several patients complained of mild transient sedation, but impaired school performance was not noted among children.

In a multicenter, double-blind trial comparing the efficacy and toxicity of four antiepileptic drugs in the treatment of partial and secondarily generalized tonic-clonic seizures in 622 adults, Mattson et al. (29) noted that overall treatment success was highest with carbamazepine or phenytoin, intermediate with phenobarbital, and lowest with primidone. Retention time in the study was best for phenobarbitals, phenytoin, and carbamazepine and worst for primidone. Retention time in the group with phenobarbital-treated tonic-clonic seizures was the same, but analysis of patients with partial seizures showed a higher retention rate for carbamazepine and phenytoin compared to phenobarbital or primidone. Phenobarbital was associated with the lowest incidence of motor disturbances and the fewest gastrointestinal side effects. Phenobarbital also caused less dysmorphic and idiosyncratic side effects (gum hypertrophy, hirsutism, acne, and rash) than did carbamazepine or phenytoin. Decreased libido and impotence were more frequently noted in patients receiving phenobarbital (16%) than in patients receiving carbamazepine (13%) or phenytoin (11%), but distinctly less frequently than in patients receiving primidone (22%). Significant leukopenia was not a problem in phenobarbital-treated patients. There was no statistically significant difference between phenobarbital and the other drugs assessed in this study as regards the number of seizures in all patients at 12, 24, and 36 months, and no difference between the time therapeutic drug levels were achieved and the first recurrence of seizures. Of note in this population, however, is that total seizure control was only 30% through the first 12 months. Complete control of tonic-clonic seizures was also similar (carbamazepine, 48%; phenobrbital, 43%; phenytoin, 43%; and primidone, 45%).

Carbamazepine, however, provided significantly better control of partial seizures (43%) than did phenobarbital (16%). Complete control of tonic-clonic seizures for 12 months was considered possible for 55% of the patients remaining in the carbamazepine group, 58% in the phenobarbital group, 48% in the phenytoin group, and 63% in the primidone group. These differences were not significant. The complete control of partial seizures, however, was significantly better with carbamazepine (65%) than phenobarbital (33%), phenytoin (34%), or primidone (26%) at 18 months.

In keeping with the observations of Schmidt et al. (38) and Feely et al. (16), Mattson et al. (29) found that phenobarbital was as successful as carbamazepine and phenytoin in the treatment of predominately tonic-clonic seizures but had a higher failure rate in the management of partial seizures. As more than half of their patients had both partial and secondarily generalized tonic-clonic seizures, phenobarbital would seem the logical drug of choice only in patients who are sensitive to the gastrointestinal and motor system effects of phenytoin and carbamazepine. In this study utilizing monotherapy, the authors noted that although more than 75% of the patients were successfully treated with carbamazepine or phenytoin for a year, the percentage maintaining complete seizure control decreased over time. Only 39% of patients begun on one drug could continue on that drug and have complete seizure control through the first 12 months. When patients were placed on a combination of two drugs, seizure frequency and severity decreased in 11% but at the cost of greater toxicity.

USE IN PREGNANCY

The use of any drug including phenobarbital during pregnancy raises concerns about both mother and fetus (45). On the one hand, seizures during pregnancy affect the fetus, and careful attention must be paid to changes in phenobarbital distribution. On the other hand, the role of phenobarbital in the production of fetus hemorrhagic disease and malformations is also of concern.

Available data indicate one should anticipate decreased levels of phenobarbital beginning late in the first trimester and continuing throughout pregnancy (27,52). Bardy et al. (3) followed the clearance of phenobarbital in 23 patients before, during, and 52 weeks after pregnancy. All patients were being treated with more than one anticonvulsant. Phenobarbital clearance increased in 12 women, decreased in one, and either remained unchanged or increased in 10. There was a great deal of interpatient variability but when plasma phenobarbital levels decreased, the magnitude was as large as 40%. Battino et al. (5) found that in 12 women being treated with phenobarbital monotherapy, plasma levels decreased in four. Plasma clearance increased during pregnancy and decreased following delivery. Phenobarbital clearance between 25 and 32 weeks and from the 33rd to 40th week of gestation was significantly larger than after delivery. Plasma levels of phenobarbital also decreased in six patients on a constant dosage of phenobarbital.

Although decreased intestinal absorption associated with decreased protein binding and decreased compliance have been postulated as mechanisms for the reduction of plasma phenobarbital concentrations during pregnancy, the most likely explanations are related to an increased volume of distribution, hepatic clearance, and renal clearance during pregnancy.

Phenobarbital does not appear to be associated with an increased risk of malformations in the fetus independent of epilepsy (41). Shapiro et al. (40) noted an incidence of 9.3% among mothers with seizures exposed to phenobarbital during months 1 through 4, compared to a 5.3% incidence in mothers exposed to phenobarbital during the same period but without a convulsive disorder. There was also no evidence in this combined Finnish and American collaborative study that phenobarbital caused fetal central nervous system injury.

A unique hemorrhagic phenomena has been reported in infants of epileptic mothers taking any anticonvulsant, including phenobarbital. The bleeding tendency is due to a deficiency of vitamin K clotting factors II, VII, IX, and X. Phenobarbital appears to be a competitive inhibitor of prothrombin precursors. The inhibition can be reversed by prophylactic administration of vitamin K_1 to mothers during the last 2 weeks of pregnancy. Intramuscular vitamin K in infants will eventually reverse the abnormality but the time required is in terms of days and during this period the child is at risk for serious hemorrhagic disease. The resultant mortality when this disorder is symptomatic approaches 30%.

USE IN RENAL AND HEPATIC DISEASES

Information regarding the disposition of phenobarbital in renal failure is unavailable but plasma half-life has been reported to be normal in uremic patients. The elimination of phenobarbital, however, is more dependent upon renal excretion than hepatic metabolism, and some accumulation of phenobarbital would be expected in the presence of advanced renal disease (2,20,35). In patients with renal disease, lower maintenance doses of phenobarbital have been recommended for patients receiving long-term therapy. Postdialysis supplemental phenobarbital is necessary for both peritoneal and hemodialysis.

Alvin et al. (1) demonstrated that the half-life of phenobarbital was significantly prolonged in patients with cirrhosis (130 ± 15 hr) compared to a control population (86 ± 3 hr). A significant reduction of conjugated hydroxyphenobarbital in the urine of these patients was noted. In patients with viral hepatitis, the prolongation of the elimination half-life was not significant and a large intersubject variation was found. In these patients with acute hepatic injury, the pattern of excretion of phenobarbital metabolites was unchanged. These latter studies are based on single-dose administration of phenobarbital and may not reflect changes that occur during long-term therapy. Adjustment of the dose in the presence of cholestasis appears unnecessary as biliary excretion of phenobarbital is not significant in man.

USE IN STATUS EPILEPTICUS

Phenobarbital has both advantages and disadvantages in the treatment of status epilepticus. The anticonvulsant action of phenobarbital is long, allowing it to be used in subsequent long-term therapy, but it may cause respiratory depression, excessive sedation, and hypotension. Theoretically, phenobarbital achieves a maximum brain-to-plasma ratio much more slowly than does diazepam and the response time in the treatment of status epilepticus therefore might be considerably slower. Until recently, however, a randomized clinical study comparing phenobarbital to a combination of diazepam and phenytoin had not been conducted.

Shaner et al. (39) in a randomized, non-blinded clinical trial evaluating 36 consecutive patients with generalized convulsive status epilepticus, compared phenobarbital to a combination of diazepam and phenytoin. There were 18 episodes of status epilepticus in each treatment group. Phenobarbital was initially administered intravenously at a rate of 100 mg/min until a dose of 10 mg/kg was achieved. If the patient continued to convulse 10 min after treatment was initiated, phenytoin was administered intravenously and additional phenobarbital delivered. Diazepam was infused at 2 mg/min intravenously and phenytoin administered simultaneously at a rate of 40 mg/min until a loading dose of 18 mg/kg was achieved. If the patient continued to convulse after delivery of an initial 20-mg dose of diazepam, a continuous diazepam infusion was administered. Convulsions were controlled in all 36 patients within 7 hr. The median cumulative convulsion time, however, was shorter for those patients receiving phenobarbital (5 min) than those receiving the combination of diazepam and phenytoin (9 min). Sixteen of the 18 patients (89%) treated with phenobarbital exhibited clinical convulsive activity for less than 10 min and no patient demonstrated activity longer than 25 min. Ten of 18 patients (56%) in the diazepam-phenytoin group convulsed for less than 10 min and five experienced a cumulative convulsion time greater than 25 min. The frequency of complications (i.e., arrhythmias, hypotension, and need for intubation) were similar among the two regimens. Sixteen of 18 patients required phenobarbital doses less than 12 mg/kg. Eleven of 18 cases were controlled with phenobarbital alone at mean serum concentrations of 18.3 μg/ml. Statistical evaluation did not demonstrate a dramatic difference between the phenobarbital and diazepam-phenytoin groups, but 95% confidence intervals demonstrated that the mean cumulative convulsion time for the phenobarbital regimen was between 0 and 14 min less than the diazepam-phenytoin regimen.

Rather than the postulated 20-min response latency noted by some investigators, Shaner et al. (39) noted a median response time of 5.5 min to phenobarbital. This finding is in keeping with experimental data demonstrating that although maximum brain-to-plasma ratios of phenobarbital may be achieved only after 60 min following administration, effective brain concentrations of phenobarbital are achieved within 3 min (25,34). Thus, despite many theoretic limitations, phenobarbital may be as effective as any other treatment regimen in the therapy of status epilepticus.

REFERENCES

1. Alvin, J., McHorse, T., Hoyumpa, A., Bush, M. T., Schenker, S. (1975): The effect of liver disease in man on the disposition of phenobarbital. *J. Pharmacol. Exper. Therapeutics*, 192:224–235.
2. Asconape, J., and Penry, J. (1982): Use of anti-epileptic drugs in the presence of liver and kidney disease: A review. *Epilepsia*, 23(Suppl 1):65–79.
3. Bardy, A. H., Teramo, K., and Hiilesmaa, C. K. (1982): Apparent plasma clearances of phenytoin, phenobarbitone, primidone and carbamazepine during pregnancy: Results of the prospective Helsinki study. In: *Epilepsy, Pregnancy and the Child*, edited by Jance, I. Bossi, M. Dam, H. Helge, A. Richens, and D. Schmidt, pp 141–145. Raven Press, New York.
4. Battino, D., Avanzini, G., Bossi, I., Canger, L., Cumo, M. L., Croci, D., and Spina, S. (1982): Monitoring of anti-epileptic plasma levels during pregnancy and the puerperium. In: *Epilepsy, Pregnancy, and the Child*, edited by D. Jan, I. Bossi, M. Dam, H. Helge, A. Richens, and D. Schmidt, pp. 147–154. Raven Press, New York.
5. Battino, D., Binelli, S., Bossi, L., Como, M. L.,

Croci, D., Cusi, C., and Avanzini, G. (1984): Changes in primidone, phenobarbitone ratio during pregnancy and the puerperium. *Clin. Pharmacokin.*, 9:252–260.

6. Buchthal, F., and Lennox-Buchthal, M. A. (1972): Relation of serum concentration to control of seizures. In: *Antiepileptic Drugs*, edited by D. M. Woodbury, J. K. Penry, and R. P. Schmidt, pp 335–343. Raven Press, New York.

7. Camfield, C. S., Chaplin, S., and Doyle, A. (1979): Side effects of phenobarbital in toddlers: Behavioral and cognitive aspects. *J. Pediatr.*, 95:361–365.

8. Danner, R., Shewmon, A., and Sherman, M. (1985): Seizures in an Atelencephalic. *Arch. Neurol.*, 42:1014–1016.

9. Diaz, J., Schain, R., and Bailey, B. G. (1977): Phenobarbital—induced brain growth retardation in artificially reared rat pups. *Biology, Neonate*, 32:77–82.

10. Dodson, W. E. (1984): Antiepileptic drug utilization in pediatric patients. *Epilepsia*, 25(Suppl 2):S132–S139.

11. Dodson, W., Prensky, A., DeVivo, D., Goldring, S., and Dodge, P. R. (1976): Management of seizure disorders. Selected aspects. Part I. *J. Pediatr.*, 89:527.

12. Donn, S., Grasela, T., and Goldstein, G. (1985): Safety of a higher loading dose of phenobarbital in the term newborn. *Pediatrics*, 75:1061–1064.

13. Eaide, M. J., Lander, C. M., Hooper, W. D., and Tyrer, J. H. (1977): Factors influencing plasma phenobarbital levels in epileptic patients. *Br. J. Clin. Pharmacol.*, 4:541.

14. Elwes, R. D. S., Johnson, A. L., Shorvon, S. C., and Reynolds, E. H. (1984): The prognosis for seizure control in newly diagnosed epilepsy. *N. Engl. J. Med.*, 311:944–947.

15. Faero, O., Kastrup, K. W., Nielsen, E., Melchior, J. C., and Thorn, I. (1972): Successful prophylaxis of febrile convulsions with phenobarbital. *Epilepsia*, 13:279–285.

16. Feely, M., O'Callagan, M., Duggan, G., and Callaghan, N. (1980): Phenobarbitone in previously untreated epilepsy. *J. Neurol. Neuros. Psych.*, 43:365–368.

17. Fischer, J., Lockman, L., Zoske, D., and Kriel, R. (1981): Phenobarbital maintenance dose requirements in treating neonatal seizures. *Neurology*, 31:1042–1044.

18. Freeman, J. (1980): Febrile seizures: A consensus of their significance, evaluation and treatment. *Pediatrics*, 6:1609.

19. Gal, P., Tobock, J., Boer, H., Erkan, N., and Wells, T. (1982): Efficacy of phenobarbital monotherapy in treatment of neonatal seizures—Relationship to blood levels. *Neurology*, 32:1401–1404.

20. Gambertoglio, J. G., and Lauer, R. M. (1981): Use of neuropsychiatric drugs. In: *Clinical Use of Drugs in Patients with Kidney and Liver Disease*, edited by R. I. Anderson and R. W. Schrier, pp 276–295. W. B. Saunders, Philadelphia.

21. Hutt, S. J., Jackson, P. M., Belsham, A. B., and Higgins, G. (1968): Perceptual/motor behavior in relation to blood phenobarbital levels. *Dev. Med. Child Neurol.*, 10:626–632.

22. Kuban, K., Leviton, A., Brown, E., Krishnamoorthy, K., Baglivo, J., Sullivan, K., and Allred, E. (1987): Respiratory complications in low birth weight infants who received phenobarbital. *A.J.D.C.*, 141:996–999.

23. Lennox, W. G. (1942): Gains against epilepsy. *J.A.M.A.*, 120:449–453.

24. Lennox, W. G., and Lennox, M. A. (1960): *Epilepsy and Related Disorders*. Boston, Little Brown.

25. Leppik, I. E., and Sherwin, A. L. (1979): Intravenous phenytoin and phenobarbital: Anticonvulsant action, brain content, and plasma binding in the rat. *Epilepsia*, 20:201–207.

26. Lesser, R. P., Luders, H., Wyllie, E., Dinner, D. S., and Morris, H. (1986): Mental deterioration in epilepsy. *Epilepsia*, (Suppl 2):105–123.

27. Levy, R., and Yerby, M. (1985): Effects of pregnancy on anti-epileptic drug utilization. *Epilepsia*, 26 (Suppl 1):52–57.

28. Lockman, L. A., Kriel, R., and Zaske, D. (1979): Phenobarbital dosage for control of neonatal seizures. *Neurology*, 29:1445–1449.

29. Mattson, R., Cramer, J., Collins, J., Smith, D., Delgado-Escueta, A., Brown, E. T., Williamson, T., Treiman, D., McNamara, J., McCutchen, C., Homan, R., Crill, W., Lubozynski, M., Rosenthal, N., and Mayersdorf, A. (1985): Comparison of carbamazepine, phenobarbital, phenytoin and primidone in partial and secondarily generalized tonic-clonic seizures. *N. Engl. J. Med.* 313:145–151.

30. Mitchell, W., and Chavez, J. (1987): Carbamazepine versus phenobarbital for partial onset seizures in children. *Epilepsia*, 28:56–60.

31. Mizrahi, E., and Kelloway, P. (1987): Characterization and classification of neonatal seizures. *Neurology*, 37:1837–1844.

32. Painter, M. J., Minnigh, B., Mollica, L., and Alvin, J. (1987): Binding profiles of anticonvulsants in neonates with seizures. *Ann. Neurol.* 22:413.

33. Painter, M. J., Pippenger, C., Wasterlain, C., Barmada, M., Pitlick, W., Carter, G., and Abern, S. (1981): Phenobarbital and phenytoin in neonatal seizures: Metabolism and tissue distribution. *Neurology*, 31:1107–1112.

34. Ramsey, R. E., Hammond, E. J., Perchalski, R. J., and Wilder, J. (1979): Brain uptake of phenytoin, phenobarbital and diazepam. *Arch. Neurol.*, 36:535–539.

35. Reidenberg, M. M., and Drayer, D. E. (1978): Effects of renal disease upon drug disposition. *Drug Metab. Rev.*, 8:293–302.

36. Robertson, M., Trimble, M., and Townsend, H. (1987): Phenomenology of depression in epilepsy. *Epilepsia*, 28:364–372.

37. Rossi, L. N. (1979): Correlation between age and plasma level/dosage for phenobarbital in infants and children. *Acta Paediatr. Scan.*, 68:431.

38. Schmidt, D., Einicke, I., and Haenel, F. (1986): The influence of seizure type on the efficacy of

plasma concentrations of phenytoin, phenobarbital and carbamazepine.

39. Shaner, M. D., McCurdy, S., Herring, M., and Gabor, A. (1988): Treatment of status epilepticus: A prospective comparison of diazepam and phenytoin versus phenobarbital and optional phenytoin. *Neurology*, 38:202–207.

40. Shapiro, S., Hartz, S., Siskind, V., Mitchell, A., Slone, D., Rosenberg, L., Monson, R., Heinonen, O., Idanpaan-Heikkila, J., Saxen, L., and Sakari, H. (1976): Anticonvulsants and parental epilepsy in the development of birth defects. *Lancet*, 272–275.

41. Stumpf, D. (1985): Anticonvulsant use during pregnancy. *Clin. Ther.*, 7:258–265.

42. Svenningson, N. W., Blennow, G., Landroth, M., Gaddlin, P., and Ahlstorm, H. (1982): Brain oriented intensive care treatment in severe neonatal asphyxia. *Arch. Dis. of Childh.*, 57:176–183.

43. Tchicaloff, M., and Gaillard, F. (1970): Quelques effets indesirables des medicaments, anti-epileptiques, sur le rendements intellectuales. *Rev. Neuropsych. Infant*, 18:599–602.

44. Theodore, W. H., and Porter, R. J. (1983): Removal of sedative hypnotic anti-epileptic drugs from the regimens of patients with intractable epilepsy. *Ann. Neurol.*, 13:320–324.

45. Thilbert, A., and Dam, M. (1982): The epileptic mother and her child. *Epilepsia*, 23:85–99.

46. Thompson, P. J., Sander, J. W. A. S., and Oxley, J. (1985): Intellectual deterioration in severe epilepsy. Presented at Epilepsy International Symposium, Hamburg, West Germany. September 6–9.

47. VanOrman, C. B., and Darrvish, H. Z. (1985): Efficacy of phenobarbital in neonatal seizures. *Can. J. Neurol. Sci.*, 12:95–99.

48. Vining, E. P. G., Mellits, E. D., and Cataldo, M. F. (1983): Effects of phenobarbital and sodium valproate on neuropsychological function and behavior. (Abstract) *Ann. Neurol.*, 14:360.

49. Watson, P. D. (1980): Once daily doses of phenobarbital in children. *J. Pediatr.*, 97:303.

50. Wolf, S., and Forsythe, A. (1978): Behavior disturbance, phenobarbital, and febrile seizures. *Pediatrics*, 61:728–731.

51. Yanai, J., and Bergman, I. (1981): Neuronal deficits after neonatal exposure to phenobarbital. *Exper. Neurol.*, 73:199–208.

52. Yerby, M. (1987): Problems in management of the pregnant woman with epilepsy. *Epilepsia*, 28 (Suppl 3):29–36.

53. Young, R. S. K., Alger, P. M., Bauer, L., and Lauderbaugh, D. (1986): A randomized, double-blind, crossover study of phenobarbital and methobarbital. *J. of Child Neurology*, 1:361–363.

Antiepileptic Drugs, Third Edition, edited by
R. Levy, R. Mattson, B. Meldrum,
J. K. Penry, and F. E. Dreifuss.
Raven Press, Ltd., New York © 1989.

23

Phenobarbital

Toxicity

Richard H. Mattson and Joyce A. Cramer

Worldwide use of phenobarbital for almost a century has allowed the accumulation of considerable knowledge of its toxicity. Phenobarbital enjoys a reputation of safety because serious systemic side effects are very uncommon. Unfortunately, annoying neurological and psychological toxicity is frequent, and systemic toxicity has been noted more commonly in recent years. This chapter focuses on problems associated with single-dose and long-term use of the drug in doses producing serum concentrations considered effective in antiepileptic drug therapy.

New information about single-dose and long-term neurological and systemic toxicity is available from the recently completed VA Epilepsy Cooperative Study (48). Phenobarbital was initiated as sole antiepileptic drug in 177 adults who were followed a mean of 36 months, with some followed for as long as 6 years.

NEUROTOXICITY

With the long-term use of phenobarbital, even at the usual dosage-producing serum concentrations of the drug in the broad therapeutic range of 15 to 40 µg/ml, adverse changes in affect, behavior, and cognitive function are often encountered. High serum concentrations cause neurological signs of "drunkenness," including nystagmus, dysarthria, incoordination, and ataxia. Often, the neurotoxic side effects occur together in different degrees.

Sedation

The hallmark of barbiturate toxicity in adults is sedation. In the VA study, 2 of 3 patients complained of sedation at one or more visits in the first year. Interestingly, phenobarbital produced no more acute sedation than the other drugs tested, probably because of cautious dose increases.

Complaints of fatigue and tiredness are difficult to quantify and are often variable and subtle. The patient and family may describe listlessness or lack of spontaneity even when excessive sleeping time is not observed. As dosage is increased, overt sleepiness is observable and often apparent by difficulty in arousal in the morning and naps after school or work. An associated loss of interest, particularly in social activity or playing with friends, is common. Drowsiness usually accompanies the initiation of phenobarbital and may persist for days or weeks in many patients.

Butler et al. (10) noted that patients complained of sedation at the onset of treatment when phenobarbital concentrations were only 5 µg/ml. Two weeks later, there were few complaints despite a fivefold increase in the serum levels. Others have also reported that sedation occurred primarily during the first few days of treatment and cleared rapidly as tolerance developed (8,31). Somnolence was even briefer if phenobarbital was restarted after a withdrawal period (8). It was also found that a dose that caused sedation during initiation of therapy in adults no longer caused sleepiness after 1 or 2 weeks of treatment (8). After tolerance was acquired, adverse effects of phenobarbital were not observed when the serum concentration was less than 30 μg/ml. A subgroup of 58 patients taking phenobarbital in the VA Cooperative Study were examined at every visit for the first 3 months (1,2,4,8,12 weeks) to assess the incidence of acute adverse effects and development of tolerance (46). Of the subgroup studied for tolerance, 33% of patients started on phenobarbital reported initial sedation, declining significantly to 24% by 12 weeks ($p < .04$). Development of tolerance was evidenced by decreasing symptoms despite increasing phenobarbital concentrations from 18 μg/ml at 2 weeks to 24 μg/ml at 12 weeks.

Mattson et al. (51), however, found many exceptions to the correlation between serum phenobarbital concentrations and complaints of tiredness. The variation among individuals was evident in that some patients were asymptomatic when serum phenobarbital levels were as high as 50 μg/ml, whereas others complained of feeling "drugged" when levels were as low as 15 μg/ml. It should be noted that the tolerable range of serum concentrations when phenobarbital is used as sole drug is 15 to 30 μg/ml.

Neurological Side Effects

Increasing the dosage of phenobarbital eventually leads to neurological signs similar to those found with the use of other antiepileptic drugs. Dysarthria, incoordination, ataxia, dizziness, and nystagmus appear as serum levels exceed 40 μg/ml. The VA study found at lower levels and at initiation of therapy that these signs and symptoms were significantly less frequent with use of phenobarbital than with carbamazepine, phenytoin, or primidone ($p < .03$).

Behavior

Instead of the sedative effect of phenobarbital common in adults, a paradoxical effect of the drug in children and the elderly may produce insomnia and hyperkinetic activity. Ounsted (61), reviewing the hyperkinetic syndrome in epileptic children, found that 79% of the children receiving antiepileptic drug therapy were overactive. Phenobarbital commonly exacerbated aggressiveness and overactivity. The pattern of behavior included signs of distractibility, shortened attention span, fluctuation of mood, and aggressive outbursts. It is of interest that 79% of the children were boys. Wolf and Forsythe (87) found a higher incidence of behavioral disturbances. Forty-two percent of 109 children receiving daily phenobarbital therapy to prevent recurrence of febrile seizures developed these problems. Surprisingly, 64% of the 38 children exhibiting hyperactivity had serum phenobarbital concentrations of less than 15 μg/ml, indicating such problems can be seen even in what would be considered the low or subtherapeutic range. When phenobarbital therapy was stopped, behavior returned to normal in 16 children and improved in six. Only two of the improved children had a history of behavioral problems prior to the use of phenobarbital. Three of eight different children who exhibited other nonhyperkinetic behavioral disturbances during treatment also returned to normal after stopping the drug. The authors (87) concluded that behavioral disturbances associated with phenobarbital use are more likely to become evident in children in the presence of organic brain disease or deficits.

In contrast, Camfield et al. (11) assessed 35 toddlers given phenobarbital and 30 given placebo, finding no differences in hyperactivity between the groups after a year. Dose-related irritability and erratic sleep were common in the phenobarbital group without frank hyperactivity. Reduction from 4 to 5 mg/kg/day to 2 to 3 mg/kg/day resolved these problems in four children. Elderly patients with organic brain disease may also become agitated rather than sedated with use of phenobarbital.

Affect

Phenobarbital therapy can produce alteration of affect, particularly depression. It is difficult to determine whether such mood changes are a reaction to the often newly diagnosed illness, the addition of another drug to treat severe seizures, or a direct neurotoxic effect of phenobarbital. Clinical observations suggest a direct effect of phenobarbital, because changes to carbamazepine therapy have been associated with improved mood scores (70). Despite these findings in children, studies have not revealed statistically significant changes over time among adults on phenobarbital compared to other drugs (48). Early psychological problems including affect, mood, and cognition were reported by 13% of patients in the VA study at 1 month and 12% at 3 months (46). This was not significantly different in phenobarbital-treated patients than for carbamazepine, phenytoin, or primidone treatment. However, 40 of 56 patients treated for at least 1 year reported some psychological effect of phenobarbital during the first year.

Cognition

A side effect of phenobarbital of considerable potential importance, especially in children, is a possible disturbance in cognitive function. Problems with memory or compromised work and school performance may develop independent of sedation and hyperkinetic activity, although these factors may play a contributory role. Lennox (39) observed a marked impairment in affect and cognitive function in patients whose capacity had already been compromised: "Many physicians in attempting to extinguish seizures only succeed in drowning the finer intellectual processes of their patients." Such effects are often subtle and difficult to measure despite reports by patients, families, and teachers.

Changes in cognitive function have been measured by various standardized neuropsychological tests. Interestingly, in early reports, institutionalized epileptic patients showed some improvement in intelligence testing after treatment with antiepileptic drugs. Improved tests scores could be attributed to decreased seizure frequency or practice effect from repeated testing. Lennox (39) found 58% of his patients unchanged on subjective evaluation of mentality while using phenobarbital. He separated the improvement of patients because of diminished seizure frequency from the effect of the medication on mentality. A more detailed study by Somerfeld-Ziskind and Ziskind (75) showed no overall change in IQ after phenobarbital therapy for a year. Twelve patients actually showed increased IQ scores whereas 10 patients had lower scores (maximum change, 11 points); 79% had fewer seizures while receiving phenobarbital.

Stores (78) reviewed studies of the effect of phenobarbital on intellectual function. He commented that the educational problem for these children appears to be that their attainments fail to match their capacities as measured by standardized tests. Formal studies have not been able to assess this disparity. On careful testing, children treated with phenobarbital can perform at appropriate levels. It is difficult to assess subjective complaints unless the children are treated with a different medication and tested before and after the change from barbiturate therapy.

A recent double-blind crossover comparison of psychological and behavioral effects of phenobarbital and valproate was performed in 21 children (ages 6–15 years) (83). Cognitive function and behavior were significantly diminished during phenobarbital therapy ($p < .01$), although differences were subtle. Overall intelligence assessed by the Wechsler Intelligence Scale for Children (Revised) showed significantly lower performance and full-scale IQ scores for phenobarbital than for valproate treatment periods. Differences were seen both in verbal and nonverbal tasks, particularly for complex tests. The extensive neuropsychological testing showed important problems with epilepsy and developmental problems in children (83). The comparison with valproate, a drug not considered likely to cause cognitive impairments, provided information suggesting that phenobarbital can affect childhood learning and behavior. Camfield et al. (11) found a trend toward decreased memory and concentration scores in children taking phenobarbital compared to a placebo group ($p < .07$) that correlated well with serum levels ($p < .05$). They suggested caution in long-term exposure of children to phenobarbital, particularly at high dosage.

In a careful study of children receiving an average daily dose of 1.8 mg/kg of phenobarbital, Wapner et al. (84) compared learning behavior and intelligence before therapy and 6 weeks later. Phenobarbital did not affect the function of the children in the classroom situation. Although seizure control was incomplete, there was not significant change in learning or intellect compared with a control group.

When carbamazepine was substituted for phenobarbital in children, several mental functions were improved. Schain et al. (70) found a statistically significant difference in

intelligence (as measured by WISC) and results of three problem-solving tests of attentiveness and impulse control. Parents and teachers also reported a significant improvement in alertness and attentiveness. These drug changes improved seizure control but the psychological improvements were considered to be a function of removal of the sedating drug.

Specific psychological testing has been done to sample sectors of performance thought to be more sensitive to subtle compromise by drug effects. Mirsky and Kornetsky (55) showed that barbiturates can impair performance on vigilance tests. These investigators suggested that barbiturate therapy may be related to learning difficulties in children. However, they did not take into consideration the fact that tolerance to barbiturate therapy develops very quickly. Therefore, the single-dose effects measured in their study could be expected to diminish with prolonged administration. Other investigators (31) studied adults who had received phenobarbital for 2 weeks, allowing the development of tolerance before performance testing. They found that phenobarbital did not diminish performance on simple tasks requiring attention but did affect tasks requiring sustained effort. It is interesting to note that even the tasks requiring sustained effort showed improvement when patients were stimulated during the testing. Others also showed the difference between self-paced tests and tests in which sustained attention was necessary (37). Impaired vigilance and sensory perception during phenobarbital usage have been noted in patients of average intelligence (44).

Hutt (31) tested the effects of phenobarbital after tolerance had developed. Although sedation was lessened at the time of testing compared with early acute effect, performance of perceptual-motor tests was significantly impaired in proportion to serum phenobarbital concentration. Tests requiring sustained vigilance were affected negatively. The author defined several factors that were significantly correlated with test performance: (a) serum phenobarbital concentration; (b) difficulty and duration of the task; and (c) tester interaction with the subject (i.e., external stimulation).

A closely related but separate issue is the question of memory impairment, which is a common complaint from epileptic patients and which unquestionably is related, in part, to the brain lesion (20). In detailed studies of patients tested when phenobarbital concentrations were at moderate and then high therapeutic levels, MacLeod et al. (42) compared short-term versus long-term memory storage. They found short-term memory scanning significantly impaired when phenobarbital levels were high, but retrieval of information stored in long-term memory was undiminished. Although this study was unfortunately brief in its 1-week trial at each dose, the data suggest that phenobarbital impairs access to information in short-term memory but not long-term memory. The authors suggested that impaired short-term memory may be an important influence in acquisition of new information because of impaired attention span. Oxley (62) indicated that a significant improvement in memory function can be achieved following a reduction in phenobarbital dose. This report was of interest because the patients experienced increased seizure frequency when the barbiturate level dropped, indicating that it is not seizure activity that impairs memory. In summary, the assessment indicated that phenobarbital has a deleterious effect on short-term memory with test performance related to dose. Even when serum concentration is within the therapeutic range, ability to concentrate and perform simple tasks is reduced.

Barbiturate Overdose

Frank overdose of phenobarbital causing serum levels in excess of 50 to 60 μg/ml leads to progressive neurological dysfunction and depression in levels of consciousness, even in patients on long-term therapy. Excessively high dose first produces ataxia, dysarthria, nystagmus, incoordination, and uncontrollable sleepiness. As the serum levels rise, these effects progress to stupor and coma. Ultimately, depression of cardiorespiratory function may lead to death. A level of 80 μg/ml is considered potentially lethal (5). The severity of central nervous system depression is much greater in the drug-naive patient. Because of tolerance, the occasional individual on prolonged therapy may remain almost unaffected by serum levels that cause unconsciousness in the naive individual. Nonetheless, concentrations above 70 μg/ml can be expected to compromise levels of consciousness in almost all individuals. Details of treatment will be considered below.

Dependence, Habituation, and Withdrawal

Physical dependence on phenobarbital must be considered an aspect of barbiturate neurotoxicity. Phenobarbital shares the properties of other barbiturates in that prolonged usage produces physical dependence: abrupt discontinuation after high dosage produces abstinence symptoms. Such symptoms include anxiety, emotional lability, insomnia, tremors, diaphoresis, confusion, and possible seizures for several days (29,32). These symptoms can be reversed by reinstituting the drug.

Isbell (32) described drug intoxication and withdrawal in terms of barbiturate abuse rather than its controlled use as an antiepileptic drug. If a decision is made to stop phenobarbital therapy, the drug should be tapered slowly to avoid withdrawal seizures.

Because phenobarbital can cross the placenta and enter the fetal system, special care must be taken during the neonatal period of children born to mothers who received phenobarbital. The neonatal withdrawal syndrome was described by Desmond et al. (21) for infants born to epileptic mothers. The infants were allowed to withdraw from phenobarbital postpartum. Hyperexcitability, tremor, irritability, and gastrointestinal upset continued for several days to several months. Although the withdrawal syndrome is similar among infants born to heroin addicts, barbiturate addicts, and epileptic mothers, the babies of women on antiepileptic doses of phenobarbital have a milder and briefer withdrawal experience with good results for all infants (6,38). There is no apparent residual damage after withdrawal. In order to calculate the probable length of withdrawal in neonates, it should be noted that the phenobarbital concentration in umbilical cord serum is approximately equal to the maternal serum concentration (54). The rate of elimination of phenobarbital in neonates is probably slower than in adults, possibly because neonatal liver is not fully capable of metabolizing barbiturates until enzyme induction has occurred (24,54).

Some evidence suggests that discontinuation of phenobarbital in epileptic patients may lead to exacerbation of seizures not only because of the underlying epilepsy but also because of an additional barbiturate withdrawal mechanism (8). Even with abrupt discontinuation, the slow elimination of phenobarbital results in slowly decreasing plasma drug levels. Even so, gradual tapering may be advisable.

Libido and Potency

A side effect of phenobarbital not documented in the literature and too little appreciated by treating physicians is impotence (48). Although primidone has been associated with this problem, there are no similar case reports of impotence caused by phenobarbital. In clinical practice, we have found that response to specific questions will reveal numerous complaints from men receiving phenobarbital. It is difficult to assess whether the problem is organic or related to psychological depression. Occasionally, dosage reduction will improve the problem. Although the effect may be associated with phenobarbital-induced metabolism of steroids (40) and specifically testosterone, the results of the VA study suggest a direct central nervous system action. Fifteen percent of patients in the VA study complained of decreased libido and/or potency, and this problem was found to be more common in patients treated with phenobarbital or primidone than those receiving carbamazepine or phenytoin ($p <$ .06) (48). Fourteen percent of 56 patients treated for 1 year with phenobarbital reported a transient or continuous decrease in sexual function. The reports increased over time, indicating that this is neither an acute problem nor one for which tolerance develops. Lowering the dose allowed improvement in some instances, but that drug was discontinued for patients who did not improve.

As noted above, multiple mechanisms, including altered metabolism of testosterone (82) and psychosocial factors (81), may be responsible for these complaints. However, the problem usually disappeared when carbamazepine or phenytoin was substituted for phenobarbital, but not when phenobarbital was changed to another barbiturate. Psychosocial factors were comparable, testosterone levels (both total and free) were equal, and enzyme-inducing properties are similar for all drugs in the four treatment groups. Consequently, we concluded that the changes in sex behavior may be a direct, neurogenic effect.

LONG-TERM DEVELOPMENTAL EFFECTS

Schain and Watanabe (71) reported that young rats were found to have retardation of brain growth and changes in behavior after long-term administration of phenobarbital. Hillesmaa et al. (28) subsequently reported decreased fetal head growth associated with maternal use of antiepileptic drugs and suggested a phenobarbital effect. Several groups have found disturbed neuronal development in cultures containing phenobarbital comparable or greater than is found with other antiepileptic drugs (3,57,73). These experimental findings may not be directly applicable to human use but raise special concern because phenobarbital is currently a drug of choice in pregnancy and treatment of neonates (see Chapter 22).

SYSTEMIC TOXICITY

Hematological

Phenobarbital is particularly benign in its likelihood to produce serious hematological changes other than during use in combination with other antiepileptic drugs. Sole therapy with phenobarbital does not require numerous blood tests in anticipation of leukopenia, agranulocytosis, thrombocytopenia, or aplastic anemia (22). Mild and clinically unimportant leukopenia (3,000–5,000 white blood count) may occur following initiation of treatment, as is also observed with use of other antiepileptic drugs (48).

Megaloblastic Anemia

Megaloblastic anemia has been described during treatment with phenobarbital alone or, more commonly, when it is used with other antiepileptic drugs, particularly phenytoin. Anticonvulsant megaloblastic anemia probably occurs in less than 1% of patients; the incidence was 0.15 to 0.75% in one report (27). The etiology and pathogenesis of macrocytosis and megaloblastic anemia during antiepileptic drug therapy are

unknown, but these conditions usually respond to folate therapy.

Folate Deficiency

Frank serum and red blood cell folate deficiency is relatively common. Reynolds (63) surveyed 16 reports ranging from 27% to as high as 91% subnormal serum folate levels, averaging 52%, in patients receiving long-term therapy with phenytoin, phenobarbital, or primidone. The significance of low folate levels is controversial.

Reynolds and Travers (65) reported improvement in psychiatric abnormalities in patients whose low serum folate concentrations were treated with folate therapy. However, such subjective observations are difficult to assess. Controlled trials have not confirmed that replacement folate therapy in patients receiving phenobarbital or phenytoin either aggravates the disease or improves patients' psychological status (35,50).

Reynolds (8) has postulated that antiepileptic drug-induced folate deficiency diminishes seizure control and that administration of folate therapy exacerbates seizures. Mattson et al. (50) found that serum phenobarbital and phenytoin concentrations decreased when folic acid was given in very high doses. It is possible that reports of seizure exacerbation resulted in part from the decrease in drug concentration rather than from an epileptogenic activity of folate, although the mechanism of this interaction is unknown.

The significance of folate deficiency remains speculative. Other than in cases of obvious megaloblastic anemia, subnormal serum folate probably requires no therapeutic intervention. Except perhaps during pregnancy, proper nutritional balance is sufficient to maintain adequate folate levels during antiepileptic drug therapy.

Although an inverse correlation exists between folate and phenobarbital levels in both serum and cerebrospinal fluid (CSF) (64), Mattson et al. (50) found no change in CSF folate concentration during folic acid therapy. In fact, animal studies (36) show clearly that even in severe folate deprivation, the brain maintains sufficient folate.

Vitamin K

Another hematological abnormality caused by antiepileptic drug therapy affects vitamin K. Phenobarbital and phenytoin, which enter the liver of the fetus, can compete with vitamin K to prevent production of vitamin K-dependent clotting factors. This can occur even in the presence of normal clotting factors in mothers receiving drug therapy. Mountain et al. (56) reported seven neonates with a severe coagulation defect in a series of 16 neonates whose mothers received various antiepileptic drugs (including 13 receiving barbiturates). The neonate can suffer from intraperitoneal, intrathoracic, or intracranial bleeding if vitamin K-dependent coagulation factors are deficient. These signs occur within the first day or two postpartum. Vitamin K administered to mothers prepartum will prevent this coagulation deficiency (56).

Bone Disorders

Antiepileptic drug therapy may affect calcium and vitamin D metabolism, leading to hypocalcemia or, rarely, osteomalacia (13). Despite a high incidence of subnormal calcium levels, only 10% of epileptic patients were found to have osteomalacia, with these developing only after many years of drug therapy (77). The incidence of this disorder may relate to climate (i.e., lack of sunshine) and diet.

Induction of liver enzymes leading to increased hydroxylation of vitamin D is a probable mechanism for altered calcium metabolism (67). Reversing signs of deficiency can be accomplished with less than 125 µg of vitamin D_3 per week (60).

CONNECTIVE TISSUE DISORDERS

A higher incidence of Dupuytren's contractures with palmar nodules, frozen shoulder, lederhose syndrome (plantar fibromas), Peyronie's disease, heel and knuckle pads, and general joint pain have been noted in patients taking antiepileptic drugs than in the general population. These connective tissue disorders were first linked to epilepsy patients in 1925 when Maillard and Renard (43) called attention to joint pain associated with the use of the newly introduced barbiturates, especially phenobarbital (Gardenal). Soon thereafter, Beriel and Barbier (4) termed this disorder "rheumatism gardenalique." Until recently, little evidence was available to differentiate among probable etiologic agents. Data from the VA study (49) provided evidence of a statistically significant association between use of phenobarbital and primidone for at least 6 months and onset of all 10 cases of connective tissue disorders (49). None of the 107 patients receiving solely carbamazepine or the 121 on phenytoin developed a problem ($p < .001$). Critchley et al. (18) were able to define phenobarbital as a common cause in contractures, and Janz and Piltz (33) associated primidone with frozen shoulder.

Incidence of barbiturate-related disorders ranges from 5% to 38% depending on the population studied. Froscher and Hoffman (25) noted that their general outpatient epilepsy patients had a 5% incidence of contractures, similar to that found in the outpatient VA study patients, but a higher incidence, 20%, in patients with severe epilepsy. Noble (59) reported a surgeon's point of view, having seen Dupuytren's contractures in 10% to 38% of institutionalized epilepsy patients. Duration of treatment probably increases the incidence of disorders.

Reversibility has occurred during continued drug use (33) but improvement is most likely when the barbiturate is stopped (30). Mattson et al. (49) also described clearing of signs and symptoms when carbamazepine, phenytoin, or valproate were substituted for the barbiturate.

HEPATIC DISORDERS

Phenobarbital is a hepatotoxin only in unusual susceptible individuals. Liver disease induced by antiepileptic drugs, particularly phenobarbital or phenytoin, appears not to be dose-dependent and has a low incidence. Most drugs are indirect hepatotoxins, selectively blocking metabolic pathways and producing structural changes by precise biochemical lesions (90). Idiosyncratic acute hepatic injury may be cytotoxic, cholestatic, or mixed. Cytotoxicity can lead to liver necrosis or cholestasis. These drugs probably produce hepatocellular injury, e.g., liver necrosis or cholestasis (90) (see "Hypersensitivity Reactions").

Enzymatic Effects

Antiepileptic drugs, particularly phenobarbital, are potent inducers of hepatic microsomal enzymes, which can lead to enhanced metabolism of other drugs or endogenous substances (66). Although some of these effects are considered drug interactions, the basis of these interactions must be considered a hepatic side effect of phenobarbital therapy. When metabolism of other compounds is accelerated, the end effect of drugs or substances can be diminished or negated, or pathways modified to produce different potentially effective or toxic metabolites. For example, the induction of microsomal valproate metabolism increased the concentration of the 4-en-VPA, hepatotoxic metabolite (2). Phenobarbital probably affects hydroxylation

pathways related to numerous endogenous and exogenous substances.

Phenobarbital increases the excretion of 6B-hydroxycortisol, leading to decreased plasma cortisol half-life (9). It has also been shown to increase the rate of metabolism of dexamethasone and prednisone. The resulting lower serum concentrations of these drugs used by patients with bronchial asthma disturbed the treatment of their pulmonary disorder. Withdrawal of phenobarbital allowed these changes to reverse (7). Enhanced hormone metabolism can cause failure of oral contraceptives, particularly with low-dose pills (34,40). Interference with the anticoagulation activity of coumarin drugs has been related to phenobarbital therapy (41). Erratic control of anticoagulation with decreased prothrombin time was noted during phenobarbital therapy, and increased dosage with the anticoagulant drug was necessary. However, if phenobarbital is withdrawn, allowing decreased enzyme stimulation, the other drug also requires dosage reduction or bleeding may occur.

Porphyria

Because phenobarbital can induce synthesis of liver enzymes, it has been shown to enhance the synthesis of δ-aminolevulinic acid (ALA) synthetase, which can cause chemical porphyria. Granick (26) hypothesized that drugs such as barbiturates may interact with heme, thereby diminishing inhibition of enzymes controlling ALA synthase production. Hereditary acute porphyria can be exacerbated when barbiturates are used.

Hyperbilirubinemia

Bilirubin conjugation has been induced by phenobarbital to treat neonatal hyperbilirubinemia (89). Because of induced action of hepatic microsomal enzymes, bilirubin excretion is enhanced through glucuronidation.

Ethanol and Other Drugs

Cramer (16) has reviewed the interactions between ethanol and antiepileptic drugs, noting several characteristics shared by phenobarbital ,and ethanol. Both compounds lead to hypertrophy of hepatic smooth endoplasmic reticulum, inducing nonspecific increase in numerous hepatic drug-metabolizing enzymes and cytochrome P-450. Both compounds are oxidized by NADH microsomal systems (15,68). Barbiturate-hydroxylating enzymes are increased in men given alcohol (69). Enzyme induction allows for increased clearance of drugs in alcoholic patients as well as in those receiving barbiturates. It is interesting to note that phenobarbital used with other drugs of abuse significantly affects their metabolism. In addition to altered ethanol metabolism, phenobarbital increases the rate of heroin deacetylation. This increase in detoxification is dose-related, parallel to increased enzyme induction (17). Conversely, barbiturates can reduce alcohol dehydrogenase activity, allowing high levels of alcohol to occur when both compounds are used concurrently. The synergy of barbiturate and ethanol toxicity can cause respiratory depression, leading to unexpected death (29).

GASTROINTESTINAL DISTURBANCES

Gastrointestinal complaints were significantly less frequent in patients treated with phenobarbital in the VA study (46). Early problems occurred in 2% to 3% of patients compared to 7% to 18% of patients on carbamazepine, phenytoin, or primidone. Although probably of central origin when nausea and vomiting occur acutely, as with primidone, some local gastrointestinal irritation is possible.

ONCOGENICITY

Animal studies have shown liver tumors appearing with the use of phenobarbital and other drugs that activate liver enzymes. Although enzyme induction causes an increase in liver size, it may also protect against the carcinogenicity of other compounds (i.e., known chemical carcinogens) by enhancing their metabolism.

There is no evidence of an increased frequency of liver tumors in patients taking phenobarbital. In fact, Clemmensen et al. (14) found a decrease in tumor incidence in patients receiving anticonvulsants. White et al. (86) found an increase in cancer deaths for epileptic patients, but this was not statistically significant.

HYPERSENSITIVITY REACTIONS

Phenobarbital causes various types of skin reactions. These usually are mild maculopapular, morbilliform, or scarlatiniform rashes that fade rapidly when drug administration is stopped. The incidence has been reported to be as low as 1% to 3% of all patients receiving barbiturates (72). Overall, hypersensitivity reaction to phenobarbital occurred in 9% of patients in the VA study. The rash was transient and did not require a change in treatment in five of 13 patients. None required hospitalization. Considering the universal usage of this drug, reports of exfoliative dermatitis, erythema multiforme, Stevens-Johnson syndrome, or toxic epidermal necrolysis are impressively rare. Welton (85) reported a case of exfoliative dermatitis with hepatitis caused by phenobarbital.

Hypersensitivity reactions are characterized by rash, eosinophilia, and fever (90). Histological changes in the liver show eosinophilic or granulomatous inflammation

(90). McGeachy and Bloomer (53) reviewed 17 instances of fatal sensitivity to phenobarbital. Another half-dozen cases of acute reaction to barbiturates and details of treatment were reported by Yatzidis (88). Corticosteroids are of value in treatment (53,79). Once sensitivity has been documented, only rarely should the patient be reexposed to the barbiturate (79).

Systemic lupus erythematosus (SLE) can develop with use of antiepileptic drugs. Alarcon-Segovia (1) suggests that the drugs elicit production of antinuclear antibodies by altering nuclear components. This may unmask SLE in predisposed individuals and can be reversed by prompt discontinuation of the drug.

TERATOGENICITY

With the current awareness that some antiepileptic drugs have teratogenic effects, counseling for the patient who wishes to become pregnant is indicated. It is difficult to correlate specific teratogenic effects with individual drug use in clinical studies of teratogenicity because of the frequent use of multiple drugs as well as other independent environmental and genetic risk factors. Animal studies suggest that all antiepileptic drugs have some potential for teratogenicity. However, when Chatot et al. (12) grew rat embryos in a media containing human serum from patients taking antiepileptic drugs, malformed embryos were less common for phenobarbital than carbamazepine, phenytoin, or valproate.

A variety of malformations have been observed in the offspring of six women who used only phenobarbital during their pregnancy: tracheo-esophageal fistula, ileal atresia, diaphragmatic hernia with pulmonary hypoplasia, thumb and radius aplasia, congenital heart lesion with microcephaly, mental retardation, hypospadias, and meningomyelocele (76). In this report and a similar retrospective survey by Nelson et al.

(58), the lack of characteristic malformation associated with sole phenobarbital use suggests coincidence rather than causal relationship (as with phenytoin and cleft palate).

Fedrick (23) found phenytoin far more teratogenic than phenobarbital, but when the two drugs were used in combination, teratogenicity was even more pronounced. Only 4.9% of infants born to mothers who received only phenobarbital during the first trimester were known to have birth defects. This is much lower than incidence rates of 15.2% for sole phenytoin therapy and 22% for combined. Surprisingly, in the same study there was a 10.5% incidence of malformation when mothers with epilepsy took no drugs during pregnancy. A large cooperative study in the United States and Finland (74) implicated phenytoin as a teratogen but gave no evidence of an association between birth defects whether the mothers used the drug for seizure prevention or for other indications (i.e., nonepileptic mothers). The question was raised whether fetal damage was attributable to antiepileptic drugs or to epilepsy. Statistically subtracting drug use, the malformation rate in children born to mothers with epilepsy was increased by 60%. A key factor associated with increased risk of fetal malformation may be the presence of epilepsy in either parent.

The Italian Multicentric Cohort Study (45) found reduced birth weight and head circumference in offspring of women treated with phenobarbital compared to other drugs. However, a maternal connection was suggested because children of untreated epileptic women had the same outcome. The major drawback in all of these studies of antiepileptic drug teratogenicity is the difficulty in obtaining information about maternal drug use. There is some evidence that higher drug dose and serum concentration correlate with increasing risk of malformation (19).

In summary, although gross malformations appear to be less common with pheno-barbital use, changes in neuronal development as described earlier may be a subtle but potentially important effect. Phenobarbital, when used alone, has occasionally been associated with fetal malformations but is thought to potentiate teratogenic effects when used with other drugs. Whether malformations occurring in offspring of epileptic parents are caused by epilepsy, antiepileptic drug therapy, other environmental problems, or a combination of these and other factors remains controversial. The available information suggests that if antiepileptic drug therapy is clearly indicated, phenobarbital, in comparison with phenytoin or valproate, may be considered a reasonably safe drug or perhaps a drug of choice during pregnancy.

TREATMENT

Many neurotoxic side effects improve with a simple reduction in dosage. Of course, improvement is gradual because of the slow elimination of phenobarbital. Such lowering of serum concentration provides less protection against seizures (80). In the past when seizure control could be achieved only at the cost of neurotoxic side effects, sedation and/or hyperactivity were sometimes ameliorated with concomitant administration of amphetamines. The additional complications attendant with the use of these stimulants are less necessary today. A change to treatment with an alternative antiepileptic drug may be equally effective and spare some side effects.

Recommendations for altered treatment when toxicity is apparent vary with the severity of the problem. The drug should be discontinued if a hypersensitivity reaction develops. Other acute toxicity early in the initiation of treatment should be viewed cautiously. Dosage can be held constant while symptoms abate, and increases should be slow thereafter. If decreased li-

bido is reported, lowering the serum phenobarbital concentration might improve the problem.

In cases where reversing side effects and lowering serum concentration must be rapid, elimination can be accelerated by alkalinization and induction of forced diuresis (52). Approximately one-third of an oral dose of phenobarbital is found in the urine unchanged. When necessary, administration of parenteral fluids up to 5 mg/kg/hr can increase excretion severalfold (10). If some of the fluid given is 1.25% sodium bicarbonate, the alkalinization of blood and urine further enhances elimination after overdose. At pH 7.4, 60% of phenobarbital is ionized. This polar compound poorly crosses cellular membranes. Penetration into and out of tissue is possible for the 40% of the drug that is un-ionized. When acidosis occurs, a higher percentage of phenobarbital is un-ionized, allowing passage into the intercellular space. This effectively increases tissue concentrations without any change in total body phenobarbital. Alkalosis has an opposite effect and leads to movement of phenobarbital out of brain and other tissues. Similarly, shifts in urinary pH can greatly modify the rate of phenobarbital elimination. Phenobarbital is cleared from the kidney and at the usually acid pH is largely in the un-ionized form. It is readily reabsorbed from the kidney tubule back into the circulation. In alkaline urine, the excreted phenobarbital becomes ionized and is not reabsorbed. By this mechanism alkalinization can appreciably increase elimination of phenobarbital from the body.

Changes due to systemic effects reverse more slowly. Reversal of enzyme induction effects may take days to weeks (47). Some changes, such as connective tissue disorders, may not reverse for months, or in the case of Dupuytren's contractures, may require surgery. Finally, if changes occur early in fetal or neonatal development, the toxic effects may be irreversible.

ACKNOWLEDGMENTS

This work was supported by the Veterans Administration Medical Research Service and NINCDS Grant No. NSO6208-22.

REFERENCES

1. Alarcon-Segovia, D. (1966): Drug-induced lupus syndromes. *Mayo Clin. Proc.*, 44:664–681.
2. Baillie, T. A. (1988): Metabolic activation of valproic acid and drug-mediated hepatotoxicity. Role of the terminal olefin, 2-*n*-propyl-4-pentenoic acid. *Chem. Res. Toxicol.*, 1:195–199.
3. Bergey, G. K., Swaiman, K. F., Schreir, B. K., et al. (1981): Adverse effects of phenobarbital on morphological and biochemical development of fetal mouse spinal cord neurons in culture. 9:584–589.
4. Beriel, L., and Barbier, J. (1934): Le rhumatisme gardenalique. *Presse Med.*, 42:67–69.
5. Berman, L. B., Jeghers, H. J., Schreiner, G. E., and Pallotta, A. J. (1956): Hemodialysis, an effective therapy for acute barbiturate poisoning. *J.A.M.A.*, 161:820–827.
6. Bleyer, W. A., and Marshall, R. E. (1972): Barbiturate withdrawal syndrome in a passively addicted infant. *J.A.M.A.*, 221:185–186.
7. Brooks, S. M., Werk, E. E., Ackerman, S. J., Sullivan, I., and Thrasher, K. (1972): Adverse effects of phenobarbital on corticosteroid metabolism in patients with bronchial asthma. *N. Eng. J. Med.*, 286:1125–1128.
8. Buchthal, F., Svensmark, O., and Simonsen, H. (1968): Relation of EEG and seizures to phenobarbital in serum. *Arch. Neurol.*, 19:567–572.
9. Burstein, S., and Klaiber, E. (1965): Phenobarbital induced increase in 6B-hydroxycortisol excretion: Clue to its significance in human urine. *J. Clin. Endocrinol. Metab.*, 25:293–296.
10. Butler, T. C., Mahafee, C., and Waddell, W. J. (1954): Studies of elimination accumulation, tolerance and dosage schedules. *J. Pharmacol. Exp. Therap.*, 111:425–435.
11. Camfield, C. S., Chaplin, S., Doyle, A. B., Shapiro, S. H., Cummings, C., and Camfield, P. R. (1979): Side effects of phenobarbital in toddlers; Behavioral and cognitive aspects. *J. Pediatr.*, 95:361–365.
12. Chatot, C. L., Klein, N. W., Clapper, M. L., Resor, S. R., Singer, W. D., Russman, B. S., Holmes, G. L., Mattson, R. H., and Cramer, J. A. (1984): Human serum teratogenicity studied by rat embryo culture: Epilepsy, anticonvulsant drugs, and nutrition. *Epilepsia*, 25:205–216.
13. Christiansen, C., Rodbro, P., and Lund, M. (1973): Incidence of anticonvulsant osteomalacia and effect of vitamin D: Controlled therapeutic trial. *Br. Med. J.*, 4:695–701.
14. Clemmensen, J., Fuglsang-Frederiksen, V., and Plum, C. M. (1974): Are anticonvulsants oncogenic? *Lancet* 1:705–707.
15. Conney, A. H., Jacobson, M., Schneidman, K., and Kuntzman, R. (1965): Induction of liver microsomal cortisol 6B-hydroxylase by diphenylhydantoin or phenobarbital. An explanation for the increased excretion of 6-hydroxycortisol in humans treated with these drugs. *Life Sci.*, 4:1091–1098.
16. Cramer, J. A. (1989): Ethanol metabolism and interactions with antiepileptic drugs. In: *Alcohol and Seizures*, edited by R. J. Porter, R. H. Mattson, J. A. Cramer, and I. Diamond, F. A. Davis, Philadelphia (*in press*).
17. Cramer, J. A., Cohn, G., and Meggs, L. (1975): Effect of phenobarbital and heroin metabolism in the rat. *Fed. Proc.*, 34:814.
18. Critchley, E. M. R., Vakil, S. D., Hayward, H. W., and Owen, V. M. H. (1976): Dupuytren's disease in epilepsy: Result of prolonged administration of anticonvulsants. *J. Neurol. Neurosurg. Psychiat.*, 39:498–503.
19. Dansky, L., Andermann, N. C., Sherwin, A., Andermann, F., and Kinch, R. A. (1980): Maternal epilepsy and congenital malformation: A prospective study with monitoring of plasma anticonvulsant levels during pregnancy. *Neurology*, 30:438.
20. Delaney, R. C., Rosen, A. J., Mattson, R. H., and Novelly, R. A. (1980): Memory function in focal epilepsy: A comparison of nonsurgical, unilateral temporal lobe and frontal lobe samples. *Cortex*, 16:103–117.
21. Desmond, M. M., Schwanecke, R. P., Wilson, G., Yasunaga, S., and Burgdorff, I. (1972): Maternal barbiturate utilization and neonatal withdrawal symptomatology. *J. Pediatr.*, 80:190–197.
22. DeVries, S. I. (1965): Haematological aspects during treatment with anticonvulsant drugs. *Epilepsia*, 6:1–15.
23. Fedrick, J. (1973): A report from the Oxford record linkage study. *Br. Med. J.*, 1:442–448.
24. Fouts, J. R., and Adamson, R. H. (1959): Drug metabolism in the newborn rabbit. *Science*, 129:897–898.
25. Froscher, W., and Hoffman, F. (1983): Dupuytren's contracture in patients with epilepsy: Follow-up study. In: *Antiepileptic Therapy: Chronic Toxicity of Antiepileptic Drugs*, edited by J. Oxley et al., pp. 147–154. Raven Press, New York.
26. Granick, S. (1965): Hepatic porphyria and drug-induced or chemical porphyria. *Ann. N. Y. Acad. Sci.*, 123:188–197.
27. Hawkins, C. F., and Meynell, M. J. (1958): Macrocytosis and macrocytic anemia caused by anticonvulsant drugs. *Am. J. Med.*, 27:45–63.
28. Hillesmaa, V. K., Teramo, K., Granstrom, M. L., and Bardy, A. H. (1981): Fetal head growth retardation associated with maternal antiepileptic drugs. *Lancet*, 1:165–167.
29. Hollister, L. E. (1965): Nervous system reactions to drugs. *Ann. N.Y. Acad. Sci.*, 123:342–353.
30. Horton, P., and Gerster, J. C. (1984): Reflex sympathetic dystrophy syndrome and barbiturates. A study of 25 cases treated with barbiturates com-

pared with 124 cases treated without barbiturates. *Clin. Rheumatol.*, 3:493–500.

31. Hutt, S. J., Jackson, P. M., Belsham, A., and Higgins, G. (1968): Perceptual motor behaviour in relation to blood phenobarbitone level: A preliminary report. *Dev. Med. Child Neurol.*, 10:626–632.

32. Isbell, H., and Fraser, H. F. (1950): Addiction to analgesics and barbiturates. *Pharmacol. Rev.*, 2:355–397.

33. Janz, D., and Piltz, U. (1983): Frozen shoulder induced by primidone. In: *Antiepileptic Therapy: Chronic Toxicity of Antiepileptic Drugs*, edited by J. Oxley, et al., pp. 155–159. Raven Press, New York.

34. Janz, D., and Schmidt, D. (1974): Antiepileptic drugs and failure of oral contraceptives. *Lancet*, 1:1113.

35. Jensen, O. N., and Olesen, O. V. (1970): Subnormal serum folate due to anticonvulsive therapy. *Arch. Neurol.*, 22:181–182.

36. Klipstein, F. A. (1964): Subnormal serum folate and macrocytosis associated with anticonvulsant drug therapy. *Blood*, 23:68–86.

37. Kornetsky, C., and Orzack, M. H. (1964): A research note on some of the critical factors on the dissimilar effects of chlorpromazine and secobarbital on the digit symbol substitution and continuous performance tests. *Psychopharmacology*, 6:79–86.

38. Kuhnz, W., Koch, H., Helge, H., and Nau, H. (1988): Primidone and phenobarbital during lactation period in epileptic women: Total and free drug serum levels in the nursed infants and their effects on neonatal behavior. *Dev. Pharmacol. Ther.*, 11:147–154.

39. Lennox, W. G. (1942): Brain injury, drugs and environment as causes of mental decay in epilepsy. *Am. J. Psychiatry*, 99:174–180.

40. Levin, W., Kuntzman, R., and Conney, A. H. (1979): Stimulatory effect of phenobarbital on the metabolism of the oral contraceptive 17a-ethynylestradiol-3-methyl ether (Mestranol) by rat liver microsomes. *Pharmacol.*, 19:294–255.

41. MacDonald, M. G., and Robinson, D. S. (1968): Clinical observations of possible barbiturate interference with anticoagulation. *J.A.M.A.*, 204:95–100.

42. MacLeod, C. M., Dekaban, A. S., and Hunt, E. (1978): Memory impairment in epileptic patients: Selective effects of phenobarbital concentration. *Science*, 202:1102–1104.

43. Maillard, G., and Renard, G. (1925): Un nouveau traitement de l'épilepsie: La phenylethylmalonyturée. *Presse Med.*, 33:315–317.

44. Marchesi, G. F. (1979): Effect of anticonvulsants on psychological tests in patients of normal intelligence. *Epilepsy Int., Florence, Italy* (abs).

45. Mastroiacovo, P., et al., (1988): Fetal growth in the offspring of epileptic women: Results of an Italian multicentric cohort study. *Acta Neurol. Scand.*, 78:110–114.

46. Mattson, R. H. (1986): Early tolerance to antiepileptic drug side effects: A controlled trial of 247 patients. In: Tolerance to beneficial and/or adverse

effects of antiepileptic drug. In: *Recent Advances in Epilepsy*, edited by Koella W. P., Raven Press, New York.

47. Mattson, R. H., and Cramer, J. A. (1989): Antiepileptic drug interactions in clinical use: An overview. In: *Drug Interactions*, edited by W. Pitlick et al., pp. 75–85. Demos Press, New York.

48. Mattson, R. H., Cramer, J. A., Collins, J. F., et al. (1985): Comparison of carbamazepine, phenobarbital, phenytoin, and primidone in partial and secondary generalized tonic-clonic seizures. *N. Engl. J. Med.*, 313:145–151.

49. Mattson, R. H., Cramer, J. A., McCutchen, C. B., and VA Epilepsy Cooperative Study Group. (1989): Barbiturate related connective tissue disorders. Arch. Int. Med., (*in press*).

50. Mattson, R. H., Gallagher, B. B., Reynolds, E. H., and Glass, D. (1973): Folate therapy in epilepsy: A controlled study. *Arch. Neurol.*, 29:78–81.

51. Mattson, R. H., Williamson, P. D., and Hanahan, E. (1976): Eterobarb therapy in epilepsy. *Neurol.*, 26:1014–1017.

52. Mawer, G. E., and Lee, H. A. (1968): Value of forced diuresis in acute barbiturate poisoning. *Br. Med. J.*, 2:790–792.

53. McGeachy, T. E., and Bloomer, W. E. (1953): The phenobarbital sensitivity syndrome. *Am. J. Med.*, 14:600–604.

54. Melchior, J. C., Svensmark, O., and Trolle, D. (1967): Placental transfer of phenobarbitone in epileptic women, and elimination in newborns. *Lancet*, 2:860–861.

55. Mirsky, A. F., and Kornetsky, C. (1964): On the dissimilar effects of drugs on the digit symbol substitution and continuous performance tests: A review and preliminary integration of behavioral and physiological evidence. *Psychopharmacology*, 5:161–177.

56. Mountain, K. R., Hirsh, J., and Gallus, A. S. (1970): Neonatal coagulation defect due to anticonvulsant drug treatment in pregnancy. *Lancet*, 1:265–268.

57. Neale, E. A., Sher, P. K., Graubard, B. I., et al. (1985): Differential toxicity of chronic exposure to phenytoin, phenobarbital, or carbamazepine in cerebral cortical cell cultures. *Pediatr. Neurol.*, 1:143–150.

58. Nelson, M. M., and Forfar, J. O. (1971): Associations between drugs administered during pregnancy and congenital abnormalities of the fetus. *Br. Med. J.*, 1:523–527.

59. Noble, J. (1983): Connective tissue disorders: Discussion. In: *Antiepileptic Therapy: Chronic Toxicity of Antiepileptic Drugs*, edited by J. Oxley et al., pp. 169–173. Raven Press, New York.

60. Offermann, G., Pinto, V., and Kruse, R. (1979): Antiepileptic drugs and vitamin D supplementation. *Epilepsia*, 20:3–15.

61. Ounsted, C. (1955): The hyperkinetic syndrome in epileptic children. *Lancet*, 1:303–311.

62. Oxley, J. (1979): The effect of antiepileptic drugs on psychological performance. *Epilepsy Int., Florence, Italy* (abs).

63. Reynolds, E. H. (1974): Chronic antiepileptic toxicity: A review. *Epilepsia,* 16:319–352.
64. Reynolds, E. H., Mattson, R. H., and Gallagher, B. B. (1972): Relationships between serum and cerebrospinal fluid anticonvulsant drug and folic acid concentrations in epileptic patients. *Neurology,* 22:841–844.
65. Reynolds, E. H., and Travers, R. D. (1974): Serum anticonvulsant concentrations in epileptic patients with mental symptoms: A preliminary report. *Br. J. Psychiat.,* 124:440–445.
66. Richens, A. (1974): The clinical consequences of chronic hepatic enzyme induction by anticonvulsant drugs. *Br. J. Clin. Pharmacol.,* 1:185–187.
67. Richens, A., Rowe, D. J. F. (1970): Disturbance of calcium metabolism by anticonvulsant drugs. *Br. Med. J.,* 4:73–76.
68. Rubin, E., Hutterer, F., and Lieber, C. S. (1968): Ethanol increases hepatic smooth endoplasmic reticulum and drug-metabolizing enzymes. *Science,* 159:1469–1470.
69. Rubin, E., and Lieber, C. S. (1968): Hepatic microsomal enzymes in man and rat: Induction and inhibition by ethanol. *Science,* 162:690–691.
70. Schain, R. J., Ward, J. W., and Guthrie, D. (1977): Carbamazepine as an anticonvulsant in children. *Neurology,* 27:476–480.
71. Schain, R. J., and Watanabe, K. (1976): Origin of brain growth retardation in young rats treated with phenobarbital. *Exp. Neurol.,* 50:806–809.
72. Schmidt, R. P., and Wilder, B. J. (1968): *Epilepsy.* F. A. Davis, Philadelphia.
73. Serrano, E. E., Kunis, D. M., and Ransom, B. R. (1988): Effects of chronic phenobarbital exposure on cultured mouse spinal cord neurons. *Ann. Neurol.,* 24:429–438.
74. Shapiro, S., Hartz, S. C., Siskind, V., Mitchell, A. A., Slone, D., Rosenberg, L., Monson, R. R., and Heinonen, O. P. (1976): Anticonvulsants and parental epilepsy in the development of birth defects. *Lancet,* 1:272–275.
75. Somerfeld-Ziskind, E., and Ziskind, E. (1940): Effect of phenobarbital on the mentality of epileptic patients. *Arch. Neurol. Psychol.,* 43:70–79.
76. Speidel, B. D., and Meadow, S. R. (1972): Maternal epilepsy and abnormalities of the fetus and newborn. *Lancet,* 2:839–843.
77. Stamp, T. C. B. (1974): Effects of long-term anticonvulsant therapy on calcium and vitamin D metabolism. *Proc. R. Soc. Med.,* 67:64–68.
78. Stores, G. (1975): Behavioral effects of antiepileptic drugs. *Dev. Med. Child Neurol.,* 17:647–658.
79. Stuttgen, G. (1973): Toxic epidermal necrolysis provoked by barbiturates. *Br. J. Dermatol.,* 88:291–293.
80. Svensmark, O., and Butchthal, F. (1963): Accumulation of phenobarbital in man. *Epilepsia,* 4:199–206.
81. Taylor, D. C. (1969): Sexual behavior and temporal lobe epilepsy. *Arch. Neurol.,* 21:510–516.
82. Toone, B. K., Wheeler, M., and Fenwick, P. B. C. (1980): Sex hormone changes in male epileptics. *Clin. Endocrinol.,* 12:391–395.
83. Vining, E. P. G., Mellits, E. D., Dorsen, M. M., Cataldo, M. F., Quaskey, S. A., Spielberg, S. P., and Freeman, J. M. (1987): Psychologic and behavioral effects of antiepileptic drugs in children: A double-blind comparison between phenobarbital and valproic acid. *Pediatrics,* 80:165–174.
84. Wapner, I., Thurston, D. L., and Holowach, J. (1962): Phenobarbital: Its effect on learning in epileptic children. *J.A.M.A.,* 182:937.
85. Welton, D. G. (1950): Exfoliative dermatitis and hepatitis due to phenobarbital. *J.A.M.A.,* 143:232–234.
86. White, S. J., McLean, A. E. M., and Howland, C. (1979): Anticonvulsant drugs and cancer: A cohort study in patients with severe epilepsy. *Lancet,* 2:458–461.
87. Wolf, S. M., and Forsythe, A. (1977): Psychology, pharmacotherapy and new diagnostic approaches. In: *Advances in Epileptology,* edited by H. Meinardi and A. J. Rowan, pp. 124–127. Swets & Zeitlinger, Amsterdam.
88. Yatzidis, H. (1971): The use of ion exchange resins and charcoal in acute barbiturate poisoning. In: *Acute Barbiturate Poisoning,* edited by H. Matthew, pp. 223–232. Excerpta Medica, Amsterdam.
89. Yeung, C. Y., Tam, L. S., Chan, A., and Lee, K. H. (1971): Phenobarbitone prophylaxis for neonatal hyperbilirubinemia poisoning. *Pediatrics,* 48:372–376.
90. Zimmerman, H. J. (1978): Drug-induced liver disease. *Drugs,* 16:25–45.

Antiepileptic Drugs, Third Edition, edited by
R. Levy, R. Mattson, B. Meldrum,
J. K. Penry, and F. E. Dreifuss.
Raven Press, Ltd., New York © 1989.

24

Other Barbiturates

Methylphenobarbital and Metharbital

Mervyn J. Eadie

Over the past half century, two *N*-methyl derivatives of barbituric acid have been employed as antiepileptic agents. Neither drug has come into any widespread use. Metharbital, which was introduced into therapeutics in 1948 (36), appears to have been little prescribed. Virtually nothing has been published concerning its clinical pharmacology. However methylphenobarbital, which began to be used in 1932 (1), does enjoy a certain popularity, at least in some countries. Thus, in Australia, National Health Service prescription numbers over several years for methylphenobarbital have remained reasonably similar to those for phenobarbital itself, and for primidone. Methylphenobarbital is reputed, at least by word of mouth, to be as effective as phenobarbital as an antiepileptic agent in humans, with the advantage that it is less sedative. Over the years a certain amount of information has accumulated about the pharmacokinetics and pattern of metabolism of methylphenobarbital, and there has been recent interest in stereospecific aspects of its biotransformation (25,28). It is now possible to provide a coherent picture of the clinical pharmacology of this drug, though not of metharbital.

CHEMISTRY

Methylphenobarbital (mephobarbital, methylphenobarbitone, Mebaral), chemi-

cally 5-ethyl-1-methyl-5-phenylbarbituric acid (Fig. 1) is the *N*-methylated analog of phenobarbital. It is a white crystalline powder, weakly acidic, with a pK_a value of 7.8 and a molecular weight of 246.26 daltons. It is more lipid soluble than phenobarbital. As usually supplied, methylphenobarbital is a racemic mix of R- and S-isomers.

Metharbital (*N*-methylbarbitone, Gemonil), chemically is 5, 5-diethyl-1-methylbarbituric acid (Fig. 2). It also is a weak acid with a pK_a value of 8.45 and a molecular weight of 198.22 daltons. Like methylphenobarbital, it is less polar and more lipid soluble than its *N*-desmethylated analog.

The general method for barbiturate synthesis involves condensation of an appropriate malonic acid derivative with urea. In the case of the *N*-methylbarbiturates, methylurea is used in place of urea (43). The reactions may be carried out in alkaline, neutral, or acidic media. Alternative synthetic pathways exist, e.g., condensations of (a) cyanoacetic esters with methyl urea, (b) malonamides with ethylcarbamate, or (c) malonylnitrile derivatives with methylurea (4).

METHODS OF DETERMINATION

Various methods have been used to measure the *N*-methyl barbiturates and their

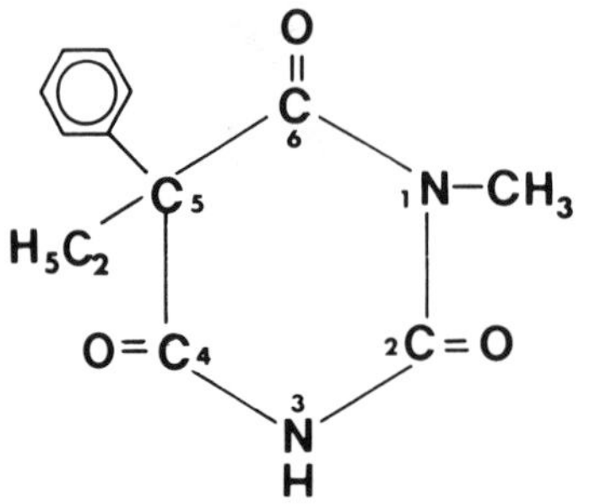

FIG. 1. Structure of methylphenobarbital.

desmethylated metabolites in biological material. The earliest methods appear to be those of Butler (4,5), who devised ultraviolet spectrophotometric assays, first for methylphenobarbital and its metabolite phenobarbital and subsequently for metharbital and barbital. The principles underlying such assays were reviewed by Bush and Sanders-Bush (3).

Nitration, followed by thin-layer chromatography, was used to resolve methylphenobarbital from phenobarbital (24). The nitrated residues were subsequently reduced, diazotized, and then diazo-coupled to yield products which were measured spectrophotometrically.

A number of gas-liquid chromatographic techniques have been developed for measuring methylphenobarbital and phenobarbital. Summary details of many of the methods and references to the original papers are

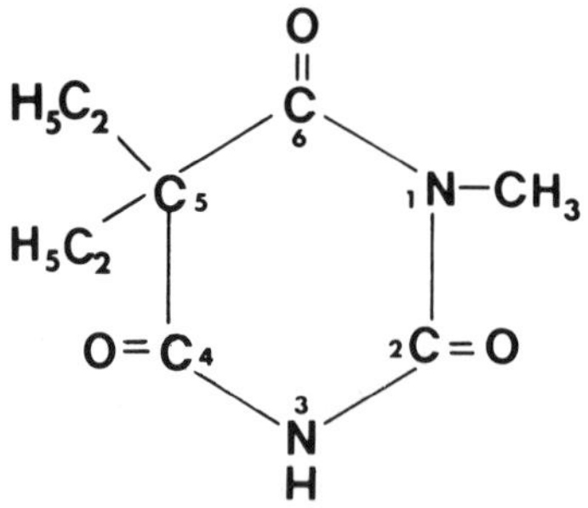

FIG. 2. Structure of metharbital.

given by Rambeck and Meijer (37). The two substances can be measured without derivatization (11), but derivatization provides more satisfactory chromatographic results. However, the most commonly used derivatization technique for anticonvulsant work, i.e., formation of methyl derivatives, yields the same product from both methylphenobarbital and phenobarbital. Thus, the parent substance and its metabolite cannot be quantitated individually. To overcome this difficulty, MacGee (33) formed ethyl rather than methyl derivatives. In this situation phenobarbital forms the N,N^1-diethyl compound, whereas methylphenobarbital yields N-ethyl-N-methylphenobarbital, and the two derivatives can be resolved from each other and measured separately. Higher alkyl derivatives might also be made and this should permit separate gas chromatographic quantitation of methylphenobarbital and phenobarbital. Hooper et al. (19) described a gas-liquid chromatographic assay for methylphenobarbital and phenobarbital which depended on formation of different butyl derivatives of the two substances.

Gas chromatography-mass spectrometry can be used for specific measurement of methylphenobarbital and phenobarbital in the same sample of biological material (22,29).

It is possible to measure methylphenobarbital and phenobarbital at biological concentrations without prior derivatization by the use of high-performance liquid chromatography with ultraviolet detection. This method (27) has proved quite satisfactory for routine assays in the author's laboratory, and, with the use of chiral columns, permits the measurement of the individual stereoisomers of the drug and its metabolites.

Various types of immunoassay method, such as the enzyme-multiplied immunoassay technique (EMIT) and radioimmunoassay, have been used to measure phenobarbital at biologically applicable concentrations. The antibodies used, at least for EMIT tests, are not completely specific for phenobarbital and measure methylphenobarbital as phenobarbital (40). Consequently, for patients taking methylphenobarbital (who are likely to have both the parent drug and phenobarbital simultaneously present in plasma), such assays will probably measure only the sum of concentrations of the two substances, and not the individual concentrations. Quantitation would be feasible only if completely specific antibodies were available, or if preliminary chromatographic separations were carried out prior to application of the immunoassay.

It appears likely that the methods discussed above for measuring methylphenobarbital and its desmethylated metabolite could be applied, with minor modification, to the measurement of metharbital and barbital. However, there has been little interest in measuring the latter substances. Flynn and Spector (16) did describe an antibody which they claimed was specific for barbital in the presence of metharbital. This antibody was employed in a radioimmunoassay that was used only in *in vitro* metabolic studies.

ABSORPTION, DISTRIBUTION, AND ELIMINATION

It should be recognized that, until quite recently, all pharmacokinetic work on methylphenobarbital was carried out using analytical methods that did not distinguish between the two stereoisomers of the drug. In the sections that follow the data apply to a racemic mix of the isomers, except where specifically indicated.

Absorption

Extent of Absorption

There is a long-standing clinical tradition that the dose of methylphenobarbital required to produce a given biological effect is approximately twice that of phenobarbital. Molecular weight differences cannot account for this discrepancy. Butler and Waddell (8), in studies on urine from three humans, could account for only 50% to 60% of a methylphenobarbital dose as the parent substance plus derived phenobarbital. On the basis of this finding, it has sometimes been suggested that only about 50% of an oral methylphenobarbital dose is absorbed. However, Butler and Waddell (8) and also Maynert (34) raised the possibility that part of the drug dose might be excreted as an unknown metabolite or metabolites. In this case, absorption of the orally administered drug might be more complete than was believed.

It has been suggested that the greater lipid solubility and lower aqueous solubility of methylphenobarbital, as compared with that of phenobarbital, might explain the incomplete absorption of methylphenobarbital from the alimentary tract. However, methylphenobarbital is not totally insoluble in cold water, and its greater lipid solubility as compared with phenobarbital might easily mean that it is better absorbed than the latter. It is now known that a significant proportion (some 35%) of a dose of racemic methylphenobarbital in man is excreted in urine as a previously unidentified *p*-hydroxyphenyl glucuronide derivative of the parent drug (21). A study with two volunteers, using a specially prepared intravenous formulation of racemic methylphenobarbital, found a 75% absolute bioavailability for the orally administered drug (20).

No quantitative data on the bioavailability of orally administered metharbital have been traced. It has been implied that the drug is likely to be better absorbed than methylphenobarbital because it is more water soluble, but this argument is suspect.

No information is available on the absorption of these *N*-methylated barbiturates after intramuscular administration.

Rate of Absorption

Except for data on three subjects, there does not appear to be published information on the absorption rate constants of orally administered methylphenobarbital or metharbital. Eadie et al. (13) carried out single-dose pharmacokinetic studies on orally administered racemic methylphenobarbital in eight human subjects. Unfortunately, in only one subject were sufficient data points obtained on the rising phases of the plasma drug level-time curves to permit calculation of absorption rate parameters for the drug. However, the times at which peak plasma concentrations occurred could be measured in all subjects. In seven of the eight, peak plasma methylphenobarbital levels occurred between 2.5 and 7 hr from the time of drug intake and, in the eighth subject, 26.5 hr after intake. Such T_{max} values are sometimes taken as a measure of a drug's absorption rate. However, the T_{max} is determined by both absorption and elimination rates, since it is the time when elimination rate first exceeds absorption rate after a drug dose. In the one subject in the series in whom an absorption rate constant could be measured, the absorption half-time was comparatively brief (1.4 hr). Later, in an oral bioavailability study in two volunteers, Hooper et al. (20) calculated absorption rate constants for the racemic drug corresponding to absorption half-times of 0.48 and 0.38 hr, respectively.

Factors Influencing Absorption

There does not appear to be any information published concerning factors that have been shown to modify the absorption of orally administered methylphenobarbital or metharbital in humans.

Distribution

Tissue Distribution

The literature contains little experimental data on the actual patterns of distribution of methylphenobarbital or metharbital in the various tissues and body fluids of humans. Buch et al. (2) published values for the uptake of the individual stereoisomers of methylphenobarbital by the brain of Wistar rats. The (+) isomer was more readily taken up than the (−) isomer, though the latter was the more potent anesthetic. The calculated apparent volume of distribution of racemic methylphenobarbital in man (13) and the dog (4) proves greater than the volume of total body water. Such values, and the known lipophilicity of the drug, suggest that it may achieve higher concentrations in tissues (particularly adipose tissue and brain) than in plasma. In rats, Craig and Shideman (11) found that brain methylphenobarbital levels were eight times those of the drug simultaneously measured in blood.

Apparent Volume of Distribution

Eadie et al. (13) calculated that the value of the apparent volume of distribution (V_d) of racemic methylphenobarbital in human adults was between 49 and 246 liters (mean, 132 liters). These values depended on the assumption that the orally administered drug was fully bioavailable. However, after intravenous administration of the drug to two volunteers, Hooper et al (20) obtained comparable V_d values of 153.5 and 188.3 liters, respectively. Butler's (4) earlier work in two dogs had provided V_d values of 1.9 and 2.1 liters kg^{-1} for methylphenobarbital, which are consistent with the values obtained in humans for this parameter. In one human subject (13) the V_d of phenobarbital (administered separately on another occasion) was 25.9 liters, whereas the V_d of methylphenobarbital was 246 liters. As mentioned above, the V_d figures suggest that methylphenobarbital achieves higher concentrations in tissues than in plasma.

There do not appear to be human data available for the V_d of metharbital. In the dog, Butler (5) found that the V_d was 1.22 liters kg^{-1}, whereas the V_d value of barbital itself was 0.6 liters kg^{-1}.

Plasma Protein Binding

There do not seem to be any direct measurements or indirect indications of the extent of the plasma protein binding of methylphenobarbital or metharbital, or any information concerning factors influencing the binding, with the exception of some *in vitro* data for methylphenobarbital which indicated that 58% to 68% of the drug in solution was bound to human serum albumin (at a concentration of 40 gram/liter) (2).

Elimination

Half-Life

After intravenous administration of racemic methylphenobarbital to two previously unmedicated volunteers, Hooper et al. (20) obtained terminal half-life values of 47.9 and 52.2 hr, respectively. Horning et al. (23) found half-lives of 34 and 47 hr in two subjects. In four adults not being treated with other drugs, the mean half-life of racemic methylphenobarbital after the first oral dose of this substance was 49.0 ± 18.8 (SD) hr (13). However, in five adults who were already being treated with a variety of drugs, mainly anticonvulsants, the mean elimination half-life of racemic methylphenobarbital was significantly shorter (19.6 ± 5.0 [SD] hr). The latter five subjects included one member of the first group of four subjects. This patient's only previous treatment at the time of the second half-life measurement comprised the single dose of methylphenobarbital given for the earlier pharmacokinetic study. In this subject, the half-life of methylphenobarbital fell from 35.2 hr in the first study to 18.7 hr in the second study. Continued methylphenobarbital intake leads to the formation of con-

siderable amounts of phenobarbital (a known hepatic microsomal mono-oxidase-inducing agent). It therefore seems likely that continued intake of methylphenobarbital would lead to autoinduction of the body's capacity to biotransform it. Thus, in patients receiving chronic methylphenobarbital therapy, it might be reasonable to anticipate that the racemic drug's own half-life would lie in the range of 12 to 24 hr.

Lim and Hooper (32) used a stereospecific analytical method to study the pharmacokinetics of the two enantiomers of methylphenobarbital in six previously untreated volunteers who were known to be extensive metabolizers of the drug. After oral intake, the mean half-life of the S-isomer was 65.01 ± 3.98 (SD) hr and that of the R-isomer was 7.75 ± 1.03 (SD) hr.

In keeping with the elimination rate constant (i.e., the half-life) data, the total body clearance of racemic methylphenobarbital averaged 1.85 ± 0.70 (SD) liters hr^{-1} in the noninduced subjects and 5.8 ± 2.70 (SD) liters hr^{-1} in the presumably induced subjects after oral administration of the drug (13). After intravenous dosage of racemic methylphenobarbital, clearance values of 2.21 and 2.50 liters hr^{-1} were obtained in two subjects (20). In their six noninduced volunteers, Lim and Hooper (32) calculated a mean clearance of 33.95 ± 6.65 (SD) liters hr^{-1} for the R-isomer and 1.26 ± 0.09 (SD) liters hr^{-1} for the S-isomer.

No data are available for the half-life or clearance of metharbital in humans.

Renal Excretion

Maynert and van Dyke (35) stated that no methylphenobarbital was excreted unchanged in urine. In three human subjects, Eadie et al. (13) found that renal excretion of unmetabolized racemic methylphenobarbital accounted for approximately 1.5% to 3.0% of the dose of drug administered orally. Even if only 50% to 60% of the drug was bioavailable, these renal excretion data would suggest that methylphenobarbital is cleared from the human body almost entirely by means of biotransformation. In the same three subjects referred to immediately above, approximately 8% to 25% of the dose of racemic methylphenobarbital was excreted in urine as phenobarbital (and it is possible that the urine may not have been collected long enough to determine the full amount of phenobarbital that was ultimately excreted via this route). The investigation of Hooper et al. (20) showed that, at least in the acute single-dose situation in noninduced human subjects, p-hydroxy-methylphenobarbital (5-ethyl-5-p-hydroxy-phenyl-1-methylbarbituric acid) is a major urinary metabolite of racemic methylphenobarbital, accounting for 30% to 35% of the drug dose. This hydroxy derivative is excreted in human urine mainly as a phenolic glucuronide conjugate. Small amounts of the p-hydroxyphenyl derivative of phenobarbital are found, as are traces of the m-hydroxyphenyl isomer of methylphenobarbital. However, this m-hydroxy isomer was thought to have occurred in these circumstances as a methodological artifact.

No detailed studies of the renal mechanisms involved in handling methylphenobarbital and its phenolic metabolite are available. From its physical properties, one might anticipate that the drug would be filtered through the renal glomerulus and then resorbed passively as water resorbs during its passage down the renal tubules. The pK_a value of methylphenobarbital is probably high enough for changes in urine pH to have little influence on the extent of urinary excretion of the drug. One might anticipate that p-hydroxymethylphenobarbital glucuronide, like other glucuronides, would be actively secreted into proximal tubular urine as well as filtered from plasma water into the renal glomerulus. Factors influencing the renal handling of phenobarbital itself are discussed in Chapter 22.

There does not appear to be any pub-

lished information regarding factors involved in the renal handling of metharbital and its metabolite, barbital. It is belived that metharbital is extensively converted to barbital, and the latter is said not to undergo further metabolic transformation (17). In dogs, barbital is filtered through the renal glomerulus and extensively resorbed during the passage of urine down the renal tubules (17). Similar considerations probably apply in humans.

Hepatic Metabolism

Methylphenobarbital appears to be cleared from the body mainly by biotransformation. In rats, the demethylation of the drug, producing phenobarbital, is known to occur in the liver (7,9,41). It seems likely that the liver is also the main site of metabolism of the drug in humans. It is not known whether disease alters the liver's capacity for biotransformation of the drug.

In the rat, metharbital is oxidatively demethylated in the liver (9,41). The analogous biotransformation in humans is presumed to occur in this organ. No information is available regarding factors in humans that may influence the hepatic handling of the drug.

Other Routes of Elimination

It is not known whether methylphenobarbital is excreted from the human body in significantly quantities in feces or various bodily secretions, e.g., sweat, tears, and milk. Whether the drugs or their glucuronide metabolites undergo an enterohepatic circulation is also unknown.

BIOTRANSFORMATION

Chemical Aspects of Metabolism

That methyphenobarbital is biotransformed to phenobarbital has been known since 1939 (6). This was originally thought to be the major biotransformation pathway of the drug in humans, leading to the presence in urine of further stage biotransformation products, e.g., *p*-hydroxyphenobarbital and the dihydrodiol metabolite of phenobarbital (18). However, the data of Kunze et al. (27) and Hooper et al. (21) demonstrated that there was an alternative major biotransformation pathway for the drug in man, viz. aromatic hydroxylation. This finding was based on urinary excretion data in humans. Thus urine from patients taking methylphenobarbital was heated with hydrochloric acid to hydrolyze any glucuronide or sulfate conjugates, and both the *meta* and the *para* isomers of 5-ethyl-5-hydroxypenyl-1-methylbarbituric acid could be identified. However, if the hydrolysis was carried out by incubation with β-glucuronidase, only the *para* isomer was found. By analogy with what happens to the aromatic hydroxylation products of phenytoin, it might be inferred that a dihydrodiol metabolite initially forms from methylphenobarbital (perhaps via an epoxide), and that the dihydrodiol then preferentially converts to the *p*-hydroxyphenyl isomer in the human liver. The postulated dihydriodiol has not yet been identified in the urine of patients taking methylphenobarbital. If the dihydrodiol was present in urine, acid hydrolysis might be expected to convert it to both *p*- and *m*-hydroxyphenyl isomers. Recently Treston et al. (42) have identified small amounts of an *O*-methyl-catechol derivative of the drug in urine. A tentative scheme of methylphenobarbital metabolism in humans can be proposed (Fig. 3).

The current interest in stereoselective drug metabolism has led to some investigation of the preferential biotransformation pathways for the enantiomers of methylphenobarbital. Kupfer and Branch (28) and Jacqz et al. (25) have shown that the drug undergoes a polymorphic pattern of metabolism that appears to be coregulated with that of the more intensively studied hydan-

toin derivative, mephenytoin (methoin). In a group of subjects categorized either as extensive or as poor metabolizers of mephenytoin, Kupfer and Branch (28) showed that over 8 hr the extensive metabolizers excreted 2.5% to 48% of a racemic methylphenobarbital dose in urine as its *p*-hydroxyphenyl derivative, whereas the poor metabolizers excreted less than 1% of the dose in this form. It appears that the S-isomer of methylphenobarbital is cleared mainly by demethylation, whereas the R-isomer is rapidly eliminated by both aromatic hydroxylation and demethylation in extensive metabolizers of the drug, but only by the latter route in poor metabolizers (who cannot readily hydroxylate the drug).

As far as can be ascertained, there is no direct published evidence of the metabolic fate of metharbital in humans. It is generally assumed that the drug is oxidatively demethylated to barbital, as it is in the dog (5). Barbital is said to probably undergo no further metabolic degradation (35).

Pharmacological Aspects of Metabolism

p-Hydroxymethylphenobarbital (in the form of its phenolic glucuronide) is the major urinary metabolite present after the initial dose of racemic methylphenobarbital, but would be expected to possess little biological activity. From the standpoint of pharmacological activity, phenobarbital appears to be the more significant biotransformation product. In patients receiving long-term anticonvulsant therapy, including therapy with methylphenobarbital itself, there is some evidence that the human body's capacity for conversion of methylphenobarbital to phenobarbital is increased (13). One patient who had taken multiple anticonvulsants over several years excreted almost 25% of an initial methylphenobarbital dose as phenobarbital during the 75-hr period following the dose, whereas two subjects not previously exposed to drugs ex-

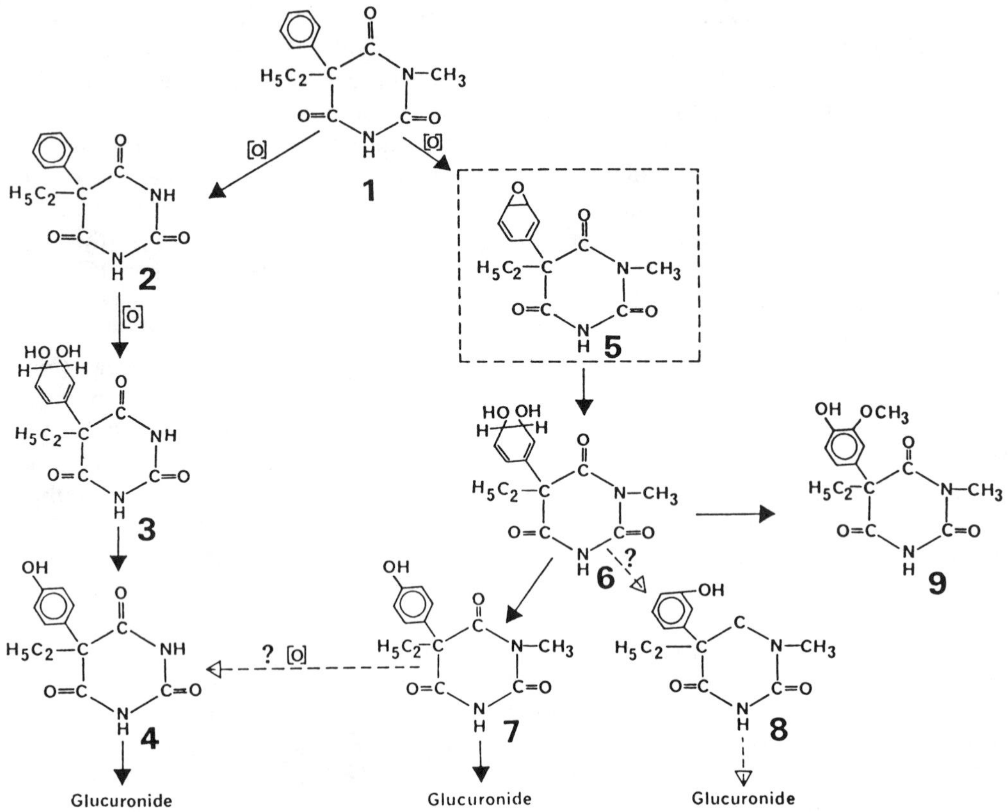

FIG. 3. Tentative scheme of methylphenobarbital metabolism: **1**, methylphenobarbital; **2**, phenobarbital; **3**, dihydrodiol metabolite of phenobarbital; **4**, *p*-hydroxyphenobarbital; **5**, postulated epoxide metabolite of methylphenobarbital; **6**, dihydrodiol metabolite of methylphenobarbital; **7**, *p*-hydroxymethylphenobarbital; **8**, *m*-hydroxymethylphenobarbital; **9**, **O**-methyl catechol metabolite of methylphenobarbital. (From Eadie and Tyrer, ref. 15, with permission.)

creted only 8% and 11% of their initial methylphenobarbital doses as phenobarbital in the 200 hr following dosage. Not only was methylphenobarbital cleared faster in patients on long-term anticonvulsant therapy, but in these patients phenobarbital appeared earlier in the blood and tended to achieve higher peak plasma levels (Fig. 4). However, this work was carried out in small numbers of patients before the significance of stereoselective metabolism of the drug was appreciated. Fortuitous study of a few subjects who were poor hydroxylators of

the drug may have confused the interpretation of the findings, though there is evidence (cited above) that methylphenobarbital dealkylation may be increased in subjects previously exposed to anticonvulsants.

Eadie et al. (13) studied areas under the plasma phenobarbital level–time curves in a patient who, on separate occasions, took a first dose of phenobarbital and a first dose of methylphenobarbital. Using this approach, it could be calculated that some 52% of the racemic methylphenobarbital

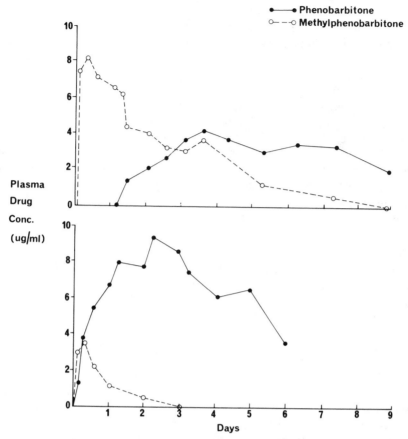

FIG. 4. Time-courses of plasma concentrations of methylphenobarbital and derived phenobarbital after an initial oral dose of racemic methylphenobarbital in a previously untreated patient (**top panel**) and in a patient already treated with other antiepileptic drugs (**bottom panel**). (From Eadie et al., ref. 13, with permission.)

dose was converted to phenobarbital. No metabolic balance studies were carried out to account for the remainder of the dose.

No quantitative data on metharbital biotransformation in man are available.

INTERACTIONS WITH OTHER DRUGS

Pharmacodynamic Interactions

As indicated above, in humans a significant portion of a methylphenobarbital dose is converted to phenobarbital. The latter is more slowly cleared than the former and has a smaller volume of distribution. Therefore, under the conditions of prolonged methylphenobarbital intake, plasma phenobarbital levels (but not necessarily tissue phenobarbital levels) come to be almost an order of magnitude higher than simultaneous plasma methylphenobarbital levels. There are no pharmacokinetic data or results of plasma level monitoring available to indicate whether similar considerations apply to metharbital in humans. However, it seems not unreasonable to suspect that they may. Because of the presence of biologically active dealkyl metabolites, unless plasma levels of all the relevant substances are measured, it may be difficult to know whether pharmacodynamic type drug–drug interactions apparently involving methylphenobarbital or metharbital are related primarily to the parent drug, to its metabolite, or to both.

It seems likely that any interaction that has been described for phenobarbital (see Chapter 23) may also occur when methylphenobarbital is the source of phenobarbital. Such interactions will not be dealt with in detail here. Methylphenobarbital itself acts as a central nervous system depressant and sedative. If it is prescribed combined with other drugs with sedative actions, e.g., tricyclic antidepressants, antipsychotics, benzodiazepines, or various hypnotics, it might be anticipated that the overall degree of depression of central nervous system function would be increased.

Methylphenobarbital probably possesses antiepileptic activity in its own right (see below), as well as by virtue of the phenobarbital it produces. It may have additive antiepileptic effects if combined with other anticonvulsants that are appropriate for the patient's type of seizure disorder. The degree of antiepileptic effect of the individual enantiomers of the drug is not yet known.

Pharmacokinetic Interactions

Phenobarbital is a well-known inducer of the hepatic microsomal mono-oxidase system. Methylphenobarbital intake might be expected to lead to similar induction by virtue of the phenobarbital to which it is biotransformed, and possibly by a direct effect also. It is therefore conceivable that methylphenobarbital intake might alter the plasma concentrations of co-administered drugs that undergo microsomal oxidations. Lander et al. (30) used a multiple-variable, linear-regression technique on data from a population of epileptic patients to see whether interactions could be detected in which methylphenobarbital altered plasma levels of phenytoin and carbamazepine taken concurrently. No such interactions were found.

In a group of patients receiving methylphenobarbital, Eadie et al. (13) carried out a multiple-variable, linear-regression analysis of plasma methylphenobarbital and derived phenobarbital levels on methylphenobarbital dose to try to trace interactions in which other anticonvulsants might have altered the body's handling of methylphenobarbital. Dosage of phenytoin, carbamazepine, and sulthiame, the three drugs most widely combined with methylphenobarbital in the patients studied, had no statistically significant effects on the regressions for the plasma levels of parent drug or phenobarbital on methylphenobarbital dose. This failure to detect interactions in a population study does not necessarily mean that interactions do not occur in individual members of the population studied. If an interaction raises plasma drug levels in some patients and lowers them in others, the effects may cancel out to such an extent that mean plasma levels in the population do not change appreciably.

The present author has not seen instances of pharmacokinetic-type interactions in individual patients taking methylphenobarbital with other antiepileptic drugs, except when the drug was taken with valproate. On several occasions, the introduction of valproate to the therapeutic regimen of a patient taking methylphenobarbital has resulted in a progressive and sustained rise of considerable magnitude in plasma phenobarbital levels and in a lesser rise in plasma methylphenobarbital levels. Such an interaction has been illustrated by Eadie and Tyrer (15).

There appears to be nothing published on the interactions of metharbital, though it is likely that the expected pharmacodynamic-type interactions of the drug would occur if the drug were used in practice.

RELATIONSHIP OF PLASMA CONCENTRATION TO SEIZURE CONTOL

Therapeutic Plasma Concentrations

Phenobarbital is more slowly eliminated than methylphenobarbital so that when methylphenobarbital is taken on a long-term basis, steady-state plasma concentrations of the pharmacologically active metabolite come to exceed plasma levels of the administered drug. For practical purposes, it often seems sufficient to use plasma phenobarbital levels as a guide to the therapeutic situation and to ignore simultaneous plasma methylphenobarbital levels. This is possible largely because the therapeutic range of plasma phenobarbital levels is wide (10–40 mg/L), its limits are not sharply demarcated, and relatively little methylphenobarbital is present in plasma relative to phenobarbital. However, to ignore plasma methylphenobarbital levels is to overlook a measure of one active antiepileptic substance present in the body. Further, the antiepileptic agent that is neglected is one that, because of its high apparent volume of distribution relative to that of phenobarbital and its lipid solubility, probably has substantially higher brain levels relative to plasma levels than has phenobarbital. The present author has seen a patient taking multiple antiepileptic drugs who failed to develop a further increase in plasma phenobarbital level beyond 20 mg/L when his daily methylphenobarbital dose was increased from 180 to 300 mg, although he became exceedingly drowsy and ataxic. Despite the failure of his plasma phenobarbital level to increase, his plasma methylphenobarbital level had risen from 2 to 8 mg/L. Reduction in the methylphenobarbital dose relieved the toxicity. This patient probably exhibited an unusual saturation of his capacity to demethylate methylphenobarbital and his alternative major biotransformation pathway (aromatic hydroxylation) could not cope with the increased metabolic load. Nevertheless, this case history illustrates the point that methylphenobarbital is not devoid of direct biological effect, and that it is occasionally important to be able to measure its plasma concentrations. It may be sufficient to measure plasma phenobarbital levels to monitor the therapeutic situation in most patients taking methylphenobarbital and to recognize that one may be underestimating the total anticonvulsant activity present though one has a reasonably valid measure of it. However, the simultaneous specific measurement of methylphenobarbital and phenobarbital levels provides even more useful, and occasionally critical, information. If phenobarbital is measured by a nonspecific assay that measures methylphenobarbital as phenobarbital, potentially misleading results may occasionally be obtained. Whether it will be necessary to measure the individual enantiomers of the drug routinely is a question for the future.

There does not appear to be any information available regarding plasma metharbital or barbital levels in humans, or the relationship of these levels to therapeutic or toxic effects. Therefore, the remaining information pertains only to methylphenobarbital.

Relationship of Dose to Plasma Concentration

Figure 5 shows the linear relationship that was found between simultaneous steady-state plasma concentrations of both methylphenobarbital and derived phenobarbital, and the dose of racemic methylphenobarbital in populations of treated patients (13). Steady-state plasma phenobarbital levels correlate more closely with methylpheno-

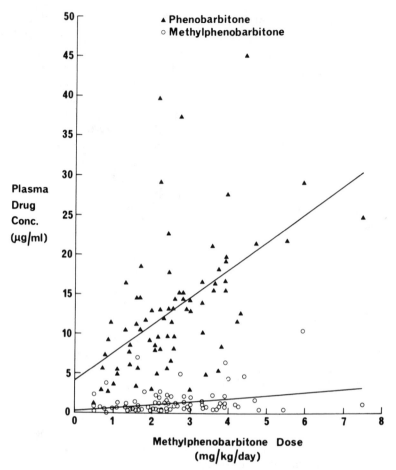

FIG. 5. Relationship between steady-state plasma levels of methylphenobarbital and derived phenobarbital and dose of racemic methylphenobarbital in a group of treated epileptic patients. (From Eadie et al., ref. 13, with permission.)

barbital dose than do plasma levels of the parent substance. However, the increased relative scatter in methylphenobarbital levels, as compared with the scatter in phenobarbital levels, may have resulted from difficulty measuring with equal precision plasma concentrations that usually differ by an order of magnitude. The assay used had been arranged to provide optional precision in measuring phenobarbital. Methylphenobarbital doses of 3 to 4 mg/kg per day produced a mean plasma phenobarbital level of 15 mg/L, and a dose of 5 mg/kg per day produced a mean level of 20 mg/L.

The relationship between simultaneous steady-state plasma phenobarbital and methylphenobarbital levels in the same patients is shown in Fig. 6. Plasma phenobarbital levels averaged 7 to 10 times those of methylphenobarbital when plasma levels of the former were between 10 and 20 mg/L, values commonly encountered in treating epilepsy. At higher plasma methylphenobarbital levels, however, there was a tendency for plasma phenobarbital levels to be proportionately less than at lower methylphenobarbital levels. This finding raises the possibility that the demethylation of meth-

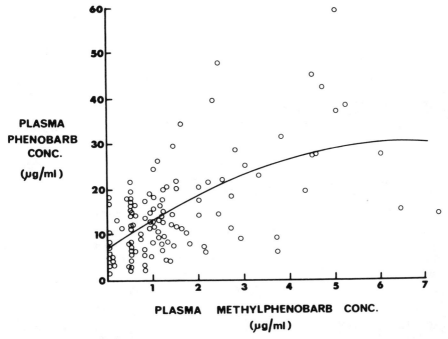

FIG. 6. Relationship between simultaneous steady-state plasma levels of methylphenobarbital and derived phenobarbital in epileptic patients treated with racemic methylphenobarbital. (From Eadie et al., ref. 13, with permission.)

ylphenobarbital may tend to become rate-limited at higher values of plasma concentrations of the drug that are encountered therapeutically. However, the interpretation of this finding may have to be revised in light of contemporary awareness of the possibilities implicit in stereoselective metabolism of the drug. Kupferberg and Longacre-Shaw (29) found in a small series of patients that plasma phenobarbital levels averaged 20 times those of methylphenobarbital.

In addition to knowing the relationships between steady-state plasma methylphenobarbital and phenobarbital levels and methylphenobarbital dose in treated populations, it is desirable to know the steady-state plasma level–dose relationship in treated individuals who have had plasma levels measured while receiving different methylphenobarbital doses at different times. As shown in Fig. 7, at least for

plasma phenobarbital levels up to 30 mg/L, the relationship between plasma phenobarbital levels and methylphenobarbital dose usually appears linear (14). The relationship between methylphenobarbital plasma level and dose also appears linear (12). It should be noted that when phenobarbital itself is taken, the relationship in the individual between steady-state plasma phenobarbital level and phenobarbital dose appears curvilinear (14). This difference in the behavior of plasma phenobarbital levels when the drug is supplied directly or is supplied indirectly via methylphenobarbital suggests that plasma phenobarbital levels may be adjusted more predictably when using methylphenobarbital than when using phenobarbital itself.

Population studies (14) have shown that the slope of the regression for steady-state plasma phenobarbital level on drug dose changes with age. The effect of this change

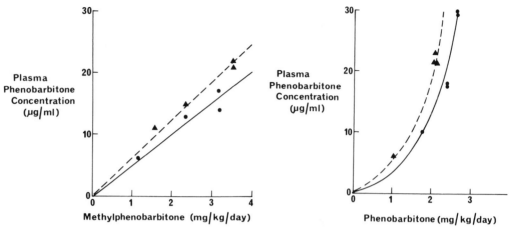

FIG. 7. Relationship between steady-state plasma level of phenobarbital and racemic methylphenobarbital dose (**left**) and between steady-state phenobarbital level and phenobarbital dose (**right**), each in two subjects who took different doses of the drugs at different times. (From Eadie et al., ref. 14, with permission.)

is such that the methylphenobarbital dose required to produce a given plasma phenobarbital level tends to decrease with age, if doses are expressed relative to body weight, Thus, to achieve a plasma phenobarbital level of 15 mg/L, a person under 15 years would require a mean daily methylphenobarbital dose of 4 mg/kg, and a person over 40 years would require a mean daily dose of 2 mg/kg. Regression analysis shows that the patient's sex also influences the relationship between steady-state plasma phenobarbital level and methylphenobarbital dose. For a given methylphenobarbital dose (corrected for body weight), males tend to have average plasma phenobarbital levels some 5 mg/L higher than females.

Relationship of Plasma Concentrations to Therapeutic Effect

It has already been mentioned that in clinical practice it is desirable to measure simultaneous plasma levels of both methylphenobarbital and phenobarbital in patients receiving methylphenobarbital. However there is no information available on the

therapeutic range of plasma methylphenobarbital levels. It seems that the conventional therapeutic range of plasma phenobarbital levels (15–30 or 10–40 mg/L) usually proves a reasonable guide to the antiepileptic effects of methylphenobarbital, although it does tend to underestimate the total antiepileptic activity present.

Toxic Effects Related to Plasma Concentrations

As with anticonvulsant effects, toxic effects of administered methylphenobarbital tend to correlate reasonably well with plasma phenobarbital levels. Since plasma phenobarbital levels tend to parallel plasma methylphenobarbital levels, the latter are also likely to correlate with toxic effects of the drug. Toxic effects of phenobarbital (apart from idiosyncratic reactions) are mostly consequences of depression of central nervous functions. In some individuals, such unwanted effects may appear with plasma phenobarbital levels as low as 10 to 15 mg/L, particularly if these levels are achieved early in the course of therapy.

Many patients, however, show no clinically obvious depression of nervous system functions at plasma phenobarbital levels as high as 40 mg/L, particularly if these levels have been achieved slowly.

One has the impression that true pharmacological tolerance to phenobarbital, as distinct from time-related autoinduction of phenobarbital elimination, does occur, although no absolute proof of this phenomenon appears to exist. The existence of such pharmacological tolerance would, however, explain some of the difficulty that exists in designating any sharp toxicity threshold for plasma phenobarbital concentrations. It is, of course, possible, and indeed likely, that tests of psychological function may detect a progressive impairment of performance that correlates with rising plasma levels of phenobarbital and methylphenobarbital when methylphenobarbital is taken, even though there may be no sharp concentration threshold at which obvious toxicity appears. Such a progressive decline in measured intellectual performance has been shown to exist when orally administered phenobarbital itself is prescribed (39).

As mentioned above, the demethylation of methylphenobarbital may occasionally appear to become saturated under clinical conditions. In these circumstances, significant central nervous system depression may occur at plasma phenobarbital concentrations that would usually be regarded as nontoxic, though at plasma methylphenobarbital levels above 5 or 6 mg/L.

Tolerance and Dependence

The possibility of a true pharmacological tolerance developing to the effects of phenobarbital and perhaps methylphenobarbital has been discussed above when the question of a therapeutic range for both phenobarbital and methylphenobarbital was considered. Sufficient information is not yet available to determine if a degree of apparent tolerance to the effects of methylphenobarbital develops because of a time-related increase in its elimination parameters. In patients taking the drug on a long-term basis methylphenobarbital clearance appears to be increased, with more of the drug being converted to phenobarbital. Any tolerance, in the sense of a decrease in biological effect relative to drug dose, that might result from falling methylphenobarbital levels might be offset by higher phenobarbital levels.

There are reports in the psychiatric literature of dependence developing, particularly in the elderly, to various barbiturates. However, well-authenticated reports of dependence on methylphenobarbital or metharbital have not been traced.

Pharmacological Aspects of Clinical Use

Time to Steady-State Plasma Levels

For a drug eliminated by processes that follow exponential kinetics and that is taken regularly, a clinically adequate approximation to a steady state is achieved after the lapse of four or five terminal elimination half-lives. Therefore, plasma levels of racemic methylphenobarbital ($T_{1/2}$, approximately 2 days) should attain steady-state values some 8 to 10 days after the commencement of therapy or after the most recent dosage change, though steady-state conditions for the two enantiomers of the drug may develop at quite different times. However, if autoinduction of biotransformation occurs, or if the patient's drug-metabolizing oxidative enzymes are already induced by prior exposure to other anticonvulsants, the steady state for methylphenobarbital may be achieved earlier, perhaps in as little as 4 days. From the practical clinical point of view, however, the plateau pharmacological effect of methylphenobarbital is determined by the time to achieve steady-state plasma levels of the phenobarbital derived from it. This substance has an elimination half-life of 3 to 4 days so that its steady state is likely to take some 2 to 3 weeks to develop after a methylphenobarbital dosage change, or perhaps even longer after the first dose of the drug if one allows for delay in the rate of production of phenobarbital to stabilize, should autoinduction of methylphenobarbital and phenobarbital biotransformation occur.

There is a further practical consideration that may determine when a plateau seizure-control state applies after methylphenobarbital therapy is commenced. If a dose of the drug that is calculated as likely to produce a mid-therapeutic range steady-state plasma level is prescribed as soon as therapy is started, patients often complain of such drowsiness within a few days that they are reluctant to continue therapy. If half, or less than half, of the expected dose is used for the first 1 or 2 weeks of therapy and the dose is then increased, this problem is usually obviated. However, there will be a corresponding delay in achieving steady-state therapeutic plasma levels of derived phenobarbital.

Variation in Steady-State Plasma Levels

In view of the relatively slow eliminations of both racemic methylphenobarbital and phenobarbital, steady-state plasma levels of both the prescribed racemic drug and its metabolite would be expected to show relatively little fluctuation over 12-hr or even 24-hr dosage intervals, even when the drug is taken only once a day. This expectation is borne out in practice, as illustrated by Eadie and Tyrer (15). However the half-life data for the enantiomers of the drug suggest that the plasma levels of the more rapidly eliminated R-isomer may show an appreciable degree of interdosage fluctuation under steady-state conditions, should the appropriate measurements be made.

Metabolism During Pregnancy

Alterations in Plasma Levels During Pregnancy

Lander et al. (31) showed that in women taking constant daily methylphenobarbital doses, plasma phenobarbital levels tended to fall during the course of pregnancy and to rise again in the puerperium. In the case of methylphenobarbital, the mechanisms involved in this phenomenon have not yet been determined.

Teratogenesis

It is not known whether methylphenobarbital and metharbital are teratogens in man. The evidence as to whether the metabolite phenobarbital is a teratogen is considered in Chapter 25.

Breast Milk

It was reported (10) that methylphenobarbital could not be found in the breast milk of women taking the drug. This finding is somewhat surprising, but perhaps the assay used was not sufficiently sensitive. Phenobarbital, administered as such, also was reportedly not found in milk in this study, but it is certainly detectable in milk when phenobarbital itself is taken by lactating women (26).

Dose Required to Achieve a Given Plasma Concentration

Loading Dose

There does not appear to be any published information on loading doses of methylphenobarbital that have proved satisfactory in practice. Although the drug is almost certainly an anticonvulsant in its own right, its therapeutic range of plasma levels when it acts as the sole antiepileptic substance present at the outset of therapy is unknown. Therefore, one does not have this information as a basis on which to predict a suitable loading dose of methylphenobarbital. If one aimed to attain a plasma phenobarbital level of 15 mg/L (a reasonable initial therapeutic level) in an adult, the data shown in Fig. 5 suggest that a daily methylphenobarbital dose of 3 mg/kg would suffice, so that a single loading dose of perhaps 6 mg/kg could be used initially. However, it would take so many days for the phenobarbital to form from methylphenobarbital and achieve something approaching steady-state conditions that it seems clinically unrealistic to consider the question of a loading dose determined on this basis.

A loading dose of methylphenobarbital that would have an adequate antiepileptic effect within a few hours could be determined empirically. However, this dose would probably make the patient very drowsy indeed. The drowsiness might persist for several days if the usual proportion of the methylphenobarbital dose is converted to phenobarbital. Methylphenobarbital is better suited to long-term use than to single-dose use, by virtue of both its chemical properties and its handling by the human body.

Oral Therapy

The data of Eadie et al. (13) suggest that to produce a therapeutic plasma phenobarbital level of 15 mg/L, children require an average methylphenobarbital dose of 5 mg/kg per day, young adults an average dose of 4 mg/kg per day, and adults over 40 years of age an average dose of 2 mg/kg per day. Slightly higher doses might be needed in females than in males. As mentioned above, the use of half the calculated daily methylphenobarbital dose for the first 2 weeks of therapy reduces the incidence of early drowsiness, although it may delay achieving a therapeutic effect.

When Plasma Concentrations are Too High or Too Low

When plasma concentrations of either methylphenobarbital or phenobarbital are too high, patients experience drowsiness and mental slowing. Some become irritable or depressed. Ataxia of gait, slowed speech, and nystagmus may occur at high plasma levels of drug and metabolite.

Subtherapeutic plasma levels of methylphenobarbital and derived phenobarbital (levels of the latter below 10 mg/L) are likely to be associated with failure to control the types of epilepsy that might be expected to respond to the drug. Very occasionally, patients fail to tolerate even such low plasma drug levels.

Guidelines to Dosage Adjustment

Methylphenobarbital dosage may need adjustment in at least three circumstances.

1. When plasma phenobarbital levels are subtherapeutic and the patient has a type of epilepsy in which seizures occur only at long intervals, so that it is reasonable to anticipate that the methylphenobarbital dose will ultimately prove inadequate if one waits long enough.

2. Irrespective of plasma methylphenobarbital and phenobarbital levels, if seizures continue and the patient is free from toxic manifestations of the therapy.

3. Irrespective of plasma methylphenobarbital and phenobarbital levels if the patient has toxic manifestations that prove a greater disadvantage than the epileptic seizures for which the drug is prescribed.

In adjusting methylphenobarbital doses, at least while plasma phenobarbital levels are in or below the therapeutic range, steady-state plasma phenobarbital levels in the individual usually change in direct proportion to the methylphenobarbital dose alteration. Therefore, so long as the steady-state plasma phenobarbital level is known at one methylphenobarbital dose, changes in drug dose are likely to produce proportionate changes in plasma phenobarbital levels. It is this property of methylphenobarbital that confers on it a significant advantage over prescribed phenobarbital. As indicated earlier, when phenobarbital itself is used and its dose is increased, plasma phenobarbital levels tend to increase more than in proportion to the dose increment, with consequent risk of unexpected overdosage manifestations.

After a methylphenobarbital dose is altered, the passage of some 2 or 3 weeks may be required for new steady-state plasma phenobarbital levels to be achieved. Plasma level monitoring prior to this time may provide results that mislead the clinician. Making further dosage adjustments within this 2- to 3-week period risks the development of a confused therapeutic situation.

Methylphenobarbital is cleared chiefly by the liver rather than by the kidneys, and its clearance is limited by hepatic metabolic capacity rather than by hepatic blood flow. The derived phenobarbital undergoes significant renal clearance. Methylphenobarbital dosages are unlikely to need much adjustment in cardiac failure. However, dosages may need to be reduced if liver cell or renal function deteriorates.

Synergism

The possibility of synergism between methylphenobarbital and other antiepileptic drugs was mentioned in the discussion of drug–drug interactions above. Clinicians generally accept the fact that additive antiepileptic effects may occur if two appropriate anticonvulsants are combined. However, it is often difficult to obtain rigid proof of the phenomenon and it has not been possible to trace published experimental evidence of it in relation to the methylbarbiturate anticonvulsants. It is even more difficult to prove that true synergism occurs in these circumstances.

It is, of course, irrational to combine methylphenobarbital with phenobarbital or primidone. The use of such combinations is tantamount to raising methylphenobarbital doses in a pharmacokinetically complicated way.

TOXICITY

It is difficult to make firm statements about the direct toxicity of methylphenobarbital or metharbital in man, since both drugs form biologically active metabolites. The toxic manifestations of phenobarbital are described in Chapter 25, and the account will not be repeated here. There seems to be no *a priori* reason why any of the known toxic manifestations of phenobarbital should not occur in patients taking methylphenobarbital. In practice, most of the toxic effects seen in patients taking methylphenobarbital involve depression of central nervous system function which is usually manifested as drowsiness, intellectual blunting, decreased concentration, and irritability. As mentioned above, such symptoms may be direct toxic effects of methylphenobarbital itself as well as consequences of the presence of excess phenobarbital. Metharbital (and probably the barbital to which it is converted) may also produce similar manifestations of depression of central nervous system function. There do not appear to be any characteristic toxic effects of any particular one of these four barbiturate anticonvulsants.

PHARMACODYNAMICS

As with so many other aspects of the clinical pharmacology of the methylated barbiturate anticonvulsants, interpretation of studies of the pharmacodynamics of these drugs is often ambiguous, since investigators have usually not determined whether biotransformation has produced the demethylated congener of the drug in the experimental system studied. Perhaps the clearest evidence is that of Craig and Shideman (11) who showed that after single doses of methylphenobarbital in rats, immediate protection against maximal electroshock seizures correlated better with brain levels of methylphenobarbital than with levels of phenobarbital. With the exception of the work of Buch et al. (2), the biological effects of the individual enantiomers of methylphenobarbital are still to be explored.

Other studies have demonstrated antiepileptic effects of methylphenobarbital and metharbital in various experimental preparations. However, in such investigations the biotransformation products phenobarbital or barbital may have had significant effects. Reinhard and Reinhard (38) tabulated the results of a number of studies in which methylphenobarbital appeared to protect against maximal electroshock seizures in the mouse, rat, and cat and against minimal electroshock seizures and pentylenetetrazol-induced seizures in the mouse and rat. Metharbital has appeared to protect against both maximal electroshock and pentylenetetrazol seizures in the mouse (44).

There does not appear to have been any study of the actions of methylphenobarbital or metharbital in any experimental system of lesser complexity than that of the whole experimental animal. The drugs do not seem to have been studied by modern cellular electrophysiological or neurochemical techniques.

Details of the pharmacodynamics of phenobarbital are provided in Chapter 19 and elsewhere (15), and will not be considered here.

THERAPEUTIC USE

Methylphenobarbital (with the phenobarbital derived from it) is an antiepileptic agent with a reasonably broad spectrum of action against a variety of seizure patterns. It is useful in all types of partial seizure and in generalized seizures manifesting as convulsive attacks (including benign febrile convulsions of infancy) or as myoclonic attacks in adolescence or adult life. The drug does not appear to be sufficiently potent to control the more active types of myoclonic epilepsy that develop in earlier life, and it is not effective in absence (petit mal) seizures. The drug's relatively long half-life and the even longer half-life of the derived phenobarbital make methylphenobarbital suitable for once- or twice-daily administration during long-term therapy. At the same time, the long half-life of phenobarbital means that there is a 2- or 3-week delay before any dosage change produces its maximal effects. Therefore, it is best not to adjust methylphenobarbital dosage more frequently than this.

Methylphenobarbital is thus suited to long-term therapeutic purposes and unhurried dosage manipulations, but it is less well suited to clinical situations that require rapid anticonvulsant effects and frequent dosage adjustments. Methylphenobarbital possesses the advantage that none of the other antiepileptic drugs in common use (with the exception of valproic acid) affects its plasma levels, or those of the phenobarbital derived from it, when the drugs are administered in combination.

Metharbital appears to have been very little used as an antiepileptic drug in recent times. Both its spectrum of activity against different types of epilepsy and its relative efficacy compared with other antiepileptic drugs are unknown.

CONCLUSIONS

Methylphenobarbital has often been regarded merely as a pro-drug for phenobarbital with the disadvantages of being somewhat more expensive and less reliably absorbed after oral administration. The pharmacokinetic and clinical pharmacological data that have become available suggest that methylphenobarbital may be reason ably well absorbed after oral administration, that it may enter the brain more readily than phenobarbital and there exert a useful antiepileptic effect in its own right, and that it has a peculiar advantage over phenobarbital in that it produces plasma phenobarbital levels that vary in direct proportion to drug dose. Despite its rather higher price, some might now regard methylphenobarbital as an advantageous way of providing phenobarbital for patients. If the pharmacological activity of methylphenobarbital should prove to reside in only one of its stereoisomers, new treatment practices and dosage regimens may be developed in the future.

Little is known of metharbital. Whether it has a real role as an antiepileptic drug in contemporary practice is debatable.

ACKNOWLEDGMENTS

The writer wishes to thank Dr. W. D. Hopper both for making available data from his as yet unpublished studies on the pharmacokinetics of the enantiomers of methylphenobarbital in man, and for his careful review of this manuscript. He is grateful to the editors and copyright owners of the *British Journal of Clinical Pharmacology* and *Clinical and Experimental Neurology* for permission to reproduce Figs. 4-7 from previously published work and to Churchill-Livingstone of Edinburgh for permission to reproduce Fig. 3.

CONVERSIONS

Methylphenobarbital

Conversion factor:

$$CF = \frac{1000}{mol.\ wt.} = \frac{1000}{246.3} = 4.06$$

Conversion:

(mg/L) or (μg/ml) × 4.06 = (μmoles/liter)

(μmoles/liter)/4.06 = (mg/L) or (μg/ml)

Metharbital

Conversion factor:

$$CF = \frac{1000}{mol.\ wt.} = \frac{1000}{198.4} = 5.04$$

Conversion:

(mg/L) or (μg/ml) × 5.04 = (μmoles/liter)

(μmoles/liter)/5.04 = (mg/L) or (μg/ml)

Barbital

Conversion factor:

$$CF = \frac{1000}{mol.\ wt.} = \frac{1000}{184.2} = 5.43$$

Conversion:

(mg/L) or (μg/ml) × 5.43 = (μmoles/liter)

(μmoles/liter)/5.43 = (mg/L) or (μg/ml)

REFERENCES

1. Blum, E. (1932): Die Bekampfung epileptischer Anfalle und iher Folgeer scheinungen mit Prominal. *Dtsch. Med.Wochenscher.* 58:230–236.
2. Buch, H., Knabe, J., Buzello, W., and Rummel, W. (1970): Stereospecificity of anaesthetic activity, distribution, inactivation and protein binding of the optical antipodes of two N-methylated barbiturates. *J. Pharmacol. Exp. Ther.*, 176:709–716.
3. Bush, M. T., and Sanders-Bush, E. (1972): Phenobarbital, mephobarbital and metharbital and their metabolites: Chemistry and methods for determination. In: *Antiepileptic Drugs*, 1st edition edited by D. M. Woodbury, J. K. Penry, and R. P. Schmidt, pp. 293–302. Raven Press, New York.
4. Butler, T. C. (1952): Quantitation studies of the metabolic fate of mephobarbital (N-methylphenobarbital). *J. Pharmacol. Exp. Ther.*, 106:235–245.
5. Butler, T. C. (1953): Quantitative studies of the demethylation of N-methyl barbital (metharbital, Gemonil). *J. Pharmacol. Exp. Ther.*, 108:474–480.
6. Butler, T. C., and Bush, M. T. (1939): The metabolic fate of N-methylphenobarbituric acids. *J. Pharmacol. Exp. Ther.*, 65:205–213.
7. Butler, T. C., Mahaffee, D., and Mahaffee, C. (1952): The role of the liver in the metabolic disposition of mephabarbital. *J. Pharmacol. Exp. Ther.*, 106:364–369.
8. Butler, T. C., and Waddell, W. J. (1958): N-Methylated derivatives of barbituric acids, hydantoin

and oxazolidine used in the treatment of epilepsy. *Neurology (Minneap.)*, 8(Suppl. 1):106–112.

9. Butler, T. C., Waddell, W. J., and Poole, D. T. (1965): Demethylation of trimethadione and metharbital by rat liver microsomal enzymes: Substrate concentration—yield relationships and competition between substrates. *Biochem. Pharmacol.*, 85:937–942.

10. Coradello, H. (1973): Ueber dieAusscheidung von Antiepileptika in die Muttermilch. *Wien. Klin. Wochenschr.*, 85:695–697.

11. Craig, C. R., and Shideman, F. E. (1971): Metabolism and anticonvulsant properties of mephobarbital and phenobarbital in rats. *J. Pharmacol. Exp. Ther.*, 176:35–41.

12. Eadie, M. J. (1976): Plasma level monitoring of anticonvulsants. *Clin. Pharmacokinet.* 1:52–66.

13. Eadie, M. J., Bochner, F., Hooper, W. D., and Tyrer, J. H. (1978): Preliminary observations on the pharmacokinetics of methylphenobarbitone. *Clin. Exp. Neurol.*, 15:131–144.

14. Eadie, M. J., Lander, C. M., Hooper, W. D., and Tyrer, J. H. (1977): Factors influencing plasma phenobarbitone levels in epileptic patients. *Br. J. Clin. Pharmacol.*, 4:541–547.

15. Eadie, M. J., and Tyrer, J. H. (1989): *Anticonvulsant Therapy. Pharmacological Basis and Practice*, 3rd edition. Churchill-Livingstone. Edinburgh, New York.

16. Flynn, E. J., and Spector, S. (1974): Radioimmunoassay for hepatic *N*-demethylation of metharbital *in vitro. J. Pharmacol. Exp. Ther.*, 189:550–556.

17. Giotti, A., and Maynert, E. W. (1951): The renal clearance of barbital and the mechanism of its reabsorption. *J. Pharmacol. Exp. Ther.*, 101:296–309.

18. Harvey, D. J., Glazener, L., Stratton, C., Nowlin, J., Hill, R. M., and Horning, M. G. (1972): Detection of a 5-(3,4-dihydroxy-1,5-cyclohexadien-1-yl)-metabolite of phenobarbital and mephobarbital in rat, guinea pig and human. *Research Commu. Chem. Path. Pharmacol.*, 3:557–566.

19. Hooper, W. D., Dubetz, D. K., Eadie, M. J., and Tyrer, J. H. (1975): Simultaneous assay of methylphenobarbitone and phenobarbitone using gas-liquid chromatography with on-column butylation. *J. Chromatogr.*, 110:206–209.

20. Hooper, W. D., Kunze, H. E., and Eadie, M. J. (1981): Pharmacokinetics and bioavailability of methylphenobarbital in man. *Ther. Drug Monitor.*, 3:39–44.

21. Hooper, W. D., Kunze, H. E., and Eadie, M. J. (1981); Qualitative and quantitative studies of methylphenobarbital metabolism in man. *Drug Metab. Dispos.*, 9:381–385.

22. Hooper, W. D., Kunze, H. E., and Eadie, M. J. (1981): Simultaneous assay of methylphenobarbital or phenobarbital in plasma using GC-MS with selected ion monitoring. *J. Chromatog.*, 223:426–431.

23. Horning, M. G., Nowlin, J., Butler, C. M., Lertratanangkoon, K., Sommer, K.,and Hill, R. M. (1975): Clinical applications of gas chromatograph/mass spectrometer/computer systems. *Clin. Chem.*, 21:1281–1287.

24. Huisman, J. W. (1966): The estimation of some important anticonvulsant drugs in serum. *Clin. Chim. Acta*, 13:323–328.

25. Jacqz, E., Hall, S. D., Branch, R. A., and Wilkinson, G. R. (1986): Polymorphic metabolism of mephenytoin in man: Pharmacokinetic interaction with a co-regulated substrate, mephobarbital. *Clin. Pharmacol. Therap.*, 39:646–653.

26. Kaneko, S., Fukushima, Y., Sato, T., Ogawa, Y., Nomura, Y., and Shinagawa, S. (1984): Breast feeding in epileptic mothers. In: *Antiepileptic Drugs and Pregnancy*, edited by T. Sato and S. Shinagawa, pp. 38–45. Excerpta Medica. Amsterdam.

27. Kunze, H. E., Hooper, W. D., and Eadie, M. J. (1981): High performance liquid chromatographic assay of methylphenobarbital and metabolites in urine. *Ther. Drug Monitor.*, 3:45–49.

28. Kupfer, A., and Branch, R. A. (1985): Stereoselective mephobarbital hydroxylation cosegregates with mephenytoin hydroxylation. *Clin. Pharm. Ther.*, 38:414–418.

29. Kupferberg, H. J., and Longacre-Shaw, J. (1979): Mephobarbital and phenobarbital plasma concentrations in epileptic patients treated with mephobarbital. *Ther. Drug Monitor.*, 1:117–122.

30. Lander, C. M., Eadie, M. J., and Tyrer, J. H. (1975): Interactions between anticonvulsants. *Proc. Aust. Assoc. Neurol.*, 12:111–116.

31. Lander, C. M., Edwards, V. E., Eadie, M. J., and Tyrer, J. H. (1977): Plasma anticonvulsant concentrations during pregnancy. *Neurology (Minneap.)*, 27:128–131.

32. Lim, W., and Hooper, W. D. (*in press*): Stereoselective metabolism of methylphenobarbitone (MPB) in man. *Clin. Exp. Pharm. Physiol.*

33. MacGee, J. (1971): Rapid identification and quantitation of barbiturates and glutethimide in blood by gas-liquid chromatography. *Clin. Chem.*, 17:587–591.

34. Maynert, E. W. (1972): Phenobarbital, mephobarbital, and metharbital: Absorption, distribution and excretion. In: *Antiepileptic Drugs*, 1st edition, edited by D. M.Woodbury, J. K. Penry, and R. P. Schmidt, pp. 303–310. Raven Press, New York.

35. Maynert, E. W., and van Dyke, H. B. (1949): The metabolism of barbiturates. *Pharmacol. Rev.*, 1:217–242.

36. Peterman, M. G. (1948): Epilepsy in childhood: Newer methods of diagnosis and treatment. *J.A.M.A.*, 138:1012–1019.

37. Rambeck, B., and Meijer, J. W. A. (1980): Gas chromatographic methods for the determination of antiepileptic drugs: A systematic review. *Ther. Drug Monitor.*, 2:385–396.

38. Reinhard, J. F., and Reinhard, J. F., Jr. (1977): Experimental evaluation of anticonvulsants. In: *Anticonvulsants*, edited by J. A. Vida, pp. 57–111. Academic Press, New York.

39. Reynolds, E. H., and Travers, R. D. (1974): Serum anticonvulsant concentrations in epileptic patients

with mental symptoms. A preliminary report. *Br. J. Psychiatry*, 124:440–445.

40. Schottelius, D. D. (1978): Homogeneous immunoassay system (EMIT) for quantitation of antiepileptic drugs in biological fluids. In: *Antiepileptic Drugs: Quantitative Analysis and Interpretation*, edited by C. E. Pippenger, J. K. Penry, and H. Kutt, pp. 95–108. Raven Press, New York.

41. Smith, J. A., Waddell, W. J., and Butler, T. C. (1963): Demethylation of *N*-methyl derivatives of barbituric acid, hydantoin and 2,4-oxazolidinedione by rat liver microsomes. *Life Sci.*, 7:486–492.

42. Treston, A. M., Phillipides, A., Jacobsen, N. W., Eadie, M. J., and Hooper, W. D. (1987): Identification and synthesis of *O*-methylcatechol metabolites of phenobarbital and some *N*-alkyl derivatives. *J. Pharm.Sci.*, 76:496–501.

43. Vida, J. A., and Gerry, E. H. (1977): Cyclic ureides. In: *Anticonvulsants*, edited by J. A. Vida. pp. 151–291. Academic Press, New York.

44. Vida, J. A., Hooker, M. L., Samour, C. M., and Reinhard, J. F. (1973): Anticonvulsants. 4. Metharbital and phenobarbital derivatives. *J. Med. Chem.*, 16:1378–1381.

Antiepileptic Drugs, Third Edition, edited by
R. Levy, R. Mattson, B. Meldrum,
J. K. Penry, and F. E. Dreifuss.
Raven Press, Ltd., New York © 1989.

25

Primidone

Chemistry and Methods of Determination

Helmut Schäfer

Primidone (Mysoline) is an important anticonvulsant used for the treatment of generalized tonic–clonic seizures with complex symptomatology. The pharmacological profile of primidone (PRM) was first described by Bogue and Carrington (3). In man, PRM is mainly metabolized to phenylethylmalonamide (PEMA) and phenobarbital (PB), as shown in Fig. 1. Therefore, in the course of antiepileptic therapy with PRM, PEMA and PB will also be present in any body fluid. Consequently, each treatment with PRM will be a simultaneous treatment with PEMA and PB.

CHEMISTRY AND SYNTHESIS

Primidone

Primidone is 5-ethyldihydro-5-phenyl-4,6[1H,5H]-pyrimidine-dione (C.A. registry number 125-33-7), $C_{12}H_{14}N_2O_2$, and has a molecular weight of 218.25. It is a nonhygroscopic, colorless, crystalline powder with a slightly bitter taste; its melting point is 286 to 287°C, and it can be crystallized from acetone (1). Crystal structure analysis of PRM, which shows a certain steric similarity between PRM and PB, was performed by Yeates and Palmer (70). Differences were shown in the pyrimidine parts of the molecule: the dioxopyrimidine ring of PRM

is fixed in a flat boat conformation, whereas the trioxopyrimidine part of PB is rather planar. The fixed flat boat conformation of PRM may be the basis of its weak acidic properties: from UV data we assume that PRM has a pK_a of approximately 13.

The approximate solubility of PRM is as follows: in methanol and ethanol (95%), about 6 mg/liter; in acetone, 2 mg/liter; in chloroform, ether, and benzene, <0.1 mg/liter (10). The solubility of PRM in aqueous mixtures is shown in Table 1. As a weakly acidic cyclic amide, PRM is better soluble in 1 N NaOH than in water of pH 6.5.

The dipole moment of PRM was found to be 1.04 (69), whereas that of PB was measured as 0.73. The higher polarity of PRM (and PEMA) results in distinctly lower partition coefficients, $k(c_{lipophil}/c_{hydrophil})$, of PRM compared with that of PB (Table 2). Goedhart et al. (17), using ^{14}C-PRM and ^{14}C-PB (New England Nuclear, Boston, Mass.), found high partition coefficients for PRM and PB at pH 7.4 of the aqueous phase in ethyl acetate (PRM, 3.30; PB, 52.0), and lower coefficients in chloroform (PRM, 0.603; PB, 2.25) and in toluene (PRM, 0.06; PB, 0.552). The highest partition coefficients of more than 400 were found in the system acetone/ammonium sulfate-saturated water at pH 6.6. Further values given by Alvin and Bush (1), and Schäfer (51) demonstrated that previous knowledge of

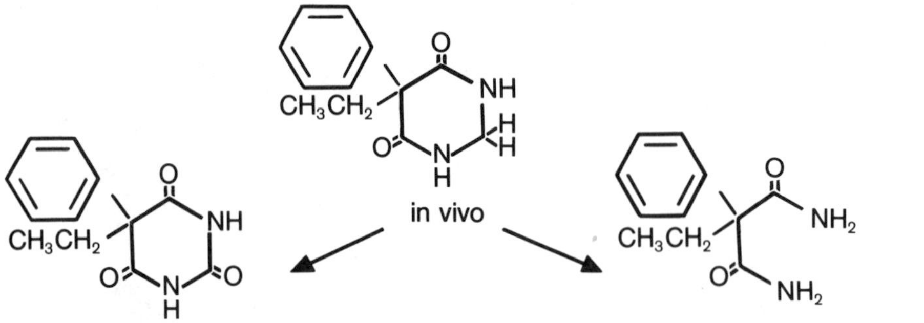

FIG. 1. Structural formulas of primidone and its main metabolites, phenylethylmalonamide and phenobarbital.

these data is indispensable in developing convenient extraction procedures suitable especially for PRM and PEMA.

The UV absorption spectrum of PRM shows maxima at 264, 258, and 252 nm when scanned in a rather high concentration of about 50 mg/100 ml methanol. There are no other maxima above 210 nm (10). The IR spectrum of PRM was compared with that of PB (5). Infrared spectra of two crystal forms of PRM as mineral oil mulls between KBr plates (10) and the NMR spectrum of PRM with characteristic resonances at 3.96 and 4.12 ppm (caused by the fragment -NH-CH$_2$-NH-) are discussed by Daley (10). Mass spectra of PRM are covered in several reports (1,10,18,21,23, 42,62). Mass spectra of PRM and 5-^{2}H$_5$-PRM recorded in the chemical ionization (CI) mode using isobutane at 65 to 133 Pa

(0.5 to 1.0 torr) show the peaks of the protonated molecular ions (62). Bourgeois et al. (6) discussed the electron impact (EI) mass spectra of PRM with its base peak of m/e 146 (C$_{10}$H$_{10}$O), which can also be observed as a minor peak during the fragmentation of PB.

Synthetic routes for preparation of PRM are (a) ring closure of PEMA with formamide/formic acid at 190°C (4,13) and (b) hydrogenolysis of 2-imino-(or cyanimino-) phenobarbital or of 2-thiophenobarbital with Raney nickel (4), zinc, and formic acid (4), or zinc and hydrochloric acid (1,4). We believe that hydrogenolysis of 2-thiophenobarbital or its homologs with zinc and hydrochloric acid is the most convenient method of preparing PRM or its derivatives for use as internal standards (11,51) in the laboratory.

TABLE 1. *Solubility and stability of PRM, PB, and PEMA in aqueous solutions*

	Solubility (mg/liter) in				% Stability of 50 mg/liter 0.5 N NaOH after	
	H$_2$O (37°)	H$_2$O (20°)	Serum (37°)	1 N (20°) NaOH	1 hr	24 hr
PRM	0.6	0.4	0.7	4.6	100	100
PB	1.8	—[a]	—[a]	—[a]	100	79
PEMA	4.1	1.6	3.8	1.4	100	100

[a] Not determined.

TABLE 2. *Partition coefficients[a] of PRM, PB, and PEMA (10 mg/liter each) in five systems*

	A[b]	B	C	D	E
PRM	2.90	2.05	0.68	0.71	<0.03
PB	49.80	10.01	2.72	2.05	<0.01
PEMA	1.004	0.822	0.64	0.64	0.17

[a] Partition coefficient = $C_{lipophilic}/C_{hydrophilic}$.
[b] Systems used: **A**, ethyl acetate-chloroform (210:40, v:v)/0.25 N HCL; **b**, ethyl acetate-chloroform (210:40, v:v)/phosphate buffer (pH 5.2); **C**, chloroform/phosphate buffer (pH 5.2); **D**, chloroform/phosphate buffer (pH 7.1); **E**, chloroform/1 N NaOH.

Phenylethylmalonamide

Phenylethylmalonamide is 2-ethyl-2-phenyl propandiamide (C.A. registry number 7206-76-0), $C_{11}H_{14}N_2O_2$, and has a molecular weight of 206.24. It is a colorless crystalline powder with a bitter taste, melting point 117° to 118°C, and can be crystallized from methanol/water. These crystals, dried at 50°C and 2,600 Pa (approximately 20 torr), contain about 6% crystal H_2O. Phenyl-ethylmalonamide behaves as a nonacidic compound. Its solubility in ethanol (95%) is 125 mg/liter and in chloroform is 18 mg/liter, which is greater than that of PRM. Solubilities and partition coefficients are given in Tables 1 and 2. Spectral data are available for UV (45), IR (45), NMR (45), and mass spectra (18,21,45).

Phenylethylmalonamide may be synthesized from diethylphenylethylmalonate, formamide, and sodium methoxide (1). We prefer to prepare PEMA by hydrolysis of phenylethylcyanacetamide with sulfuric acid (98%). Dudley et al. (13) specified an interesting possibility for preparing PEMA and its homolog *p*-methyl-PEMA via the hydrogenolysis of a 4,4-disubstituted pyrazolidine-3,5-dione.

METHODS OF DETERMINATION

Procedures for the determination of PRM, PB, and other anticonvulsants par-

tially including PEMA have been reviewed elsewhere (2,7,9,18,27,39–41,47,52). As mentioned above, PRM therapy results in therapeutic plasma levels of PEMA and PB, as well as PRM levels. This chapter covers isolated assays of PRM (especially immunoassay methods), isolated assays of PEMA, and the simultaneous determination of PRM and PEMA with regard to PB and other drugs or metabolites in body fluids. Streete et al. (58) reviewed the conflicting reports on the contribution of PEMA to the pharmacodynamic action of PRM therapy and concluded that the determination of PEMA did not seem to be essential in PRM assays. However, the PEMA concentration should be determined, if possible, as metabolic disturbances or compliance problems are occasionally diagnosed from comprehensive therapeutic drug monitoring (B. Rambeck, *personal communication*). Unfortunately, the PEMA concentration has sometimes been ignored in gas-liquid chromatographic (GLC) or high-performance liquid chromatographic (HPLC) determination of PRM and other antiepileptic drugs. It ought to be established whether or not PEMA will be separated from PRM, PB, or other drugs or metabolites, as the chromatographic methods can supply within a single run a complete pattern of drugs and metabolites. This superiority, in contrast with the single-drug determination in immunoassays, should also be discussed whenever a new determination technique is to be established in a laboratory (48).

Chromatography

As the result of recent advances in HPLC, it has replaced GLC as a routine tool for the determination of PRM, PEMA, PB, and other drugs in common practice. On the other hand, GLC methods are still efficient enough, both economically and technically, to remain acceptable. An efficient GLC method is especially required to separate complex mixtures of drugs and metabolites when GLC-MS coupling is performed. Thin-layer chromatography (TLC) has seldom been used to quantitate PRM, PEMA, and PB, subsequently or simultaneously (15,52). TLC methods seem to be no longer performed routinely.

Sample Preparation

As a first step in any GLC or HPLC determination of drugs in body fluids, it is generally imperative to prepare the samples in such a way that the subsequent chromatographic runs will result in sharp peaks and/or that the quality of the columns will not deteriorate too quickly. At the beginning of drug determination in body fluids by chromatographic techniques, liquid-liquid extraction procedures have been optimized and may still be the preferred method of sample extraction. Of all the antiepileptic drugs to be determined, PRM and PEMA are usually the most difficult ones to extract. On the basis of the drugs' partition coefficients, acetone is the most effective solvent for extracting PRM, PEMA, PB, and other antiepileptic drugs from aqueous body fluids when saturated with ammoniumsulfate (46). Ethylacetate also seems to be a suitable solvent, resulting in excellent absolute recoveries (19,32,36,65). From our experience, it is recommended that 1 ml of an acidified body fluid be extracted with 5 ml of ethylacetate-chloroform (210:40, v:v). We assume that the precipitation of the protein layer may be improved by the addition of some chloroform to the essential solvent ethylacetate.

Many of the published determination procedures do not include a step for purification of the extracts of the body fluids. However, such purification becomes more important the longer the time between sampling and analysis.

Primidone, PEMA, and PB in serum are stable when stored (67,68). However, degradation products from native serum contents caused by bacterial or fungal overgrowth (68) may contribute to extraneous peaks during GLC of nonpurified extracts. Furthermore, the peaks from the equipment and cholesterol from serum may interfere with the peaks of PRM, PEMA, and PB; we prefer a method similar to those described elsewhere (36,46,51). The dried serum extract is dissolved in 0.5 ml methanol, 75 μl water is added, and the solution is extracted twice with 2 ml *n*-hexane. In this way fatty acids, plasticizers, and, above all, cholesterol are removed. PRM, PEMA, PB, and other antiepileptic drugs remain almost completely in the methanolic phase. After the evaporation, the residue is redissolved in methanol or acetone and injected into the gas chromatograph.

Juergens et al. (30) systematically compared three basic methods of sample pretreatment for HPLC of antiepileptic drugs, including PRM, PEMA, and PB; protein precipitation with acetonitrile, liquid–liquid extraction with ethylacetate and liquid–liquid extraction after having partitioned the sample over the surface of kieselguhr. In our experience the pretreatment, which includes the partition of the sample over the surface of an Extrelut tube, is a very practicable one: to the filling of an Extrelut-1 tube, add 0.5 ml serum, 50 μl internal standard solution, 0.5 ml phosphate buffer pH 5.2, and 1 ml of a solvent mixture dichlormethane/n-propanol (97:3, v/v). After standing for 10 min, the sample is eluted with another 5 ml of the dichlormethane/*n*-propanol mixture and the eluate is evaporated to dryness under vacuum. A favorable pretreatment method is also the adsorption of the sample onto a solid material, preferably C_{18} reversed-phase material, from which the drugs can be eluted after cleaning the sample (26,27,31). Instead of these single extraction columns (Bondelut®), cassettes of 10 samples are used in an advanced automated sample processor (AASP) (26).

Internal Standards

Because of their similarity in chemical behavior as well as in physical properties, derivatives of PRM, PEMA, and PB are best suited for use as internal standards in HPLC or GLC. The *p*-methyl derivatives [5 - ethyl-dehydro - 5 - (p-tolyl)-4,6(1H,3H, 5H)-pyrimidinedione (p-methyl-PRM) and 2-ethyl-2-(p-tolyl)malonamide (p-methyl-PEMA)] are commercially available.

High-Performance Liquid Chromatography

High-performance liquid chromatography (HPLC) on reversed-phase (RP) columns is the most widely performed chromatographic technique for the routine determination of antiepileptic drugs and their metabolites in body fluids. The main problem in the identification and quantification of PRM, PEMA, and PB in mixtures of drugs and metabolites is the exact separation of PRM and PEMA. Because of their high polarity and their low partition coefficients in a lipophilic-stationary, hydrophilic-mobile RP system, PRM and PEMA usually appear near the beginning of the chromatogram. Furthermore, any overlapping peaks of PEMA or PRM with the carbamazepine (CBZ) metabolite 10,11-dihydro-CBZ-10,11-diol (CBZ diol) should be avoided by means of optimal chromatographic conditions. Riedmann et al. (49) obtained good separation of PEMA and PRM from other polar drugs and metabolites, including CBZ diol. The chromatographic conditions were the result of a systematic method of development in liquid chromatography (48) that included relevant sample constituent data, dependence of pH of the mobile phase on peak area, elution strength of organic solvents on RP mobile phases, and a basic knowledge of liquid chromatographic (LC) theory. Unfortunately, the chromatographic run took more than 20 min to determine eight drugs and metabolites.

Using a column packed with 3 μm particle size C_{18} RP packing, a mobile phase consisting of methanol/acetonitrile/phosphat-buffer at a rate of 3 ml/min at 50°C, and a detector with a very fast response time, a similar LC analysis was performed within about 3 min (31). However, it is uncertain whether or not the method ensures exact separation between PEMA or PRM and CBZ diol. These methods were performed in an isocratic mode of elution.

We are also familiar with an HPLC method that can quantitate PEMA, PRM, PB, CBZ diol, CBZ, phenytoin (PHT) and metabolites within about 13 min. Equipment and operating conditions include: 125×4.6 mm column filled with 5 μm RP 18, mobile phase (pH 5.3): acetonitrile 1945 ml/phosphate buffer pH 6.9 0.01 molar, 8055 ml/3.75 ml 85% H_3PO_4, 4-methyl-PRM and 4-methyl-PB are used as internal standards. Retention times (min): PEMA (0.75), PRM (1.16), CBZ diol (1.39), 4-methyl-PRM (2.33), CBZ epoxide (4.11), 4-methyl-PB (6.59), CBZ (10.30), PHT (12.22). It has been proposed by Riedmann et al. (49) that we recycle the mobile phase during routine work. We prepare 10-liter batches of the above-mentioned mixture. After about 1,000 injections of serum samples, there appears to be no deterioration of the mobile phase that would influence base-line noise or other parameters.

Depending on the available equipment, the following very promising courses of HPLC development have been recommended: column switching techniques enable the analyst to perform chromatographic runs after direct injections of untreated serum or plasma samples (25,28,33). Although being a rather polar substance, PEMA is not eluted from the precolumn during the washing cycle. On the contrary, PEMA gives quantitative recovery (33). Gradient elution techniques at elevated column temperatures improve the separation of a greater amount of substances in a complex mixture of drugs and metabolites, which results in sharp peaks from the beginning to the end of a chromatogramm (26,29,30,33,65). Wad (65) separated CBZ diol and 11 antiepileptic compounds, PRM and PEMA included, using an acetonitrile/water mixture at 35°C. Finally, the use of microbore columns (27,29) can help economize the HPLC procedure: the costs of solvents are reduced as much as 70% because the flow rate is lowered from 1.0 to 0.3 ml/min (27). Thus, Juergens (27) demonstrated that 14 compounds, including PEMA, PRM, and CBZ diol, are well separated within about 12 min at 65°C using two different mixtures of acetonitrile and water, adjusted to pH 4 with diluted perchloric acid (27).

Gas-Liquid Chromatography

Pippenger and Gillen (44) first described a GLC method for simultaneous determination of free PRM, PEMA, and PB. In today's view, their results seem to be unsatisfactory. At that time, however, highly efficient columns were not available. This led to interactions between the rather polar PRM and a polar support or the liquid phase. On less polar columns, free PRM, PEMA, and PB were inadequately resolved from each other and from other drugs. Therefore, derivatives of PRM, PEMA, and PB were made to decrease their polarity and to increase their volatility, resulting in sharp peaks with little or no tailing. However, the simultaneous determination of PRM, PEMA, PB, and other antiepileptic drugs is best performed by injecting the free drugs into a suitable column (47). For this purpose, highly efficient column fillings such as 3% Dexsil on Supelcoport (34), 3% OV 225 on Chromosorb G-HPAW (46), and 2% SP 2510 DA on Supelcoport® (20,36) are available. A mixed phase of 2% SP 2110/1% SP 2510 DA on Supelcoport (60) is suitable for an efficient isothermal separation at

230°C of PEMA, PB, *p*-methyl-PB, CBZ, PRM, *p*-methyl-PRM, PHT, and *p*-methylphenyl hydantoin (MPPH) in order of increasing retention times. Recently in the course of a study on the GLC determination of PEMA, Streete and Berry (57) selected two phases, namely, 2% SP 2510 and a specially prepared CDMS/WG11, from among 10 different liquid phases as best suited for the simultaneous determination of PEMA, PRM, PB, and other drugs, including the internal standard, *p*-methyl-PEMA.

Presently, a derivatization step prior to GLC seems to be unnecessary, since highly suitable columns for the determination of PRM, PEMA, and PB are available. However, in special cases like GLC-MS coupling with or without the use of capillary columns and for determination of low quantities of drugs or metabolites by means of special detectors (e.g., electron capture detector), derivatization of the substances to be measured may be indicated. In the course of on-column methylation of PRM, PEMA, and PB, the extracted drugs are dissolved in methanolic tetramethylammonium hydroxide (TMAH) or trimethylphenylammonium hydroxide (TMPAH) solutions. Within the high temperature of the injection port of the gas chromatograph, a rapid Hoffmann degradation reaction proceeds, yielding nearly quantitatively *N,N'*-dimethyl-PRM and *N,N'*-dimethyl-PB, for instance. Because of their instability in strong alkaline solutions such as TMAH or TMPAH, decomposition products are formed. The main decomposition product of PB is *N*-methyl-2-phenylbutyramide, which has a high probability of also being the on-column methylation product of PEMA. During flash-heater methylation, PRM yields about 5% of a decomposition product, the structure of which we found not to be identical with PEMA, *N,N'*-dimethyl-PEMA, or *N*-methyl-2-phenylbutyramide. The amounts of *N*-methyl-2-phenylbutyramide formed during flash-heater methylation of PB are related directly to the concentration of TMAH or TMPAH and to the length of time the drug is in contact with the base prior to injection into the column.

To overcome this problem, the use of p-methyl-PRM and p-methyl-PB as suitable internal standards has been shown to be an important improvement (17,18). These compounds are similar in structure to PRM and PB, respectively, and therefore undergo similar decomposition. Alkylation of PRM before injection into the gas chromatograph offers an alternative to the on-column alkylation technique. Thus, Roseboom and Hulshoff (50) proposed the butylation of PRM and PB with butyl iodide, Vandemark and Adams (63) methylated them, and Kapetanovic and Kupferberg (32) used ethyl iodide or propyl iodide in acetonitrile as alkylation agents. The alkylation of PEMA was not mentioned. The trimethylsilylation of PRM and PEMA (14,37,42) is not suitable for PB because of the instability of its trimethylsilyl derivative (37). Derivatives of PRM and PEMA suitable for determination by electron-capture gas chromatography were prepared by Wallace et al. (62,63). Primidone was acylated with pentafluorobenzoyl chloride. The resulting N,N'dipentafluorobenzoyl-PRM was extremely sensitive to the electron-capture detector of a gas chromatograph. Therefore, only microliter amounts of serum were required in the analysis. Phenylethylmalonamide was dehydrated by trifluoroacetic anhydride, yielding phenylethylcyanacetamide, which was also very sensitive to electron-capture detection. With p-methyl-PRM and p-methyl-PEMA used as internal standards, PRM and PEMA may be quantitated from one sample. The ethyl acetate/benzene extract is divided into separate aliquots prior to derivatization with pentafluorobenzyl chloride and trifluoroacetic anhydride, respectively. Perchalski and Wilder (43) prepared the N,N-dimethylaminomethylene derivative of PEMA by its reaction with dimethylformamide dimethylacetal.

Gas-Liquid Chromatography-Mass Spectrometry

Nitrogen-selective and electron-capture detectors substantially enhance the sensitivity and specificity of GLC procedures. However, mass spectrometry (MS) yields a significant improvement in detection of charged ions of a specific molecular weight. Depending on the MS technique, mass fragmentography, selected- or single-ion monitoring (SIM) using computer capabilities may be performed. Thus, Horning et al. (21), employing the chemical ionization mode, separated PRM, PEMA, and PB in a single analysis by SIM. The ions m/e 363, 351, and 261 corresponded, respectively, to trimethylsilyl-PRM, trimethylsilyl-PEMA, and dimethyl-PB MH$^+$ ions. The MH$^+$ of dimethyl-PB-2,4,5-^{13}C with m/e 264 was used as internal standard.

Johnson et al. (23) described SIM chromatography in a case of overdosage with PRM. Alvin and Bush (1) described mass fragmentation patterns of PRM, ethyl-1,1-^{2}D$_2$-PRM, and a mixture of the two, in preparation for GLC-MS studies with SIM using stable isotope-labeling of PRM, PEMA, and PB. Truscott et al. (62) described the determination of PRM simultaneously with PHT, CBZ, PB, and mephobarbital (MPB) in serum using direct chemical ionization MS without prior chromatographic separation. Corresponding stable isotope-labeled drugs, e.g., 5-^{2}H$_5$-PRM, for quantitation of PRM were used as internal standards. Concentrated chloroform extracts of serum samples were transferred to a probe tip, evaporated, and admitted to the mass spectrometer. Immediately after insertion of the sample into the ion source, the instrument, operating in the

CI mode, was programmed to scan repetitively for a total of 30 scans as the sample was warmed by induction from the source. During a clinical study, Nau et al. (42) evaluated the placental transfer and the neonatal disposition of PRM and its metabolites PEMA, *PB*, and *p*-OH-PB by means of a newly developed microassay using SIM-MS. The ions of m/z = 218 (22) and = 273 (32) of methylated and propylated PRM, respectively, were monitored during GC/MS analyses of body fluids.

Immunoassays

Over the last 10 years or more, many immunological techniques have become available for therapeutic drug monitoring (9,39,53). The techniques do not require prior extraction of the drugs and, when coupled to optimizing instrumentation, offer excellent assay speed, simplicity, and reliability. The immunoassay methods used most frequently for PRM determination by the participants of two quality control programs in 1986 in the United States and the United Kingdom were the enzyme-mediated immunoassay technique (EMIT, Syva), fluorescence polarization immunoassay (FPIA, Abbott), substrate-labeled fluorescence immunoassay (SLFIA, Ames), and nephelometric inhibition immunoassay (NIIA, Beckman). These proved to be the most accepted immunoassay methods in the clinical laboratories: EMIT, 44.2% (USA), 44.6% (UK); FPIA, 47.3%, 44.6%; SLFIA, 4.4%, 7.6%; NIIA, 2.0%, 3.2% (J. W. A. Meijer, *personal communication*). These methods, on the basis of antibodies employed, are quite specific for PRM, and the specificity of EMIT relative to GLC (41,53) and HPLC methods for PRM was confirmed (41). Improved EMIT systems may increase the assay's economy (35,59). In a microvolume EMIT adapted to a CentrifiChem analyzer, only a 3-μl sample is needed (59).

FPIA seems to be the most frequently used immunoassay technique, and methods have involved the use of complex, automated equipment such as the TDx system (24). A comparative PRM determination was performed (16) using different automated equipment for FPIA and SLFIA. The SLFIA for PRM is based on the cross reaction of an antibody with the fluorogenic galactosyl-umbelliferone derivative of PRM (8,38,54,61). The fluorescence assay is rapid and simple, and only small volumes (10 μl) of serum are needed. SLFIA has been compared to GLC (41,61), HPLC (41), and, also in fully automated systems, to EMIT (8,38,59). SLFIA shows few problems with lipemic, icteric, or uremic specimens, and any interferences are reduced considerably by the dilution of plasma by reagent (61).

Sidki et al. (55) proposed a direct determination of PRM by a magnetizable solid-phase fluoroimmunoassay. This separation technique has the advantage that appropriate assay design enables the removal of interfering components of serum or plasma before the endpoint determination is made. A dual-label fluoroimmunoassay allows the simultaneous determination of PRM and PB in a single 10 μl sample (56) using mixed immunochemical reagents. Because the excitation and emission spectra of rhodamin 101 do not overlap with those of fluorescein, fluorescein isothiocyanate was used to label PB and an isothiocyanate derivative of rhodamine 101 to label PRM; the excitation maxima are separated by 85 nm.

Radioimmunoassay procedures for PRM, PB, and PHT were developed by Cook et al. (9), who also described the synthetic route to PRM antigens and to the radiolabeled *p*-tritium-PRM used for the competitive binding assay. The cross reactivity with antibodies of 1- and 5-substituted PRM-protein conjugates, respectively, to PEMA and PB or *p*-hydroxyphenobarbital appears to be minimal. Immunoassays for the determination of PEMA have not yet been described.

CONVERSION

Primidone

Conversion factor:

$$CF = \frac{1000}{\text{mol. wt.}} = \frac{1000}{218.3} = 4.58$$

Conversion:

$$(\mu g/ml) \times 4.58 = (\mu moles/liter)$$

$$(\mu moles/liter) \div 4.58 = (\mu g/ml)$$

PEMA

Conversion factor:

$$CF = \frac{1000}{\text{mol. wt.}} = \frac{1000}{206.2} = 4.85$$

Conversion:

$$(\mu g/ml) \times 4.85 = (\mu moles/liter)$$

$$(\mu moles/liter) \div 4.85 = (\mu g/ml)$$

REFERENCES

1. Alvin, J. D., and Bush, M. T. (1975): Synthesis of millimole amounts of [14]C- and [2]D-labelled primidone, phenylethylmalonamide and phenobarbital of high sensitivity detection in biological materials. *Mikrochim. Acta (Wien)*, 1:685–696.
2. Bente, H. B. (1978): Nitrogen selective detectors: Application to quantitation of antiepileptic drugs. In: *Antiepileptic Drugs: Quantitative Analysis and Interpretation*, edited by C. E. Pippenger, J. K. Penry, and H. Kutt, pp. 139–146. Raven Press, New York.
3. Bogue, J. Y., and Carrington, H. C. (1953): The evaluation of "Mysoline"—a new anticonvulsant drug. *Br. J. Pharmacol.*, 8:230–236.
4. Boon, W. R., Carrington, H. C., Greenhalgh, N., and Vasey, C. H. (1954): Some derivatives of tetra- and hexa-hydro-4:6-dioxopyrimidine. *J. Chem. Soc.*, 8:3263–3272.
5. Bouché, R. (1973): Proposition d'attribution des bandes d'absorption des barbituriques dans la région de 1700 cm^{-1}. *Chim. Ther.*, 6:676–681.
6. Bourgeois, G., Brachet-Liermain, A., and Ferrus, L. (1974): Etude comparée de la fragmentation de trois composés médicamenteux à structure hétérocyclique: La primaclone, le glutethimide et le phenobarbital. *Organ. Mass Spectrom.*, 9:53–57.
7. Burke, J. T., and Thénot, J. P. (1985): Determi-nation of antiepileptic drugs. *J. Chromatogr.*, 340:199–241.
8. Carl, G. F., Smith, D. B., and Bridges, G. (1982): Comparison of fluorescent immunoassay and EMIT® for assay of serum primidone concentration. *Ther. Drug. Monit.*, 4:325–328.
9. Cook, C. E., Christensen, H. D., Amerson, E. W., Kepler, J. A., Tallent, C. R., and Taylor, G. F. (1976): Radioimmunoassay of anticonvulsant drugs: Phenytoin, phenobarbital and primidone. In: *Quantitative Analytic Studies in Epilepsy*, edited by P. Kellaway and I. Petersén, pp. 39–58. Raven Press, New York.
10. Daley, R. D. (1973): Primidone. *Anal. Profiles Drug Subst.*, 2:409–437.
11. Dudley, K. H. (1978): Internal standards in gas-liquid chromatographic determination of antiepileptic drugs. In: *Antiepileptic Drugs: Quantitative Analysis and Interpretation*, edited by C. E. Pippenger, J. K. Penry, and H. Kutt, pp. 19–34. Raven Press, New York.
12. Dudley, K. H., Bius, D. L., Kraus, B. L., and Boyles, L. W. (1977): Gaschromatographic on-column methylation technique for the simultaneous determination of antiepileptic drugs in blood. *Epilepsia*, 18:259–275.
13. Dudley, K. H., Bius, D. L., and Maguire, J. H. (1978): Synthesis of internal standards for analytical determinations of primidone and its metabolite, phenylethylmalonamide (PEMA). *J. Heterocyclic Chem.*, 15:923–926.
14. Gallagher, B. B., and Baumel, I. P. (1972): Primidone, chemistry and methods for determination. In: *Antiepileptic Drugs*, 1st edition, edited by D. M. Woodbury, J. K. Penry, and R. P. Schmidt, pp. 353–356. Raven Press, New York.
15. Garceau, Y., Philopoulos, Y., and Hasegawa, J. (1973): Quantitative TLC Determination of primidone, phenylethylmalonediamide, and phenobarbital in biological fluids. *J. Pharm. Sci.*, 62:2032–2034.
16. George, H., Fisher, S. J., Dimarzio, J. M., Horton, Ch. M., and Kurtz, S. R. (1985): Comparative evaluation of the Optimate® and TDX® analyzers using NCCLS guidelines. *Am. J. Clin. Pathol.*, 84:730–736.
17. Goedhart, D. M., Driessen, O. M. J., and Meijer, J. W. A. (1978): The extraction of antiepileptic drugs. *Arzneim. Forsch.*, 28:19–21.
18. Gudzinowicz, B. J., and Gudzinowicz, M. J. (1977): Analysis of drugs and metabolites by gas chromatography-mass spectrometry. Vol. 2: *Hypnotic, Anticonvulsants and Sedatives*. Marcel Dekker, New York.
19. Gupta, R. N., Dobson, K., and Keane, P. M. (1977): Gas-liquid chromatographic determination of primidone in plasma. *J. Chromatogr.*, 132:140–144.
20. Hewitt, T. E., Sievers, D. L., and Kessler, G. (1978): Improved gas-chromatographic analysis for anticonvulsants. *Clin. Chem.*, 24:1854–1856.
21. Horning, M. G., Lertratanangkoon, K., Nowlin, J., Stillwell, W. G., Stillwell, R. N., Zion, T. E., Kellaway, P., and Hill, R. M. (1974): Anticonvul-

sant drug monitoring by GC-MS-COM techniques. *J. Chromatogr. Sci.*, 12:630–635.

22. Inotsume, N., Higashi, A., Konshita, E., Matsuoka, T., and Nakano, M. (1986): Rapid and sensitive determination of ethotoin as well as carbamazepine, phenobarbital, phenytoin and primidone in human serum. *J. Chromatogr.*, 383:166–171.

23. Johnson, G. F., Least, C. J., Jr., Serum, J. W., Solow, E. B., and Solomon, H. M. (1976): Monitoring drug concentrations in a case of combined overdosage with primidone and methsuximide. *Clin. Chem.*, 22:915–921.

24. Jolley, M. E. (1981): Fluorescence polarization immunoassay for the determination of therapeutic drug levels in human plasma. *J. Anal. Toxicol.*, 5:236–240.

25. Juergens, U. (1984): Routine determination of eight common anti-epileptic drugs and metabolites by high-performance liquid chromatography using a column-switching system for direct injection of serum samples. *J. Chromatogr.*, 310:97–106.

26. Juergens, U. (1986): High-performance liquid chromatographic determination of antiepileptic drugs by an advanced automated sample processor. *J. Chromatogr.*, 371:307–312.

27. Juergens, U. (1987): HPLC analysis of antiepileptic drugs in blood samples: Microbore separation of fourteen compounds. *J. Liquid Chromatogr.*, 10:507–532.

28. Juergens, U. (1986): Pre-column switching techniques for the determination of drugs and metabolites in body fluids in research and routine analysis. *Intern. J. Environ. Anal. Chem.*, 25:221–233.

29. Juergens, U. (1987): Simultaneous determination of Zonisamide and nine other anti-epileptic drugs and metabolites in serum. A comparison of microbore and conventional high-performance liquid chromatography. *J. Chromatogr.*, 385:233–240.

30. Juergens, U., May, T., Hillenkötter, K., and Rambeck, B. (1984): Systematic comparison of three basic methods of sample pretreatment for high-performance liquid chromatographic analysis of antiepileptic drugs using gas chromatography as a reference method. *Ther. Drug Monit.*, 6:334–343.

31. Kabra, P. M., Nelson, M. A., and Marton, L. J. (1983): Simultaneous very fast liquid-chromatographic analysis of ethosuximide, primidone, phenobarbital, phenytoin, and carbamazepine in serum. *Clin. Chem.*, 29:473–476.

32. Kapetanovic, I. M., and Kupferberg, H. J. (1981): GC and GC-mass spectrometric determination of *p*-hydroxyphenobarbital extracted from plasma, urine, and hepatic microsomes. *J. Pharm. Sci.*, 70:1218–1224.

33. Kuhnz, W., and Nau, H. (1984): Automated high-pressure liquid chromatographic assay for antiepileptic drugs and their major metabolites by direct injection of serum samples. *Ther. Drug Monit.*, 6:478–483.

34. Külpmann, W. R. (1980): Eine gaschromatographische Methode zur Bestimmung von Carbamazepin, Phenobarbital, Phenytoin und Primidon im

gleichen Serumextrakt. *J. Clin. Chem. Clin. Biochem.*, 18:227–232.

35. Lacher, D. A., Sinn, J. A., Wills, M. R., and Savory, J. (1980): Rapid centrifugal analyzer enzyme immunoassays for phenytoin, phenobarbital, and primidone. *Am. J. Clin. Pathol.*, 74:205–208.

36. Leal, K. W., Lilensky, A. J., and Rapport, R. L. (1978): Simultaneous analysis of primidone, phenobarbital, and phenylethylmalonamide in plasma and brain. *J. Anal. Toxicol.*, 2:214–218.

37. Least, C. J., Jr., Johnson, G. F., and Solomon, H. M. (1975): Therapeutic monitoring of anticonvulsant drugs: Gas chromatographic simultaneous determination of primidone, phenylethylmalonamide, carbamazepine, and diphenylhydantoin. *Clin. Chem.*, 21:1658–1662.

38. Li, Th. M., Robertson, St. P., Crouch, Th. H., Pahuski, E. E., Bush, G. A., and Hydo, St. J. (1983): Automated fluorometer/photometer system for homogeneous immunoassays. *Clin. Chem.*, 29:1628–1634.

39. Marks, V. (1981): Immunoassays for drugs. In: *Therapeutic Drug Monitoring*, edited by A. Richens and V. Marks, pp. 155–182. Churchill Livingstone, Edinburgh.

40. Meijer, J. W. A. (1981): Antiepileptic drugs: Analytical techniques. In: *Therapeutic Drug Monitoring*, edited by A. Richens and V. Marks, pp. 349–369. Churchill Livingstone, Edinburgh.

41. Meijer, J. W. A., Rambeck, B., and Riedmann, M. (1983): Antiepileptic drug monitoring by chromatographic methods and immunotechniques—Comparison of analytical performance, practicability, and economy. *Ther. Drug. Monit.*, 5:39–53.

42. Nau, H., Jesdinsky, D., and Wittfoht, W. (1980): Microassay for primidone and its metabolites phenylethylmalondiamide, phenobarbital and *p*-hydroxyphenobarbital in human serum, saliva, breast milk and tissues by gas chromatography-mass spectrometry using selected ion monitoring. *J. Chromatogr.*, 182:71–79.

43. Perchalski, R. J., and Wilder, B. J. (1978): Gas-liquid chromatographic determination of carbamazepine and phenylethylmalonamide in plasma after reaction with dimethylformamide dimethylacetate. *J. Chromatogr.*, 145:97–103.

44. Pippenger, C. E., and Gillen, H. W. (1969): Gas chromatographic analysis for anticonvulsant drugs in biologic fluids. *Clin. Chem.*, 15:582–590.

45. Pirl, J. N., Spikes, J. J., and Fitzloff, J. (1977): Isolation, identification, and quantitation of 2-ethyl-2-phenylmalondiamide, a primidone metabolite. *J. Anal. Toxicol.*, 1:200–203.

46. Rambeck, B., and Meijer, J. W. A. (1979): Comprehensive method for the determination of antiepileptic drugs using a novel extraction technique and a fully automatic gas chromatograph. *Arzneim. Forsch.*, 29:99–103.

47. Rambeck, B., and Meijer, J. W. A. (1980): Gas chromatographic methods for the determination of antiepileptic drugs: A systematic review. *Ther. Drug Monit.*, 2:385–396.

48. Rambeck, B., Riedmann, M., and Meijer, J. W. A. (1981): Systematic method of develop-

ment in liquid chromatography applied to the determination of antiepileptic drugs. *Ther. Drug Monit.*, 3:377–395.

49. Riedmann, M., Rambeck, B., and Meijer, J. W. A. (1981): Quantitative simultaneous determination of eight common antiepileptic drugs and metabolites by liquid chromatography. *Ther. Drug Monit.*, 3:397–413.

50. Roseboom, H., and Hulshoff, A. (1979): Rapid and simple cleanup and derivatization procedure for the gas chromatographic determination of acidic drugs in plasma. *J. Chromatogr.*, 173:65–74.

51. Schäfer, H. R. (1975): Some problems concerning the quantitative assay of primidone and its metabolites. In: *Clinical Pharmacology of Anti-Epileptic Drugs*, edited by H. Schneider, D. Janz, C. Gardner-Thorpe, H. Meinardi, and A. L. Sherwin, pp. 124–129. Springer-Verlag, Berlin, Heidelberg, New York.

52. Schäfer, H. R. (1982): Primidone. Chemistry and methods of determination. In: *Antiepileptic Drugs*, 2nd edition, edited by D. M. Woodbury, J. K. Penry, and C. E. Pippenger, pp. 395–404. Raven Press, New York.

53. Schottelius, D. D. (1978): Homogeneous immunoassay system (EMIT) for quantitation of antiepileptic drugs in biological fluids. In: *Antiepileptic Drugs: Quantitative Analysis and Interpretation*, edited by C. E. Pippenger, J. K. Penry, and H. Kutt, pp. 95–108. Raven Press, New York.

54. Sheehan, M., and Caron, G. (1985): Evaluation of an automated system (optimate) for substrate-labelled fluorescent immunoassays. *Ther. Drug Monit.*, 7:108–114.

55. Sidki, A. M., Rowell, F. J., and Landon, J. (1983): Direct determination of primidone in serum or plasma by a magnetizable solid-phase fluoroimmunoassay. *Am. Clin. Biochem.*, 20:227–232.

56. Sidki, A. M., Smith, D. S., and Landon, J. (1985): Dual-label fluoroimmunoassay for simultaneous determination of primidone and phenobarbital. *Ther. Drug. Monit.*, 7:101–107.

57. Streete, J. M., and Berry, D. J. (1987): Gas chromatographic analysis of phenylethylmalonamide in human plasma. *J. Chromatogr.*, 416:281–291.

58. Streete, J. M., Berry, D. J., Newberry, J. E., and Crome, P. (1987): Pharmacokinetics of phenylethylmalonamide (PEMA) in elderly men. *Eur. J. Clin. Pharmacol.*, 33:431–434.

59. Studts, D., Haven, G. T., and Kiser, E. J. (1983): Adaptation of microvolume EMIT® assays for theophylline, phenobarbital, phenytoin, carba-

mazepine, primidone, ethosuximide, and gentamicin to a centrifichem® chemistry analyzer. *Ther. Drug Monit.*, 5:335–340.

60. Thoma, J. J., Ewald, T., and McCoy, M. (1978): Simultaneous analysis of underivatized phenobarbital, carbamazepine, primidone, and phenytoin by isothermal gas-liquid chromatography. *J. Anal. Toxicol.*, 2:219–225.

61. Toseland, P. A., Wicks, J. F. C., and Newall, R. G. (1983): Application of substrate-labelled fluorescent immunoassay to the measurement of anticonvulsant and antiasthmatic drug levels in plasma and serum. *Ther. Drug Monit.*, 5:501–505.

62. Truscott, R. J. W., Burke, D. G., Korth, J., Halpern, B., and Summons, R. (1978): Simultaneous determination of diphenylhydantoin, mephobarbital, carbamazepine, phenobarbital and primidone in serum using direct chemical ionization mass spectrometry. *Biomed. Mass Spectrom.*, 5:477–482.

63. Vandemark, F. L., and Adams, R. F. (1976): Ultramicro gas-chromatographic analysis for anticonvulsants, with use of a nitrogen-selective detector. *Clin. Chem.*, 22:1062–1065.

64. Varma, R. (1978): Simultaneous gas chromatographic determination of diphenylhydantoin, carbamazepine (Tegretol), phenobarbital and primidone in presence of Kemadrin (procyclidine) and Prolixin (fluphenazine) in plasma of psychiatric patients. *J. Chromatogr.*, 155:182–186.

65. Wad, N. (1984): Simultaneous determination of eleven antiepileptic compounds in serum by highperformance liquid chromatography. *J. Chromatogr.*, 305:127–133.

66. Wallace, J. E., Hamilton, H. E., Shimek, E. L., Jr., Schwertner, H. A., and Blum, K. (1977): Determination of primidone by electron-capture gas chromatography. *Anal. Chem.*, 49:903–906.

67. Wallace, J. E., Hamilton, H. E., Shimek, E. L., Jr., Schwertner, H. A., and Haegele, C. D. (1977): Determination of phenylethylmalonamide by electroncapture gas chromatography. *Anal. Chem.*, 49:1969–1973.

68. Wilensky, A. J. (1978): Stability of some antiepileptic drugs in plasma. *Clin. Chem.*, 24:722–723.

69. Wollmann, H., Skaletzki, B., and Schaaf, A. (1974): Zur Bestimmung der Polarität von Arzneistoffen. *Pharmazie*, 29:708–711.

70. Yeates, D. G. R., and Palmer, R. A. (1975): The crystal structure of primidone. *Acta Crystalogr.*, 31:1077–1082.

Antiepileptic Drugs, Third Edition, edited by
R. Levy, R. Mattson, B. Meldrum,
J. K. Penry, and F. E. Dreifuss.
Raven Press, Ltd., New York © 1989.

26

Primidone

Absorption, Distribution, Excretion

James C. Cloyd and Ilo E. Leppik

Primidone (PRM) remains an important agent in the treatment of epilepsy despite the introduction of newer antiepileptic drugs. It is as effective as carbamazepine (CBZ), phenobarbital (PB), or phenytoin (PHT) in controlling partial or generalized tonic-clonic seizures, although it has a higher incidence of side effects such as dizziness, sedation, nausea, and vomiting (25). Rational use of primidone requires an understanding of its pharmacokinetics, which are complicated by the presence of two active metabolites: phenobarbital and phenylethylmalonamide (PEMA).

PHARMACOKINETICS

Primidone pharmacokinetics are influenced by its physical-chemical characteristics (see Chapter 27). It is very slightly soluble in water and most organic solvents, which accounts for the absence of a commercially available parenteral formulation. Primidone is weakly acidic with a pK_a of 13 and lipophilic partition coefficients that are 5% to 25% of those for phenobarbital. These properties contribute to primidone's low plasma protein binding and relatively slow distribution to nonvascular tissues.

Extent and Rate of Absorption

Direct measurement of PRM bioavailability is not possible due to the absence of a commercially available parenteral formulation. Kaufman et al. (19) indirectly estimated the extent of PRM absorption under pseudo steady-state conditions in four children on monotherapy and eight on PHT and PRM. Over a 24-hr period they recovered from urine 92% (range, 75–123%) of the daily dose as either PRM (42.3 ± 15.2%), PEMA (45.2 ± 13.9%), or PB (4.9 ± 2.1%). The fraction absorbed can also be roughly estimated by comparing either distribution volumes or clearances calculated following oral administration versus values determined from i.v. data. Significantly greater oral distribution volumes or clearances would indicate that the fraction absorbed is less than 100%. In a study involving 10 patients on combination therapy, Zavadil and Gallagher (39) used a C^{14}-labeled PRM parenteral formulation to measure distribution volume. They reported a mean volume of 0.74 L/Kg, which is consistent with values determined following oral administration, which range from 0.64 to 0.86 L/Kg (10,28). The similarity of distribution volumes obtained from intravenous and oral routes of administration provides indirect evidence that the fraction absorbed approaches 100%.

Primidone absorption remains constant over a range of clinically relevant dosages. On average a 500 mg (7.2 mg/Kg) dose produces a C_{pmax} that is twice that from a 250 mg (3.6 mg/Kg) dose: 8 to 10 mg/L versus 4 to 5 mg/L, respectively (10,28,8). However, there is poor correlation between initial PRM dose and C_{pmax} due to variability among patients in absorption, distribution, and elimination. Present bioavailability data suggest, but do not prove, that PRM is well absorbed. Further studies are needed to determine what effect factors such as age, disease state, or concomitant therapy have on extent of absorption.

The absorption rate for PRM is intermediate among antiepileptic drugs when data from similar dosage forms are compared. In a majority of patients the observed time to maximum concentration (T_{max}) following administration of a 250 mg tablet ranges from 2 to 6 hr with a mean of 3 hr (8,10,14,19,28,39). Co-administration of other antiepileptic drugs does not significantly alter T_{max}, but does produce slightly lower maximum concentrations (10). There is a tendency for T_{max} to occur somewhat later during maintenance therapy, although values vary widely (14,6).

The presence of neurological toxicity following an initial PRM dose is highly correlated with both rate and extent of absorption. The onset of side effects parallels appearance of PRM in blood. The most severe side effects occur at T_{max} and are associated with concentrations at or below the therapeutic range (23). Tolerance develops within hours after initial exposure; thereafter much greater PRM concentrations are required to produce neurological side effects (see Chapter 32) (8,23). The influence of absorption on toxicity during maintenance therapy is obscured by the accumulation of PB and PEMA (see Chapter 25).

Both the extent and rate of absorption may be influenced by differences in formulation. Primidone (Mysoline, Wyeth-Ayerst Laboratories) suspension and 250 mg tablets are similar with respect to T_{max} and C_{pmax}, suggesting comparable bioavailability (Wyeth-Ayerst, *personal communication*). However, Bielmann et al. (7) compared the rate and extent of absorption of two lots of primidone 250 mg tablets (Mysoline) with different *in vitro* dissolution characteristics. The study involved 12 patients on maintenance PRM monotherapy. Subjects were randomly assigned to receive drug from one lot for 7 days, then crossed over to the alternate lot. There were no differences in PRM concentrations, but both PB (30 versus 20 mg/L) and PEMA (9 versus 7 mg/L) concentrations were significantly higher during the second week in patients taking the lot with slow *in vitro* dissolution characteristics. Although the authors offered several hypotheses to explain the differences they observed, it is difficult to conceive of a mechanism that accounts for stable PRM concentrations while PB and PEMA concentrations increase. Nevertheless, this study does suggest that differences in the rate of absorption may influence PRM metabolism and PB and PEMA concentrations. More recently Wylie et al. (38) reported a single case in which a hospitalized patient was switched from Mysoline tablets to a similar dosage form and strength made by a generic manufacturer. Substitution of the generic product was associated with decreased serum PRM and Pb concentrations and an increase in seizure frequency. The authors attributed the decrease in drug concentrations and loss of seizure control to differences in bioavailability. Subsequently, a Food and Drug Administration review of this case concluded that the patient's seizures had not been controlled on either product and that a bioequivalence problem could not be confirmed (12). Well-controlled, systematic studies in patients comparing the relative PRM bioavailability of products from various manufacturers are needed to determine if clinically significant differences in rate or extent of absorption exist.

Absorption following PRM overdose is prolonged and erratic. Plasma primidone concentrations ranging from 95 to 300 mg/L have been reported following acute overdose. The time-course of PRM concentrations may show a biphasic pattern with maximum concentrations occurring within hours after ingestion and a second, lower peak concentration 24 to 48 hr after ingestion (26,37,9). This phenomenon is due to the formation and subsequent break-up of multitablet concretions in the intestine. Crystalluria has occurred following PRM overdoses and is due to PRM's limited aqueous solubility (37,9).

There is limited information on the effect drugs such as antacids have on PRM absorption. Syversen et al. (34) described three patients in whom both plasma and urine PRM concentrations were significantly reduced when acetazolamide was given concurrently.

The absolute bioavailability of PEMA has been determined in humans. Pisani and Richens (29), using investigational formulations, gave six healthy volunteers 500 mg doses of PEMA intravenously and orally. Following oral administration, T_{max} averaged 3 hr (range, 0.5–4 hr) with maximum serum concentrations of 55.4 ± 10.2 mg/L. The mean bioavailability of oral PEMA was 91% (range, 86.5–95.9%). Time to maximum concentration occurs earlier and C_{pmax} is approximately 20% less in patients receiving enzyme-induced antiepileptic drugs (11). There are no reports describing the rate and extent of PEMA absorption under steady-state conditions.

Distribution

Primidone distributes throughout body tissues and fluids in a similar pattern and to the same extent as phenobarbital (36). Penetration into brain tissue lags behind the serum concentration-time profile. Following a single 50 mg/kg oral PRM dose given to mice, serum and brain T_{maxs} were 0.6 and 1.0 hr respectively (21). Maximum brain concentrations in rats occur approximately 2 hr after drug administration and 1 hr after

maximum plasma concentrations. The brain-to-plasma PRM concentration ratio averaged 0.4 within 2 hr after drug administration and remained stable thereafter. In man the onset of central nervous system side effects following an initial dose parallels the appearance of PRM in blood (23). This suggests rapid equilibrium between plasma and brain in humans when PRM is given orally. There is some disagreement on the extent to which PRM penetrates human brain tissue. Houghton et al. (22) found an extremely high correlation (0.96) between plasma and temporal lobe PRM concentrations in 11 patients on maintenance therapy who had undergone temporal lobe resection. Brain concentrations averaged 87% of plasma values. In contrast, Leal et al. (21) reported that brain PRM concentrations averaged 40% of those in plasma among six patients on long-term therapy. Discrepancies in PRM brain-to-plasma concentration ratios may be due to one or more reasons, including extraction methods, or the timing of specimen collections relative to administration of the dose. Holler and Penin (16) investigated intracerebral PRM metabolism in isolated rat brains. They found that substantial quantities of PEMA and PB are formed during a 2 hr PRM perfusion.

The rate at which PRM derived PEMA and PB penetrate brain tissue is dependent upon their rate of biotransformation and physicochemical properties. Data from animal studies demonstrate that both PB and PEMA reached maximum plasma and brain concentrations 6 to 8 hr after an orally administered PRM dose (5,18). The brain-to-plasma ratios for PB and PEMA vary from 0.46 to 0.98 and 0.28 to 1.0, respectively, depending upon species and experimental conditions (5,18).

Primidone does not bind significantly to plasma proteins. Measurements of PRM binding, using either equilibrium dialysis or ultrafiltration, range from 0 to 20% (6,35,32,20). There is good agreement between total or unbound (free) plasma PRM concentrations and either cerebrospinal fluid (CSF) or saliva concentrations, with most reported correlation coefficients ranging from 0.9 to 0.99 (17,20,31,15,24). Several investigators have shown that saliva PRM concentrations are equivalent to total and unbound PRM concentrations, although others have reported saliva values equal to 70% to 80% of total plasma concentrations (20,15,24,2). Primidone concentration in the CSF averages 70% to 100% of that in plasma (6,17,31,32,35). Variance in CSF or saliva-to-plasma PRM ratios may be due to the time required for PRM to equilibrate between these fluids. Schottelius (35) reported a CSF-to-plasma PRM ratio of 0.6 if samples were collected within 4 hr following a dose, but the ratio reached unity (1.0) when samples were collected 7 hr after the dose. Bartels et al. (32) noted that stimulation of salivary flow resulted in a decrease in the saliva-to-plasma ratio. The relatively slow penetration of PRM across lipid membranes could account for time- and flow-related differences in CSF or saliva-to-plasma ratios. Saliva PRM concentrations are suitable for estimating either CSF or plasma concentrations, but attention must be paid to time after dose and the manner in which the specimen is collected.

Zavadil and Gallagher (39) characterized PRM distribution volume in 10 patients with epilepsy, seven of whom were receiving other antiepileptic drugs. They found a mean value of 0.72 L/Kg (range, 0.44–1.02 L/Kg). Concurrent administration of antiepileptic drugs had no affect on distribution volume. We studied PRM pharmacokinetics in 18 patients following a single 250 mg dose (4). Distribution volume ranged from 0.37 to 1.1 L/Kg, with a mean of 0.64 L/Kg. Pisani (28) reported somewhat larger values in seven healthy volunteers and seven nonepileptic patients with viral hepatitis: 0.97 ± 0.32 L/Kg.

Baumel et al. (6), using equilibrium dialysis, found that unbound serum PEMA and CSF concentrations represented 91%

and 76% of the total plasma concentration. The distribution volume for PEMA is similar to that of PRM (29).

Elimination Half-Life

Primidone, when given experimentally to patients as a rapid intravenous injection, displays a biphasic log concentration-time curve reflecting both a rapid distribution (minutes) and prolonged elimination (hours) (39). Following oral administration the distribution phase is obscured because of prolonged absorption. Primidone elimination half-life in patients is reported to range from 3.3 to 22.4 hr with factors such as age and concomitant therapy accounting for much of the variability (6,8,10,14,19,28,39). Booker et al. (8) found a half-life ranging from 10 to 12 hr in six volunteers given a single 500 mg dose of PRM. We found a mean half-life of 15.2 hr (range, 8.9–22.4 hr) in nine patients receiving an initial 250 mg dose of PRM as monotherapy (10). Similar results are reported by Pisani et al. (28) using a 500 mg PRM dose. These data indicate that PRM half-life following a single dose is independent of dose or plasma concentration, which is consistent with a first order, linear pharmacokinetic model.

Theoretically, long-term PRM therapy could alter its half-life. Accumulation of PB could decrease PRM half-life as a result of microsomal enzyme induction. Alternatively, the structural similarity between PB and PRM might result in inhibition of PRM metabolism, thus extending its half-life. The effect of PEMA on microsomal enzymes is not known, but could exert an effect in the same manner as PB. Frey et al. (13) in a study involving dogs have shown that PRM half-life decreases by as much as 65% after 18 days of treatment. Studies in man are conflicting. Baumel et al. (6) studied two patients on long-term PRM monotherapy which had half-lives of 5.3 and 7 hr, values that are below the range reported following an initial dose. In contrast, Gallagher et al. (14) reported PRM half-lives of 7.2 and 19.2 hr in two patients on long-term monotherapy. We measured serum concentrations over an 8-hr dosing interval in seven patients on maintenance monotherapy (10). The study design precluded determination of half-life, but the decline from peak to trough PRM concentrations averaged 40%. This was a much greater decrease than predicted using each patient's own half-life data obtained from a single dose. These results, in combination with information on the time-dependent changes in PRM clearance (see below), suggest that PRM half-life becomes shorter during maintenance therapy. This may necessitate 6 or 8 hr dosing intervals in some patients to avoid excessively high or low plasma PRM concentrations.

Concurrent administration of other antiepileptic drugs significantly decreases PRM half-life. We found that PRM half-life in patients on combination antiepileptic drug therapy was approximately half that of patients on monotherapy: 8.3 ± 2.9 hr versus 15.2 ± 4.77 hr, $p < 0.05$ (10). Studies by Gallagher et al. (14) and Zavadil and Gallagher (39) reported PRM half-lives ranging from 3.3 to 11 hr in patients on polytherapy. In a study of 12 children age 7 to 14 years on long-term PRM therapy, Kaufman et al. (19) found that eight patients taking PHT had somewhat shorter half-lives than those on PRM alone: 7.9 versus 10.25 hr.

There are limited data on time-dependent alterations in PRM half-life in patients on concomitant antiepileptic drugs. Zavadil and Gallagher (39) characterized PRM half-life in five patients on concomitant antiepileptic drugs following an initial 500 mg dose and after 2 months of maintenance therapy. In three patients there was no change (8.8 versus 9.2 hr), but in two patients on phenytoin and phenobarbital, PRM half-life increased from 8.3 to 25 and 5 to 9 hr, respectively.

When PEMA is administered directly to man, its half-life ranges from 10 to 25 hr (11,29). Results obtained following an oral dose of PRM may be biased because formation of PEMA is often incomplete during the time period of the study. Hunt and Miller (18) found that PEMA half-life decreased by 22% and 75% in two rabbits pretreated with PHT. In a study involving six healthy volunteers and six patients receiving enzyme-inducing antiepileptic drugs, PEMA half-life was 20% faster in patients: 16.7 versus 21 hr (11).

Clearance

There is poor correlation between PRM daily dose and steady-state plasma concentrations. This is due in large measure to the two- to fourfold range in PRM clearance found in patients. Measurements of primidone clearance obtained after oral administration are affected by bioavailability, age, duration of PRM therapy, concomitant drugs, and medication compliance. One must consider these factors when interpreting data and comparing results from different studies.

Primidone clearance following an initial dose varies from 11.5 to 70 ml/hr/kg with a mean value of 37.4 ml/hr/kg (10,28). Clearance is not affected by the size of the dose, but is altered by concomitant antiepileptic drug therapy. We found that co-administration of enzyme-inducing antiepileptic drugs increases PRM clearance by approximately 50% compared to patients on monotherapy: 52.1 ± 15.5 versus 35.5 ± 18.6 ml/hr/kg, $p < 0.05$ (10). Concomitant antiepileptic drugs were withdrawn in four patients who remained on PRM. Clearance decreased to values comparable to those observed in patients on monotherapy following an initial dose.

Changes in PRM clearance may also be time dependent. Figure 1 shows differences in PRM clearance in nine patients after an initial dose and under steady-state condi-

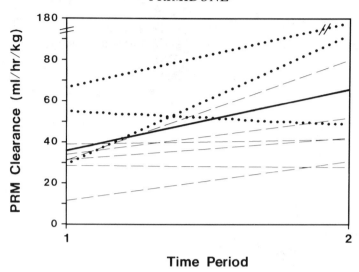

FIG. 1. Changes in PRM clearance over time. Clearance was measured in nine patients following an initial dose (Period 1) and during maintenance therapy 0.5 to 8 months later (Period 2). Patients on PRM and PHT are represented by the dotted line. Patients on monotherapy are represented by the dashed line. The mean clearance value (solid line) increases from 36.3 to 66 ml/hr/kg.

tions 0.5 to 8 months later (10). Four of six monotherapy patients and two of three on other enzyme-inducing antiepileptic drugs had increases in clearance ranging from 30% to 200%. Streete et al. (33) have proposed that PB-mediated induction of microsomal enzymes involved in PRM metabolism is responsible for the increase in PRM clearance during maintenance therapy. The presence of time-dependent changes in clearance means that increases in the daily dosage are needed to maintain stable PRM concentrations. However, since both PB and PEMA concentrations often rise over time due to induction of PRM metabolism, changes in the PRM dose should be made cautiously.

PEMA clearance in humans varies fourfold with values from 18 to 60 mg/hr/kg (34,29). As with half-life, clearance is altered by concurrent use of enzyme-inducing antiepileptic drugs (11,18). Cottrell et al. (11) found that patients on antiepileptic drug had PRM clearances 65% greater than those on monotherapy: 39.1 versus 23.8 ml/hr/kg,

suggesting that PEMA has a nonrenal pathway of elimination that can be induced.

RELATIONSHIP AMONG PRM, PEMA, AND PB CONCENTRATIONS

The appearance of PEMA and PB following initiation of PRM is influenced by the presence of other antiepileptic drugs. Among patients on monotherapy, 24 to 48 hr must elapse before detectable (>1.0 mg/L) quantities of PEMA and PB appear in plasma (10,28). Patients taking enzyme-inducing drugs produce PEMA and PB within 2 to 24 hr after the first PRM dose (6,10).

The relationship among steady-state PRM, PEMA, and PB concentrations is influenced by their respective pharmacokinetic characteristics, patient's age, and concomitant drug therapy. Battino et al. (3), in a large retrospective study, reported that children had higher PB/PRM plasma concentration ratios than adults. In all age groups, concurrent administration of PHT

TABLE 1. *Effect of enzyme-inducing antiepileptic drugs on serum concentrations of primidone and primidone-derived phenobarbital*

Treatment[a]	Patients	PRM (mg/L)	PB (mg/L)
PRM + PHT and/or CBZ	10	9 (7–14)	37 (27–58)
PRM[b]	10	18 (13–30)	19 (7–28)

[a] In both regimens, the mean daily PRM dose was 925 mg (range, 500–1,250 mg).

[b] a minimum of 3 weeks elapsed between determination of PRM and PB concentrations and the last dose of PHT and/or CBZ.

Data from B. J. Wilder, *personal communication.*

PRM, primidone; PB, phenobarbital; PHT, phenytoin; CBZ, carbamazepine.

TABLE 2. *Change in PB/PRM and PEMA/PRM ratios over an 8-hr dosing interval*

Metabolite	Minimum[a]	Ratio		
		Mean	Maximum
PB	1.8	1.4	1.1
PEMA	0.7	0.5	0.4

[a] Ratios were calculated using PRM, PB, and PEMA concentrations obtained over an 8-hr dosing interval. PRM concentrations were the measured minimum, mean, and maximum values. PB and PEMA concentrations did not change significantly. $N = 7$.

PB, phenobarbital; PRM, primidone; PEMA, phenylethylmalonamide.

or CBZ significantly increased the PB/PRM ratio compared with patients on monotherapy: 2.5 versus 4.3, $p < 0.003$. Wilder (1988, *personal communication*) studied 10 patients on PRM just prior to and at least 3 weeks after discontinuation of PHT and/or CBZ. He found that while on enzyme-inducing antiepileptic drugs the patients had PRM concentrations 50% less and PB concentrations 200% greater than values resulting from comparable PRM doses given as monotherapy (Table 1). The PB/PRM ratio decreased from 4.1:1 during combination therapy to approximately 1:1 when PRM was given alone. Schmidt (30) found that co-administration of ethosuximide, in contrast to enzyme-inducing antiepileptic drugs, did not alter the PB/PRM ratio. PEMA concentrations are equal to 70% of trough PRM values (PEMA/PRM = 0.7) when PRM is given as monotherapy (10,33). The effect of other antiepileptic drugs on PEMA/PRM ratios is not clear. Streete et al. (33) found that PB produced a significant increase in PEMA concentrations without affecting PRM concentrations: PEMA/PRM = 1.1. The addition of PHT results in a PEMA/PRM ratio of approximately 1.0, but does so by significantly decreasing PRM concentrations while PEMA concentrations remain unchanged relative to monotherapy

values. Since the percentage of PRM excreted as PEMA markedly increases in the presence of PHT, the findings reported by Streete (33) can be explained by simultaneous induction of the metabolic pathways responsible for the formation and elimination of PEMA.

The variance in PB and PEMA-to-PRM ratios is partially due to the differences in elimination half-life among the three compounds. The relatively long half-lives for PB and PEMA mean that there is minimal fluctuation in plasma concentrations over an 8 or 12 hr dosing interval. In contrast, PRM concentrations can decline by 25% to 75% over the same period due to its relatively fast half-life. As shown in Table 2, the metabolite-to-PRM ratios will vary twofold depending upon the time in the dosing interval that a blood sample is obtained (10). Timing of blood sample collection must be carefully controlled in order to properly interpret PB-to-PRM and PEMA-to-PRM ratios. Use of metabolite-to-PRM ratios to guide therapy, assess medication compliance, or estimate rates of metabolism should be done cautiously, keeping in mind the factors that influence these ratios.

ROUTES OF EXCRETION

Primidone and its metabolites are primarily eliminated by renal excretion. Zavadil and Gallagher (39) reported that 75% to 77% of an intravenously administered PRM dose appeared in urine as PRM or metabolites during a 5-day collection period (Fig. 2). Since the elimination half-life for PB ranges from 3 to 6 days, it is possible that a higher fraction of the dose could have been recovered as PB or PB metabolites had the collection period been extended. Patients on monotherapy excreted 64% of the dose as PRM, 6.6% as PEMA, and 5.1% as PB products. During the same period, patients receiving combination therapy excreted substantially more PEMA and PB (27.9% and 9.9%, respectively), whereas the amount excreted as PRM decreased to 40%. In children on long-term PRM therapy, the daily dose found as PRM, PEMA, and PB in urine was 42.3%, 45.2%, and 4.9%, respectively (19).

There is limited information on the manner in which PEMA is eliminated. Hunt and Miller (18) recovered from urine 62% of an intravenous PEMA dose given to rabbits. This percentage increased to 71% when urine was incubated with β-glucuronidase.

In humans, approximately 81% of a single, oral PEMA dose can be recovered from urine; treatment with β-glucuronidase had no effect on the fraction recovered (11).

ALTERED PHYSIOLOGICAL STATES

The effect of pregnancy on PRM disposition is variable. Clearance in some women exhibits a trend toward greater values during the last trimester although in others there is either no change or a slight decrease (1,4). Phenobarbital concentrations derived from PRM decrease during the latter part of pregnancy resulting in a lower PB-to-PRM ratio; after delivery PB concentrations increase (4). Frequent monitoring of PRM and PB concentrations is warranted due to the unpredictable nature of PRM pharmacokinetics during and immediately after pregnancy.

Nau et al. (27) found that both PRM and PEMA appear in breast milk, reaching concentrations that range from 40% to 96% (mean, 75%) of maternal steady-state serum

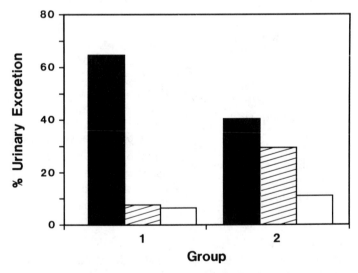

FIG. 2. The effect of enzyme induction on PRM [solid bar], PEMA [hatched bar] and PB [open bar] urinary excretion patterns. Group 1 consists of patients on PRM monotherapy. Group 2 consists of patients on combination therapy with enzyme-inducing antiepileptic drugs.

values. In the same study, they found that neonates of mothers taking PRM have concentrations of PRM and PEMA that are similar to maternal serum concentrations.

Pisani et al. (28) found that PRM pharmacokinetics following a single oral dose in seven patients with acute viral hepatitis were similar to those observed in seven healthy control patients. Renal failure is likely to result in the accumulation of PRM, PEMA, and PB since all three are partially eliminated via the kidney. Both hemodialysis and hemoperfusion are effective in removing PRM from blood (22,26).

SUMMARY

Effective use of primidone requires an understanding of its pharmacokinetics, which are complicated by the presence of active metabolites. Primidone appears to be well absorbed, although differences in patient characteristics and formulation may alter bioavailability. Time to maximum concentration typically occurs 3 to 4 hr after a dose. Primidone is poorly bound to plasma proteins with the free fraction representing 80% or more of the total plasma concentration. Primidone distributes into saliva and CSF, but equilibration occurs over a period of hours. Saliva concentrations, when properly collected, are strongly correlated with unbound plasma and CSF concentrations. Elimination occurs by the renal and hepatic routes and is influenced by age, duration of treatment, and concomitant drug therapy. Interpretation of PRM concentrations (plasma, saliva, and CSF) and PB or PEMA-to-PRM ratios should be done cautiously and include consideration of the method and timing of sample collection as well as the factors that alter PRM pharmacokinetics.

ACKNOWLEDGMENTS

We thank Kenneth Miller, Ph.D., for his many contributions to our primidone stud-

ies cited in this chapter, and B. J. Wilder, M.D., for patient data.

REFERENCES

1. Bardy, A., Teramo, K., and Hiilesmaa, V. (1982): Apparent plasma clearances of phenytoin, phenobarbitone, primidone, and carbamazepine during pregnancy: Results of the prospective Helsinki Study. *Epilepsia, Pregnancy, and the Child*, edited by D. Janz et al., pp. 141–145. Raven Press, New York.
2. Bartels, H., Gunther, E., and Wallis, S. (1979): Flow-dependent salivary primidone levels in epileptic children. *Epilepsia*, 20:431–436.
3. Battino, D., Avanzini, G., Bossi, L., Croci, D., Cusi, C., Gomeni, C., and Moise, A. (1983): Plasma levels of primidone and its metabolite phenobarbital: Effect of age and associated therapy. *Ther. Drug Monit.*, 5:73–79.
4. Battino, D., Binelli, S., Bossi, L., Como, M., Croci, D., Cusi, C., and Avanzini, G. (1984): Changes in primidone/phenobarbitone ratio during pregnancy and the puerperium. *Clin. Pharmacokin.*, 9:252–260.
5. Baumel, I. P., Gallagher, B. B., DiMicco, J., and Goico, H. (1973): Metabolism and anticonvulsant properties of primidone in the rat. *J. Pharmacol. Exp. Ther.*, 186:305–314.
6. Baumel, I., Gallagher, B., and Mattson, R. (1972): Phenylethylmalonamide (PEMA), an important metabolite of primidone. *Arch. Neurol.*, 27:34–41.
7. Bielmann, P., Levac, T., Langlois, Y., and Tetreault, L. (1974): Bioavailability of primidone in epileptic patients. *Int. J. Clin. Pharmacol.*, 9:132–137.
8. Booker, H., Hosokowa, K., Burdette, R., and Darcey, B. (1970): A clinical study of serum primidone levels. *Epilepsia*, 11:395–402.
9. Brillman, J., Gallagher, B., and Mattson, R. (1974): Acute primidone intoxication. *Arch. Neurol.*, 30:255–258.
10. Cloyd, J. C., Miller, K. W., and Leppik, I. E. (1981): Primidone kinetics: Effects of concurrent drugs and duration of therapy. *Clin. Pharmacol. Ther.*, 29(3):402–407.
11. Cottrell, P. R., Streete, J. M., Berry, D. J., et al. (1982): Pharmacokinetics of phenylethylamlonamide (PEMA) in normal subjects and in patients treated with antiepileptic drugs. *Epilepsia*, 23:307–313.
12. Food and Drug Administration. Therapeutic Inequivalency Action Coordinating Committee (1988): Therapeutic Inequivalency—Primidone Tablets, 250 tablets, Bolar Pharmaceuticals, Inc., summary report. Report No. 87-TI-01.
13. Frey, H., Gobel, W., and Loscher, W. (1979): Pharmacokinetics of primidone and its active metabolites in the dog. *Arch. Int. Pharmacodyn.*, 242:14–30.
14. Gallagher, B., Baumel, I., and Mattson, R. (1972):

Metabolic disposition of primidone and its metabolites in epileptic subjects after single and repeated administration. *Neurology*, 22:1186–1192.

15. Goldsmith, R. F., and Ouvrier, R. A. (1981): Salivary anticonvulsant levels in children: A comparison of methods. *Ther. Drug Monit.*, 3:151–157.

16. Holler, M., and Penin, H. (1984): Studies on the intracerebral metabolism of anticonvulsant drugs. I. Perfusion of primidone through the isolated brain of the rat. *Biochem. Pharmacol.*, 33:1753.

17. Houghton, G., Richens, A., Toseland, P., Davidson, S., and Falconer, M. (1975): Brain concentrations of phenytoin, phenobarbitone and primidone in epileptic patients. *Europ. J. Clin. Pharmacol.*, 9:73–78.

18. Hunt, R., and Miller, K. (1978): Disposition of primidone, phenylethylmalonamide, and phenobarbital in the rabbit. *Drug Metab. and Disp.*, 6(1):75–81.

19. Kauffman, R. E., Habersang, R., and Lansky, L. (1977): Kinetics of primidone metabolism and excretion in children. *Clin. Pharmacol. Ther.*, 22:200–205.

20. Knott, C., and Reynolds, F. (1984): The place of saliva in antiepileptic drug monitoring. *Ther. Drug Monit.*, 6:35–41.

21. Leal, K., Rapport, R., Wilensky, A., and Friel, P. (1978): Single-dose pharmacokinetics and anticonvulsant efficacy of primidone in mice. *Ann. Neurol.*, 5:470–474.

22. Lee, C., Marbury, T., Perchalski, R., and Wilder, B. (1982): Pharmacokinetics of primidone elimination by uremic patients. *J. Clin. Pharmacol.*, 22:301–308.

23. Leppik, I. E., Cloyd, J. C., and Miller, K. W. (1984): Development of tolerance to the side effects of primidone. *Ther. Drug Monit.*, 6:189–191.

24. MacAulife, J. J., Sherwin, A. L., Leppik, I. E., Fayle, S. A., and Pippenger, C. E. (1977): Salivary levels of anticonvulsants: A practical approach to drug monitoring. *Neurology*, 27:409–413.

25. Mattson, R. H., Cramer, J. A., Collins, J. F., et al. (1985): Comparison of carbamazepine, phenobarbital, phenytoin and primidone in partial and generalized tonic-clonic seizures. *N. Eng. J. Med.*, 313:145–151.

26. Matzke, G. R., Cloyd, J. C., and Sawchuk, R. J. (1981): Acute phenytoin and primidone intoxication—A pharmacokinetic analysis. *J. Clin. Pharmacol.*, 21:92–99.

27. Nau, H., Rating, D., Hauser, I., et al. (1980): Placental transfer and pharmacokinetics of primidone and its metabolites phenobarbital, PEMA and hydroxyphenobarbital, in neonates and infants of epileptic mothers. *Eur. J. Clin. Pharmacol.*, 18:31–42.

28. Pisani, F., Perucca, E., Primerano, G., D'Agostino, A., Petrelli, R., Fazio, A., Oteri, G., and Di Perri, R. (1984): Single-dose kinetics of primidone in acute viral hepatitis. *Eur. J. Clin. Pharmacol.*, 27:465–469.

29. Pisani, F., and Richens, A. (1983): Pharmacokinetics of phenylethylmalonamide (PEMA) after oral and intravenous administration. *Clin. Pharmacol.*, 8:272–276.

30. Schmidt, D. (1975): The effect of phenytoin and ethosuximide on primidone metabolism in patients with epilepsy. *J. Neurol.*, 209:115–123.

31. Schmidt, D., and Kupferberg, H. J. (1975): Diphenylhydantoin, phenobarbital and primidone in saliva, plasma and cerebrospinal fluid. *Epilepsia*, 16:735–741.

32. Schottelius, D. D. (1982): Primidone: Absorption, distribution and excretion. In: *Antiepileptic Drugs*, 2nd edition, edited by D. M. Woodbury, J. K. Penry, and C. E. Pippenger, pp. 405–413. Raven Press, New York.

33. Streete, J., Berry, D., Pettit, L., and Newbery, J. (1986): Phenylethylmalonamide serum levels in patients treated with primidone and the effects of other antiepileptic drugs. *Ther. Drug Monit.*, 8:161–165.

34. Syverson, G., Morgan, J., Weintraub, M., and Myers, G. (1977): Acetazolamide-induced interference with primidone absorption. *Arch. Neurol.*, 34:80–84.

35. Troupin, A. S., and Friel, P. (1975): Anticonvulsant level in saliva serum and cerebrospinal fluid. *Epilepsia*, 16:223–227.

36. van der Klein, E., Guelen, P. J. M., Van Wijk, C., and Baars, I. (1975): Clinical pharmacokinetics in monitoring chronic medication with anti-epileptic drugs, in *Clinical Pharmacology of Antiepileptic Drugs*, edited by J. Schneider, D. Janz, D. Gardner-Thorpe et al. Springer Verlag, Berlin.

37. van Heijst, A., de Jong, W., Sledenrijk, R., and van Dijk, A. (1983): Coma and crystalluria: A massive primidone intoxication treated with haemoperfusion. *J. Toxicol.—Clin. Toxicol.*, 20(4):307–318.

38. Wylie, E., Pippenger, C. E., and Rothner, A. D. (1987): Increased seizure frequency with generic primidone. *J.A.M.A.*, 258:1216–1217.

39. Zavadil, P., and Gallagher, B. (1976): Metabolism and excretion of ^{14}C-primidone in epileptic patients. In: *Epileptology*, edited by D. Jang. George Thieme Verlag KG, Stuttgart.

Antiepileptic Drugs, Third Edition, edited by
R. Levy, R. Mattson, B. Meldrum,
J. K. Penry, and F. E. Dreifuss.
Raven Press, Ltd., New York © 1989.

27

Primidone

Biotransformation and Mechanisms of Action

Blaise F. D. Bourgeois

The particular relevance of the metabolic conversion of primidone *in vivo* is related to the fact that primidone typically illustrates the complexities involved when a drug with pharmacological activity of its own is converted into active metabolites. Thus, any consideration of primidone's mechanisms of action will also have to question the relative contribution of the metabolites. This emphasizes the relevance of quantitative aspects of biotransformation and of factors that will influence the extent of conversion to these metabolites.

METABOLIC PATHWAYS

The primary and most relevant metabolic pathways of primidone biotransformation, as they are known today, are illustrated in Fig. 1. They involve the formation of phenylethylmalonamide (PEMA) by cleavage of the pyrimidine ring, and the formation of phenobarbital by oxidation of the methylene group. Phenobarbital then undergoes hydroxylation to *p*-hydroxyphenobarbital (see Chapter 20). Soon after the introduction of primidone into clinical use in 1952 (30), PEMA was first identified as a metabolite in rats by Bogue and Carrington (10), and it was subsequently found in all species studied for its presence. The second metabolite of primidone to be identified was

phenobarbital. In 1956, Butler and Waddell (15) reported that they had identified phenobarbital as well as *p*-hydroxyphenobarbital in the urine and in the plasma of a dog and of a patient receiving primidone. Plaa et al. (47) also identified phenobarbital in patients and in rats treated with primidone and were the first to attribute intoxication from primidone to the presence of phenobarbital. The conversion of primidone to phenobarbital could also be demonstrated in all species studied, although the biotransformation was found to be very slow in guinea pigs (22).

Minor metabolites of primidone identified so far include α-phenylbutyramide (20), *p*-hydroxyprimidone (32,33) and α-phenyl-γ-butyrolactone (2). There is no evidence at this time that these metabolites have any importance during therapy with primidone. All metabolites identified so far, as well as primidone itself, are excreted in the urine. Crystalluria has long been recognized as a sign of primidone intoxication in man (14,16,39,43,55). The hexagonal crystals present in the urine were found to consist mostly of primidone itself (3,14).

QUANTITATIVE ASPECTS OF BIOTRANSFORMATION

Several studies have addressed the question of the relative amounts of primidone

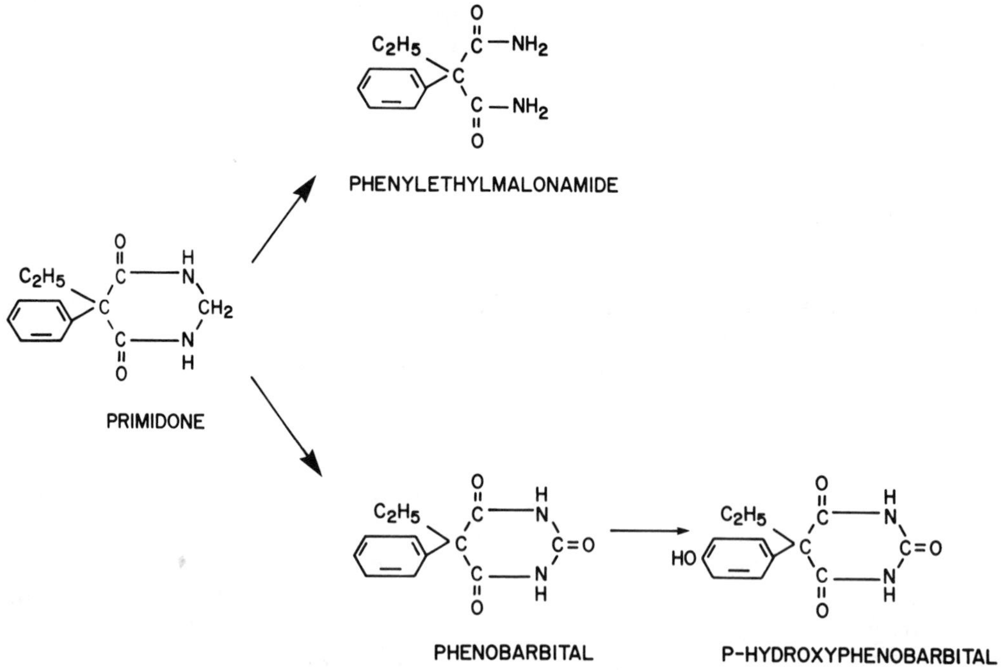

FIG. 1. The main biotransformation pathways of primidone consist of formation of PEMA by ring scission and oxidation to phenobarbital, which is then parahydroxylated.

converted to its metabolites after single or multiple doses. After single and multiple oral doses of primidone in rabbits (25), the amount of primidone excreted unchanged in urine was calculated to be about 20% of a single dose, whereas 48% was excreted as PEMA and 10% as phenobarbital and p-hydroxyphenobarbital. The results also suggested that the conversion to PEMA occurred earlier and more rapidly than the conversion to phenobarbital. This led the authors to suspect a rate-limited formation of phenobarbital from primidone. In a later study in rabbits, primidone was administered intravenously and, on the basis of plasma and urinary measurements, it was concluded that approximately 20% of the dose was excreted as unchanged primidone, 40% was metabolized to PEMA, and another 40% was metabolized to phenobarbital (34). Both PEMA and phenobarbital were detectable in plasma within 5 min of

the intravenous administration of primidone. All three compounds disappeared from the plasma in a manner that could be described by a biexponential equation and the plasma concentrations could be fitted by using a four-compartment pharmacokinetic model, consisting of two compartments for primidone and one compartment each for PEMA and phenobarbital. The discrepancy between the finding that phenobarbital accounted for 40% of the dose as compared with 10% of the dose in the study by Fujimoto et al. (25) was interpreted as possibly being due to the difference in dose (10 mg/kg versus 400 mg/kg in the earlier study) and saturable biotransformation of primidone to phenobarbital. Pretreatment with phenytoin for 5 days increased the total body clearance of primidone, PEMA, and phenobarbital, and accelerated the rate of formation of the metabolites. After oral administration of primidone to rats (7), levels of primidone reached their peak in plasma after 1 hr and in brain after 2 hr. Both PEMA and phenobarbital were detected in plasma 30 min after doses of 250 mg/kg or more and 1 hr after doses of 62.5 mg/kg or more. Neither PEMA nor phenobarbital was detected throughout a 24-hr period after doses of primidone below 62.5 mg/kg. Rapid conversion of primidone to phenobarbital and PEMA could also be shown in mice. After a single oral dose of 50 mg/kg, both metabolites were detectable in plasma after 30 min and their concentration peaked in plasma and brain after about 6 hr (37). The rate of conversion of primidone to its metabolites appears to be increased during pregnancy in mice (42) as can be concluded from higher ratios of metabolites to parent drug and relatively lower values of primidone at the later sampling times.

Conversion of primidone to its two main metabolites also was demonstrated in domestic fowl (35) and gerbils (24). In fowl, phenobarbital could be detected within 1 hr of intraperitoneal administration. In gerbils, both phenobarbital and PEMA could be detected in plasma 1 hr after oral administration of a single dose, but only phenobarbital and primidone could be detected in the brain.

There is good experimental evidence that the liver is responsible for the enzymatic biotransformation of primidone. In a study in which 98% of ^{14}C-primidone perfused through isolated rat liver could be recovered in the perfusate, the liver, and the bile (1), primidone and PEMA could be found in the first sample at 30 min. After 120 min, phenobarbital production was equivalent to 15% of the metabolized primidone, whereas PEMA accounted for 79% of metabolism and was therefore by far the most important metabolite from a quantitative point of view. Another 3% of the recovered radioactivity was unidentified. PEMA had a weak inhibitory effect on primidone biotransformation, whereas no such effect was observed with phenobarbital.

Acceleration of primidone metabolism was observed in the livers of rats pretreated with primidone and particularly with phenobarbital, suggesting a certain degree of autoinduction. Evidence pointing toward the importance of the liver for the biotransformation of primidone had already been derived from studies showing that liver damage in rats increased the potency and duration of action of primidone (52). In the same studies, nephrectomy also increased potency and duration of action of primidone, suggesting that this organ might also be involved in primidone metabolism. Additional evidence for primidone biotransformation in the liver is provided by the observation that pretreatment of fowl and mice with the inhibitor of liver mixed-function hydroxylases SKF 525A inhibits the conversion of primidone to its metabolites (12,35,37).

The quantitative aspects of primidone biotransformation in man have been assessed in numerous studies. Olesen and Dam (44) compared the level-to-dose ratios for phenobarbital and primidone in patients who had taken either drug for at least 6 months. By comparing the two ratios they concluded that, on the average, 24.5% of the primidone administered was converted to phenobarbital. There was a tendency toward a dose-dependent effect, with a lower conversion percentage at the higher doses. Similarly, Bogan and Smith (9) found that in order to achieve the same blood phenobarbital levels, the primidone dose (in mg/kg) had to be about five times higher than the corresponding dose of phenobarbital. The time course of appearance in plasma was found to be different for phenobarbital and PEMA, the latter being detectable within the first 24 hr after primidone administration (500–750 mg) in epileptic patients previously treated with phenytoin and/or phenobarbital, whereas the appearance of phenobarbital was characterized by a delay of at least 24 hr and up to 96 hr (26). In another study of epileptic patients,

PEMA could be detected within 2 hr of a first dose of 500 mg of primidone (6). In contrast, after a 500 mg dose in volunteers, no phenobarbital could be detected in the serum throughout a 48-hr period (8).

Quantitative aspects of primidone biotransformation were studied in adults with epilepsy, using the intravenous infusion of a ^{14}C-primidone dose over 3 to 5 min (57). The patients were divided into two groups depending on whether they had no previous exposure to anticonvulsants (group I) or were taking other anticonvulsants (group II). The plasma half-life and urinary excretion of primidone and its metabolites were measured. In patients with no previous exposure to anticonvulsants, the mean plasma half-life of primidone was about twice as long as in patients taking other antiepileptic drugs (14.4 versus 7.33 hr). The amount of drug excreted in the urine during the first 24 hr after the ^{14}C-primidone infusion was 46.7% of the dose in group I and 45.5% in group II, but the relative amounts of primidone, phenobarbital, and PEMA were different in the two groups: 42% unchanged primidone, 2% PEMA, 1.2% phenobarbital, and 1.5% unidentified product in untreated patients (group I) as opposed to 31% unchanged primidone, 10% PEMA, 1.3% phenobarbital, and 2.8% unidentified product in group II. By the end of the fifth day, 75.5% of the dose had been recovered in group I and 77.4% in group II. The relative amount of unchanged primidone was 64% and 39.6%, respectively, for groups I and II, the values for PEMA being 6.6% and 27.9%, for phenobarbital 2.1% and 3.3%, and for unidentified products 3% and 6.5%, respectively. The unidentified products were considered to be mainly free and conjugated p-hydroxyphenobarbital.

The metabolic profile of primidone and the rate of production of its two main metabolites during long-term dosing was studied in a group of 12 children (36). They had all been on a constant dose of primidone for more than 3 months and eight of them were also taking phenytoin. Blood samples and urine were collected for 24 hr after the total daily dose was administered as a single dose. The previous primidone dose had been given 16 hr earlier. The mean elimination half-life of primidone was 8.7 hr, a value similar to that reported in adults. On the average, 92% of the primidone dose was recovered in the 24-hr urine collection with 42.3% as unchanged primidone, 45.2% as PEMA, and 4.9% as phenobarbital, including p-hydroxyphenobarbital and 3,4-hydroxyphenobarbital. Interpatient variability with regard to half-life and urinary excretion was quite pronounced. It should be pointed out that strict steady-state conditions were not met in view of the changes in dosing intervals. Indeed, inspection of the data provided indicates that the average primidone level was lower at the end of the 24-hr period than before the test dose. Thus, the values for urinary excretion of primidone are likely to represent an overestimation.

A different approach to the quantitative assessment of primidone biotransformation in patients is the determination of steady-state blood concentration ratios between primidone and its two main metabolites. Since other antiepileptic drugs can markedly affect these ratios, this aspect is closely related to the issue of drug interactions. Specific interactions between primidone and other drugs are discussed in Chapter 28. Because of its relatively short half-life, the levels of primidone fluctuate more than the levels of the metabolites, and the concentration ratios are therefore not constant. The primidone levels are lowest before the first morning dose. The phenobarbital-to-primidone (PB-to-PRM) ratio in patients on primidone monotherapy was found to be 1.84 (17) and 2.14 (41) at the time of minimum primidone values, and 1.07 at the time of maximum primidone values (17). The PB-to-PRM ratio was 1.45 4 hr after the dose of primidone (50) and 1.05 between 2 and 4 hr after the last dose (19). In contrast, a PB-to-PRM ratio of 4.35 (19), and 4.2 (49) 2 to 4 hr after the primidone dose was determined in patients on combination therapy.

Values for the blood PEMA-to-PRM ratio have also been reported. In patients on combination therapy, Haidukewych and Rodin (29) found values of 1.16 to 1.55, depending on the type of drug combinations. In another study (51), the serum PEMA-to-PRM ratio was 0.66 in 56 patients on primidone monotherapy and 0.94 to 1.18 in various groups of patients on combination therapy. Blood samples were drawn at various times after the last primidone dose. Table 1 summarizes the relationship between primidone dose and the serum concentrations of primidone, phenobarbital, and PEMA, as well as the serum concentration ratios before the first morning dose in hospitalized patients and under steady-state conditions (*unpublished results*). All doses and concentrations were converted to μmol/kg and μmol/l, respectively. The ratio between phenobarbital concentration and primidone dose was increased by a factor of 1.6 in the presence of comedication. This value of 1.6 would represent the extent of induction of the conversion of primidone to phenobarbital, under the assumption that phenobarbital elimination is not affected by comedication. Although the PEMA-to-PRM ratio is markedly increased by comedication, the PEMA concentration in relation to the primidone dose is not affected to the same extent.

Other factors besides concomitant drug therapy can influence the biotransformation of primidone. One of them is age. The conversion of primidone to phenobarbital and to PEMA was found to be very limited or even absent in neonates (48). The effect of age on the PB/PRM ratio in children was evaluated in a study that demonstrated a progressive decline of this ratio after infancy, a minimum value being reached between 10 and 15 years of age, with a subsequent rise during adolescence and into adulthood (4).

The effect of pregnancy on primidone metabolism was studied in nine patients taking constant doses of primidone, six of whom were on monotherapy (5). Pregnancy caused a significant decrease in the PB-to-PRM ratio, as well as a significant decrease in the concentration of derived phenobarbital. Changes in primidone concentrations were not significant. The decrease in primidone-derived phenobarbital concentration could have been related to decreased conversion as well as to accelerated phenobarbital elimination since, in the same study, the phenobarbital levels also decreased, although not significantly, in patients taking phenobarbital.

The effect of acute viral hepatitis on primidone metabolism was studied by administering a single dose of 500 mg to seven patients and seven control subjects (46). On the average, PEMA was measurable in the serum of controls within 9 hr. In contrast, during 60 hr of observation, PEMA could be detected in the serum of only one patient

TABLE 1. *Serum concentration/primidone dose ratios and serum concentration ratios of primidone, phenobarbital, and PEMA at steady state*

	N	Serum concentration/primidone dose (Kg·d/l, molar ratio)			Serum concentration ratio (molar ratio)	
		PRM	PB	PEMA	PB/PRM	PEMA/PRM
Monotherapy	10	0.78 ± 0.25	1.38 ± 0.50	0.68 ± 0.41	1.55 ± 0.70	0.74 ± 0.38
Comedication[a]	53	0.4 ± 0.15	2.26 ± 0.92	0.79 ± 0.44	5.48 ± 2.46	1.81 ± 0.79

[a] Combination therapy included primidone, phenytoin, and/or carbamazepine.
Values are expressed as mean ± SD. All blood samples were drawn before the first morning dose in hospitalized patients.

after 48 hr. Despite this evidence for impaired biotransformation in patients with hepatitis, the serum half-life of primidone in patients did not differ significantly from the values in controls. In a case of renal insufficiency, elevated levels of primidone and PEMA were found (31). This is in good agreement with the observation described earlier in this chapter that substantial amounts of both primidone and PEMA are excreted in the urine, and with the fact that primidone has been shown to be dialyzable (38).

MECHANISMS OF ACTION

Although the effectiveness of primidone in epileptic patients is well established, the identification by Butler and Waddell in 1956 (15) of phenobarbital as a metabolite of primidone in man raised the question of whether primidone has independent antiepileptic activity or should merely be considered as a pro-drug. The issue became even more complex when Baumel et al. (6) demonstrated independent anticonvulsant activity in rats for PEMA, the other major metabolite of primidone in man. With regard to mechanisms of action, the presence of active metabolites distinguishes primidone from most other conventional antiepileptic drugs. First, it is more difficult to study the action of primidone alone because of the presence of the metabolites, and second, the pharmacological effect *in vivo* will always be a combined effect. Thus, if primidone, phenobarbital, and PEMA indeed have independent activity, primidone is not a drug but an obligate drug combination, and it will have to be considered as such in any discussion of the mechanisms of action. No information is available on the biochemical mechanisms by which primidone and PEMA exert their action, and the mechanisms of action of phenobarbital are discussed in detail in Chapter 17. Therefore, the following discussion will focus on the

available evidence regarding the qualitative and quantitative pharmacodynamic properties of primidone, phenobarbital, and PEMA.

The anticonvulsant effect of PEMA was first demonstrated by Baumel et al. (6), who tested it against the convulsant hexafluorodiethyl ether in rats. PEMA was much less potent than phenobarbital in this model. In the same study, it could be demonstrated that PEMA potentiated the anticonvulsant activity of phenobarbital in this experimental model and that it also potentiated the hexobarbital sleeping time in rats. In mice, PEMA was shown to be effective against maximal electroshock seizures, although it was approximately 30 times less potent than phenobarbital in this model (37).

In view of its conversion to two active metabolites, unequivocal demonstration of the independent anticonvulsant activity of primidone has been a difficult task. A comparison between therapy with primidone and with phenobarbital has been attempted in various clinical studies. Several authors concluded that an independent antiepileptic effect of primidone could not be demonstrated (28,44,56). In a more recent clinical study, primidone therapy was found to be more effective than phenobarbital against generalized tonic-clonic seizures (45). Primidone and phenobarbital were administered in a crossover design to 21 epileptic patients for 12 months each. Doses were adjusted to achieve similar phenobarbital levels with both drugs. The mean serum phenobarbital level was 138 ± 59 μmol/l during treatment with primidone and 137 ± 53 μmol/l during treatment with phenobarbital. The monthly seizure frequency was significantly higher during treatment with phenobarbital than during the primidone period. These results were independent of the treatment sequence.

The first experimental evidence in favor of independent antiepileptic activity of primidone was provided by Frey and Hahn

(22) who demonstrated protection against pentylenetetrazol-induced seizures in dogs at lower plasma phenobarbital concentrations when primidone was also present. Further experimental evidence of an independent anticonvulsant activity of primidone came from a study in rats by Baumel et al. (7), which also suggested a difference in anticonvulsant spectrum between primidone and phenobarbital. Complete protection against electroshock seizures was observed early after drug administration when only primidone was detectable in the brain. At these low primidone concentrations, however, protection against hexafluorodiethyl ether or pentylenetetrazol seizures was minimal or absent. Protection against these two systemic convulsants was related to the appearance of phenobarbital and PEMA. Independent activity of primidone was also clearly demonstrated against seizures induced by intermittent photic stimulation in epileptic fowl (35). The conversion of primidone to phenobarbital was prevented by the administration of the metabolic inhibitor SKF 525A. No anticonvulsant activity could be demonstrated for PEMA in this model when administered at the same doses as primidone. By using the metabolic inhibitor SKF 525A in mice, Leal et al. (37) also demonstrated independent activity of primidone against maximal electroshock. However, by analyzing the relationship between seizure protection and brain concentrations of primidone, phenobarbital, and PEMA after single doses of primidone without SKF 525A pretreatment, these authors concluded that most of the anticonvulsant effect under these circumstances was derived from phenobarbital.

Another study on the effect of primidone, phenobarbital, and PEMA on the electroconvulsant threshold in mice indicated that primidone was independently effective, but 1.7 times less potent than phenobarbital (21). Measurements of brain concentrations of the three compounds suggested that primidone had accounted for more than 80% of the total anticonvulsant effect at the time of the test. The anticonvulsant effect of primidone was also studied in gerbils in which seizures were elicited by a blast of compressed air (24). Determination of plasma and brain concentrations indicated that primidone itself was responsible for most of the anticonvulsant effect during the first hours after its administration. An analysis based on available data on individual anticonvulsant potency of primidone and its metabolites in dogs, and on their relative concentrations during long-term therapy, led to the conclusion that phenobarbital was probably responsible for more than 85% of the total anticonvulsant activity during long-term therapy with primidone in this species (23). Another study in dogs suggested that at comparable serum phenobarbital concentrations, only one of 15 dogs experienced improved seizure control after therapy was changed from phenobarbital to primidone (18).

The effects of primidone, phenobarbital, and PEMA were compared in a model of nerve-stimulated transmitter release in the frog neuromuscular junction (53,54). Transmitter release was not consistently affected by PEMA in this model. In contrast to phenobarbital, primidone required stimulation of the preparation for its presynaptic effect to become apparent. Thus, the effects of primidone, phenobarbital, and PEMA differed in this *in vitro* model.

So far, we have seen that primidone possesses independent antiepileptic activity against electroshock seizures, that its anticonvulsant effect against chemical convulsants is weak or absent in contrast to phenobarbital, and that PEMA has a low anticonvulsant potency. A series of experiments addressed the question of the neurotoxicity of primidone and its metabolites, and of the pharmacodynamic interactions among the three compounds with regard to antiepileptic potency and neurotoxicity (12,13). For this purpose, seizure protection, neurotoxicity, and therapeutic indices of primidone, phenobarbital, and PEMA individually and in varying combinations were assessed quantitatively in mice. All results were expressed in terms of brain concentrations to eliminate any possible pharmacokinetic interaction from the analysis. Neurotoxicity by the rotorod test, anticonvulsant efficacy, and therapeutic index of the three compounds tested individually are summarized in Table 2 (12). Phenobarbital has a similar potency against maximal electroshock and against pentylenetetrazol. The median neurotoxic concentration is much higher for primidone than for phenobarbital, indicating that primidone is 2.5 times less neurotoxic than phenobarbital in this model. Based on brain concentrations, primidone is as potent as phenobarbital against electroshock seizures, and primidone has therefore a substantially higher therapeutic index because of its lower neurotoxicity. No protection against the clonic seizures induced by pentylenetetrazol or bicuculline could be achieved with primidone, even at brain concentrations as high as 81.7 and 103.3 μg per gram, respectively. These differences in anticonvulsant spectrum and neurotoxic potency suggest that phenobarbital and primidone are two different anticonvulsants with different mechanisms of action. Based on its anticonvulsant spectrum, primidone is comparable to phenytoin and carbamazepine, both of which are effective against maximal electroshock but not against chemically induced seizures. In contrast to primidone, PEMA has the same anticonvulsant spectrum as phenobarbital, but is 16 times less potent than phenobarbital against both electroshock and pentylenetetrazol seizures. With regard to its neurotoxicity, PEMA is eight times less potent than phenobarbital and its therapeutic indices are therefore one-half as high as those of phenobarbital.

Since therapy with primidone is an obligate combination therapy, as stated earlier, the same experimental model was used to assess anticonvulsant effect and neurotoxicity when combining the three active compounds (13). Combined administration of phenobarbital and PEMA revealed that the anticonvulsant effect of phenobarbital against pentylenetetrazol was potentiated by PEMA, but the neurotoxicity of phenobarbital was potentiated to the same extent, leaving the therapeutic index unchanged. When primidone and phenobarbital were tested together at a brain concentration ratio of approximately 1:1 and in the absence of PEMA, their effect against electroshock seizures was supra-additive (i.e., potentiated), whereas their neurotoxicity as measured by the rotorod test was infra-additive. When PEMA was added as a third drug, it potentiated the combined neurotoxicity of primidone and phenobarbital, but did not increase the anticonvulsant effect. These results are summarized in Fig. 2.

TABLE 2. *Toxicity, anticonvulsant efficacy, and therapeutic index of PB, PRM, and PEMA*

	TC_{50}	EC_{50} MES	TI MES	EC_{50} PTZ	TI PTZ
PB	35.8 (31.4–40.7)	13.6 (12.8–14.4)	2.63	17.0 (15.0–19.3)	2.1
PRM	88.3 (80.4–97.1)	12.1 (11.2–13.1)	7.30	No protection	
PEMA	283.2 (261.4–306.7)	221.9 (195.4–252.0)	1.28	276.0 (251.5–302.9)	1.03

The median toxic brain concentration (TC_{50}) and the median effective brain concentration (EC_{50}) against maximal electroshock (MES) and pentylenetetrazol (PTZ) seizures are indicated in μg per gram wet brain weight. TI is equal to TC_{50}/EC_{50}. The 95% confidence limits are indicated in parentheses.
From Bourgeois et al., ref. 12, with permission.

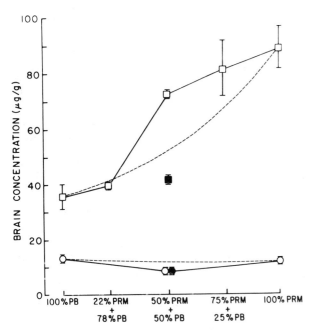

FIG. 2. The median toxic brain concentrations (TC$_{50}$, squares) and the median effective brain concentrations (EC$_{50}$) against MES-induced seizures (circles) are represented for phenobarbital (PB), primidone (PRM), and the sum of both in various combinations of PB + PRM in the absence of PEMA (open symbols) and in the presence of PEMA (closed symbols). Dashed lines indicate expected values for an additive interaction between PRM and PB. From Bourgeois et al., ref. 13, with permission.

These experimental results suggest that the optimal brain concentration ratio for primidone and phenobarbital would be approximately 1:1. This is far from the ratio usually present in patients undergoing prolonged treatment with primidone. We have seen that serum concentrations of phenobarbital are almost always in excess of primidone concentrations, by a factor of up to 5 during combination therapy. It has been shown that brain penetration is better for phenobarbital than for primidone, in humans as well as in animals (37). In our experiments (12,13), brain phenobarbital concentrations were two times higher than brain primidone concentrations at equal plasma concentrations. Thus, the PB/PRM concentration ratio is likely to be even higher in brain than in serum. Therefore, if primidone and phenobarbital are indeed approximately equipotent, the contribution of primidone to the total antiepileptic effect during long-term primidone therapy would be at best one-third at the time of peak primidone concentrations during monotherapy, and it is probably negligible during combi-

nation therapy. Also, if neurotoxicity is also lower for primidone than for phenobarbital in humans, an upper therapeutic limit for serum primidone concentrations is meaningless at naturally occurring PB-to-PRM ratios. Since phenobarbital concentrations are almost always higher than those of primidone, the latter would be unlikely to reach toxic values and, in patients who have tolerated primidone well initially, dosage increases are likely to be limited only by the occurrence of toxicity from phenobarbital, not from primidone.

Most experimental data on primidone and its metabolites were obtained from single-dose studies. The effect of long-term administration of phenobarbital on anticonvulsant and neurotoxic potencies of primidone and phenobarbital was studied in mice (11). Pretreatment with phenobarbital for 2 weeks induced tolerance to the anticonvulsant effect and neurotoxicity of phenobarbital as well as cross-tolerance of a similar magnitude to the effects of primidone. The phenobarbital-induced tolerance was more pronounced for the anticonvul-

sant than for the neurotoxic effect of phenobarbital and of primidone, which resulted in
a lower therapeutic index for both drugs
after pretreatment. These results of cross-
tolerance to the neurotoxic effects of primidone after pretreatment with phenobarbital
provide experimental support for the clinical observation suggesting that patients previously treated with phenobarbital have
fewer side effects when first exposed to
primidone (27,40). As stated earlier, phenobarbital and primidone are likely to have
different mechanisms of action. In that
case, the cross-tolerance between the two
drugs might indicate that cross-tolerance
does not necessarily imply a common mechanism of action, and that the mechanisms
involved in the development of tolerance
are not as specific as the individual drug
actions.

ACKNOWLEDGMENT

Original data presented in this chapter
were obtained in collaboration with Mr. N.
Wad at the Swiss Epilepsy Center in Zürich,
Switzerland.

REFERENCES

1. Alvin, J., Gohr, E., and Bush, M. T. (1975): Study
   of the hepatic metabolism of primidone by improved technology. *J. Pharmacol. Exp. Ther.*,
   194:117–125.
2. Andresen, B. D., Davis, F. T., Templeton, J. L.,
   Hammer, R. H., and Panzik, H. L. (1976): Synthesis and characterization of alpha-phenyl-
   gamma-butyrolactone, a metabolite of glutheti-
   mide, phenobarbital and primidone in human urine.
   Res. Commun. Chem. Pathol. Pharmacol., 15:21–
   30.
3. Bailey, D. N., and Jatlow, P. I. (1972): Chemical
   analysis of massive crystalluria following primidone overdose. *Am. J. Clin. Pathol.*, 58:583–589.
4. Battino, D., Avanzini, G., Bossi, L., Croci, D.,
   Cusi, C., Gomeni, C., and Moise, A. (1983):
   Plasma levels of primidone and its metabolite
   phenobarbital: Effect of age and associated therapy. *Ther. Drug Monit.*, 5:73–79.
5. Battino, D., Binelli, S., Bossi, L., Como, M. L.,
   Croci, D., Cusi, C., and Avanzini, G. (1984):
   Changes in primidone/phenobarbitone ratio during

pregnancy and the puerperium. *Clin. Pharmacokin.*, 9:252–260.
6. Baumel, I. P., Gallagher, B. B., and Mattson, R.
   H. (1972): Phenylethylmalonamide. An important
   metabolite of primidone. *Arch. Neurol.*, 27:34–41.
7. Baumel, I. P., Gallagher, B. B., DiMicco, J., and
   Goico, H. (1973): Metabolism and anticonvulsant
   properties of primidone in the rat. *J. Pharmacol.
   Exp. Ther.*, 186:305–314.
8. Boer, H. E., Hosokowa, K., Burdette, R. D., and
   Darcey, B. (1970): A clinical study of serum primidone levels. *Epilepsia*, 11:395–402.
9. Bogan, J., and Smith, H. (1968): The relation between primidone and phenobarbitone blood levels.
   J. Pharm. Pharmac., 20:64–67.
10. Bogue, J. Y., and Carrington, H. C. (1952): Per-
    sonal communication cited by Goodman, L. S.,
    Swinyard, E. A., Brown, W. C., Schiffman, D. O.,
    Grewal, M. S., and Bliss, E. L. (1953): Anticon-
    vulsant properties of 5-phenyl-ethyl hexahydro-
    pyrimidine-4-6-dione (Mysoline), a new antiepilep-
    tic. *J. Pharmacol. Exp. Ther.*, 108:428–436.
11. Bourgeois, B. F. D. (1986): Individual and crossed
    tolerance to the anticonvulsant effect and neuro-
    toxicity of phenobarbital and primidone in mice.
    In: *Tolerance to Beneficial and Adverse Effects of
    Antiepileptic Drugs*, edited by H. H. Frey, W.
    Fröscher, W. P. Koella, and H. Meinardi, pp. 17–
    24. Raven Press, New York.
12. Bourgeois, B. F. D., Dodson, W. E., and Ferren-
    delli, J. A. (1983): Primidone, phenobarbital and
    PEMA: I. Seizure protection, neurotoxicity and
    therapeutic index of individual compounds in
    mice. *Neurology*, 33:283–290.
13. Bourgeois, B. F. D., Dodson, W. E., and Ferren-
    delli, J. A. (1983): Primidone, phenobarbital and
    PEMA: II. Seizure protection, neurotoxicity and
    therapeutic index of varying combinations in mice.
    Neurology, 33:291–295.
14. Brillman, J., Gallagher, B. B., and Mattson, R. H.
    (1974): Acute primidone intoxication. *Arch. Neu-
    rol.*, 30:255–258.
15. Butler, T. C., and Waddell, W. J. (1956): Metabolic
    conversion of primidone (Mysoline) to phenobar-
    bital. *Proc. Soc. Exp. Biol. Med.*, 93:544–546.
16. Cate, J. C., and Tenser, R. (1975): Acute primi-
    done overdosage with massive crystalluria. *Clin.
    Toxicol.*, 8:385–389.
17. Cloyd, J. C., Miller, K. W., and Leppik, I. E.
    (1981): Primidone kinetics: Effects of concurrent
    drugs and duration of therapy. *Clin. Pharmacol.
    Ther.*, 29:402–407.
18. Farnbach, G. C. (1984): Efficacy of primidone in
    dogs with seizures unresponsive to phenobarbital.
    J. Am. Vet. Med. Assoc., 185:867–868.
19. Fincham, R. W., Schottelius, D. D., and Sahs, A.
    L. (1974): The influence of diphenylhydantoin on
    primidone metabolism. *Arch. Neurol.*, 30:259–
    262.
20. Foltz, R. L., Couch, M. W., Greer, M., Scott, K.
    N., and Williams, C. M. (1972): Chemical ioni-
    zation mass spectrometry in the identification of
    drug metabolites. *Biochem. Med.*, 6:294–298.
21. Frey, H. H., Göbel, W., and Löscher, W. (1979):

Pharmacokinetics of primidone and its active metabolites in the dog. *Arch. Int. Pharmacodyn.*, 242:14–30.

22. Frey, H. H., and Hahn, I. (1960): Untersuchungen über die Bedeutung des durch Biotransformation gebildeten Phenobarbital für die antikonvulsive Wirkung von Primidon. *Arch. Int. Pharmacodyn. Ther.*, 128:281–290.

23. Frey, H. H., and Löscher, W. (1980): Kann primidon mehr als phenobarbital? *Nervenarzt*, 51:359–362.

24. Frey, H. H., Löscher, W., Reiche, R., and Schultz, D. (1984): Anticonvulsant effect of primidone in the gerbil. Time course and significance of the active metabolites. *Pharmacology*, 28:329–335.

25. Fujimoto, J. M., Mason, W. H., and Murphy, M. (1968): Urinary excretion of primidone and its metabolites in rabbits. *J. Pharmacol. Exp. Ther.*, 159:379–388.

26. Gallagher, B. B., Baumel, I. P., and Mattson, R. H. (1972): Metabolic disposition of primidone and its metabolites in epileptic subjects after single and repeated administration. *Neurology*, 22:1186–1192.

27. Gallagher, B. B., Baumel, I. P., Mattson, R. H., and Woodbury, S. G. (1973): Primidone, diphenylhydantoin and phenobarbital. Aspects of acute and chronic toxicity. *Neurology*, 23:145–149.

28. Gruber, C. M., Brock, J. T., and Dyken, M. (1962): Comparison of the effectiveness of primidone, mephobarbital, diphenylhydantoin, ethotoin, metharbital, and methylphenylethylhydantoin in motor seizures. *Clin. Pharmacol. Ther.*, 3:23–28.

29. Haidukewych, D., and Rodin, E. A. (1980): Monitoring 2-ethyl-2-phenylmalonamide in serum by gas-liquid chromatography: Application to retrospective study in epilepsy patients dosed with primidone. *Clin. Chem.*, 26:1537–1539.

30. Handley, R., and Stewart, A. S. R. (1962): Mysoline: A new drug in the treatment of epilepsy. *Lancet*, 1:742–744.

31. Heipertz, R., Guthoff, A., and Bernhardt, W. (1979): Primidone metabolism in renal insufficiency and acute intoxication. *J. Neurol.*, 221:101–104.

32. Hooper, W. D., Treston, A. M., Jacobsen, N. W., et al. (1983): Identification of *p*-hydroxyprimidone as a minor metabolite of primidone in rat and man. *Drug Metab. Dispos.*, 11:607–610.

33. Horning, M. G., Nowlin, J., Buller, C. M., Lertratanangkoon, K., Sommer, K., and Hill, R. M. (1975): Clinical applications of gas chromatograph/mass spectrometer/computer systems. *Clin. Chem.*, 21:1282–1287.

34. Hunt, R. J., and Miller, K. W. (1978): Disposition of primidone, phenylethylmalonamide, and phenobarbital in the rabbit. *Drug Metab. Dispos.*, 6:75–81.

35. Johnson, D. D., Davis, H. L., Crawford, R. D. (1978): Epileptiform seizures in domestic fowl. VIII. Anticonvulsant activity of primidone and its metabolites, phenobarbital and phenylethylmalonamide. *Can. J. Physiol. Pharmacol.*, 56:630–633.

36. Kauffman, R. E., Habersang, R., and Lansky, L. (1977): Kinetics of primidone metabolism and excretion in children. *Clin. Pharmacol. Ther.*, 22:200–205.

37. Leal, K. W., Rapport, R. L., Wilensky, A. J., and Friel, P. N. (1979): Single dose pharmacokinetics and anticonvulsant efficacy of primidone in mice. *Ann. Neurol.*, 5:470–474.

38. Lee, C. C., Marbury, T. C., Perchalski, R. T., and Wilder, B. J. (1982): Pharmacokinetics of primidone elimination in uremic patients. *J. Clin. Pharmacol.*, 22:301–308.

39. Lehmann, D. F. (1987): Primidone crystalluria following overdose. A report of a case and an analysis of the literature. *Med. Toxicol. Adverse Drug Exp.*, 2:383–387.

40. Leppik, I. E., Cloyd, J. C., and Miller, K. (1984): Development of tolerance to the side effects of primidone. *Ther. Drug Monit.*, 6:189–191.

41. Lesser, R. P., Pippenger, C. E., Lüders, H., and Dinner, D. S. (1984): High-dose monotherapy in treatment of intractable seizures. *Neurology*, 34:707–711.

42. McElhatton, P. R., Sullivan, F. M., and Toseland, P. A. (1977): The metabolism of primidone in nonpregnant and 14-day pregnant mice. *Xenobiotica*, 7:611–615.

43. Morley, D., and Wynne, N. A. (1957): Acute primidone intoxication. *Br. Med. J.*, 1:90.

44. Olesen, O. V., and Dam, M. (1967): The metabolic conversion of primidone (Mysoline) to phenobarbitone in patients under long-term treatment. *Acta Neurol. Scand.*, 43:348–356.

45. Oxley, J., Hebdige, S., Laidlaw, J., Wadsworth, J., and Richens, A. (1980): A comparative study of phenobarbitone and primidone in the treatment of epilepsy. In: *Antiepileptic Therapy. Advances in Drug Monitoring*, edited by S. I. Johannessen, P. L. Morselli, C. E. Pippenger, A. Richens, D. Schmidt, and H. Meinardi, pp. 237–245. Raven Press, New York.

46. Pisani, F., Perucca, E., Primerano, G., D'Agostino, A. A., Petrelli, R. M., Fazio, A., Oteri, G., and Di Perri, R. (1984): Single-dose kinetics of primidone in acute viral hepatitis. *Eur. J. Clin. Pharmacol.*, 27:465–469.

47. Plaa, G. L., Fujimoto, J. M., and Hine, C. H. (1958): Intoxication from primidone due to its biotransformation to phenobarbital. *J.A.M.A.*, 168:1769–1770.

48. Powell, C., Painter, M. J., and Pippenger, C. E. (1984): Primidone therapy in refractory neonatal seizures. *J. Pediatr.*, 105:651–654.

49. Schmidt, D. (1975): The effect of phenytoin and ethosuximide on primidone metabolism in patients with epilepsy. *J. Neurol.*, 209:115–123.

50. Schottelius, D. D. (1982): Primidone—Biotransformation. In: *Antiepileptic Drugs*, 2nd edition, edited by D. M. Woodbury, J. K. Penry, and C. E. Pippenger, pp. 415–420. Raven Press, New York.

51. Streete, J. M., Berry, D. J., Pettit, L. I., and Newbery, J. E. (1986): Phenylethylmalonamide serum levels in patients treated with primidone and the

effects of other antiepileptic drugs. *Ther. Drug Monit.*, 8:161–165.

52. Swinyard, E. A., Tedeschi, D. H., and Goodman, L. S. (1954): Effects of liver damage and nephrectomy on anticonvulsant activity of Mysoline and phenobarbital. *J. Am. Pharm. Assoc.*, 43:114–116.

53. Talbot, P. A., and Alderdice, M. T. (1982): Primidone but not phenylethylmalonamide, a major metabolite, increases nerve-evoked transmitter release at the frog neuromuscular junction. *J. Pharmacol. Exp. Ther.*, 222:87–93.

54. Talbot, P. A., and Alderdice, M. T. (1984): Effects of primidone, phenobarbital and phenylethylmalonamide in the stimulated frog neuromuscular junction. *J. Pharmacol. Exp. Ther.*, 228:121–127.

55. Turner, C. R. (1980): Primidone intoxication and massive crystalluria. *Clin. Pediatr.*, 19:706–707.

56. White, P. T., Plott, D., and Norton, J. (1966): Relative anticonvulsant potency of primidone. A double blind comparison. *Arch. Neurol.*, 14:31–35.

57. Zavadil, P., and Gallagher, B. B. (1976): Metabolism and excretion of ^{14}C-primidone in epileptic patients. In: *Epileptology*, edited by D. Janz, pp. 129–139. Georg Thieme, Stuttgart.

Antiepileptic Drugs, Third Edition, edited by
R. Levy, R. Mattson, B. Meldrum,
J. K. Penry, and F. E. Dreifuss.
Raven Press, Ltd., New York © 1989.

28

Primidone

Interactions with Other Drugs

Richard W. Fincham and Dorothy D. Schottelius

Primidone (PRM) may provide effective therapy for patients who are refractory to or intolerant of other antiepileptic drugs, and its combination with other drugs is rarely necessary. Primidone's biotransformation to phenobarbital (PB) and phenylethylmalonamide (PEMA) allows for interactions of these compounds, and polypharmacy amplifies these possibilities.

Primidone, in common with most of the other antiepileptic drugs, has a narrow therapeutic range and in order to control seizures, it is often necessary to prescribe a dose nearly as high as one that produces dose-related toxic effects. Unlike many of the other antiepileptic drugs, PRM requires that we be concerned about the therapeutic ranges of two other substances (the metabolites), their toxic manifestations, and their possible contribution to the total therapeutic and toxic activity of the parent compound. In this chapter there is discussed the clinical and experimental studies of interactions involving PRM, PB, PEMA, and other drugs that may influence this compound. Also considered is the influence of PRM on the efficacy of other drugs. Since PRM and PB appear to induce enzyme activity, their influence on other drugs may be important.

PHARMACOLOGICAL INTERACTIONS

Alterations in plasma drug concentrations, whether accompanied by clinical manifestations or not, may be reliable indicators of drug interactions in the case of PRM. Increased seizure frequency when plasma PRM levels are low or disturbance of corticai and cerebellar function when plasma drug levels increase may be immediately manifested clinically or may be delayed for variable lengths of time. The same drug combinations can cause varying effects in different patients because of individual variability. Individuals have different genetically determined efficiencies in biotransformation, and environmental agents can further modify these responses. It is necessary in the case of PRM to consider not only the interactions of the parent drug, but also those of the two active metabolites, PEMA and PB.

Pharmaceutical and Pharmacodynamic Interactions

Although there are no specific examples of pharmaceutical incompatibility between PRM and other drugs, it should not be overlooked when considering the physical and chemical properties of the drug. Interference at the site(s) of action (pharmacodynamic interactions) with altered drug effects have not been shown with PRM specifically. However, the potentiation of sedation from barbiturates by alcohol and of the antiepileptic activity of PB by nicotinamide (6) could be involved when PRM is used.

Pharmacokinetic Interactions

As with the other antiepileptic drugs, far more pharmacokinetic interactions have been reported between PRM and other drugs. These interactions can be beneficial as well as potentially damaging. The rate of absorption or total amount of drug absorbed or both may be altered in all routes of drug administration. Since only an oral preparation of PRM is available, only drugs that might affect the gastrointestinal tract need to be considered. The mechanisms involved include changes in pH and motility of the gastrointestinal tract and the possible formation of insoluble complexes, which would delay or prevent absorption.

Distribution, including protein binding, has not been involved in interactions of either PRM or its main metabolites. The amount of protein binding of PRM is relatively small (approximately 20%), so displacement by other compounds is not significant.

The main pharmacokinetic interactions concern the biotransformation or metabolism of PRM and its metabolites. Several factors are important. Most significant may be the influence of other drugs on the metabolic conversion of PRM to PEMA and PB. The induction of microsomal enzymes by the barbiturates, especially PB, is well known and this inducibility is influenced by a variety of factors, including genetics, age, and disease processes.

Finally, interactions that influence the excretion of a drug should be considered and may involve the competition of drugs in active renal tubular secretion. Clearance of the drug (weak organic acids) is lower in acid urine than in alkaline urine, and alkaline diuresis may remove excess PB.

INTERACTIONS OF PRM, PB, AND PEMA

The possibility that the total activity of PRM might be influenced by the interaction of PB and PEMA was suggested by studies of the effect of combinations of these two substances on seizure thresholds in rats (4,14,15). It was noted that in doses normally without anticonvulsant activity, PEMA augmented the activity of PB on two experimental measures of seizure threshold. Since the effect was not equal, it was suggested that either separate neural mechanisms are involved or PEMA exerts quantifiably disparate effects in diverse areas of the central nervous system. Additional evidence that PEMA has an effect on hepatic microsomal enzymes was the finding that it significantly prolonged hexabarbital sleeping time. These results suggested a possible synergistic interaction between PEMA and PB.

Studies in the rat (3) gave some indications of interaction among PRM, PEMA, and PB with respect to anticonvulsant potency. In mice, PRM has been shown to be equal to PB in potency against the electroshock model of epilepsy while being markedly less neurotoxic (7,8). Its lack of potency against pentylenetetrazol-induced seizures was also noted in this model.

Clinical studies also indicate the possibility of substance interactions. The delayed appearance of PEMA and PB in plasma (4,5) and the influence of repeated administration on that delay (3,13,17) suggest that the enzyme systems responsible for the biotransformation of PRM may be altered by interactions among all three of these compounds. Adverse effects on the central nervous system occurring with initiation of therapy were nonexistent or greatly alleviated when the patient was previously treated with PRM or PB (14). Our findings of a different relationship in the PB-to-PRM ratio when the steady-state serum PB levels were above or below 15 μg/ml may be indicative of interactions at the level of enzyme systems responsible for biotransformation of PRM (Fig. 1). PEMA levels are influenced not only by the dose of primidone, but also by the serum levels of other antiepileptic drugs present, particularly PB (28).

These clinical findings are supported by the observations of Alvin et al. (1) of isolated perfused rat liver. Rats were pretreated with daily doses (50 mg/kg, intraperitoneal injection) of either PRM or PB for 4 days prior to removal of the liver for perfusion studies. Phenobarbital pretreatment greatly accelerated the rate of PRM metabolism, and pretreatment with PRM increased it to a lesser extent. There was no indication of a differential induction of the pathways. In addition, when PEMA or PB (50 μg/ml) was added directly to liver perfusates, PEMA reduced the rate of PRM metabolism but PB had no effect. The authors concluded that biotransformation of PRM may be simultaneously influenced by the processes of metabolite induction (PB) and metabolite inhibition (PEMA). Although it is unwise to extrapolate findings from experimental animals to man, the probability of such interactions in man is supported by the earlier findings of possible interactions. Until more definitive clinical information is obtained, we can only speculate that some of the interindividual variability in half-lives, plasma concentrations, and excretory patterns of PRM, PEMA, and PB are the result of the interactions of these three substances.

INTERACTIONS OF PRIMIDONE WITH OTHER DRUGS

Phenytoin

Fincham et al. (13) reported that phenytoin (PHT) apparently promoted induction of the enzyme system responsible for the oxidation of PRM to PB. The possibility that PHT interfered with the hydroxylation or renal excretion of PB was also entertained. We have continued to examine this interaction and our findings are shown in Figs. 2 and 3 and Table 1. All patients involved in these studies were in steady state with respect to PRM, PB, and PHT, having been on the same dose of drugs for many

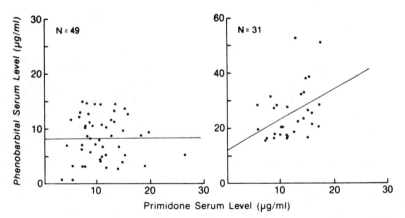

FIG. 1. Serum phenobarbital levels as a function of serum primidone levels from patients taking primidone as sole medication. Patients were maintained for a sufficient length of time to achieve steady state of both drugs. **Left:** data from individuals whose serum PB levels never exceeded 15 μg/ml; serum PB level = 8.2 + 0.02 serum primidone levels; correlation coefficient = 0.02. **Right:** data from individuals whose serum PB levels varied from 15.5 to 51.6 μg/ml; serum PB level = 12.5 + 1.08 serum primidone levels; correlation coefficient = 0.39.

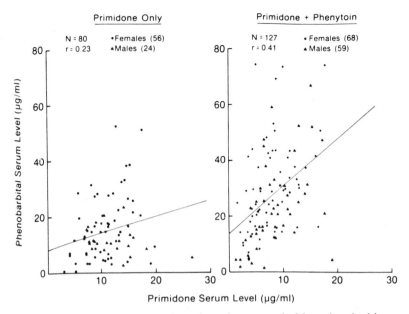

FIG. 2. Serum phenobarbital levels as a function of serum primidone levels. Linear regression analysis for PRM only, serum PB level = 8.3 + 0.6 serum PRM level; for PRM + PHT, serum PB level = 13.6 + 1.7 serum PRM level.

months and, in some instances, years. Blood samples were obtained 2 to 4 hr after the last dose of PRM. In contrast to the PB-to-PRM ratios of Reynolds et al. (23,24) (1.57 ± 0.17, PRM only; 2.20 ± 0.12, PRM and PHT), our original data (13) did not show a correlation between the PB-to-PRM ratio and serum PHT levels. Unlike our patients, some of the patients in their studies (23,24) were taking other anticonvulsant or psychotropic drugs which may have influenced the PB-to-PRM ratio and correlation with serum PHT levels.

In the 127 patients we have currently analyzed, there may be a weak correlation between these two factors. When the PB-to-PRM ratio was plotted versus the serum PHT level, the linear regression line indicated PB/PRM = 3.2 ± 0.05 serum PHT level, with a correlation coefficient of 0.19. This comparison shows a great deal of interindividual variability, as do the comparisons illustrated in Figs. 2 and 3. As previously reported (13), the primidone dosage

did not influence the PB-to-PRM ratio in either the group treated with PRM only or the group treated with PRM and PHT.

Schmidt (26) also examined the interaction of PHT and PRM in 28 patients receiving primidone alone and in 16 patients receiving both PRM and PHT, and found a similar difference in PB-to-PRM ratios between the two groups (1.6 ± 0.2, PRM alone; 4.2 ± 0.7, PRM and PHT). Also undertaken was a longitudinal study of patients on PRM therapy in which PHT was added to the regimen. In both cases, serum PB levels increased with rising serum PHT levels, although the PRM levels remained unchanged; consequently, the resulting rise in PB-to-PRM ratio was caused by increasing PB concentrations. This increase in the PB-to-PRM ratio persisted during the 30 to 70 days of observation and was considered to result from inhibition of the metabolism and/or excretion of PB and not from induction of the enzymes that oxidize PRM to PB.

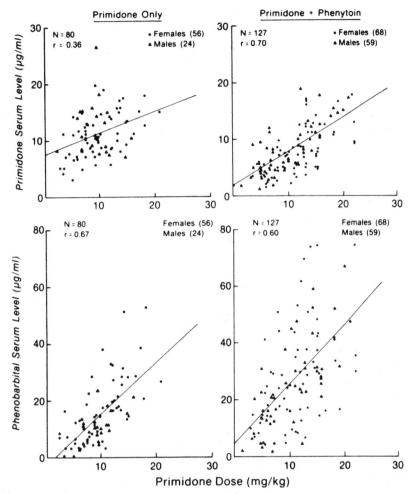

FIG. 3. Serum phenobarbital and primidone concentrations as a function of primidone dose. PRM only; **upper left,** serum PRM level = 7.6 + 0.38 PRM dose; **lower left,** serum PB level = −3.0 + 1.8 PRM dose. PRM + PHT; **upper right,** serum PRM level = 1.6 + 0.6 PRM dose; **lower right,** serum PB level = 4.9 + 2.07 PRM dose.

There is clinical and experimental evidence (22,25) that PHT may inhibit the metabolism or impair the renal excretion of PB. This effect of PHT on PB metabolism or excretion was not confirmed in a later investigation (10) in which comparable serum PB levels were found between two groups of patients when PHT was present and when it was absent. The investigators found an increase in PB levels and an increase in the PB-to-PRM ratio when comparing patients taking PRM only or PRM and PHT. There was no significant relationship between serum PHT levels and the PB-to-PRM ratio in the patients taking both medications.

There is a contrast in the urinary excretion pattern of patients taking PRM only and PRM plus a variety of comedications (33). The latter group excreted less unchanged PRM and more PEMA and PB, and a large percentage of the dose was excreted at a

TABLE 1. *Effect of phenytoin on primidone biotransformation*

	Primidone only (N = 80)	Primidone and phenytoin (N = 127)
PRM dose (mg/kg)	9.7 ± 0.2	10.6 ± 0.4
PHT dose (mg/kg)	—	4.8 ± 0.1
Serum PHT level (μg/ml)	—	12.1 ± 0.1
Serum PRM level (μg/ml)	11.3 ± 0.2	8.1 ± 0.4
Serum PB level (μg/ml)	15.0 ± 0.4	27.2 ± 1.4
PB/PRM	1.45 ± 0.10	3.82 ± 0.24

Values are expressed as mean ± standard error.

later time (days 4 and 5). Both of these findings suggest that the biotransformation of PRM to PEMA and PB is enhanced by comedications and that disposal of the metabolites is not inhibited.

Only scattered reports are available concerning the interaction of PRM and PHT in children. One report (31) suggested that there is a decrease in serum PHT levels with concomitant administration of PRM and PHT; the possible alteration in PB levels in these instances was not investigated. Kauffman et al. (20) stated that this interaction between PHT and PRM was not found in children, and there was no correlation between the rate constant for metabolism and the presence or absence of concomitant PHT therapy. The calculated mean values for the children treated with PRM only or PRM and PHT are as follows: PB production, PRM only 0.0037, PRM and PHT 0.0049; PEMA production, PRM only 0.0310, PRM and PHT 0.0480. The ratio of PB-to-PRM in children cannot be calculated or compared to adults because of the difference in sampling time in relation to the last dose of PRM and lack of data.

The effects of phenytoin pretreatment on the metabolism of primidone have been investigated in the rabbit (19). Rabbits were treated for 5 days with PHT (40 mg/day, intravenous) and then with PRM (10 mg/kg, intravenous), with each animal serving as its own control in a crossover fashion. Primidone was eliminated more rapidly after PHT pretreatment, and a smaller fraction was excreted unchanged in the urine. Pretreatment with PHT appeared to accelerate the rate of formation of PB and PEMA, and both were eliminated more rapidly. The total body clearance of PRM was increased almost twofold in the rabbit, a finding that appears to be similar to clearance in man (10). It was thought that this finding in the rabbit conflicted with the mechanism of interaction in man in which PB levels increase and PRM levels remain constant with PHT treatment (10,13). The clinical findings, however, are based on long-term administration of PRM, whereas the experimental data are from a single intravenous injection of PRM.

From all of the evidence obtained in these various investigations under widely varying experimental conditions, the findings are somewhat more in favor of altered PRM biotransformation with PHT treatment than inhibition of metabolism or impaired renal excretion of PB or PEMA. Observations of the effect of isoniazid and nicotinamide provide further support for this concept (6,29).

Determining which mechanism is responsible for the increased PB-to-PRM ratio is not critical before deciding that this is a clinically significant finding. We have observed several instances of PB intoxication when PRM and PHT were used at usual or reduced therapeutic dosages, and the marked interindividual variability in serum drug levels indicated in Fig. 3 makes it impossible to predict a "standard" regimen when these drugs are combined. The presence of renal or liver disease could contribute to an exaggeration of this interaction. It is possible that the interaction could be useful clinically to obtain therapeutic concentrations of three anticonvulsant substances, but it can only be achieved by careful and continuous monitoring of serum drug levels.

Succinimides

The combination of ethosuximide and PRM was investigated by Schmidt (26), who found no difference in the PB-to-PRM ratio. In contrast, methsuximide, was shown by Browne et al. (9) to increase PRM by 33% and PB by 17% when added to a PRM regimen.

Carbamazepine

Reports on both animals (12) and humans (2,10,33) have indicated that carbamazepine (CBZ) increases the metabolism of primidone to its metabolites. An apparent opposite effect was found with the reported increase in serum PRM levels in patients taking CBZ (11), but the study was not continued long enough to provide a definitive answer concerning increases or decreases in metabolism of PRM. Primidone has been reported to lower the serum level of CBZ (27). This interaction may be clinically significant since the two drugs are frequently used together. Insufficient data are available to prove an increased conversion of PRM to PB, but this possibility, along with lower CBZ levels than expected, indicates that monitoring serum drug levels is necessary to achieve maximum therapeutic benefit when these drugs are used in combination.

Isoniazid

A clinical case of inhibition of PRM biotransformation by isoniazid was thoroughly studied by Sutton and Kupferberg (29). The steady-state PRM levels increased an average of 12.2 µg/ml when the two drugs were given simultaneously, and the plasma half-life of PRM increased from 8.7 hr to 14 hr. Serum levels of PB and PEMA fell during simultaneous treatment. There was some indication that sodium aminosalicylate may have potentiated the inhibition of PRM metabolism.

Valproic Acid

Windorfer et al. (32) observed marked increases in serum PRM levels only a few days after valproic acid (VPA) was added to the regimen, but in most cases, the levels returned to original values after 1 to 3 months. The report gave no information concerning the dose-sample interval or PB levels, so it is difficult to interpret these alterations. We have examined the influence of the addition of VPA to the regimens of 16 patients in whom all medications were in steady state and doses of all other medications remained the same. Only two of these patients were taking PRM as a sole medication; the other 14 were also taking PHT and/or carbamazepine. None were taking PB. Blood samples were obtained between 1.5 and 4 hr after the PRM dose, and the same dose-sample interval was utilized in the samples obtained before and after the addition of VPA to the regimen. There were no significant changes in PRM or PB levels (PRM before VPA, 9.4 ± 0.7 µg/ml; PRM after VPA 8.6 ± 0.6 µg/ml, PB before VPA, 26.7 ± 1.5 µg/ml; PB after VPA, 29.2 ± 2.0 µg/ml). The mean PB-to-PRM ratios were 3.01 ± 0.31 before VPA and 3.56 ± 1.4 after VPA. Interindividual variability was great; some patients showed marked changes in serum PRM and PB levels and the PB-to-PRM ratio, which indicated an increase in biotransformation of PRM. A greater number of patients who are taking PRM alone must be investigated to determine if this may become a clinically significant interaction.

Nicotinamide

Bourgeois et al. (6,7,8) demonstrated that nicotinamide decreased the conversion of PRM to PB in mice and in humans. The PB-

TABLE 2. *Drug interactions with primidone*

Interaction	Severity	Onset	Documentation	Effect	Mechanism
Effect on primidone by:					
Carbamazepine	Minor	Delayed	Possible	Increase PB	Increase biotransformat
Acetazolamide	Moderate	Delayed	Possible	Decrease PRM levels	Decrease PRM absorpti
Phenytoin	Moderate	Delayed	Established	Decrease PRM levels	Increase PRM biotransformation
Isoniazid	Minor	Delayed	Possible	Increase PRM levels	Decrease PRM biotransformation
Nicotinamide	Minor	Delayed	Possible	Increase PRM levels	Decrease PRM biotransformation
Methsuximide	Minor	Delayed	Possible	Increase PRM levels	Altered PRM metabolisr
Valproic acid	Moderate	Delayed	Established	Increase PRM, PB levels	Altered PRM metabolisr
Clonazepam	Moderate	Delayed	Probable	Increase PRM	Altered metabolism
Carbamazepine	Minor	Delayed	Possible	Decrease CBZ levels	
Corticosteroids	Moderate	Delayed	Established	Decrease steroid effect	Increase steroid metabo
Oral contraceptives	Moderate	Delayed	Suspect	Decrease in effect	Increase estrogen metabolism
Quinidine	Moderate	Delayed	Probable	Decrease in effect	Increase quinidine ?
Clonazepam	Moderate	Delayed	Probable	Decrease clonazepam levels	Increase clonazepam metabolism
Effect on primidine metabolites by:					
Charcoal	Moderate	Delayed	Probable	Decrease PB levels	Physical adsorption
Chloramphenicol	Minor	Delayed	Possible	Increase PB levels	Altered metabolism
Ethanol	Moderate	Instant	Established	Increase PB levels	Decreased PB metaboli
Phenacemide	Minor	Delayed	Possible	Increase PB effect	Decrease PB metabolisr
Propoxyphene	Minor	Delayed	Possible	Increase PB level	Decrease PB metabolisr
Pyridoxine	Minor	Delayed	Possible	Decrease PB level	Altered metabolism
Rifampin	Minor	Delayed	Possible	Decrease PB level	Increase PB metabolisr
Effect of PRM Metabolites on:					
Acetaminophen	Moderate	Delayed	Possible	Decreased	Increased metabolism
Coumarin anticoagulants	Major	Delayed	Established	Decrease coumarin	Delayed absorption, increased metabolism
β-adrenergic blockers	Moderate	Instant	Suspect	Decreased	Increased metabolism
Chloramphenicol	Minor	Delayed	Possible	Decreased antibiotic	Altered hepatic metabo
Cimetidine	Minor	Delayed	Possible	Decrease cimetidine	Delayed absorption, increased metabolism
Cyclosporine	Moderate	Delayed	Possible	Decreased	Increased metabolism
Digitoxin	Moderate	Delayed	Possible	Decreased	Increased metabolism
Doxorubicin	Moderate	Delayed	Probable	Decreased	Increased metabolism
Doxycycline	Moderate	Delayed	Probable	Decreased	Increased metabolism
Estrogens	Minor	Delayed	Possible	Decreased	Increased metabolism
Fenoprofen	None	Delayed	Probable	Decreased	Increased metabolism
Furosemide	Minor	Daleyed	Probable	Decrease diuresis	?
Griseofulvin	Minor	Delayed	Probable	Decrease antifungal	Increased metabolism
Haloperidol	Minor	Delayed	Possible	Decreased	Increased metabolism
Meperidine	Minor	Delayed	Possible	Increased	Additive CNS depressio
Methyldopa	None	Delayed	Doubtful	Decreased	?
Metoxyflurane	Moderate	Instant	Suspect	Increased nephrotoxics	Increase toxic metaboli
Metronidazole	Minor	Delayed	Possible	Decreased antimicrobial	Increased metabolism
Phenothiazines	Minor	Delayed	Possible	Decreased	Increased metabolism
Theophylline	Moderate	Delayed	Suspect	Decreased	Increased metabolism
Tricyclics	Minor	Delayed	Possible	Decreased	Increased metabolism ?

Some data from Mangini, ref. 21.

to-PRM ratio was increased in three patients, and the effect appears to be dose-related. They postulate that this interaction of nicotinamide with PRM is due to inhibition of the cytochrome P-450 enzyme system. Since seizure control was better in these three patients, nicotinamide might be used to increase the effectiveness of PRM in refractory patients.

Clonazepam

Windorfer and Sauer (31) found a significant increase in the PRM concentration when clonazepam and PRM were administered together, which contrasts with the result when PRM is administered with other antiepileptic drugs.

Other Drugs

When added to PRM therapy, ethylphenacemide resulted in both an increase and a decrease in serum PRM levels in two patients (18), but interpretation of these findings is difficult because other medications were also used. Methylphenidate (16) was implicated in the alteration of PRM biotransformation in a child in whom serum PRM levels increased from 4.4 to 21.5 µg/ml when this drug was added to a regimen of PRM and PHT. Serum PB levels also increased from 23.0 to 34.4 µg/ml.

Absorption may have been impaired in one of three patients tested when PRM and acetazolamide were given simultaneously (30). When these two drugs were administered together, only trace amounts of PRM and its metabolites were detectable in serum and urine; when PRM was given alone, expected levels of both were found in serum and urine.

Table 2 summarizes most of the reported interactions of primidone and its metabolites. All of the information presented concerning the interactions of PRM, whether between the parent compound and its metabolites or between PRM and other drugs, clearly points out the necessity and benefits of serum drug level monitoring to prevent intoxications and to gain maximum therapeutic effect.

SUMMARY

Considering that polypharmacy is widespread and many of the drugs utilized have been shown to be capable of inducing liver enzymes responsible for biotransformation, it is not surprising that more and more drug interactions are observed. Of those we have considered with PRM, the PHT interaction has had the most investigation and is clearly important clinically because of the frequency with which these two compounds are combined in therapeutic regimens. This does not imply that the interaction will always occur to the same magnitude, and indeed it does not, as is apparent from the interindividual variability noted. It also does not imply that the other interactions are not important clinically because the frequency with which they occur may not be as prevalent as the interaction between PRM and PHT.

REFERENCES

1. Alvin, J., Goh, E., and Bush, M. T. (1975): Study of the hepatic metabolism of primidone by improved methodology. *J. Pharmacol. Exp. Ther.,* 194:117–125.
2. Baciewicz, A. M., (1986): Carbamazepine drug interactions. *Therap. Drug Monit.,* 8:305–317.
3. Baumel, I. P., Gallagher, B. B., DiMicco, J., and Goico, H. (1973): Metabolism and anticonvulsant properties of primidone in the rat. *J. Pharmacol. Exp. Ther.,* 180:305–314.
4. Baumel, I. P., Gallagher, B. B., and Mattson, R. H. (1972): Phenylethylmalonamide (PEMA). An important metabolite of primidone. *Arch. Neurol.,* 27:34–41.
5. Booker, H. E., Hosokowa, K., Burdette, R. D., and Darcey, B. (1970): A clinical study of serum primidone levels. *Epilepsia,* 11:395–402.
6. Bourgeois, B. F. D., Dodson, W. E., and Ferrendelli, J. A. (1982): Interactions between primidone, carbamazepine and nicotinamide. *Neurology,* 32:1122–1126.

7. Bourgeois, B. F. D., Dodson, W. E., and Ferrendelli, J. A. (1983): Primidone, phenobarbital, and PEMA: I. Seizure protection, neurotoxicity, and therapeutic index of individual compounds in mice. *Neurology, 33*:283–290.

8. Bourgeois, B. F. D., Dodson, W. E., and Ferrendelli, J. A. (1983): Primidone, phenobarbital, and PEMA: II. Seizure protection, neurotoxicity, and therapeutic index of varying combinations in mice. *Neurology, 33*:291–295.

9. Browne, T. R., Feldman, R. G., Buchanan, R. A., Allen, N. C., Fawcett-Vickers, L., Szabo, G. K., Mattson, G. F., Norman, S. E., and Greenblatt, D. J. (1983): Methsuximide for complex partial seizures: Efficacy, toxicity, clinical pharmacology, and drug interactions. *Neurology, 33*:414–418.

10. Callaghan, N., Feeley, M., Duggan, F., O'Callaghan, M., and Sheldrup, J. (1977): The effect of anticonvulsant drugs which induce liver microsomal enzymes on derived and ingested phenobarbital levels. *Acta Neurol. Scand., 56*:1–6.

11. Cereghino, J. J., Van Meter, J. C., Brock, J. T., Penry, J. K., Smith, L. D., and White, B. G. (1973): Preliminary observations of serum carbamazepine concentration in epileptic patients. *Neurology (Minneap.), 23*:357–366.

12. DiMicco, J. A., and Gallagher, B. B. (1975): Induction of primidone metabolism in rat liver by anticonvulsants. *Fed. Proc., 34*:726.

13. Fincham, R. W., Schottelius, D. D., and Sahs, A. L. (1974): The influence of diphenylhydantoin on primidone metabolism. *Arch. Neurol., 30*:259–262.

14. Gallagher, B. B., and Baumel, I. P. (1972): Primidone: Interaction with other drugs. In: *Antiepileptic Drugs,* 1st edition, edited by D. M. Woodbury, J. K. Penry, and R. P. Schmidt, pp. 367–371. Raven Press, New York.

15. Gallagher, B. B., Baumel, I. P., and Mattson, R. H. (1972): Metabolic disposition of primidone and its metabolites in epileptic subjects after single and repeated administration. *Neurology (Minneap.), 22*:1186–1192.

16. Garrettson, L. K., Perel, J. M., and Dayton, P. G. (1969): Methylphenidate interaction with both anticonvulsants and ethyl biscoumacetate. *J.A.M.A., 207*:2053–2056.

17. Huisman, J. W. (1969): Disposition of primidone in man: An example of autoinduction of a human enzyme system? *Pharm. Weekbl., 104*:799–802.

18. Huisman, J. W., vanHeycopten, H., and van Zijl, C. H. (1970): Influence of ethylphenacemide on serum levels of other antiepileptic drugs. *Epilepsia, 11*:207–215.

19. Hunt, R. J., and Miller, K. W. (1978): Disposition of primidone, phenylethylmalonamide, and phenobarbital in the rabbit. *Drug. Metab. Dispos., 6*:75–81.

20. Kauffman, R. E., Habersang, R., and Lansky, L. (1977): Kinetics of primidone metabolism and excretion in children. *Clin. Pharmacol. Ther., 22*:200–205.

21. Mangini, R. J. (ed). (1988): *Drug Interaction Facts.* J. P. Lippincott, St. Louis, MO.

22. Morselli, P. L., Rizzo, M., and Garratin, S. (1971): Interaction between phenobarbital and diphenylhydantoin in animals and in epileptic patients. *Ann. N.Y. Acad. Sci., 179*:88–107.

23. Reynolds, E. H. (1975): Longitudinal studies of antiepileptic drug levels. Preliminary observations: Interaction of phenytoin and primidone. In: *Clinical Pharmacology of Antiepileptic Drugs,* edited by H. Schneider, D. Janz, C. Gardner-Thorpe, H. Meinardi, and A. L. Sherwin, pp. 79–85. Springer-Verlag, Berlin, Heidelberg, New York.

24. Reynolds, E. H., Fenton, G., Fenwick, P., Johnson, A. L., and Laundy, M., (1975): Interaction of phenytoin and primidone. *Br. Med. J., 14*:594–595.

25. Rizzo, M., Morselli, P. L., and Garratin, S. (1971): Further observations on the interactions between phenobarbital and diphenylhydantoin during clinical treatment in the rat. *Biochem. Pharmacol., 18*:449–454.

26. Schmidt, D. (1975): The effect of phenytoin and ethosuximide on primidone metabolism in patients with epilepsy. *J. Neurol., 209*:115–123.

27. Schneider, H. (1975): Carbamazepine: The influence of other antiepileptic drugs on its serum level. In: *Clinical Pharmacology of Antiepileptic Drugs,* edited by H. Schneider, D. Janz, C. Gardner-Thorpe, H. Meinardi, and A. L. Sherwin, pp. 189–196. Springer-Verlag, Berlin, Heidelberg, New York.

28. Streete, J. M., Berry, D. J., Pettit, L. I., and Newberry, J. E. (1986): Phenylethylmalonamide serum levels in patients treated with primidone and the effects of other antiepileptic drugs. *Therap. Drug Monit., 8*:161–165.

29. Sutton, G., and Kupferberg, H. J. (1975): Isoniazid as an inhibitor of primidone metabolism. *Neurology (Minneap.), 25*:1179–1181.

30. Syverson, G. B., Morgan, J. P., Weintraub, M., and Myers, G. J. (1977): Acetozolamide-induced interference with primidone absorption. *Arch. Neurol., 34*:80–84.

31. Windorfer, A., and Sauer, W. (1977): Drug interactions during anticonvulsant therapy in childhood: Diphenylhydantoin, primidone, phenobarbitone, clonazepam, nitrazepam, carbamazepine and dipropylacetate. *Neuropaediatrie, 8*:29–41.

32. Windorfer, A., Sauer, W., and Gadeke, R. (1975): Elevation of diphenylhydantoin and primidone serum concentrations by addition of dipropylacetate, a new anticonvulsant drug. *Acta Paediatr. Scand., 64*:771–772.

33. Zavadil, P., and Gallagher, B. B. (1976): Metabolism and excretion of ^{14}C-primidone in epileptic patients. In: *Epileptology,* edited by D. Janz, pp. 129–138. Georg Thieme, Stuttgart.

Antiepileptic Drugs, Third Edition, edited by
R. Levy, R. Mattson, B. Meldrum,
J. K. Penry, and F. E. Dreifuss.
Raven Press, Ltd., New York © 1989.

29

Primidone

Clinical Use

Dennis B. Smith

Primidone (PRM) was first synthesized in 1949 by Bogue and Carrington (7) and shown to be effective against both electrically and chemically induced convulsions in laboratory animals, including monkeys. It had extremely low toxicity and virtually no hypnotic effects, even at doses many times those required to protect against maximal electroshock (MES) seizures. Handley and Stewart (33) published the first clinical trial in 1952. In that study, PRM was added to existing drugs in 40 patients with intractable "major attacks." Of these, 37.5% became seizure-free, and an additional 25% showed a greater than 66% reduction in seizure frequency. Doses ranged from 0.8 to 2 g. Toxicity, occurring as dizziness and drowsiness, was noted only at doses above 1.6 g.

Several clinical reports followed (72–74), all of which found that PRM as add-on therapy for refractory epilepsy produced a notable reduction in seizure frequency in the majority of patients. The reports uniformly commented on the lack of serious toxicity, specifically hypnotic side effects. In 1954, however, Wilson and Hodgson (87) reported a deterioration in seizure control in eight of nine patients when PRM was substituted for phenobarbital (PB). In addition, at an average dose of 750 mg per day, they found that the drug was "overtly toxic," and produced intolerable drowsiness and ataxia, as well as an alarming fall in the

white blood cell count in 50% of their patients. All other reports on PRM between 1953 and 1956 agreed that it was an effective drug, particularly for generalized tonic-clonic seizures, when used either alone or in combination with other antiepileptic drugs (1,2,7,8,16,18,19,23,37,46,52,70, 83,86).

In 1956, Butler and Waddell (17) demonstrated for the first time that PRM was prominently converted to PB in both dogs and humans. They emphasized that the *in vivo* conversion of PRM to PB generated plasma PB levels sufficiently high to produce anticonvulsant effects, and suggested that the anticonvulsant properties of PRM were in fact due to its derived PB. Following this demonstration, Gruber et al. (31) reported that PB and PRM were equally effective as anticonvulsants and that the dose of PRM required to produce an anticonvulsant effect comparable to PB was greater than five times the dose of PB.

The first double-blind comparison of the anticonvulsant properties of PRM and PB was done by White et al. in 1966 (85). Twenty patients were studied in a complex crossover design with treatment periods of 14 days and various combinations of PRM, placebo, PB, and phenytoin (PHT). There was no significant difference in the anticonvulsant efficacy of PRM, PB, or PHT, and toxicity was comparable among the three drugs. Unfortunately, the treatment period was too short to draw meaningful comparisons, and, as in all previous studies of PRM, plasma levels of PRM and PB were not obtained. In 1967, Olesen and Dam (55) concluded that PRM had no independent antiepileptic properties and that its effectiveness was entirely due to its conversion to PB. They based their conclusion on a study of 47 patients who had been treated with PRM for longer than a year. They compared plasma PB levels and "clinical state" in these patients, with 41 patients taking PB alone. Despite comparable PB levels in the two groups, they found no significant differences in clinical state. Millichap and Aymat in 1968 (50) conducted a double-blind comparison of PRM and PHT, each used as monotherapy in 40 children aged 3 to 14. A parallel design was used, and the dose of each drug was pushed to complete seizure control or toxicity. Each drug was given for 7 to 9 months. Although the anticonvulsant effectiveness of the drugs was comparable, the side effects of PHT were more troublesome than those of PRM.

The early clinical studies reported a great deal of clinical success with the use of PRM, particularly as add-on therapy, but enthusiasm was tempered in the late '50s and '60s by the demonstration that PB is a major metabolite of PRM and by several comparative studies indicating that PRM was not appreciably more effective than either PB or PHT (50,55,65,85). With the appearance of those reports, the controversy over whether PRM is simply a pro-drug for PB was born. That controversy persists today. In fact, Shorvon (71) concludes that the major antiepileptic effect of PRM is due to the derived PB and that any differences in efficacy between the two drugs, "if they exist at all," are slight.

This chapter reviews the experimental and clinical evidence that PRM has antiepileptic properties in addition to those that can be attributed to the derived PB.

ANTIEPILEPTIC EFFECTS

Animal Studies

Following Bogue and Carrington's report (7) that PRM was more effective than PB against MES seizures and somewhat less effective than PB against chemically induced seizures, numerous studies have cataloged the antiepileptic properties of PRM. In fact, within a year of that report, a comprehensive study of the antiepileptic characteristics of PRM was published by Goodman et al. (30). This group examined the effects of PRM on MES and pentylenetetrazol (PTZ) seizures as well as hyponatremic, and minimal electroshock seizure threshold in both mice and rats. Maximal electroshock seizures and PTZ seizures were also used as models in cats and rabbits to study the effects of PRM. They also studied the antiepileptic potency of PRM in humans by examining its effect on seizures induced by electroconvulsive therapy in psychiatric patients. From the results of this extensive and diverse battery of tests, they concluded that PRM is considerably more effective than PB in protecting against MES seizures in mice, rats, cats, and rabbits, and that it "is very much less toxic than PB." The spectrum of antiepileptic drug activity was more similar to that of PHT than PB. The superior effects of PRM on MES seizures was later confirmed (81).

The first study to control for PB levels was performed by Frey and Hahn (26). They found that PRM had greater effects than PB in PTZ-induced seizures in both dogs and mice, despite lower plasma PB levels in the PRM-treated animals. They concluded that at least 50% of the effectiveness of PRM was due to the parent compound and not to the derived PB. Gallagher et al. (29) examined the effects of comparable blood levels of PB derived from PRM or from PB, using the volatile convulsant hexafluorodiethyl ether in rats. Although there was significant conversion of PRM to

PB, PRM apparently had antiepileptic properties independent of PB. The tonic-clonic seizure threshold was different for PB-treated rats compared with PRM-treated rats. The animals receiving PRM had higher thresholds for tonic-clonic seizures at all plasma PB levels up to 50 μg/ml (Fig. 1). This study demonstrated that PRM had antiepileptic effects clearly independent of its derived PB. Because Bogue et al. (8) had previously shown that phenylethylmalonamide (PEMA) had little antiepileptic properties, it is likely that PRM itself, and not PEMA or any other metabolite, was responsible for the results.

Several years later, in a paper that rekin-

dled a great deal of controversy about the clinical usefulness of PRM, Leal et al. (42) concluded that PRM had no antiepileptic properties against MES seizures in mice, apart from its derived PB. Their conclusions were in direct conflict with the earlier exhaustive study of Goodman et al. (30), which also used an MES seizure model in mice, and with the study of Gallagher et al. (29) in rats. Leal et al. (42) used SKF-525A as a metabolic inhibitor to prevent the conversion of PRM to PB or PEMA. The results showed that PB was four times more potent than PRM alone in an MES seizure model and that brain concentrations of PRM seemed randomly related to the ef-

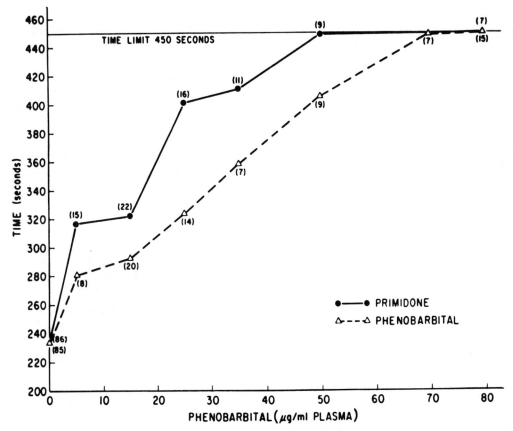

FIG. 1: Seizure threshold measured to the appearance of a tonic-clonic seizure. Difference between mean thresholds are significant (P < .05; *t* test) at 0–10, 10–20, 20–30, 30–40, and 40–50 μg/ml. (From Gallagher et al., ref. 29, with permission.)

fectiveness of PRM against MES seizures. Nonetheless, even though the study was unable to show a correlation with brain concentrations of PRM, mice treated with PRM and SKF-525A *were* protected against MES seizures. The results did not support the conclusions and were, in fact, consonant with the results of previous studies (29,30).

Leal et al. (42) also reported that they could find only "negligible or absent PRM concentration in the brains of patients on PRM therapy who were undergoing surgery for intractable epilepsy" and used this evidence to support their conclusion that PRM per se had no antiepileptic properties independent of its derived PB. Yet Guelen and van der Kleijn (32), using autoradiographic methods, demonstrated a high accumulation of PRM in the brain of squirrel monkeys and in the same uniform distribution pattern as PB. More importantly, an earlier paper by Houghton et al. (36) had reported significant brain concentrations of PRM in 11 patients and found that brain levels of PRM showed a high correlation with plasma levels.

In a more recent study in mice, Bourgeois et al. (12,13) demonstrated that PRM has a different spectrum of activity than PB and is relatively less toxic than PB. The combination of PRM and PB appeared more effective than either one alone in terms of the spectrum of antiepileptic activity and relative toxicity. In contrast with the report of Leal et al. (42), brain concentrations of PRM showed a linear relationship to plasma concentrations of PRM, although brain concentrations correlated poorly with oral doses of the drug. Further, the absorption of PRM appeared to be nonlinear in mice. The studies also confirmed previous reports that PRM and PEMA are both efficacious against MES seizures and that PRM alone is ineffective against PTZ-induced seizures. The EC_{50} of PB against MES seizures *in the presence of PRM* was substantially lower than with PB alone, but the combination provided no additional protection against PTZ seizures. The toxicity of PRM and PB was less than expected from a purely additive interaction. These findings suggest that PRM has a spectrum of antiepileptic activity more similar to PHT and carbamazepine (CBZ) (both of which are effective against MES seizures, but ineffective against PTZ-induced seizures) than to PB. Phenylethylmalonamide was found to potentiate the protective effects of PB against PTZ, even at low plasma concentrations.

The combined results of these studies (12,13) demonstrate that in mice, PB and PRM potentiate each other against MES seizures while showing little additive toxicity, and that the combination of PB and PRM is "superior to either one alone." The presence of PEMA apparently provides no additional benefit. In addition, the most potentiation of PB and PRM occurs when brain concentrations of PRM and PB are nearly equal. They also showed that a PRM-to-PB brain ratio of 1:1 can be best achieved by plasma ratios of 1.5:1 to 2:1. This is a condition rarely seen clinically, where the average PRM-to-PB ratio is closer to 0.9:1 or less.

The preponderance of evidence from animal studies indicates that PRM has antiepileptic effects independent of metabolically derived PB. The spectrum of antiepileptic activity of PRM resembles that of CBZ and PHT. When brain concentrations of PRM and PB are approximately equal, the combination produces a better therapeutic response. Metabolically derived PEMA contributes little to the antiepileptic properties of PRM, and its toxicity probably is additive. Some discrepancies in the results of various studies may be explained by variables such as unpredictable oral absorption and failure to study effects of PRM relative to plasma and brain concentrations.

Clinical Studies

The first clinical reports of the antiepileptic efficacy of PRM were uniformly enthusiastic about its potential clinical usefulness (18,19,23,33,37,46,52,72–74). Most studies, however, used PRM as add-on therapy and were not prospective or controlled. Following the documentation that PB was a major metabolite of PRM, negative reports appeared, with one study (87) even indicating that PRM was less effective than PB or PHT and that serious complications, including reduction in white blood cell count, were common. This worrisome report has never been confirmed, however.

Early double-blind comparative studies such as that of White et al. (85) showed that PRM and PB were equally effective, but did not control for plasma PB levels. Olesen and Dam (55) did control for plasma PB levels, and although they reported no clinical difference between PB and PRM, they studied a population of institutionalized refractory epilepsy patients—a difficult population upon which to base meaningful conclusions of comparative efficacy. In addition, careful review of their data reveals that a small number of patients showed deterioration in seizure control when PB was substituted for PRM. Because plasma PB levels remained constant, this finding (also noted by Booker [9]) suggests that in some patients PRM has antiepileptic effects beyond those attributable to PB.

Booker et al. (10) documented the half-life of PRM in normal volunteers and studied the range of therapeutic levels in over 100 epileptic patients. Significantly, no difference in half-life (T½ = 10 to 12 hr) was found between untreated subjects and patients who had been on long-term PB or PRM therapy. The mean PRM level in 30 patients taking PRM but no other barbiturate was 9.2 µg/ml, and the mean PB level in the same patients was 31 µg/ml, producing a PB-to-PRM ratio of 3-to-1. No difference in clinical state was observed between patients taking PRM and patients taking PB despite comparable PB levels. The authors also observed that PB was undetectable in normal volunteers up to 48 hr following a single dose of PRM and theorized that the difference in half-life of the two drugs accounted for this finding. Side effects in normal volunteers were similar to those attributed to PB, although two of six subjects had marked side effects, including a lightheaded, giddy feeling, slurred speech, and difficulty with concentration. Because no PB was present in plasma at the time of these symptoms, it is likely that the side effects were the result of PRM effects on the brain.

Further clarification of the metabolic distribution of PRM and its metabolites in humans resulted from a series of studies by Baumel et al. (6) and Gallagher et al. (27,28). They reported that PRM has a somewhat shorter biological half-life than the values Booker (10) reported. After a single dose of PRM, patients receiving long-term therapy with PRM or another antiepileptic drug had a PRM half-life of 3.3 to 25 hr (mean, 8.0 ± 1.1 hr), with peak concentrations occurring in 2.7 ± 0.4 hr. They did not find any clear association with time of peak concentration or half-life and the patients' medication regimen at the time of study, although all patients were taking some combination of antiepileptic drugs prior to the metabolic studies and some had been on long-term PRM therapy. Two patients who were acutely withdrawn from PRM experienced widely different half-lives. One patient had a half-life of 7.2 hr with no PRM being detected in plasma after 48 hr, and another patient had a half-life of 19.2 hr.

Figure 2 shows the variation in PRM levels over 96 hr in a patient receiving PRM for the first time. Even though the levels fluctuate widely with dosing at 24-hr intervals, they remain well within the accepted therapeutic range after 60 hr. With closer dosing intervals (every 8 hr) in another patient on PRM monotherapy, there was little fluctuation in plasma PRM levels.

In a study correlating EEG paroxysms, seizure frequency, and plasma PRM and PB

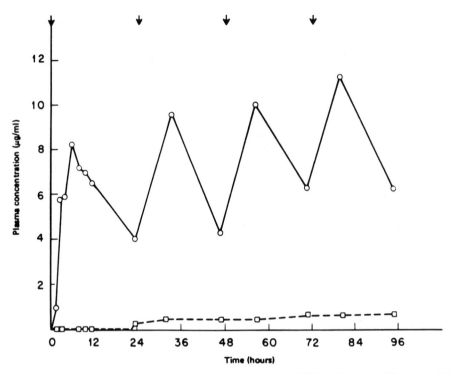

FIG. 2: Plasma concentration of primidone (○——○) and PEMA (□————□) in a subject receiving primidone for the first time. Arrow indicates 500-mg oral dose of primidone. (From Gallagher et al. ref. 27, with permission.)

levels, Rowan et al. (67), using 24-hr video-EEG monitoring, showed that peak PRM and PB levels were associated with periods of decreased clinical seizure activity and with fewer EEG paroxysms. Although it cannot be concluded that the EEG changes and seizure frequency decrease were due to the changes in PRM levels per se, the fluctuations in PRM levels were more abrupt than PB, and the rapid change in PRM levels correlated somewhat better with the EEG and clinical changes than the slower variations in PB levels.

A number of comparative clinical studies of PRM and other antiepileptic drugs have been performed within the last two decades (48,50,56,57,66,77), but only one has shown evidence that PRM is superior in efficacy. Oxley et al. (56) reported a study of 21 patients residing at the Chalfont Centre for Epilepsy who were taking either PRM or PB for at least a year in combination with a variety of other antiepileptic drugs. While holding the dose of concomitant antiepileptic drugs constant, they adjusted the dose of PRM or PB until comparable plasma PB levels were obtained both in the group of patients taking PRM and in the group of patients taking PB. After 1 year, those patients taking PRM were changed over to PB, and patients taking PB were switched to PRM. Doses were again adjusted until plasma PB levels were similar in both groups. Fourteen of the 21 patients experienced better control of generalized tonic-clonic seizures while taking PRM, while four had more frequent seizures. There were no differences between the two groups in the observed frequency of complex partial or generalized absence seizures.

In a recently completed nationwide Veterans Administration (VA) Cooperative Study (48,77) in which CBZ, PHT, PB, and PRM were compared in a double-blind prospective study design, overall treatment success was highest for CBZ and PHT, and lowest for PRM. Six hundred and twenty-two patients were entered into the study, randomized to one of the four drugs, and then followed for a minimum of 1 year or until toxicity or unacceptable seizure frequency intervened. One of the end points for evaluating the relative efficacy of the four study drugs was the length of time a patient remained on the drug. This end point (patient retention time) was affected by seizure control and toxicity. Retention rates were better for patients taking CBZ or PHT than for patients taking PRM ($p < 0.001$). Patients taking PB also had a better retention rate than patients taking PRM ($p < 0.05$). The major reason for the low retention rate of patients taking PRM in this trial was the appearance of intolerable acute side effects such as nausea, vomiting, sedation, and dizziness. These side effects occurred within the first month, and usually within the first week of therapy with PRM. In fact, after the first month, the retention rate for patients taking PRM was virtually identical to the retention rate for patients taking CBZ or PHT. These side effects occurred despite a conservative initial dosing schedule (125 µg PRM at bedtime).

Another end point in the study was comparison of the percentage of patients who were seizure-free on each of the four drugs. There were no significant differences between the drugs in control of tonic-clonic seizures: 63% of patients remained seizure-free after a year on PRM, 58% on PB, 55% on CBZ, and 48% on PHT.

When the behavioral effects of the four drugs were compared, PRM appeared to have fewer adverse effects, as measured by the total behavioral toxicity battery (BTB), than either PHT or PB (75). The BTB score was derived by combining scores of indi-

TABLE 1. *Total number of best and worst scores on subtests of the behavioral toxicity battery at 1 month, 3 months, 6 months, and 12 months after therapy*

Treatment group	POMS[a]	Motor	Attention/concentration
	Best score		
CBZ	11	4	10
PHT	2	1	2
PRM	9	3	1
PB	2	1	0
	Worst score		
CBZ	0	0	1
PHT	13	4	0
PRM	2	5	6
PB	9	0	5

Best and worst scores indicate scores that are significantly different from scores attained by two or more other groups for the same subtest in the same rating period.
[a] POMS, profile of mood states.

vidual subtests, which were transformed into weighted ordinal units of change based on published norms (76). On the subtests of the BTB and on the total BTB score, PRM showed a very different behavioral profile than PB (Table 1). The difference in toxicity between PRM and PB strongly suggests that PRM has effects (both positive and negative) that are independent of PB.

Figure 3 shows the mean PB level after 1 week, 1 month, 3 months, and 12 months of monotherapy with PRM. At each period, the mean PB level is shown for four different therapeutic ranges of plasma PRM levels (low, 4 to 6.9 µg/ml; medium, 7 to 9.9 µg/ml; high, 10 to 12.5 µg/ml; highest, >12.5 µg/ml). As expected, PB was barely detectable at 1 week, but by 1 month, PB levels stabilized and did not change appreciably at 3 months and 12 months. As importantly, plasma PB levels did not appear to bear any consistent relationship to plasma PRM levels. Figure 4 emphasizes this poor correlation, although there is a tendency for higher PB levels to be associated with higher PRM levels. The mean PB-to-PRM ratio over the first 12 months

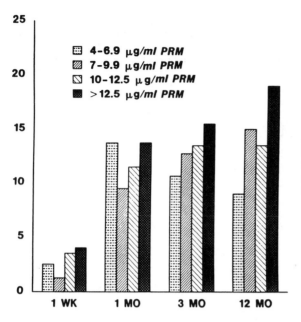

FIG. 3: Mean plasma PB levels in μg/ml for each of four different therapeutic ranges of plasma PRM after 1 week, 1 month, 3 months, and 12 months of PRM monotherapy.

was 1.2:1, which is close to the optimal ratio predicted by Bourgeois et al. (13) in mice.

The poor correlation between dose and plasma PRM or PB levels found in the VA cooperative study is shown in Table 2. Not only is there a wide range of dose evident in the high standard deviation associated with each range of plasma PRM levels, but the mean dose bears no consistent relation-

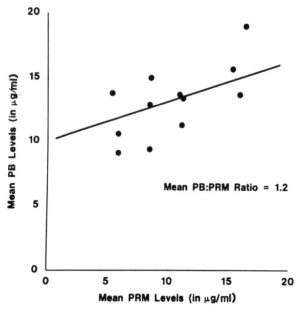

FIG. 4: Mean plasma PB levels over the first 12 months of study plotted against mean plasma PRM levels.

TABLE 2. *The relationship of PRM dose to plasma PRM and PB levels after 12 months of monotherapy with PRM*

PRM level (therapeutic range)	PRM dose (mg/kg)	PRM level (μg/ml)	PB level (μg/ml)
Low (4–6.9 μg/ml)	720 ± 350[a]	5.9 ± 1.0	9.9 ± 8.2
Medium (7–9.9 μg/ml)	820 ± 250	8.6 ± 0.8	15.0 ± 8.0
High (10–12.5 μg/ml)	650 ± 180	11.3 ± 0.7	13.4 ± 9.1
Highest (>12.5 μg/ml)	756 ± 150	16.4 ± 3.8	19.0 ± 12.2

[a] Mean ± standard deviation.

ship to the mean PRM levels. Plasma PB levels are highly variable and show poor correlation with either plasma PRM levels or with the PRM dose. These results are similar to those reported by Fincham and Schottelius (24), who also showed that PB levels correlated poorly with either PRM dose or plasma PRM levels. They based their findings on 80 patients studied over 8 years on monotherapy with PRM. Because excellent seizure control was found in 29 patients who had PB levels of less than 15 μg/ml, they concluded that PRM per se was probably responsible for the antiepileptic effects. In our patients on monotherapy with PRM, the mean derived PB level for the first 12 months of the study was 13.4 μg/ml and ranged from 12.1 μg/ml at 1 month to 15.4 μg/ml at 12 months. All of these levels are below the accepted therapeutic range for PB. In contrast, the mean PB level for patients on PB monotherapy for 12 months was 24.4 μg/ml, which is well within the accepted therapeutic range.

Further evidence for the independent antiepileptic properties of PRM comes from a case report by Wyllie et al. (88). A 16-year-old girl with one or two generalized tonic-clonic and atonic seizures per week suddenly developed a dramatic rise in seizure frequency after a generic form of PRM was substituted. With reinstatement of Mysoline, seizure frequency returned to base line. Three months later, during a hospitalization, generic PRM was again substituted and again associated with an increase in seizure frequency. A dramatic fall in the plasma PRM of 53% and a fall in plasma PB of only 16% occurred. It is unlikely that the relatively small change in plasma PB (from 19.1 μg/ml to 15.9 μg/ml) can account for the dramatic change in seizure frequency observed.

Clinical studies of PRM confirm animal experimental work and indicate that the drug has considerable efficacy against tonic-clonic seizures that cannot be explained solely on the basis of conversion to PB. The neurotoxicity and behavioral toxicity of PRM and PB are distinct. Acute systemic and central nervous system (CNS) toxicity is greater with initial use of PRM, whereas long-term behavioral effects appear to be less.

Poor correlation exists between PRM dose and levels of PRM or PB. The elimination half-life of PRM is also quite variable but averages 8 hr, making it advisable to administer PRM twice or three times a day. When PRM is used as monotherapy, the mean ratio of PB-to-PRM in plasma is 1.2, but this is sufficiently variable to make it useful to test for both levels as a guide to management.

TREATMENT GUIDELINES

On the basis of both animal and clinical data, PRM should be considered primary therapy for partial and secondarily generalized tonic-clonic seizures. If PB has failed to achieve adequate seizure control, it should not be assumed that PRM will also fail because PRM is also a barbiturate. Primidone has antiepileptic properties independent of PB, and its spectrum of activity in both animals and humans is different from that of PB.

Initiation of Therapy

Evidence from both animal and human studies indicates that the early systemic and CNS toxicity observed with PRM therapy is a result of a rapid build-up of a brain PRM concentration. Primidone is not significantly bound to plasma protein and penetrates readily into brain tissue. Phenylethylmalonamide also is not significantly bound, but concentrations rise more slowly in plasma and are very low when the first signs of toxicity appear. Phenobarbital is usually not detectable at all for the first 24 to 48 hr. Seizure protection against MES seizures in animals occurs before either PEMA or PB appear in plasma or brain, giving further evidence for the rapid penetration of PRM into brain tissue.

Clinically, the rapid rise in plasma and brain PRM levels following oral doses can lead to intolerable side effects, including nausea, vomiting, giddiness, lightheadedness, and difficulty concentrating. To avoid these troublesome side effects, it is advisable to initiate treatment slowly by giving 125 mg (1.8 mg/kg) only at bedtime for 3 days, and then increasing the dose by 125 mg increments every 3 days. In some patients, even lower dosage of 50 mg may be necessary if early side effects are a problem. If the patient is already taking PB, an abrupt switch can be made, substituting 250 mg of PRM for each 60 mg of PB. In this circumstance, toxicity during switchover is usually not a problem. A switchover from PHT or CBZ to PRM should be done more cautiously, and initiation of therapy with PRM should begin with 1.8 mg/kg given only at bedtime for the first 3 days. Tapering of the other drug should not begin until a trough PRM level of 6 μg/ml or greater has been achieved (usually in less than a week). It is not clear why patients can be abruptly switched from PB to PRM without experiencing significant toxicity, but require a more conservative approach to avoid toxicity when switching from either CBZ or PHT to PRM. Induction of PRM metabolism by PB is not a reasonable explanation because PHT and CBZ are also powerful hepatic enzyme inducers. It is likely that PB produces some tolerance to the CNS toxicity of PRM (28), probably at a membrane receptor level.

Maintenance Therapy and Relation of Plasma Concentration to Seizure Control

It is clear from both animal studies and clinical investigations that there is a poor correlation between the oral dose of PRM and plasma levels of PRM or its derived PB. It is also clear that there is a very good correlation between plasma PRM levels and brain concentrations of PRM. The clinical importance of these observations cannot be overemphasized: it is essential to base dosing decisions in each patient on plasma PRM levels. Plasma PB levels are not predictive of plasma PRM levels, but are helpful to the extent that they give information about the PRM-to-PB ratio. It may be that the PRM-to-PB ratio is the most important factor in predicting the likelihood of clinical success, but further study is needed. Available evidence suggests that it is important to adjust the dose of PRM on the basis of both plasma PRM and plasma PB levels. The VA cooperative study (48) suggests that the optimal mean plasma PRM level is 12 μg/ml with an associated mean derived PB level of 15 μg/ml, resulting in a PRM-to-PB ratio of 0.8, but much variation can be expected among patients. The likelihood of increased toxicity on long-term therapy with PRM appears to be associated with low PRM-to-PB ratios and high plasma PB levels, such as found when PRM is co-administered with PHT.

A high interindividual variability in PRM-to-PB ratios was reported by Cornaggia et al. (22), but the ratio of PRM to PB remains relatively constant over time, suggesting that autoinduction on monotherapy with PRM does not occur to any clinically significant degree. In addition, in rare patients, enzyme induction apparently does not occur at all (25).

The half-life of PRM in humans is quite variable and ranges from 3 hr to over 20 hr (10,21,24,27). The short half-life in some patients and the wide intersubject variability in the metabolic rate of PRM makes the assessment of PRM levels alone difficult. Without performing detailed pharmacokinetic studies in each patient, the timing of a trough level is complex and leads to inaccuracies (69). In the absence of individual pharmacokinetic data, it is reasonable to assume a half-life of 8 hr, although on monotherapy the half-life is frequently much closer to 15 hr (21). Based on the conservative assumption of a half-life of 8 hr, a thrice a day dosing schedule is recommended and trough levels (obtained just before the next dose) should be no less than 6 μg/ml. If the patient experiences toxicity at this level, a peak level measured 1 to 2 hr after dosing with a concomitant plasma PB level may be helpful in adjusting the dose and dose frequency.

Effect of Drug Interaction on Plasma PRM Levels and Antiepileptic Efficacy

Carbamazepine and phenytoin both are powerful hepatic enzyme inducers (21,39,44,60) and can be expected to shorten the half-life of PRM, although the interaction between CBZ and PRM appears to be minimal, with some authors (11,20,21) reporting no change in plasma PRM or PB levels after CBZ was added to PRM. In fact, Cereghino et al. (20) noted that both PRM

and PB appeared to *increase* in some patients during treatment with CBZ.

The effects of PHT on PRM metabolism are better documented and appear more consistent (21,24,41,60,63,79). The ratio of derived PB to PRM is consistently raised in patients taking PHT in addition to PRM (69). Fincham et al. (24) reported that the PB-to-PRM ratio was increased from 1.05 in patients on monotherapy with PRM to 4.35 in patients taking PHT and PRM (PRM-to-PB ratios have been mentioned above; PB-to-PRM ratios of 1.05 and 4.35 correspond to PRM-to-PB ratios of 0.95 and 0.22, respectively). Porro et al. (60) and Reynolds et al. (63) reported similar changes in the PRM-to-PB ratio associated with PHT therapy.

The effects of valproate are less predictable. Valproate tends to inhibit PRM metabolism, but it also inhibits PB metabolism. Therefore, less PRM may be converted to PB, but the PB still accumulates (1,14,43). In fact, increased sedation caused by accumulated PB after addition of valproate to a PRM regimen can occur (34,64). The effects of valproate on plasma PRM levels are negligible, in part because of the low protein binding of PRM (14).

Acetazolamide has been reported to interfere with the absorption of PRM, leading to low PRM levels (82). Interactions with benzodiazepines and other antiepileptic drugs appear not to be clinically significant (40).

An intriguing interaction is the effect of nicotinamide on PRM metabolism. Nicotinamide is a nontoxic, water soluble vitamin that produces inhibition of hepatic cytochrome P-450 enzymes. Use of this compound can increase the half-life of PRM, decrease the conversion of PRM to PB, and increase the plasma PRM concentration (11). Because of this interaction, it has been suggested that nicotinamide may be a useful adjuvant to PRM therapy for achieving optimal PRM-to-PB ratios (11,80).

Because of the importance and variability

of the conversion of PRM to PB and the unpredictable interactive effects of other antiepileptic drugs on PRM metabolism, measurement of both PRM and PB levels whenever PRM is used in conjunction with any other antiepileptic drug is essential.

Effects of Age on Primidone Pharmacokinetics and Dosing

Clinical treatment may need to be modified in different age populations. The metabolism of PRM in children has not been studied as extensively as it has been in adults. Painter (58) has studied 16 neonates in whom PRM was used in addition to PB or PHT. Phenobarbital was discontinued in four of these neonates, allowing some observations of PRM metabolism while the infants were on PRM monotherapy. The metabolism of PRM in all these infants was highly variable, but significant conversion of PRM to PB was delayed for 30 days or more. Absorption of PRM in infants is faster than in adults with corresponding earlier peaks in PRM levels.

The effectiveness and toxicity of PRM in the treatment of febrile seizures has been studied by Herranz et al. (35). They concluded that PRM was slightly more effective than PB in the prophylactic treatment of febrile seizures, and that fewer side effects were associated with PRM therapy. Phenobarbital levels were less than 15 μg/ml on PRM therapy.

In children over the age of 7, despite a tendency toward more efficient metabolism, the half-life of PRM is similar to that of adults, although plasma concentrations tend to be lower on equivalent mg/kg doses (4,59). In addition, steady-state PRM concentrations are even more variable in children than in adults (3). During adolescence, the metabolic rate decreases quite rapidly to adult values (84). Plasma PRM and PB levels may change quite rapidly during puberty, and frequent drug level monitoring is necessary.

In the elderly, even though the metabolism of PRM may be slower, and the half-life of PRM may be somewhat prolonged, PB still accumulates (15). This population may be more sensitive to the hypnotic effects of PB and may not tolerate usual doses of PRM for that reason.

In both children and the elderly, the dosage of PRM needs to be closely monitored, with frequent plasma PRM and PB determinations. In both population age extremes, plasma PRM and PB levels should be obtained no less than every 3 months.

Use in Pregnancy

The metabolism of PRM changes during pregnancy, as does the metabolism of most other antiepileptic drugs. The levels of PB and PEMA tend to decrease during the first trimester, although the plasma levels of PRM tend to remain fairly stable (62) or may even be slightly increased (5). Levy and Yerby (45) reported large decreases in plasma concentrations of PB during pregnancy with a rapid rise occurring immediately after delivery. Increased seizure activity was not associated with these changes in PB concentration.

Transplacental passage of PRM is well documented (47,49,53). In fact, a syndrome of tremulousness, jitteriness, disturbance of sleep rhythm, and unmotivated crying has been reported in neonates exposed to PRM *in utero*. At the onset of the syndrome, no PRM levels are detectable although PEMA and PB concentrations are still considerable (54,61), providing convincing evidence that the syndrome is related specifically to PRM withdrawal and not PB withdrawal. The poor ability of the infant to metabolize PRM and PB is discussed in the previous section.

The possibility of specific PRM teratogenicity has been raised in several reports (38,49,51,68). McElhatton et al. (49) found an increase in palatal defects in fetal mice exposed to PRM, and several case reports have suggested that PRM was implicated in birth defects, including cranial facial abnormalities and delayed development. The effect of PRM on chromosomes of human leukocytes has also been studied (78), and no significant increase in breaks, gaps, or abnormal forms was found compared with control cultures. Data are still too insufficient to allow meaningful assessment of the specific teratogenicity of PRM independent of its derived PB.

SUMMARY

There is now ample evidence from multiple animal and clinical studies that PRM has antiepileptic properties independent of PB and that it is a clinically useful and unique antiepileptic drug. Some portion of its antiepileptic activity is assumed to be due to the derived PB and PRM appears to be most successful with a PRM-to-PB ratio of 1, at which time PB levels are usually well below the accepted therapeutic range for PB. The importance of monitoring both plasma PRM and PB levels during therapy with PRM is emphasized by the poor correlation between the dose of PRM and plasma PRM levels, and by the high interpatient variability in the PRM-to-PB ratio. Another advantage of measuring both PRM and PB levels is that the large difference in half-lives between the parent drug and its metabolite, PB, makes it easy to assess compliance. For example, a PRM-to-PB ratio of greater than 2-to-1, or no detectable PB level with plasma PRM levels greater than 6 μg/ml strongly suggests noncompliance.

Because of the relatively short half-life of PRM, which averages between 8 and 10 hr, the timing of the plasma level determinations is complex. The blood needs to be drawn at the same time of day, and just before the next dose. For the same reason, multiple daily doses are necessary in most patients. An accepted therapeutic range is difficult to determine for PRM, but levels between 8 and 12 μg/ml seem appropriate. Many individuals tolerate much higher levels without side effects, and dosage increases must be determined by clinical response.

The early toxicity associated with initiation of PRM therapy is the most limiting factor in the use of PRM as a primary antiepileptic drug. In most patients, a gradual dosage increment, beginning with 1.8 mg/kg (usually 125 mg) or less at bedtime, will avoid this troublesome toxicity.

When used as monotherapy and with careful monitoring of plasma PRM and PB concentrations, PRM can be very effective against generalized tonic-clonic and partial seizures.

REFERENCES

1. Adams, D. J., Luders, H., and Pippenger, C. (1978): Sodium valproate in the treatment of intractable seizure disorders: A clinical and electroencephalographic study. *Neurol.*, 28:152–157.
2. Adderly, D. S., and Monro, A. B. (1953): Mysoline in the treatment of epilepsy. *Lancet*, 1:1154.
3. Armijo, J. A., Herranz, J. L., Arteaga, R., and Valiente, R. (1986): Poor correlation between single-dose data and steady-state kinetics for phenobarbitone, primidone, carbamazepine and sodium valproate in children during monotherapy: Possible reasons for the lack of correlation. *Clin. Pharmacokinet.*, 11:323–335.
4. Battino, D., Avanzini, G., Bossi, L., Croci, D., Cusi, C., Gomeni, C., and Moise, A. (1983): Plasma levels of primidone and its metabolite phenobarbital: Effect of age and associated therapy. *Ther. Drug Monit.*, 5:73–79.
5. Battino, D., Binelli, S., Bossi, L., Como, M. L., Croci, D., Cusi, C., and Avanzini, G. (1984): Changes in primidone/phenobarbitone ratio during pregnancy and the puerperium. *Clin. Pharmacokinet.*, 9:252–260.
6. Baumel, I. P., Gallagher, B. B., and Mattson, R. H. (1972): Phenylethylmalonamide (PEMA). An important metabolite of primidone. *Arch. Neurol.*, 27:34–41.
7. Bogue, J. Y., and Carrington, H. C. (1953): The evaluation of Mysoline—A new anticonvulsant drug. *Br. J. Pharmacol.*, 8:230–236.
8. Bogue, J. Y., Carrington, H. C., and Bentley, S. (1956): L'activité anticonvulsive de la Mysoline. *Acta Neurol. Psychiatr. Belg.*, 56:640–650.
9. Booker, H. E. (1972): Primidone: Relation of plasma levels to clinical control. In: *Antiepileptic*

Drugs, 1st edition, edited by D. Woodbury, K. Penry, and R. Schmidt, pp. 373–376. Raven Press, New York.

10. Booker, H. E., Hosokowa, K., Burdette, R. D., and Darcey, B. (1970): A clinical study of serum primidone levels. *Epilepsia,* 11:395–402.

11. Bourgeois, B. F. D., Dodson, W. E., and Ferrendelli, J. A. (1982): Interactions between primidone, carbamazepine, and nicotinamide. *Neurol.,* 32:1122–1126.

12. Bourgeois, B. F. D., Dodson, W. E., and Ferrendelli, J. A. (1983): Primidone, phenobarbital, and PEMA: I. Seizure protection, neurotoxicity, and therapeutic index of individual compounds in mice. *Neurol.,* 33:283–290.

13. Bourgeois, B. F. D., Dodson, W. E., and Ferrendelli, J. A. (1983): Primidone, phenobarbital, and PEMA: II. Seizure protection, neurotoxicity, and therapeutic index of varying combinations in mice. *Neurol.,* 33:291–295.

14. Bruni, J. (1981): Valproic acid and plasma levels of primidone and derived phenobarbital. *Le J. Canadien des Sci. Neurol.,* 8:91–92.

15. Bruni, J., and Albright, P. S. (1984): The clinical pharmacology of antiepileptic drugs. *Clin. Neuropharm.,* 7:1–34.

16. Burton-Bradley, B. G. (1953): Report on Mysoline in treatment of mental hospital epileptics. *Med. J. Aust.,* 2:705–706.

17. Butler, T. C., and Waddell, W. J. (1956): Metabolic conversion of primidone (Mysoline) to phenobarbital. *Proc. Soc. Exp. Biol. Med.,* 93:544–546.

18. Butter, A. J. M. (1953): Mysoline in treatment of epilepsy. *Lancet,* 1:1024.

19. Calnan, W. L., and Borrell, Y. M. (1953): Mysoline in the treatment of epilepsy. *Lancet,* 2:42–43.

20. Cereghino, J. J., Van Meter, J. C., Brock, J. T., Penry, J. K., Smith, L. D., and White, B. G. (1973): Preliminary observations of serum carbamazepine concentration in epileptic patients. *Neurol.,* 23:357–366.

21. Cloyd, J. C., Miller, K. W., and Leppik, I. E. (1981): Primidone kinetics: Effects of concurrent drugs and duration of therapy. *Clin. Pharmacol. Ther.,* 29:402–407.

22. Cornaggia, C. M., Altamura, A. C., Bianchi, M., Canger, R., Polana, P., and Pruneri, C. (1983): PB:PRM ratio in patients with epilepsy treated with primidone. *Int. J. Clin. Pharm. Res.,* 3:185–193.

23. Doyle, P. J., and Livingston, S. (1953): Use of Mysoline in treatment of epilepsy. *J. Pediatr.,* 43:413–416.

24. Fincham, R. W., and Schottelius, D. D. (1982): Primidone: Relation of plasma concentration to seizure control. In: *Antiepileptic Drugs,* 2nd edition, edited by D. M. Woodbury, J. K. Penry, and C. E. Pippenger, pp. 429–440. Raven Press, New York.

25. Fincham, R. W., Schottelius, D. D., and Sahs, A. L. (1974): The influence of diphenylhydantoin on primidone metabolism. *Arch. Neurol.,* 30:259–262.

26. Frey, H. H., and Hahn, I. (1960): Untersuchungen uber die Bedentung des durch biotransformation gebildeten Phenobarbital fur die antikonvulsive Wirkung von Primidon. *Arch. Int. Pharmacodyn.,* 128:281–290.

27. Gallagher, B. B., Baumel, I. P., and Mattson, R. H. (1972): Metabolic disposition of primidone and its metabolites in epileptic subjects after single and repeated administration. *Neurology (Minneap.),* 22:1186–1192.

28. Gallagher, B. B., Baumel, I. P., Mattson, R. H., and Woodbury, B. S. (1973): Primidone, diphenylhydantoin and phenobarbital. Aspects of acute and chronic toxicity. *Neurology (Minneap.),* 23:145–149.

29. Gallagher, B. B., Smith, D. B., and Mattson, R. H. (1970): The relationship of the anticonvulsant properties of primidone to phenobarbital. *Epilepsia,* 11:293–301.

30. Goodman, L. S., Swinyard, E. A., Brown, W. C., Schiffman, D. O., Grewal, M. S., and Bliss, E. L. (1953): Anticonvulsant properties of 5-phenyl-5-ethyl-hexahydropyrimidine-4, 6-dione (Mysoline). A new antiepileptic. *J. Pharmacol. Exp. Ther.,* 108:428–436.

31. Gruber, C. M., Jr., Mosier, J. M., and Grant, P. (1957): Objective comparison of primidone and phenobarbital in epileptics. *J. Pharmacol. Exp. Ther.,* 120:184–187.

32. Guelen, P. J. M., and van der Kleijn, E. (eds.) (1978): *Rational Anti-Epileptic Drug Therapy,* pp. 15–44. Elsevier/North-Holland, New York.

33. Handley, R., and Stewart, A. S. R. (1952): Mysoline: A new drug in the treatment of epilepsy. *Lancet,* 1:742–744.

34. Harvey, C. D., Sherwin, A. L., and van der Kleijn, E. (1977): Distribution of anticonvulsant drugs in gray and white matter of human brain. *Can. J. Neurol. Sci.,* 4:89–92.

35. Herranz, J. L., Armijo, J. A., and Arteaga, R. (1984): Effectiveness and toxicity of phenobarbital, primidone, and sodium valproate in the prevention of febrile convulsions, controlled by plasma levels. *Epilepsia,* 25:89–95.

36. Houghton, G. W., Richens, A., Toseland, P. A., Davidson, S., and Falconer, M. A. (1975): Brain concentrations of phenytoin, phenobarbitone, and primidone in epileptic patients. *Eur. J. Clin. Pharmacol.,* 9:73–78.

37. Jorgenson, G. (1953): Mysoline in the treatment of epilepsy. *Lancet,* 2:835.

38. Krauss, C. M., Holmes, L. B., VanLang, Q. N., and Keith, D. A. (1984): Four siblings with similar malformations after exposure to phenytoin and primidone. *J. Pediatr.,* 105:750.

39. Kutt, H. (1975): Interactions of antiepileptic drugs. *Epilepsia,* 16:393–402.

40. Kutt, H. (1984): Interactions between anticonvulsants and other commonly prescribed drugs. *Epilepsia,* 25(Suppl 2):S118–S131.

41. Lambie, D. G., and Johnson, R. H. (1981): The effects of phenytoin on phenobarbitone and primidone metabolism. *J. Neurol. Neurosurg. Psych.,* 44:148–151.

42. Leal, K. W., Rapport, R. L., Wilensky, A. J., and

Friel, P. N. (1979): Single-dose pharmacokinetics and anticonvulsant efficacy of primidone in mice. *Ann. Neurol.,* 5:470–474.

43. Levy, R. H., and Koch, K. M. (1982): Drug interactions with valproic acid. *Drugs,* 24:543–556.

44. Levy, R. H., and Pitlick, W. H. (1982): Carbamazepine: Interactions with other drugs. In: *Antiepileptic Drugs,* 2nd edition, edited by D. M. Woodbury, J. K. Penry, and C. E. Pippenger, pp. 497–505. Raven Press, New York.

45. Levy, R. H., and Yerby, M. S. (1985): Effects of pregnancy on antiepileptic drug utilization. *Epilepsia,* 26(Suppl 1):S52–S57.

46. Livingston, S., and Petersen, D. (1956): Primidone (Mysoline) in the treatment of epilepsy. *N. Engl. J. Med.,* 254:327–329.

47. Martinez, G., and Snyder, R. D. (1973): Transplacental passage of primidone. *Neurol.,* 23:381–383.

48. Mattson, R. H., Cramer, J. A., Collins, J. F., Smith, D. B., Delgado-Escueta, A. V., Browne, T. R., Williamson, P. D., Treiman, D. M., McNamara, J. O., McCutchen, C. B., Homan, R. W., Crill, W. E., Lubozynski, M. F., Rosenthal, N. P., and Mayersdorf, A. (1985): Comparison of carbamazepine, phenobarbital, phenytoin, and primidone in partial and secondarily generalized tonic-clonic seizures. *N. Engl. J. Med.,* 313:145–151.

49. McElhatton, P. R., Sullivan, F. M., and Toseland, P. A. (1977): Teratogenic activity and metabolism of primidone in the mouse. *Epilepsia,* 18:1–11.

50. Millichap, J. C., and Aymat, F. (1968): Controlled evaluation of primidone and diphenylhydantoin sodium. Comparative anticonvulsant efficacy and toxicity in children. *J.A.M.A.,* 204:738–739.

51. Myhre, S. A., Williams, R. (1981): Teratogenic effects associated with maternal primidone therapy. *J. Pediatr.,* 99:160–162.

52. Nathan, P. W. (1954): Primidone in treatment of nonidiopathic epilepsy. *Lancet,* 1:21–22.

53. Nau, H., Kuhnz, W., Egger, H.-J., Rating, D., and Helge, H. (1982). Anticonvulsants during pregnancy and lactation: Transplacental, maternal and neonatal pharmacokinetics. *Clin. Pharmacokinet.,* 7:508–543.

54. Nau, H., Schmidt, D., Beck-Mannagetta, G., Rating, D., Koch, S., and Helge, H. (1981): Pharmacokinetics of primidone and metabolites during human pregnancy. In: *Epilepsy, Pregnancy and the Child,* edited by Janz et al., pp. 121–130. Raven Press, New York.

55. Olesen, O. V., and Dam, M. (1967): The metabolic conversion of primidone to phenobarbitone in patients under long-term treatment. *Acta Neurol. Scandinav.,* 43:348–356.

56. Oxley, J., Hebdige, S., Laidlaw, J., Wadsworth, J., and Richens, A. (1980): A comparative study of phenobarbitone and primidone in the treatment of epilepsy. In: *Antiepileptic Therapy: Advances in Drug Monitoring,* edited by S. I. Johannessen et al., pp. 237–245. Raven Press, New York.

57. Oxley, J., Hebdige, S., and Richens, A. (1979): A comparison of phenobarbitone and primidone in the control of seizures in chronic epilepsy. *Br. J. Clin. Pharmacol.,* 7:414P.

58. Painter, M. J. (1983): How to use primidone. In: *Antiepileptic Drug Therapy in Pediatrics,* edited by P. L. Morselli, C. E. Pippenger, and J. K. Penry, pp. 263–270. Raven Press, New York.

59. Pippenger, C. E. (1978): Pediatric clinical pharmacology of antiepileptic drugs: A special consideration. In: *Antiepileptic Drugs: Quantitative Analysis and Interpretation,* C. E. Pippenger, J. K. Penry, and H. Kutt, pp. 315–319. Raven Press, New York.

60. Porro, M. G., Kupferberg, H. J., Porter, R. J., Theodore, W. H., and Newmark, M. E. (1982): Phenytoin: An inhibitor and inducer of primidone metabolism in an epileptic patient. *Br. J. Clin Pharmac.,* 14:294–297.

61. Rating, D., Jager-Roman, E., Koch, S., Nau, H., and Helge, H., (1981): Enzyme induction in neonates due to antiepileptic therapy during pregnancy. In: *Epilepsy, Pregnancy and the Child,* edited by Janz et al., pp. 349–355. Raven Press, New York.

62. Rating, D., Nau, H., Jager-Roman, E., Gopfert-Geyer, I., Koch, S., Beck-Mannagetta, G., Schmidt, D., and Helge, H. (1982): Teratogenic and pharmacokinetic studies of primidone during pregnancy and in the offspring of epileptic women. *Acta Paediatr. Scand.,* 71:301–311.

63. Reynolds, E. H., Fenton, G., Fenwick, P., Johnson, A. L., and Laundy, M. (1975): Interaction of phenytoin and primidone. *Br. Med. J.,* 2:594–595.

64. Richens, A., and Ahmad, S. (1975): Controlled trial of sodium valproate in severe epilepsy. *Br. Med. J.,* 4:255–256.

65. Rodin, E. A. (1968): *The Prognosis of Patients wtih Epilepsy,* p. 202. Charles C Thomas, Springfield, Illinois.

66. Rodin, E. A., Choo, S. R., Hideki, K., Lewis, R., and Rennick, P. M. (1976): A comparison of the effectiveness of primidone versus carbamazepine in epileptic outpatients. *J. Nerv. Ment. Dis.,* 163:41–46.

67. Rowan, A. J., Pippenger, C. E., McGregor, P. A., and French, J. H. (1975): Seizure activity and anticonvulsant drug concentration. 24 hour sleep waking studies. *Arch. Neurol.,* 32:281–288.

68. Rudd, N. L., and Freedom, R. M. (1979): A possible primidone embryopathy. *J. Pediatr.,* 94:835–837.

69. Schottelius, D. D., and Fincham, R. W. (1978): Clinical application of serum primidone levels. In: *Antiepileptic Drugs: Quantitative Analysis and Interpretation,* edited by C. E. Pippenger, J. K. Penry, and H. Kutt, pp. 273–282. Raven Press, New York.

70. Sciarra, D., Carter, S., Vicale, C. T., and Merritt, H. H. (1954): Clinical evaluation of primidone (Mysoline), a new anticonvulsant drug. *J.A.M.A.,* 154:827–829.

71. Shorvon, S. (1987): The treatment of epilepsy by drugs. In: *Epilepsy,* edited by A. Hopkins, pp. 229–282. Demos Publications, New York.

72. Smith, B., and Forster, F. M. (1953): The role of

some experimental anticonvulsants, Mysoline, Milontin and 1461L. *M. Ann. District of Columbia,* 22:279–282.

73. Smith, B., and Forster, F. M. (1954): Mysoline and Milontin: Two new medicines for epilepsy. *Neurology (Minneap.),* 4:137–142.

74. Smith, B. H., and McNaughton, F. L. (1953): Mysoline, new anticonvulsant drug: Its value in refractory cases of epilepsy. *Can. Med. Assoc. J.,* 68:464–467.

75. Smith, D. B. (1986): *Unpublished data* from VA Cooperative Study #118.

76. Smith, D. B., Craft, B. R., Collins, J., Mattson, R. H., Cramer, J. A., and the VA Cooperative Study Group 118 (1986): Behavioral characteristics of epilepsy patients compared with normal controls. *Epilepsia,* 27:760–768.

77. Smith, D. B., Mattson, R. H., Cramer, J. A., Collins, J. F., Novelly, R. A., Craft, B. and the V.A. Epilepsy Cooperative Study Group (1987): Results of a nationwide Veterans Administration cooperative study comparing the efficacy and toxicity of carbamazepine, phenobarbital, phenytoin, and primidone. *Epilepsia,* 28(Suppl. 3):S50–S58.

78. Stenchever, M. A., and Allen, M. (1973): The effect of selected antiepileptic drugs on the chromosomes of human lymphocytes *in vitro. Am. J. Obstet. Gynecol.,* 116:867–870.

79. Streete, J. M., Berry, D. J., Pettit, L. I., and Newbery, J. E. (1986): Phenylethylmalonamide serum levels in patients treated with primidone and the effects of other antiepileptic drugs. *Ther. Drug Monitor.,* 8:161–165.

80. Sutton, G., and Kupferberg, H. J. (1975): Isoniazid as an inhibitor of primidone metabolism. *Neurol.,* 25:1179–1181.

81. Swinyard, E. A., Tedeschi, D. H., and Goodman, L. S. (1954): Effect of liver damage and nephrectomy on anticonvulsant activity of Mysoline and phenobarbital. *J. Am. Pharm. Assoc.,* 43:114–116.

82. Syversen, G. B., Morgan, J. P., Weintraub, M., and Myers, G. J. (1977): Acetazolamide-induced interference with primidone absorption. *Arch. Neurol.,* 34:80–84.

83. Timberlake, W. H., Abbott, J. A., and Schwab, R. S. (1955): Mysoline: An effective anticonvulsant with initial problems of adjustment. *N. Engl. J. Med.,* 252:304–307.

84. Vajda, F. J. E., and Aicardi, J. (1983): Reassessment of the concept of a therapeutic range of anticonvulsant plasma levels. *Dev. Med. Child Neurol.,* 25:660–671.

85. White, P. T., Plott, D., and Norton, J. (1966): Relative anticonvulsant potency of primidone. A double blind comparison. *Arch. Neurol.,* 14:31–35.

86. Whitty, C. W. M. (1953): Value of primidone in epilepsy. *Br. Med. J.,* 2:540–541.

87. Wilson, W. E., and Hodgson, O. E. F. (1954): Mysoline in epilepsy: A comparison with older methods of treatment. *J. Ment. Sci.,* 100:250–261.

88. Wyllie, E., Pippenger, C. E., and Rothner, A. D. (1987): Increased seizure frequency with generic primidone. *J.A.M.A.,* 258:1216–1217.

Antiepileptic Drugs, Third Edition, edited by
R. Levy, R. Mattson, B. Meldrum,
J. K. Penry, and F. E. Dreifuss.
Raven Press, Ltd., New York © 1989.

30

Primidone

Toxicity

Ilo E. Leppik and James C. Cloyd

Although primidone (PRM) was rated as being less toxic than phenobarbital (PB) in the original laboratory trials (8) and in more recent studies evaluating brain concentrations of the drugs in rodents (11), many patients experience symptoms of toxicity related to use of this drug (24,37,38,56,58,60). Primidone is metabolized to PB and phenylethylmalonamide (PEMA) and is often used in combination with other antiepileptic drugs. Side effects present at initiation of treatment are attributable to the parent compound, but those present later may be caused by PB. This metabolite is present in high concentrations during PRM therapy and may be the cause of adverse reactions (see Chapter 23). Levels of PEMA may equal those of the parent drug, but PEMA plays a small role, if any, in toxicity (6). With comedication, some of the observed toxicity may result from the addition of another depressant drug to those already present, so studies using monotherapy provide the best indication of toxicity (38). This chapter emphasizes the adverse effects of PRM on patients receiving PRM only or on those in which PRM could be implicated because of the reversal of toxicity with its withdrawal in the presence of continued therapy with other agents.

NERVOUS SYSTEM TOXICITY

Symptoms involving the central nervous system (CNS) are the most common side effects of PRM therapy (Table 1), and may be perceived by as many as 43% to 85% of patients (31,37,38,57,58,59,60). Primidone may have to be discontinued in some 9% to 32% of patients because of side effects (37,38,57). Indeed, in the Veteran's Administration (VA) cooperative study (38), side effects were the single most important factor in the poor outcome of persons treated with PRM.

Persons receiving their initial PRM dose often experience drowsiness, weakness, dizziness, and a feeling of intoxication within 1 to 2 hr after ingesting the drug. In a study of 13 patients who were hospitalized during the initiation of therapy with PRM and had frequent examinations during the first day, all were affected to some degree (35). Mean peak serum PRM levels were approximately 6 µg/ml. These side effects were attributable to PRM alone, as they occurred before any metabolites were present (35).

Occasionally these symptoms are severe and incapacitating, with gradual improvement occurring over a few days (2,26). The intolerance of some patients to a PRM dose often tolerated by others has been designated an idiosyncratic reaction (26). However, the signs and symptoms resemble those occurring after PRM overdose (12), and were encountered to a lesser degree in volunteers taking 500 mg and attaining peak PRM levels of approximately 10 µg/ml (10).

TABLE 1. *Primidone side effects and adverse reactions*

System	Signs and symptoms
Nervous system	Acute: sedation, ataxia, nystagmus
	Chronic: decreased psychometric performance
	Personality change
	Impotence
	Polyradiculitis (R)[a]
Metabolic	Folic acid deficiency
Hematological	Megaloblastic anemia
	Leukopenia (R)
	Thrombocytopenia (R)
	Hemorrhagic disease of newborn
Hepatic and renal	Enzyme induction
	Edema (R)
Hypersensitivity reactions	Benign maculopapular rash
	Systemic lupus erythematosus (R)
	Lymphadenopathy, malignant (R)

[a] R = rare: fewer than five well-documented cases.

Acute symptoms appear to be related to the plasma concentration of the drug, with individual variability in degree of sensitivity to PRM accounting for the spectrum of discomfort encountered. Since these severely disturbing reactions may occur in as many as 14% of patients during initiation of therapy (61), some physicians use a test dose of 50 mg and initiate treatment according to the reaction (10).

Most patients develop tolerance to the CNS side effects of PRM. In a study of the pharmacokinetics of PRM, we observed significant toxicity during the first exposure to the drug. Side effects included ataxia, nystagmus, and mental symptoms, which were rated on a 4-unit scale. The time course of the toxicity rating paralleled the PRM concentrations at a time when no phenobarbital was present (Fig. 1). Rapid tolerance to the effects of primidone developed. The ratio of the toxicity rating to the PRM concentration was significantly greater during the first 6 hr after the initial

250-mg dose (35), which demonstrates a rapid pharmacodynamic development of tolerance to the drug. The time course of development of tolerance to PRM is similar to that seen with alcohol. Previous use of PB reduces symptoms on initiation of therapy with PRM, but exposure to phenytoin or carbamazepine (CBZ) does not (24,35).

Personality changes have been observed during the use of PRM (37,46,58,59). Patients had significantly higher scores on the psychopathic deviate scale of the Minnesota Multiphasic Inventory when they were treated with PRM than when they were receiving CBZ, and also tended to become progressively more depressed while on PRM, as judged by psychometric rating (53). Occasionally, paranoid reactions to PRM occur, and in one patient, appeared three times as the PRM dose was increased (58). Acute confusional and schizophrenia-like psychoses were observed when PRM was combined with phenytoin (20).

Impotence and decreased libido have been mentioned in some instances, but most reports give few details regarding their severity or time of onset (53,57,61). Impotence was clearly documented in a recent multicenter study (38). In a study comparing CBZ with PRM in 60 patients, there was one instance of decreased libido with PRM but none with CBZ (53).

Many persons, especially those who are active and employed, complain of nonspecific difficulties with memory, concentration, and energy during long-term PRM therapy. These effects may be documented by psychometric testing. In a study comparing PRM with CBZ as an adjunct to phenytoin, the patients had significantly more impairment on the cognitive perceptual-motor battery during the PRM phase of treatment (53). Significant negative correlations were found between PB and PRM concentrations and 11 neuropsychological subtests measuring general mental function, concentration, and fine motor performance (30).

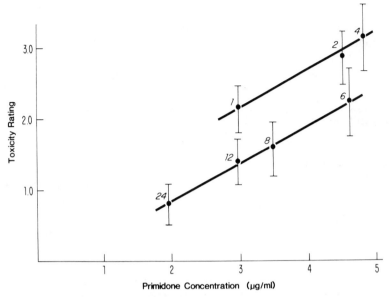

FIG. 1. Primidone concentrations and toxicity rating (mean ± SEM) during 24 hr after the initial dose. Hours 1, 2, and 4 are the absorptive phase and hours 6, 8, 12, and 24 the post-absorptive phase. The y intercepts of these two lines are significantly different ($p < 0.05$) although the slopes are similar, demonstrating the development of tolerance by a pharmacodynamic mechanism.

The nystagmus described with PRM use usually does not differ from that seen with use of other antiepileptic medication (61). Three cases of partial or total external ophthalmoplegia associated with PRM and phenytoin use have been reported (48). Two cases of downbeat nystagmus during phenytoin and PRM use have been observed, and PRM was implicated as a contributing factor because phenytoin concentrations were below 20 µg/ml (3). However, in both patients, the abnormal ocular findings cleared after the phenytoin dose was decreased.

Polyradiculitis and ataxia following a single dose of PRM have been observed in two children (62). Remission of the radiculitis occurred after treatment with corticosteroids (9).

Changes in the electroencephalogram attributable to PRM consist of beta activity superimposed on alpha activity. With serum levels of 15 to 100 µg/ml attained after an overdose, slow activity was intermingled with background activity (12).

OVERDOSE

Clinical findings of PRM overdose consist of CNS depression, flaccidity, and depression of deep tendon reflexes (32). With serum PRM levels of 90 to 100 µg/ml, patients exhibit somnolence and lethargy (12,39). Symptoms correlate with plasma and cerebrospinal fluid concentrations of PRM but not with levels of PEMA or PB, which often increase as the patient improves (12). Although fatal cases of PRM overdose have been reported (7), as much as 22 g may be ingested without permanent sequelae, and PRM appears to have a wide range of safety (12). Crystalluria is a prominent feature of PRM overdose and has been reported in most cases; it should serve to direct attention to the possibility of PRM overdose in comatose patients (4,7,14,34). Overdose should be treated with gastric lavage and supportive measures (39). Analeptic drugs have been used unsuccessfully (18) and are not generally recommended for treatment of PRM overdose (32).

HEMATOLOGICAL TOXICITY

Data from clinical trials conducted shortly after the introduction of PRM indicated that the drug was not associated with serious hematological abnormalities (13,28,29,50,57,58,61). Subsequently, the most commonly reported disorder has been megaloblastic anemia. Fewer than 1% of patients receiving antiepileptic drugs develop megaloblastic anemia (19), and it is most commonly observed in patients receiving phenytoin alone or in combination with other drugs. However, PRM was implicated as the causative agent in several cases (5). In one case, a patient had been treated with phenytoin and PB for 4 years; PRM was substituted for phenytoin, and severe megaloblastic anemia developed 2 months later (15). In two other instances, PRM was the only antiepileptic drug being used when megaloblastic anemia occurred in a patient 4 months after substitution of PRM for PB and in another patient 2 years after initiation of PRM therapy (22). In the fourth case, discontinuation of PRM was accompanied by a reticulocytosis of 16% and resolution of anemia in a patient whose phenytoin and PB were continued (17). When PRM was reinstituted the anemia recurred, but was treated with folate and resolved without the need to stop the drug. In the last case, involving a patient taking PRM only, a folate-responsive anemia developed in the presence of normal folic acid clearance, a state compatible with normal tissue stores of folate (16). Nevertheless, the anemia responded quickly to oral doses of folic acid.

When present during PRM treatment, macrocytic anemia usually responds to folic acid (25); however, in some cases it has been responsive to vitamin B_{12} (43,47).

Hemorrhagic disorders involving the use of PRM are rare. Maternal use of this drug has been linked to one case of neonatal coagulation defect (42) and suspected in others (45,60). Prophylactic use of vitamin K is indicated in women receiving PRM during pregnancy.

Well-documented thrombocytopenia has been reported in one patient who was placed on PRM after phenytoin-induced bone marrow depression (49). The thrombocytopenia cleared with the discontinuation of PRM, although PB was still being given. The PRM concentration was 10 μg/ml. One case of thrombocytopenic purpura has been associated with PRM (10). Leukopenia may be an occasional complication. One patient on both PRM and mephobarbital experienced a drop in the white blood cell (WBC) count to 3,000 with 50% neutrophils, which returned to normal after both drugs were discontinued (61). Neither drug alone produced the drop in the WBC count. Most studies found only transient or minor decreases in the WBC count (36,63).

Lymphadenopathy in conjunction with folate deficiency anemia has been observed in a patient taking PRM (33).

HEPATIC AND RENAL TOXICITY

No report linking PRM to hepatitis has been published. However, PRM is capable of inducing the hepatic enzyme system, and this must always be considered when the drug is given in combination with others.

A striking crystalluria has been observed after massive primidone overdose (4,12,39,44), but no hematuria or acute or chronic renal failure developed. Occasional cases of edema with no definite renal or hepatic involvement have been associated with PRM use (27).

BONE AND CONNECTIVE TISSUE DISORDERS

In a survey of calcium metabolism in nine patients with epilepsy in a residential center, subnormal levels of calcium were found in 22.5% of patients, and increased alkaline phosphatase in 29% (52). Although patients were receiving multiple antiepileptic drugs, there was a trend toward lower calcium values in patients receiving PRM or phenacemide as part of triple-drug therapy. Similar results were reported in a population of institutionalized children, with patients receiving PRM having the lowest levels of calcium and 25-hydroxy vitamin D (64). Patients receiving PRM, however, also received the largest number of other antiepileptic drugs and had the longest duration of therapy, so these findings may be attributable to the total exposure to drugs rather than to PRM specifically.

Frozen shoulder and Dupuytren's contracture related to PB and PRM use are discussed in reports by Critchley and Blanquart, as reviewed by Schmidt (56). The frozen shoulder syndrome was initially reported in 1928 in association with PB use, but subsequently has been reported with PRM. Other antiepileptic drugs do not appear to cause this syndrome. Dupuytren's contracture occurs independent of the frozen shoulder, appears to be dose related, and may clear after PB withdrawal. It is not clear if PRM itself causes the connective tissue problems or if the derived PB is the culprit.

TERATOGENICITY

Primidone administered to mice in doses of 100 to 250 mg/kg during days 6 to 16 of pregnancy and giving peak levels of 43 μg/ml was associated with a significant incidence of cleft palate as compared with control animals (41). Folic acid itself was not teratogenic but, when it was given in combination with PRM, there was a much higher incidence of malformations than occurred with PRM alone (40). Although PRM has been linked to human fetal malformations only occasionally (21), the number of instances in which PRM has been used as the sole agent are too few to make definitive statements regarding its ultimate teratogenicity in comparison with other antiepileptic drugs.

HYPERSENSITIVITY REACTIONS

Dermatological side effects of PRM are infrequent and usually occur at the onset of therapy. Of 96 patients, four had transient rashes that cleared in a day or two after the drug was discontinued and did not recur when PRM was reinstituted (61). In contrast to these benign reactions, a fatal case of dermatitis bullosa has been reported (54). An unusually hypersensitive patient experienced severe mucocutaneous eruptions from PRM, PB, phenytoin, CBZ, and mephenytoin (51). Eosinophilia of 10%, edema, and rash were observed in a patient who began taking PRM during the first month of pregnancy. Symptoms cleared when PB was substituted for PRM (23).

Primidone has been associated with systemic lupus erythematosus (SLE) in only one well-documented case (1). This occurred in a patient initially taking phenytoin who was later placed on PRM; symptoms of SLE developed, and LE smears were positive. Phenytoin was substituted for PRM, and symptoms cleared. The incidence of this reaction to PRM is apparently much less frequent than its appearance with the use of other antiepileptic drugs.

SUMMARY

Many patients experience side effects of drowsiness, weakness, and dizziness when PRM therapy is initiated. These symptoms are usually tolerable but occasionally may be quite severe and last for a few days. Tolerance to these symptoms usually develops, but some chronic CNS effects may be detected by psychometric testing. Primidone has only rarely been implicated in severe hematological or idiosyncratic reactions.

It shares with the other antiepileptic drugs the problem of folate and vitamin D disturbance.

ACKNOWLEDGMENTS

This work was supported in part by Grant No. 1-P50-NS-16308-08 from the National Institute of Neurological and Communicative Disorders and Stroke, Bethesda, Maryland.

REFERENCES

1. Ahuja, G. K., and Schumacher, G. A. (1966): Drug induced systemic lupus erythematosus. Primidone as a possible cause. *J.A.M.A.*, 198:669–671.
2. Ajax, E. T. (1966): An unusual case of primidone intoxication. *Dis. Nerv. Syst.*, 27:660–661.
3. Alpert, J. (1978): Downbeat nystagmus due to anticonvulsant toxicity. *Ann. Neurol.*, 4:471–473.
4. Bailey, D. N., and Jatlow, P. I. (1972): Chemical analysis of massive crystalluria following primidone overdose. *Am. J. Clin. Pathol.*, 58:583–589.
5. Baker, H., Frank, O., Huter, S., Aaronson, S., Ziffer, H., and Sobotka, H. (1962): Lesions in folic acid metabolism induced by primidone. *Experientia*, 18:224–226.
6. Baumel, I. P., Gallagher, B. B., and Mattson, R. H. (1972): Phenylethylmalonamide (PEMA). An important metabolite of primidone. *Arch. Neurol.*, 27:34–41.
7. Bogan, J., Rentoul, E., and Smith H. (1965): Fatal poisoning by primidone. *J. Forensic Sci. Soc.*, 5:97–98.
8. Bogue, J. Y., and Carrington, H. C. (1953): Evaluation of mysoline: New anticonvulsant drug. *Br. J. Pharmacol.*, 8:230–236.
9. Booker, H. E. (1972): Primidone toxicity, In: *Antiepileptic Drugs*, 1st edition, edited by D. M. Woodbury, J. K. Penry, and R. P. Schmidt, pp. 377–383. Raven Press, New York.
10. Booker, H. E., Hosokowa, K., Burdette, R. D., and Darcy, B. (1970): A clinical study of serum primidone levels. *Epilepsia*, 11:395–402.
11. Bourgeois, B. F., Dodson, W. E., and Ferrendelli, J. A. (1983): Primidone, phenobarbital, and PEMA: I. Seizure protection, neurotoxicity, and therapeutic index of individual compounds in mice. *Neurology*, 33(3):283–290.
12. Brillman, J., Gallagher, B. B., and Mattson, R. (1974): Acute primidone intoxication. *Arch. Neurol.*, 30:255–258.
13. Butter, A. J. M. (1953): Mysoline in the treatment of epilepsy. *Lancet*, 1:1024.
14. Cate, J. C., and Tenser, R. (1975): Acute primidone overdosage with massive crystalluria. *Clin. Toxicol.*, 8:385–389.
15. Chalmers, J. N. M., and Boheimer, K. (1954): Megaloblastic anemia and anticonvulsant therapy. *Lancet*, 2:920–921.
16. Chanarin, I., Elmes, P. C., and Mollin, D. L. (1958): Folic acid studies in megaloblastic anemia. *Br. Med. J.*, 2:80–82.
17. Christenson, W. N., Ultman, J. E., and Roseman, D. M. (1957): Megaloblastic anemia during primidone (Mysoline) therapy. *J.A.M.A.*, 163:940–942.
18. Dotevall, G., and Herner, B. (1957): Treatment of acute primidone poisoning with bemegride and amiphenazole. *Br. Med. J.*, 3:451–452.
19. Flexner, J. M., and Hartmann, R. C. (1960): Megaloblastic anemia associated with anticonvulsant drugs. *Am. J. Med.*, 28:386–396.
20. Franks, R. D., and Richter, A. J. (1979): Schizophrenia-like psychosis associated with anticonvulsant toxicity. *Am. J. Psychiatry*, 136:973–974.
21. Fredrick, J. (1973): Epilepsy and pregnancy: A report from the Oxford record linkage study. *Br. Med. J.*, 1:442–448.
22. Fuld, H., and Moorhouse, E. H. (1956): Observations on megaloblastic anemias after primidone. *Br. Med. J.*, 1:1021–1023.
23. Gabriel, R. M. (1957): Delayed reaction to PRM in pregnancy. *Br. Med. J.*, 1:344.
24. Gallagher, B. B., Baumel, I. P., Mattson, R. H., and Woodbury, S. G. (1973): Primidone, diphenylhydantoin and phenobarbital: Aspects of acute and chronic toxicity. *Neurology*, 23:145–149.
25. Girdwood, R. H., and Lenman, J. A. R. (1956): Megaloblastic anemia occurring during primidone therapy. *Br. Med. J.*, 1:146–147.
26. Goldin, S. (1954): Toxic effects of primidone. *Lancet*, 1:102–103.
27. Goodman, L. S., Swinyard, E. A., Brown, W. C., Schiffman, D. O., Grewal, M. S., and Bliss, E. L. (1953): Anticonvulsant properties of 5-phenyl-5-ethyl-hexahydropyrimidine-4,6 dione (Mysoline), a new antiepileptic. *J. Pharmacol. Exp. Ther.*, 108:248–436.
28. Greenstein, L., and Sapirstein, M. R. (1953): Treatment of epilepsy with Mysoline. *Arch. Neurol.*, 70:469–473.
29. Handley, R., and Stewart, A. S. R. (1952): Mysoline: A new drug in the treatment of epilepsy. *Lancet*, 1:742–744.
30. Hartlage, L. C., Stovall, K., and Kocack, B. (1980): Behavioral correlates of anticonvulsant blood levels. *Epilepsia*, 21:185.
31. Herranz, J. L., Armijo, J. A., and Atreaga, R. (1984): Effectiveness and toxicity of phenobarbital, primidone, and sodium valproate in the prevention of febrile convulsions, controlled by plasma levels. *Epilepsia*, 25(1):89–95.
32. Kappy, M. S., and Buckley, J. (1969): Primidone

intoxication in a child. *Arch. Dis. Child,* 44:282–284.

33. Langlands, A. O., MacLean, N., Pearson, J. G., and Williamson, E. R. D. (1967): Lymphadenopathy and megaloblastic anemia in patients receiving primidone. *Br. Med. J.,* 1:215–217.

34. Lehman, D. F. (1987): Primidone crystalluria following overdose. A report of a case and an analysis of the literature. *Med. Toxicol. Adverse Drug Exp.,* 2(5):383–387.

35. Leppik, I. E., Cloyd, J. C., and Miller, K. (1984): Development of tolerance to the side effects of primidone. *Ther. Drug Mon.,* 6(2):189–191.

36. Livingston, S. (1966): *Drug Therapy for Epilepsy.* Charles C Thomas, Springfield, Illinois.

37. Livingston, S., and Petersen, D. (1956): Primidone (Mysoline) in the treatment of epilepsy. *N. Engl. J. Med.,* 254:327–329.

38. Mattson, R. H., Cramer, J. A., Collins, J. F., Smith, D. B., Delgado-Escueta, A. V., Browne, T. R., Williamson, P. D., Treiman, D. M., McNamara, J. O., and McCutchen, C. B. (1985): Comparison of carbamazepine, phenobarbital, phenytoin, and primidone in partial and secondarily generalized tonic-clonic seizures. *N. Engl. J. Med.,* 313(3):145–151.

39. Matzke, G. R., Cloyd, J. C., and Sawchuk, R. J. (1981): Acute phenytoin and primidone intoxication: A pharmacokinetic analysis. *J. Clin. Pharmacol.,* 21:92–99.

40. McElhatton, P. R., and Sullivan, F. M. (1975): Teratogenic effects of primidone in mice. *Br. J. Pharmacol.,* 54:267P–268P.

41. McElhatton, P. R., Sullivan, F. M., and Toseland, P. A. (1977): Teratogenic activity and metabolism of primidone in the mouse. *Epilepsia,* 18:1–11.

42. Monnet, P., Rosenberg, D., and Bovier-Lapierre, M. (1968): Therapeutique anticomitiale administrée pendant la grossesse et maladie hemorragique du nouveau—V^e. Remarques critiques à propos de trois observations personnelles. *Rev. Fr. Gynaecol. Obstet.,* 63:695–702.

43. Montgomery, D., and Craig, J. (1958): Megaloblastic anemia during primidone therapy. Report of a case responding to vitamin B$_{12}$. *Scott. Med. J.,* 3:460.

44. Morley, D., and Wynne, N. A. (1957): Acute primidone poisoning in a child. *Br. Med. J.,* 1:90.

45. Mountain, K. R., Hirsh, J., and Gallus, A. S. (1970): Neonatal coagulation defects due to anticonvulsant drug treatment in pregnancy. *Lancet,* 1:265–268.

46. Nathan, P. W. (1954): Primidone in treatment of nonidiopathic epilepsy. *Lancet,* 1:21.

47. Newman, M. J. D., and Sumner, D. W. (1957): Megaloblastic anemia following the use of primidone. *Blood,* 12:183–188.

48. Orth, D. N., Almedia, H., Walsh, F. B., and

Honda, M. (1967): Ophthalmoplegia resulting from diphenylhydantoin and primidone intoxication. *J.A.M.A.,* 201:485–487.

49. Parker, W. A. (1974): Primidone thrombocytopenia. *Ann. Intern. Med.,* 81:559–560.

50. Poch, G. F. (1955): Estudio critico de valor de la primidona en el tratamiento de las epilepsias. *Arq. Bras. Med.,* 45:171–182.

51. Pollack, M. A., Burk, P. G., and Nathanson, G. (1979): Mucocutaneous eruptions due to antiepileptic drug therapy in children. *Ann. Neurol.,* 5:262–267.

52. Richens, A., and Rowe, D. J. F. (1970): Disturbances of calcium metabolism by anticonvulsant drugs. *Br. Med. J.,* 4:73–76.

53. Rodin, E. A., Rim, C. S., Kitano, H., Lewis, R., and Rennick, P. M. (1976): A comparison of the effectiveness of primidone versus carbamazepine in epileptic outpatients. *J. Nerv. Ment. Dis.,* 163:41–46.

54. Rodriguez, V. L. E., and Ovideo, S. G. V. (1957): Dermatitis ampollosa mortal desencadenada por la primidona (Mysoline). *Rev. Esp. Pediatr.,* 13:737–747.

55. Rose, M., and Johnson, I. (1978): Reinterpretation of the haematological effects of anticonvulsant treatment. *Lancet,* 1:1349–1350.

56. Schmidt, D. *Adverse Effects of Antiepileptic Drugs.* Raven Press, New York, 1982.

57. Sciarra, D., Carter, S., Vicale, C. T., and Merritt, H. H. (1954): Clinical evaluation of primidone (Mysoline), a new anticonvulsant drug. *J.A.M.A.,* 154:827–829.

58. Smith, B., and Forster, F. M. (1954): Mysoline and milotoin: Two new medicines for epilepsy. *Neurology,* 4:137–142.

59. Smith, B. H., and McNaughton, F. L. (1953): Mysoline, a new anticonvulsant drug. Its value in refractory cases of epilepsy. *Can. Med. Assoc. J.,* 68:464–467.

60. Stevenson, M. M., and Gilbert, E. G. (1970): Anticonvulsants and hemorrhagic disease of the newborn. *J. Pediatri.,* 77:516.

61. Timberlake, W. H., Abbott, J. A., and Schwab, R. S. (1955): An effective anticonvulsant with initial problems of adjustment. *N. Engl. J. Med.,* 252:304–307.

62. Verdura, G., and Lupi, G. (1969): La prevenzione e la terpaia degli effetti "neurotossici" acuti de "primidone." *Aggoir. Pediatr.,* 20:81–86.

63. Wilson, W. E. J., and Hodgson, E. E. F. (1954): Mysoline in epilepsy: A comparison with older methods of treatment. *J. Ment. Sci.,* 100:250–261.

64. Winnacker, J. L., Yeager, H., Saunders, J. A., Russell, B., and Anast, S. (1977): Rickets in children receiving anticonvulsant drugs. *Am. J. Dis. Child.,* 131:286–290.

Antiepileptic Drugs, Third Edition, edited by
R. Levy, R. Mattson, B. Meldrum,
J. K. Penry, and F. E. Dreifuss.
Raven Press, Ltd., New York © 1989.

31

Carbamazepine

Mechanisms of Action

Robert L. Macdonald

INTRODUCTION

Carbamazepine (CBZ) is an iminostil-bene and a structural congener of the tricyclic antidepressant drug imipramine (Fig. 1). CBZ has been shown to be effective in the treatment of simple partial, complex partial, and generalized tonic-clonic seizures but is ineffective against generalized absence seizures (4,50,53,61). CBZ and the antiepileptic drug phenytoin (PHT) (Fig. 1) have been shown to have equivalent efficacy in treatment of partial seizures and tonic-clonic seizures when used alone or as initial therapy (26,48), and both CBZ and PHT are drugs of first choice in the treatment of these seizure disorders (35). CBZ is an effective anticonvulsant in experimental animals (15,60) and has an anticonvulsant profile similar to PHT's (23,27). It is effective against maximal electroshock seizures at nontoxic doses but is not active against subcutaneous pentylenetetrazol-induced seizures. CBZ may also be effective in the single dose and long-term treatment of manic-depressive illness (43) and is the drug of choice for treatment of trigeminal neuralgia (2). CBZ is a lipid-soluble drug that is 65% to 80% bound to plasma proteins (22) and is administered to adults in doses of 10 to 20 mg per kg per day to achieve total plasma concentrations of 4 to 12 μg/ml (16–48 μM) (3,29). The lower range of plasma concentrations are adequate to control seizures in patients with tonic-clonic seizures alone, but the higher plasma concentrations are required to treat seizures in patients with partial seizures with or without tonic-clonic seizures (52). Cerebrospinal fluid (CSF) concentrations vary from 19% to 33% of total plasma concentrations (11). Assuming that 25% of total plasma CBZ is unbound, free plasma and CSF concentrations are likely to be 1 to 3 μg/ml (4.2–12.6 μM(22).

Multiple mechanisms of action of CBZ have been proposed. These can be divided into two basic mechanisms of drug action: an action of CBZ on neuronal sodium channels to reduce sustained, high frequency repetitive firing of action potentials, and actions of CBZ on synaptic transmission. Although evidence supporting both of these mechanisms has been reported, the weight of current experimental evidence suggests that CBZ's major mechanism of action is to modify the ability of neurons to fire at high frequency by producing an enhancement of sodium channel inactivation.

REDUCTION OF SUSTAINED HIGH FREQUENCY REPETITIVE FIRING BY CBZ

In early studies, CBZ was shown to reduce the excitability of peripheral nerves

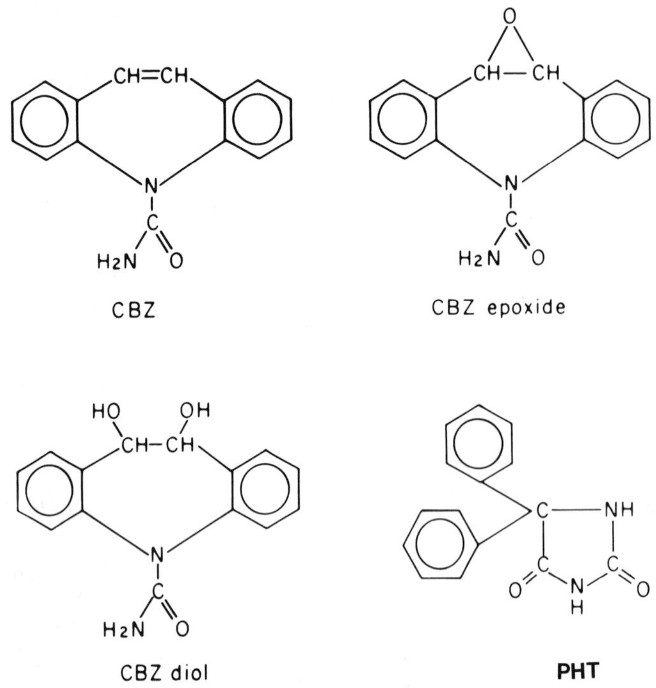

FIG. 1. Structures of CBZ, CBZ metabolites, CBZ epoxide, CBZ diol, and PT.

(20,28). These original observations suggested that CBZ directly reduced the sodium conductance underlying the action potential since there was an increased threshold, decreased conduction velocity, and decreased action potential height. However, it is likely that CBZ concentrations used in these experiments were supratherapeutic. Schauf et al. (51) demonstrated directly that CBZ reduced sodium current in *Myxicola* giant axons. This effect was not specific for sodium currents since potassium currents were also reduced. The CBZ effect occurred only at very high CBZ concentrations (0.25 to 1.0 mM). Thus, early studies demonstrated that CBZ directly affected sodium channels, but only at supratherapeutic concentrations.

Early studies also suggested that CBZ may have some effect on spontaneous or evoked repetitive firing recorded from peripheral nerves. Honda and Allen (20) demonstrated that CBZ reduced spontaneous firing of action potentials recorded from peripheral nerves immersed in isotonic sodium oxalate or phosphate solutions. Hershkowitz and Raines (18) studied the effect of CBZ on muscle spindle discharges. They correlated effects on spindle discharges with blood levels and demonstrated that CBZ depressed several aspects of muscle spindle discharges at concentrations that had little or no effect on nerve conduction velocity. They demonstrated that CBZ depressed muscle spindle activity in a manner similar to that produced by local anesthetics. The sustained and prolonged repetitive firing of spontaneous activity and the static stretch response were sensitive to CBZ block but the brief response to muscle stretch was spared. In addition, CBZ was demonstrated to reduce repetitive afterdischarges originating from small unmyelinated nerves in production of neuromuscular posttetanic potentiation in the cat soleus neuromuscular preparation at CBZ concentrations similar to those suppressing spontaneous activity in static stretch responses of muscle spindles (17). This effect on posttetanic repetitive after discharges recorded from isolated ventral root filaments occurred at concentrations that did not effect conduction velocity of the motor nerves (17).

The effect of CBZ on repetitive firing was not limited to neuromuscular preparations. CBZ reduced high frequency repetitive firing of action potentials recorded from mouse spinal cord (Fig. 2), neocortical and hippocampal pyramidal neurons grown in primary dissociated cell culture (30,36, 39,40), and from hippocampal pyramidal neurons in the slice (21). When depolarized, spinal cord and cortical neurons sustain high frequency repetitive discharges. In the presence of CBZ at therapeutic free serum concentrations [above 1 μM (4.2 μg/ml)], there was a concentration-dependent reduction in the number of action potentials evoked with 500 msec depolarizing pulses and in the percent of neurons manifesting sustained repetitive firing. No effect was produced on single action potentials at concentrations of CBZ below 10.6 μM (2.5 μg/ml). In addition to CBZ, its active metabolite, CBZ epoxide (Fig. 1), was also effective in limiting high frequency repetitive firing at concentrations comparable to those of CBZ (Fig. 2). However, an inactive metabolite of CBZ, CBZ diol (Fig. 1), did not affect high frequency repetitive firing until concentrations were an order of magnitude higher than those effective for CBZ (Fig. 2). Thus, CBZ and its active metabolite limited sustained high frequency repetitive firing of action potentials at therapeutic free serum

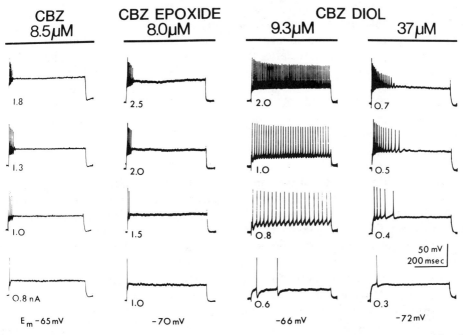

FIG. 2. CBZ, CBZ epoxide, and CBZ diol reduced sustained high-frequency repetitive firing in spinal cord neurons. Each column shows recordings from a single spinal cord neuron bathed in a high magnesium salt solution. Sustained high frequency repetitive firing was limited by CBZ and CBZ epoxide at low, clinically relevant concentrations. CBZ diol had no effect at a clinically relevant concentration but did limit sustained repetitive firing at a high nontherapeutic concentration (39).

concentrations that did not modify single action potentials.

The effect of CBZ on repetitive firing had three major properties. First, the effect was *voltage-dependent*. The reduction of sustained repetitive firing by CBZ could be enhanced by evoking the action potentials from a reduced membrane potential and could be reversed by evoking the repetitive train following membrane hyperpolarization. Second, the effect was *use-dependent* (8). When limitation of repetitive firing was produced, the first action potential in the action potential train was unaffected. However, with successive action potential in the train, there was a reduction in the maximal rate of rise of the action potentials and in the action potential heights until there was firing failure. Third, the effect was *time-dependent*. After a train of action potentials was evoked to produce a reduced firing in the presence of CBZ, subsequent action potentials evoked following the train were also reduced in amplitude and maximum rate of rise. This reduction in action potential properties lasted several hundred msec after the initial conditioning train.

These results suggested that CBZ was affecting sodium channels. However, the effect was likely to be on the inactivation process of sodium channels. It was proposed that CBZ bound to sodium channels only in the inactive state and, therefore, would limit repetitive firing only when the membrane was depolarized so that a fraction of the channels was in the inactive state (39). Blockade of repetitive firing could be reversed by hyperpolarizing the membrane to remove all sodium channel inactivation. Furthermore, since inactivation was enhanced by CBZ, initial action potentials in the train were unaffected, but subsequent action potentials in the train were more affected due to the prolonged inactivation of sodium channels opened during early action potentials in the train. Finally, recovery of sodium channels from inactivation was thought to be prolonged and, therefore, the

reduction in action potentials produced in a train would persist for several hundred msec. Thus, it was proposed that CBZ limited high frequency repetitive firing by binding to sodium channels in the inactive state and by slowing the rate of recovery from inactivation of these channels. In addition to CBZ, several other antiepileptic drugs that are effective against generalized tonic–clonic and partial seizures block high frequency repetitive firing (30,31,32) including phenytoin and valproic acid (38), possibly by a similar mechanism.

The action of CBZ on inactivated sodium channels has been confirmed using voltage clamp techniques. In studies of peripheral nerve and muscle (9) and neuroblastoma cells in culture (66), CBZ was shown to produce a frequency- and voltage-dependent block of sodium channels and to shift the voltage-dependency of steady state inactivation to more negative voltages. The block appeared to be selective for the inactive form of the closed channel. Thus, it is likely that CBZ binds preferentially to the inactive form of the sodium channel, an action consistent with the modulated receptor hypothesis of local anesthetic drug action proposed by Hille (19) (see Chapter 4).

In addition to its effect on sodium action potentials and currents, CBZ has been demonstrated to reduce veratridine-stimulated calcium flux (10,12), and batrachotoxin activated sodium influx in N18 neuroblastoma cells and rat brain synaptosomes (67). Veratridine and batrachotoxin both bind to voltage-dependent sodium channels. Therefore, the block of either calcium or sodium transport activated by either veratridine or batrachotoxin suggests an action of CBZ on voltage-dependent sodium channels. Furthermore, CBZ inhibited binding of [^{3}H]batrachotoxinin A 20-α-benzoate to sodium channels of rat brain synaptosomes (65). Interestingly, batrachotoxin causes persistent activation, not block, of sodium channels by binding to high affinity states of the channel.

The effect of CBZ has also been studied in a more organized neuronal preparation, the hippocampal slice. In this preparation, CBZ has been demonstrated to reduce spontaneous bursts recorded from the CA_1 region of the rat hippocampal slice in a low calcium, high magnesium solution (14,21, 41). This effect was produced in the absence of synaptic transmission since the slices were bathed in a low calcium solution. These results were produced at CBZ concentrations that did not block single antidromically evoked action potentials. Since the effect on paroxysmal bursting in hippocampal pyramidal neurons was produced when chemical synaptic transmission was blocked, the antiepileptic effect of CBZ was likely to reduce directly membrane excitability of pyramidal neurons. CBZ eliminated repetitive afterdischarges in immature rat CA_3 hippocampal pyramidal neurons produced by penicillin without altering epileptiform bursts, also suggesting an effect on neuronal excitability (57).

Thus, it appears that CBZ blocks high frequency sustained repetitive firing of action potentials and spontaneous burst discharges, veratridine and batrachotoxin-induced sodium flux, and [^{3}H]batrachotoxinin binding by binding to sodium channels and enhancing voltage-dependent sodium channel inactivation.

SYNAPTIC ACTIONS OF CBZ

In spinal cord, CBZ did not alter monosynaptic reflex discharges at systemic doses that depressed polysynaptic discharges and posttetanic potentiation (PTP) (23,28, 59,60). However, the blood levels required to reduce PTP were supratherapeutic (23), and CBZ failed to alter PTP in the rat hippocampal slice (21). CBZ also reduced synaptic transmission in the spinal trigeminal nucleus of cats (2,13,16,49) and in the nucleus centrum medianum of the thalamus (16). Similarly, the extracellular excitatory postsynaptic potential field potential (PSP) recorded in hippocampal CA_1 apical dendrites and evoked by stratum radiatum stimulation were reduced by CBZ at moderate concentrations (10–100 μM) (21). These studies suggest that CBZ may decrease excitatory synaptic transmission, but they do not clarify whether the effect of CBZ is presynaptic or postsynaptic.

In addition to the effects on the process of synaptic transmission, CBZ has been reported to alter neurotransmitter levels, metabolism, and receptors. The primary neurotransmitters studied include adenosine, monoamines, acetylcholine, γ-aminobutyric acid (GABA), and glutamate.

A role for CBZ in modifying adenosine receptors was suggested by the finding that CBZ modified the specific binding of adenosine agonists to rat brain membranes (62,34,54,55,56). CBZ specifically displaced the adenosine agonist, [^{3}H]cyclohexyl adenosine (CHA), and antagonist, [^{3}H]diethylphenylxanthine (DPX), binding (33,34,62). CBZ also inhibited adenosine-stimulated adenylate cyclase activity. The DPX binding was displaced by CBZ with a K_I of 3.5 μM while CHA binding was displaced with a K_I of 24.5 μM. The inhibition of adenosine receptor binding by CBZ was competitive (34). However, despite a clearly described interaction of CBZ with adenosine receptors, it is unlikely that this interaction is responsible for the antiepileptic properties of CBZ. There was no correlation between the potency of a series of CBZ analogs as inhibitors of either agonist or antagonist binding and their ability to inhibit maximal electroshock seizures (34). Furthermore, adenosine antagonists did not block the anticonvulsant effect of CBZ on amygdala-kindled seizures (63). It was reported, however, that theophylline pretreatment decreased the antiepileptic effects of CBZ on pentylenetetrazol-induced tonic hind limb extension. However, in studies with hippocampal slice, CBZ did not appear to have an action mediated by adenosine receptors. The depressant effect of adenosine on the population spike recorded in CA_1 was completely blocked by caffeine but the depressant effect of CBZ was not modified by caffeine (41). Furthermore, a role of adenosine receptors in CBZ action could not be supported in the immature rat hippocampus *in vitro* (57). Thus, although it appears established that CBZ binds to adenosine receptors and acts as an adenosine receptor antagonist, it is unlikely that antiepileptic properties of CBZ are derived from actions at adenosine receptors.

It has been suggested that monoamines may be involved in the actions of CBZ. The threshold for inducing electroshock seizures was reduced following administration of drugs that deplete brain monoamines (1,5,24,25,47). In contrast, the threshold for inducing electroshock seizures was elevated by administration of monoamine precursors or inhibitors of monoamine catabolism (6,24,44). Following an intraventricular injection of 6-hydroxy dopamine (6-OHD) that reduced forebrain catecholamines, CBZ was less effective in raising the electroconvulsive threshold current (46,47). Pretreatment with desipramine, which protected noradrenergic neurons from 6-OHD toxicity, blocked the 6-OHD effect on the CBZ anticonvulsant effect. Reduction of brain serotonin levels by destruction of raphe neurons did not alter the CBZ anticonvulsant effect (46). Purdy et al. (45) demonstrated that 100 μM CBZ inhibited both the uptake and release of [^{3}H]norepinephrine from brain synaptosomes. These results suggested that norepinephrine may be involved in the action of CBZ. However, Westerink et al. (64) found no change in 3,4-dihydroxyphenyl acidic acid and homovanillic acid, the metabolites of dopamine, in corpus striatum, nucleus accumbens, and tuberculum olfactorium of the rat following CBZ treatment. Furthermore, CBZ did not alter the firing rate of noradrenergic neurons in the locus coeruleus (42). A role of CBZ on catechola-

mine metabolism, therefore, remains uncertain.

An effect of CBZ on cholinergic responses in the brain has also been reported. Consolo et al. (7) found a selective increase in striatal acetylcholine and a decrease in choline levels of rat brain after the injection of CBZ. Neither choline acetyltransferase nor cholinesterase activity were effected by CBZ. However, this finding has not been confirmed.

A number of antiepileptic drugs have been demonstrated to enhance $GABA_A$ synaptic transmission (31). However, on spinal cord neurons in cell culture, no effect of CBZ was found on postsynaptic responses to iontophoretically applied GABA (39). Furthermore, CBZ did not alter GABAergic inhibition in the hippocampal slice (21). These results suggest that CBZ does not modify $GABA_A$ receptor mechanisms.

CBZ is unlikely to modify acidic amino acid excitatory action. CBZ did not modify postsynaptic responses to glutamate in a normal magnesium solution, suggesting that quisqualate- and kainate-like responses are not effected by CBZ (39). In addition, CBZ (400 μM) failed to affect sodium-dependent or [^{3}H]L-glutamate binding to hippocampal synaptic membranes (21), suggesting that CBZ does not modify postsynaptic glutamate action.

CONCLUSION

CBZ and its active metabolite CBZ epoxide both limit sustained high frequency repetitive firing of sodium-dependent action potentials. It is likely that they do so by binding to the inactive form of sodium channels, producing use- and voltage-dependent block of sodium channels. Thus CBZ will be more effective in reducing high frequency repetitive firing when neurons are depolarized since more channels are in the inactive state. Under normal physiological conditions, it is likely that vertebrate myelinated and unmyelinated axons have a large negative membrane potential, therefore propagated action potentials are relatively resistant to the action of CBZ. In contrast, the cell body of neurons is subject to synaptic depolarization and inward currents that produce burst firing. This is particularly true in neurons undergoing epileptic discharge. CBZ is effective, therefore, in limiting high frequency action potentials generated in bursting neurons.

In addition to altering neuronal excitability, CBZ may alter the process of synaptic transmission by affecting presynaptic sodium channels. It has been demonstrated that (^{3}H)BTX-B binding sites are not restricted to cell bodies and axons but are present in synaptic zones with a heterogeneous distribution in the nervous system (68). In the hippocampal slice, stimulation of stratum radiatum elicited extracellular field potentials recorded from the CA_1 pyramidal cell layer. The field potentials consisted of a fiber spike, which reflects axonal propagation, and a population spike, which reflects effective synaptic transmission. Veratridine, which displaces (^{3}H)BTX-B binding, produced a specific reduction in the synaptically evoked population spike without affecting the fiber spike. This effect of veratridine was antagonized by CBZ. It is likely, therefore, that CBZ blocks presynaptic sodium channels and the firing of action potentials; this would secondarily reduce voltage-dependent calcium entry and synaptic transmission. In summary, CBZ is likely to act both presynaptically to block release of neurotransmitter by blocking firing of action potentials and postsynaptically by blocking the development of high frequency repetitive discharge initiated at cell bodies. This combined pre- and postsynaptic effect is likely to form the basis for the antiepileptic actions of CBZ.

REFERENCES

1. Azzaro, A. J., Wenger, G. R., Craig, C. R., and Stitzel, R. E. (1972): Reserpine-induced alterations in brain amines and their relationship to changes in the incidence of minimal electro- shock seizures in mice. *J. Pharmac. Exp. Ther.*, 180:558–568.
2. Blom, S. (1963): Tic douloureau treated with a new anticonvulsant: Experiences with G 32883. *Arch. Neurol.*, 2:357–366.
3. Cereghino, J. J. (1982): Carbamazepine: Relation of plasma concentration to seizure control. In: *Antiepileptic Drugs*, edited by D. M. Woodbury, J. K. Penry, and C. E. Pippenger, pp. 507–519. Raven Press, New York.
4. Cereghino, J. J., Brock, J. T., Van Meter, J. C., Penry, J. K., Smith, L. D., and White, B. G. (1974): Carbamazepine for epilepsy. A controlled prospective evaluation. *Neurology*, 24:401–410.
5. Chen, G., Ensor, C. R., and Bohner, B. (1954): A facilitation action of reserpine on the central nervous system. *Proc. Soc. Exp. Biol. Med.*, 86:507–510.
6. Chen, G., Ensor, C. R., and Bohner, B. (1968): Studies of drug effects on electrically induced extensor seizures and clinical implications. *Arch. Int. Pharmacodyn. Ther.*, 172:183–218.
7. Consolo, S., Bianchi, S., and Ladinski, H. (1976): Effect of carbamazepine on cholinergic parameters in rat brain areas. *Neuropharmacology*, 15:653.
8. Courtney, K. R. (1975): Mechanism of frequency-dependent inhibition of sodium currents in myelinated nerve by the lidocaine derivative GEA 968. *J. Pharmacol. Exp. Therap.*, 195:225–236.
9. Courtney, K. R., and Etter, E. G. (1983): Modulated anticonvulsant block of sodium channels in nerve and muscle. *Eur. J. Pharm.*, 88:1–9.
10. Crowder, J. M., and Bradford, H. F. (1987): Common anticonvulsants inhibit Ca^{2+} uptake and amino acid neurotransmitter release *in vitro. Epilepsia*, 28:378–382.
11. Eadie, M. J., and Tyrer, J. H. (1980): *Anticonvulsant Therapy*, chapter 7, Carbamazepine, pp. 132–161. Churchill Livingstone, Edinburgh.
12. Ferrendelli, J. A., and Daniels-McQueen, S. (1982): Comparative actions of phenytoin and other anticonvulsant drugs on potassium- and veratridine-stimulated calcium uptake in synaptosomes. *J. Pharmacol. Exp. Ther.*, 220:29–34.
13. Fromm, G. H., and Killian, J. M. (1967): Effect of some anticonvulsant drugs on the spinal trigeminal nucleus. *Neurology*, 17:275–280.
14. Heinemann, U., Feranceschetti, S., Hamon, B., Honnerth, A., and Yaari, Y. (1985): Effects of anticonvulsants on spontaneous epileptiform activity which develops in the absence of chemical synaptic transmission in hippocampal slices. *Brain Res.*, 325:349–353.
15. Hernandez-Peon, R. (1964): Anticonvulsant action of G32883. *Third Proc. Int. Neuropsychopharmacologicum.*, 3:303–311.
16. Hernandez-Peon, R. (1965): Central action of G32883 upon transmission of trigeminal pain impulses. *Med. Pharmacol. Exp. (Basel)*, 12:73–80.
17. Hershkowitz, N., Dretchen, K. L., and Raines, A. (1978): Carbamazepine suppression of post-tetanic potentiation at the neuromuscular junction. *J. Pharmacol. Exp. Therap.*, 207:810–816.

18. Hershkowitz, N., and Raines, A. (1978): Effects of carbamazepine on muscle spindle discharges. *J. Pharmacol. Exp. Therap.*, 204:581–591.

19. Hille, B. (1977): Local anesthetics: Hydrophilic and hydrophobic pathways for the drug-receptor reaction. *J. Gen. Physiol.*, 69:497–515.

20. Honda, H., and Allen, M. (1973): The effect of an iminostilbene derivative (G32883) on peripheral nerve. *J. Med. Assoc. Ga.*, 62:38–42.

21. Hood, T. W., Siegfried, J., and Haas, H. L. (1983): Analysis of carbamazepine actions in hippocampal slices of the rat. *Cell. Molec. Neurobiol.*, 3:213–222.

22. Johannessen, S. I., Gerna, M., Bakke, J., Strandjord, R. E., and Marselli, P. L. (1976): CSF concentrations and serum protein binding of carbamazepine and carbamazepine 10,11-epoxide in epileptic patients. *Br. J. Clin. Pharmac.*, 3:575–582.

23. Julien, R. M., and Hollister, R. P. (1975): Carbamazepine: Mechanism of action. *Adv. Neurol.*, 11:263–277.

24. Kilian, M., and Frey, H.-H. (1973): Central monoamines and convulsive thresholds in mice and rats. *Neuropharmacology*, 12:681–692.

25. Koe, B. K., and Weissman, A. (1968): The pharmacology of para-chlorophenylalanine, a selective depletor of serotonin stores. *Adv. Pharmac.*, 6B:29–47.

26. Kosteljanetz, M., Christiansen, J., Dam, A. M., Hansen, B. S., Lyon, B. B., Pedersen, H., and Dam, M. (1979): Carbamazepine vs phenytoin. *Arch. Neurol.*, 36:22–24.

27. Krall, R. L., Penry, J. K., White, B. G., Kupferberg, H. J., and Swinyard, E. A. (1978): Antiepileptic drug development: II. Anticonvulsant drug screening. *Epilepsia*, 19:409–428.

28. Krupp, P. (1969): The effect of Tegretol on some elementary neuronal mechanisms. *Headache*, 9:42–46.

29. Kutt, H. (1978): Clinical pharmacology of carbamazepine. In: *Antiepileptic Drugs: Quantitative Analysis and Interpretation*, edited by C. E. Pippenger, J. K. Penry, and H. Kutt, pp. 307–314. Raven Press, New York.

30. Macdonald, R. L. (1983): Mechanisms of anticonvulsant drug action. In: *Recent Advances in Epilepsy*, edited by B. S. Meldrum and T. A. Pedley, pp. 1–23. Churchill Livingston, New York.

31. Macdonald, R. L., and McLean, M. J. (1986): Anticonvulsant drugs: Mechanisms of action. *Adv. Neurol.*, 44:713–735.

32. Macdonald, R. L., McLean, M. J., and Skerritt, J. H. (1985): Anticonvulsant drug mechanisms of action. *Fed. Proc.*, 44:2634–2639.

33. Marangos, P. J., Patel, J., Smith, K. D., and Post, R. M. (1987): Adenosine antagonist properties of carbamazepine. *Epilepsia*, 28:387–394.

34. Marangos, P. J., Post, R. M., Patel, J., Zander, K., Parma, A., and Weiss, S. (1983): Specific and potent interactions of carbamazepine with brain adenosine receptors. *Eur. J. Pharmacol.*, 93:175–182.

35. Mattson, R. H., Cramer, J. A., Collins, J. F., Smith, D. B., Delgado-Escueta, A. V., Browne, T. R., Williamson, P. D., Treiman, D. M., McNamara, J. O., McCutchen, C. B., Homan, R. W., Crill, W. E., Lubozynski, M. F., Rosenthal, N. P., and Mayersdorf, A. (1985): Comparison of carbamazepine, phenobarbital, phenytoin, and primidone in partial and secondarily generalized tonic-clonic seizures. *N. Eng. J. Med.*, 313:145–151.

36. McLean, M. J., and Macdonald, R. L. (1983a): Selective effects of anticonvulsant drugs on high frequency repetitive firing of action potentials in mouse spinal cord neurons in cell culture. *Neurology*, 33:213.

37. McLean, M. J., and Macdonald, R. L. (1983b): Multiple actions of phenytoin on mouse spinal cord neurons in cell culture. *J. Pharmacol. Exp. Therap.*, 227:779–789.

38. McLean, M. J., and Macdonald, R. L. (1986a): Sodium valproate, but not ethosuximide, produces use- and voltage-dependent limitation of high frequency repetitive firing of action potentials of mouse central neurons in cell culture. *J. Pharmacol. Exp. Ther.*, 237:1001–1011.

39. McLean, M. J., and Macdonald, R. L. (1986b): Carbamazepine and 10, 11-epoxycarbamazepine produce use- and voltage-dependent limitation of rapidly firing action potentials of mouse central neurons in cell culture. *J. Pharmacol. Exp. Ther.*, 228:727–738.

40. McLean, M. J., Taylor, C. P., and Macdonald, R. L. (1984): Phenytoin and carbamazepine limit sustained high frequency repetitive firing of action potentials of hippocampal neurons in cell culture and tissue slices. *Soc. Neurosci. Abs.*, 10:873.

41. Olpe, H.-R., Baudry, M., and Jones, R. S. G. (1985): Electrophysiological and neurochemical investigations on the action of carbamazepine on the rat hippocampus. *Eur. J. Pharmacol.*, 110:71–80.

42. Olpe, H.-R., and Jones, R. S. G. (1983): The action of anticonvulsant drugs on the firing of locus coeruleus neurons: Selective activating effect of carbamazepine. *Eur. J. Pharmacol.*, 91:107.

43. Post, R. M., Uhde, T. W., and Wolff, E. A. (1984): Profile of clinical efficacy and side effects of carbamazepine in psychiatric illness: Relationship to blood and CSF levels of carbamazepine and its 10,11-epoxide metabolite. *Acta Psychiatria Scand.*, 69:104–120.

44. Prockop, D. J., Shore, P. A., and Brodie, B. B. (1959): An anticonvulsant effect of monoamine oxidase inhibitors. *Experientia*, 15:145–147.

45. Purdy, R. E., Julien, R. M., Fairhurst, A. S., and Terry, M. D. (1977): Effect of carbamazepine on the *in vitro* uptake and release of norepinephrine in adrenergic nerves of rabbit aorta and in whole brain synaptosomes. *Epilepsia*, 18:251.

46. Quattrone, A., Crunelli, V., and Samanin, R. (1978): Seizure susceptibility and anticonvulsant activity of carbamazepine, diphenylhydantoin and phenobarbital in rats with selective depletions of brain monoamines. *Neuropharmacol.*, 17:643–647.

47. Quattrone, A., and Samanin, R. (1977): Decreased

anticonvulsant activity of carbamazepine in 6-hydroxydopamine-treated rats. *Eur. J. Pharmacol.*, 41:333–336.

48. Ramsay, R. E., Wilder, B., Berger, J., and Bruni, J. (1983): A double-blind study comparing carbamazepine with phenytoin as initial seizure therapy in adults. *Neurology*, 33:904–910.

49. Rasmussen, P., and Rushede, J. (1970): Facial pain treated with carbamazepine (Tegretol). *Acta Neurol. Scand.*, 46:385–408.

50. Rodin, E. A., Rim, C. S., and Rennick, P. M. (1974): The effects of carbamazepine on patients with psychomotor epilepsy: Results of a double blind study. *Epilepsia*, 15:547–561.

51. Schauf, C. L., Floyd, A. D., and Marder, J. (1974): Effects of carbamazepine in the ionic conductances of myxicola giant axons. *J. Pharmacol. Exp. Therap.*, 189:538–543.

52. Schmidt, D., Einicke, I., and Haenel, F. (1986): The influence of seizure type on the efficacy of plasma concentrations of phenytoin, phenobarbital, and carbamazepine. *Arch. Neurol.*, 43:263–265.

53. Simonsen, J., Zander Olsen, P., Kuhl, V., Lund, M., and Wendelboe, J. (1976): A comparative controlled study between carbamazepine and diphenylhydantoin in psychomotor epilepsy. *Epilepsia*, 17:169–176.

54. Skerritt, J. H., Davies, L. P., and Johnston, G. A. R. (1982): A purinergic component in the anticonvulsant action of carbamazepine? *Eur. J. Pharmacol.*, 82:195–197.

55. Skerritt, J. H., Davies, L. P., and Johnston, G. A. R. (1983a): Interactions of the anticonvulsant carbamazepine with adenosine receptors: 1. Neurochemical studies. *Epilepsia*, 24:642–643.

56. Skerritt, J. H., Davies, L. P., and Johnston, G. A. R. (1983b): Interactions of the anticonvulsant carbamazepine with adenosine receptors: 2. Pharmacological studies. *Epilepsia*, 24:643–650.

57. Smith, K. L., and Swann, J. W. (1985): Does carbamazepine act via an adenosine receptor? *Epilepsia*, 26:524.

58. Smith, K. L., and Swann, J. W. (1987): Carbamazepine suppresses synchronized afterdischarging in disinhibited immature rat hippocampus *in vitro*. *Brain Res.*, 400:371–376.

59. Theobald, W., Krupp, P., and Levin, P. (1970): Neuropharmacologic aspects of the therapeutic action of carbamazepine in trigeminal neuralgia. In: *Trigeminal Neuralgia: Pathogenesis and Pathophysiology*, edited by R. Hassler and A. E. Walker, pp. 107–114. Thieme, Stuttgart.

60. Theobald, W., and Kunz, H. A. (1963): Zur pharmacologie des Antiepileptikums 5-carbmyl-5H-dibenzo b,f azepin. *Arznei. Forsch.*, 13:122–125.

61. Troupin, A., Ojemann, L. M., Halpern, L., Dodrill, C., Wilkus, R., Friel, P., and Feigl, P. (1977): Carbamazepine—A double-blind comparison with phenytoin. *Neurology*, 27:511–519.

62. Weir, R. L., Padgett, W., Daly, J. W., and Adderson, S. M. (1984): Interaction of anticonvulsant drugs with adenosine receptors in the central nervous system. *Epilepsia*, 25:492–498.

63. Weiss, S. R. B., Post, R. M., Marangos, P. J., and Patel, J. (1985): Adenosine antagonists, lack of effect on the inhibition of kindled seizures in rats by carbamazepine. *Neuropharmacol.*, 24:535–638.

64. Westerink, B. H. C., Lejeune, B., Korf, J., and Van Pragg, H. M. (1977): On the significance of regional dopamine metabolism in the rat brain for the classification of centrally acting drugs. *Eur. J. Pharmacol.*, 42:179–190.

65. Willow, M., and Caterall, W. A. (1982): Inhibition of binding of [^{3}H]batrachotoxin A 20-α-benzoate to sodium channels by the anticonvulsant drugs diphenylhydantoin and carbamazepine. *Molec. Pharmacol.*, 22:627–635.

66. Willow, M., Gonoi, T., and Catterall, W. A. (1985): Voltage clamp analysis of the inhibitory actions of diphenylhydantoin and carbamazepine on voltage-sensitive sodium channels in neuroblastoma cells. *Molec. Pharmacol.*, 27:549–558.

67. Willow, M., Kuenzel, E. A., and Caterall, W. A. (1984): Inhibition of voltage-sensitive sodium channels in neuroblastoma cells and synaptosomes by the anticonvulsant drugs diphenylhydantoin and carbamazepine. *Molec. Pharmacol.*, 25:228–234.

68. Worley, P. F., and Baraban, J. M. (1987): Site of anticonvulsant action on sodium channels: Autoradiographic and electrophysiological studies in rat brain. *Neurobiol.*, 84:3051–3055.

Antiepileptic Drugs, Third Edition, edited by
R. Levy, R. Mattson, B. Meldrum,
J. K. Penry, and F. E. Dreifuss.
Raven Press, Ltd., New York © 1989.

32

Carbamazepine

Chemistry and Methods of Determination

Henn Kutt

INTRODUCTION

Carbamazepine (Tegretol) was developed in the laboratories of J. R. Geigy AG (Basel, Switzerland) in the late 1950s. Its synthesis was described by Schindler (57) in 1961 (U.S. patent 2,948,718), and its anticonvulsant properties, demonstrated by testing in animals, were reported by Theobald and Kunz (63) in 1963.

Historically, iminodibenzyl (10,11-dihydro-5H-dibenzo(b,f)azepine), shown in Fig. 1A and first described by Thiele and Holzinger (64) in 1899, may be considered the precursor of carbamazepine. Synthesis of a number of iminodibenzyl derivatives was reported by Schindler and Hafliger (58) in 1954. These compounds possessed local anesthetic as well as antihistaminic properties but only modest antiepileptic activity. Considerable anticonvulsant effect, however, occurred when a carbamyl (carboxamide) group was added at the 5 position of iminodibenzyl. The carbamyl side chain combined with iminostilbene (Fig. 1B), a structure analogous to iminodibenzyl but having a double bond between the 10 and 11 positions, showed the strongest anticonvulsant properties and became known as carbamazepine (Fig. 1C). In comparison with the succinimide, hydantoin, barbiturate, and benzodiazepine anticonvulsants, carbamazepine (CBZ) lacks a saturated carbon

atom, and the amide group is in the side chain rather than in the ring. It differs from imipramine only by having a double bond between positions 10 and 11 and by having a shorter side chain.

CHEMISTRY

Carbamazepine (5-carbamyl-5H-dibenzo[b,f]azepine; 5H-dibenzo[b,f]azepine-5-carboxamide) (Fig. 1C) is an iminostilbene derivative with an empirical formula $C^{15}H^{12}N^{20}$ and molecular weight of 236.26. It is a white crystalline compound with a melting point between 190°C and 193°C. Carbamazepine can be prepared by treating iminostilbene with carbonyl chloride followed by the addition of ammonia to a boiling mixture of the latter product in absolute ethanol (57). Carbamazepine behaves as a neutral lipophilic substance; it dissolves in ethanol, chloroform, dichloromethane, and other solvents but is virtually insoluble in water. The solubility in phosphate buffer pH 7.4 is 72 mg/liter. Aqueous solution can be made with propylene glycol in which the solubility is enhanced by moderate heating.

The ultraviolet spectrum of CBZ shows a major peak at around 220 nm and a smaller one at 288 to 290 nm. Acid hydrolysis will result in a major ultraviolet absorption peak at 255 nm. Treatment with perchloric acid

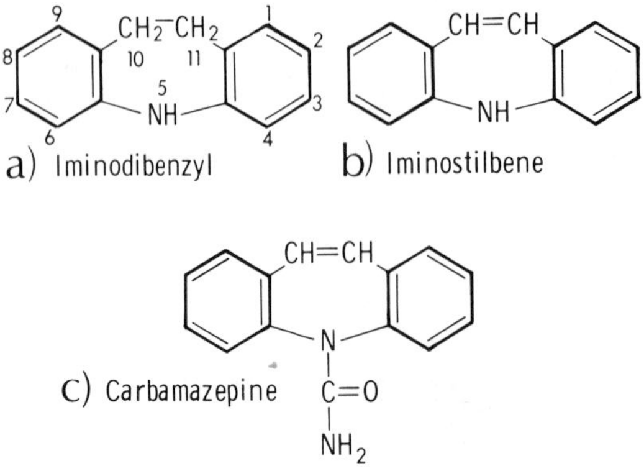

FIG. 1. Carbamazepine and its precursors.

CBZ to imipramine is also obvious in the steric parameters except for the torsion angle which is 20° for imipramine (19).

Separation of the carbamyl group from position 5, yielding iminostilbene, is thought to occur as a result of the action of biotransformation enzymes (16). Breakdown of CBZ to iminostilbene also occurs pyrolytically in the course of gas-liquid chromatography (16,28). Another pyrolysis product of CBZ is 9-methylacridine, shown in Fig. 2C. The pyrolytic breakdown product of CBZ epoxide and CBZ-dihydroxide is 9-acridinecarboxaldehyde (3,16).

The double bond between positions 10 and 11 in the CBZ molecule is somewhat unstable and provides a site of action for the biotransformation enzyme(s) of the epoxidation pathway. The products of this series are CBZ-10,11-dihydro-10,11-epoxide (CBZ-epoxide), (Fig. 2D), and CBZ-*trans*-10,11-dihydro-10-,11-dihydroxide (*trans*-CBZ-diol) (Fig. 2E), and as an end-product of epoxy pathway, 9-hydroxy-methyl-10-carbamoylacridane (9-OH-CBZ) (Fig. 2F). Aromatic hydroxylation also takes place at positions 1, 2, or 3, resulting

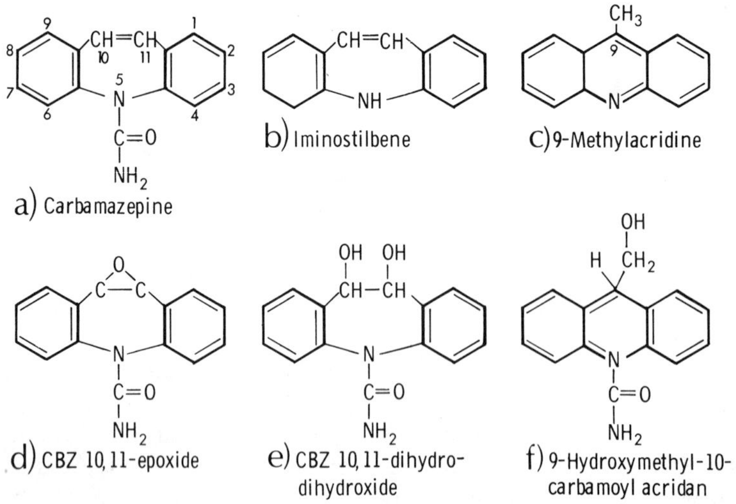

will render CBZ highly fluorescent (excitation max 366 nm, emission max 498 nm). The mass spectrum of CBZ shows a molecular ion at m/e 236 and a base peak at m/e 193 (16,49). Studies of CBZ by X-ray diffraction have revealed that in the three-dimensional structure the angle of flexure alpha is 53°, the angle of annelation beta is 30°, and the angle of torsion gamma is 3°. The distance between the centers of benzene rings measured 4.85 Å. These measurements are characteristic of tricyclic psychoactive drugs, and the similarity of

FIG. 2. Carbamazepine and its metabolites and breakdown products.

in OH-carbamazepines as well as the catechols at these positions (3,13,14).

The pharmacologically active CBZ epoxide is found in blood in concentrations 10% to 50% of that of CBZ, and the inactive *trans*-CBZ-diol concentrations in blood exceed those of CBZ-epoxide. The presumably inactive 2-OH-CBZ and 3-OH-CBZ appear in blood only in trace amounts. The *trans*-CBZ-diol is the major urinary endproduct constituting up to 50% of the dose, whereas 2-OH-CBZ, 3-OH-CBZ, and 9-OH-CBZ make up each 3% to 6% of the dose (3,13).

METHODS OF DETERMINATION

Various techniques have been used to determine the concentration of CBZ in biological fluids. These include: (a) ultraviolet spectrophotometry; (b) spectrophotometry in the visible light spectrum; (c) fluorometry, often combined with thin-layer chromatography; (d) gas-liquid chromatography; (e) immunoassays: enzyme-mediated immunoassay technique, fluorescence polarization immunoassay, substrate labeled fluorescence immunoassay; and (f) high-pressure liquid chromatography.

Sample Handling and Storage

CBZ and CBZ epoxide are relatively stable in clinical materials. Early decay was seen only in putrefied samples. Short time storage for days or a week at room temperature is safe as is longer storage for weeks or a month at 4°C or several months at −20°C. In samples kept at room temperature for 2 months, CBZ epoxide was reduced by 50% but CBZ was still essentially unchanged (41). Therefore, when mailing a sample to the laboratory it is not necessary to pack it in dry ice or refrigerate. Refrigeration for short-term storage serves mainly to deter bacterial growth.

Serum and plasma are both suitable study materials. Whole blood also can be used, but a correction factor (approximately 1.1) is necessary to make the result comparable to plasma and serum.

Ultraviolet Spectrophotometry

Historically, ultraviolet (UV) spectrophotometry of solvent extract was the earliest technique for measuring CBZ (18). Absorbance of untreated CBZ is measured at the secondary absorption peak of 290 nm or 288 nm rather than at the maximum absorbance peak of 220 nm to eliminate major interference from other common anticonvulsants, which have maximum absorption in the range of 220 nm but considerably less in the 290 nm range. Heating the starting material with hydrochloric acid shifted the 290-nm absorption peak to 255-nm but increased the specific extinction fivefold by formation of 9-methylacridine (4).

Spectrophotometry in the Visible Light Spectrum

A spectrophotometric method in which the measurement is carried out at 400 nm was developed in the Geigy laboratory by Herrmann in 1966 (23). Carbamazepine was extracted by neutral pH with dichloroethane and then treated with sodium nitrite and nitric acid. A yellow product formed. Since the metabolites of CBZ will also give a yellow color with this method, the measurement represents the sum total of CBZ and the metabolites.

Fluorometry

Fluorometric determination of CBZ and its metabolites has usually been employed in combination with thin-layer chromatography (TLC) (7). Biological materials (cerebrospinal fluid, plasma, urine, bile) or their dichloroethane extracts were applied to silica plates, which were then developed with carbon tetrachloride: methanol (7:1). The spots were visualized under UV light, scraped off, and eluted with 70% perchloric acid followed by heating at 120°C for 20 min. The resulting fluorescence was determined with a fluorescence spectrometer using excitation wavelength of 358 nm and emission wavelength of 498 nm (29).

Gas-Liquid Chromatography

Gas-liquid chromatography (GLC) has been one of the methods widely used for CBZ determination, as it offers high specificity and sensitivity. Numerous GLC techniques have been described, which indicates the difficulties of finding an ideal procedure. Some of the methods measure only the parent compound (28,49,51), but others measure both the parent compound and its epoxy metabolite (46,52,67). Still others allow simultaneous determination of other antiepileptic drugs from the same sample preparation and application (53,56). The combination of GLC with mass spectrometry (GC/MS selected ion monitoring) extends the sensitivity of the procedure to the low nanogram range for CBZ determination (49,67,68).

The major problem in the GLC method is that CBZ tends to decompose to various extents at the high temperatures necessary for gas chromatography. To deal with this problem, the following approaches have been used: (a) formation of a stable derivative of CBZ (2), (b) creation of conditions under which it is hoped that complete and reproducible breakdown takes place and then measurement of the breakdown product, e.g., iminostilbene (56); (c) creation of conditions that prevent or minimize the breakdown of underivatized CBZ in the gas chromatograph (46).

Formation of a Stable Derivative of CBZ Prior to Gas Chromatography

In the method of Kupferberg (28), cyheptamide was used as an internal standard and the plasma samples were extracted at pH 7.2 with chloroform. The final extract containing CBZ was dried and reacted with TRI-SIL/BSA in pyridine or Regisil. The column packing was OV-17. In this technique, it is important to remove phenytoin prior to derivatization and chromatography, since it has a retention time similar to that of cyheptamide. Least et al. (32) used benzylmalonate methylester monoamide (BMMA) as internal standard and Regis silylation mix to form stable derivatives. Most of the major antiepileptic drugs could be determined simultaneously by this technique, using OV-17 as column packing.

Perchalski and Wilder (51) also used cyheptamide as internal standard. The plasma sample was extracted and then derivatized with dimethylformamide dimethylacetal. Millner and Taber (43) used the same system for derivatization but used benzamide as internal standard and OV-1 as column packing. The advantage of this modification is that the derivatized internal standard remains stable longer. A recent modification of an analogous technique reported by Bathia (2) employs dimethylformamide diethylacetal.

In the method of Gerardin et al. (20), 10-methoxycarbamazepine was used as internal standard. The alkalinized sample was extracted with ethyl ether, evaporated to dryness, and treated with triethylamine and trifluoroacetic anhydride to dehydrate CBZ into stable CBZ cyanamide which was then injected into the gas chromatograph in carbon disulfide.

Conversion of CBZ to Iminostilbene

Measuring iminostilbene as a representative of CBZ was utilized by Roger et al.

(56). Solvent extract of antiepileptic drugs including CBZ, to which 5-(p-methyl-phenyl)-5-phenylhydantoin (MPPH) is added as internal standard and which has been purified by hexane washings, is dried and reconstituted in trimethylphenylammonium hydroxide (TMPAH). This effects methylation of phenytoin, phenobarbital, and primidone, if present, and leads to nearly complete breakdown of CBZ in the column packed with OV-17. Iminostilbene is the major product and, other conditions such as the speed of injection being stable, the iminostilbene peak is reasonably proportional to CBZ concentration.

This technique has been used successfully for the determination of anticonvulsants, including CBZ, in clinical material in our laboratory using a gas chromatograph equipped with an automatic liquid sampler. One of the limitations of this technique under our operating conditions is relatively low sensitivity, as the response with CBZ concentrations of less than 1 μg/ml is not linear and CBZ epoxide is not measured by this technique.

Gas-Liquid Chromatography of Underivatized CBZ

The technique of Morselli et al. (46) required daily silanization of the column. A dichloroethane extract of the sample, with N-desmethyldiazepam as an internal marker, was reconstituted in acetone and injected into the gas chromatograph. The column was packed with 3% OV-17 and operated at 250°C. This procedure allows measurement of CBZ and its epoxide. It has been ascertained by mass spectrometry that CBZ appears as such rather than as the breakdown product. With their technique, Pynnönen et al. (52) also measure CBZ and its epoxide.

Other column packings used for CBZ determination without derivatization are SP 2510 DA or a mixture of SP 2510 DA and SP 2110 (65), and DL-LSX-3-0295, among others. The breakdown of CBZ with these packings is not thought to be extensive, and reasonable accuracy and reproducibility can be achieved. All allow determination of other major antiepileptic drugs simultaneously with CBZ, but not the CBZ epoxide.

Selected Ion Monitoring

The GC/MS method of Palmer et al. (49) provided high sensitivity. A linear response was seen with amounts as low as 0.05 μg/ml. As internal standard, 10,11-dihydrocarbamazepine was used in part because it breaks down at the same rate as CBZ. Samples extracted with ethyl acetate were injected into a short (35 cm) column packed with 5% SE-52 and maintained at 210°C. An LKB 9000 gas chromatograph-mass spectrometer equipped with a multiple ion detector adjusted to record the intensity of the molecular ion of carbamazepine (m/e 236) and dihydrocarbamazepine (m/e 238) was used. The peak height ratios of m/e 236 and m/e 238 were calculated and plotted against CBZ concentration. The CBZ epoxide was not measured by this technique.

Using [9-13C]carboxyacridine and [10-13C]-5-H-dibenz[b,f]azepine as internal standard, Trager et al. (67) applied selected ion monitoring (SIM) to the determination of both CBZ and CBZ epoxide. Pantrotto et al. (50) also measured CBZ and the epoxide. Permethylated metabolites of CBZ were determined by GC/MS by Lynn et al. (34). Truscott et al. (68) used direct chemical ionization mass spectrometry without gas chromatography for determination of CBZ simultaneously with other antiepileptic drugs.

Immunoassays

The immunoassays are widely used for monitoring CBZ levels in clinical practice

in part because they require less complicated apparatus than is needed for gas-liquid or high-pressure liquid chromatography, and because the new automated
immunoassay instruments are relatively
simple to operate (40). The assay time is
usually short: a few to 25 mins, and only 50
to 100 μl of sample is needed. On the minus
side, adverse conditions such as hemolysis,
lipemia, and bilirubinemia may reduce the
validity of results with some systems (59).
There are no reagents presently specific to
CBZ epoxide or other metabolites. The antibodies generated to be specific to CBZ
crossreact with the metabolites, notably
CBZ epoxide to various extent in ratios of
6:1 to 10:1 (8,45). This adds relatively little
to the reading in patients receiving monotherapy and having CBZ epoxide concentrations 10% to 15% of the parent compound.
In patients who receive other drugs which
may cause CBZ epoxide levels to rise to up
to 50% of CBZ's, the error is greater. The
overestimation becomes sizable with very
high levels occurring with CBZ overdose
(10). Nevertheless, it is felt generally that
CBZ levels measured by immunoassays are
adequate for clinical management and therapeutic monitoring of patients (40). The
error caused by the crossreactivity becomes a problem when measuring free (nonprotein-bound) CBZ in clinical samples because low binding of CBZ epoxide (see
section on measuring free CBZ, pps. 465
and 466).

The currently popular and practical immunoassays are: (a) enzyme-mediated immunoassay technique (EMIT) developed by
the Syva Co., Palo Alta, California; (b) substrate-labeled fluorescence immunoassay
developed by Ames Division, Miles Laboratories, Indianapolis Indiana; and (c) fluorescence polarization immunoassay (TDx
developed by Abbott Laboratories, North
Chicago, Illinois). Non- or minimal-instru-
mental procedures potentially usable in office that utilize antibody-treated strips are
being developed.

Enzyme-Mediated Immunoassay Technique

EMIT was the groundbreaker in the im
munomethodology for antiepileptic drugs.
It utilizes antibodies grown in sheep im-
munized with CBZ-protein complex. The
antibodies are reacted with CBZ in the test
material (plasma, serum, cerebrospinal
fluid, saliva, tears), and the amount of drug-
antibody complex is indicated by an enzyme (glucose-6-phosphate dehydrogenase) and substrate (glucose-6-phosphate)
reaction, which in turn is quantitated by
measuring spectrophotometrically the rate
of a cofactor (NAD) utilization (59).

The earlier instrumentation consisted of
a spectrophotometer, a semiautomatic pi-
pettor-dilutor, and a calculator-printer. The
manipulative steps consisted of placing the
sample into a mixing cuvette with the pipettor, adding reagent A (antibody) and reagent B (enzyme), and aspirating the mixture into the spectrophotometer. The NAD
utilization rate was followed for 30 sec. The
unknown sample concentration was then interpolated from the previously constructed
calibration curve. Samples with high concentrations need to be diluted and reas-
sayed. For assaying very low concentration, dilute calibrators are available.

The more recent apparatus is nearly fully
automated and reduces the manipulative
steps to placing some sample into cuvettes
and setting the tray with cuvettes as well as
the reagents into the instrument. Thus
EMIT assay is basically rapid (2–3 min for
a single assay) and requires small amounts
of test material (50 μl or less). The disadvantages are that hemolyzed, icteric, or lipemic plasma samples tend to give erroneous results and need to be analyzed by
other techniques (59). There are no immu-
noreagents specific to CBZ epoxide only;
and the crossreactivity hampers the validity
to some extent, particularly in the estimations of unbound CBZ.

Substrate-Labeled Fluorescence Immunoassay

In the substrate-labeled fluorescence immunoassay (SLFIA) an enzyme-substrate reaction mediates the quantitation (47). In the system presented by Ames Division of Miles Laboratories there are three main reagents: (a) a combination of a fluorescent compound with a sugar and CBZ covalently bound in which the fluorescence is masked until the sugar is cleaved off; (b) antibodies reactive to CBZ; and (c) sugar-cleaving enzyme. In performing the assay, study material is first reacted with the antibody reagent (b) and some of the antibody binds with CBZ if the latter was present. Reagent A is then added and the remaining antibody binds with the CBZ which is incorporated into Reagent A; but a portion of Reagent A molecules (equal to the amount of CBZ in study material) remains free from the antibody. Adding now the cleaving enzyme reagent (c) will remove the sugar from the free Reagent A unmasking the fluorescence. The fluorescence is read in fluorometer and values calculated from standard curves. Several of these steps are automated.

Fluorescence Polarization Immunoassay

In the fluorescence polarization immunoassays (FPIA), of which the prototype is TDx, (TM)) the antibody-antigen complex directly influences the readout and quantitation (25,47). The main reagents in this system are (a) fluorescent-labeled CBZ (tracer) and (b) the antibody reactive to CBZ. After the tracer binds with antibody in the reaction cuvette, the rotation of the fluorophore becomes limited and linearly polarized light will have a greater effect on the receiving photocell. In the free tracer the molecules rotate and are randomly oriented and the emitted light is depolarized reducing the read out. The tracer competes with CBZ of the study sample for the antibody, thus in the reaction mixture the amount of unbound tracer is parallel to the amount of CBZ in the sample. Standards with known amounts are used to construct a curve from the polarization readouts and the concentration of the unknown is interpolated.

Performing the assay with the TDx system consists of placing a few drops of study material into sample cuvettes and placing the carouselle with cuvettes as well as the reagent package into the automatic analyzer which will give readouts in about 20 min. The antibody crossreacts with CBZ epoxide, but the system is not greatly influenced by hemolysis, lipemia, and bilirubin.

Non- or Minimal-Instrumental Immunoassays

Acculevel by Syntex Medical Diagnostics is based on enzyme immunopaper chromatography. A paperstrip coated with antibodies is placed into developing solution that contains enzyme-labeled CBZ as well as the sample of 13 µl of whole blood. CBZ migrates up and the height of the column is proportional to the amount of CBZ in the sample. The column is visualized by developing a blue color. Assay time is about 20 min and the results are found to compare favorably with other immunomethods (9).

An immuno-spot test for CBZ (Spectralyser ARIS) employs an antibody-treated strip upon with 10 µl of whole blood or plasma is placed. The spot is treated to develop color which is then eluted and read in a colorimeter. The results could be used in clinical monitoring (48).

High-Pressure Liquid Chromatography

High-pressure liquid chromatography (HPLC) is the most practical overall method for the determination of CBZ and its metabolites. It circumvents the problems of thermal instability of these compounds inherent in GLC and usually requires less elaborate sample preparation than is necessary for GC/MS. It is free of the problems of crossreactivity associated with the immunoassays.

The early HPLC methods concentrated on measuring CBZ and a reference internal standard, often another drug such as a benzodiazepine, that was unlikely to be taken when CBZ was prescribed. In the later techniques the metabolites were measured along with the parent-compound and in some modifications, other antiepileptic drugs were measured simultaneously as well. For internal standard, nondrug chemicals are used in the more recently reported HPLC techniques.

In most practical methods, CBZ and the metabolites are extracted with dichloroethane or -methane. The selected pH at extraction determines whether other drugs are also recovered. Slightly acid pH (5 or 6) allows recovery of most other weak acids such as phenobarbital and phenytoin, whereas modestly alkaline pH is used when CBZ and metabolites alone are desired. Such preselection is practiced to avoid other drug peaks interfering with CBZ. The interfering peaks can sometimes be shifted by slight modifications in the formula of the mobile phase by increasing or decreasing the concentration of the organic component or altering the ionic concentration of the aqueous component (buffer). Reversed-phase techniques using C-8 or C-18 column packings have been the most successful applications. The chromatograms are usually monitored with UV detectors set at 210 or 254 nm.

Methods for Measuring CBZ and CBZ Epoxide

One of the early practical methods was described by Eichelbaum and Bertilsson (12) for measuring both CBZ and its epoxide. Purified sample extract dissolved in mobile phase was injected into the chromatograph equipped with a column packed with Durapak Carbowax 400 Corasil. The mobile phase was n-hexane-dichloromethane-dimethyl sulfoxide, and the UV detector was set at 254 nm. At that wavelength, the detector response to CBZ epoxide, which lacks the double bond between positions 10 and 11, was more than 10 times less than the response to the parent compound, which necessitated resetting of sensitivity when the epoxide eluted. As the internal standard, 10,11-dihydrocarbamazepine (CBZ-H_2) was used. Other antiepileptic drugs needed to be removed, as they would interfere with the internal standard and the epoxide.

MacKichan (35) used lorazepam and nordiazepam for internal standards and measured both CBZ and CBZ epoxide, but other drugs were excluded by alkaline extraction. The column was Bondapak-CN and mobile phase consisted of acetonitril:water 30:70. Similar procedures were described by Chan (5) and Grasela and Rocci (21) except for using C-18 packing in the analytical column. In a procedure thought to be particularly suitable for determination of CBZ and CBZ epoxide in saliva, Hoogewigs and Massart (24) used octylsulphate as counter-ion in ion-pair extraction and a CN column for chromatography.

Methods for Measuring CBZ without Metabolites but with Other Drugs

In the method of Adams and Vandermark (1), phenacetin was used as internal standard. Column packing was ODS-Sil XI, and the mobile phase was acetonitrile:water. Most major antiepileptic drugs were determined simultaneously with CBZ, but CBZ epoxide was not. Similar reversed-phase techniques have been reported by Helmsing et al. (22), Kabra et al. (26), and Soldin and Hill (61), among others, again measuring other drugs simultaneously but not the metabolites. Recently, a technique was reported by Messina (42) in which an electrochemical detector was used to monitor the chromatogram, and imipramine and doxepine could be measured along with CBZ but not the CBZ epoxide.

Methods for Measuring CBZ, CBZ Epoxide, and Other Drugs

The method reported by Westenberg and De Zeeuw (69) used nitrazepam as the internal standard and Li Chrosorb SI 100 as column packing. The mobile phase was tetrahydrofuran in dichloromethane. Carbamazepine and its epoxide, along with other antiepileptic drugs, could be measured.

Methods for Measuring CBZ, CBZ Epoxide, trans-CBZ-diol

A multipurpose technique was described by Meatherall and Ford (38) in which CBZ, CBZ epoxide, and *trans*-CBZ-diol are measured along with other antiepileptic drugs, and by slightly modifying the conditions, hypnotic barbiturates and some antibiotics can also be assayed. Extraction pH is 6.8, column Supelco C-1 and mobile phase consists of methanol:acetonitrile:phosphate buffer in ratio of 17.5:17.5:5.65. Paramethyl phenobarbital, a nondrug, serves as internal standard.

Another newly reported procedure by Chelberg et al. (6) is well suited for measuring CBZ, CBZ epoxide, *trans*-CBZ-diol, and 2-OH-CBZ and 3-OH-CBZ. The compounds are extracted from plasma with methyl-butyl-ether at alkaline pH to exclude interference by other antiepileptic drugs. The analytical column is C-18 and mobile phase consists of acetonitrile:water 28:72. With a flow rate of 2.0 ml/min, the compounds of interest elute within 10 min. Recoveries are reported 85% to 95% for hydroxy compounds and 100% for CBZ and CBZ epoxide. For measuring metabolites in

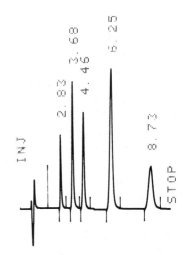

FIG. 3. HPLC tracing of carbamazepine and its metabolites. Peak 2.83 is *trans*-CBZ-diol, peak 3.68 is CBZ epoxide, peak 4.46 is alphenal (IS-1), peak 6.25 is *p*-tolyl-phenobarbital (IS-2), and peak 8.78 is CBZ. Column C-18, mobile phase methanol:0.1 molar H2KPO4:triethylamine 45:55:0.01. UV 210 nm, AUFs 0.1. Drug concentration 10 mg/l.

urine, the sample is first hydrolyzed with β-glucuronidase.

House Method

A versatile procedure for CBZ and metabolites as well as other antiepileptic drugs used in our laboratory is a modification of a procedure illustrated in a sales catalog of Supelco (Catalog #26, 1988, p. 160). Our main column is 7.5 cm long packed with 3 micron Supelcosil C-8. Mobile phase is methanol:0.1 molar KH2PO4:triethylamine (45:55:0.01). With a flow rate of 1.2 ml/min, CBZ elutes in 8 min, CBZ epoxide in 4, and *trans*-CBZ-diol in 3 min. Two nondrug internal standards are used: alphenal (IS-1) and para-tolyl-phenobarbital (IS-2); the latter is used for calculations (see Fig. 3). Phenylethylmalonamide and primidone elute in less than 2 min, phenobarbital shortly before CBZ epoxide, and phenytoin between CBZ and IS-2. The 2-OH-CBZ elutes between CBZ epoxide and pheno-barbitol and 3-OH-CBZ shortly after the IS-1. The UV detector is set at 210 nm, Absorption Units Fullscale (AUFs) 0.1; 0.05 if low concentrations are measured. Usually 0.1 ml of plasma is extracted with dichloromethane at pH 5.0, evaporated to dryness and reconstituted for injection with 20 µl. Mobile phase is recirculated. The exact concentration of methanol in the mobile phase is empirically adjusted with new column and readjusted as the column ages.

Techniques for Measuring CBZ Metabolites in Urine

Measuring CBZ metabolites in urine usually starts with liberating the conjugates by hydrolyzing an aliquot of acidified urine a few hours or overnight with β-glucuronidase. The neutralized hydrolysate is then extracted with a polar solvent for chromatography. In the Robbins et al. procedure (55) the urine was hydrolyzed for 1 to 4 hr and extracted with ethyl acetate. The analytical column was C-8 using acetonitrile:water as mobile phase. They found that *trans*-CBZ-diol was stable at least for 20 days stored at −20°C. In the method of Chelberg et al. (6), urine samples were hydrolyzed overnight and extracted with methyl-butyl-ether. A C-18 column was used for separation with 2-methyl-CBZ as internal standard; *trans*-CBZ-diol, 2-OH-CBZ, and 3-OH-CBZ were assayed.

Measuring CBZ Metabolites

Measuring active CBZ metabolite is generally helpful when evaluating unexpected clinical responses in CBZ therapy caused, for example, by accumulation of CBZ epoxide. Measuring the inactive metabolites may contribute to understanding the mechanisms of drug–drug interactions or changes of CBZ kinetics from other causes. Measuring the metabolites is also useful in balance studies and in evaluations of bioavailability.

CBZ Epoxide

The need to measure CBZ epoxide concentrations has been emphasized by several investigators (3,13). Its antiepileptic activity is nearly equal to that of the parent compound in animal testing (15). CBZ epoxide was also shown to suppress pain in patients with trigeminal neuralgia (66) and was observed to contribute to carbamazepine intoxication in patients (30,39). CBZ epoxide concentration in human plasma usually ranges from 10% to 20% in monotherapy and 20% to 50% of that of CBZ in some polytherapy combinations (3). Inducing drugs (phenytoin, phenobarbital) increase the percent of CBZ epoxide relative to CBZ by mostly reducing CBZ concentrations while variable but smaller change occurs in CBZ epoxide. Drugs reducing CBZ epoxide clearance such as valproate (31), progabide (30), and particularly valpromide (39) can markedly increase CBZ epoxide but change CBZ concentration little if any. This phenomenon has caused signs and symptoms of CBZ intoxication with unchanged, previously well-tolerated CBZ levels in epileptic patients after addition of the interacting drug (30,31,39).

As indicated in the preceding descriptions of assay techniques, several GLC and HPLC methods measure both the parent compound and the epoxide. The GLC or GC/MS SIM methods measuring both compounds include those of Trager et al. (67), and Pantrotto et al. (50). The HPLC techniques measuring CBZ and its epoxide are those of Eichenbaum and Bertilsson (12), Westenberg and De Zeeuw (69), MacKichan (35), Chan (5), Grasela and Hill (21), Meatherall and Ford (38), and Chelberg et al. (6) among others. The immunoassays currently do not measure CBZ epoxide separately. An attempt to use the immuno system to measure CBZ epoxide was described by Sidki et al. (60). The total of immunoreactive material was determined first; then a second sample of the same source was treated with acid to destroy the immunoreactivity of CBZ epoxide and the remaining immunoreactive material assayed. Theoretically, the difference represented CBZ epoxide concentration of the sample.

Trans-*CBZ-Diol and 2,3,9-Hydroxy Metabolites*

Trans-CBZ-diol is considered to be pharmacologically inactive, it occurs in plasma in concentrations somewhat exceeding those of CBZ epoxide, and it constitutes the major end product of the epoxy pathway; thus it serves as a marker for the changes in epoxy pathway due to interactions or changes in bioavailability. In the urine 20% to 30% of the dose appears as *trans*-CBZ-diol during monotherapy whereas 50% to 60% is seen in polytherapy. The 2-, 3-, and 9-OH-CBZ occur in the blood only in trace amounts but are found in urine representing 6%, 9%, and 5% of the dose, respectively, during monotherapy with somewhat smaller proportions during polytherapy. This suggests that induction affects mostly the epoxy pathway (3,13,14). Methods that measure *trans*-CBZ-diol in plasma include Meatherall and Ford's (38), Chelberg's et al. (6), and our house method, among others. For urinary *trans*-CBZ-diol, the procedure of Robbins et al. (55), and Chelberg's et al. (6) modification for urine are applicable.

Measuring Free (Nonprotein-bound) CBZ and CBZ Epoxide

The concentration of unbound CBZ ranges from 70% to 80% of the total plasma CBZ and unbound CBZ epoxide is approximately 50% of the total plasma CBZ epoxide in the majority of patients. Arguments in favor of measuring free CBZ include that observing variations in the free fraction might contribute to insight for intra- and interindividual variations in the clinical response with similar total concentration (3,62). Furthermore, the free fraction has been shown to be increased by displacement by strongly binding drugs such as valproate (37). Reduced binding is expected to occur in hepatic or renal disease to some extent. Generally, however, the need for free CBZ and CBZ epoxide determination in clinical management of epileptic patients has not been found compelling (3,17,62). The main interest in assaying free CBZ and CBZ epoxide lies in research of basic mechanisms in pharmacokinetics and drug–drug interactions.

Estimating the unbound fractions has been performed with the help of equilibrium dialysis or with ultrafiltration. Some investigators have offered saliva levels as indicators of free CBZ (27,36) (see also p. 466). For critical work with free CBZ and CBZ epoxide, however, currently the most practical technique is to generate ultrafiltrate from clinical plasma samples with a commercially available device that contains YMT filter membrane such as Centrifree by Amicon Corporation. Parenthetically, improved filter and membrane design has essentially eliminated problems with protein leaks or clogged filters seen in earlier years. Low force/speed centrifugation 1,000 to 2,000xg (about 1,500 rpm) for 15 min is best to avoid heating samples in centrifuge. For best reproducibility it is essential to use the same centrifuge setting and even the same instrument. The quantitation is best performed chromatographically using some HPLC method that measures both the parent compound and the metabolites and is set to cover low concentrations. These include the MacKichan (35), Chan (5), Grasela and Rocci (21), and Chelberg et al. (6) procedures, among others. Immunomethods are less suitable for reliable quantitation because the crossreactivity with CBZ epoxide as the latter occurs in disproportionally higher concentration in the ultrafiltrate as a result of its lower binding. Levy et al. (33) have shown that ultrafiltrate from clinical samples assayed with EMIT reagents gave values on the average 16% higher than GC-MS; EMIT overestimations up to 35% have been observed by others (8).

Measuring CBZ in Saliva

Measurements of CBZ in saliva have shown that the CBZ concentration is considerably lower than in plasma but somewhat higher than the unbound CBZ concentration in plasma (5,36). In a study by Knott and Reynolds (27), saliva content of CBZ was 25% of plasma CBZ levels in patients on monotherapy and 29% in those receiving other drugs as well, while the CBZ concentration in ultrafiltrate was 21% of plasma levels. Quite high values were observed when the saliva samples were collected soon after ingestion of CBZ (11). The overestimation generally is greater when quantitation is made using immunoassays. Additional factors contributing to the content of CBZ in saliva in excess of the unbound fraction in plasma are that saliva is a complex fluid consisting of glandular secretions that include mucus and proteins as well as tooth crevice fluid and some inflammatory gingival exudate with plasma protein leakage.

Before starting collection of saliva for CBZ determination, it is important to rinse the mouth very thoroughly since residues from recent ingestion of tablets, and crushed tablets or suspension in children, may persist in the mouth for an hour or longer (11). Saliva flow can be stimulated by chewing paraffin or with citric acid. The sample should be centrifuged at speeds of 3,500 rpm and the clear supernatant analyzed. The managing physician will benefit from knowing whether the sample was assayed by immunoassay or chromatography.

Measuring CBZ in Tears

Concentration of CBZ in tears has been mentioned by some investigators as an approximation of free CBZ concentration (44). Tears are easily available even from the very young, but may be contaminated by conjunctival irritation or infections; and some concentration of the ingredients invariably takes place through evaporation. The tear data may be useful in clinical management if other materials for measuring CBZ concentration are not available. Sensitive chromatographic methods or immunoassays would be used for quantitation.

CONVERSION

Carbamazepine

Conversion factor:

$$CF = \frac{1000}{\text{mol. wt.}} = \frac{1000}{236.3} = 4.23$$

Conversion:

$$(\mu g/ml) \times 4.23 = (\mu moles/liter)$$

$$(\mu moles/liter) \div 4.23 = (\mu g/ml)$$

Carbamazepine-10,11-epoxide

Conversion factor:

$$CF = \frac{1000}{\text{mol. wt.}} = \frac{1000}{252.3} = 3.96$$

Conversion:

$$(\mu g/ml) \times 3.96 = (\mu moles/liter)$$

$$(\mu moles/liter) \div 3.96 = (\mu g/ml)$$

REFERENCES

1. Adams, R. F., and Vandermark, F. L. (1976): Simultaneous high-pressure liquid-chromatographic determination of some anticonvulsants in serum. *Clin. Chem.*, 22:25–31.
2. Bathia, H. M. (1986): Improved gas-chromato-

graphic determination of carbamazepine. *Clin. Chem.*, 32:563–564.

3. Bertilsson, L., and Tomson, T. (1986): Clinical pharmacokinetics and pharmacological effects of carbamazepine and carbamazepine-10,11-epoxide: An update. *Clin. Pharmacokinet.*, 11:177–198.

4. Beyer, K. H., Bredenstein, O., and Schenck, G. (1971): Isolierung und Identifizierung eines Carbamazepine Reaktionproduktes. *Arzneim. Forsch.*, 1:1033–1034.

5. Chan, K. (1985): Simultaneous determination of carbamazepine and carbamazepine-10,11-epoxide metabolite in plasma and urine by high-performance liquid chromatography. *J. Chromat.*, 342:341–347.

6. Chelberg, R. D., Gunawan, S., Treiman, D. M. (1988): Simultaneous high-performance liquid chromatographic determination of carbamazepine and its principal metabolites in human plasma and urine. *Ther. Drug Monit.* 110:188–193.

7. Christiansen, J. (1973): Assay of carbamazepine and metabolites in plasma by quantitative thin-layer chromatography. In: *Methods of Analysis of Anti-Epileptic Drugs*, edited by J. W. A. Meijer, H. Meinardi, C. Gardner-Thorpe, and E. van der Kleijn, pp. 87–90. Excerpta Medica, Amsterdam.

8. Contin, M., Riva, R., Albani, F., Perucca, E., and Baruzzi, A. (1985): Determination of total and free plasma carbamazepine concentrations by enzyme multiplied immunoassay: Interference with the 10,11-epoxide metabolite. *Ther. Drug Monit.*, 7:46–50.

9. Cramer, J., Toftness, B., Massey, K., Phelps, S., Denio, L., and Drake, M. (1987): Carbamazepine whole blood/plasma ratio determined by a non-instrumental assay. *Epilepsia*, 28:580.

10. Deng, J. F., Shipe, J. R. J., Rogol, A. D., Donowitz, L., and Spyker, D. A. (1986): Carbamazepine toxicity: Comparison of measurements of drug levels by HPLC and EMIT and model of carbamazepine kinetics. *J. Toxicol. Clin. Toxicol.*, 34:281–294.

11. Dickinson, R. G., Hooper, W. D., King, A. R., and Eadie, M. J. (1985): Fallacious results from measuring salivary carbamazepine concentrations. *Ther. Drug Monit.*, 7:41–45.

12. Eichelbaum, M., and Bertilsson, L. (1975): Determination of carbamazepine and its epoxide metabolite in plasma by high-speed liquid chromatography. *J. Chromatogr.*, 103:135–140.

13. Eichelbaum, M., Tomson, T., Tybring, G., and Bertilsson, L. (1985): Carbamazepine metabolism in man. Induction and pharmacogenetic aspects. *Clin. Pharmacokinet.*, 10:80–90.

14. Faigle, J. W., Brechbuhler, S., Feldmann, K. F., and Richter, W. J. (1976): The biotransformation of carbamazepine. In: *Epileptic Seizures—Behaviour—Pain*, edited by W. Birkmayer, pp. 127–140. Huber Publishers, Bern.

15. Faigle, J. W., Feldmann, K. F., and Baltzer, V. (1977): Anticonvulsant effect of carbamazepine. An attempt to distinguish between the potency of the parent drug and its epoxide metabolite. In: *Antiepileptic Drug Monitoring*, edited by C. Gardner-Thorpe, D. Janz, H. Meinardi, and C. E. Pippenger, pp. 104–109. Pitman Medical, Tunbridge Wells, Kent.

16. Frigerio, A., and Morselli, P. L. (1975): Carbamazepine: Biotransformation. In: *Complex Partial Seizures and Their Treatment*, edited by J. K. Penry and D. D. Daly, pp. 295–308. Raven Press, New York.

17. Fröscher, W., Burr, W., Penin, H., Vohl, J., Bulau, P., and Kreiten, K. (1985): Free level monitoring of carbamazepine and valproic acid: Clinical significance. *Clin. Neuropharmacol.*, 8:362–371.

18. Fuhr, J. (1964): Untersuchungen uber die Vertraglichkeit und Ausscheidung eines neuartiges Antiepilepticums. *Arzneim. Forsch.*, 14:74–75.

19. Gagneux, A. R. (1976): The chemistry of carbamazepine. In: *Epileptic Seizures—Behaviour—Pain*, edited by W. Birkmayer, pp. 120–126. Huber Publishers, Bern.

20. Gerardin, A., Abadie, F., and Laffont, J. (1975): GLC determination of carbamazepine suitable for pharmacokinetic studies. *J. Pharm. Sci.*, 64:1940–1942.

21. Grasela, D. M., and Rocci, M. L., Jr. (1984): Liquid chromatographic microassay for carbamazepine and its 10,11-epoxide in plasma. *J. Pharm. Sci.*, 73:1874–1875.

22. Helmsing, P. J., van der Woude, J., and van Eupen, O. M. (1978): A micromethod for simultaneous estimation of blood levels of some commonly used antiepileptic drugs. *Clin. Chim. Acta*, 89:301–309.

23. Herrmann, B. (1966): *Tegretol G 32883 Determination in Serum, Plasma and CSF.* Geigy Pharmaceuticals, Ardsley, New York.

24. Hoogewigs, G., and Massart, D. L. (1984): Development of a standardized analysis strategy for basic drugs, using ion-pair extraction and high-pressure liquid chromatography. VI. Drug level determination in saliva. *J. Chromat.*, 309:329–337.

25. Jolley, M. E., Stroupe, S. D., Wang, C. H. J., Panas, H. N., Keegan, C. L., Schmidt, R. L., and Schwenzer, K. S. (1981): Fluorescence polarization immunoassay. I. Monitoring aminoglycoside antibodies in serum and plasma. *Clin. Chem.*, 27:1190–1197.

26. Kabra, P. M., McDonald, D. M., and Marton, L. J. (1978): A simultaneous high-performance liquid chromatographic analysis of the most common anticonvulsants and their metabolites in serum. *J. Anal. Toxicol.*, 2:127–133.

27. Knott, C., and Reynolds, F. (1984): The place of saliva in antiepileptic drug monitoring. *Ther. Drug Monit.*, 6:35–41.

28. Kupferberg, H. J. (1972): GLC determination of carbamazepine in plasma. *J. Pharm. Sci.*, 61:284–286.

29. Kutt, H. (1975): Carbamazepine: Chemistry and methods of determination. In: *Complex Partial Seizures and Their Treatment*, edited by J. K. Penry and D. D. Daly, pp. 249–261. Raven Press, New York.

30. Kutt, H., Solomon, G. E., Dhar, A. K., Resor,

S. R. Jr., Krall, R. L., and Morselli, P. L. (1984): Effects of progabide on carbamazepine epoxide and carbamazepine concentrations in plasma. *Epilepsia*, 25:674.

31. Kutt, H., Solomon, G., Peterson, H., Dhar, A., Caronna, J. (1985): Accumulation of carbamazepine epoxide caused by valproate contributing to intoxication syndromes. *Neurology*, 35 (Suppl #1):286–287.

32. Least, C. J., Johnson, G. F., and Solomon, H. M. (1975): Therapeutic monitoring of anticonvulsant drugs: Gas-chromatographic simultaneous determination of primidone, phenylethylmalonamide, carbamazepine and diphenylhydantoin. *Clin. Chem.*, 21:1658–1662.

33. Levy, R. H., Friel, P. N., Johno, I., Linthicum, L. M., Colin, L., Koch, K., Raisys, V. A., Wilensky, A. J., and Temkin, N. R. (1984): Filtration for free drug level monitoring: Carbamazepine and valproic acid. *Ther. Drug Monit.*, 6:67–76.

34. Lynn, R. K., Smith, R. G., Thompson, R. M., Deiner, M. L., Griffin, D., and Gerber, N. (1978): Characterization of glucuronide metabolites of carbamazepine in human urine by gas chromatography and mass spectrometry. *Drug Metab. Dispos.*, 6:494–501.

35. MacKichan, J. J. (1980): Simultaneous liquid chromatographic analysis for carbamazepine and carbamazepine-10,11-epoxide in plasma and saliva by use of double internal standardization. *J. Chromatogr.*, 181:373–383.

36. MacKichan, J. J., Duffner, P. K., and Cohen, M. E. (1981): Salivary concentrations and plasma protein binding of carbamazepine and carbamazepine-10,11-epoxide in epileptic patients. *Br. J. Clin. Pharmacol.*, 12:31–37.

37. Mattson, G. F., Mattson, R. H., and Cramer, J. A. (1982): Interaction between valproic acid and c arbamazepine: An in vitro study of protein binding. *Ther. Drug Monit.*, 4:181–184.

38. Meatherall, R., and Ford, D. (1988): Isocratic liquid chromatographic determination of theophylline, acetaminophen, chloramphenicol, caffeine, anticonvulsants and barbiturates in serum. *Ther. Drug Monit.*, 10:101–115.

39. Meijer, J. W. A., Binnie, C. D., Debets, R. M. C., van Parys, J. A. P., and De Beer-Pawlikowski, N. K. B. (1984): Possible hazard of valpromide-carbamazepine combination therapy in epilepsy. *Lancet*, 1:802.

40. Meijer, J. W. A., Rambeck, B., and Riedman, M. (1983): Antiepileptic drug monitoring by chromatographic methods and immunotechniques—Comparison of analytical performance, practicability and economy. *Ther. Drug Monit.*, 5:39–53.

41. Mendez-Alvarez, E., Soto-Otero, R., and Sierra-Marcuno, G. (1986): The effect of storage conditions on the stability of carbamazepine and carbamazepine-10,11-epoxide in plasma. *Clin. Chim. Acta*, 154:243–246.

42. Messina, F. S. (1986): Determination of carbamazepine by HPLC electrochemical detection and application for estimation of imipramine, desipramine, doxepine and nordoxepine. *Alcohol*, 3:135–138.

43. Millner, S. N., and Taber, C. A. (1979): Rapid gas chromatographic determination of carbamazepine for routine therapeutic monitoring. *J. Chromatogr.*, 163:96–102.

44. Monaco, F., Mutiani, R., Mastropaolo, C., and Tondi, M. (1979): Tears as the best practical indicator of the unbound fraction of an anticonvulsant drug. *Epilepsia*, 20:705–710.

45. Monaco, F., and Piredda, S. (1980): Carbamazepine-10,11-epoxide determined by EMIT carbamazepine reagent. *Epilepsia*, 21:475–477.

46. Morselli, P. L., Biandrate, P., Frigerio, A., Gerna, M., and Tognoni, G. (1973): Gas chromatographic determination of carbamazepine and carbamazepine-10,11-epoxide in human body fluids. In: *Methods of Analysis of Anti-Epileptic Drugs*, edited by J. W. A. Meijer, H. Meinardi, C. Gardner-Thorpe, and E. van der Kleijn, pp. 169–175. Excerpta Medica, Amsterdam.

47. Nakamura, R. M. (1983): Advances in analytical fluorescence immunoassays: Methods and clinical application. In: *Clinical Laboratory Assays*, edited by R. M. Nakamura, W. R. Dito, E. S. Tucker III, pp. 33–60. Masson Publishing USA, Inc.

48. Oles, K. S., Penry, J. K., Leppik, I. E., Regan, A., Sheehan, M., and Parker, D. R. (1987): An epoenzyme immunoassay system for carbamazepine. *Epilepsia*, 28:579.

49. Palmer, L., Bertilsson, K., Collste, P., and Rawlins, M. (1973): Quantitative determination of carbamazepine in plasma by mass fragmentography. *Clin. Pharmacol. Ther.*, 15:827–832.

50. Pantrotto, C., Crunelli, V., Lanzoni, J., Frigerio, A., and Quattrone, A. (1979): Quantitative determination of carbamazepine and carbamazepine-10,11-epoxide in rat brain areas by multiple ion detection mass fragmentography. *Anal. Biochem.*, 93:115–123.

51. Perchalski, R. J., and Wilder, B. J. (1974): Rapid gas-liquid chromatographic determination of carbamazepine in plasma. *Clin. Chem.*, 20:492–493.

52. Pynnonen, S., Sillanpaa, M., Frey, H., and Iisalo, E. (1976): Serum concentration of carbamazepine: Comparison of Herrmann's spectrophotometric method and a new GLC method for determination of carbamazepine. *Epilepsia*, 17:67–72.

53. Rambeck, B., and Meijer, J. W. A. (1979): Comprehensive method for the determination of antiepileptic drugs using a novel extraction technique and a fully automated gas chromatography. *Arzneim. Forsch.*, 29:99–103.

54. Riva, R., Contin, M., Albani, F., Perucca, E., Ambrosetto, G., Gobbi, G., Cortelli, P., Procaccianti, G., and Baruzzi, A. (1984): Free and total plasma concentration of carbamazepine and carbamazepine-10,11-epoxide in epileptic patients: Diurnal fluctuation and relationship to side effects. *Ther. Drug Monit.*, 6:408–413.

55. Robbins, D. K., Shih-Ling Chang, Baumann, R. J., and Wedlund, P. J. (1987): Quantitation of *trans*-10,11-dihydroxy-10,11-dihydrocarbamazepine. *J. Chromat.*, 415:208–213.

56. Roger, J. C., Rodgers, G., Jr., and Soo, A. (1973): Simultaneous determination of carbamazepine (Tegretol®) and other anticonvulsants in human plasma by gas-liquid chromatography. *Clin. Chem.*, 19(6):590–592.

57. Schindler, W. (1961): 5H-Dibenz[b,f]azepines. *Chem. Abstr.*, 55:1671.

58. Schindler, W., and Hafliger, F. (1954): Uber Derivate des Iminodibenzyls. *Helv. Chim. Acta*, 37:472–483.

59. Schottelius, D. D. (1978): Homogeneous immunoassay system (EMIT) for quantitation of antiepileptic drugs in biological fluids. In: *Antiepileptic Drugs: Quantitative Analysis and Interpretation*, edited by C. E. Pippenger, J. K. Penry, and H. Kutt, pp. 95–108. Raven Press, New York.

60. Sidki, A. M., Smith, D. S., and Landon, J. (1986): Direct homogeneous phosphoroimmunoassay for carbamazepine in serum. *Clin. Chem.*, 32:53–56.

61. Soldin, S. J., and Hill, J. G. (1976): Rapid micromethod for measuring anticonvulsant drugs in serum by high-performance liquid chromatography. *Clin. Chem.*, 22:856–859.

62. Svensson, C. K., Woodruff, M. N., Baxter, J. G., and Lalka, D. (1986): Free drug concentration monitoring in clinical practice. Rationale and current status. *Clin Pharmacokinet.*, 11:450–469.

63. Theobald, W., and Kunz, H. A. (1963): Zur Pharmacologie des Antiepilepticums 5-Carbamyl-5H-dibenzo[b,f]azepin. *Arzneim. Forsch.*, 13:122–125.

64. Thiele and Holzinger (1899): Cited by W. Schindler and F. Hafliger (reference 58).

65. Thoma, J. J., Ewald, T., and McCoy, M. (1978): Simultaneous analysis of underivatized phenobarbital, carbamazepine, primidone and phenytoin by isothermal gas-liquid chromatography. *J. Anal. Toxicol.*, 2:219–225.

66. Tomson, T., and Bertilsson, L. (1984): Potent therapeutic effect of carbamazepine-10,11-epoxide in trigeminal neuralgia. *Arch. Neurol.*, 41:598–601.

67. Trager, W. F., Levy, H., Patel, I. H., and Neal, J. M. (1978): Simultaneous analysis of carbamazepine and carbamazepine-10,11-epoxide by GC/CI/MS stable isotope methodology. *Anal. Lett.* [B], 11:119–133.

68. Truscott, R. J. W., Burke, D. G., Korth, J., and Halpern, B. (1978): Simultaneous determination of diphenylhydantoin, mephobarbital, carbamazepine, phenobarbital and primidone in serum using direct chemical ionization mass spectrometry. *Biomed. Mass Spectrom.*, 5:477–482.

69. Westenberg, H. G., and De Zeeuw, R. A. (1976): Rapid and sensitive liquid chromatographic determination of carbamazepine suitable for use in monitoring multiple-drug anticonvulsant therapy. *J. Chromatogr.*, 118:217–224.

Antiepileptic Drugs, Third Edition, edited by
R. Levy, R. Mattson, B. Meldrum,
J. K. Penry, and F. E. Dreifuss.
Raven Press, Ltd., New York © 1989.

33

Carbamazepine

Absorption, Distribution and Excretion

Paolo L. Morselli

INTRODUCTION

Carbamazepine (CBZ) (5-H-dibenzo-[b,f]azepine-]-carbazamide; Tegretol is currently considered the drug of first choice for the treatment of partial seizures with and without complex symptomatology as well as of generalized tonic-clonic seizures. The clinical effectiveness of CBZ has been improved considerably in the last 10 years by increased information on its pharmacokinetic profile and on the factors capable of modifying its concentration in body fluids and tissues.

ABSORPTION

Experimental Studies

When administered intraperitoneally CBZ is rapidly absorbed, and peak plasma concentrations are attained within 30 to 60 min (41,88,99). However, when administered by the oral route, CBZ is absorbed relatively slowly, and in the rat and the monkey, maximal concentrations are reached 3 to 8 hr after administration (109). The absorption rate is faster in the dog, with peak concentrations attained 1 to 2 hr after dosing (55). In the rat, peak plasma levels are proportional to the dose up to 150 mg/kg, but for higher doses, a reduction in peak

concentrations is observed (53). In the monkey the bioavailability varies from 58% to 86% depending on the dose (82).

The time of administration (morning or evening) and the vehicle used for the oral dose may have a significant effect on the absorption rate and the total amount absorbed (24,85,109). Addition of Tween or propylene glycol to the solution or suspension used for the oral administration of the drug accelerates the absorption rate with peak plasma levels achieved at 2 hr, and doubles the area under the curve of plasma concentrations over time (109).

In the rat the active metabolite of carbamazepine, the carbamazepine epoxide, is well and rapidly absorbed (52,57).

Clinical Studies

The gastrointestinal absorption of the commercially available CBZ formulation is rather slow, erratic, and unpredictable (97,108,109,110). The absorption rate in epileptic patients may be more rapid than in healthy volunteers (28,74,97,166). Peak plasma concentrations are generally attained between 4 and 8 hr after ingestion, but peaks as late as 24 and 26 hr have been reported (19,36,45,62,69,84,108,109,129, 154,155,166). Absorption of the drug is apparently slower after the evening dose (41).

If frequent blood sampling is performed during the absorptive phase, secondary and tertiary peaks are frequently observed during a long-term regimen (157,159), suggesting that the absorption of CBZ does not follow a simple first-order process.

The causes behind such irregular absorption may be related to the physicochemical properties of the molecule, involving a very slow dissolution rate in the gastrointestinal fluid, or to the anticholinergic properties of the drug, which may become more evident during prolonged treatment, modifying the gastrointestinal transit time. A recent paper by Riad et al. (143) suggests that in man CBZ undergoes a simultaneous first-order and zero-order absorption, with about 35% of the available dose absorbed at a zero-order rate. The available data indicate, in fact, constant prolonged absorption in the upper and lower part of the intestine. This hypothesis explains the numerous secondary peaks and the rather flat plasma concentration curves obtained over 24 hr with the slow-release preparation. The phenomenon is probably due to incomplete or very slow dissolution of high doses of CBZ in the gastrointestinal fluid. Therefore, with use of the regular, commercially available tablets, three or four daily doses are preferred to twice-a-day administration.

Because of the lack of an injectable formulation, no precise data exist on the absolute bioavailability of CBZ. A value, estimated from studies conducted with the ^{14}C-labeled molecule, ranges from 75% to 85% (51). In cases of massive overdose (12–34 g), peak plasma CBZ concentrations were reached during the second or third day after drug ingestion (65,118,168). Peak concentrations ranged from 33 to 77 μg/ml for CBZ and from 10 to 20 μg/ml for CBZ epoxide, and were followed in a few cases by a plateau lasting 150 to 180 hr (168).

Solutions, suspensions, syrups, and the newly developed chewable and slow-release formulations seem to have similar bioavailability (2,16,30,36,69,87,129,135).

With long-term treatment, the syrup form does not appear to present a real advantage over the tablet form (102), although increased bioavailability and a faster absorption rate have been observed with the syrup in healthy volunteers following single oral doses (19,69,110,115,169). However, the slow-release formulations give rise to more stable and less fluctuating plasma CBZ concentrations (2,112).

The effect of food on the absorption rate of CBZ is variable (84,104,159) and of low clinical significance. However, the size of both the daily and the unitary doses may significantly influence the absorption rate, as well as the total amount absorbed. As first shown by Johannessen et al. (71), daily doses higher than 20 mg/kg are less efficiently absorbed, with an inverse relationship between absorption and doses above 20 to 25 mg/kg. Further recent data suggest optimal absorption rates at 14 to 16 mg/kg (15,36,63,79,84,135,155,171).

In contrast with CBZ, CBZ epoxide when given as such is readily absorbed with peak plasma concentrations attained between 1 and 2 hr after administration (157,162).

DISTRIBUTION

Experimental Studies

Studies conducted in mice, rats, and monkeys indicate that CBZ distributes rapidly and quite uniformly to various organs and tissues, with higher concentrations achieved in high blood flow areas such as liver, kidney, and brain (50,53,97,109, 167,173). Tissue concentrations parallel plasma concentrations without any evident accumulation in specific organs (53,173) after both single dose and repeated administration.

In the rat, brain CBZ concentrations are 1.1 to 1.6 times the plasma concentrations, whereas the ratio of the CBZ epoxide ranges from 0.4 to 0.8, suggesting reduced brain penetration (53,97,109). Threshold levels for protection against maximal electroshock seizures are on the order of 3.5 to 4.5 µg/g for both CBZ and CBZ epoxide concentrations in the brain (52,53,103,109).

Studies on the regional brain distribution show CBZ concentrations in the cortex, thalamus, and hippocampus shortly after dosing (115). With time, there is a progressive leveling of drug concentrations in various areas, and later subcortical structures have the highest relative drug concentrations. Such distribution is very similar to that observed for other lipophilic drugs (104,125) and reflects vascularity and cerebral blood flow. CBZ epoxide, too, appears to have a uniform distribution (115).

In the rat, CBZ at concentrations of 3 to 30 µg/ml is 74% to 80% bound to plasma proteins (24). In the dog, the plasma protein binding is of 70% to 72% for CBZ (K_a = 2.7 × 10^3M^{-1}) and about 40% for CBZ epoxide (55,86). In the rhesus monkey, the plasma protein binding is 65% to 71% for CBZ and 41% to 60% for CBZ epoxide.

The apparent volume of distribution in the rat ranges from 1.4 to 1.7 L/kg without significant differences between adult, young, old, and pregnant animals (34,53,97). In the rhesus monkey, similar values (0.8–1.6 L/kg) have been reported for CBZ and CBZ epoxide (82,116).

Clinical Studies

In vitro and *in vivo* studies with healthy volunteers have shown that CBZ at concentrations of 3 to 30 µg/ml is 75% to 78% bound to plasma proteins (42,107,108). Proteins other than albumin are implicated in the CBZ binding (42). For the CBZ-albumin complex, only one group of binding sites is involved and the complex has a relatively low association constant (K_a = 1.30 × 10^3M^{-1}). A similar association constant (K_a = 0.93 × 10^3M^{-1}) has been found for CBZ epoxide, which is 48% to 53% bound

(162). Similar values have been reported for adult epileptics and patients with other diseases (10,68,71,72,83,108,120,139,161), as well as in case of massive overdose (118,168), whereas a lower plasma protein binding has been observed in patients with hepatic diseases (68). All data indicate that the interindividual variability in plasma protein binding of CBZ and its two metabolites may be high in the various series of patients tested so far. A partial explanation of this phenomenon may be found in a recent report by Baruzzi et al. (10). These authors underline the important role played by alpha$_1$acid-glycoprotein in the binding of CBZ and show that the free fraction of CBZ is inversely correlated with serum alpha$_1$acid-glycoprotein concentration. However, it is known that alpha$_1$acid-glycoprotein levels are often altered in presence of inflammation, mild infections (bronchitis, tonsillitis, angina), or trauma, and they do change as a function of age (10,35).

The apparent volume of CBZ ranges from 0.8 to 2.0 L/kg (45,47,97,106,108,140,154, 157,174). The real figures are probably somehow lower because of possible incomplete bioavailability. The apparent volume of distribution for CBZ epoxide is 0.59 to 1.50 L/kg (157,162), which is in good agreement with its reduced liposolubility.

Patients whose epilepsy was treated neurosurgically because of poor response to pharmacological treatment had brain-to-plasma ratios of 0.8 to 1.6, which were similar to those observed in experimental animals (9,58,59,66,97,102,111). In most of the brain specimens analyzed so far, CBZ epoxide has also been found at concentrations similar to those present in plasma, with brain-to-plasma ratios of 0.5 to 1.5.

Cerebrospinal fluid (CSF) concentrations of CBZ may range from 17% to 31% of those in plasma (43,71,72,73,74,92,103). CSF concentrations of CBZ epoxide and carbamazepine-10,11-diol are 45% to 55% of the corresponding total plasma levels (42,72,

130). These data on CBZ and its metabolites are in good agreement with what is known about their plasma protein binding in man.

Saliva concentrations of CBZ and CBZ epoxide also reflect the free fraction of the drug, and under steady-state conditions they may represent a useful and easy tool for measuring unbound drugs (3,8,18,29, 126,150,161,165,174). However, saliva concentrations cannot be used for kinetic evaluation following repeated or single doses of the drug (40,69). Saliva concentrations range from 25% to 30% of the plasma concentrations for CBZ and from 30% to 40% for CBZ epoxide. Similar values have been reported for tears (94,163).

The biliary excretion of carbamazepine in man is rather limited. Only 1% of a single 400-mg dose was eliminated in bile as unconjugated metabolites within 72 hr (160). Bile-to-plasma ratios were variable (0.24–0.84) and apparently related to the bile cholesterol content. These findings do not exclude the possibility of consistent biliary excretion of metabolites, such as glucuronide derivates.

Erythrocyte-to-plasma ratios of 0.14 to 0.38 indicate a rather limited penetration into red blood cells. No CBZ epoxide could be measured in erythrocytes (68,130,134).

EXCRETION AND ELIMINATION

Experimental Studies

Carbamazepine is extensively metabolized in all species studied so far. In the rat, about 70% of the injected drug administered as ^{14}C-CBZ is recovered within 120 hr in urine (30%) and feces (38%) (37,97,107). There are significant differences in drug clearances between male (0.96 L/kg/hr) and female (0.56 L/kg/hr) rats, as well as between young (0.72 L/kg/hr) and old (0.32 L/kg/hr) rats (34,53). The phenomenon reflects a higher metabolic rate constant in

adult male rats and young rats, since no differences could be observed in apparent volume of distribution (V_d).

In the rhesus monkey, the plasma disappearance rate of CBZ is 1 to 2 hr with a total body clearance of 0.43 to 0.59 L/kg/hr (82,117,147,172). The clearance of CBZ epoxide is apparently 10% to 15% faster than that of the parent compound (83,116,117). In the dog, the apparent plasma half-life of CBZ following a single dose is 1.1 to 1.9 hr. The decrease in plasma CBZ concentrations is accompanied by a very high formation rate of CBZ epoxide, whose apparent plasma half-life has been estimated to be of 1.6 to 7.0 hr (55).

Repeated CBZ administration leads to a marked and significant increase in the clearance of the drug and a decrease in steady-state levels in all species tested so far (50,53,55,103,116,123,172). The increased total body clearance is mainly due to increased activity of the hepatic microsomal monooxygenase systems. Subsequent to repeated CBZ treatment, an increases in liver cytochrome P-450, NADPH-cytochrome reductase activity, and N-demethylase activity have been observed (50,170), as well as increased *in vitro* formation of CBZ epoxide (44). Furthermore, other studies indicate that epoxide hydrases also are increased and that *in vivo*, following repeated treatment in animals, there is no demonstrable rise in plasma CBZ epoxide levels (50,116).

Circadian oscillations in plasma CBZ concentrations have been observed in rhesus monkeys under constant infusion (83,172). According to the authors, the phenomenon is not due to variations in metabolic activity, but could be linked to the circadian rhythmicity of several physiological processes (e.g., plasma protein concentrations, hemodynamics, day/night changes, motor activity). In the monkey, increased drug clearance is accompanied by increased urinary excretion of D-glucaric acid (82,83).

All above-mentioned data indicate that

CBZ is a strong metabolic inducer and that it induces its own metabolism. Unmetabolized CBZ is found in urine only in traces (37,50,82,107). The autoinduction also has a very definite effect on brain CBZ concentrations (103).

Several metabolic products have been identified and are discussed in detail in Chapter 36. Among the major products, representing about 60% of the urinary excreted material are CBZ-10,11-epoxide, *trans*-CBZ-10,11-dihydroxide, 9-hydroxy-carbamyol acridane, iminostilbene, and the derivates hydroxylated in the aromatic ring in either 2, 4, or 6 positions (5,6,37,50,51, 56,57,97,107). The remaining 35% to 40% of the urinary excreted products consists of very polar compounds not yet completely identified.

In the monkey, measurable amounts of CBZ have been found in the feces after intravenous infusion (82). These data and those previously mentioned in the rat suggest the existence of important enterohepatic recycling in the experimental animals. Such enterohepatic recycling could explain some of the fluctuations in plasma CBZ concentrations often observed during the early phase of intravenous infusion.

Clinical Studies

The elimination of CBZ is well described in most cases by a one-compartment open model. The rate of disappearance from plasma may be variable. In healthy young volunteers, following a single dose the CBZ half-life may range from 18 to 55 hr with corresponding clearance values of 0.021 to 0.011 L/kg/hr (45,47,51,84,101,108,140, 157). Half-lives of 34 to 36 hr have been reported in elderly subjects (67). Following repeated treatment in volunteers and epileptic patients, the apparent plasma half-life of carbamazepine may vary from 5 to 26 hr, with clearance values of 0.540 to 0.025 L/hr/kg (41,44,45,46,47,91,105, 108,124,157,166).

The large interindividual differences in apparent plasma half-life and total body clearance are linked to the autoinduction phenomenon, which reaches different levels in different individuals. The auto-inducing effect of CBZ on liver microsomal enzymes leads in effect to what has been defined as time dependent kinetics, a situation where clearance values increase with time and higher doses are needed to maintain the same plasma concentrations (81,91,158). It has been estimated that in healthy volunteers, although a certain induction is present after 2 to 4 days of treatment, a plateau for autoinduction is reached only after 20 to 30 days. The situation and the time course of the autoinduction may be totally different in epileptic patients already induced by other antiepileptic or nonantiepileptic drugs (14,15,16).

The poststeady-state apparent plasma half-life of CBZ epoxide ranges from 3 to 23 hr (45,108,174). With the shorter half-life of the epoxide compared with the parent compound, it is difficult to understand reports of a higher epoxide-to-CBZ ratio in induced patients (31,39) unless an inhibitory effect on epoxide-hydrase activities is exerted by the associated drugs. In fact, the epoxide-to-CBZ ratio is not increased by drugs such as phenytoin or phenobarbital (76,95,96). However, the ratio is increased by valproate (see Chapter 36) and progabide (see Chapter 64) or by increasing the total daily CBZ doze (71). A decreased epoxide-to-CBZ ratio has been observed in elderly patients (67).

Carbamazepine is almost completely metabolized in man (see Chapter 36). The epoxidation of the molecule followed by enzymatic hydrolysis to give *trans*-10,11-dihydroxycarbamazepine is the major metabolic pathway (5,15,46,47,48,56,162). In healthy volunteers, the urinary excretion of unmetabolized carbamazepine accounts for 1% of the dose (50,51,108), the major portion of the urinary excreted material being represented by the *trans*-diol which is present both in free and conjugated forms (15,48,50,52,97,101,102,105,108,162). Other compounds identified in smaller amounts are described in detail in Chapter 36. Following oral intake of ^{14}C-CBZ, about 28% of the labeled dose was found in the feces, suggesting both incomplete absorption and/or a non-negligible biliary excretion of unidentified (conjugated?) metabolites (50,51).

In epileptic patients undergoing long-term treatment with CBZ, 20% to 60% of the daily dose is excreted as the *trans*-diol, 5% to 11% as 9-hydroxymethyl-10-carbamoylacridane, 5% to 10% as phenolic derivatives (2,4, 6-OH), 1% to 2% as CBZ epoxide, and 0.5% as unmetabolized carbamazepine (23,46,47,48). The same percentages have been observed in cases of massive overdoses (168).

The estimated renal clearances in epileptic patients and healthy volunteers are 8 to 10 ml/min for CBZ epoxide and 60 to 70 ml/min for the *trans*-diol (23,163). Evaluating the renal excretion of CBZ after massive overdoses, Vree et al. (168) observed that the renal clearance of free carbamazepine and free CBZ epoxide (1 ml/min and 8 ml/min, respectively) was flow dependent, but the clearance of the *trans*-diol (60–350 ml/min) was flow independent.

The total body clearance of the *trans*-diol may vary from 4.3 ml/hr/kg in volunteers to 58.6 ml/hr/kg in patients (48). When CBZ epoxide is administered to healthy volunteers, its disappearance rate is characterized by an apparent plasma half-life of 4.6 to 7.6 hr with a total body clearance of 63 to 178 ml/hr/kg (157,162).

Carbamazepine is nearly completely (80–90%) metabolized to the *trans*-diol, which is found in the urine mostly in the unconjugated form (162). The above data and the different percentages of *trans*-diol found in urine after CBZ or CBZ epoxide administration indicate that the epoxidation is the rate-limiting step to the *trans*-diol formation and that the disposition of the epoxide, after

CBZ administration follows a flip-flop model where the formation rate is the rate limiting step (157).

PREGNANCY

Experimental Studies

In pregnant rats the absorption of CBZ is delayed, with peak plasma levels attained 2 to 3 hr after intrapetoneal administration (53,54). In this series of observations, the apparent volume of distribution was not different from that computed for control rats, whereas total body clearance was significantly reduced. These data confirm the slower disposition rate in pregnant animals observed for other compounds. Equilibrium between maternal and fetal tissues was reached within 30 to 60 min, suggesting a rapid transfer of the drug across the placenta. There was no evidence of selective accumulation in any fetal tissue. The disappearance rate of CBZ from fetal tissues follows that of maternal plasma concentrations.

Clinical Studies

There are no specific data on the absorption of CBZ during pregnancy. However, judging from the plasma CBZ concentrations usually observed in pregnant women, there are no reasons to suspect modified absorption during the first 6 months of the pregnancy. Lower plasma CBZ concentrations during the last 3 months of pregnancy have been reported by some authors (11,21,32,38,80), but not others (77,114). Further, the drop in plasma concentrations of other antiepileptic drugs (21,38) during pregnancy is still unexplained.

The binding of CBZ and CBZ epoxide does not vary significantly, and free fractions of 20% to 30% for CBZ and 30% to 55% for CBZ epoxide have been reported (32,38,78,175). Moreover, two recent studies (114,175) report that no changes in the intrinsic clearance of CBZ occur during pregnancy if the free fraction and changes in maternal body weight are taken into consideration. The increased epoxide-to-CBZ ratio, accompanied by a reduction in the *trans*-diol concentration, is probably the result of inhibition of the epoxide hydrases rather than increased epoxidation of CBZ (175,176).

In early pregnancy, the placental transfer of CBZ is extensive and rapid (128). The drug distributes to various tissues and organs of the fetus homogeneously, and the reported fetal brain-to-plasma ratios are similar to those observed in adults (59,100,128). CBZ epoxide also has been found in fetal tissues and amniotic fluid at concentrations similar to those observed in adults tissues and CSF (32,128). It is interesting to note that the human fetal liver at 15 to 21 weeks gestation is able to metabolize CBZ to CBZ epoxide *in vitro* (122).

Carbamazepine and CBZ epoxide are present in breast milk at concentrations that are 25% to 60% of plasma concentrations (160). Estimations of the possible daily amount transferred to the newborn by lactating epileptic mothers with therapeutic concentrations of carbamazepine (4–8 μg/ml) suggest that a newborn of 3 to 3.5 kg would receive about 0.5 to 0.7 mg/kg/day (60,90,99,113,131). Whether such a dose has any effect on the newborn has never been evaluated.

PEDIATRIC PATIENTS

Newborns

In neonates from epileptic mothers undergoing prolonged treatment, the plasma CBZ concentrations at birth are similar to those present in the mother's plasma (22,70,77,78,137). Transplacentally acquired CBZ is cleared according to first-order kinetics. For gestational ages of 32 to 42 weeks, the half-life ranges from 8 to 37 hr for CBZ (22,77,88,137) and 20 to 24 hr for CBZ epoxide (77). These values are very close to those reported in epileptic patients, and induction of fetal liver drug metabolizing enzymes *in utero* is very probable (98,106). In newborns older than 2 days CBZ is absorbed rather rapidly, with peak levels attained in 2 to 6 hr (88,142) and plasma concentrations comparable to those observed in adults.

Protein binding is moderately decreased with a free fraction of 30% to 35% for CBZ and 58% to 63% for CBZ epoxide (64,78). According to Rey et al. (142), the apparent V_d in the neonate is 1.5 to 2.0 times greater than in adults. The apparent CBZ half-life in the newborn of 1 to 7 weeks of age (and sometimes pretreated with phenobarbital) may vary from 4.6 to 15.2 hr (88,142). Such a high rate of elimination is in keeping with the rate observed for other drugs in newborns after the first week of age (98,99,106).

Infants

There appear to be no major differences in absorption, protein binding, and distribution of CBZ between infants and adults. From autopsy observations, Pynnönen et al. (128) described a more or less even distribution of CBZ in various tissues and organs, and CSF concentrations of about 24% of the plasma concentrations. Plasma protein binding of CBZ and CBZ epoxide in infants is within the adult ranges (35,146).

The apparent V_d is 1.5 to 2 times greater than in grown-up children and adults (133,142). The values relative to the disappearance rate of CBZ refer either to single doses (two cases) or to infants also receiving other antiepileptic drugs (four cases) (133,142) and range from 12 to 36 hr. In a recent study of a large group of infants, children, and adolescents, Battino et al. (12) described a significant positive correlation between the plasma level-to-dose ratio and age. According to a recent report (146), the epoxide-to-CBZ ratio in infants is comparable to that observed in adults.

Children

The absorption of CBZ in children is as poor and erratic as in adults. Peak plasma levels are attained 4 to 8 hr after dosing, with large interindividual variations and frequent secondary peaks (110,147,150), suggesting that as in adults, absorption of the drug in children does not follow a first-order process. In children there is also an inverse relationship between dose and absorption rate, with impaired absorption at doses over 25 mg/kg (12). Data from CBZ concentrations in saliva and tears suggest that CBZ and CBZ epoxide free fractions are slightly higher in children than in adults, with values of 30% to 35% and 40% to 45%, respectively (1,4,8,35,49,132,146,148,149,150,161,163). Brain-to-plasma ratios are similar to those observed in adults (58), and the apparent V_d (computed assuming complete bioavailability) is larger than in adults (14,133,142).

The apparent plasma half-life of CBZ in children ranges from 3 to 32 hr (14,133,136,138,142). The variability may be explained by age of the child, associated treatment, and length of treatment (95,96,98,102,110,136,138,139). A recent report (14) has shown that in children 10 to 13 years of age, the CBZ half-life may decline from 25 to 32 hr after a single dose, to 18 to 22 hr after 4 to 6 days of treatment, and to 10 to 14 hr after 4 weeks of therapy with the drug. The CBZ epoxide-to-CBZ ratio is quite variable (0.16–0.66) and tends to be higher in children according to some authors (23,49,90,138,152), but not others (146,149,161). However, as in adults, there seems to be agreement that the higher CBZ epoxide levels are found during co-treatment with valproate (49,83,152,161). Furlanut et al. (61) recently reported that girls appear to have a lower CBZ clearance than

boys. The apparent plasma half-life of CBZ epoxide in children is 13 to 22 hr, which is similar to that in adults (133).

Globally, the available information in children indicates that as for other drugs (98,106), the clearance of CBZ is age-dependent, with the highest disposition rates during infancy and early childhood. The clearance rate then decreases progressively to reach adult values at the age of 15 to 17 years. As a consequence of the increased clearance, children need relatively larger total daily doses and smaller, more frequent unitary doses (3–4 times/day) to avoid wide fluctuations in plasma levels, which can cause disturbing intermittent side effects (98,144).

Carbamazepine absorption may be greatly reduced in children suffering from protein energy malnutrition, because of alteration of the absorptive intestinal surface and disturbed gastric emptying. According to a recent report (7), the bioavailability may be one-third of that observed in control children.

CARBAMAZEPINE PHARMACOKINETICS IN DISEASE STATES OTHER THAN EPILEPSY

Epileptic patients may suffer from concomitant disease and require treatment with other drugs that may lead to important variations of the physiological variables determining the extent of drug distribution as well as the rates of absorption and elimination. The interactions of CBZ with other drugs are extensively described in Chapter 38 and will not be discussed here. However, it is important to emphasize the possible consequences of various pathological conditions on the disposition of CBZ and its metabolites and the possible risks of increased drug toxicity or loss of efficacy. Although there are no specific studies available on the influence of cardiac, renal, or liver diseases on the kinetics of CBZ, it is possible to estimate with reasonable certainty the type of alteration in the disposition of CBZ that could be encountered in these disease states by considering information on other drugs (105) and the physicochemical properties of CBZ and its pharmacokinetic profile under normal conditions.

Cardiac Failure

In cardiac failure, reduced cardiac output is accompanied by increased filling pressure, congestion of major vital organs, edema and expansion of blood volume, tissue hypoxemia, and acidosis (13). Such a condition may easily lead to edema of the intestinal epithelium, reduction of liver blood flow, impairment of microsomal hepatic enzyme activities, altered glomerular filtration and tubular resorption rates, and lower plasma and tissue protein binding. As a consequence, the already erratic and slow carbamazepine absorption will be further impaired and the drug will very probably be metabolized and cleared at a lower rate.

Factors such as reduced renal excretion rates and reduced plasma protein binding should not play an important role for carbamazepine, but they could be important for the clearance of the epoxide and of the *trans*-diol. Furthermore, it is difficult to estimate the possible clinical significance of modified redistribution phenomena caused by differences in pH and relative blood flow to various organs. In practical terms, depending on the prevalence of impairment at absorptive or elimination phases, there may be either loss of effects or increased risk of adverse reactions. Also, CBZ may cause increased water and sodium retention (105,121), which may significantly aggravate an already compromised hemodynamic condition.

Liver Diseases

No significant alterations in CBZ pharmacokinetics should be expected in cases of moderate alterations of liver function (127). Significant alterations may be expected with severe cirrhosis, hepatitis, and obstructive conditions. These are all situations where a portocaval shunt, a decreased rate of protein synthesis, reduced microsomal activity, high circulating bilirubin, diffuse edemas, and a trend to reduction in renal function (17,20) may significantly modify the pharmacokinetic profile. For CBZ, the reduction in hepatic microsomal activity appears more important than a reduced plasma protein binding. In severe liver disease, the risk of CBZ toxicity is greatly increased and careful monitoring should be maintained.

Renal Diseases

The effect of impaired kidney function on the kinetic profile of drugs may be quite variable. In general, the pathological picture may be accompanied by a modified hematocrit, a reduction in glomerular and/or tubular functions, a rise in total body water with increased extracellular water, variable degrees of hypoalbuminemia, electrolyte imbalance, increased uremia, and functional changes in the gastrointestinal tract (106,141). These alterations may modify drug bioavailability, reduce plasma protein binding of an acidic drug, increase the apparent volume of distribution, lead to accumulation of polar metabolites, and have different effects on drug clearance rates, depending on the physicochemical properties and the prevalent elimination process. In the case of CBZ, no modification in either bioavailability or clearance rates has been reported up to now. It should be stressed, however, that CBZ may exert a significant antidiuretic effect with increased danger of fluid retention.

Other Pathological States

The disposition of antiepileptic drugs may be altered in situations such as malnutrition syndromes, pulmonary disease, fever, and postoperative sequelaes (105). No alteration in CBZ pharmacokinetics is observed in thyroid disorders (93), but the kinetics of the drug may be altered in malnutrition syndromes (reduced absorption) (7), fever (increased catabolism), and pulmonary diseases (reduced catabolism). In postoperative states, the major modification may be a reduction in plasma protein binding affecting mainly acidic compounds.

CARBAMAZEPINE AND CBZ EPOXIDE PLASMA CONCENTRATIONS IN LONG-TERM TREATMENT

During long-term treatment, plasma concentrations of CBZ and CBZ epoxide show great interindividual variability associated with large intraindividual fluctuations. There is no evident relationship between the dose and plasma concentration of either CBZ or CBZ epoxide. For the same daily dose, fivefold to sevenfold interindividual differences have been reported (4,23,25, 27,28,43,63,71,95,96,108,119,135,139,144, 145,146,149,151,161). With the currently used doses of 600 to 1,200 mg/day, though plasma concentrations of CBZ plus CBZ epoxide may vary from 2 to 20 µg/ml without a clear relationship between concentration of the parent compound and of the metabolite. Apparently, the epoxide-to-CBZ ratio may vary with age, associated treatment, physiological status, dose regimens, and dosage schedule (1,23,25,41,43,71,72, 108,135,139,149,155,156,159,161). Furthermore, it has been clearly shown that plasma concentrations of both compounds oscillate considerably during the dosing intervals (23,89,90,119,144,146,149,161). Fluctuations of 40% to 150% for carbamazepine and 40% to 500% for the epoxide have been described (49,89,119,149).

The relationship of the CBZ plasma concentration to the drug's effect is treated in detail in Chapter 39. According to various reports, efficacious concentrations of CBZ may range from 4 to 12 µg/ml (26,27,39, 102,108,144,145,153,164). It may be interesting to recall that animal data appear to be in agreement since minimal brain threshold concentrations against maximal electroshock seizures are 3.5 to 4.5 µg/g in the rat (33,53,109) and similar minimal protective concentrations have been described for cats (75) and monkeys (85).

CONCLUSIONS AND IMPLICATIONS FOR DOSAGE REGIMENS

The pharmacokinetics of carbamazepine appear rather complex, and the molecule cannot be described as easy to handle. Furthermore, other factors such as age and concomitant drug treatment may further complicate the picture, especially with regard to the absorptive and the elimination processes. Because of the evident relationship between drug concentration in body fluids and its effects, a precise dosing schedule appears to be an important prerequisite for a correct therapeutic approach. However, because of the lack of a relationship between daily doses and trough plasma levels, the wide intraindividual fluctuations in plasma concentrations, the time-dependent kinetics, and the variable and apparently dose-dependent rate of absorption, CBZ dose schedules are difficult to define without the aid of plasma drug level monitoring. (This procedure should always include the measurement of the CBZ epoxide.)

In the case of patients requiring combined treatment with other antiepileptic drugs, daily CBZ dosages of 14 to 20 mg/kg are needed in most subjects to achieve plasma levels of 6 to 10 µg/ml. In patients treated with CBZ alone, daily doses of 8 to 12 mg/kg may be sufficient to obtain therapeutic plasma concentrations.

In practical terms, it is useful to start the therapy with 200 mg of CBZ given twice a day, and to increase the dose progressively to 800 to 1,000 mg/day, if needed. Because of the dose effect on drug absorption, it may be useful to divide a daily dose of 800 mg or higher into three or four doses.

During long-term treatment, food does not appear to have any significant influence on either the rate of absorption or the amount of CBZ absorbed. Hence, the drug may be taken either before or after meals.

The future availability of slow-release preparations permitting once-a-day administration will surely facilitate patient compliance and, in most cases, the physician's decisions. It will, however, complicate individualization of the dosage regimen for difficult patients.

Because of the age-dependent disposition rate of CBZ in children, relatively higher doses should be prescribed with more frequent daily administrations. In both adults and children, because of the time-dependent kinetics, plasma concentrations should be monitored at least twice during the first month of treatment and the dose adjusted as a function of both clinical response and plasma concentrations.

ACKNOWLEDGMENTS

The author expresses gratitude to Mrs. B. Chapelier Boullie and Ms. M. P. Vignaud for their valuable assistance and help in the preparation of the manuscript.

REFERENCES

1. Agbato, O. A., Elyas, A. A., Patsalos, P. N., Brett, E. M., and Lascelles, P. T. (1986): Total and free serum concentrations of carbamazepine and carbamazepine-10,11-epoxide in children with epilepsy. *Arch. Neurol.,* 43:1111–1116.
2. Aldenkamp, A. P., Alpherts, W. C. J., Moerland, M. C., Ottevanger, N., and Van Parys, J. A. P. (1987): Controlled release carbamazepine: Cognitive side effects in patients with epilepsy. *Epilepsia,* 25(5):507–514.
3. Aucamp, A. K., and Hundt, H. K. L. (1978): A study of carbamazepine and its epoxy and hydroxymetabolites in serum and saliva of male and female epileptic patients. In: *Advances in Epilep-*

tology 1977. Psychology, Pharmacotherapy and New Diagnostic Approaches, edited by H. Meinardi and A. J. Rowan, pp. 280–284. Swets & Zeitlinger, Amsterdam, Lisse.
4. Bäckman, E., Dahlström, G., Eeg-Olofsson, O., and Bertler, A. (1987): The 24 hour variation of salivary carbamazepine and carbamazepine-10,11-epoxide concentrations in children with epilepsy. *Pediatr. Neurol.,* 3:327–330.
5. Baker, K. M., Csetenyi, J., Frigerio, A., Morselli, P. L., and Paravicini, F., and Pifferi, G. (1973): 10,11-Dihydro-10,11-dihydroxy-5H-dibenz(b,f)asepine-5-carboxamide, a metabolite of carbamazepine isolated from human and rat urine. *J. Med. Chem.,* 16:703–705.
6. Baker, K. M., Frigerio, A., Morselli, P. L., and Pifferi, G. (1973): Identification of a rearranged degradation product from carbamazepine-10,11-epoxide. *J. Pharm. Sci.,* 62:475–476.
7. Bano, G., Raina, R. K., and Sharma, D. B. (1986): Pharmacokinetics of carbamazepine in protein energy malnutrition. *Pharmacology,* 32:232–236.
8. Bartels, H., Oldigs, H. D., and Gunter, E. (1977): Use of saliva in monitoring carbamazepine medication in epileptic children. *Eur. J. Pediatr.,* 126:37–44.
9. Baruzzi, A., Cabrini, G. P., Gerna, M., Sironi, V. A., and Morselli, P. L. (1977): Anticonvulsant plasma level monitoring in epileptic patients undergoing stereo-EEG. In: *Antiepileptic Drug Monitoring,* edited by C. Gardner-Thorpe, D. Janz, H. Meinardi, and C. E. Pippenger, pp. 317–334. Pitman Medical, Tunbridge Wells, Kent.
10. Baruzzi, A., Contin, M., Perucca, E., Albini, F., and Riva, R. (1986): Altered serum protein binding of carbamazepine in disease states associated with an increased α_1-acid glycoprotein concentration. *Eur. J. Clin. Pharmacol.,* 31:85–89.
11. Battino, D., Binelli, S., Bossi, L., Canger, R., Croci, D., Cusi, C., De Giambattista, M., and Avanzini, G. (1985): Plasma concentrations of carbamazepine and carbamazepine-10,11-epoxide during pregnancy and after delivery. *Clin. Pharmacokinet.,* 10:279–284.
12. Battino, D., Bossi, L., Croci, D., Franceschetti, Gomeni, S., Moise, A., Vittali, A., and Breschi, F. (1980): Carbamazepine plasma levels in children and adults: Influence of age and associated therapy. *Therapeutic Drug Monitoring,* 2:315–322.
13. Benowitz, N. L., and Meister, W. (1976): Pharmacokinetics in patients with cardiac failure. *Clin. Pharmacokinet.,* 1:389–405.
14. Bertilsson, L., Höjer, B., Tybring, G., Osterloh, J., and Rane, A. (1980): Autoinduction of carbamazepine metabolism in children examined by a stable isotope technique. *Clin. Pharmacol. Ther.,* 27:83–88.
15. Bertilsson, L., and Tomson, T. (1986a): Clinical pharmacokinetics and pharmacological effects of carbamazepine and carbamazepine-10,11-epox-

ide. An update. *Clin. Pharmacokinet.*, 11:177–198.

16. Bertilsson, L., Tomson, T., and Tybring, G. (1986b): Pharmacokinetics: Time-dependent changes—Autoinduction of carbamazepine epoxidation. *J. Clin. Pharmacol.*, 26:459–462.

17. Blaschke, T. F. (1977): Protein binding and kinetics of drugs in liver diseases. *Clin. Pharmacokinet.*, 2:32–44.

18. Blom, F. G., and Guelen, P. J. M. (1977): The distribution of antiepileptic drugs between serum, saliva and cerebrospinal fluid. In: *Antiepileptic Drug Monitoring*, edited by C. Gardner-Thorpe, D. Janz, H. Meinardi, and C. E. Pippenger, pp. 287–296. Pitman Medical, Tunbridge Wells, Kent.

19. Bloomer, D., Dupuis, L. L., MacGregor, D., and Soldin, S. J. (1987): Palatability and relative bioavailability of an extemporaneous carbamazepine oral suspension. *Clinical Pharmacy*, 6:646–649.

20. Bond, W. S. (1978): Clinical relevance of the effect of hepatic disease on drug disposition. *Ann. J. Hosp. Pharm.*, 35:406–414.

21. Bossi, L., Avanzini, G., Assael, B. M., Battino, D., Caccamo, M. L., Canger, R., Como, M. L., De Giambattista, M., Franceschetti, S., Masini, A., Pardi, G., Piffarotti, G., Porro, M. G., Rovei, V., Sanjuan, M., Soffientini, M. E., Spina, S., and Spreafico, R. (Milan Collaborative Group) (1980): Plasma levels and clinical effects of antiepileptic drugs in pregnant epileptic patients and their newborn. In: *Antiepileptic Therapy—Advances in Drug Monitoring*, edited by S. I. Johannessen, P. L. Morselli, C. E. Pippenger, A. Richens, D. Schmidt, and H. Meinardi, pp. 9–14. Raven Press, New York.

22. Bossi, L., Battino, D., Caccamo, M. L., De Giambattista, M., Latis, G. O., Oldrini, A., and Spina, S. (1981): Pharmacokinetics and clinical effects of antiepileptic drugs in newborns of chronically treated epileptic mothers. In: *Epilepsy, Pregnancy and the Child*, edited by D. Janz, L. Bossi, M. Dam, H. Helge, A. Richens, and D. Schmidt, pp. 373–383. Raven Press, New York.

23. Bourgeois, B. F. D., and Wad, N. (1984): Carbamazepine-10,11-diol steady-state serum levels and renal excretion during carbamazepine therapy in adults and children. *Therapeutic Drug Monitoring*, 6:259–265.

24. Brueguerolle, B., Valli, M., Bouyard, L., Jadot, G., and Bouyard, P. (1981): Circadian effect on carbamazepine kinetics in rat. *European Journal of Drug Metabolism and Pharmacokinetics*, 6(3):189–193.

25. Callaghan, N., O'Callaghan, M., Duggan, B., and Feely, M. (1978): Carbamazepine as a single drug in the treatment of epilepsy. A prospective study of serum levels and seizure control. *J. Neurol. Neurosurg. Psychiatry*, 11:309–329.

26. Cereghino, J. J. (1975): Serum carbamazepine concentration and clinical control. *Adv. Neurol.*, 41:907–912.

27. Cereghino, J. J., Brock, J. T., Van Meter, J. C., Penry, J. K., Smith, L. D., and White, B. G. (1974): Carbamazepine for epilepsy. A controlled prospective evaluation. *Neurology (Minneap.)*, 24:401–410.

28. Cereghino, J. J., Van Meter, J. C., Brock, J. T., Penry, J. K., Smith, L. D., and White, B. G. (1973): Preliminary observations of serum carbamazepine concentration in epileptic patients. *Neurology (Minneap.)*, 23:357–366.

29. Chambers, R. E., Homeida, M., Hunter, K. R., and Teague, R. H. (1977): Salivary carbamazepine concentration. *Lancet*, 1:656–657.

30. Chan, K. K. H., Sawchuk, R. J., Thompson, T. A., Redalieu, E., Wagner, W. E., Lesher, A. R., Weeks, B. J., Hall, N. R., and Gerardin, A. (1985): Bioequivalence of carbamazepine chewable and conventional tablets: Single-dose and steady-state studies. *Journal of Pharmaceutical Sciences*, 74(8):866–870.

31. Christiansen, J., and Dam, M. (1975): Drug interaction in epileptic patients. In: *Clinical Pharmacology of Antiepileptic Drugs*, edited by H. Schneider, D. Janz, C. Gardner-Thorpe, H. Meinardi, and A. L. Sherwin, pp. 197–200. Springer-Verlag, Berlin.

32. Christiansen, J., and Dam, M. (1977): Plasma and salivary levels of carbamazepine and carbamazepine-10,11-epoxide during pregnancy. In: *Antiepileptic Drug Monitoring*, edited by C. Gardner-Thorpe, D. Janz, H. Meinardi, and C. E. Pippenger, pp. 128–135. Pitman Medical, Tunbridge Wells, Kent.

33. Chu, N. S. (1979): Carbamazepine: Prevention of alcohol withdrawal seizures. *Neurology (Minneap.)*, 29:1397–1401.

34. Conti, I., Guiso, G., Urso, R., and Caccia, S. (1987): Inhibitory and inducing effects of denzimol on carbamazepine metabolism in the rat. *Pharmacology*, 35:241–248.

35. Contin, M., Riva, R., Albani, F., Perucca, E., Lamontanara, G., and Baruzzi, A. (1985): Alpha$_1$-acid glycoprotein concentration and serum protein binding of carbamazepine and carbamazepine-10,11-epoxide in children with epilepsy. *Eur. J. Clin. Pharmacol.*, 29:211–214.

36. Cotter, L. M., Eadie, L. J., Hooper, W. D., Lander, C. M., Smith, G. A., and Tyrer, J. H. (1977): The pharmacokinetics of carbamazepine. *Eur. J. Clin. Pharmacol.*, 12:451–456.

37. Csetenyi, J., Baker, K. M., Frigerio, A., and Morselli, P. L. (1973): Iminostilbene—A metabolite of carbamazepine isolated from rat urine. *J. Pharm. Pharmacol.*, 25:340–341.

38. Dam, M., Christiansen, J., Munck, O., and Mygind, K. I. (1979): Antiepileptic drugs: Metabolism in pregnancy. *Clin. Pharmacokinet.*, 4:53–62.

39. Dam, M., Jensen, A., and Christiansen, J. (1975): Plasma level and effect of carbamazepine in grand mal and psychomotor epilepsy. *Acta Neurol. Scand. (Suppl.)*, 60:33–38.

40. Dickinson, R. G., Hooper, W. D., King, A. R., and Eadie, M. J. (1985): Fallacious results from

measuring salivary carbamazepine concentrations. *Therapeutic Drug Monitoring*, 7:41–45.

41. Diehl, L. W., Müller-Oelinghausen, B., and Riedel, E. (1976): The importance of individual pharmacokinetic data for treatment of epilepsy with carbamazepine. *Int. J. Clin. Pharmacol.*, 14:144–148.

42. Di Salle, E., Pacifici, G. M., and Morselli, P. L. (1974): Studies on plasma protein binding of carbamazepine. *Pharmacol. Res. Commun.*, 6:193–202.

43. Eichelbaum, M., Bertilsson, L., Lund, L., Palmer, L., and Sjöqvist, F. (1976): Plasma levels of carbamazepine and carbamazepine-10,11-epoxide during treatment of epilepsy. *Eur. J. Clin. Pharmacol.*, 9:417–421.

44. Eichelbaum, M., Bertilsson, L., Rane, A., and Sjöqvist, F. (1976): Autoinduction of carbamazepine metabolism in man. In: *Anticonvulsant Drugs and Enzyme Induction*, edited by A. Richens and B. Woodford, pp. 147–158. Associated Scientific Publishers, Amsterdam.

45. Eichelbaum, M., Ekbom, K., Bertilsson, L., Ringberger, V. A., and Rane, A. (1975): Plasma kinetics of carbamazepine and its epoxide metabolite in man after single and multiple doses. *Eur. J. Clin. Pharmacol.*, 8:337–341.

46. Eichelbaum, M., Köthe, K. W., Hoffmann, F., and Von Unruh, G. E., (1979): Kinetics and metabolism of carbamazepine during combined antiepileptic drug therapy. *Clin. Pharmacol. Ther.*, 26:366–371.

47. Eichelbaum, M., Köthe, K. W., Hoffmann, F., and Von Uruh, G. E. (1982): Use of stable labelled carbamazepine to study its kinetics during chronic carbamazepine treatment. *Eur. J. Clin. Pharmacol.*, 23:241–244.

48. Eichelbaum, M., Tomson, T., Tybring, G., and Bertilsson, L. (1985): Carbamazepine metabolism in man: Induction and pharmacogenetic aspects. *Clin. Pharmacokinet.*, 10:80–90.

49. Eylas, A. A., Patsalos, P. N., Agbato, O. A., Brett, E. M., and Lascelles, P. T. (1986): Factors influencing simultaneous concentrations of total and free carbamazepine and carbamazepine-10,11-epoxide in serum of children with epilepsy. *Therapeutic Drug Monitoring*, 8:288–292.

50. Faigle, J. W., Brechbuher, S., Feldmann, K. F., and Richter, W. J. (1976): The biotransformation of carbamazepine. In: *Epileptic seizure, behaviour, pain*, edited by W. Birkmayer, pp. 127–140. Huber Publishers, Bern.

51. Faigle, J. W., and Feldmann, K. F. (1975): Pharmacokinetic data of carbamazepine and its major metabolites in man. In: *Clinical Pharmacology of Antiepileptic Drugs*, edited by H. Schneider, D. Janz, C. Gardner-Thorpe, H. Meinardi, and H. Sherwin, pp. 159–165. Springer-Verlag, Berlin.

52. Faigle, J. W., Feldmann, K. F., and Baltzer, V. (1977): Anticonvulsant effect of carbamazepine. An attempt to distinguish between potency of the parent drug and its epoxide metabolite. In: *Antiepileptic Drug Monitoring*, edited by C. Gardner-Thorpe, D. Janz, H. Meinardi, and C. E. Pip-

penger, pp. 104–109. Pitman Medical, Tunbridge Wells, Kent.

53. Farghali-Hassan, Assael, B. M., Bossi, L., Garattini, S., Gerna, M., Gomeni, R., and Morselli, P. L. (1976): Carbamazepine pharmacokinetics in young, adult and pregnant rats. Relation to pharmacological effects. *Arch. Int. Pharmacodyn. Ther.*, 220:125–139.

54. Farghali-Hassan, Assael, B. M., Bossi, L., and Morselli, P. L. (1975): Placental transfer of carbamazepine in the rat. *J. Pharm. Pharmacol.*, 27:956–957.

55. Frey, H. H., and Löscher, W. (1985): Pharmacokinetics of anti-epileptic drugs in the dog: A review. *J. Vet. Pharmacol. Therap.*, 8:219–233.

56. Frigerio, A., Fanelli, R., Biandrate, P., Passerini, G., Morselli, P. L., and Garattini, S. (1972): Mass spectrometric characterization of carbamazepine-10,11-epoxide, a carbamazepine metabolite isolated from human urine. *J. Pharm. Sci.*, 61:1044–1047.

57. Frigerio, A., and Morselli, P. L. (1975): Carbamazepine: Biotransformation. *Adv. Neurol.*, 11:295–308.

58. Friis, M. L., and Christiansen, J. (1978): Carbamazepine, carbamazepine-10,11-epoxide and phenytoin concentrations in brain tissue of epileptic children. *Acta Neurol. Scand.*, 58:104–108.

59. Friis, M. L., Christiansen, J., and Hvidberg, E. F. (1978): Brain concentration of carbamazepine and carbamazepine-10,11-epoxide in epileptic patients. *Eur. J. Clin. Pharmacol.*, 14:47–51.

60. Froescher, W., Eichelbaum, M., Niesen, M., Dietrich, K., and Rausch, P. (1984): Carbamazepine levels in breast milk. *Therapeutic Drug Monitoring*, 6:266–271.

61. Furlanut, M., Montanari, G., Bonin, P., and Casara, G. L. (1985): Carbamazepine and carbamazepine-10,11-epoxide serum concentrations in epileptic children. *J. Pediatr.*, 106:491–495.

62. Gérardin, A. P., Abadie, F. V., Campestrini, J. A., and Theobald, W. (1976): Pharmacokinetic of carbamazepine in normal humans after single and repeated oral doses. *J. Pharmacokinet. Biopharm.*, 4:521–535.

63. Ghose, K., Fry, D. E., and Christfides, J. A. (1983): Effect of dosage frequency of carbamazepine on drug serum levels in epileptic patients. *Eur. J. Clin. Pharmacol.*, 24:375–381.

64. Groce III, J. B., Casto, D. T., and Gal, P. (1985): Carbamazepine and carbamazepine-epoxide serum protein binding in newborn infants. *Therapeutic Drug Monitoring*, 7:274–276.

65. Gruska, H., Beyer, K. H., Kubicki, S., and Schneider, H. (1971): Klinik, Toxikologie und Therapie einer schweren carbamazepine-vergiftung. *Arch. Toxicol.*, 27:193–203.

66. Harvey, C. D., Sherwin, A. L., and Van der Kleijn, E. (1977): Distribution of anticonvulsant drugs in gray and white matter of human brain. *Can. J. Neurol. Sci.*, 4:89–92.

67. Hockings, N., Pall, A., Moody, J., Davidson, A. V. M., and Davidson, D. L. W. (1986): The effects of age on carbamazepine pharmacokinet-

ics and adverse effects. *Br. J. Clin. Pharmac.*, 22:725–728.

68. Hooper, W. D., Dubetz, D. K., Bochner, F., Cotter, L. M., Smith, G. A., Eadie, M. J., and Tyrer, J. H. (1975): Plasma protein binding of carbamazepine. *Clin. Pharmacol. Ther.*, 17:433–440.

69. Hooper, W. D., King, A. R., Patterson, M., Dickinson, R. G., and Eadie, M. J. (1985): Simultaneous plasma carbamazepine and carbamazepine-epoxide concentrations in pharmacokinetic and bioavailability studies. *Therapeutic Drug Monitoring*, 7:36–40.

70. Hoppel, C., Rane, A., and Sjöqvist, F. (1975): Kinetics of phenytoin and carbamazepine in the newborn. In: *Basic and Therapeutic Aspects of Perinatal Pharmacology*, edited by P. L. Morselli, S. Garattini, and F. Sereni, pp. 341–345. Raven Press, New York.

71. Johannessen, S. I., Baruzzi, A., Gomeni, R., Strandjord, R. E., and Morselli, P. L. (1977): Further observations on carbamazepine and carbamazepine-10,11-epoxide kinetics in epileptic patients. In: *Antiepileptic Drug Monitoring*, edited by C. Gardner-Thorpe, D. Janz, H. Meinardi, and C. E. Pippenger, pp. 110–124. Pitman Medical, Tunbridge Wells, Kent.

72. Johannessen, S. I., Gerna, M., Bakke, J., Strandjord, R. E., and Morselli, P. L. (1976): CSF concentrations and serum protein binding of carbamazepine and carbamazepine-10,11-epoxide in epileptic patients. *Br. J. Clin. Pharmacol.*, 3:575–582.

73. Johannessen, S. I., and Strandjord, R. E. (1972): The concentration of carbamazepine (Tegretol®) in serum and in cerebrospinal fluid in patients with epilepsy. *Acta Neurol. Scand.* (Suppl.), 51:445–446.

74. Johannessen, S. I., and Strandjord, R. E. (1975): Absorption and protein binding in serum of several antiepileptic drugs. In: *Clinical Pharmacology of Antiepileptic Drugs*, edited by H. Schneider, D. Janz, C. Gardner-Thorpe, H. Meinardi, and A. L. Sherwin, pp. 262–273. Springer-Verlag, Berlin.

75. Julien, R. M., and Hollister, R. P. (1975): Carbamazepine: Mechanisms of action. *Adv. Neurol.*, 11:263–277.

76. Korczyn, A. D., Ben-Zvi, Z., Kaplanski, J., Danon, A., and Berginer, V. V. (1978): Plasma levels of carbamazepine and metabolites: Effect of enzyme inducers. In: *Advances in Epileptology 1977. Psychology, Pharmacotherapy and New Diagnostic Approaches*, edited by H. Meinardi and A. J. Rowan, pp. 278–279. Swets & Zeitlinger, Amsterdam, Lisse.

77. Kuhnz, W., Jäger-Roman, E., Rating, D., Deichl, A., Kunze, J., Helge, H., and Nau, H. (1983): Carbamazepine and carbamazepine-10,11-epoxide during pregnancy and postnatal period in epileptic mothers and their nursed infants: Pharmacokinetics and clinical effects. *Pediatric Pharmacology*, 3:199–208.

78. Kuhnz, W., Steldinger, R., and Nau H. (1984): Protein binding of carbamazepine and its epoxide

in maternal and fetal plasma at delivery: Comparison to other anticonvulsants. *Dev. Pharmacol. Ther.*, 7:61–72.

79. Kumps, A. H. (1981): Dose-dependency of the ratio between carbamazepine serum level and dosage in patients with epilepsy. *Therapeutic Drug Monitoring*, 3:271–274.

80. Lander, C. M., Edwards, V. E., Eadie, M. J., and Tyrer, J. H. (1977): Plasma anticonvulsant concentrations during pregnancy. *Neurology (Minneap.)*, 27:128–131.

81. Levy, R. H., and Lane, E. A. (1978): Biological halflives of antiepileptic drugs: Linearity and nonlinearity. In: *Advances in Epileptology, 1977*, edited by H. Meinardi and A. J. Rowan, pp. 186–196. Swets & Zeitlinger, Amsterdam, Lisse.

82. Levy, R. H., Lockard, J. S., Gree, J. R., Friel, P., and Martis, L. (1975): Pharmacokinetics of carbamazepine in monkeys following intravenous and oral administration. *J. Pharm. Sci.*, 64:302–307.

83. Levy, R. H., Moreland, T. A., Morselli, P. L., Guyot, M., Brachet-Liermain, A., and Loiseau, P. (1984): Carbamazepine/valproic acid interaction in man and rhesus monkey. *Epilepsia*, 25(3):338–345.

84. Levy, R. H., Pitlick, W. H., Troupin, A. S., Green, J. R., and Neal, J. M. (1975): Pharmacokinetics of carbamazepine in normal man. *Clin. Pharmacol. Ther.*, 17:657–668.

85. Lockard, J. S., Levy, R. H., Uhlir, V., and Farmuhar, J. A. (1974): Pharmacokinetic evaluation of anticonvulsants prior to efficacy testing exemplified by carbamazepine in epileptic monkey model. *Epilepsia*, 15:351–359.

86. Löscher, W. (1979): A comparative study of the protein binding of anticonvulsant drugs in serum of dog and man. *J. Pharmacol. Exp. Ther.*, 208:429–435.

87. Maas, B., Garnett, W. R., Pellock, J. M., and Comstock, T. J. (1987): A comparative bioavailability study of carbamazepine tablets and a chewable tablet formulation. *Therapeutic Drug Monitoring*, 9:28–33.

88. MacKintosh, D. A., Baird-Lampert, J., and Buchanan, N. (1987): Is carbamazepine an alternative maintenance therapy for neonatal seizures? *Dev. Pharmacol. Ther.*, 10:100–106.

89. Macphee, G. J. A., Butler, E., and Brodie, M. J. (1987): Intradose and circadian variation in circulating carbamazepine and its epoxide in epileptic patients: A consequence of autoinduction of metabolism. *Epilepsia*, 28(3):286–294.

90. McKauge, L., Tyrer, J. H., and Eadie, M. J. (1981): Factors influencing simultaneous concentrations of carbamazepine and its epoxide in plasma. *Therapeutic Drug Monitoring*, 3:63–70.

91. McNamara, P. J., Colburn, W. A., and Gibaldi, M. (1979): Time course of carbamazepine self-induction. *J. Pharmacokinet. Biopharm.*, 7:63–68.

92. Miyamoto, K., Seino, M., and Ikeda, Y. (1975): Consecutive determination of the levels of twelve antiepileptic drugs in blood and cerebrospinal

fluid. In: *Clinical Pharmacology of Antiepileptic Drugs*, edited by H. Schneider, D. Janz, C. Gardner-Thorpe, H. Meinardi, and A. L. Sherwin, pp. 323–330. Springer-Verlag, Berlin.

93. Molholm Hansen, J., Skovsted, L., Kampmann, J. P., Lumholtz, B. I., and Siersbaek-Nielsen, K. (1978): Unrelated metabolism of phenytoin in thyroid disorders. *Acta Pharmacol. Toxicol.* (Kbh.), 42:343–346.

94. Monaco, F., Mutani, R., Mastropaolo, C., and Tondi, M. (1979): Tears as the best practical indicator of the unbound fraction of an anticonvulsant drug. *Epilepsia*, 20:705–710.

95. Monaco, F., Riccio, A., Benna, P., Covacich, A., Durelli, L., Fantini, M., Furlan, P. M., Gilli, M., Mutani, R., Troni, W., Gerna, M., and Morselli, P. L. (1976): Further observations on carbamazepine plasma levels in epileptic patients. Relationships with therapeutic and side effects. *Neurology (Minneap.)*, 26:936–943.

96. Monaco, F., Riccio, A., Fantini, M., Baruzzi, A., and Morselli, P. L. (1979): A month-by-month longterm study on carbamazepine: Clinical, EEG and pharmacological evaluation. *J. Int. Med. Res.*, 7:152–157.

97. Morselli, P. L. (1975): Carbamazepine: Absorption, distribution and excretion. *Adv. Neurol.*, 11:297–293.

98. Morselli, P. L. (1977): Antiepileptic drugs. In: *Drug Disposition During Development*, edited by P. L. Morselli, pp. 311–360. Spectrum, New York.

99. Morselli, P. L. (1978): Problems of antiepileptic drugs administration in the neonatal period. In: *Barneepilepsi*, edited by A. W. Munthe-Kass and S. I. Johannessen, pp. 173–192. Ciba Geigy, Hassle.

100. Morselli, P. L., Baruzzi, A., Gerna, M., Bossi, L., and Porta, M. (1977): Carbamazepine and carbamazepine-10,11-epoxide concentration in human brain. *Br. J. Clin. Pharmacol.*, 4:535–540.

101. Morselli, P. L., Biandrate, P., Frigerio, A., Gerna, M., and Tognoni, G. (1973): Gas chromatographic determination of carbamazepine and carbamazepine-10,11-epoxide in human bloody fluids. In: *Methods of Analysis of Antiepileptic Drugs*, edited by J. W. A. Meijer, H. Meinardi, C. Gardner-Thorpe, and E. Van der Kleijn, pp. 169–175. Excerpta Medica, Amsterdam.

102. Morselli, P. L., Bossi, L., and Gerna, M. (1976): Pharmacokinetic studies with carbamazepine in epileptic patients. In: *Epileptic Seizures, Behaviour, Pain*, edited by W. Birkmayer, pp. 141–150. Huber Publishers, Bern.

103. Morselli, P. L., Calderini, G., Consolazione, A., Riva, E., and Altamura, C. Effect of Carbamazepine on brain mediators in control and cobalt-treated rats (1977). In: *Advances in Epileptology: XIIIth Congress of the International League Against Epilepsy and IXth Symposium of the International Bureau for Epilepsy*, edited by H. Meinardi, A. J. Rowan, pp. 176–182. Swets & Zeitlinger B. V., Amsterdam, Lisse.

104. Morselli, P. L., Cassano, G. B., Placidi, G. F.,

Muscettola, G. B., and Rizzo, M. (1973): Kinetics of the distribution of ^{14}C-diazepam and its metabolites in various areas of cat brain. In: *The Benzodiazepines*, edited by S. Garattini, E. Mussini, and O. Randall, pp. 129–143. Raven Press, New York.

105. Morselli, P. L., and Franco-Morselli, R. (1980): Clinical pharmacokinetics of antiepileptic drugs in adults. *Pharmacol. Ther.*, 10:65–101.

106. Morselli, P. L., Franco-Morselli, R., and Bossi, L. (1980): Clinical pharmacokinetics in newborns and infants. *Clin. Pharmacokinet.*, 5:485–527.

107. Morselli, P. L., and Frigerio, A. (1975): Metabolism and pharmacokinetics of carbamazepine. *Drug Metab. Rev.*, 4:97–113.

108. Morselli, P. L., Gerna, M., de Mayo, D., Zanda, G., Viani, F., and Garattini, S. (1975): Pharmacokinetic studies on carbamazepine in volunteers and in epileptic patients. In: *Clinical Pharmacology of Antiepileptic Drugs*, edited by H. Schneider, D. Janz, C. Gardner-Thorpe, H. Meinardi, and A. L. Sherwin, pp. 166–180. Springer-Verlag, Berlin.

109. Morselli, P. L., Gerna, M., and Garattini, S. (1971): Carbamazepine plasma and tissue levels in the rat. *Biochem. Pharmacol.*, 20:2043–2047.

110. Morselli, P. L., Monaco, F., Gerna, M., Recchia, M., and Riccio, A. (1975): Bioavailability of two carbamazepine preparations during chronic administration to epileptic patients. *Epilepsia*, 16:759–764.

111. Munari, C., Bossi, L., Stoffels, C., Brunet, P., Bancaud, J., Talairach, J., and Morselli, P. L. (1982): Concentrations cérébrales des médicaments anti-comitiaux chez les malades ayant une épilepsie tumorale. *Re. E.E.G. Neurophysiol.*, 12:38–43.

112. Neuvonen, P. J. (1985): Bioavailability and central side effects of different carbamazepine tablets. *International Journal of Clinical Pharmacology, Therapy and Toxicology*, 23(4):226–232.

113. Niebyl, J. R., Blake, D. A., Freeman, J. M., and Luff, R. D. (1979): Carbamazepine levels in pregnancy and lactation. *Obstet. Gynecol.*, 53:139–140.

114. Otani, K. (1985): Risk factors for the increased seizure frequency during pregnancy and puerperium. *Folia Psychiatrica Neurologica Japonica*, 39:33–41.

115. Pantarotto, C., Crunelli, V., Lanzoni, J., Frigerio, A., and Quattrone, A. (1979): Quantitative determination of carbamazepine and carbamazepine-10,11-epoxide in rat brain areas by multiple ion detection mass fragmentography. *Annals Biochem.*, 93:115–123.

116. Patel, I. H., Levy, R. H., and Trager, W. F. (1978): Pharmacokinetics of carbamazepine-10,11-epoxide before and after autoinduction in rhesus monkeys. *J. Pharmacol. Exp. Ther.*, 206:607–613.

117. Patel, I. H., Wedlund, P., and Levy, R. H. (1981): Induction effect of phenobarbital on the carbamazepine to carbamazepine-10,11-epoxide path-

way in rhesus monkeys. *J. Pharmacol. Exp. Ther.*, 217:555–558.

118. Patsalos, P. N., Krishna, S., Elyas, A. A., and Lascelles, P. T. (1987): Carbamazepine and carbamazepine-10,11-epoxide pharmacokinetics in an overdose patient. *Human Toxicol.*, 6:241–244.

119. Paxton, J. W., Aman, M. G., and Werry, J. S. (1983): Fluctuations in salivary carbamazepine and carbamazepine-10,11-epoxide concentrations during the day in epileptic children. *Epilepsia*, 24:716–724.

120. Pena, M. I. A., and Lope, E. S. (1987): Can a single measurement of carbamazepine suffice for therapeutic monitoring? *Clin. Chem.*, 33-6:812–813.

121. Perucca, E., Garratt, A., Hebdige, S., and Richens, A. (1978): Water intoxication in epileptic patients receiving carbamazepine. *J. Neurol. Neurosurg. Psychiatry*, 41:713–718.

122. Piafsky, K. M., and Rane, A. (1978): Formation of carbamazepine epoxide in human fetal liver. *Drug Metab. Dispos.*, 6:502–503.

123. Pitlick, W. H., and Levy, R. H. (1977): Time-dependent kinetics I: Exponential autoinduction of carbamazepine in monkeys. *J. Pharm. Sci.*, 66:647–649.

124. Pitlick, W. H., Levy, R. H., Troupin, A. S., and Green, J. R. (1976): Pharmacokinetic model to describe self-induced decreases in steady-state concentrations of carbamazepine. *J. Pharm. Sci.*, 65:462–463.

125. Placidi, G. F., Tognoni, G., Pacifici, G. M., Cassano, G. B., and Morselli, P. L. (1976): Regional distribution of diazepam and its metabolites in the brain of cat after chronic treatment. *Psychopharmacologia*, 48:133–137.

126. Pynnönen, S. (1977): The pharmacokinetics of carbamazepine in plasma and saliva of man. *Acta Pharmacol. Toxicol.* (Kbh.), 41:465–471.

127. Pynnönen, S., Björkquist, S. E., and Pekkarinen, A. (1978): The pharmacokinetics of carbamazepine in alcoholics. In: *Advances in Epileptology 1977. Psychology, Pharmacotherapy and New Diagnostic Approaches*, edited by H. Meinardi and A. J. Rowan, pp. 285–289. Swets & Zeitlinger, Amsterdam, Lisse.

128. Pynnönen, S., Kanto, J., Sillanpää, M., and Erkkola, R. (1977): Carbamazepine: Placental transport, tissue concentrations in foetus and newborn and level in milk. *Acta Pharmacol. Toxicol.* (Kbh.), 41:244–253.

129. Pynnönen, S., Mäntylä, R., and Iisalo, E. (1978): Bioavailability of four different pharmaceutical preparations of carbamazepine. *Acta Pharmacol. Toxicol.* (Kbh.), 43:306–310.

130. Pynnönen, S., Siirtola, T., Mölsä, P., and Aaltonen, L. (1978): On the distribution of carbamazepine in blood, plasma, saliva, cerebrospinal fluid and plasma water. *Acta Neurol. Scand.* (Suppl.), 67:266–267.

131. Pynnönen, S., and Sillanpää, M. (1975): Carbamazepine and mother's milk. *Lancet*, 1:563.

132. Pynnönen, S., Sillanpää, M., Frey, H., and Iisalo, E. (1977): Carbamazepine and its 10,11-epoxide in children and adults with epilepsy. *Eur. J. Clin. Pharmacol.*, 11:129–133.

133. Pynnönen, S., Sillanpää, M., Iisalo, E., and Frey, H. (1977): Elimination of carbamazepine in children after single and multiple doses. In: *Epilepsy, the Eighth International Symposium*, edited by J. K. Penry, pp. 191–196. Raven Press, New York.

134. Pynnönen, S., and Yrjänä, T. (1977): The significance of the simultaneous determination of carbamazepine and its 10,11-epoxide from plasma and human erythrocytes. *Int. J. Clin. Pharmacol.*, 15:222–226.

135. Rambeck, B., May, T., and Juergens, U. (1987): Serum concentrations of carbamazepine and its epoxide and diol metabolites in epileptic patients: The influence of dose and comedication. *Therapeutic Drug Monitoring*, 9:298–303.

136. Rane, A., and Bertilsson, L. (1980): Kinetics of carbamazepine in epileptic children. In: *Antiepileptic Therapy: Advances in Drug Monitoring*, edited by S. I. Johannesen, P. L., Morselli, C. E. Pippenger, A. Richens, D. Schmidt, and H. Meinardi, pp. 49–54. Raven Press, New York.

137. Rane, A., Bertilsson, L., and Parmer, L. (1975): Disposition of placentally transferred carbamazepine (Tegretol®) in the newborn. *Eur. J. Clin. Pharmacol.*, 8:283–284.

138. Rane, A., and Wilson, J. T. (1976): Plasma level monitoring of diphenylhydantoin and carbamazepine in the pediatric patient. In: *Clinical Pharmacy and Clinical Pharmacology*, edited by W. A. Gouveia, G. Tognoni, and E. van Der Kleijn, pp. 295–302. Elsevier/North Holland Biomedical Press, Amsterdam.

139. Rapeport, W. G. (1985): Factors influencing the relationship between carbamazepine plasma concentration and its clinical effects in patients with epilepsy. *Clinical Neuropharmacology*, 8(2):141–149.

140. Rawlins, M. D., Collste, P., Bertilsson, L., and Palmer, L. (1975): Distribution and elimination kinetics of carbamazepine in man. *Eur. J. Clin. Pharmacol.*, 8:91–96.

141. Reidenberg, M. M., and Drayer, D. E. (1978): Effects of renal diseases upon drug disposition. *Drug Metab. Rev.*, 8:293–302.

142. Rey, E., d'Athis, P., de Lauture, D., Dulac, O., Aicardi, J., and Olive, G. (1979): Pharmacokinetics of carbamazepine in the neonate and in the child. *Int. J. Clin. Pharmacol. Biopharm.*, 17:90–96.

143. Riad, L. E., Chan, K. K. H., Wagner, W. E., and Sawchuk, R. J. (1986): Simultaneous first- and zero-order absorption of carbamazepine tablets in humans. *Journal of Pharmaceutical Sciences*, 75(9):897–900.

144. Riva, R., Albani, F., Ambrosetto, G., Contin, M., Cortelli, P., Perucca, E., and Baruzzi, A. (1984): Diurnal fluctuations in free and total steady-state plasma levels of carbamazepine and correlation with intermittent side effects. *Epilepsia*, 25(4):476–481.

145. Riva, R., Contin, M., Albani, F., Perucca, E.,

Ambrosetto, G., Procaccianti, G., Santucci, M., and Baruzzi, A. (1985a): Lateral gaze nystagmus in carbamazepine-treated epileptic patients: Correlation with total and free plasma concentrations of parent drug and its 10,11-epoxide metabolite. *Therapeutic Drug Monitoring*, 7:277–282.

146. Riva, R., Contin, M., Albani, F., Perucca, E., Lamontanara, G., and Baruzzi, A. (1985): Free and total serum concentrations of carbamazepine and carbamazepine-10,11-epoxide in infancy and childhood. *Epilepsia*, 26(4):320–322.

147. Ronfeld, R. A., and Benet, L. Z. (1975): Dose dependent kinetics of carbamazepine in the monkey. *Res. Commun. Chem. Pathol. Pharmacol.*, 10:303–314.

148. Rylance, G. W., Butcher, G. M., and Moreland, T. (1977): Saliva carbamazepine levels in children. *Br. Med. J.*, 3:1481.

149. Rylance, G. W., Edwards, C., and Gard, P. R. (1984): Carbamazepine 10,11-epoxide in children. *Br. J. Clin. Pharmac.*, 18:935–939.

150. Rylance, G. W., Moreland, T. A., and Butcher, G. M. (1978): Individualisation of anticonvulsant medication: A new approach with carbamazepine levels in children. *Arch. Dis. Child.*, 53:690.

151. Sanchez, A., Duran, J. A., and Serrano, J. S. (1986): Steady-state carbamazepine plasma concentration-dose ratios in epileptic patients. *Clin. Pharmacokinet.*, 11:411–414.

152. Schoeman, J. F., Elyas, A. A., Brett, E. M., and Lascelles, P. T. (1984): Altered ratio of carbamazepine-10,11-epoxide/carbamazepine in plasma of children: Evidence of anticonvulsant drug interaction. *Developmental Medicine & Child Neurology*, 26:749–755.

153. Simonsen, N., Zander Olsen, P., Kühl, V., Lund, M., and Wendelboe, J. (1976): A comparative controlled study between carbamazepine and diphenylhydantoin in psychomotor epilepsy. *Epilepsia*, 17:169–176.

154. Smith, G. A., Hooper, W. D., Tyrer, J. H., Eadie, M. J., and Werth, B. (1979): The comparative bioavailability of carbamazepine in 100 mg and 200 mg tablets. *Clin. Exp. Pharmacol. Physiol.*, 6:37–40.

155. Strandjord, R. E., and Johannessen, S. I. (1975): A preliminary study of serum carbamazepine levels in healthy subjects and in patients with epilepsy. In: *Clinical Pharmacology of Antiepileptic Drugs*, edited by H. Schneider, D. Janz, C. Gardner-Thorpe, H. Meinardi, and A. L. Sherwin, pp. 181–188.

156. Strandjord, R. E., and Johannessen, S. I. (1978): Monoterapi und Karmabazepin. In: *Barnepilepsy*, edited by A. W. Munthe-Kaas and S. I. Johannessen, pp. 77–82. Ciba-Geigy, Basel.

157. Sumi, M., Watari, N., Umezawa, O., and Kaneniwa, N. (1987): Pharmacokinetic study of carbamazepine and its epoxide metabolite in humans. *J. Pharmacobio. Dyn.*, 10:652–661.

158. Suzuki, K., Kaneko, S., and Sato, T. (1978): Time-dependency of serum carbamazepine concentration. *Foli Psychiatr. Neurol. Jpn.*, 32:199–209.

159. Tedeschi, G., Cenraud, B., Guyot, M., Gomeni, R., Morselli, P. L., Levy, R. H., and Loiseau, P. Influence of food on carbamazepine absorption. In: *Advances in Epileptology: XIIth Epilepsy International Symposium*, edited by M. Dam, L. Gram, and J. K. Penry, pp. 563–568, Raven Press, New York.

160. Terhaag, B., Richter, K., and Diettrich, H. (1978): Concentration behavior of carbamazepine in bile and plasma of man. *Int. J. Clin. Pharmacol.*, 16:607–609.

161. Tomlin, I., McKinlay, Smith, (1986): A study on carbamazepine levels, including estimation of 10-11-epoxy-carbamazepine and levels in free plasma and saliva. *Developmental Medicine & Child Neurology*, 28:713–718.

162. Tomson, T., Tybring, G., and Bertilsson, L. (1983): Single-dose kinetics and metabolism of carbamazepine-10,11-epoxide. *Clinical Pharmacology and Therapeutics*, 133(1):58–65.

163. Tondi, M., Mutani, R., Mastropaolo, C., and Monaco, F. (1978): Greater reliability of tear versus saliva anticonvulsant levels. *Ann. Neurol.*, 4:154–155.

164. Troupin, A. S. (1978): Carbamazepine in epilepsy. In: *Clinical Neuropharmacology*, vol. 3, edited by H. L. Klawans, pp. 15–40. Raven Press, New York.

165. Troupin, A. S., and Friel, P. (1978): Anticonvulsant level in saliva, serum and cerebrospinal fluid. *Epilepsia*, 16:223–227.

166. Troupin, A. S., Green, J. R., and Levy, R. H. (1974): Carbamazepine as an anticonvulsant: A pilot study. *Neurology (Minneap.)*, 24:863–869.

167. Van der Kleijn, E., Guelen, P. J. M., Van Wijk, C., and Baars, I. (1975): Clinical pharmacokinetics in monitoring chronic medication with antiepileptic drugs. In: *Clinical Pharmacology of Antiepileptic Drugs*, edited by H. Schneider, D. Janz, C. Gardner-Thorpe, H. Meinardi, and A. L. Sherwin, pp. 11–33. Springer-Verlag, Berlin.

168. Vree, T. B., Janssen, T. J., Hekster, Y. A., Termond, E. F. S., van de Dries, A. C. P., and Wijnands, W. J. A. (1986): Clinical pharmacokinetics of carbamazepine and its epoxy and hydroxy metabolites in humans after an overdose. *Therapeutic Drug Monitoring*, 8:297–304.

169. Wada, J. A., Troupin, A. S., Friel, P., Remick, R., Leal, K., and Pearmain, J. (1978): Pharmacokinetic comparison of tablet and suspension dosage forms of carbamazepine. *Epilepsia*, 19:251–255.

170. Wagner, J., and Schmid, K. (1987): Induction of microsomal enzymes in rat liver by oxcarbazepine, 10,11-dihydro-10-hydroxy-carbamazepine and carbamazepine. *Xenobiotica*, 17(8):951–956.

171. Watanabe, S., Kuyama, C., Yokoyama, S., Kubo, S., and Iwai, H. (1977): Distribution of plasma carbamazepine in epileptic patients. *Folia Psychiatr. Neurol. Jpn.*, 31:587–595.

172. Wedlund, P. J., and Levy, R. H. (1983): Time-dependent kinetics VII: Effect of diurnal oscillations on time course of carbamazepine autoin-

duction in the rhesus monkey. *Journal of Pharmaceutical Sciences*, 72(8):905–908.

173. Westenberg, H. G. M., Jonkman, J. H. G., and Van der Kleijn, E. (1977): The distribution of carbamazepine and its metabolites in squirrel monkey and mouse. *Acta Pharmacol. Toxicol.* (Suppl.) (Kbh.), 41:136–137.

174. Westenberg, H. G. M., Van der Kleijn, E., Oei, T. T., and de Zeeuw, R. (1978): Kinetics of carbamazepine and carbamazepine-epoxide, determined by use of plasma and saliva. *Clin. Pharmacol. Ther.*, 23:320–328.

175. Yerby, M. S., Friel, P. N., and Miller, D. Q. (1985): Carbamazepine protein binding and disposition in pregnancy. *Therapeutic Drug Monitoring*, 7:269–273.

176. Yerby, M. S. (1987): Problems and management of the pregnant women with epilepsy. *Epilepsia*, 28(suppl. 3):29–36.

Antiepileptic Drugs, Third Edition, edited by
R. Levy, R. Mattson, B. Meldrum,
J. K. Penry, and F. E. Dreifuss.
Raven Press, Ltd., New York © 1989.

34

Carbamazepine

Biotransformation

J. W. Faigle and K. F. Feldmann

INTRODUCTION

Carbamazepine (CBZ), the active ingredient of Tegretol, belongs to the series of tricyclic compounds. Its chemical name is 5-carbamoyl-5H-dibenz[b,f]azepine or 5H-dibenz[b,f]azepine-5-carboxamide. In its ring structure it differs from the other established antiepileptics, but is related to some antidepressants such as imipramine or clomipramine (21). Owing to the nature of their side chains, however, these antidepressants are basic compounds, whereas CBZ is a neutral substance (Fig. 1).

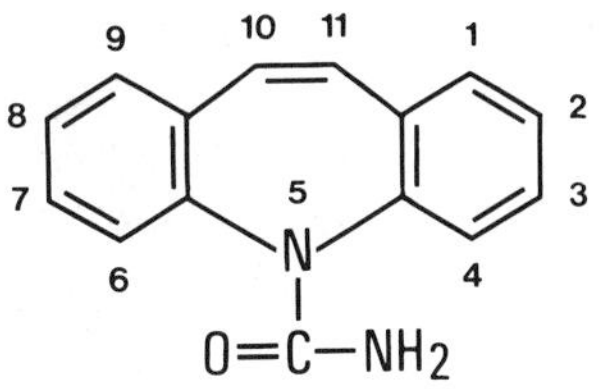

Being a liposoluble neutral substance, CBZ can easily pass through the blood-brain barrier and other membranes of the body (11). Yet, CBZ is not eliminated as such in the urine or bile. The mammalian body possesses no mechanism by which exogenous lipophilic compounds, including especially those of a neutral character, can readily be excreted in unchanged form (2). A family of enzymes converts such compounds ultimately into hydrophilic metabolites that are easily removed by the normal routes of waste disposal.

CBZ does indeed undergo almost complete biotransformation in both humans and animals (13,32). A large number of metabolites is formed by parallel or consecutive

FIG. 1. Structural formula of CBZ, 5-carbamoyl-5H-dibenz[b,f]azepine, and numbering of positions in the tricyclic skeleton of the molecule.

reactions. A few of the intermediate products possess anticonvulsant activities of their own. The kinetics of CBZ and its active metabolites in the patient's body are determined by the rates of the pertinent enzymatic reactions. All these processes have a direct influence on the efficacy and tolerability of antiepileptic treatment. In this chapter, therefore, we also wish to consider some enzymological, pharmacological, and toxicological aspects of CBZ biotransformation, in addition to the pure chemistry of the metabolic reactions.

CHEMICAL ASPECTS OF METABOLISM

Mass Balance and Structures of Metabolites

In a key study with ^{14}C-labeled CBZ in healthy volunteers, urinary metabolites were isolated and identified by liquid chromatographic and spectroscopic techniques. With measurement of radioactivity, it was possible to establish a mass balance of the metabolic end products (11,12,13). In this study, 72% of a 400-mg oral dose of CBZ was recovered in urine and the remainder was recovered in feces. Only about 3% of the total radioactivity present in urine, corresponding to 2% of the dose, was identified as unchanged CBZ.

The structures of the metabolites isolated disclose that biotransformation of CBZ in humans proceeds by four major pathways (Fig. 2).

Taking the total urinary radioactivity as 100%, the following approximate percentages are attributable to products of these pathways: oxidation of the 10,11-double bond of the azepine ring, 40%; hydroxylation of the six-membered aromatic rings, 25%; direct *N*-glucuronidation at the carbamoyl side chain, 15%; and substitution of the six-membered rings with sulfur-containing groups, 5%. This adds to a mass balance of about 90% of total urinary radioactivity.

In an independent detailed study, Lertratanangkoon and Horning (32) found most of the metabolites shown in Fig. 2 also in the urine of patients receiving long-term treatment with CBZ. In addition, they identified several products formed by more than one of the known metabolic reactions, e.g., by 10,11-oxidation and aromatic hydroxylation. Such products, which also occur in healthy subjects, further add to the metabolic balance in urine.

Partial findings on CBZ biotransforma-

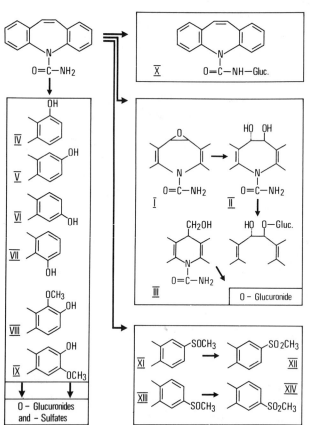

FIG. 2. Structures of metabolites of CBZ isolated from human urine and major pathways of biotransformation.

tion are available from numerous other sources. By and large, they all confirm what is known from the above studies (for review see refs. 5,9,13,54). Some rearrangement and degradation products that had been isolated in very early investigations were later recognized as artifacts (13).

The Epoxide Pathway

In CBZ biotransformation, the epoxide pathway is quantitatively the most important one. That is true for normal subjects, and even more so for patients with induced liver enzymes (10,13). The first actually tangible product of this pathway is 10,11-epoxy-carbamazepine (epoxy-CBZ, I). Being an aliphatic rather than aromatic epoxide, it is chemically stable under physiological conditions. Yet, only little of epoxy-CBZ is excreted as such (about 1% of the dose), with most being enzymatically converted to the corresponding diol, 10,11-dihydro-10,11-di-hydroxy-carbamazepine (10,11-di-H-10,11-di-OH-CBZ, II). The hydroxyl groups of II are *trans* to each other, as was shown by spectroscopic analysis in comparison with the synthetic *cis* and *trans* isomers (12). The diol is formed in an enantiomeric excess of 80%, the prevalent enantiomer having the (−)-10S,11S configuration (4). In urine, the diol is partly present as such and partly as its mono-*O*-glucuronide (48).

9-Hydroxymethyl-10-carbamoyl acridan (III) is a minor metabolite related to the epoxide pathway (see Fig. 2). It is almost completely conjugated with glucuronic acid at the hydroxymethyl group before excretion (10,13). Originally, we postulated the epoxide I and/or the diol II as intermediary precursors of III, but this hypothesis has to be revised in light of more recent findings. Bertilsson and co-workers administered epoxy-CBZ to humans (5,55) and recovered 90% of the dose as free plus conjugated diol metabolite II in urine. The amount of III, in relation to the diol, was only about one-tenth of that found after CBZ administration, however (10).

Independent studies on metabolic oxidation of carbon-carbon double bonds offer a ready explanation. According to Loew and co-workers (29,45), cytochrome P-450 mediated oxidation begins with the addition of a single oxygen to one of the C-atoms of the double bond. The first intermediate may give rise to an epoxide or, alternatively, to rearrangement products. Based on these findings and on known mechanisms of azepine ring contraction (47), we propose the reaction scheme displayed in Fig. 3.

Reaction (a) involves an oxidative attack at the 10,11-double bond of CBZ. The oxygen-containing intermediate is formulated as a biradical, because radical pathways are preferred over ionic ones in epoxide formation (29). The main processes (b) and (c) do in fact result in epoxy-CBZ (I) and 10,11-di-H-10,11-di-OH-CBZ (II). As a side path, the first intermediate undergoes the consecutive rearrangements (d), (e), and (f), yielding 10-carbamoyl acridan-9-carboxaldehyde. Eventually, metabolic reduction converts this aldehyde into the hydroxymethyl compound III.

For readers involved in metabolic and kinetic studies with CBZ, it may be noteworthy that the essential products (I, II, III) of the epoxide pathway have been prepared synthetically. For the respective methods of preparation see Bellucci et al. (4) and Heckendorn (24).

Aromatic Hydroxylation

Oxidations at various positions of the six-membered aromatic rings represent an additional pathway of CBZ biotransformation. Quantitatively, it is less important than oxidation in the central azepine ring. Single substitution results in all four possible phenols, i.e., 1-, 2-, 3-, and 4-hydroxycarbamazepine (IV to VII in Fig. 2). Two other products of this pathway carry a hydroxyl

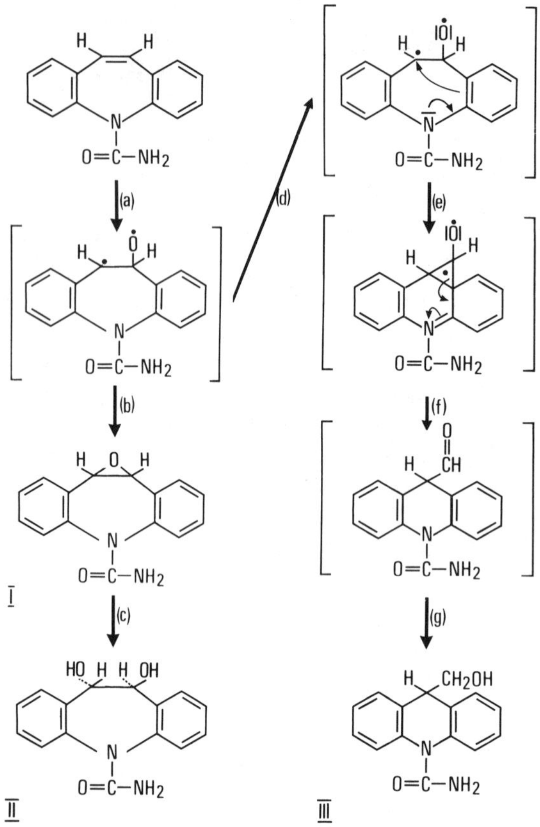

FIG. 3. Metabolites resulting from enzymatic oxidation of the 10,11-double bond of CBZ: proposed pathways and mechanisms. (The intermediates in brackets are hypothetic.)

group in position 2 and, additionally, a methoxy group in position 1 or 3 (13). Only trace amounts of these phenols are excreted unconjugated by the kidneys, the bulk being converted to the *O*-glucuronides and *O*-sulfates in a ratio of about 2:1. Additional products of twofold aromatic oxidation were described by Lynn et al. (35), and Lertratanangkoon and Horning (32). They include hydroxymethoxy as well as dihydroxy metabolites of CBZ, most of them carrying the substituents *ortho* to each other.

The true mechanism by which the phenolic metabolites of CBZ are formed is still unexplored. Arene oxides are conceivable intermediates arising from cytochrome P-450 mediated oxidation. In accordance with known mechanisms (29), arene oxides

would presumably be formed by the biradical pathway (h) and (i) illustrated in Fig. 4. Rearrangement (k) would lead to a monofunctional phenol. Hydrolysis of the arene oxide, followed by aromatization of the dihydro dihydroxy intermediate, would result in bifunctional phenols with vicinal groups (32).

Reaction (l) in Fig. 4 represents another possible pathway of enzymatic oxidation. The first product is a cation, which would yield the phenol by water-assisted deprotonation (m). This reaction has a particularly low enthalpy of activation (29). Bifunctional phenols would then emerge from consecutive oxidative attacks. Future studies are needed to find out which of the pathways is actually operative in the aromatic hydroxylation of CBZ.

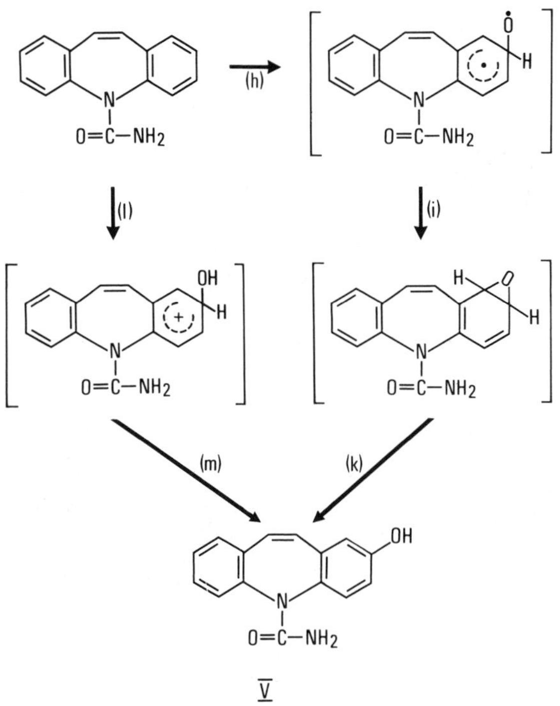

FIG. 4. Possible mechanisms of enzymatic oxidation at the aromatic rings of CBZ, formation of the phenol V serving as an example. (The intermediates in brackets are hypothetic.)

Conjugation Reactions

Direct conjugation of CBZ with glucuronic acid is the third important route of biotransformation (13,35). In the conjugate, the ligand is bound to the amino group of the carbamoyl side chain (X in Fig. 2). A possible binding to the hydroxyl group of the isourea structure is ruled out by the infrared spectrum of the pure metabolite (48). It is interesting to note that the conjugate cannot be cleaved with β-glucuronidase, although it possesses β-D-configuration.

Glucuronidation also occurs as a secondary metabolic process. Virtually all of the CBZ metabolites carrying free hydroxyl groups are converted to their O-glucuronides, at least to some extent (10,13,35,54). This includes the diol II, the hydroxymethyl compound III, and the mono- and bifunctional phenols. The O-glucuronides encountered in CBZ biotransformation are susceptible to hydrolysis with β-glucuronidase.

Conjugation of the phenolic metabolites with sulfuric acid is an additional secondary process, which is less prominent than glucuronidation, however (13).

Last but not least is the formation of sulfur-containing conjugates of CBZ. They include the 2- and 3-substituted methylsulfinyl and methylsulfonyl compounds XI to XIV in Fig. 2 (13), and some isomers with undefined sites of substitution (32). So far, no intermediates of this pathway of CBZ biotransformation have been traced. Therefore, the underlying mechanisms can only be deduced from general knowledge obtained with other aromatic compounds.

In all likelihood, the metabolites in question result from oxidation of the respective methylthio intermediates. The latter may arise from at least two pathways (52). Direct metabolic transfer of the methylthio group of methionine to an aromatic nucleus is possible, but it is encountered in a few special cases only. Another and well established pathway includes the conjugation of a reactive intermediate, e.g., an arene oxide (see Fig. 4), with glutathione or acetylcysteine. The resulting conjugate is broken down to a thiophenol, which then undergoes enzymatic methylation yielding the methylthio analog. We assume that the methylsulfinyl and methylsulfonyl conjugates of CBZ are derived from the latter reaction sequence. Schemes showing details of this sequence have been published elsewhere (32,52).

ENZYMOLOGICAL ASPECTS OF METABOLISM

Enzymes Involved in Major Pathways

CBZ is not subject to any first-pass metabolism. This is evident from a pharmacokinetic comparison of the oral and intravenous routes of CBZ administration in healthy subjects, which showed complete bioavailability of the oral dose (A. Gérardin, *unpublished data*). Thus, metabolic attack by enzymes of the gastric or intestinal walls can be ruled out. Animal studies suggest that another metabolically active site, i.e., the lung, contributes only marginally to the total body clearance of CBZ (61). Human liver microsomes, on the other hand, are able to metabolize CBZ *in vitro*, epoxy-CBZ being the major product (56,58). For the most part, therefore, biotransformation of CBZ appears to be localized in the liver.

Oxidative attack at the 10,11-double bond is the major process controlling the elimination of the drug from the human body. The initial reaction (see Fig. 3) is catalyzed by hepatic microsomal cytochrome P-450 (49,56,57,62). Although the isoenzyme actually involved is still unexplored, certain indications as to its nature do exist. It is known that the enzyme in question is strongly induced by repeated administration of CBZ to both humans and animals

(46,54,56). The type of induction is the same as that produced by phenobarbital (60). We therefore conclude that 10,11-oxidation of CBZ is brought about by one of the phenobarbital-inducible isoenzymes of the P-450IIB or P-450IIC subfamily, as defined in the new standardized nomenclature (39).

According to Sumi et al. (51), enzymatic formation of epoxy-CBZ in man follows Michaelis-Menten kinetics. However, the K_m-value is well above the therapeutic plasma concentration of CBZ. In the relevant concentration range, therefore, CBZ kinetics appear linear.

Epoxy-CBZ is almost completely converted to the *trans*-diol II (see Figs. 2 and 3). The respective epoxide hydrolase is inducible by repeated doses of CBZ, although to a lesser extent than the P-450 isoenzyme which produces epoxy-CBZ (6,10,56). This hydrolase is located in the microsomal fraction of the liver cell (27,56). Cytosolic epoxide hydrolases also exist, but they are not inducible by substances of the phenobarbital type (37).

Aromatic hydroxylation is catalyzed by hepatic cytochrome P-450, regardless of whether it proceeds by the cationic or the biradical mechanism (29) (see Fig. 4). The isoenzyme mediating the attack at the aromatic rings of CBZ is not the same as that responsible for 10,11-oxidation. This is clearly demonstrated by the differential effects of CBZ administration on the rate of the two processes in man: whereas 10,11-oxidation is strongly induced, aromatic hydroxylation remains virtually unchanged (10).

Glucuronidation is involved in several steps of CBZ metabolism (see above). Nevertheless, only the conversion of CBZ into its direct *N*-glucuronide X is a primary reaction actually influencing the rate of CBZ elimination. This reaction requires a UDP-glucuronyltransferase, which is a microsomal enzyme system located in the liver and other organs. Several isoenzymes have been described (8,43), but the essential one for CBZ conjugation is yet unidentified. However, direct glucuronidation of CBZ is only a minor pathway (13).

Enzyme Induction and Inhibition

CBZ is cleared from the human body almost exclusively by hepatic metabolism. Thus, the plasma clearance values can be taken as a direct measure of the activity of the metabolizing enzymes. In Table 1, such values are listed for three groups of subjects, i.e., healthy volunteers after single CBZ doses, epileptic patients receiving monotherapy with CBZ, and patients receiving CBZ in combination with other anticonvulsants (10). Compared to the first group, total plasma clearance of CBZ is increased about threefold in the second and sixfold in the group group.

Among the individual pathways investigated, it is 10,11-oxidation (leading eventually to the diol II and the hydroxymethyl compound III) that is most strongly enhanced. Aromatic hydroxylation (leading to phenols such as V and VI) is induced by the other drugs, but not by CBZ alone. As a consequence of differential enzyme induction, the amount of diol recovered in urine of individual subjects is closely correlated

with the total plasma clearance of CBZ. In strongly induced patients, the diol may account for up to 60% of the dose (10,54).

Preliminary findings suggest that the metabolic clearance of epoxy-CBZ is approximately 75 to 85 $ml \cdot hr^{-1} \cdot kg^{-1}$ in normal subjects, compared to 165 $ml \cdot hr^{-1} \cdot kg^{-1}$ in patients receiving antiepileptic drugs (10,44). This would imply a doubling of the rate of epoxide hydrolysis, which is considerably lower than the enhancement of 10,11-oxidation (see Table 1). In patients, therefore, the concentration ratio of epoxy-CBZ to CBZ in plasma is higher than in non-induced volunteers.

Several drugs are known to interfere with the metabolism of CBZ in man by inhibiting cytochrome P-450 enzyme systems. Examples of such drugs are danazol, diltiazem, erythromycin, isoniazid, nafimidone, propoxyphene, triacetyloleandomycin, verapamil, and viloxazine. They increase the plasma concentration of CBZ when they are added to an existing therapeutic treatment with CBZ. For reviews of clinical implications see Baciewicz (3), Kraemer et al. (30), and Chapter 36. In a few cases, the underlying mechanism has been studied and recognized as a reversible inhibition of enzymatic 10,11-oxidation of CBZ (31,49).

Another drug, valpromide, is known to

TABLE 1. *Total plasma clearances of CBZ (Cl_p), and clearances to individual metabolites (Cl_{II}, Cl_{III}, Cl_V, Cl_{VI}) in healthy volunteers and epileptic patients[a]*

Subjects	Cl_p	Cl_{II}	Cl_{III}	Cl_V	Cl_{VI}
Healthy volunteers ($N = 6$); single doses of CBZ	19.8 ± 2.7	4.3 ± 1.3	0.9 ± 0.2	1.2 ± 0.5	1.1 ± 0.4
Epileptic patients ($N = 4$); monotherapy with CBZ	54.6 ± 6.7	14.5 ± 2.7	4.6 ± 1.5	1.3 ± 0.4	1.6 ± 0.7
Epileptic patients ($N = 5$); polytherapy with CBZ and other drugs	133.3 ± 33.4	58.6 ± 26.5	7.8 ± 2.9	3.6 ± 1.7	4.3 ± 1.5

[a] Clearances are given in terms of $ml \cdot hr^{-1} \cdot kg^{-1}$ (mean values ± SD), as reported by Eichelbaum et al. (10).

II, 10,11-di-H-10,11-di-OH-CBZ; III, 9-Hydroxymethyl-10-carbamoyl acridan; V, 2-Hydroxycarbamazepine; VI, 3-Hydroxycarbamazepine.

competitively inhibit the hepatic microsomal epoxide hydrolase (36,40,44). In patients receiving CBZ, concomitant administration of valpromide leads to an increase of epoxy-CBZ concentrations in plasma. This inhibition is a specific effect of valpromide; it is not produced by its analog, valproic acid.

Pharmacogenetics

As mentioned above, 10,11-oxidation and aromatic hydroxylation are the two major pathways of CBZ elimination in man. They are mediated by two different isoenzymes of the cytochrome P-450 complex. The metabolic capacities of the two pathways do not correlate with 4-hydroxylation of debrisoquine or oxidation of sparteine (10). This is consistent with the general classification of the P-450 isoenzymes: debrisoquine 4-hydroxylase is assigned to the P-450IID subfamily (39), whereas the isoenzymes involved in CBZ oxidation belong to other subfamilies, presumably P-450IIB and/or P-450IIC.

From these findings, we infer that the genetic polymorphism related to debrisoquine and sparteine oxidation has no effect on the kinetics of CBZ in man. However, we cannot exclude the possibility that there are other genetic factors that influence the individual's metabolism of CBZ or the inducibility of the metabolizing enzymes.

In this context it seems noteworthy that CBZ clearance by the epoxide pathway in man does not correlate with several other metabolic reactions. They include 3- and 4-hydroxylation of antipyrine, demethylation of amitriptyline, and total metabolic clearance of theophylline (10).

PHARMACOLOGICAL AND TOXICOLOGICAL ASPECTS OF METABOLISM

Metabolites Present in Blood and Brain

Knowledge of the structures and the mass balance of urinary metabolites is essential when the pathways of biotransformation of

CBZ are to be deduced (see Fig. 2). However, when the pharmacological and toxicological effects of CBZ are discussed, it is more important to consider the drug-related products present in blood.

The radiotracer experiment mentioned earlier (11,12) yielded a mass balance of CBZ and its metabolites in the plasma of healthy volunteers after single oral doses of 400 mg. On the basis of the areas under the concentration-time curves (AUC, 0–96 hr), the unchanged drug accounts for about 75% of the total radioactivity present in plasma, epoxy-CBZ for 10%, and the sum of all other metabolites for only 15%. These findings suggest that the bulk of metabolites, including the strongly hydrophilic end products, is rapidly removed from the circulation by the kidneys.

The elimination of CBZ from the blood is controlled by the primary metabolic reactions rather than by renal or biliary excretion of unchanged drug. These reactions particularly include 10,11-oxidation, aromatic hydroxylation, and N-glucuronidation, all of which are mediated by hepatic enzymes. The kinetics of the major intermediary metabolite, epoxy-CBZ, are likewise under enzymatic control. There is no indication that the enzymes involved are saturated within the clinically relevant dose range of CBZ. In a given subject, the kinetics of both CBZ and epoxy-CBZ are in fact linear. This applies to healthy volunteers after single doses as well as to patients receiving long-term treatment (5,11,55). Only after the intake of massive overdoses, i.e., up to 18 g of CBZ, might saturation kinetics show up (59).

The preferential induction of 10,11-oxidation by prolonged exposure to CBZ (see Table 1) leads to an increase of the plasma concentrations of epoxy-CBZ relative to those of CBZ. This is even more pronounced when other anticonvulsants such as phenytoin, phenobarbital, or primidone are co-administered. Hundt et al. (25), for instance, reported plasma concentration ratios derived from more than 2,000 measurements in epileptic patients. All patients were under long-term treatment with CBZ, and most of them also with other drugs. Expressed as a percentage of the respective CBZ concentration, the values for epoxy-CBZ averaged about 30% and those for the diol 50%. After single doses of CBZ, none of the metabolites exceeded 20% (13).

Epoxy-CBZ possesses anticonvulsant activities of its own, whereas the diol metabolite does not (see below). Therefore, among the drug-related compounds reaching sizeable concentrations in plasma, only CBZ and epoxy-CBZ are of clinical interest. Both compounds readily pass into the central nervous system, presumably by passive diffusion (11,34,38). The concentrations in the cerebrospinal fluid of humans reflect the free, nonprotein bound fractions in plasma, i.e., about 25% and 50% of the total plasma concentration of CBZ and epoxy-CBZ, respectively (26). The concentrations in the brain are higher, as a result of binding to brain proteins or phospholipids (23). According to Friis et al. (19), the actual brain-to-plasma concentration ratio is 1.5 for CBZ and 1.1 for epoxy-CBZ. These data represent mean values in epileptic patients receiving long-term treatment with CBZ.

In the same patients, the absolute mean concentrations in brain amount to about 8 $\mu g/g$ for CBZ and 3 $\mu g/g$ for epoxy-CBZ (19). This agrees fairly well with the range of brain concentrations found to protect animals against electroshock-induced convulsions (7,14,63). In the mouse, for instance, the effective brain concentration (EC_{50}) of CBZ is 6 $\mu g/g$. Epoxy-CBZ is somewhat less active in terms of brain concentrations, but the effects of the two compounds are additive (7).

Biological Activities of Metabolites

The results from several independent studies clearly show that epoxy-CBZ possesses intrinsic pharmacological activities. For instance, it is a potent anticonvulsant in animals (7,14), and it is effective in the treatment of trigeminal neuralgia in patients (5). For more details on the significance of epoxy-CBZ, see Chapter 35. For several other metabolites of CBZ, the anticonvulsant properties in animal models are known as well. The compounds are listed in Table 2 together with the doses (ED_{50}) required to protect 50% of the animals against convulsions induced by electroshock or pentylenetetrazol (13). The values for CBZ and epoxy-CBZ are also included in the table. In those cases where no ED_{50} was obtained, the table specifies the highest dose examined and the corresponding percentage of protected animals.

On the basis of the ED_{50} values, the efficacy of epoxy-CBZ is similar to that of the parent drug (although in terms of concentrations the epoxide appears somewhat less

TABLE 2. *Anticonvulsant activities of CBZ and metabolites in animals, measured after single oral doses of the synthetic products (13)*

Compound	ED_{50} in three animal models[a]		
	Electroshock-mice	Electroshock-rats	PTZ-mice[b]
CBZ	10–13	7–10	21–60
Epoxy-CBZ (I)	12–16	13–15	8–24
10,11-di-H-10,11-di-OH-CBZ (II)	100 (0%)	—[c]	—
9-Hydroxymethyl-10-carbamoyl acridan (III)	17–39	50	100 (20–40%)
2-Hydroxycarbamazepine (V)	300 (0%)	—	—
3-Hydroxycarbamazepine (VI)	38	100 (10%)	100 (0%)
3-Methylsulfonylcarbamazepine (XIV)	300 (0%)	—	—

[a] ED_{50}, dose (mg/kg) required to protect 50% of the animals.
[b] PTZ, pentylenetetrazol test in mice.
[c] not tested.

active; see above). 9-Hydroxymethyl-10-carbamoyl acridan, which is another product of 10,11-oxidation, is considerably less active than CBZ, and 10,11-di-H-10,11-di-OH-CBZ is inactive. Two products of aromatic hydroxylation, 2- and 3-hydroxy-carbamazepine, show only little or no activity in the tests used. A representative of the metabolites carrying sulfur-containing substituents, 3-methylsulfonyl-carbamazepine, is again devoid of anticonvulsant effects.

The activity data in Table 2 confirm what has already been indicated by the concentration pattern in human plasma: of all the metabolites, it is only epoxy-CBZ that can significantly add to the antiepileptic effects of CBZ. The other metabolites do not essentially contribute because of their low potency or low concentration, or both. Thus, plasma level monitoring in patients who receive CBZ treatment should always include the epoxide metabolite.

In view of their similar activity spectrum, it is to be expected that CBZ and epoxy-CBZ also resemble each other regarding their side effects. This assumption is indeed supported by some clinical observations. For instance, addition of valpromide to an existing treatment with CBZ in epileptic patients led to symptoms typical of CBZ intoxication, although the serum concentration of the unchanged drug remained constant (36). In these patients, however, the epoxy-CBZ levels were markedly increased, because valpromide interferes with the hydrolysis of the epoxide (40,44). In animals, the brain concentration required to precipitate neurotoxicity is also virtually the same for CBZ and epoxy-CBZ, but is three to four times above the pharmacologically effective concentration (7).

Prenatal exposure to some combinations of antiepileptic drugs can result in an increased rate of congenital anomalies in the infant. It has been speculated that this effect may be attributable to enzyme induction and enhanced formation of epoxy-CBZ or of epoxides of other drugs (33,41). In animal

models, CBZ shows no or only a slight teratogenic potential. In a special study, two strains of mice were included, one having a low and the other having a high level of epoxide hydrolase activity (16). Long-term administration of CBZ resulted in largely different plasma concentrations of epoxy-CBZ in these two strains. Elevation of the epoxide was not correlated with the incidence of fetal abnormality and, therefore, epoxy-CBZ appears devoid of any special teratogenic risk.

Several products of oxidative biotransformation of CBZ may be considered as potentially reactive metabolites. This includes particularly the biradical, the cationic, and the arene oxide intermediates postulated in Figs. 3 and 4. Theoretically, such reactive intermediates may cause toxic effects through spontaneous covalent binding to macromolecules, such as protein, DNA, and RNA. The bacterial mutagenicity test of Ames et al. (1) is a sensitive method for the detection of covalent binding, because in situ metabolite formation is ensured by adding mammalian microsomal enzymes. However, both CBZ and epoxy-CBZ were shown to be negative in the Ames test under various experimental conditions (22). We assume that the reactive intermediates generated in CBZ biotransformation do not substantially bind to macromolecules, but rather react along the sequences outlined in Figs. 3 and 4. The stable products of CBZ oxidation, e.g., the metabolites I, II, III, V, and VI, do not produce mutagenic effects either (28).

SPECIES DIFFERENCES IN METABOLISM

Rates of Metabolic Elimination

In all animal species studied so far, CBZ is largely eliminated by metabolism. Direct excretion of unchanged CBZ in urine and bile is quantitatively unimportant (13). In this respect, there is close similarity between animals and man. However, the overall rate of biotransformation in man is drastically different from that in the animal species, as reflected by the elimination half-lives of CBZ determined in plasma.

Table 3 shows that the mean half-lives in noninduced rats, gerbils, rabbits, dogs, and rhesus monkeys are all in the range of 0.7 to 1.8 hr (15,17,18,42,50). In noninduced human subjects, however, the half-life is 36 hr (13). Consequently, the metabolic clearance of CBZ in these animal species is higher by more than a power of 10 than in man. To maintain a certain concentration of CBZ in plasma, a correspondingly higher specific dose is needed in the animals. Therefore, the same plasma concentration of CBZ, though possibly equal in pharmacological effectiveness, may toxicologically imply a higher burden to the animals than to man.

Male rats eliminate CBZ more rapidly than females do, the half-life being about 50% longer in the latter case (see Table 3) (15). For humans, no such comparison of half-life exists, but the available clinical data suggest that the kinetics of CBZ and epoxy-CBZ in male and female patients or healthy volunteers do not differ significantly (20; G. Menge et al., *unpublished data*).

Pretreatment of the animals with CBZ or phenobarbital results in an enhanced elimination of CBZ from the body. Actually, the half-life is reduced by one-third to one-half, which again is in agreement with the observations made in healthy subjects (see Table 3). This effect is caused by induction of microsomal enzymes in the liver, as demonstrated in independent animal studies (46,56,60,62).

Pathways of Elimination

With regard to structural identification of CBZ metabolites in animals, the rat is the only species for which results have been reported (13,32). From the available information we infer that the metabolites formed in the rat are essentially the same as those in man (see Fig. 2). The rat, too, excretes the bulk of metabolites in conjugated form. Therefore, in spite of the largely different rate of biotransformation in rat and man, the major pathways are qualitatively similar in both species. Several additional metabolites found in the rat are also derived from the known reaction sequences. Some of these products carry substituents introduced by more than one pathway.

The quantities and structures of the me-

TABLE 3. *Plasma elimination half-lives of CBZ in various animal species and in man, measured before and after induction of enzymes*

Species	N	Dose (mg/kg) and route	Elimination half-life (hr)[a]		Refs.
			Noninduced	Induced	
Rat, male	(4)[b]	25, i.v.	1.2(1.0–1.3)	0.8(0.6–1.0)[c]	(15)
Rat, female	(4)[b]	25, i.v.	1.8(1.5–2.2)	1.0(0.8–1.2)[c]	(15)
Gerbil, male, female	(2)[b]	40, p.o.	1.8[d]	[d]	(18)
Rabbit[d]	(8)	10, i.v.	0.7 ± 0.1	0.4 ± 0.1[e]	(50)
Dog, male, female	(≤6)	40, p.o.	1.5(1.1–1.9)	0.7(0.6–0.7)[c]	(17)
Rhesus monkey[d]	(7)	[d], i.v.	1.0 ± 0.2	0.6 ± 0.2[e]	(42)
Healthy human subjects[d]	(≥22)	<15, p.o.	36.0 ± 3.9	23.9 ± 4.1[c]	(13)

[a] Mean values, and range or standard deviation.
[b] Number of animals used for each sampling time.
[c] Induction by repeated administration of CBZ.
[d] Not specified or not measured.
[e] Induction by repeated administration of phenobarbital.

tabolites identified in rat bile and rat urine imply that 10,11-oxidation of CBZ accounts for a higher percentage of the dose than does any of the other pathways (13). However, the epoxide intermediate is transformed to the diol metabolite only to a comparatively low rate in the rat. The activity of hepatic epoxide hydrolase is in fact lower in the rat than in man (37).

Although the biotransformation of CBZ has not been specifically investigated in other species, some conclusions can be drawn from pharmacokinetic findings. They show that epoxy-CBZ is an important plasma metabolite in mice (7,16,53), rats (11,49), rabbits (50), dogs (11,17), and rhesus monkeys (42). Thus, 10,11-oxidation of CBZ is a pathway common to all these species. Interestingly, the epoxide is not detectable in the plasma of gerbils, which is an animal occasionally used as a model in epilepsy research (18).

In animals, the epoxide metabolite has a longer elimination half-life than CBZ itself (14,17,50). The respective values reported for the rabbit are 2.5 and 0.7 hr, for instance, and those for the dog are 2.2 and 1.5 hr. In noninduced humans, in contrast, the half-life of epoxy-CBZ (6 hr) (44,51,55) is considerably shorter than that of CBZ (36 hr; see Table 3). The different rates of the metabolic reactions are reflected by the concentration profiles in plasma in that the ratio of epoxy-CBZ to CBZ is generally higher in animals than in man.

Induction of microsomal enzymes by CBZ or phenobarbital affects the epoxide pathway of CBZ in all animal species investigated. Both 10,11-oxidation of CBZ and hydrolysis of the epoxide metabolite become accelerated (17,42,50,56). Another metabolic pathway, i.e., the one leading to sulfur-containing conjugates (see Fig. 2), has recently been suspected of being inducible as well. Pretreatment of rats with CBZ resulted in increased recovery of thioethers in the urine (46). However, the analytical method used was specific for the

thioether group only, but not for CBZ-related products. Thus it is conceivable that CBZ simply enhanced the formation of endogenous sulfur-containing metabolites.

In conclusion, the standard laboratory species seem to metabolize CBZ by the same basic mechanisms as do humans. Therefore, it is permissible to extrapolate those pharmacological and biochemical findings, which can only be elaborated in animal models, to man. Considering the species differences in metabolic rates, however, any interpretation obtained from animals *in vivo* should be based on the pharmacokinetics of the essential molecules, particularly CBZ and epoxy-CBZ.

REFERENCES

1. Ames, B. N., McCann, J., and Yamasaki, E. (1975): Methods for detecting carcinogens and mutagens with the Salmonella/mammalian-microsome mutagenicity test. *Mutat. Res.*, 31:347–364.
2. Armstrong, R. N. (1987): Enzyme-catalyzed detoxication reactions: Mechanisms and stereochemistry. *CRC Crit. Rev. Biochem.*, 22:39–88.
3. Baciewicz, A. M. (1986): Carbamazepine drug interactions. *Ther. Drug Monit.*, 8:305–317.
4. Bellucci, G., Berti, G., Chiappe, C., Lippi, A., and Marioni, F. (1987): The metabolism of carbamazepine in humans: Steric course of the enzymatic hydrolysis of the 10,11-epoxide. *J. Med. Chem.*, 30:768–773.
5. Bertilsson, L., and Tomson, T. (1986): Clinical pharmacokinetics and pharmacological effects of carbamazepine and carbamazepine-10,11-epoxide. An update. *Clin. Pharmacokinet.*, 11:177–198.
6. Bourgeois, B. F. D., and Wad, N. (1984): Carbamazepine-10,11-diol steady-state serum levels and renal excretion during carbamazepine therapy in adults and children. *Ther. Drug Monit.*, 6:259–265.
7. Bourgeois, B. F. D., and Wad, N. (1984): Individual and combined antiepileptic and neurotoxic activity of carbamazepine and carbamazepine-10,11-epoxide in mice. *J. Pharmacol. Exp. Ther.*, 231:411–415.
8. Coughtrie, M., Jackson, M., Harding, D., Corser, R., Hume, R., and Burchell, B. (1988): Molecular probes for human UDP-glucuronosyltransferases. *Biochem. Soc. Trans.*, 16:157–158.
9. Eichelbaum, M., Jensen, C., von Sassen, W., Bertilsson, L., and Tomson, T. (1984): *In vivo* and *in vitro* biotransformation of carbamazepine in man and rat. In: *Metabolism of Antiepileptic Drugs*, edited by R. H. Levy, W. H. Pitlick, M. Eichelbaum, and J. Meijer, pp. 27–34. Raven Press, New York.

10. Eichelbaum, M., Tomson, T., Tybring, G., and Bertilsson, L. (1985): Carbamazepine metabolism in man. Induction and pharmacogenetic aspects. *Clin. Pharmacokinet.*, 10:80–90.

11. Faigle, J. W., Brechbuehler, S., Feldmann, K. F., and Richter, W. J. (1976): The biotransformation of carbamazepine. In: *Epileptic Seizures-Behaviour-Pain*, edited by W. Birkmayer, pp. 127–140. Hans Huber Publishers, Berne, Stuttgart, Vienna.

12. Faigle, J. W., and Feldmann, K. F. (1975): Pharmacokinetic data of carbamazepine and its major metabolites in man. In: *Clinical Pharmacology of Anti-Epileptic Drugs*, edited by H. Schneider, D. Janz, C. Gardner-Thorpe, H. Meinardi, and A. L. Sherwin, pp. 159–165. Springer-Verlag, Berlin, Heidelberg, New York.

13. Faigle, J. W., and Feldmann, K. F. (1982): Carbamazepine: Biotransformation. In: *Antiepileptic Drugs*, 2nd edition edited by D. M. Woodbury, J. K. Penry, and C. E. Pippenger, pp. 483–495. Raven Press, New York.

14. Faigle, J. W., Feldmann, K. F., and Baltzer, V. (1977): Anticonvulsant effect of carbamazepine: An attempt to distinguish between the potency of the parent drug and its epoxide metabolite. In: *Antiepileptic Drug Monitoring*, edited by C. Gardner-Thorpe, D. Janz, H. Meinardi, and C. E. Pippenger, pp. 104–109. Pitman Medical, Kent.

15. Farghali-Hassan, Assael, B. M., Bossi, L., Gerna, M., Garattini, S., Gomeni, G., and Morselli, P. L. (1976): Carbamazepine pharmacokinetics in young, adult and pregnant rats. Relation to pharmacological effects. *Arch. Int. Pharmacodyn. Ther.*, 220:125–139.

16. Finnell, R. H., Mohl, V. K., Bennett, G. D., and Taylor, S. M. (1986): Failure of epoxide formation to influence carbamazepine-induced teratogenesis in a mouse model. *Teratogenesis Carcinog. Mutagen.*, 6:393–401.

17. Frey, H. H., and Loescher, W. (1980): Pharmacokinetics of carbamazepine in the dog. *Arch. Int. Pharmacodyn. Ther.*, 243:180–191.

18. Frey, H. H., Loescher, W., Reiche, R., and Schultz, D. (1981): Pharmacology of antiepileptic drugs—I. Pharmacokinetics. *Neuropharmacology*, 20:769–771.

19. Friis, M. L., Christiansen, J., and Hvidberg, E. F. (1978): Brain concentrations of carbamazepine and carbamazepine-10,11-epoxide in epileptic patients. *Eur. J. Clin. Pharmacol.*, 14:47–51.

20. Froescher, W., Stoll, K.-D., Hildenbrand, G., and Eichelbaum, M. (1988): Investigations on the intraindividual constancy of the ratio of carbamazepine to carbamazepine-10,11-epoxide in man. *Arzneimittelforschung*, 38:724–726.

21. Gagneux, A. R. (1976): The chemistry of carbamazepine. In: *Epileptic Seizures-Behaviour-Pain*, edited by W. Birkmayer, pp. 120–126. Hans Huber Publishers, Berne, Stuttgart, Vienna.

22. Glatt, H. R., Oesch, F., Frigerio, A., and Garattini, S. (1975): Epoxides metabolically produced from some known carcinogens and from some clinically used drugs. I. Differences in mutagenicity. *Int. J. Cancer*, 16:787–797.

23. Goldberg, M. A., and Todoroff, T. (1980): Brain binding of anticonvulsants: Carbamazepine and valproic acid. *Neurology*, 30:826–831.

24. Heckendorn, R. (1987): Synthesis of *trans*-10,11-dihydro-10,11-dihydroxy-5H-dibenz[b,f]azepine-5-carboxamide, a major metabolite of carbamazepine. *Helv. Chim. Acta*, 70:1955–1962.

25. Hundt, H. K. L., Aucamp, A. K., Mueller, F. O., and Potgieter, M. A. (1983): Carbamazepine and its major metabolites in plasma: A summary of eight years of therapeutic drug monitoring. *Ther. Drug. Monit.*, 5:427–435.

26. Johannessen, S. I., Baruzzi, A., Gomeni, R., Strandjord, R. E., and Morselli, P. L. (1977): Further observations on carbamazepine and carbamazepine-10,11-epoxide kinetics in epileptic patients. In: *Antiepileptic Drug Monitoring*, edited by C. Gardner-Thorpe, D. Janz, H. Meinardi, and C. E. Pippenger, pp. 110–127. Pitman Medical, Kent.

27. Jung, R., Bentley, P., and Oesch, F. (1980): Influence of carbamazepine 10,11-oxide on drug metabolizing enzymes. *Biochem. Pharmacol.*, 29:1109–1112.

28. Koenigstein, M., Larisch, M., and Obe, G. (1984): Mutagenicity of antiepileptic drugs. I. Carbamazepine and some of its metabolites. *Mutat. Res.*, 139:83–86.

29. Korzekwa, K., Trager, W., Gouterman, M., Spangler, D., and Loew, G. H. (1985): Cytochrome P450 mediated aromatic oxidation: A theoretical study. *J. Am. Chem. Soc.*, 107:4273–4279.

30. Kraemer, G., Besser, R., and Theisohn, M. (1987): Interaktionen von Carbamazepin mit anderen Medikamenten. In: *Carbamazepin in der Neurologie*, edited by G. Kraemer and H. C. Hopf, pp. 70–90. Georg Thieme Verlag, Stuttgart, New York.

31. Kraemer, G., Theisohn, M., von Unruh, G. E., and Eichelbaum, M. (1986): Carbamazepine-danazol drug interaction: Its mechanism examined with a stable isotope technique. *Ther. Drug Monit.*, 8:387–392.

32. Lertratanangkoon, K., and Horning, M. G. (1981): Metabolism of carbamazepine. *Drug. Metab. Dispos.*, 10:1–10.

33. Lindhout, D., Hoeppener, R. J. E. A., and Meinardi, H. (1984): Teratogenicity of antiepileptic drug combinations with special emphasis on epoxidation (of carbamazepine). *Epilepsia*, 25:77–83.

34. Loescher, W., and Frey, H. H. (1984): Kinetics of penetration of common antiepileptic drugs into cerebrospinal fluid. *Epilepsia*, 25:346–352.

35. Lynn, R. K., Smith, R. G., Thompson, R. M., Deinzer, M. L., Griffin, D., and Gerber, N. (1978): Characterization of glucuronide metabolites of carbamazepine in human urine by gas chromatography and mass spectrometry. *Drug Metab. Dispos.*, 6:494–501.

36. Meijer, J. W. A., Binnie, C. D., Debets, R. M. C., van Parys, J. A. P., and de Beer-Pawlikowski, N. K. B. (1984): Possible hazard of valpromide-carbamazepine combination therapy in epilepsy (letter). *Lancet*, i:802.

37. Meijer, J., and Depierre, J. W. (1988): Cytosolic

epoxide hydrolase. *Chem. Biol. Interact.,* 64:207–249.

38. Monaco, F., Sechi, G. P., Russo, A., Traccis, S., and Mutani, R. (1985): Brain distribution of carbamazepine and phenobarbital given in combination in experimental epilepsy. *Epilepsia,* 26:103–108.

39. Nebert, D. W., and Gonzalez, F. J. (1987): P450 genes: Structure, evolution and regulation. *Ann. Rev. Biochem.,* 56:945–993.

40. Pacifici, G. M., Franchi, M., Bencini, C., and Rane, A. (1986): Valpromide inhibits human epoxide hydrolase. *Br. J. Clin. Pharmacol.,* 22:269–274.

41. Pacifici, G. M., Tomson, T., Bertilsson, L., and Rane, A. (1985): Valpromide/carbamazepine and risk of teratogenicity. *Lancet,* i:397–398.

42. Patel, I. H., Wedlund, P., and Levy, R. H. (1981): Induction effect of phenobarbital on the carbamazepine to carbamazepine-10,11-epoxide pathway in Rhesus monkeys. *J. Pharmacol. Exp. Ther.,* 217:555–558.

43. Peters, W. H. M., and Jansen, P. L. M. (1988): Immunocharacterization of UDP-glucuronyltransferase isoenzymes in human liver, intestine and kidney. *Biochem. Pharmacol.,* 37:564–567.

44. Pisani, F., Fazio, A., Oteri, G., Spina, E., Perucca, E., and Bertilsson, L. (1988): Effect of valpromide on the pharmacokinetics of carbamazepine-10,11-epoxide. *Br. J. Clin. Pharmacol.,* 25:611–613.

45. Pudzianowski, A. T., and Loew, G. H. (1982): Quantum chemical studies of model cytochrome P450 hydrocarbon oxidation mechanisms. II. Mechanisms and relative kinetics of oxene reactions with alkenes. *J. Mol. Catal.,* 17:1–22.

46. Regnaud, L., Sirois, G., and Chakrabati, S. (1988): Effect of four-day treatment with carbamazepine at different dose levels on microsomal enzyme induction, drug metabolism and drug toxicity. *Pharmacol. Toxicol.,* 62:3–6.

47. Renfroe, B., and Harrington, C. (1984): Dibenzazepines and other tricyclic azepines. In: *Heterocyclic Compounds,* Vol. 43, Part 1, edited by A. Rosowsky, pp. 528–529. John Wiley and Sons, New York, Chichester, Brisbane, Toronto, Singapore.

48. Richter, W. J., Kriemler, P., and Faigle, J. W. (1978): Newer aspects of the biotransformation of carbamazepine: Structural characterization of highly polar metabolites. In: *Recent Developments in Mass Spectrometry in Biochemistry and Medicine,* Vol. 1, edited by A. Frigerio, pp. 1–14. Plenum Press, New York.

49. Salmona, M., Conti, I., Testa, R., Fracasso, C., and Caccia, S. (1987): Interaction of the anticonvulsants, denzimol and nafimidone, with liver cytochrome P450 in the rat. *J. Pharm. Pharmacol.,* 40:17–21.

50. Sumi, M., Watari, N., Naito, H., Umezawa, O., and Kaneniwa, N. (1987): Influence of phenobarbital on pharmacokinetics of carbamazepine and

its epoxide metabolite in the rabbit. *Yakugaku Zasshi,* 107:984–991.

51. Sumi, M., Watari, N., Umezawa, O., and Kaneniwa, N. (1987): Pharmacokinetic study of carbamazepine and its epoxide metabolite in humans. *J. Pharmacobiodyn.,* 10:652–661.

52. Tateishi, M. (1983): Methylthiolated metabolites. *Drug Metab. Rev.,* 14:1207–1234.

53. Taylor, S. M., Bennett, G. D., Abbott, L. C., and Finnell, R. H. (1985): Seizure control following administration of anticonvulsant drugs in the quaking mouse. *Eur. J. Pharmacol.,* 118:163–170.

54. Theisohn, M., Sigmund, M., Demant, L., Roth, B., Heimann, G., Gesenhues, K., Kraemer, G., and Besser, R. (1987): Metabolisierung von Carbamazepin bei einmaliger und wiederholter Gabe. In: *Carbamazepin in der Neurologie,* edited by G. Kraemer and H. C. Hopf, pp. 28–43. Georg Thieme Verlag, Stuttgart, New York.

55. Tomson, T., Tybring, G., and Bertilsson, L. (1983): Single-dose kinetics and metabolism of carbamazepine-10,11-epoxide. *Clin. Pharmacol. Ther.,* 33:58–65.

56. Tybring, G., von Bahr, C., Bertilsson, L., Collste, H., Glaumann, H., and Solbrand, M. (1981): Metabolism of carbamazepine and its epoxide metabolite in human and rat liver *in vitro.* *Drug Metab. Dispos.,* 9:561–564.

57. Van Boxtel, C. J., Rane, A., Brown, R. D., and Wilson, J. T. (1981): The formation of carbamazepine epoxide by rat liver microsomes: An investigation of the biphasic kinetic profile. *Life Sci.,* 29:2575–2584.

58. Von Bahr, C., Groth, C.-G., Jansson, H., Lundgren, G., Lind, M., and Glaumann, H. (1980): Drug metabolism in human liver *in vitro*: Establishment of a human liver bank. *Clin. Pharmacol. Ther.,* 27:711–725.

59. Vree, T. B., Janssen, T. J., Hekster, Y. A., Termond, E. F. S., van de Dries, A. C. P., and Wijnands, W. J. A. (1986): Clinical pharmacokinetics of carbamazepine and its epoxy and hydroxy metabolites in humans after an overdose. *Ther. Drug Monit.,* 8:297–304.

60. Wagner, J., and Schmid, K. (1987): Induction of microsomal enzymes in rat liver by oxcarbazepine, 10,11-dihydro-10-hydroxy-carbamazepine and carbamazepine. *Xenobiotica,* 17:951–956.

61. Wedlund, P. J., Chang, S. L., and Levy, R. H. (1983): Steady-state determination of the contribution of lung metabolism to the total body clearance of drugs: Application to carbamazepine. *J. Pharm. Sci.,* 72:860–862.

62. Wedlund, P. J., Nelson, S. D., Nickelson, S., and Levy, R. H. (1982): Linear relationship between cytochrome P-450 and carbamazepine clearance in Rhesus monkeys. *Drug Metab. Dispos.,* 10:480–485.

63. Wimbish, G. H., Jones, G. L., Amato, R. J., and Peyton, G. A. (1980): Anticonvulsant activities and brain concentrations of cyheptamide and carbamazepine. *Proc. West. Pharmacol. Soc.,* 23:75–79.

Antiepileptic Drugs, Third Edition, edited by
R. Levy, R. Mattson, B. Meldrum,
J. K. Penry, and F. E. Dreifuss.
Raven Press, Ltd., New York © 1989.

35

Carbamazepine

Carbamazepine Epoxide

Bradley M. Kerr and René H. Levy

INTRODUCTION

Carbamazepine (CBZ) was recognized to be effective for the treatment of epilepsy and trigeminal neuralgia in the early 1960s (80,84), but it was not until 1972 that carbamazepine-10,11-epoxide (CBZ epoxide) was identified as a metabolite of CBZ (24). There have been numerous investigations of CBZ epoxide, not only because of its quantitative significance in the parent drug's metabolism, but also because it is pharmacologically active and accumulates in the plasma of CBZ-treated patients. Although CBZ epoxide has not been tested for anticonvulsant activity in man, its well-established anticonvulsant effect in animals (2,9,21) suggests that it must contribute to the clinical effects of CBZ in man. The neuropharmacological activity of the epoxide in man is substantiated by drug interaction reports in which symptoms of intoxication are associated with pronounced elevations of plasma CBZ epoxide levels while CBZ concentrations remain unchanged (39,52,66). In view of the interest in CBZ epoxide as a pharmacologically active entity, this chapter provides an overview of its chemical, biochemical, and pharmacological properties.

CHEMISTRY AND METHODS OF DETERMINATION

Carbamazepine-10,11-epoxide is synthesized by epoxidation of CBZ with *m*-chloroperoxybenzoic acid (3,4,24). A yield of epoxide as high as 65% has been reported for this procedure (4). Purified CBZ epoxide is a white crystalline compound with the empirical formula $C_{15}H_{12}N_2O_2$, a molecular weight of 252.27, and a melting point with decomposition at 200 to 205°C (3,4).

The ultraviolet spectrum of CBZ epoxide shows an absorbance maximum at approximately 210 nm (4,24). The proton nuclear magnetic resonance spectrum of CBZ epoxide with deuterated chloroform as the solvent shows multiplet peaks at $\delta = 7.2$–7.6 parts per million (ppm) for the eight aromatic protons, a broad singlet peak at $\delta = 4.5$ ppm for the two carboxamide protons, and a sharp singlet peak at $\delta = 4.3$ ppm for the two protons in the 10- and 11-positions (4). The positive ion electron impact mass spectrum of CBZ epoxide shows a molecular ion at $m/z = 252$, the base peak at $m/z = 180$, and other major fragments at $m/z = 207$ and 223 (24,35).

Carbamazepine epoxide is a neutral, lipophilic compound that, like the parent drug, readily dissolves in organic solvents such as diethyl ether, dichloromethane, and ethanol, and has a very limited solubility in aqueous solution. The stability of the epoxide has been evaluated in aqueous solution at pH 2, 5, and 7 (83). Over a period of 5 hr no degradation was detectable at pH 5 or 7. The degradation half-life of CBZ epoxide is approximately 1 hr at pH 2. The acid catalyzed degradation of the epoxide is reported to lead preferentially to formation of ring contracted products rather than to formation of the *trans*-dihydrodiol through hydrolysis of the epoxide (4).

The assay of CBZ epoxide in biological fluids has been carried out by gas chromatography (GC) and high-performance liquid chromatography (HPLC). A number of these assay procedures can be used to simultaneously quantitate CBZ and CBZ epoxide. Liquid/liquid extraction of the metabolite from the biological matrix, with a recovery of 90% or greater, is typically accomplished with an organic solvent such as chloroform or dichloromethane (19,53,75,88). Solid-phase extraction of CBZ and CBZ epoxide has also been described (30).

Carbamazepine epoxide undergoes complete thermal degradation during analysis by GC (3,23). The compound that elutes from the GC column following injection of CBZ epoxide has a molecular weight of 207, rather than the CBZ epoxide's molecular weight of 252. Comparison of the mass spectrum and physical properties of the eluted compound with an authentic standard confirmed that this degradation product is 9-acridinecarboxaldehyde (Fig. 1) (3). Certain GC conditions have also been reported to catalyze the degradation of carbamazepine-10,11-*trans*-dihydrodiol to 9-acridinecarboxaldehyde (23). Despite the thermal stability problems associated with carbamazepine epoxide, several GC assay procedures have been described for quantitation of this compound (12,56,62,67,68, 85). The chemical species that is actually detected and quantified in each of these procedures is the 9-acridinecarboxaldehyde thermal degradation product. Detection is achieved by means of flame ionization detection (56,67), nitrogen-phosphorous detection (12,68), and mass spectrometry (62,85). The mass spectrometric methods of detection provide the most sensitivity for quantitative assay of CBZ epoxide by GC.

Carbamazepine epoxide is currently assayed on a routine basis by HPLC, which has two advantages over GC: (a) the problem of thermal degradation of the epoxide is not encountered in HPLC, and (b) good sensitivity is achieved by HPLC assays without the need for elaborate mass spectrometric detection systems. Detection of CBZ epoxide in conjunction with HPLC is most frequently carried out by ultraviolet absorption at or near a wavelength of 210 nm (19,30,45,53,75,88). Chromatographic separation of the epoxide has been performed with both normal-phase (17,35,90) and reversed-phase systems (19,30,37,45, 49,53,54,75,88). The most frequently reported procedures utilize either a C_8 or C_{18} reversed-phase column with a mobile phase consisting of acetonitrile and/or methanol in water (19,30,37,45,53,54,75,88).

The principal metabolite of carbamazepine-10,11-epoxide in man is carbamazepine-10,11-*trans*-dihydrodiol (Fig. 2), which was first characterized in 1972 (29). Physicochemical properties of the *trans*-dihydrodiol allow it to be readily distinguished from its *cis*-dihydrodiol isomer (20,40,86). Quantitation of the *trans*-dihydrodiol in urine and plasma has been accomplished by GC and HPLC. The GC analysis of the *trans*-dihydrodiol is preceded by the conversion of the *trans*-dihydrodiol and the *cis*-dihydrodiol internal standard to trimethylsilyl (TMS) derivatives. Mass spectrometric detection of these TMS derivatives has been carried out by select ion monitoring of the M/Z 486 molecular ion (35,83,87). Several reversed-phase HPLC procedures have been described for quantitation of the *trans*-dihydrodiol in plasma or urine (37,53,74,

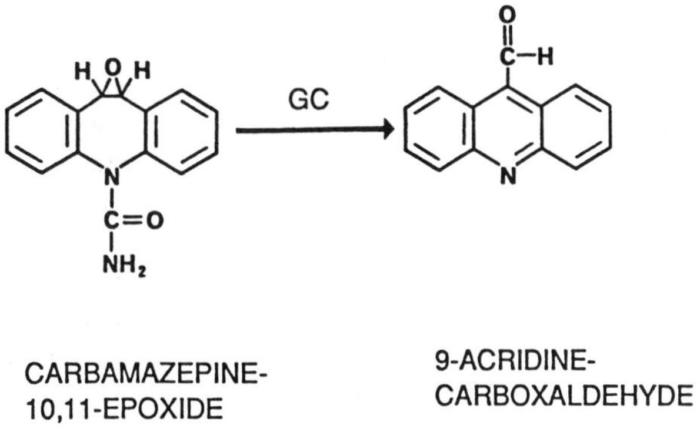

FIG. 1. Rearrangement of CBZ epoxide during analysis by gas chromatography.

CARBAMAZEPINE-
10,11-EPOXIDE

9-ACRIDINE-
CARBOXALDEHYDE

86,88). Chromatography is carried out on a C_8 or C_{18} column with a mobile phase consisting of methanol and/or acetonitrile in water, and detection is typically by means of ultraviolet absorption at or near a wavelength of 210 nm. Resolution of the (S,S)- and (R,R)-*trans*-dihydrodiol enantiomers as *bis*-MTPA ester derivatives was accomplished through normal-phase HPLC (4).

PHARMACOLOGY

The accumulation of CBZ epoxide in the plasma of CBZ treated patients used to be of concern because nothing was initially known about the potential of the epoxide for eliciting serious toxic effects often associated with epoxide exposure, such as mutagenesis, carcinogenesis, teratogenesis, and cytotoxicity. Subsequent studies have shown CBZ epoxide to be neither cytotoxic nor mutagenic (25,28,33), and the lethal dose (LD_{50}) has been reported to be the same as that of CBZ (25). Thus, CBZ epoxide appears to be free of the serious toxicities often associated with epoxides, most likely because it is not highly reactive. The chemical stability of CBZ epoxide is demonstrated by its presence in blood and urine, indicating that it is not likely to be very reactive toward cellular nucleophiles. The lack of reactivity of CBZ epoxide toward the nucleophilic agent 4-(*p*-nitrobenzyl)-pyridine is further evidence of its chemical stability (10). *In vitro* studies show that the epoxide has little or no capacity to inhibit the activities of epoxide hydrolase or glutathione transferase (31), suggesting that metabolic detoxification of reactive, toxic epoxides is not likely to be impaired by CBZ epoxide.

Carbamazepine epoxide has never been tested as an anticonvulsant in man, but it does exhibit anticonvulsant activity in rodents. On the basis of the ED_{50} (the dose required to protect 50% of a group of animals against seizures), CBZ epoxide is equipotent to CBZ in protecting against seizures induced by electroshock, strychnine, and pentylenetetrazol in mice (21,25), and in protecting against electroshock and amygdala-kindled seizures in rats (2,21). On the basis of brain concentrations, CBZ epoxide is slightly less potent than the parent drug in protecting against maximal electroshock-induced seizures in mice (9). Other metabolites of CBZ possess anticonvulsant activity in rodents (21), but the epoxide is the only one that accumulates to therapeutically relevant concentrations in CBZ treated patients. Carbamazepine-10,11-*trans*-dihydrodiol, the principal metabolite of CBZ epoxide in man, also accumulates to detectable levels in the plasma of CBZ-treated patients, but this metabolite lacks anticonvulsant activity in mice (9), perhaps because of an inability to penetrate into the brain.

The accumulation of CBZ epoxide to plasma concentrations approximating those of CBZ raises the question as to which molecular species is responsible for the pharmacological effects observed during CBZ therapy. Faigle et al. (22) compared the time course of anticonvulsant effect in rats with the time course of blood concentrations of CBZ and the epoxide metabolite following a single dose of CBZ. It was concluded that anticonvulsant activity was associated with unchanged CBZ, but that the epoxide metabolite reinforces this anticonvulsant effect in rats. Attempts to assess the contribution of CBZ epoxide to the pharmacological effects associated with CBZ administration in man have led to ambiguous results (6). However, in view of its well-established anticonvulsant effect in animals, and because of the significant accumulation of the epoxide in patients treated with CBZ, it is likely that the epoxide metabolite reinforces the anticonvulsant actions of the parent drug in man.

An unequivocal evaluation of the pharmacological effects of CBZ epoxide requires that the epoxide be directly administered to patients. The efficacy of the epoxide in the treatment of trigeminal neuralgia has been evaluated through direct administration of the epoxide to a group of six patients (81). Carbamazepine epoxide therapy was substituted for CBZ for 3 to 6 days, with patients blinded to the change in therapy. Similar doses of CBZ epoxide and CBZ resulted in comparable control of pain. Plasma concentrations of CBZ epoxide associated with pain relief during treatment with the epoxide were lower than concentrations of CBZ associated with pain relief during CBZ therapy, suggesting that the epoxide may have a higher pain-relieving potency than the parent drug.

Carbamazepine epoxide appears to have the potential to contribute to neurological side effects as well as to therapeutic effects in patients treated with CBZ. The neurotoxic potency of CBZ epoxide has been evaluated and compared with that of CBZ in the rotorod toxicity test (9), which is a test of the ability of an animal to maintain its equilibrium. Following separate administrations of CBZ and CBZ epoxide to mice, it was found that similar brain concentrations of the two compounds were required to produce signs of neurological deficit by the rotorod test. Drug interaction reports in epileptic patients substantiate the ability of the epoxide to elicit neurological side effects. In patients stabilized on CBZ therapy, the addition of either valpromide (52,66) or progabide (39) to the drug regimen was often observed to produce symptoms of CBZ intoxication. Surprisingly, these symptoms were associated with pronounced elevations in the plasma concentrations of CBZ epoxide (3–20 µg/mL), whereas plasma levels of CBZ were unchanged. Although the relationship of CBZ epoxide to neurological side effects during routine CBZ therapy has been debated (64,77,82), the drug interaction reports with valpromide and progabide clearly indicate that there are some circumstances under which CBZ epoxide concentrations can be elevated to the point of producing symptoms of intoxication.

The threshold concentration of CBZ epoxide for producing neurological side effects in man has not been established. Following administration of the epoxide in the absence of CBZ to four healthy volunteers and to four patients with trigeminal neuralgia, Tomson et al. (81,83) reported that concentrations of CBZ epoxide up to 4 µg/mL were tolerated without side effects. In our own studies involving 69 separate administrations of 100-mg single doses of CBZ epoxide, maximal blood epoxide concentrations of up to 2.7 µg/mL produced no drowsiness, dizziness, blurred vision, or other indications of neurotoxicity

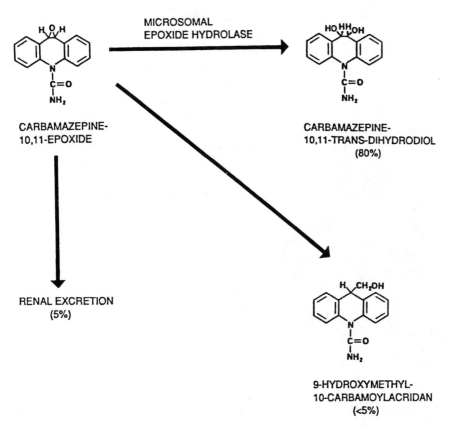

FIG. 2. Disposition of CBZ epoxide in man.

(32,36,42,43,46). Although side effects were not encountered in our studies and those of Tomson et al., Sumi et al. (79) reported that four of six volunteers who received 150 mg of CBZ epoxide as a single dose complained of drowsiness, malaise, and dizziness up to 10 hr following administration, while maximal epoxide concentrations were less than 3 μg/mL.

BIOTRANSFORMATION

Clinical Studies

Carbamazepine epoxide is almost completely hydrolyzed in man prior to excretion into the urine as the 10,11-*trans*-dihydrodiol metabolite. Tomson et al. (83) reported that after administration of single oral doses of CBZ epoxide to healthy volunteers, the portion of the dose recovered in urine as the *trans*-dihydrodiol (unconjugated plus *O*-glucuronidated) ranged from 73% to 100%, indicating that alternative pathways of CBZ epoxide elimination must be quantitatively minor. The results of our own single-dose CBZ epoxide studies confirm that the hydrolysis of CBZ epoxide is extensive in man. We found up to 80% of an oral dose of the epoxide in urine as the *trans*-dihydrodiol, and an additional 5% as unchanged CBZ epoxide (Fig. 2) (32,46). The high urinary recovery of the *trans*-dihydrodiol relative to unchanged CBZ epoxide in the single-dose studies is consistent with the high ratio of *trans*-dihydrodiol to epoxide (20:1) in the urine of patients treated with CBZ (18).

The *in vivo* hydrolysis of CBZ epoxide has often been speculated to be mediated by the epoxide hydrolase enzyme system. An early report indicating that the *trans*-dihydrodiol recovered from urine is optically active provided evidence that at least a portion of the *in vivo* hydrolysis is through enzymatic processes (20), a conclusion later strengthened by the finding that the *trans*-dihydrodiol in the urine of CBZ-treated patients is in an enantiomeric excess of 80% (4). The prevalent *trans*-dihydrodiol enantiomer was reported to have the (-) -10S, 11S absolute configuration (4). The biotransformation of CBZ epoxide to the *trans*-dihydrodiol has been reported to occur in both human and rat liver microsomal preparations (86), suggesting that this hydrolytic reaction is catalyzed by microsomal epoxide hydrolase. It has subsequently been found in our laboratory that preparations of pure human liver microsomal epoxide hydrolase catalyze the hydrolysis of CBZ epoxide at a rate much higher than that observed in microsomes (Table 1) (32). These data lend support to the hypothesis that microsomal epoxide hydrolase is responsible for the *in vivo* hydrolysis of CBZ epoxide.

The only metabolite other than the *trans*-dihydrodiol that has been identified in urine following administration of CBZ epoxide in man is 9-hydroxymethyl-10-carbamoylacridan (Fig. 2). This metabolite accounts for less than 4% of the epoxide dose (18). It is of interest that experimental evidence has never been published to confirm the existence of a sulfur-containing derivative of carbamazepine-10,11-epoxide, although 10-hydroxyl-11-methylsulfonyl-10,11-dihydro-carbamazepine was reportedly recovered in rat bile after CBZ administration (21). Thus, it is unlikely that conjugation of CBZ epoxide with glutathione represents a quantitatively significant metabolic pathway in man.

Experimental Studies

The disposition of CBZ epoxide has been investigated in rats and monkeys, with the finding that the metabolite profile in these two animal species is quite different from that observed in humans (Table 2) (32). Whereas urinary excretion of the 10,11-*trans*-dihydrodiol accounts for roughly 75% of an oral dose of CBZ epoxide in humans, urinary excretion of this metabolite only accounts for 10% to 20% and 1% of an intravenous dose of CBZ epoxide in monkeys and rats, respectively. In humans, mon-

TABLE 1. *Carbamazepine-10,11,-*trans-*dihydrodiol formation rate (pmol/min/mg protein) from carbamazepine-10,11-epoxide (0.25 mM) at pH 7.4, 37°C. Mean ± std. dev. of four determinations*[a]

Human liver identification no.	Carbamazepine-10,11-*trans*-dihydrodiol (pmol/min/mg protein)	
	Microsomes	Pure microsomal epoxide hydrolase
101	44.1 ± 1.58	—
102	51.0 ± 1.49	351 ± 65.5
103	38.2 ± 0.74	—
107	—	912 ± 51.2
108	—	262 ± 2.38

[a] From B. M. Kerr, ref. 32.

TABLE 2. *Urinary excretion of carbamazepine-10,11-epoxide (CBZ-E) and carbamazepine-10,11-*trans-*dihydrodiol (*trans-*diol) in adult man and other animals*

Species	N	Body weight	Drug	Percent of dose in urine		Percent of trans-diol unconjugated in urine	trans-diol half-life (hr)
				CBZ-E	trans-diol		
Man	5	77 ± 13 kg	CBZ-E 100 mg, p.o.	3–7%	75–81%	80–87%	12.7 ± 0.95
Rhesus monkey	4	7.3 ± 1.1 kg	CBZ-E 1.2 mg/kg, i.v.	2–3%	8–18%	41–74%	3.46 ± 0.35
Sprague-Dawley rat	6	266 ± 11 g	CBZ-E 4 mg, i.v.	9–15%	0.7–1.0%	76–98%	6.30 ± 1.16
Sprague-Dawley rat	4	250 ± 7 g	trans-diol 4 mg, i.v.	—	61–67%	92–98%	4.80 ± 0.61

i.v., intravenous; p.o., *per os*.
From B. M. Kerr, ref. 32.

keys, and rats, the *trans*-dihydrodiol is found in urine primarily in the unconjugated form, with lesser amounts excreted as a glucuronide conjugate (20,32,48,72,83). The percent of a CBZ epoxide dose excreted unchanged ranges up to 15% among these three animal species (Table 2) (32).

The low urinary recovery of the *trans*-dihydrodiol in rats and monkeys could be due to extensive elimination of the dihydrodiol by pathways other than urinary excretion. Alternatively, formation of the *trans*-dihydrodiol may be a minor pathway of CBZ epoxide metabolism in these animal species. The *trans*-dihydrodiol was directly administered to rats in order to assess the fraction of the *trans*-dihydrodiol that is excreted into urine unchanged or as a conjugate (32). It was found that about 64% of the administered dose of carbamazepine-10,11-*trans*-dihydrodiol was recovered in rat urine unchanged or conjugated to glucuronic acid (Table 2). Therefore, the low recovery of *trans*-dihydrodiol in rat urine following administration of CBZ epoxide is likely due to extensive elimination or metabolism of the epoxide by pathways other than hydrolysis to the *trans*-dihydrodiol.

An alternative pathway for CBZ epoxide metabolism is hydrolysis of the carboxamide moiety to yield iminostilbene epoxide.

Iminostilbene-10,11-epoxide and iminostilbene-10,11-*trans*-dihydrodiol were both reported to be urinary metabolites of CBZ epoxide in rats on the basis of GC-mass spectrometric data (5). However, it has never been independently confirmed that these iminostilbene derivatives are genuine metabolites of CBZ epoxide in any animal species. Carbamazepine is known to thermally degrade to iminostilbene during GC analysis (38), suggesting that the iminostilbene epoxide and iminostilbene *trans*-dihydrodiol may have been artifacts of the GC procedure. In order to determine if iminostilbene epoxide is a genuine metabolite, CBZ epoxide was administered to rats, urine extracts were derivatized with trifluoroacetic anhydride in the presence of triethylamine at 60°C, and analysis was carried out in our laboratory by means of GC-FID and GC-MS (32). The nitrile-derivative of CBZ epoxide was an expected reaction product (27) and was readily detected, but the trifluoroacetyl derivative of iminostilbene epoxide was absent in these derivatized urine extracts. Thus, we were unable to confirm that iminostilbene epoxide is a genuine metabolite of CBZ epoxide in rats.

The fate of 80% of a CBZ epoxide dose remains unaccounted for in rats and monkeys. The metabolic profile of CBZ

(21,40,48,72) suggests that CBZ epoxide may be subject to *N*-glucuronidation or aromatic hydroxylation by cytochrome P-450, but there is still no evidence that these metabolic pathways are operative for the epoxide metabolite in any animal species.

PHARMACOKINETICS

Carbamazepine epoxide has been directly administered to human subjects as an oral suspension (32,36,41,42,43,46,79, 81,83). According to the dosing protocol developed by Tomson (81,83), antacid (10 ml Novaluzid) is administered immediately before, and again at 15 and 30 min after ingestion of the CBZ epoxide suspension. The antacid is administered to minimize acid-catalyzed degradation of CBZ epoxide by gastric juice. This dosing strategy results in rapid, extensive, and reproducible absorption of CBZ epoxide. The ultimate recovery of 80% to 100% of the epoxide dose in urine as the *trans*-dihydrodiol metabolite indicates that absorption of the epoxide from the gastrointestinal tract is essentially complete (83). Peak plasma concentrations of CBZ epoxide, which are typically achieved in 2 hr or less, are proportional to the dose of epoxide (83) and are predictable. In our own single-dose CBZ epoxide studies involving both healthy adult volunteers and adult epileptic patients (32,36,42,43,46), the administration of 100 mg of CBZ epoxide with antacid (three doses of 12.5 ml Maalox Therapeutic Concentrate) on 69 different occasions has resulted in peak blood CBZ epoxide concentrations of 1 to 2 µg/mL on 63 occasions. The range of the maximum epoxide concentration was 0.8 to 2.7 µg/mL and the overall mean was 1.54 ± 0.35 µg/mL. The reproducibility of the maximum blood level of CBZ epoxide provides evidence of good bioavailability from the oral suspension dosage form.

The distribution and elimination charac-teristics of CBZ epoxide show a low degree of intersubject variability in healthy, normal adult subjects. In a group of four volunteers, Tomson et al. (83) reported a CBZ epoxide half-life of 6.1 ± 0.88 hr (range, 4.6 to 6.9), an oral clearance of 1.44 ± 0.42 mL/min/kg (range, 1.06 to 2.26), and a volume of distribution of 0.74 ± 0.13 L/kg (range, 0.59 to 0.92). It was noted that administration of up to 200 mg of CBZ epoxide resulted in no indication of dose-dependent kinetics of the epoxide. In six volunteers, Sumi et al. (79) reported a CBZ epoxide half-life of 6.4 ± 0.7 hr (range, 5.8 to 7.7), an oral clearance of 1.88 ± 0.61 mL/min/kg (range, 1.15 to 2.98), and a volume of distribution of 0.98 ± 0.29 L/kg (range, 0.71 to 1.53). In our own single-dose studies, we administered CBZ epoxide to healthy adults in the absence of enzyme inducers and inhibitors on 24 occasions (32,36,42,43,46). With the exception of one subject, the half-life and clearance of CBZ epoxide fell within narrow ranges (Figs. 3 and 4). The mean values for half-life, clearance, and volume of distribution were 6.7 ± 1.2 hr (range, 5.2 to 11.4), 1.63 ± 0.25 mL/min/kg (range, 0.88 to 2.05), and 0.93 ± 0.13 L/kg (range, 0.75 to 1.22), respectively. As indicated in the following section on drug interactions, metabolic inducers and inhibitors can have pronounced effects on the clearance and half-life of CBZ epoxide. The half-life of CBZ epoxide following administration of the epoxide is shorter than the epoxide terminal half-life after administration of CBZ (79,83). Because the half-life of CBZ is longer than the actual half-life of CBZ epoxide, the epoxide metabolite will display formation rate limited kinetics in the presence of the parent drug, and the terminal elimination phase of the epoxide in plasma will simply parallel that of CBZ.

The pharmacokinetics of CBZ epoxide have been characterized in the rat (13,14) and rhesus monkey (32,63) in our laboratory following intravenous administration of the epoxide in a solution of polyethylene glycol

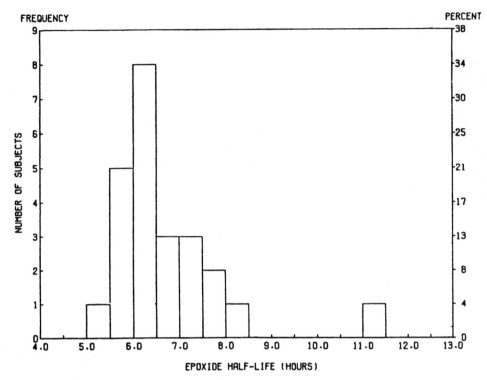

FIG. 3. Distribution of CBZ epoxide half-life in 24 healthy volunteers. The subject with the longest half-life also had the lowest clearance.

400. The disposition of intravenous doses of CBZ epoxide in the rabbit has been investigated bySumi et al. (78). The results of these studies, in addition to the results of the single-dose studies in 24 healthy adults, are summarized in Table 3. Although the volume of distribution is similar in all four species, the clearance of CBZ epoxide is considerably higher in the rabbit, rat, and monkey than in man. The half-life of the epoxide is much shorter in rabbit, rat, and monkey than in man, most likely because of higher clearance values in the three animal species. Plasma free fractions of CBZ epoxide are similar in various animal species, with free fraction values of 0.45 in monkey (45), 0.60 in rat (14), and about 0.35 to 0.45 in man (1,15,57,73). The blood-to-plasma ratio in rat, monkey, and man is slightly greater than one (14,89). Urinary excretion data indicates that the half-life of

carbamazepine-10,11-*trans*-dihydrodiol is longer than that of the epoxide in man, monkey, and rat (Table 2) (32,83).

The low fraction of a CBZ epoxide dose recovered unchanged in urine in rat, monkey, and man (32) indicates that the clearance of the epoxide is principally reflective of nonrenal elimination processes. These nonrenal elimination processes have not been well elucidated in the rat and monkey. However, extensive recovery of the *trans*-dihydrodiol in human urine suggests that the clearance and half-life of CBZ epoxide are measures of *in vivo* epoxide hydrolase activity in man.

DRUG INTERACTIONS

The ratio of CBZ epoxide to CBZ in plasma is decreased by several compounds

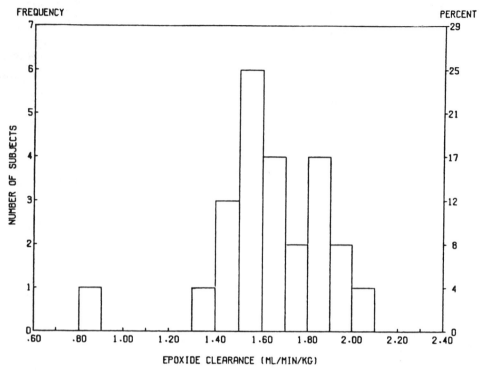

FIG. 4. Distribution of CBZ epoxide clearance in 24 healthy volunteers. The subject with the lowest clearance also had the longest half-life.

known to be inhibitors of cytochrome P-450, such as propoxyphene (16), verapamil (50), and stiripentol (32,43,44). In these interactions, the epoxide-to-CBZ ratio is likely decreased through inhibition of CBZ epoxide formation clearance, although an enhanced or induced elimination clearance of the epoxide could also decrease that ratio. The effect of stiripentol on the disposition of single oral doses of CBZ epoxide (100 mg) was investigated in healthy volunteers (32,43), but neither the half-life nor clearance of the epoxide was significantly affected by stiripentol at concentrations of stiripentol known to inhibit CBZ elimination. There was a tendency for the elimination of the epoxide to be induced by stiripentol, but this effect was not pronounced under the conditions of the study (stiripentol doses of 1,200 mg/day for 7 days). Therefore, the decreased epoxide-to-CBZ ratio in

the presence of the cytochrome P-450 inhibitors appears to be principally the result of a reduced formation clearance of CBZ epoxide. The lack of effect of a cytochrome P-450 inhibitor on CBZ epoxide disposition *in vivo* also confirms that cytochrome P-450 does not significantly contribute to the *in vivo* metabolism of the epoxide metabolite in man.

Co-administration of CBZ with other anticonvulsants such as phenobarbital or phenytoin is associated with an increased plasma ratio of the epoxide to CBZ (8,11,26,34,51,55,70,91) because cytochrome P-450 induction results in an enhanced formation clearance of the epoxide (18). However, phenobarbital and phenytoin are known to induce epoxide hydrolase (58,71,86), and it is likely that these drugs also induce the *in vivo* elimination of CBZ epoxide. The disposition of single oral

TABLE 3. *Comparative* in vivo *pharmacokinetics of carbamazepine-10,11-epoxide in man and other animals*

Species	N	Route of administration	V_d(L/kg)	CL(mL/min/kg)	$T_{1/2}$(hr)
Human[a]	24	Oral	0.93 ± 0.13	1.63 ± 0.25	6.68 ± 1.22
Rhesus monkey[b]	8	i.v.	1.33 ± 0.21	18.9 ± 3.9	0.85 ± 0.14
Sprague-Dawley rat[c]	8	i.v.	1.07 ± 0.08	4.82 ± 0.94	2.64 ± 0.48
Rabbit[d]	6	i.v.	1.02 ± 0.14	5.67 ± 3.5	2.57 ± 1.04

[a] References 32, 36, 42, 43, 46.
[b] References 32, 63.
[c] References 13, 14.
[d] Reference 78.

doses of CBZ epoxide (100 mg) was evaluated in epileptic patients treated with phenobarbital and/or phenytoin (32,42), and it was found that the epoxide half-life was shortened and the clearance enhanced relative to the corresponding values in healthy subjects (Table 4). Therefore, phenobarbital and phenytoin induce both the formation and elimination clearance of CBZ epoxide, but the increased epoxide-to-CBZ plasma ratio indicates that the formation clearance is induced to a larger extent.

Administration of the anticonvulsant valproic acid with CBZ has been widely reported to increase the ratio of epoxide to CBZ in plasma (11,45,47,51,66,69,76). However, the amide analog of valproic acid, valpromide, has a more pronounced effect than valproic acid itself on the plasma levels of CBZ epoxide. The substitution of valpromide therapy for valproic acid in seven patients receiving CBZ resulted in large increases in plasma CBZ epoxide concentrations, and produced symptoms of intoxication in five patients even though CBZ concentrations were unchanged (52). It was subsequently confirmed that similar doses of valproic acid and valpromide elevate the epoxide-to-CBZ ratio, but valpromide increases it to a much greater extent (66). The differential effects of valproic acid and valpromide on CBZ epoxide concentration are striking because valpromide is extensively converted to valproic acid *in vivo*, with similar doses of valproate and valpromide yielding essentially equivalent plasma concentrations of valproic acid (65,66). Furthermore, plasma valpromide concentrations are reported to be either undetectable or only transiently detectable following oral administration of the drug (7,65).

The mechanism by which valproic acid and valpromide increase the epoxide-to-CBZ ratio is not obvious because, unlike phenobarbital and phenytoin, neither valproic acid nor valpromide are known to induce cytochrome P-450 or the formation clearance of CBZ epoxide. The alternative explanation is that the elimination clearance of CBZ epoxide is inhibited, with valprom-

TABLE 4. *Comparative* in vivo *pharmacokinetics of carbamazepine-10,11-epoxide in uninduced healthy volunteers versus epileptic patients induced with phenytoin and/or phenobarbital*

	N	$T_{1/2}$(hr)	CL(mL/min/kg)	V_d(L/kg)
Uninduced[a]	24	6.68 ± 1.22	1.63 ± 0.25	0.93 ± 0.13
Induced[b]	6	3.97 ± 0.84	2.89 ± 0.78	0.96 ± 0.18

[a] References 32, 36, 42, 43, 46.
[b] References 32, 42.

ide behaving as a more potent inhibitor. This hypothesis was tested in two parallel studies (32,41). Carbamazepine epoxide was administered orally as a 100-mg suspension to healthy volunteers on two occasions separated by 1 week. One dose served as a control, and the other dose was administered during treatment with either sodium valproate (500 mg/day) or valpromide (400 mg/day). The trough blood levels of valproic acid after administration of valproate (0.11 ± 0.05 mM) were comparable to those following administration of valpromide (0.12 ± 0.04 mM), whereas valpromide itself was only detectable in one subject at trace levels (<10 μM) in the valpromide-treated group. Both valproic acid and valpromide were found to inhibit the elimination of CBZ epoxide, as indicated by a reduced clearance and prolonged half-life, but the effect of valpromide was much more pronounced than the effect of valproic acid (Table 5). These results are consistent with the differential effects of valproate and valpromide on plasma levels of CBZ epoxide in CBZ-treated patients.

It can be hypothesized that the mechanism by which valproic acid and valpromide inhibit CBZ epoxide elimination is through inhibition of the hydrolysis of the epoxide by epoxide hydrolase. However, reports of the inhibition of epoxide hydrolase activity in microsomes appear inconsistent with the in vivo inhibition of CBZ epoxide elimination by valproic acid and valpromide. Valpromide has been reported to inhibit micro-somal epoxide hydrolase activity (59,61), but only at concentrations ($K_I \approx 500$ μM) far in excess of valpromide concentrations found in the plasma of valpromide-treated patients (<10 μM). Furthermore, valproic acid has been reported to be ineffective as an inhibitor of epoxide hydrolase activity at concentrations (10 mM) much greater than therapeutic concentrations of valproic acid (0.3 to 0.7 mM) (59,60,61). The apparent discrepancy between in vitro and in vivo inhibitory potencies of valproic acid and valpromide prompted further in vitro investigations in our laboratory (32). It was found that the hydrolysis of both CBZ epoxide and styrene oxide in human liver microsomes was inhibited by therapeutically relevant concentrations of valproic acid (K_I values < 0.7 mM) and valpromide (K_I values < 10 μM). These results were confirmed in preparations of purified human liver microsomal epoxide hydrolase (32). Therefore, inhibition of CBZ epoxide elimination in vivo is probably due to direct inhibition of microsomal epoxide hydrolase by valproic acid and valpromide, with valpromide behaving as a very potent inhibitor.

A reported drug interaction between the anticonvulsant progabide and CBZ epoxide shows striking similarities to the interaction between valpromide and CBZ epoxide. Progabide produced elevations of plasma CBZ epoxide concentrations and increased the epoxide-to-CBZ ratio in seven CBZ-treated patients, with symptoms of intoxication oc-

TABLE 5. *Inhibition of elimination of carbamazepine-10,11-epoxide (100 mg, oral dose) by sodium valproate (500 mg/day) or valpromide (400 mg/day) in healthy adult men*[a]

Treatment	N	$T_{1/2}$(hr)	CL(mL/min/kg)	V_d(L/kg)
Control		6.27 ± 0.51	1.56 ± 0.15	0.84 ± 0.15
Valproate	6	7.55 ± 1.22	1.30 ± 0.20	0.84 ± 0.07
Paired-T		P < .01	P < .01	P = .96
Control		6.92 ± 0.77	1.68 ± 0.16	1.01 ± 0.09
Valpromide	6	15.4 ± 2.55	0.64 ± 0.12	0.83 ± 0.09
Paired-T		P < .01	P < .01	P = .027

[a] References 32, 41.

curring in two of the patients despite no change in CBZ levels (39). Single-dose studies with CBZ epoxide in our laboratory have confirmed that progabide inhibits the *in vivo* elimination of CBZ epoxide (36), and human liver microsomal studies indicate that progabide inhibits epoxide hydrolase activity with a potency approximating that of valpromide (32).

CONCLUSION

Carbamazepine-10,11-epoxide is a pharmacologically active and chemically stable epoxide metabolite of the anticonvulsant carbamazepine. Carbamazepine epoxide is not commercially available for direct administration to epileptic patients, but the epoxide has been administered to human subjects for experimental purposes. Single-dose studies have confirmed that the elimination of CBZ epoxide is controlled by the activity of epoxide hydrolase. Administration of epoxide hydrolase inhibitors, such as valpromide or progabide, to patients receiving CBZ can lead to intoxication with CBZ epoxide, illustrating the clinical significance of this metabolite.

REFERENCES

1. Agbato, O. A., Elyas, A. A., Patsalos, P. N., Brett, E. M., and Lascelles, P. T. (1986): Total and free serum concentrations of carbamazepine and carbamazepine-10,11-epoxide in children with epilepsy. *Arch. Neurol.*, 43:1111–1116.
2. Albright, P. S., and Bruni, J. (1984): Effects of carbamazepine and its epoxide metabolite on amygdala-kindled seizures in rats. *Neurology*, 34:1383–1386.
3. Baker, K. M., Frigerio, A., Morselli, P. L., and Pifferi, G. (1973): Identification of a rearranged degradation product from carbamazepine-10,11-epoxide. *J. Pharm. Sci.*, 62:475–476.
4. Bellucci, G., Berti, G., Chiappe, C., Lippi, A., and Marioni, F. (1987): The metabolism of carbamazepine in humans: Steric course of the enzymatic hydrolysis of the 10,11-epoxide. *J. Med. Chem.*, 30:768–773.
5. Belvedere, G., Pantarotto, C., and Frigerio, A. (1975): Carbamazepine-10,11-epoxide metabolites in rat urine. *Res. Commun. Chem. Pathol. Pharmacol.*, 11:221–232.
6. Bertilsson, L., and Tomson, T. (1986): Clinical pharmacokinetics and pharmacological effects of carbamazepine and carbamazepine-10,11-epoxide. *Clin. Pharmacokinet.*, 11:177–198.
7. Bialer, M., Rubinstein, A., Raz, I., and Abramsky, O. (1984): Pharmacokinetics of valpromide after oral administration of a solution and a tablet to healthy volunteers. *Eur. J. Clin. Pharmacol.*, 27:501–503.
8. Bourgeois, B. F. D., and Wad, N. (1984): Carbamazepine-10,11-diol steady-state serum levels and renal excretion during carbamazepine therapy in adults and children. *Ther. Drug Monit.*, 6:259–265.
9. Bourgeois, B. F. D., and Wad, N. (1984): Individual and combined antiepileptic and neurotoxic activity of carbamazepine and carbamazepine-10,11-epoxide in mice. *J. Pharmacol. Exp. Ther.*, 231:411–415.
10. Braun, V. R., Dittmar, W., Machut, M., and Weickmann, S. (1982): Valepotriate mit Epoxidstruktur–Beachtliche Alkylantien. *Dtsch. Apoth. Z.*, 122:1109–1113.
11. Brodie, M. J., Forrest, G., and Rapeport, W. G. (1983): Carbamazepine-10,11-epoxide concentrations in epileptics on carbamazepine alone and in combination with other anticonvulsants. *Br. J. Clin. Pharmacol.*, 16:747–750.
12. Chambers, R. E. (1978): Simultaneous determination by gas-liquid chromatography of carbamazepine and carbamazepine-10,11-epoxide in plasma. *J. Chromatogr.*, 154:272–274.
13. Chang, S.-L. (1983): *Mechanism of the Interaction Between Valproic Acid and Carbamazepine in the Rat.* Ph.D. thesis, University of Washington, Seattle.
14. Chang, S.-L., and Levy, R. H. (1986): Inhibitory effect of valproic acid on the disposition of carbamazepine and carbamazepine-10,11-epoxide in the rat. *Drug Metab. Dispos.*, 14:281–286.
15. Contin, M., Riva, R., Albani, F., Perucca, E., Lamontanara, G., and Baruzzi, A. (1985): Alpha$_1$-acid glycoprotein concentration and serum protein binding of carbamazepine and carbamazepine-10,11-epoxide in children with epilepsy. *Eur. J. Clin. Pharmacol.*, 29:211–214.
16. Dam, M., Christensen, J. M., Brandt, J., Hansen, B. S., Hvidberg, E. F., Angelo, H., and Lous, P. (1980): Antiepileptic drugs: Interaction with dextropropoxyphene. In: *Antiepileptic Therapy: Advances in Drug Monitoring,* edited by S. I. Johannessen, P. L. Morselli, C. E. Pippenger, A. Richens, D. Schmidt, and H. Meinardi, pp. 299–306. Raven Press, New York.
17. Eichelbaum, M., and Bertilsson, L. (1975): Determination of carbamazepine and its epoxide metabolite in plasma by high-speed liquid chromatography. *J. Chromatogr.*, 103:135–140.
18. Eichelbaum, M., Tomson, T., Tybring, G., and Bertilsson, L. (1985): Carbamazepine metabolism in man. Induction and pharmacogenetic aspects. *Clin. Pharmacokinet.*, 10:80–90.

19. Elyas, A. A., Ratnaraj, N., Goldberg, V. D., and Lascelles, P. T. (1982): Routine monitoring of carbamazepine and carbamazepine-10,11-epoxide in plasma by high-performance liquid chromatography using 10-methoxycarbamazepine as internal standard. *J. Chromatogr.*, 231:93–101.

20. Faigle, J. W., and Feldmann, K. F. (1975): Pharmacokinetic data of carbamazepine and its major metabolites in man. In: *Clinical Pharmacology of Antiepileptic Drugs,* edited by H. Schneider, D. Janz, C. Gardner-Thorpe, H. Meinardi, and A. L. Sherwin, pp. 159–165. Springer-Verlag, Berlin, Heidelberg, New York.

21. Faigle, J. W., and Feldmann, K. F. (1982): Carbamazepine. Biotransformation. In: *Antiepileptic Drugs,* 2nd edition, edited by D. M. Woodbury, J. K. Penry, and C. E. Pippenger, pp. 483–495. Raven Press, New York.

22. Faigle, J. W., Feldmann, K. F., and Baltzer, V. (1977): Anticonvulsant effect of carbamazepine. An attempt to distinguish between the potency of the parent drug and its epoxide metabolite. In: *Antiepileptic Drug Monitoring,* edited by C. Gardner-Thorpe, D. Janz, H. Meinardi, and C. E. Pippenger, pp. 104–109. Pitman Press, Avon.

23. Frigerio, A., Baker, K. M., and Belvedere, G. (1973): Gas chromatographic degradation of several drugs and their metabolites. *Anal. Chem.*, 45:1846–1851.

24. Frigerio, A., Fanelli, R., Biandrate, P., Passerini, G., Morselli, P. L., and Garattini, S. (1972): Mass spectrometric characterization of carbamazepine-10,11-epoxide, a carbamazepine metabolite isolated from human urine. *J. Pharm. Sci.*, 61:1144–1147.

25. Frigerio, A., and Morselli, P. L. (1975): Carbamazepine: Biotransformation. In: *Advances in Neurology, Vol. II,* edited by J. K. Penry and D. D. Daly, pp. 295–308. Raven Press, New York.

26. Furlanut, M., Montanari, G., Bonin, P., and Casara, G. L. (1985): Carbamazepine and carbamazepine-10,11-epoxide serum concentrations in epileptic children. *J. Pediatr.*, 106:491–495.

27. Gérardin, A., Abadie, F., and Laffont, J. (1975): GLC determination of carbamazepine suitable for pharmacokinetic studies. *J. Pharm. Sci.*, 64:1940–1942.

28. Glatt, H. R., Oesch, F., Frigerio, A., and Garattini, S. (1975): Epoxides metabolically produced from some known carcinogens and from some clinically used drugs. I. Differences in mutagenicity. *Int. J. Cancer,* 16:787–797.

29. Goenechea, V. S., and Hecke-Seibicke, E. (1972): Beitrag zum Stoffwechsel von Carbamazepin. *Z. Klin. Chem. Klin. Biochem.*, 10:112–113.

30. Hartley, R., Lucock, M., Cookman, J. R., Becker, M., Smith, I. J., Smithells, R. W., and Forsythe, W. I. (1986): High-performance liquid chromatographic determination of carbamazepine and carbamazepine-10,11-epoxide in plasma and saliva following solid-phase sample extraction. *J. Chromatogr.*, 380:347–356.

31. Jung, R., Bentley, P., and Oesch, F. (1980): Influence of carbamazepine-10,11-oxide on drug metabolizing enzymes. *Biochem. Pharmacol.*, 29:1109–1112.

32. Kerr, B. M. (1989): *Role of epoxide hydrolase in carbamazepine epoxide drug interactions.* Ph.D. thesis, University of Washington, Seattle.

33. Königstein, M., Larisch, M., and Obe, G. (1984): Mutagenicity of antiepileptic drugs. I. Carbamazepine and some of its metabolites. *Mutat. Res.*, 139:83–86.

34. Korczyn, A. D., Ben-Zvi, Z. Kaplanski, J., Danon, A., and Berginer, V. (1977): Plasma levels of carbamazepine and metabolites: Effect of enzyme inducers. In: *Advances in Epileptology,* edited by H. Meinardi and A. J. Rowan, pp. 278–279. Swets and Zeitlinger, Amsterdam.

35. Köthe, K. W. (1980): *Chemisch-analytische Untersuchungen zur Pharmakokinetik und zum Metabolismus von Carbamazepin.* Rheinischen Friedrich-Wilhelms-Universität, Bonn.

36. Kroetz, D. L., Kerr, B. M., Loiseau, P., Guyot, M., and Levy, R. H. (1988): Is progabide an inhibitor of epoxide hydrolase in man? Meeting abstract, American Association of Pharmaceutical Scientists, Western Regional Meeting, Reno, Nevada, Jan. 31–Feb. 3, 1988.

37. Kumps, A. (1984): Simultaneous HPLC determination of oxcarbazepine, carbamazepine and their metabolites in serum. *J. Liq. Chromatogr.*, 7:1235–1241.

38. Kutt, H., and Paris-Kutt, M. (1982): Carbamazepine. Chemistry and methods of determination. In: *Antiepileptic Drugs,* 2nd edition, edited by D. M. Woodbury, J. K. Penry, and C. E. Pippenger, pp. 453–463. Raven Press, New York.

39. Kutt, H., Solomon, G. E., Dhar, A. K., Resor, S. R., Jr., Krall, R. L., and Morselli, P. L. (1984): Effects of progabide on carbamazepine epoxide and carbamazepine concentrations in plasma. *Epilepsia,* 25:674.

40. Lertratanangkoon, K., and Horning, M. G. (1982): Metabolism of carbamazepine. *Drug Metab. Dispos.*, 10:1–10.

41. Levy, R. H., Kerr, B. M., Loiseau, P., Guyot, M., and Wilensky, A. J. (1986): Inhibition of carbamazepine epoxide elimination by valpromide and valproic acid. *Epilepsia,* 27:592.

42. Levy, R. H., Loiseau, P., Guyot, M., and Kerr, B. M.: *Unpublished data.*

43. Levy, R. H., Martinez-Lage, J. M., Kerr, B. M., and Viteri, C. (1987): Effect of stiripentol on the formation and elimination of carbamazepine epoxide. Meeting abstract, 17th Epilepsy International Congress, Jerusalem, Israel, September 6–11, 1987.

44. Levy, R. H., Martinez-Lage, J. M., Tor, J., Blehaut, H., Gonzalez, I., and Bainbridge, B. (1985): Stiripentol level-dose relationship and interaction with carbamazepine in epileptic patients. *Epilepsia,* 26:544.

45. Levy, R. H., Moreland, T. A., Morselli, P. L., Guyot, M., Brachet-Liermain, A., and Loiseau, P. (1984): Carbamazepine/valproic acid interaction in man and rhesus monkey. *Epilepsia,* 25:338–345.

46. Levy, R. H., Wilensky, A. J., Chang, S.-L., and Kerr, B. M.: *Unpublished data.*

47. Lindhout, D., Höppener, R. J. E. A., and Meinardi, H. (1984): Teratogenicity of antiepileptic drug combinations with special emphasis on epoxidation (of carbamazepine). *Epilepsia,* 25:77–83.

48. Lynn, R. K., Smith, R. G., Thompson, R. M., Deinzer, M. L., Griffin, D., and Gerber, N. (1978): Characterization of glucuronide metabolites of carbamazepine in human urine by gas chromatography and mass spectrometry. *Drug Metab. Dispos.,* 6:494–501.

49. MacKichan, J. J. (1980): Simultaneous liquid chromatographic analysis for carbamazepine and carbamazepine-10,11-epoxide in plasma and saliva by use of double internal standardization. *J. Chromatogr.,* 181:373–383.

50. MacPhee, G. J. A., Thompson, G. G., McInnes, G. T., and Brodie, M. J. (1986): Verapamil potentiates carbamazepine neurotoxicity: A clinically important inhibitory interaction. *Lancet,* 1986i:700–703.

51. McKauge, L., Tyrer, J. H., and Eadie, M. J. (1981): Factors influencing simultaneous concentrations of carbamazepine and its epoxide in plasma. *Ther. Drug Monit.,* 3:63–70.

52. Meijer, J. W. A., Binnie, C. D., Debets, R. M. C., Van Parys, J. A. P., and de Beer-Pawlikowski, N. K. B. (1984): Possible hazard of valpromide-carbamazepine combination therapy in epilepsy. *Lancet,* 1984i:802.

53. Mendez-Alvarez, E., Soto-Otero, R., and Sierra-Marcuño, G. (1987): Simultaneous determination of carbamazepine, phenobarbital and their major metabolites in serum, brain tissue and urine by high-performance liquid chromatography. *Anal. Lett.,* 20:1275–1292.

54. Mihaly, G. W., Phillips, J. A., Louis, W. J., and Vajda, F. J. (1977): Measurement of carbamazepine and its epoxide metabolite by high-performance liquid chromatography, and a comparison of assay techniques for the analysis of carbamazepine. *Clin. Chem.,* 23:2283–2287.

55. Miura, H. (1981): Plasma levels and pharmacokinetics of antiepileptic drugs in children. *Folia Psychiatr. Neurol. Jpn.,* 35:305–313.

56. Morselli, P. L., Biandrate, P., Frigerio, A., Gerna, M., and Tognoni, G. (1973): Gas chromatographic determination of carbamazepine and carbamazepine-10,11-epoxide in human body fluids. In: *Methods of Analysis of Anti-epileptic Drugs,* edited by J. W. A. Meijer, H. Meinardi, C. Gardner-Thorpe, and E. van der Kleijn, pp. 169–175. Excerpta Medica, Amsterdam.

57. Morselli, P. L., Gerna, M., de Maio, D., Zanda, G., Viani, F., and Garattini, S. (1975): Pharmacokinetic studies on carbamazepine in volunteers and in epileptic patients. In: *Clinical Pharmacology of Antiepileptic Drugs,* edited by H. Schneider, D. Janz, C. Gardner-Thorpe, H. Meinardi, and A. L. Sherwin, pp. 166–180. Springer-Verlag, Berlin, Heidelberg, New York.

58. Oesch, F. (1980): Microsomal epoxide hydrolase. In: *Enzymatic Basis of Detoxification, Vol. II,* edited by W. B. Jakoby, pp. 277–290. Academic Press, New York.

59. Pacifici, G. M., Franchi, M., Bencini, C., and Rane, A. (1986): Valpromide inhibits human epoxide hydrolase. *Br. J. Clin. Pharmacol.,* 22: 269–274.

60. Pacifici, G. M., and Rane, A. (1987): Valpromide but not sodium hydrogen divalproate inhibits epoxide hydrolase in human liver. *Pharmacol. Toxicol.,* 60:237–238.

61. Pacifici, G. M., Tomson, T., Bertilsson, L., and Rane, A. (1985): Valpromide/carbamazepine and risk of teratogenicity. *Lancet,* 1985i:397–398.

62. Pantarotto, C., Crunelli, V., Lanzoni, J., Frigerio, A., and Quattrone, A. (1979): Quantitative determination of carbamazepine and carbamazepine-10,11-epoxide in rat brain areas by multiple ion detection mass fragmentography. *Anal. Biochem.,* 93:115–123.

63. Patel, I. H., Levy, R. H., and Trager, W. F. (1978): Pharmacokinetics of carbamazepine-10,11-epoxide before and after autoinduction in rhesus monkeys. *J. Pharmacol. Exp. Ther.,* 206:607–613.

64. Patsalos, P. N., Stephenson, T. J., Krishna, S., Elyas, A. A., Lascelles, P. T., and Wiles, C. M. (1985): Side-effects induced by carbamazepine-10,11-epoxide. *Lancet,* 1985ii:496.

65. Pisani, F., Fazio, A., Oteri, G., and Di Perri, R. (1981): Dipropylacetic acid plasma levels: Diurnal fluctuations during chronic treatment with dipropylacetamide. *Ther. Drug Monit.,* 3:297–301.

66. Pisani, F., Fazio, A., Oteri, G., Ruello, C., Gitto, C., Russo, F., and Perucca, E. (1986): Sodium valproate and valpromide: Differential interaction with carbamazepine in epileptic patients. *Epilepsia,* 27:548–552.

67. Pynnönen, S., Sillanpää, M., Frey, H., and Iisalo, E. (1976): Serum concentration of carbamazepine: Comparison of Hermann's spectrophotometric method and a new GLC method for the determination of carbamazepine. *Epilepsia,* 17:67–72.

68. Pynnönen, S., Sillanpää, M., Frey, H., and Iisalo, E. (1977): Carbamazepine and its 10,11-epoxide in children and adults with epilepsy. *Eur. J. Clin. Pharmacol.,* 11:129–133.

69. Ramsey, R. E., Guterman, A., Vasquez, D., Percholski, R., and Wong, P. (1983): Carbamazepine metabolism in man: The effect of concomitant anticonvulsant therapy. *Epilepsia,* 24:244.

70. Rane, A., Höjer, B., and Wilson, J. T. (1976): Kinetics of carbamazepine and its 10,11-epoxide metabolite in children. *Clin. Pharmacol. Ther.,* 19:276–283.

71. Rane, A., and Peng, D. (1985): Phenytoin enhances epoxide metabolism in human fetal liver cultures. *Drug Metab. Dispos.,* 13:382–385.

72. Richter, W. J., Kriemler, P., and Faigle, J. W. (1978): Newer aspects of the biotransformation of carbamazepine: Structural characterization of highly polar metabolites. In: *Recent Developments in Mass Spectrometry in Biochemistry and Medicine, Vol. 1,* edited by A. Frigerio, pp. 1–14. Plenum Press, New York.

73. Riva, R., Contin, M., Albani, F., Perucca, E., La-

montanara, G., and Baruzzi, A. (1985): Free and total serum concentrations of carbamazepine and carbamazepine-10,11-epoxide in infancy and childhood. *Epilepsia,* 26:320–322.

74. Robbins, D. K., Chang, S.-L., Baumann, R. J., and Wedlund, P. J. (1987): Quantitation of trans-10,11-dihydroxy-10,11-dihydrocarbamazepine in human urine by high-performance liquid chromatography. *J. Chromatogr.,* 415:208–213.

75. Sawchuk, R. J., and Cartier, L. L. (1982): Simultaneous liquid-chromatographic determination of carbamazepine and its epoxide metabolite in plasma. *Clin. Chem.,* 28:2127–2130.

76. Schoeman, J. F., Elyas, A. A., Brett, E. M., and Lascelles, P. T. (1984): Altered ratio of carbamazepine-10,11-epoxide/carbamazepine in plasma of children: Evidence of anticonvulsant drug interaction. *Dev. Med. Child. Neurol.,* 26:749–755.

77. Schoeman, J. F., Elyas, A. A., Brett, E. M., and Lascelles, P. T. (1984): Correlation between plasma carbamazepine-10,11-epoxide concentration and drug side-effects in children with epilepsy. *Dev. Med. Child. Neurol.,* 26:756–764.

78. Sumi, M., Watari, N., Naito, H., Umezawa, O., and Kaneniwa, N. (1987): Influence of phenobarbital on pharmacokinetics of carbamazepine and its epoxide metabolite in the rabbit. *Yakugaku Zasshi,* 107:984–991.

79. Sumi, M., Watari, N., Umezawa, O., and Kaneniwa, N. (1987): Pharmacokinetic study of carbamazepine and its epoxide metabolite in humans. *J. Pharmacobiodyn.,* 10:652–661.

80. Suria, A., and Killam, E. K. (1980): Carbamazepine. In: *Antiepileptic Drugs: Mechanisms of Action,* edited by G. H. Glaser, J. K. Penry, and D. M. Woodbury, pp. 563–575. Raven Press, New York.

81. Tomson, T., and Bertilsson, L. (1984): Potent therapeutic effect of carbamazepine-10,11-epoxide in trigeminal neuralgia. *Arch. Neurol.,* 41:598–601.

82. Tomson, T., and Bertilsson, L. (1985): Side-effects of carbamazepine: Drug or metabolite? *Lancet,* 1985ii:1010.

83. Tomson, T., Tybring, G., and Bertilsson, L. (1983): Single-dose kinetics and metabolism of carbamazepine-10,11-epoxide. *Clin. Pharmacol. Ther.,* 33:58–65.

84. Tomson, T., Tybring, G., Bertilsson, L., Ekbom, K., and Rane, A. (1980): Carbamazepine therapy in trigeminal neuralgia. Clinical effects in relation to plasma concentration. *Arch. Neurol.,* 37:699–703.

85. Trager, W. F., Levy, R. H., Patel, I. H., and Neal, J. N. (1978): Simultaneous analysis of carbamazepine and carbamazepine-10,11-epoxide by GC/CI/MS, stable isotope methodology. *Anal. Lett.* [B], 11:119–133.

86. Tybring, G., von Bahr, C., Bertilsson, L., Collste, H., Glaumann, H., and Solbrand, H. (1981): Metabolism of carbamazepine and its epoxide metabolite in human and rat liver *in vitro. Drug. Metab. Dispos.,* 9:561–564.

87. Von Unruh, G. E., and Paar, W. D. (1986): Gas chromatographic/mass spectrometric assays for oxcarbazepine and its main metabolites, 10-hydroxy-carbazepine and carbazepine-10,11-transdiol. *Biomed. Mass Spectrom.,* 13:651–656.

88. Wad, N. (1984): Simultaneous determination of elevation antiepileptic compounds in serum by high-performance liquid chromatography. *J. Chromatogr.,* 305:127–133.

89. Wedlund, P. J. (1981): *Carbamazepine: Mechanisms of Autoinduction of Clearance in Rhesus Monkey and Rat.* Ph.D. thesis, University of Washington, Seattle.

90. Westenberg, H. G. M., and de Zeeuw, R. A. (1976): Rapid and sensitive liquid chromatographic determination of carbamazepine suitable for use in monitoring multiple-drug anticonvulsant therapy. *J. Chromatogr.,* 118:217–224.

91. Westenberg, H. G. M., van der Kleijn, E., Oei, T. T., and de Zeeuw, R. A. (1978): Kinetics of carbamazepine and carbamazepine-epoxide determined by use of plasma and saliva. *Clin. Pharmacol. Ther.,* 23:320–328.

Antiepileptic Drugs, Third Edition, edited by
R. Levy, R. Mattson, B. Meldrum,
J. K. Penry, and F. E. Dreifuss.
Raven Press, Ltd., New York © 1989.

36

Carbamazepine

Interactions with Other Drugs

William H. Pitlick and René H. Levy

The clinical manifestations of interactions involving carbamazepine (CBZ) depend on several factors. It is necessary to consider whether CBZ is the affecter or the affected molecular species, and whether the interaction involves alteration of metabolism such as induction or inhibition of metabolism, other pharmacokinetic processes such as absorption or distribution, or pharmacodynamic factors. In addition, since CBZ is metabolized to an active species, carbamazepine-10,11-epoxide (CBZ epoxide), the effects of the interaction on concentrations of the active metabolite must also be considered.

Carbamazepine possesses enzyme-inducing properties and generally causes decreases in steady-state blood levels of other drugs. Likewise, phenytoin, phenobarbital, and primidone cause decreases in CBZ. However, the CBZ epoxide-to-CBZ ratio is concomitantly increased. Although the decrease in the CBZ level may result in breakthrough seizures, few such reports are available. In most cases, these interactions can be anticipated, and monitoring of plasma drug levels enables appropriate dosage adjustments to be made. However, certain unexpected interactions associated with serious clinical manifestations still occur.

Inhibition of CBZ metabolism by other drugs can result in CBZ intoxication. This type of interaction is now better understood because of recent advances in information on the mechanisms of cytochrome P-450 inhibition and the fate of CBZ. Thus, consideration of the chemical structure of an added drug should signal the potential of an interaction with CBZ. For example, known inhibitors of drug metabolism, such as imidazoles, can be expected to increase steady-state plasma CBZ levels, with possible toxic manifestations. Cimetidine (19,51), diltiazem (9), and denzimol (75) all increase steady-state CBZ levels in humans. Agents with a history of producing interactions should also indicate caution. Erythromycin (93), triacetyloleandomycin (24,64,71), and propoxyphene (21,22) have all produced signs of CBZ intoxication in patients with epilepsy.

PHARMACOKINETICS AND PRINCIPLES OF INTERACTIONS

The pharmacokinetic parameters of CBZ are discussed fully in Chapters 35 and 37, but salient features will be reviewed here as they pertain to drug interactions. In humans, CBZ is readily absorbed from the gastrointestinal tract, with minimal first-pass metabolism. However, bioavailability problems are possible and even suspected at high doses. Carbamazepine is completely cleared by hepatic mechanisms. Epoxidation of the 10,11 double bond and subsequent hydration of this epoxide to a dihydrodiol (*trans*-diol) is the major pathway of CBZ elimination. In epileptic patients, 30% to 60% of CBZ is converted to CBZ epoxide and subsequently excreted as the *trans*-diol in urine. Clearance of the epoxide is three times as great as that of the parent drug in healthy subjects, several times as great in patients on long-term CBZ monotherapy, and even greater in the presence of antiepileptic polytherapy. Nevertheless, CBZ epoxide accumulates and contributes to CBZ's therapeutic efficacy and toxic effects.

Increases in CBZ clearance are due principally to induction of the epoxide-*trans*-diol pathway. There is some evidence that both the epoxidation and epoxide hydrolase enzymes are subject to induction by pretreatment with inducing agents (27), and likewise subject to inhibition by metabolic inhibitors (77,78). In healthy volunteers, the plasma clearance of the epoxide is approximately four times as great as that of CBZ, with a half-life of 6.1 hr for the epoxide versus 26 hr for CBZ, and 90% of the epoxide is metabolized to the *trans*-diol (6).

As with most other antiepileptic drugs, hepatic clearance of CBZ is small relative to liver blood flow and its extraction ratio is less than 10%. It is noted in Chapter 2 that the hepatic clearance of a drug reflects the ability of the liver to extract drug from blood passing through it and can be affected by hepatic blood flow. Intrinsic clearance represents the intrinsic ability of the eliminating organs to remove drug in the absence of any flow limitations. For a drug with low intrinsic clearance and therefore a low extraction ratio, such as CBZ, hepatic clearance is relatively independent of liver blood flow (and approximates intrinsic clearance). Thus, changes in liver blood flow would not be expected to produce a change in hepatic clearance of CBZ. An increase in intrinsic clearance, as occurs during enzyme induction, results in an almost identical increase in hepatic clearance. Also, since CBZ is eliminated completely by metabolism, its hepatic and total body clearances are equal. Therefore, alterations in the intrinsic clearance of CBZ result in inversely proportional alterations in steady-state plasma drug levels and changes in half-life. The free fraction of CBZ in human plasma is approximately 25% and appears concentration-independent within therapeutic concentrations. One binding site on albumin has been proposed. The effects of protein binding interactions on free and total drug levels are described in Chapter 2. Few such interactions have been reported for CBZ.

These principles can also be used to understand the effects of CBZ on other drugs, since the major antiepileptic drugs have low extraction ratios and are extensively metabolized. However, the characteristics of each drug (e.g., protein binding) must be taken into consideration to make accurate predictions.

EFFECTS OF CARBAMAZEPINE ON ITS OWN DISPOSITION

It is widely reported that CBZ increases the total body clearance of itself and several other drugs in various animal species, including humans (5,8,26,35,38,49,56,58, 68,72,73,80,82,84,89). The preponderance of evidence indicates that the increase in clearance is caused by an increased metabolic capacity of both the epoxidation and hydration steps in formation of the *trans*-diol metabolite. The increased clearance is associated with a shortened half-life and a reduction in the total serum drug concentration at steady-state. For example, the half-life of CBZ was reduced from greater than 30 hr to less than 20 hr with long-term use (79), and the average steady-state concentration of CBZ was reduced by 50% after 3 weeks of drug administration (29).

Typically, in patients not previously exposed to CBZ, maximum plasma concentrations will be observed in 3 to 4 days after initiation of therapy. The levels tend to decrease over the next month to a steady-state approximately 50% lower than would be predicted on the basis of single-dose studies (30,35,36). Pharmacokinetic modeling of this phenomenon has been done in both humans and monkeys (35,53,79). In humans, an induction half-life of 4 days was calculated, which is consistent with a period of 3 to 4 weeks for achieving a new steady-state.

Autoinduced increases in CBZ clearance have also been studied in children by a stable isotope technique (5). In three children (10–13 years old), CBZ clearance doubled after 32 days of treatment, resulting in steady-state concentrations that were 50% less than predicted. During the next 4 months, there was no further increase in clearance or decrease in serum CBZ concentrations. These data tend to support the earlier finding that the autoinduction phenomenon is complete within 1 month.

EFFECT OF CARBAMAZEPINE ON OTHER DRUGS

Not only does CBZ induce its own metabolism, it also alters the biotransformation of other drugs, including anticonvulsants, given concomitantly.

The effect of CBZ on phenytoin administered simultaneously to epileptic patients is of variable consequence. Early reports (38) indicated that CBZ significantly decreased the serum phenytoin level and half-life. More recent data (10,11,94) indicate an inconsistent effect of variable clinical significance. In five epileptic patients before and during treatment with 600 mg of CBZ daily (38), the phenytoin half-life decreased from 10.6 hr to 6.4 hr after 9 days of CBZ therapy. In seven patients, 600 mg of CBZ daily was added to phenytoin after steady-state levels of phenytoin were measured (38). The serum phenytoin levels decreased markedly following 4 to 14 days of CBZ treatment in three patients, but were unchanged in the remaining four. Constant-rate infusion of CBZ before treatment resulted in more than a 40% decrease in the plasma half-life of phenytoin.

On the other hand, in 12 of 24 epileptic patients, the mean steady-state phenytoin concentrations nearly doubled when CBZ was added to the regimens (94). In another study of six patients (10), phenytoin pharmacokinetics were studied with a stable isotope tracer technique before and after the addition of CBZ. A marked decrease in phenytoin clearance with concomitant increases in half-life and serum concentrations were observed in addition to drug-related toxicity. In interpreting the effects of CBZ on phenytoin, it is important to evaluate the amount of phenytoin administered, the timing of the interaction, the study populations, and the pharmaceutical dosage forms. All of these variables have been shown to affect the pharmacokinetics of phenytoin. Routine therapeutic monitoring of plasma CBZ and phenytoin levels is recommended when the drugs are co-administered.

The effect of CBZ on primidone metabolism has also been studied. Phenobarbital, a byproduct of primidone metabolism, showed significant increases when CBZ was added to the regimen of four patients (13). However, evidence is lacking for an effect of CBZ on ingested phenobarbital. In one study of 25 patients taking both phenobarbital and CBZ, no change in phenobarbital clearance was observed in comparison with a group taking phenobarbital alone (25).

Several studies indicate CBZ increases plasma clearance of valproic acid, probably through induction of the metabolic processes responsible for valproic acid elimination. Six healthy subjects received 250 mg of valproic acid twice daily for 4 weeks;

CBZ 200 mg once daily, was added after 4 days of valproic acid therapy (8). A significant increase in clearance and a concomitant decrease in steady-state blood valproate levels was apparent after 2 weeks of CBZ therapy. Similar findings have also been reported in epileptic patients (1,20). In two patients receiving CBZ and valproic acid, steady-state valproate levels were 37% to 64% lower than predicted from a single dose of valproate (65). In another study, steady-state valproate levels were compared in two groups of adult patients, seven on valproate monotherapy and six also receiving CBZ. The ratio of plasma level to dose was 38% lower in the presence of CBZ (85).

The effects of CBZ on specific metabolic pathways of valproate were recently examined in epileptic patients (54). The formation of Δ^4-valproate (hepatotoxic metabolite of valproate) was increased by 105% in the presence of CBZ. The clearances of several other pathways were increased: ω and ω-1 oxidation (both cytochrome P-450 mediated) as well as glucuronidation.

Similar studies have been performed to determine the extent and time course of interaction between CBZ and clonazepam in healthy subjects (49). Seven subjects receiving a 1 mg clonazepam tablet daily were given 200 mg of CBZ daily for up to 29 days. Fifteen days after initiation of CBZ there was a marked decrease in both clonzaepam and CBZ levels. The half-life of clonazepam was reduced from 32 hr to 22 hr after CBZ was added to the regimen.

When CBZ (200 mg/day) was added to the regimen of healthy subjects maintained on 250 mg of ethosuximide a day, ethosuximide clearance increased significantly after 10 days of CBZ therapy, with a synchronous decrease in ethosuximide half-life from 54 to 45 hr (89). Carbamazepine has also been shown to affect the half-life of the antibiotic doxycycline. In five patients on long-term carbamazepine therapy, the half-life of doxycycline (8.4 hr) was significantly shorter than the mean half-life of 15.1 hr in nine control patients (76).

With the increased use of CBZ in neuropsychiatry, interactions with haloperidol have become evident. Three studies have shown that haloperidol levels are reduced by more than 50% following the addition of CBZ (2,31,46). In some cases, this effect was so pronounced that clinical worsening of the patients was observed.

Alterations in the fraction of drug bound to plasma proteins may also produce changes in total plasma drug levels. For drugs with a low extraction ratio, such as antiepileptic drugs, concentrations of free drug are independent of the free fraction, but total drug levels are inversely proportional to the free fraction. In all the above interactions, it was assumed that the mechanism involved an increase in intrinsic (metabolic) clearance. Theoretically, a protein binding displacement would also result in a decrease in steady-state levels. Such a hypothesis is unlikely for several reasons. Theoretically, CBZ should not behave as a displacer since its molar concentration is very small relative to that of albumin and its association constant is not high. In fact, the effects of CBZ on the protein binding of other drugs were investigated and no displacement effect was found. In patients treated with phenytoin, the addition of CBZ produced little or no change in the free fraction of phenytoin (39). In another study, there was no evidence of competitive binding to plasma proteins between phenytoin and CBZ (59). The ability of CBZ to reduce the steady-state levels of valproic acid, clonazepam, and ethosuximide was also demonstrated in controlled studies in rhesus monkeys (17,18,50). Carbamazepine and each of these anticonvulsants were administered intravenously, thereby excluding the possibility of a mechanism of interaction involving a reduction in fraction of dose absorbed.

EFFECTS OF OTHER DRUGS ON CARBAMAZEPINE

It appears that CBZ clearance can be altered by many other drugs, including coadministered antiepileptic drugs. In considering the consequences of such interactions, it should be kept in mind that CBZ epoxide is also active, and its clearance may also be affected. Both increases (due to inhibition of metabolism) and decreases (due to enzymatic induction) have been reported for CBZ and CBZ epoxide. However, combinations and permutations of induction and inhibition for CBZ and CBZ epoxide have also been reported. There have been few reports of significant interactions involving CBZ protein binding.

Inhibition

There are a number of conflicting reports on the effects of valproic acid on CBZ disposition. Both increases and decreases in CBZ levels have been observed following the addition of valproic acid (14,32,37,42,92). In addition, elevation of CBZ epoxide levels has been reported after the addition of valproic acid (14). Careful pharmacokinetic analysis of the effects of valproic acid on the CBZ-to-CBZ epoxide ratio clarifies the mechanism of this interaction. The interaction between valproic acid and CBZ may involve both displacement from protein binding and metabolic inhibition. Since valproic acid decreases CBZ binding *in vitro* (62) and valproic acid inhibits CBZ metabolism, CBZ levels may increase, decrease, or remain unchanged when the drugs are co-administered, depending on which effect prevails. Of seven patients maintained at steady-state levels of CBZ, five had significant decreases in steady-state CBZ levels and two showed no change after the addition of valproic acid (55). However, the CBZ epoxide-to-CBZ

ratio increased significantly in all seven patients. Animal studies have shown that valproic acid decreases protein binding of both CBZ and CBZ epoxide (67), and decreases the epoxide clearance by inhibition of epoxide hydrolase. This effect was recently verified in healthy volunteers (52) and is described in more detail in Chapter 37. Valpromide, the amide derivative of valproic acid, is associated with an even greater inhibition of epoxide hydrolase (70,77,78). In patients stabilized on regimens of valproic acid and CBZ, replacement of valproic acid with valpromide caused a striking elevation of CBZ epoxide levels with concomitant CBZ toxicity, in spite of unchanged plasma CBZ levels (63). Addition of valproic acid to CBZ regimens should be accompanied by careful monitoring of plasma drug levels.

Several drugs that inhibit drug metabolism increase plasma CBZ levels when given concomitantly with CBZ. Cimetidine was noted to cause increases in plasma CBZ concentrations principally in healthy volunteers, but later studies have shown this interaction to be of modest clinical significance. In epileptic patients stabilized on CBZ, the modest inhibition of CBZ metabolism by cimetidine is apparently compensated for by the induction of metabolism caused by CBZ (19,51). Ranitidine has no effect on the clearance of CBZ (66,90).

Calcium channel blockers have variable effects on CBZ metabolism. Verapamil nearly doubled CBZ concentrations in six epileptic patients maintained on CBZ, resulting in toxic side effects (4,60). Diltiazem, but not nifedipine, has been reported to have a similar effect on CBZ levels (9). These interactions appear to be clinically significant.

Several imidazoles have been reported to inhibit CBZ metabolism. Nicotinamide caused elevation of CBZ levels in two patients, with high correlations between CBZ clearance and nicotinamide doses (7). Isoniazid has been shown to inhibit CBZ metabolism, with resultant signs of CBZ intoxication (88). The potential antiepileptic drugs denzimol (75) and nafimidone (87), both imidazoles, and stiripentol (54) inhibit CBZ elimination. Nafimidone reduced CBZ metabolism by 76% to 87% in six epileptic patients (87).

Danazol, an antiestrogenic steroid, inhibits the epoxide-*trans*-diol elimination of CBZ, resulting in a 50% to 100% increase in steady-state plasma CBZ levels during co-administration of the two drugs (48). In eight epileptic patients, the clearance of CBZ was reduced from 6.1 ± 1.1 to 2.0 ± 0.7 L/hr after 10 weeks of stiripentol treatment. The CBZ epoxide-to-CBZ ratio was also reduced (57).

The addition of propoxyphene to a regimen of CBZ, alone or with other antiepileptic drugs, was associated with signs of CBZ intoxication: headache, dizziness, ataxia, nausea, and fatigue (23). Dam et al. (21,22) have shown that propoxyphene causes an increase in plasma CBZ levels associated with a decrease in the epoxide level.

Triacetyloleandomycin, an antibiotic widely used in France, has been shown to cause CBZ intoxication associated with elevation of plasma CBZ levels (24). Mesdjian et al. (64) reported that 17 epileptic subjects being treated with CBZ developed acute and unexpected intoxication (drowsiness, nausea, vomiting, dizziness) when triacetyloleandomycin was administered. Similar symptoms were found when erythromycin was given to two patients who were taking CBZ (64).

Induction

Several studies in the last decade have consistently demonstrated that CBZ metabolism is highly inducible by other antiepileptic drugs. Although this effect has caused no alarming clinical findings, Hvidberg and Dam (41), underlining the clinical relevance of this interaction, point out that "patients may suffer from seizures in the morning, when plasma carbamazepine is low, and show signs and symptoms of intoxication in the evening when plasma level is high."

Christiansen and Dam (15,16) showed in 123 patients that the slope of the relationship between plasma level and dose of CBZ is reduced separately by phenytoin, phenobarbital, and the combination of phenytoin and phenobarbital. Similar findings were reported by Schneider (86) in 184 patients involving eight different combinations of CBZ and other drugs. This study showed that primidone has a significant effect in decreasing the slope of the relationship between plasma level and dose, presumably as a consequence of enzymatic induction. In 142 patients, Johannessen and Strandjord (45) found also that phenytoin or phenobarbital, or a combination of both, can reduce the plasma level-to-dose ratio of CBZ. They emphasized the need to monitor CBZ levels during polytherapy to achieve the proper dosage increments. Rane et al. (83) compared the mean CBZ levels in two groups of children, one on monotherapy, the other on a combination of drugs. They found that the ratio of plasma level to dose was lower in the group on polytherapy. In that same group, however, the concentration of 10,11-epoxide metabolite was significantly higher.

Using a pulse dose of stable isotope-labeled CBZ, Eichelbaum et al. (28) were able to measure the half-life of CBZ in six patients on combined anticonvulsant therapy. The half-life ranged from 5.0 to 16 hr (mean, 8.2 hr). From those data, as well as the urinary excretion of the 10,11-*trans*-diol metabolite (approximately 50% of the dose), they concluded that concomitant therapy induces the metabolism of CBZ. Callaghan et al. (12) confirmed the findings of others that primidone causes a significant reduction in steady-state CBZ levels.

Hoppener et al. (40) compared the daily

fluctuations in CBZ levels in 19 patients on monotherapy and 43 patients on polytherapy. All patients received the drug three times a day (8 A.M., 12:30 P.M., and 8 P.M.) The fluctuation was 34.5 ± 10.9% in the group on monotherapy and 68.5 ± 21.2% in the group on polytherapy. The authors therefore recommended frequent administration of CBZ (three to four times a day) in patients on multiple-drug therapy.

A provocative analysis of the relationship between plasma level and dose of CBZ was performed by Battino et al. (3). Based on 567 determinations of plasma CBZ levels in 326 patients of all ages, these authors segregated the main variables in the plasma level-to-dose ratio as age, associated therapy, and CBZ dose. The ratio increased linearly with age between 1 and 19 years. The ratio was significantly reduced with polytherapy in several subgroups homogeneous with respect to age (0–3, 4–9, 10–15, and 19–45 years).

Numerous investigations have focused on the effects of concomitant therapy on the CBZ-10,11-epoxide metabolite. This metabolite is of interest because it has shown anticonvulsant activity in rats (33). Also, in cerebrospinal fluid its concentration is 40% to 60% that of CBZ (43,81), whereas in plasma it is 10% to 25% that of the parent drug. This difference is attributable to the lower degree of plasma protein binding of the epoxide. Several studies have found that the ratio of epoxide to CBZ at steady-state plasma levels was higher in patients taking CBZ with other antiepileptic drugs than in those taking CBZ only (16,22,83,86,91).

Korczyn et al. (47) studied the plasma levels of CBZ and the epoxide and dihydrodiol metabolites in two groups of patients (monotherapy versus polytherapy). They concluded that heteroinduction involves the epoxidation of CBZ, as well as the conversion of the epoxide to the dihydrodiol.

A recent study in rhesus monkeys examined the effect of phenobarbital on the ratio of epoxide to CBZ at steady-state levels (74). An increase in this ratio was attributed to induction of epoxide formation.

Brain-to-plasma ratios of CBZ and CBZ epoxide were determined in two studies of epileptic patients undergoing brain surgery. In one study of 21 patients with brain tumors, the ratio was 1.1 ± 0.1 for CBZ and 1.1 to 1.2 for the CBZ epoxide (68). In the other study (34), the brain-to-plasma ratios were measured in five patients undergoing unilateral temporal lobectomy. The ratio ranged from 1.4 to 1.6 for CBZ and 0.6 to 1.5 for the epoxide. For CBZ, the ratios were similar in patients treated with CBZ alone or in combination with other anticonvulsants, but for CBZ epoxide, the ratio was higher in patients on multiple-drug therapy. In the latter patients, the plasma and brain CBZ epoxide concentrations were two to three times higher than in patients receiving CBZ only.

Protein Binding

The influence of several other drugs on the plasma binding of CBZ at a concentration of 5 μg/ml was studied by ultrafiltration. It was found that phenobarbital, phenytoin, and nortriptyline had no effect on the protein binding of CBZ, whereas ethosuximide and phensuximide showed a very slight increase in the percent of CBZ bound to protein (84). As mentioned, valproic acid was found to cause an increase in the free fraction of CBZ (61,73).

In vivo studies of CBZ protein binding are relatively rare, and there is even less information on the effects of protein binding interactions. One study of 10 patients undergoing long-term CBZ therapy showed a mean cerebrospinal fluid (CSF)-to-serum ratio of 0.24 (43). In another study of 19 adult patients receiving long-term carbamazepine therapy plus other anticonvulsants, the CSF-to-serum ratio was 0.22 (44).

From these data it appears unlikely that significant interactions occur with CBZ as a result of alterations in protein binding.

THERAPEUTIC IMPLICATIONS

Interactions between CBZ and other antiepileptic drugs are prevalent. Carbamazepine tends to decrease the plasma level-to-dose ratio of other drugs. Conversely, the metabolism of CBZ is very sensitive to induction by other antiepileptic drugs, resulting also in a decrease of the plasma level-to-dose ratio. This effect is found in all age groups, including infants. Monitoring plasma CBZ levels in therapy-resistant patients should be useful in making optimal dosage adjustments. However, timing of blood sample collections becomes paramount in view of recent reports of CBZ's 6 hr half-life. This awareness has led to the development of controlled-release drug formulations. According to currently available information, there appears to be no need to distinguish between free and total levels of CBZ. However, this may not be the case for other drugs affected by CBZ, especially when three or more drugs are administered simultaneously. Thus, a low plasma level-to-dose ratio for phenytoin may be due to an increase in intrinsic clearance caused by CBZ induction or to a high free fraction caused by valproic acid. In such cases, monitoring free drug levels enables distinction between the two mechanisms. Such distinction is necessary because the induction mechanism would require a dose increment, whereas the binding phenomenon would not.

The list of drugs known to cause CBZ intoxication has increased appreciably in the last few years. In addition to the early reports associated with propoxyphene, triacetyloleandomycin, and erythromycin, recent reports include calcium channel blockers (verapamil, diltiazem), nicotinamide, isoniazid, new antiepileptic agents (nafimidone, denzimol, stiripentol), and valpromide. Much caution should be exercised when prescribing these drugs to patients on CBZ.

REFERENCES

1. Adams, D. J., Luders, H., and Pippenger, C. E. (1978): Sodium valproate in the treatment of intractable seizure disorders: A clinical and electroencephalographic study. *Neurology (Minneap.)*, 28:152–157.
2. Arana, G. W., Goff, D. C., Friedman, H., Ornsteen, M., Greenblatt, D. J., Black, B., and Shader, R. I. (1986): Does carbamazepine-induced reduction of plasma haloperidol level worsen psychotic symptoms? *Am. J. Psychiatry*, 143:650–651.
3. Battino, D., Bossi, L., Croci, D., Franceschetti, S., Gomeni, C., Moise, A., and Vitali, A. (1980): Carbamazepine plasma levels in children and adults: Influence of age, dose, and associated therapy. *Ther. Drug Monit.*, 2:315–322.
4. Beattie, B., Biller, J., Mehlhaus, B., and Murray, M. (1988): Verapamil-induced neurotoxicity. *Eur. J. Neurology*, 28:104–105.
5. Bertilsson, L., Hojer, B., Tybring, G., Osterloh, J., and Rane, A. (1980): Autoinduction of carbamazepine metabolism in children examined by a stable isotope technique. *Clin. Pharmacol. Ther.*, 27:83–88.
6. Bertilsson, L., and Tomson, T. (1982): Kinetics and metabolism of carbamazepine-10,11-epoxide in man. In: *Metabolism of Antiepileptic Drugs*, and edited by R. H. Levy, W. H. Pitlick, M. Eichelbaum, and J. Meijer, pp. 19–26. Raven Press, New York.
7. Bourgeois, B. F. D., Dodson, W. E., and Ferrendelli, J. A. (1982): Interaction between primidone, carbamazepine and nicotinamide. *Neurology*, 32:1122–1126.
8. Bowdle, T. A., Levy, R. H., and Cutler, R. E., (1979): Effects of carbamazepine on valproic acid in normal man. *Clin. Pharmacol. Ther.*, 26:629–634.
9. Brodie, M. M., and Macphee, G. J. A. (1986): Carbamazepine neurotoxicity precipitated by diltiazem. *Br. Med. J.*, 292:1170–1171.
10. Browne, T. R., Evans, J. H., and Szabo, G. K. (1984): Effect of carbamazepine on phenytoin pharmacokinetics determined by a stable isotope technique. *Neurology* [suppl.1], 35:284.
11. Browne, T. R., Szabo, G. K., Evans, J. H., Evans, B. A., Greenblatt, D. J., and Mikati, M. A. (1988): Carbamazepine increases phenytoin serum concentration and reduces phenytoin clearance. *Neurology (in press)*.
12. Callaghan, N., Duggan, B., O'Hare, J., and O'Driscoll, D. (1980): Serum levels of phenobarbitone and phenylethylmalonamide with primidone used as a single drug and in combination with

carbamazepine or phenytoin. In: *Antiepileptic Therapy: Advances in Drug Monitoring*, edited by S. I. Johannessen, P. L. Morselli, C. E. Pippenger, A. Richens, D. Schmidt, and H. Meinardi, pp. 307–313. Raven Press, New York.

13. Callaghan, N., Feely, M., Duggan, F., O'Callaghan, M., and Seldrup, J. (1977): The effect of anticonvulsant drugs which induce liver microsomal enzymes on derived and ingested phenobarbitone levels. *Acta Neurol. Scand.*, 56:1–6.

14. Chang, S. L., and Levy, R. H. (1986): Inhibitory effect of valproic acid on the disposition of carbamazepine and carbamazepine-10,11-epoxide in the rat. *Drug Metabolism and Disposition*, 14:281–286.

15. Christiansen, J., and Dam, M. (1973): Influence of penobarbital and diphenylhydantoin on plasma carbamazepine levels in patients with epilepsy. *Acta Neurol. Scand.*, 49:543–546.

16. Christiansen, J., and Dam, M. (1975): Drug interaction in epileptic patients. In: *Clinical Pharmacology of Anti-Epileptic Drugs*, edited by H. Schneider, D. Janz, C. Gardner-Thorpe, H. Meinardi, and A. L. Sherwin, pp. 197–200. Springer-Verlag, Berlin.

17. Corbisier, P. H., and Levy, R. H. (1977): Pharmacokinetics of drug interaction by enzyme induction. I. Carbamazepine and valproic acid. *APhA/Acad. Pharm. Sci. Abstr.*, 7:163.

18. Corbisier, P. H., and Levy, R. H. (1977): Pharmacokinetics of drug interaction by enzyme induction. III. Carbamazepine and ethosuximide. *APhA/Acad. Pharm. Sci. Abstr.*, 7:134.

19. Dalton, M. M., Powell, J. R., and Messenheimer, J. A. (1985): Cimetidine and carbamazepine: A complex pharmacokinetic interaction. *Drug Intell. Clin. Pharm.*, 19:456.

20. Dam, M., and Christiansen, J. (1977): Interaction of propoxyphene with carbamazepine. *Lancet*, 2:509.

21. Dam, M., Christensen, J. M., Brandt, J., Hansen, B. S., Hvidberg, E. F., Angelo, H., and Lous, P. (1980): Antiepileptic drugs: Interaction with dextropropoxyphene. In: *Antiepileptic Therapy: Advances in Drug Monitoring*, edited by S. I. Johannessen, P. L. Morselli, C. E. Pippenger, A. Richens, D. Schmidt, and H. Meinardi, pp. 299–306. Raven Press, New York.

22. Dam, M., Jensen, A., and Christensen, J. (1975): Plasma level and effect of carbamazepine in grand mal and psychomotor epilepsy. *Acta Neurol. Scand.* [Suppl.], 60:33–38.

23. Dam, M., Kristensen, C. B., Hansen, B. S., and Christiansen, J. (1977): Interaction between carbamazepine and propoxyphene in man. *Acta Neurol. Scand.*, 56:603–607.

24. Dravet, C., Mesdjian, E., Cenraud, B., and Roger, J. (1977): Interaction between carbamazepine and triacetyloleandomycin. *Lancet*, 1:810–811.

25. Eadie, M. J., Lander, C. M., Hooper, W. D., and Tyrer, J. H. (1977): Factors influencing plasma phenobarbitone levels in epileptic patients. *Br. J. Clin. Pharmacol.*, 4:541–547.

26. Eichelbaum, M., Ekbom, K., Bertilsson, L.,

Lund, L., Plamer, L., and Sjoqvist, F. (1976): Plasma levels of carbamazepine and carbamazepine-10,11-epoxide during treatment of epilepsy. *Eur. J. Clin. Pharmacol.*, 9:417–421.

27. Eichelbaum, M., Elbom, K., Bertilsson, L., Ringberger, V. A., and Rane, A. (1975): Plasma kinetics of carbamazepine and its epoxide metabolite in man after single and multiple doses. *Eur. J. Clin. Pharmacol.*, 8:337–341.

28. Eichelbaum, M., Jensen, C., von Sassen, W., Bertilsson, L., and Tomson, T. (1982): *In vivo* and *in vitro* biotransformation of carbamazepine in man and rat. In: *Metabolism of Antiepileptic Drugs.*, edited by R. H. Levy, W. H. Pitlick, M. Eichelbaum, and J. Meijer, pp. 27–34. Raven Press, New York.

29. Eichelbaum, M., Kothe, K. W., and Hoffman, F. (1979): Kinetics and metabolism of carbamazepine during combined antiepileptic drug therapy. *Clin. Pharmacol. Ther.*, 26:366–371.

30. Faigle, J. W., Brechbuhler, S., Feldman, K. F., and Richter, W. J. (1976): The biotransformation of carbamazepine. In: *Epileptic Seizures—Behavior—Pain*, edited by W. Birkkmayer, pp. 127–140. Hans Huber, Berne.

31. Fast, D. K., Jones, B. D., Kusalic, M., Erickson, M. (1986): Effect of carbamazepine on neuroleptic plasma levels and efficacy. *Am. J. Psychiatry*, 143:117–118.

32. Flachs, H., Gram, L., Wurtz-Jorgensen, A., and Parnes, J. (1979): Drug levels of other antiepileptic drugs during concomitant treatment with sodium valproate. *Epilepsia*, 20:187.

33. Frigerio, A., and Morselli, P. L. (1975): Carbamazepine: Biotransformation. *Adv. Neurol.*, 11:295–308.

34. Friis, M. L., Christiansen, J., and Hvidberg, E. F. (1978): Brain concentrations of carbamazepine and carbamazepine-10,11-epoxide in epileptic patients. *Eur. J. Clin. Pharmacol.*, 14:47–51.

35. Gerardin, A. P., Abadie, F. V., Campestrini, J. A., and Theobald, W. (1976): Pharmacokinetics of carbamazepine in normal humans after single and repeated oral doses. *J. Pharmacokinet. Biopharm.*, 4:521.

36. Gerardin, A., and Hirtz, J. (1976): The quantitative assay of carbamazepine in biological material and its application to basic pharmacokinetic studies. In: *Epileptic Seizures—Behavior—Pain*, edited by W. Birkmayer, pp. 151–164. Hans Huber, Berne.

37. Gugler, R., and von Unruh, G. E. (1980): Clinical pharmacokinetics of valproic acid. *Clin. Pharmacokinet*, 5:67–83.

38. Hansen, J. M., Siersback-Nielsen, K., and Skovsted, L. (1971): Carbamazepine-induced acceleration of diphenylhydantoin and warfarin metabolism in man. *Clin. Pharmacol. Ther.*, 12:539–543.

39. Hooper, W. D., Sutherland, J. M., Bochner, F., Tyrer, J. H., and Eadie, M. J. (1973): The effect of certain drugs on the plasma protein binding of phenytoin. *Aust. N.Z. J. Med.*, 3:377–381.

40. Hoppener, R. J., Kuyer, A., Meijer, J. W. A., and Hulsman, J. (1980): Correlation between daily

fluctuations of carbamazepine serum levels and intermittent side effects. *Epilepsia,* 21:341–350.

41. Hvidberg, E. F., and Dam, M. (1976): Clinical pharmacokinetics of anticonvulsants. *Clin. Pharmacokinet.,* 1:161–188.

42. Jeavons, P. M., and Clark, J. E. (1974): Sodium valproate in treatment of epilepsy. *Br. Med. J.,* 2:584–586.

43. Johannessen, S. I., Gerna, M., Bakke, J., Strandjord, R. E., and Morselli, P. L. (1976): CSF concentrations and serum protein binding of carbamazepine and carbamazepine-10,11-epoxide in epileptic patients. *Br. J. Clin. Pharmacol.,* 3:575–582.

44. Johannessen, S. E., and Strandjord, R. E. (1973): Concentration of carbamazepine (Tegretol®) in serum and in cerebrospinal fluid in patients with epilepsy. *Epilepsia,* 14:373–379.

45. Johannessen, S. I., and Strandjord, R. E. (1975): The influence of phenobarbitone and phenytoin on carbamazepine serum levels. In: *Clinical Pharmacology of Anti-Epileptic Drugs,* edited by H. Schneider, D. Janz, C. Gardner-Thorpe, H. Meinardi, and A. L. Sherwin, pp. 201–205. Springer-Verlag, Berlin.

46. Kidron, R., Auerbuch, I., Klein, E., and Belmaker, R. H. (1985): Carbamazepine-induced reduction of blood levels of haloperidol in chronic schizophrenia. *Biol. Psychiatry,* 20:219–222.

47. Korczyn, A. D., Ben-Zvi, A., Kaplanski, J., Danon, A., and Berginer, V. (1978): Plasma levels of carbamazepine and metabolites: Effect of enzyme inducers. In: *Advances in Epileptology,* edited by H. Meinardi and A. J. Rowan, pp. 278–279. Swets and Zeitlinger, Amsterdam.

48. Kramer, G., Theisohn, M., von Unruh, G. E., and Eichelbaum, M. (1986): Carbamazepine-danazol interaction: Its mechanism examined by a stable isotope technique. *Ther. Drug. Monit.,* 8:387–392.

49. Lai, A. A., Levy, R. H., and Cutler, R. E. (1978): Time-course of interaction between carbamazepine and clonazepam in normal man. *Clin. Pharmacol. Ther.,* 25:316–323.

50. Lai, A. A., and Levy, R. H. (1979): Pharmacokinetic description of drug interaction by enzyme induction: Carbamazepine-clonazepam in monkeys. *J. Pharm. Sci.,* 68:416–421.

51. Levine, M., Jones, M. W., and Sheppard, I. (1985): Differential effect of cimetidine on serum concentrations of carbamazepine and phenytoin. *Neurology,* 35:562–565.

52. Levy, R. H., Kerr, B., Loiseau, P., Guyot, M., and Wilensky, A. (1986): Inhibition of carbamazepine epoxide elimination by valpromide and valproic acid. *Epilepsia,* 27:592.

53. Levy, R. H., and Lai, A. A. (1980): A pharmacokinetic model for drug interaction by enzyme induction and its application to carbamazepine-clonazepam. In: *Antiepileptic Therapy: Advances in Drug Monitoring,* edited by S. I. Johannessen, P. L. Morselli, C. E. Pippenger, A. Richens, D. Schmidt, and H. Meinardi, pp. 315–323. Raven Press, New York.

54. Levy, R. H., Martinez-Lage, J. M., Tor, J., Blaut,

H., Gonzalez, I., and Bainbridge, B. (1985): Stiripentol level-dose relationship and interaction with carbamazepine in epileptic patients. *Epilepsia,* 26:544–545.

55. Levy, R. H., Morselli, P. L., Bianchetti, G., Guyot, M., Brachet-Liermain, A., and Loiseau, P. (1982): Interaction between valproic acid and carbamazepine in epileptic patients. In: *Metabolism of Antiepileptic Drugs,* edited by R. H. Levy, W. H. Pitlick, M. Eichelbaum, and J. Meijer, pp. 45–51. Raven Press, New York.

56. Levy, R. H., Pitlick, W. H., Troupin, A. S., and Green, J. R. (1976): Pharmacokinetic implications of chronic drug treatment in epilepsy: Carbamazepine. In: *The Effect of Disease States on Drug Pharmacokinetics,* edited by L. Z. Benet, pp. 87–95. APhA/Academy of Pharmaceutical Sciences, Washington.

57. Levy, R. H., Rettenmeier, A. W., Baillie, T. A., Howald, W. N., Wilensky, A. J., Priel, P. N., and Anderson, G. (1987): Formation of hepatotoxic metabolites of valproate in patients on carbamazepine or phenytoin. *Epilepsia,* 28:627.

58. Lindgren, S., Eeg-Olofsson, O., and Backman, E. (1980): The influence of carbamazepine on drug metabolic capacity in children using phenazone as model. In: *Antiepileptic Therapy: Advances in Drug Monitoring,* edited by S. I. Johannessen, P. L. Morselli, C. E. Pippenger, A. Richens, D. Schmidt, and H. Meinardi, pp. 27–36. Raven Press, New York.

59. Lunde, P. K. M., Rane, A., Yaffe, S. J., Lund, L., and Sjoqvist, F. (1970): Plasma protein binding of diphenylhydantoin in man. *Clin. Pharmacol. Ther.,* 11:846–855.

60. MacPhee, G. J., Thompson, G. G., McInnes, G. T., and Brodie, M. J. (1986): Verapamil potentiates carbamazepine neurotoxicity: A clinically important inhibitory interaction. *Lancet,* 1:700–703.

61. Mattson, G. F., Mattson, R. H., and Cramer, J. A. (1980): Valproic acid interaction with carbamazepine. *Ann. Neurol.,* 8:127.

62. Mattson, G. F., Mattson, R. H., and Cramer, J. A. (1982): Interaction between valproic acid and carbamazepine: An *in vitro* study of protein binding. *Therapeutic Drug Monitoring,* 4:181–184.

63. Meijer, J. W. A., Binnie, C. D., Debets, R. M. C., Van Parys, J. A. P., and De Beer-Pawlikowski, N. K. B. (1984): Possible hazard of valpromide-carbamazepine combination in epilepsy. *Lancet,* 1:802.

64. Mesdjian, E., Dravet, C., Cenraud, B., and Roger, J. (1980): Carbamazepine intoxication due to triacetyloleandomycin administration in epileptic patients. *Epilepsia,* 21:489–496.

65. Milhaly, G. W., Vajda, F. J., Miles, J. L., and Louis, W. J. (1979): Single and chronic dose pharmacokinetic studies of sodium valproate in epileptic patients. *Eur. J. Pharmacol.,* 15:23–29.

66. Mitchard, M., Harris, A., and Mullinger, B. M. (1987): Ranitidine drug interaction. A literature review. *Pharmacol. Ther.,* 32:293–325.

67. Moreland, T. A., Chang, S. L., and Levy, R. H. (1982): In: *Metabolism of Antiepileptic Drugs,* ed-

ited by R. H. Levy, W. H. Pitlick, M. Eichelbaum, and J. Meijer, pp. 53–60. Raven Press, New York.

68. Morselli, P. L., Baruzzi, A., Gerna, M., Bossi, L., and Porta, M. (1977): Carbamazepine and carbamazepine-10,11-epoxide concentrations in human brain. *Br. J. Clin. Pharmacol.*, 4:535–540.

69. Morselli, P. L., and Frigerio, A. (1975): Metabolism and pharmacokinetics of carbamazepine. *Drug Metab. Reb.*, 4:97–113.

70. Neuvonen, P. J., Penttila, O., Lehtovaara, R., and Oho, K. (1975): Effect of antiepileptic drugs on the elimination of various tetracycline derivatives. *Eur. J. Clin. Pharmacol.*, 9:147.

71. Pacifici, G. M., Tomson, T., Bertilsson, L., and Rane, A. (1985): Valpromide/carbamazepine and risk of teratogenicity. *Lancet*, 1:387–398.

72. Patel, I. H., and Levy, R. H. (1979): Valproic acid binding to human serum albumin and determination of free fraction in the presence of anticonvulsants and free fatty acids. *Epilepsia*, 20:85–90.

73. Patel, I. H., Levy, R. H., and Trager, W. F. (1978): Pharmacokinetics of carbamazepine-10,11-epoxide before and after autoinduction in rhesus monkeys. *J. Pharmacol. Exp. Ther.*, 206:607–613.

74. Patel, I. H., Wedlund, P., and Levy, R. H. (1981); Induction effect of phenobarbital on the carbamazepine to carbamazepine-10,11-epoxide pathway in rhesus monkeys. *J. Pharmacol. Exp. Ther.*, 217:555–558.

75. Patsalos, P. N., Shorvon, S. D., Elyas, A. A., and Smith, G. (1985): The interaction of denzimol (a new anticonvulsant) with carbamazepine and phenytoin. *J. Neurol. Neurosurg. Psychiat.*, 48:374–377.

76. Penttila, O., Neuvonen, P. J., Aho, K., and Lehtovaara, R. (1974): Interaction between doxycycline and some antiepileptic drugs. *Br. Med. J.*, 2:470–472.

77. Pisani, F., Fazio, A., Oteri, G., et al. (1986): Sodium valproate and valpromide: Differential interactions with carbamazepine in epileptic patients. *Epilepsia*, 27:548–552.

78. Pisani, F., Fazio, A., Oteri, G., Spina, E., Perucca, E., and Bertilsson, L. (1988): Effect of valpromide on the pharmacokinetics of carbamazepine-10,11-epoxide. *Br. J. Clin. Pharmacol. (in press)*.

79. Pitlick, W. H., and Levy, R. H. (1977): Time-dependent kinetics I: Exponential autoinduction of carbamazepine in monkeys. *J. Pharm. Sci.*, 66:647–649.

80. Pitlick, W. H., Levy, R. H., Troupin, A. S., and Green, J. R. (1976): Pharmacokinetic model to describe self-induced decreases in steady-state concentrations of carbamazepine. *J. Pharm. Sci.*, 65:462.

81. Pynnönen, S., Frey, H., and Sillanpää, M. (1980): The autoinduction of carbamazepine during long-

term therapy. *Int. J. Clin. Pharmacol. Ther. Toxicol.*, 18:247.

82. Pynnönen, S., Sillanpää, M., Frey, H., and Iisalo, E. (1977): Carbamazepine and its 10,11-epoxide in children and adults with epilepsy. *Eur. J. Clin. Pharmacol.*, 11:129–133.

83. Rane, A., Hojer, B., and Wilson, J. T. (1976): Kinetics of carbamazepine and 10,11-epoxide metabolite in children. *Clin. Pharmacol. Ther.*, 19:276–283.

84. Rawlins, M. D., Collste, P., Bertilsson, L., and Palmer, L. (1975): Distribution and elimination kinetics of carbamazepine in man. *Eur. J. Clin. Pharmacol.*, 8:91–96.

85. Reunanen, M. I., Luoma, P., Myllyla, V. V., and Hokkanen, E. (1980): Low serum valproic acid concentrations in epileptic patients on combination therapy. *Curr. Ther. Res.*, 28:456–462.

86. Schneider, H. (1975): Carbamazepine: The influence of other antiepileptic drugs on its serum level. In: *Clinical Pharmacology of Anti-Epileptic Drugs*, edited by H. Schneider, D. Janz, C. Gardner-Thorpe, H. Meinardi, and A. L. Sherwin, pp. 189–196. Springer-Verlag, Berlin.

87. Treiman, D. M., and Ben-Menachem, E. (1987): Inhibition of carbamazepine and phenytoin metabolism by nafimidone, a new antiepileptic drug. *Epilepsia*, 28:699–705.

88. Valsalan, V. C., and Cooper, G. L. (1982): Carbamazepine intoxication caused by interaction with isoniazid. *British Medical Journal*, 285:261–262.

89. Warren, J. W., Benmaman, J. D., Wannamaker, B. B., and Levy, R. H. (1980): Kinetics of carbamazepine-ethosuximide interaction. *Clin. Pharmacol. Ther.*, 28:646–651.

90. Webster, L. K., Mihaly, G. W., Jones, D. B., Smallwood, R. A., Phillips, J. A., Vajda, F. J. (1984): Effect of cimetidine and ranitidine on carbamazepine and sodium valproate pharmacokinetics. *Eur. J. Clin. Pharmacol.*, 27:341–343.

91. Westenberg, H. G. M., van der Kleijn, E., Oei, T. T., and de Zeeuw, R. A. (1978): Kinetics of carbamazepine and carbamazepine-epoxide, determined by use of plasma and saliva. *Clin. Pharmacol. Ther.*, 23:320–328.

92. Wilder, B. J., Willmore, I. J., Bruni, J., and Villareal, H. J. (1978): Valproic acid: Interaction with other anticonvulsant drugs. *Neurology (Minneap.)*, 28:892–896.

93. Wong, J. Y. Y., Ludden, T. M., and Bell, R. D. (1983): Effect of erythromycin on carbamazepine kinetics. *Clin. Pharmacol. Ther.*, 33:460–466.

94. Zielinski, J. J., Haidukewych, D., and Leheta, B. J. (1985): Carbamazepine-phenytoin interaction: Elevation of plasma phenytoin concentrations due to carbamazepine comedication. *Therapeutic Drug Monitoring*, 7:51–53.

Antiepileptic Drugs, Third Edition, edited by
R. Levy, R. Mattson, B. Meldrum,
J. K. Penry, and F. E. Dreifuss.
Raven Press, Ltd., New York © 1989.

37

Carbamazepine

Clinical Use

Pierre Loiseau and Berrard Duche

The efficacy of carbamazepine (CBZ) in patients with epilepsy was first demonstrated in Europe in the early 1960s (10,11,65,78,92). The possibility of serious adverse reactions (hematopoietic disturbances) delayed its use in North America (4), but these fears later proved to be exaggerated. The Food and Drug Administration approved CBZ in 1974 as an anticonvulsant for adults, in 1978 for children older than 6 years of age, and in 1987 without age limitation. It is currently approved in the United States for the treatment of complex partial seizures, generalized tonic-clonic seizures, and other minor or partial seizure disorders. Carbamazepine is now considered to be a major anticonvulsant and is increasingly prescribed because it possesses less psychological and behavioral toxicity than either phenytoin or phenobarbital.

EFFICACY

More than 2,700 citations referring to CBZ have appeared in the medical literature (26), and many of these reports have established the effectiveness of CBZ in epilepsy. Their classification is difficult, however, because of their heterogeneity (e.g., open and controlled studies; groups of children, adults, or both; different types of seizures, sometimes difficult to identify; different

trial durations; different daily dosages; CBZ administered as a single drug or in combination; CBZ given alone in some patients and as comedication in others in the same study; CBZ given in polytherapy during the first part of the trial, with tapering off of other drugs in CBZ responders). This heterogeneity of the data also would make meaningless the compilation of these reports into a single table.

Open Studies

Polytherapy

The first open studies of CBZ date back to the late 1950s. Lorgé (65) added CBZ to the therapeutic regimen of 132 adult institutionalized patients with different types of epileptic seizures. The epilepsy of some of these subjects had begun shortly before the trial, but most of them had drug-resistant seizures that had lasted for many years. The follow-up period ranged from 3 months to 3½ years. Twenty-five percent of patients became seizure-free and another 37% had a more than 50% reduction in seizure frequency. The author concluded that CBZ was effective in all seizure types except absence seizures, and was particularly effective in grand mal and psychomotor seizures.

He called attention to its psychotropic effect and its lack of serious side effects.

Pakesch (79) gave CBZ to 61 patients (children and adults) resistant to previous medications, with a follow-up period ranging from 6 months to 2 years. Because of the inclusion of relatively mild epilepsies, more than 52% of patients became seizure-free. Seizure control was achieved in 64% of patients with infrequent seizures, but in only 42% of patients with more frequent attacks. Another 30% of the subjects were improved.

Bonduelle et al. (10) reviewed the effect of CBZ in an add-on open study with a follow-up of 5 months to 3½ years. Twenty-six of the 100 patients were children. Phenobarbital (PB) was maintained, but phenytoin (PHT) and primidone (PRM) were stopped. Twenty-six patients became seizure-free and 43 others had a more than 50% reduction in seizure frequency. The efficacy of CBZ in absence seizures was considered inconstant.

Sigwald et al. (110) published the conclusion of a French trial of CBZ (160 patients) with similar results. Of patients with so-called temporal lobe seizures, 23% were controlled, 26% were almost controlled, and 24% experienced a more than 50% reduction in seizure frequency. Among patients with grand mal seizures, 23% were controlled, 27% were almost controlled, and 20% had a more than 50% reduction in seizure frequency.

Jongmans (54) added CBZ to the previous regimen of 14 children and 56 adolescents or adults with epilepsy. Among 43 patients with grand mal, 17 (39.6%) were controlled and seven (6.7%) showed a 75% reduction of seizures. Among 24 patients with psychomotor seizures, seven (29%) became seizure-free and three experienced a 75% reduction of seizures.

Arieff and Mier (4) gave CBZ as an additive drug to 26 drug-resistant epileptic patients, aged 13 to 60 years, with seizures of various types for 1 to 40 years. The authors

concluded, ''Ten of the twenty-six patients seemed to improve and had a decrease in seizures. None of these patients had a lengthy remission. . . . Tegretol is a very dangerous drug . . . it certainly should not be used routinely to replace any of the standard drugs now in use.''

Dreyer (28) observed that CBZ had the best effect in grand mal seizures alone or associated with psychomotor seizures. Thirty-three of 120 adult patients were seizure-free over a mean period of 21 months. Ten patients showed an over 75% improvement and 16 an over 50% improvement.

Gamstorp (35) gave CBZ to 58 children, 55 of whom had intractable seizures. Carbamazepine was either added to the drugs given previously or replaced one or two of these drugs. Twenty-two patients became seizure-free and eight were considerably improved. The best results were obtained in children with grand mal, brief focal motor seizures, and psychomotor seizures, alone or accompanied by grand mal. Of the 30 patients who responded well initially, six relapsed in spite of unchanged treatment 4 to 12 months after the start of therapy. In three patients, CBZ seemed to increase the number of seizures and cause a deterioration in behavior. The 24 improved patients remained under observation (36). Of the 19 controlled patients, 13 remained entirely seizure-free, eight for more than 8 years. Of the six patients who relapsed, five had mild and infrequent attacks, and only one had a severe relapse 6 months after the initial response. In 1975, Gamstorp (37) reviewed the records of 43 patients with psychomotor epilepsy who were treated with CBZ at a dose of 20 mg/kg/day. Fourteen became seizure-free and six were considerably improved. Four patients who had not responded to CBZ were controlled or almost controlled when PHT replaced CBZ or was added to the therapy. Conversely, nine children who did not respond to PHT became seizure-free when CBZ replaced PHT or was added to the therapy.

Livingston et al. (63) investigated the anticonvulsive properties of CBZ in 87 drug-resistant patients, 6.5 months to 50 years of age, with daily to weekly seizures of various types. CBZ was progressively added to the existing therapeutic regimen, which was gradually withdrawn in CBZ responders. Eighteen such patients achieved CBZ monotherapy. CBZ efficacy varied depending on the seizure type. Among the 61 patients with psychomotor seizures, 72% benefited from CBZ therapy: 29% were controlled and 43% were improved. Among the 15 patients with generalized tonic-clonic seizures only, two were controlled and four improved. CBZ was ineffective in patients with absence seizures and infantile spasms.

Dalby (19) reported the results of an open trial. Twenty-one patients received CBZ as their first treatment. In 72 uncontrolled patients, CBZ was added to the previous therapy with subsequent withdrawal or reduction of one or more drugs. The duration of epilepsy varied from 1 to 10 years or more. The frequency of psychomotor seizures varied from several daily to a few yearly. Forty-four patients also experienced grand mal attacks with a yearly to weekly frequency. Eighty-three patients had symptomatic epilepsy, 42 with a known cause and 41 with no known cause, and 10 patients had cryptogenic epilepsy. In this very heterogeneous group of patients, CBZ was considered as giving full seizure control in 33% of psychomotor attacks and 43% of grand mal attacks. Partial control was obtained in 27% of psychomotor seizures and in 20% of grand mal seizures. After initial improvement, seizures returned unabated in only eight patients.

Scheffner and Schiefer (101) treated children and adolescents with grand mal or focal epilepsy or both. The follow-up period ranged from 2 to 7 years. In the CBZ-only group, 47 of 48 children became seizure-free, but only 15 of 21 comedicated children were controlled.

Dam et al. (23), adding CBZ to PB and/or PHT in 117 patients, obtained a decrease in seizure frequency in approximately 70% of patients with grand mal seizures, and in 59% with psychomotor seizures.

Parsonage (80) reported the results of a retrospective open study of 100 drug-resistant adults with complex partial seizures in which CBZ was added to or replaced previous medication. Epilepsy duration was over 10 years in 81 patients. Eleven patients were completely controlled, 22 experienced an over 50% reduction of seizure frequency, 20 had a less than 50% reduction, 15 had increased seizure frequency, and 32 were unchanged.

Monaco et al. (74) followed 20 intractable epileptic patients for 12 months after a trial of CBZ. In the 16 patients who completed the trial, the mean number of monthly seizures decreased from 6.6 to 1.2 in one year. The authors insisted on the importance of careful month-by-month monitoring of plasma CBZ levels, with a therapeutic range of 7 to 9 $\mu g/ml$.

Hassan and Parsonage (44) reported their experience with the use of CBZ in severe epilepsy of longstanding. The results were as follows: of 53 patients with simple partial seizures, 11% became seizure-free and 70% showed an over 50% reduction in seizure frequency; of 132 patients with complex partial seizures, 13% were seizure-free and 54% had an over 50% reduction in seizure frequency; of 11 patients with partial secondarily generalized seizures, three were seizure-free and four were improved; of 17 patients with primary generalized epilepsy, 12% were seizure-free and 59% had an over 50% reduction in seizure frequency; of 45 patients with secondary generalized epilepsy, 2% were seizure-free and 44% were improved. CBZ replaced previous treatment in 62 of the 174 improved patients.

Schneider (105) made a retrospective evaluation of CBZ therapy in 70 institutionalized adults with severe epilepsy. CBZ was added to standard anticonvulsants, or replaced them. The mean follow-up period was 6 years. There was complete control in 4% and a more than 50% reduction in seizure frequency in 22% of patients with psychomotor seizures. For grand mal seizures, the results were 6% and 8%, respectively.

A great number of reports established the efficacy of CBZ [for review, see Sillanpää, (111)], but from some of them arose suspicions about the development of tolerance to the drug's efficacy (4,19,35). "It has been said, the ultimate test of the efficacy of an antiepileptic drug is how it works in the long term and under natural conditions" (81).

Parsonage et al. (81) looked into the value of CBZ in long-term therapy with of a retrospective survey of 60 patients with partial epilepsies. Thirty percent of patients with psychomotor seizures achieved complete or almost complete control of their seizures and a further 27% had a 50 to 100% reduction in seizure frequency. Just over 30% of patients having tonic-clonic seizures were controlled or almost completely controlled, whereas a further 15% had a 50 to 100% reduction in seizure frequency. Forty percent of the patients were taking CBZ alone, and 60% were also taking other drugs. Good control of seizures had been maintained in a number of patients for as long as 12 years. The daily dosage ranged from 600 to 2,400 mg (mean, 1,200 mg).

Huf and Schain (49) reported their experience with the use of CBZ over a 5-year period in 61 drug-resistant patients. When necessary, CBZ was increased to a maximum of 35 mg/kg/day. Some subjects continued to receive other anticonvulsants. Thirteen (21%) patients were controlled, and 37 (61%) had at least a 50% reduction in seizures.

Jeavons (50) prescribed CBZ to 157 patients with frequent seizures. Fifty-six percent of them had been previously treated. In 99 patients the previous medication was withdrawn. The percentages of subjects who became seizure-free on CBZ alone are as follows: primary tonic-clonic seizures, 71%; secondary tonic-clonic seizures, 56%; simple partial seizures, 59%; complex partial seizures, 46%.

Monotherapy

CBZ has been prescribed as single-drug treatment in untreated patients or in previously treated patients with chronic epilepsy. Scheffner and Schiefer (101) prescribed CBZ for 48 children. Complete control was achieved in all 24 of the children with grand mal seizures and afebrile seizures, in five with both grand mal and focal seizures, and in 18 of the 19 children with focal seizures.

Lerman and Kivity-Ephraim (59) used CBZ to treat 40 children with benign partial epilepsy of childhood with centrotemporal spikes. In 12 patients, CBZ was the first treatment; the others had been previously treated. The mean period of follow-up was 26 months. Seizures ceased in 38 patients; the other two were noncompliant. Improvement was seen in 13 of the 16 children with behavior problems.

Schain et al. (100) replaced PB, PRM, or mephobarbital with CBZ in 45 children with major motor or psychomotor seizures. Most of these children had been treated for several years. Final evaluation was carried out 4 to 6 months after initiation of CBZ. Twenty children exhibited a significant reduction in seizure frequency.

Callaghan et al. (13) gave CBZ as a single drug to 32 patients with a variety of seizures. It replaced unsuccessful polypharmacy in 19 patients, of whom three became seizure-free and nine experienced a more than 50% reduction in seizure frequency. Among the 13 previously untreated patients, 10 had complete control at follow-up 7 to 32 months later.

Standjord and Johannessen (119) evaluated CBZ monotherapy in 62 outpatients with partial or generalized seizures with a mean follow-up time of 25 months. Complete control was obtained in 20 of the 24 previously untreated patients and in 25 of the 38 patients on other drugs having no satisfactory effect.

Roger et al. (97) prescribed CBZ for 50 patients with complex partial seizures, aged 2 to 71 years. Seventeen patients were previously untreated. The follow-up period ranged from 3 months to 4.5 years (mean, 18 months). Thirty-six patients were controlled, four experienced a more than 50% reduction in seizure frequency, and 18 were CBZ failures.

Klee et al. (13,56) retrospectively reviewed the case histories of 286 outpatients on CBZ monotherapy, either as a first-choice treatment (64%) or because of inadequate previous therapy. The most common types of epilepsy were grand mal (111 patients) and psychomotor seizures (61 patients) or a combination of these seizure types (73 patients). The duration of epilepsy ranged from less than 1 month (6%) or less than 1 year (33%) to more than 5 years (33%). Of the 253 patients who had been treated for more than 3 months, 74% were seizure-free or had experienced a reduction in seizure frequency by at least 75%.

Shorvon et al. (108,109) published the results of prospective trials made by Reynolds' group (93). Forty-six previously untreated outpatients with generalized seizures or partial seizures, or both, were treated initially with PHT or CBZ (mean follow-up, 18 months). Patient characteristics and therapeutic responses were similar in the two trials. Eighty-one percent of patients on CBZ were completely controlled.

Shakir et al. (106) administered to adult outpatients, randomly divided, either sodium valproate (15 patients, 12 of them previously untreated) or CBZ (10 patients, 6 of them previously untreated). The follow-up period ranged from 3 to 20 months. Carbamazepine and valproate were considered equally effective.

Froscher et al. (34) evaluated for 3 years the effectiveness of CBZ monotherapy in 72 patients. CBZ was successful in 62% of patients with various seizure types.

Dulac et al. (29) prescribed CBZ for 68 epileptic children for a mean period of 10 months. In 13 patients, CBZ was the first therapy. The seizures disappeared in 43% and decreased in another 26.5% of the patients. Three patients with idiopathic generalized epilepsy and six patients with symptomatic generalized epilepsy were not improved. Fifty-nine of these patients had partial epilepsy. Of 17 patients with idiopathic partial epilepsies, 11 were controlled, and five had a greater than 75% reduction in seizure frequency. Of 16 patients with symptomatic partial epilepsies without known etiology, eight became seizure-free and four had a greater than 75% reduction in seizure frequency.

Keränen et al. (55), in a prospective open study, replaced polytherapy with CBZ monotherapy in 43 adults with chronic epilepsy of 20 years mean duration. In 33 patients (77%) seizures were controlled and monotherapy was achieved. Ten patients showed an improvement in seizure frequency, but the others were unchanged. Side effects were significantly reduced on monotherapy. In 10 patients (23%), the reduction of polytherapy or maintenance of monotherapy failed because of an exacerbation of seizures.

Schmidt and Richter (102) addressed the question of alternative single-drug therapy for refractory epilepsy. Adults uncontrolled by single-drug therapy with CBZ (10 patients), PHT (40 patients), or PB or PRM (19 patients) received single-drug therapy with another one of these agents. Among 24 patients shifted from PHT to CBZ, three were fully controlled, three had a 75% to 99% improvement, and 18 showed no change or an increase in seizure frequency. Among six patients shifted from CBZ to PHT, one was improved and five unchanged. Among four patients shifted from CBZ to PB, one was controlled, one improved, and two unchanged. It was concluded that in some patients, CBZ works considerably better than PHT and vice-versa.

Controlled Trials

Carbamazepine has been compared with placebo or standard antiepileptic agents. It has been given either alone or as an add-on medication in these studies.

Carbamazepine Versus Placebo

Pryse-Phillips and Jeavons (88), in a double-blind study, compared the effect of CBZ and a placebo added to the unchanged therapeutic regimen in 22 long-stay patients with epilepsy in a psychiatric hospital. The maximum CBZ daily dose was 600 mg, maintained for 8 weeks. Patients had partial or generalized seizures. No significant differences between CBZ and placebo were found. However, seven patients had no seizures during any of the treatments.

Rodin et al. (96) undertook a double-blind trial of CBZ versus placebo in 37 hospitalized adults with intractable psychomotor epilepsy. CBZ or placebo was added for 3-week periods to a base-line therapy of PB and PHT. Secondarily generalized seizures were reduced by 55% and psychomotor seizures by 83% when the patients were on CBZ.

Kutt et al. (58) assessed the efficacy of CBZ versus placebo in 23 difficult-to-control outpatients. Three had grand mal seizures, eight had psychomotor seizures, and 12 had both types of seizures. Their ages ranged from 4 to 49 years and the duration of epilepsy was over 3 years in all. During the 6.5-month study, the patients received active drug and placebo for 3 months each in a double-blind fashion. The pre-existing medication was unchanged. Carbamazepine dosage was increased, according to tolerance, up to 1,200 mg. Complete control was not achieved in any patients, but an up to 50% improvement occurred in 12 patients.

Carbamazepine Versus Phenytoin

In a double-blind study, Rajotte et al. (89) compared CBZ and PHT in institutionalized epileptic patients with behavior disorders. Twenty-four adults received successively, on a random basis, the two drugs (CBZ, 600 mg/day; PHT, 300 mg/day) as sole medication, each for a period of 6 months. There was no significant difference in the effectiveness of the two drugs.

Simonsen et al. (113) undertook a comparative double-blind study of CBZ and PHT in 38 patients (>12 years of age) with psychomotor seizures. Thirty-one had been previously treated. They received CBZ or PHT only, each for 16 weeks. The effect of the two drugs in preventing psychomotor seizures was the same. Some patients, however, responded better either to CBZ or to PHT. Side effects were equally mild and encountered as often with CBZ as PHT, with a trend in favor of CBZ.

Troupin et al. (124) compared CBZ and PHT as single anticonvulsants in 47 adult outpatients with moderately severe seizure disorders. CBZ and PHT were given in two successive 4-month study blocks. This double-blind study confirmed the conclusions of a pilot study (123): CBZ and PHT are about equally effective, but significantly fewer patients have objective side effects while taking CBZ.

Kosteljanetz et al. (57) compared the antiepileptic effects of CBZ and PHT in a double-blind, crossover trial. Nineteen adult patients completed the study. Ten patients had partial epilepsy with focal motor signs, nine of whom had secondarily generalization, four had primary generalized epilepsy, four had undetermined generalized epilepsy, and one had secondarily generalized epilepsy. Two patients suffered epileptic symptoms less than 1 year, while the mean duration for the remainder was 11 years. The patients were randomly allocated to CBZ or PHT. Each treatment period lasted 10 weeks. All medication except PB (nine patients) or PRM (four patients) was discontinued gradually while CBZ or PHT was increased to a dose of approximately 15 mg/kg for CBZ and 6 mg/kg of PHT. The dose was subsequently adjusted on the basis of plasma drug levels. No statistically significant differences were found between CBZ and PHT with regard to seizure control.

Hakkarainen (42) completed a 3-year study of 100 consecutive new cases of epilepsy in adults. During the first year, 50 patients were randomly allocated to CBZ and 50 patients to PHT treatment. After the first year, complete control of seizures was achieved in 26 patients on CBZ and 24 patients on PHT. For nonresponders, the treatment was changed from CBZ to PHT or vice-versa for the second year. Complete control of seizures was achieved in another eight patients on CBZ and in nine on PHT. For the remaining 33 patients who did not respond fully to either drugs, combined CBZ and PHT treatment was used for the third year. Only five of these patients became totally seizure-free.

Ramsay et al. (90) compared CBZ with PHT as initial therapy in a double-blind, two-compartment parallel study. Patients over 17 years of age entered the study after having two or more seizures or one seizure and an electroencephalogram (EEG) with paroxysmal abnormalities. Each patient was followed at least 6 months, and 2 years were required to complete the entire study. Patients were randomly assigned to receive either CBZ plus placebo or PHT plus placebo. Increases in dosage were made until plasma drug concentrations were adequate or seizure control was attained. Twenty-seven patients (31%) had generalized convulsive seizures, 18 (20.7%) had partial seizures secondarily generalized, and 37 (42.5%) had partial seizures only. Seventy patients completed the study. The incidence of major side effects and complete control (85%) were the same in both groups.

Carbamazepine Versus Phenobarbital

Marjerrison et al. (68) evaluated behavioral and anticonvulsant effects of CBZ versus PB in 21 chronically hospitalized adult patients. Anticonvulsant and antipsychotic medications were reduced to half-dosage, with the reduced amount being replaced by a proportionate dosage of double-blind capsules of either CBZ or PB. After 2 months, a crossover was made to the other compound for an additional 4-month period. There was no significant difference in the number of seizures per patient during the final months of each treatment phase. There was some increase in major seizures during the CBZ period, but this was not sustained.

Mitchell and Chavez (73), in a single-blind study, treated 39 children with newly diagnosed partial seizures with either CBZ or PB for 12 months. The seizure frequency ranged from a single event to multiple seizures. If necessary, the dose was gradually increased to the maximum amount tolerated or until the serum drug level was 10 to 12 μg/ml for CBZ and 32 to 40 μg/ml for PB. The children were switched to the second study drug if seizures were not controlled or if systemic adverse reactions occurred. Four children were switched from CBZ to PB (three because of systemic adverse reaction, one because of behavioral changes) and three from PB to CBZ (one because of behavioral changes, two because of poor seizure control). There was a trend toward better seizure control with CBZ, but this was not statistically significant.

Carbamazepine Versus Primidone

Rodin et al. (95) compared in a single-blind study, the effectiveness of CBZ versus PRM when added to a therapeutic dose of PHT. The 55 patients were initially stabilized on therapeutic doses of PHT and one of the test compounds, while all other medications were progressively withdrawn. After 3 months of treatment, their drugs were switched for a second 3-month period. Thirty-one patients had predominantly psychomotor seizures, 26 of whom had also ex-

perienced intermittent major attacks. Fourteen patients were considered to have
idiopathic generalized epilepsy. The results
indicated that the two drugs did not differ
in their effectiveness of seizure control.
Twenty patients had fewer seizures on
PRM, 19 had fewer on CBZ. Three patients
had no seizures on either drug, five were
controlled on PRM but not on CBZ, and the
converse was the case in three others.
There was no indication that either drug was
more or less effective in suppressing secondarily versus primary generalized seizures.

Carbamazepine Versus Clonazepam

Mikkelsen et al. (72) in a double-blind
study randomly allocated to 6-month treatment with CBZ or clonazepam, 36 newly
diagnosed and previously untreated epileptic patients, aged 6 to 72 years. Ten of 19
patients were seizure-free with CBZ and 8
of 17 were seizure-free with clonazepam.

Carbamazepine Versus Phenytoin Versus Phenobarbital

Cereghino et al. (16) evaluated the efficacy and tolerance of CBZ in a prospective
double-blind study of 45 institutionalized,
drug-resistant adults. During each of the
three 21-day treatment periods, one-third of
the patients were assigned to receive PHT
(300 mg per day), PB (300 mg per day), or
CBZ (1,200 mg per day). In this population,
CBZ was equal in efficacy to PB or PHT.

Benassi et al. (6) compared the efficacy
of CBZ, PHT, and PB in a prospective double-blind, crossover study of 18 previously
polymedicated patients with frequent complex partial seizures. CBZ and PB were
more active than PHT, with improvement
in 67%, 61%, and 33% of the patients, respectively. Side effects were less prominent
during CBZ therapy.

Carbamazepine Versus Phenytoin Versus Sodium Valproate

Callaghan et al. (12) compared the efficacy of PHT, CBZ, and valproate (VPA) in
181 new referrals with epilepsy. One of the
three drugs was initially given to all patients
on a randomized basis. If the patient failed
to respond to the first drug or developed
side effects, a second drug was randomly
allocated as single treatment, and, if necessary, a third single drug was prescribed.
The dosage was adjusted on the basis of
plasma drug levels. The patients, aged 5 to
69 years, were investigated for 14 to 24
months. In patients with generalized seizures, CBZ and VPA were equally effective, but PHT was statistically more effective in patients who achieved excellent
seizure control. In partial seizures, differences did not reach significance. Results
were as follows: patients with generalized
seizures became seizure-free in 73% of
cases on PHT, 39% on CBZ, and 59% on
VPA; a greater than 50% improvement was
noted in 8%, 36%, and 19% of cases, respectively; patients with partial seizures became seizure-free in 57% of cases on PHT,
33% on CBZ, and 44% on VPA; and a
greater than 50% improvement was noted
in 19%, 39%, and 33% of cases, respectively. Among 10 VPA- or PHT-resistant
patients, four were controlled on CBZ and
one worsened; among eight CBZ-resistant
patients, one was controlled on VPA and
four were improved on one of the other
drugs.

Carbamazepine Versus Phenytoin Versus Phenobarbital Versus Primidone

Bird et al. (8) performed a controlled,
double-blind trial of CBZ for 18 months in
45 mentally subnormal inpatients suffering
from grand mal epilepsy. They concluded
that CBZ's anticonvulsant action is equivalent to that of PB, PHT, or PRM, given
separately or in combination.

Mattson et al. (69) compared the efficacy and toxicity of CBZ, PB, PHT, and PRM in a double-blind trial involving 10 centers. In that study, 622 adult patients were randomly assigned to treatment with one of these drugs and were followed for 2 years or until the drug failed to control seizures or caused unacceptable side effects. Patients had previously been untreated (58% of them) or undertreated and had simple or complex partial seizures (265 patients) or secondarily generalized tonic-clonic seizures (357 patients) as their predominant seizure type. Overall treatment success was highest with CBZ or PHT, intermediate with PB, and lowest with PRM. Differences in failure rates were mostly explained by the fact that PRM and PB caused more toxic effects. Seizure control was only 39% at 12 months and was similar among the drugs tested. The prognosis for tonic-clonic seizure control was also similar. CBZ provided significantly better control of partial seizures.

PSYCHOTROPIC EFFECTS IN PATIENTS WITH EPILEPSY

Reports on the psychotropic effects of CBZ have been conflicting, both as to their reality and mechanisms when their existence was admitted. The first investigators using CBZ to treat patients with seizure disorders noticed in their patients a frequent and sometimes dramatic improvement of mood and behavior. Lorge (65) reported that the patients' mental status improved markedly in 30% and moderately in 20% of cases. Jongmans (54) had no doubt about CBZ's favorable psychotropic effect. Bonduelle et al. (10) found a psychic improvement in 70% of their patients. A survey of 40 published reports involving about 2,500 patients allowed Dalby (20) to state that a beneficial psychotropic effect was present in 50% of patients.

Some investigators have denied the psychotropic effect of CBZ. Bird et al. (8), on a purely clinical basis, did not find a significant change in the behavior and social attitude of patients on CBZ compared with standard therapy, but the patients were mentally subnormal and institutionalized. Later, in a double-blind study of CBZ versus placebo as add-on therapy, no behavioral effect was demonstrable (96), but the study period lasted only 3 weeks. However, a 6-month study comparing CBZ and placebo as add-on therapy in 23 difficult-to-control outpatients showed no clear-cut psychotropic effect (58). Nonetheless, even if the psychotropic effect of CBZ was based mainly on clinical impressions, it was impossible to ignore the large number of favorable reports (for review, see 111). The question of a psychotropic effect of CBZ treatment was therefore addressed by means of objective neuropsychological testing and/or rating scales.

Rajotte et al. (89) investigated the psychotropic properties of CBZ in a population of 24 institutionalized epileptic patients, aged 14 to 61 years, with behavioral disorders. In a double-blind, crossover study, they received successively either CBZ or PHT as sole medication, each for 6 months. The severity of personality disorders was evaluated by a behavioral scale before each period and then monthly for 6 months. CBZ, in comparison with PHT, significantly reduced the severity of personality disorders in this population.

Marjerisson et al. (68) used the Inpatient Multidimensional Psychiatric Scale and the Psychotropic Reaction Profile in 21 adult inpatients. Psychiatric ratings were considered at the end of the base-line period and of two double-blind periods of 2 months for patients on either CBZ or PB with constant comedication. Psychiatric interview ratings as well as nurses' inventories of ward behavior demonstrated a psychotropic effect of CBZ. During the CBZ medication period, the patients were less impaired in verbal and motor behavior and in the interview situation, and their mood and activity levels improved in the ward setting.

Cereghino et al. (16) evaluated the efficacy and tolerance of CBZ in a prospective double-blind study. A behavioral rating scale was completed by ward attendants at each treatment change in 45 institutionalized patients with a moderately severe degree of mental and physical retardation. Behavior was rated as worse most often with patients receiving PHT. It was least likely with PB. Behavior was more apt to be rated as improved with CBZ.

Rodin et al. (95) conducted a crossover study comparing CBZ and PRM added to a therapeutic dose of PHT during two 3-month periods in 45 adult patients. A repeatable neuropsychological test battery and a variety of personality tests and behavioral rating scales were administered before and after each period in a double-blind fashion. The patients showed more neuropsychological impairment on PRM than on CBZ and, when on PRM, an increase of the psychopathic deviate scale of the Minnesota Multiphasic Personality Inventory (MMPI). Depressive feelings, when present, lessened while under treatment with CBZ. The authors concluded that patients who have a history of emotional and/or intellectual disturbance may profit more from CBZ than PRM.

Dodrill and Troupin (25) administered the MMPI to 40 adults with epilepsy after 4 months of treatment with CBZ or PHT. When on CBZ, patients reported improvement in alertness and mental functioning. This was consistent with fewer errors in mental tasks requiring attention and problem-solving while on CBZ. The majority of the tests failed to identify differences in psychological parameters with CBZ administration. Those that were identified were correlated to signs of emotional difficulties, even if emotional status was very slightly improved.

Because of chronic behavioral difficulties, Schain et al. (100) replaced PB, PRM, or mephobarbital with CBZ in 45 previously treated children exhibiting major motor or psychomotor seizures. A battery of measures believed to reflect attentional and perceptual abilities was administered initially and repeated 4 to 6 months later. Parents and teachers were asked to rate attentiveness and alertness on a six-point scale. Assessment of differences between pretrial and posttrial scores on the Wechsler Intelligence Scale for Children revealed only a slight change in performance. However, substantial improvement occurred in performance of all measures dependent on cognitive styles facilitating problem-solving. Significant differences were also found between pretrial and posttrial ratings of attentiveness. At the conclusion of the study, general alertness and attentiveness were improved in 37 of the 45 children.

Singh et al. (114) assessed changes in behavioral characteristics using psychiatric rating scales in 20 adult inpatients in whom epilepsy was complicated by behavioral disorders. All the patients were taking at least two anticonvulsants, and CBZ replaced one of them. The severity of behavioral disorders was significantly reduced with CBZ.

Thompson and Trimble (120), in a study of the influence of anticonvulsants on cognitive functions, addressed the question of a less detrimental and possibly beneficial effect of CBZ in comparison with other antiepileptic agents. Besides a rating scale of mood, the following tests were used: a memory task for pictures and words, Stroop Color-Word Test, visual scanning, perceptual speed, decision-making, and motor speed. CBZ was prescribed in 15 patients, following the complete (seven patients) or partial (eight patients) withdrawal of other drugs. They were tested on three occasions, at 3-month intervals. With CBZ, a marked improvement in mental functioning in all aspects of assessed cognitive processes was found. All the changes occurred 3 months after the initiation of the drug changes with no further improvement at month six. Decreased ratings of anxiety and increased ratings of activity were also noted.

Andrewes et al. (3) compared three groups of new referrals with epilepsy: 21 on PHT, 21 on CBZ, and 21 untreated, matched for age, IQ, seizure type, and epilepsy duration. Tasks were short-term memory scanning (digit span), word-list learning, memory for prose, decision-making, tracking task, and mood adjective check list. Patients receiving PHT performed consistently less well than untreated patients or those receiving CBZ for each of the memory tasks. No significant differences were found among the groups for the decision-making task or the tracking task, although on the latter, the CBZ group performed consistently better than did the PHT group. Plasma drug levels of CBZ were negatively correlated with the measures of anxiety, depression, and fatigue.

Mitchell and Chavez (73) compared the cognitive and behavioral effects of CBZ and PB in 39 preschool and school-aged children with newly diagnosed partial onset seizures. Cognitive tests were administered by a psychologist not knowing the child's drug treatment, within 1 week of enrollment and repeated 6 and 12 months later. A behavioral questionnaire was also completed by the patient. The studies found no difference between CBZ and PB in terms of behavioral or cognitive effects. There was little change in behavior at any of the follow-up evaluations for either group, even if several individuals showed moderate to marked changes, either on CBZ or on PB. Trimble (122) questioned the adequacy of the tasks employed.

Holcombe et al. (47) performed a multicenter trial designed to evaluate the safety and efficacy of CBZ and PHT. Patients were newly diagnosed epileptic children. General developmental status, fine motor control, temperament (Carey questionnaires), memory, and attention were measured both before and after 6 months of monotherapy. Development quotient, motor control, and memory did not differ from one drug to the other. Overall attention span and difficulties in temperament were improved in patients receiving CBZ.

Smith et al. (115) presented the neuropsychological part of the multicenter Veterans Administration cooperative study of anticonvulsant drug treatment (69). A behavioral toxicity battery (the Lafayette repeatable neuropsychological battery) was performed, whenever possible, before the administration of any antiepileptic drug and at 1, 3, 6, and 12 months after initiation of monotherapy. When the effects of CBZ, PHT, PB, and PRM were compared, few statistically significant differences emerged. However, even though the results on individual subtests were not dramatically revealing, the total battery score showed that CBZ had fewer detrimental behavioral effects than did the other drugs, and this difference was present after up to 12 months of therapy.

A growing body of data thus documents mental improvement of patients treated with CBZ. Various changes have been observed. They may be summarized as (a) an increase in psychic tempo in patients with the so-called epileptic personality [i.e., less slowness, sluggishness, and stickiness; less perseverations and stereotypes; a reduction in apathy and lack of initiative; a quickening of thought and action; an improvement in attention and concentration (20)], and (b) affective changes, with reduction of dysphoric episodes, states of depression and anxiety, irritability, and aggressiveness. Three nonexclusive factors might be responsible for these changes:

1. Substitution of CBZ for sedative drugs. It is now well established that the so-called epileptic personality is a consequence of prolonged therapy with large doses of PB, PRM, and even PHT (120). Patients' greater alertness is obviously related to the alleviation or disappearance of comedication. CBZ is less toxic

than other standard anticonvulsants, with the exception of valproic acid (95,115).

2. A reduction or a control of seizures (16,63). This factor may play a role, but is not indispensable for these psychotropic effects.

3. A direct psychotropic effect of CBZ. Two series of arguments are in favor of its direct action on mood. Many investigators have noticed that patients with a history of emotional or behavioral disturbances were more prone to improve when on CBZ. Gamstorp (35) noted that "CBZ did not seem to cause any change in the behavior of patients who had seemed mentally normal before the trial." Dalby (19) found that the psychotropic effect of CBZ was most pronounced in patients with phasic mental states and especially in patients with phases of depression. On the other hand, direct evidence in support of the psychotropic effects of CBZ derives from its efficacy in patients who have neither seizure disorders nor epileptiform EEG patterns (for review, see 33,43,111). CBZ has a useful effect in the prophylaxis of manic-depressive illness (5) and is reported to compare favorably with lithium (85).

WHEN TO PRESCRIBE CARBAMAZEPINE

Comparative studies have demonstrated that there is little difference in the overall efficacy of the five major antiepileptic drugs, CBZ, PB, PHT, PRM, and valproic acid. Carbamazepine and valproic acid are less toxic, and particularly less neurotoxic, than the three of the other drugs.

CBZ is effective against the entire range of partial seizures (87) (i.e., simple and complex seizures, with or without secondary generalization). In terms of epilepsies and epileptic syndromes, it is a drug of first choice in idiopathic as well as symptomatic localization-related epilepsies.

CBZ efficacy against grand mal seizures is also documented. In terms of epileptic syndromes, it can be prescribed in idiopathic generalized epilepsies with tonic-clonic seizures and in epilepsies without unequivocal generalized or focal seizures.

It is not a drug for absence seizures.

CBZ is widely used, at least in Europe, against minor motor seizures of symptomatic generalized epilepsies. However, there have been some reports of children whose seizures were seemingly made worse by CBZ. Shields and Saslow (107) reported an explosive onset of atonic, absence and/or myoclonic seizures in five children. They previously had had generalized tonic-clonic seizures, which was the only previous seizure type in three of them. Johnsen et al. (53) reported an increase of grand mal seizures or a precipitation of atonic absence and myoclonic seizures in three young patients, aged 4 and 17 years, associated with CBZ administration. In each case, the EEG demonstrated continuous or almost continuous bilateral spike-and-wave discharges. Snead and Hosey (116) had problems with 15 of 122 patients treated with CBZ for mixed seizure disorders. Eleven had an increase of atypical absences (i.e., with atonic components or even atonic seizures) and four had increases of grand mal seizures. They stated that all the patients were thought to have elements of complex partial seizures, which had led to the CBZ prescription. In fact, all the children had shown electrical evidence of generalized symptomatic epilepsy (i.e., generalized discharges of spikes and slow waves, in most cases at 1 to 2 Hz).

HOW TO USE CARBAMAZEPINE

Choice of Dosage

Of course, there is no one dosage of CBZ appropriate for all patients. As with all antiepileptic drugs, the therapeutic response depends upon the epileptic severity and upon the greater or lesser sensitivity of a given patient to the drug. In general, there is little correlation between dosage and therapeutic efficacy (15,16,75,119). Daily doses giving seizure control ranged from 200 to 1,600 mg, commonly 600 to 1,600 mg in adults (80), 8 to 34 mg/kg (100), 3.0 to 15.9 mg/kg (119), 4 to 24 mg/kg (50), or 3.38 to 16.48 mg/kg in children (90). Since children metabolize CBZ faster than adults (77), larger doses can be recommended in children. The mean daily dosage giving seizure control was 11.61 ± 4.1 mg/kg in adults and 16.9 ± 7.6 mg/kg in children (97). The mean effective daily dosage is probably 20 mg/kg in children under 5 years of age and 10 mg/kg in other patients. However, because of the wide range of effective doses, a daily dosage of 5 to 20 mg/kg is commonly used in children as well as adults (37,12). It will be less in previously untreated patients than in previously treated, uncontrolled patients. Eighty-eight percent of newly diagnosed epileptic patients were controlled with a CBZ mean daily dose of 7.5 mg, while chronic epileptic patients were controlled only with a mean CBZ dose of 10.3 mg/kg (119).

There is no difference in absorption and steady-state levels between CBZ tablets and CBZ syrup (77).

Initiation of Therapy

The procedure of rapidly achieving a therapeutic concentration by use of loading doses is not possible with CBZ because of the transient side effects that would occur during initiation of therapy (15). They include nausea, vomiting, drowsiness, blurred or double vision, vertigo, dizziness, and ataxia. These unpleasant side effects were noted by early investigators and are well documented in a controlled study of adults by Cereghino et al. (16), with a dosage regimen of 400 mg on the first day, 800 mg on the second day, and 1,200 mg on the third day. The side effects peaked on the third day. Even if they are mild and transient, they can lead patients to stopping the medication. Therefore, it is recommended to start with an initial dosage of 100 mg daily in adults, and with a lesser dose in children depending on the patient's weight. It is increased to the full therapeutic dosage over a variable period. When the clinical situation allows it, a weekly interval is preferred (87). In case of frequent seizures, the interval should be shorter, for example, every second day, with a slower increase if side effects appear. As both low doses and low plasma concentrations may give complete seizure control in many patients, at least in many with newly diagnosed epilepsy, it is important not to hurry, with an individual adjustment based on clinical grounds. In general, dosage is increased until seizures cease or dose-related side effects occur. One must remember that "a 1,000 mg daily dose of carbamazepine is often not enough for an adult" (86). In case of side effects, the total daily dose is reduced by 100 or 200 mg.

Another important point is that CBZ induces its own metabolism during prolonged administration. This results in a decrease in steady-state concentration and elimination half-life. Its half-life is reduced from 35.6 ± 15.3 hr (31) to 20.9 ± 5.0 hr (32). In another study it was 19.8 hr (61). Using stable isotopes, Bertilsson et al. (7) demonstrated an increased clearance for CBZ from 17 to 32 days after institution of prolonged treatment and with no further change evident over the next 4 months. To maintain the same plasma drug concentration, Ramsay et al. (90) had to progressively increase the CBZ daily dosage by week 2 and continued to week 20. Thus sequential increases in dosage are necessary over the first few weeks of treatment.

Dosage Interval

The number of daily doses of CBZ is conditioned by its rate of absorption and elimination half-life. Interdosage fluctuations in plasma CBZ concentrations with high peak levels are considered to be responsible for intermittent side effects (48,94,121). Furthermore, the amount of the administered dose may play a role in the rate and extent of absorption. Difficult or incomplete dissolution of the compound in the gastrointestinal fluids is probable with high doses, resulting in a delay in peak time as well as an apparent reduced absorption (75). In patients receiving comedication with enzyme inducers, such as PHT, PRM, and PB, the CBZ elimination half-life is much shorter, ranging from 5.6 to 16 hr (mean, 8.2 hr) (32). For these reasons, some epileptologists concluded that CBZ should be administered no fewer than four or five times a day (48). Such frequent dosing would be very uncomfortable for most outpatients and would lead to poor compliance. Even a thrice daily administration, as recommended by Henriksen et al. (46), is probably unnecessary for many patients. Two or three doses give about the same amount of CBZ available in circulation, with a mean fluctuation of 57 ± 20% and 56 ± 29%, respectively (51). Troupin et al. (123) considered a twice daily dosage schedule as effective. However, they mentioned that when high doses of CBZ were given, acute toxicity could be avoided by splitting the dosage into a thrice daily pattern. Gamstorp (37) and Dulac et al. (29) gave the drug twice daily in children. Jeavons (50) gave it twice daily too, with the largest dose at night and shifting to three divided doses in case of side effects. For Porter (87), too, a twice-a-day schedule is reasonable. Ghose et al. (38) observed a profile of 24-hr serum levels within the therapeutic range in patients receiving medication in thrice, twice, and once daily dosage regimens. Higher fluctuations in CBZ concentration occurred during once daily medication, but without side effects. In conclusion, twice daily administration of CBZ is recommended, at least in single-drug treatment and in the absence of clearly peak-related side effects (i.e., transient side effects occurring 2 to 4 hr after drug intake).

Slow-Release CBZ

To minimize plasma drug level fluctuations, a CBZ formulation has been developed which has slow-release, prolonged-absorption characteristics (CBZSR). It gave higher minimum serum levels (C_{min}) and lower maximum serum levels (C_{max}). Mean daily fluctuation was 30 ± 10% with a CBZSR twice daily administration, whereas it was 61 ± 17% with CBZ thrice daily (52). A once daily evening dose of CBZSR was considered to give therapeutically efficient 24-hr levels, with a plateau-like profile during the night and morning, ranging between 6 and 12 hours, without any striking peak level (117,118). Twenty outpatients poorly controlled by previous therapy with CBZ alone or in combination with PB or PHT received CBZSR in a 12-week open trial [two 4-week periods on CBZ or CBZSR, respectively, with the same schedule and the same daily dose, and 4 weeks on CBZSR twice daily (40)]. The change did not modify the efficacy profile of the drug, and intermittent unwanted effects disappeared in 10 of the 20 patients treated with CBZSR. CBZ C_{min} were almost identical during the three periods. During periods two and three, a trend toward a decrease in C_{max} and AUC values was noted while the fluctuations of CBZ levels were significantly lower. In a multicenter, double-blind, crossover trial of CBZ versus CBZSR in 30 patients, fluctuations of CBZ and CBZ epoxide levels at steady state were significantly lower for CBZSR leading to a significant decrease in intermittent side effects. These preliminary results advocate the use of CBZSR twice daily (14).

Surveillance

The surveillance of a patient with epilepsy taking CBZ must be dual, evaluating its efficacy and its possible toxicity.

Efficacy

Three reasons may explain persisting seizures: poor compliance, an inadequate dosing regimen, and a truly CBZ-resistant epilepsy. Plasma-level determinations allow easy detection of poorly compliant patients. Because of a poor correlation between dosage and efficacy, it is recommended that CBZ dosage be adjusted by plasma-level monitoring. It was assumed that the serum CBZ level was positively correlated with the degree of seizure control (103). Optimum seizure control was reported to occur with plasma CBZ concentration in the range of 4 to 12 μg/ml (58), 6 to 10 μg/ml (113), 7 to 9 μg/ml (74), 8 to 12 μg/ml (124) or 5 to 12 μg/ml (44). Other authorities stated that such a wide range of serum levels was associated with seizure control, and that it was not possible to define a therapeutic range for CBZ (13,119). These apparent discrepancies are not peculiar to CBZ. The activity of a drug depends not only on the agent itself but also on the severity of the epilepsy. When large groups of patients are considered, it is not uncommon to find that uncontrolled patients have higher plasma CBZ levels than controlled patients. For example, Roger et al. (97) observed mean daily doses of 11.61 ± 4.1 mg/kg in controlled adults and 17.2 ± 1.5 mg/kg in refractory adults, and mean daily doses of 16.9 ± 7.6 mg/kg in controlled children and 30.73 ± 14.2 mg/kg in CBZ-resistant children.

Plasma CBZ levels are subject to great fluctuations during the day. Plasma-level monitoring necessitates the measurement of trough level, sampling being done in the morning before the morning dose of CBZ to allow comparison from day to day and week to week.

The relationship between CBZ concentration and therapeutic effect may be complicated by drug interactions and the formation of CBZ epoxide. Comedication usually decreases CBZ levels (17,18,104). It has been suggested that the measurement of both CBZ and CBZ epoxide in plasma would be more useful in the clinical management of patients than the measurement of the parent drug alone (30). Another factor that may complicate the interpretation of plasma CBZ concentration is the variability of protein binding of CBZ and its metabolite. Measurement of CBZ epoxide in the saliva might provide a reliable estimate of the pharmacologically active free concentration of these compounds in plasma (67). It could be more reliable than measurement of total CBZ concentrations as a clinical guide, especially in children (1).

During past years, attention has been repeatedly called to the statistical value and not the individual value of the established therapeutic range (or useful levels). Plasma-level monitoring is a useful tool for the clinician, but has no definitive value. "It is said that the optimum level for any patient is an individual matter which is not necessarily encompassed by any so-called therapeutic range" (94). In uncontrolled patients, it is necessary to push the drug to the maximum clinically tolerable dose, irrespective of its plasma level.

Patients remaining uncontrolled at the maximum tolerable dose of CBZ should be switched to another anticonvulsant such as PHT. Troupin et al. (123) addressed the question of this change. They demonstrated that whereas crossover from PHT to CBZ exposed a patient to a minimum risk of seizure increase because of PHT's much longer half-life, crossover from CBZ to PHT must be done carefully. If CBZ is abruptly withdrawn, its plasma level declines more rapidly than the increase to an effective level of PHT. A loading dose of PHT might avoid a seizure increase. After failure of both PHT and CBZ monotherapy, PHT and CBZ (86) or VPA and CBZ (50) can be used together. Phenytoin is recommended as an additional drug in partial seizures and VPA in generalized seizures. Withdrawal of CBZ, for failure as well as for success, should always be progressive to prevent withdrawal seizures.

Toxicity

Carbamazepine toxicity is discussed fully in Chapter 39. In patient management, the skin, the central nervous system, and the blood must be checked for evidence of toxicity.

Rashes occur in about 5% of patients (28,50,56,82). They appear in most cases 8 to 12 days after initiation of therapy. They are usually transient, but can preclude a Stevens-Johnson syndrome. Our personal policy is to stop the therapy.

In children, CBZ is known to have adverse behavioral effects (irritability, agitation, insomnia, aggressiveness, hyperactivity, emotional lability). They are infrequent [seven among 200 patients (112)] and readily reversible. The decision to stop or maintain treatment must be made case by case. At all ages, neurotoxic symptoms (blurred vision, fatigue, drowsiness, dizziness), often associated with gastrointestinal symptoms, may be observed. It is important to determine if they are peak dependent or dose dependent. When they are peak dependent, they occur 2 to 4 hr after drug intake and disappear some hours later. Subdividing the daily dosage is sufficient. When they are dose dependent, they persist all day and the daily dosage must be decreased. A wide range of serum CBZ levels was associated with these side effects (13). In a study by Froscher et al. (34), patients with clinical symptoms showed higher CBZ levels than symptom-free patients although the difference was not significant, and higher CBZ epoxide levels with the difference being almost significant. However, concentrations greater than 12 μg/ml have generally been associated with toxic signs (58,103) and checking plasma CBZ level is interesting.

Because of very rare aplastic anemias and rather common benign leukopenias,

hematologic monitoring has been recommended. It is no longer requested by many European neurologists (56). Porter (86) suggests checking the white-blood-cell count weekly for 1 month and biweekly for 6 additional weeks after initiation of therapy.

Other Factors

Recurrence of seizures after their initial control on CBZ may be due to compliance problems but also to the autoinduction of the drug after some weeks. A slight dosage increase may be sufficient to achieve prolonged seizure control.

In children, the levels were in the same range as in adults on corresponding doses when CBZ was used as single-drug therapy, and no correlation between level and dose was found in children on a combined-drug regimen (91). However, CBZ elimination is influenced by age. The younger the patient, the higher the CBZ clearance rate, hence the higher the dosage required. This statement is mainly true for infants (76). Children may need a relatively larger daily dosage than adults. During pregnancy and the postpartum period, the mean intrinsic clearance of CBZ does not change appreciably (128). Breastfeeding is not usually contraindicated (127).

Clinically, CBZ metabolism induction by other drugs is less important than inhibition of its metabolism. The patient may develop rapidly, in a few days, toxic symptoms and signs. Children most often, but also adults, receiving CBZ and macrolide antibiotic therapy—mainly troleandomycin (27,71), erythromycin (39,45,64) and to a lesser extent josamycin (126)—exhibit ataxia, lethargy, and vomiting after 3 to 5 days of coadministration. Prolonged administration of isoniazid (9,125), propoxyphene (22,24) and the antidepressant agent viloxazine (83) induce a marked increase in CBZ concentration with possible symptoms of CBZ intoxication. The interaction of CBZ and cimetidine is more complex: a transient increase in plasma CBZ levels accompanied by side effects is seen after 2 days of cimetidine treatment, but CBZ returns to the precimetidine level by the seventh day of administration (21). Patients should be advised of the possibility of transient side effects for the first 3 to 5 days after starting cimetidine therapy. However, it is preferable to prescribe ranitidine, which shows no such interaction.

Carbamazepine and VPA are frequently used in combination with beneficial results in patients with either temporal lobe epilepsy (41) or a frontal epileptogenic focus. They may have synergistic effects, CBZ acting on the focus and VPA avoiding secondary generalization of seizures. Nevertheless, the combination must be prescribed with caution. By inhibiting epoxide hydrolase, VPA increases CBZ epoxide levels (60,66,84). This may result in side effects. Another inconvenience of an increase in CBZ epoxide is the increase in formation of arene oxides with probable teratogenicity, which means that the combination of CBZ and VPA must be avoided in pregnancy. The combination of CBZ and VPA must be avoided in infants, because CBZ increases the formation of delta-4 VPA, a probably hepatotoxic metabolite (62). With the amide derivate valpromide, the elevation of plasma CBZ epoxide level is much greater than with VPA, leading to clinical toxicity (70,84). The combination of CBZ and valpromide therefore must be avoided.

There may be significant differences in the characteristics between proprietary and generic anticonvulsants, just as there are among generic anticonvulsant drugs. Their therapeutic equivalence is rarely tested. These differences could result in loss of seizure control or development of toxic effects. Sachdeo et al. reported such a loss of control in three (98), then in five (99) patients switched from Tegretol to a generic CBZ product, with subsequent recovery of control upon switching back to Tegretol.

CONCLUSION

Many studies demonstrated CBZ efficacy against idiopathic and symptomatic localization-related epilepsies, undetermined epilepsies, and some forms of idiopathic generalized epilepsies. Its efficacy in symptomatic generalized epilepsy is controversial. It is effective for single-drug therapy as well as in combination with anticonvulsant therapy. However, monotherapy is always preferable. In previously untreated patients, moderate dosage is often sufficient. In seizures that are difficult to control, CBZ has to be pushed to the maximally tolerated dose. Plasma-level monitoring is more useful in polytherapy than in monotherapy. It may be compared to a warning signal, informing the clinician that it approaches possible toxic ranges. Dose choice is determined on a clinical and not on a laboratory basis. CBZ was shown to be as effective as other antiepileptic drugs with fewer long-term side effects than PB, PHT, or PRM. It is a drug of choice because of a direct psychotropic effect or indirect beneficial effects resulting from a lack of neurotoxicity. Idiosyncratic reactions are no more frequent than those of other anticonvulsants.

REFERENCES

1. Agbato, O. A., Elyas, A. S., Patsalos, P. N., Brett, E. M., and Lascelles, P. T. (1986): Total and free serum concentrations of carbamazepine and carbamazepine-10,11-epoxide in children with epilepsy. *Arch. Neurol.*, 43:1111–1116.
2. Andersen, E. B., Philbert, A., and Gordon Klee, J. (1983): Carbamazepine monotherapy in epileptic out-patients. *Acta Neurol. Scand.*, Suppl. 94:29–34.
3. Andrewes, D. G., Bullen, J. G., Tomlinson, L., Elwes, R. D. C., and Reynolds, E. H. (1986): A comparative study of the cognitive effects of phenytoin and carbamazepine in new referrals with epilepsy. *Epilepsia*, 22:128–134.
4. Arieff, A. J., and Mier, M. (1966): Anticonvulsant and psychotic action of Tegretol: A preliminary report. *Neurology (Minneap)*, 16:107–110.
5. Ballanger, J. C., and Post, R. M. (1980): Carba-

mazepine in manic-depressive illness: A new treatment. *Am. J. Psychiat.*, 137:782–790.

6. Benassi, E., Loeb, C., Desio, G., and Tanganelli, P. (1980): Carbamazepine, diphenylhydantoin, phenobarbital: A prospective trial in 18 temporal lobe epileptics. In: *Antiepileptic Therapy: Advances in Drug Monitoring*, edited by S. I. Johannessen, P. L. Morselli, C. E. Pippenger, A. Richens, D. Schmidt, and H. Meinardi, pp. 195–202. Raven Press, New York.

7. Bertilsson, L., Höjer, B., Tybring, G., Osterloh, J., and Rane, A. (1980): Autoinduction of carbamazepine metabolism in children examined by a stable isotope technique. *Clin. Pharmacol. Ter.*, 27:83–88.

8. Bird, C. A. K., Griffen, B. P., Miklazewska, J. M., and Galbraith, A. W. (1966): Tegretol (carbamazepine): A controlled trial of a new anticonvulsant. *Br. J. Psychiat.*, 112:737–742.

9. Block, S. H. C. (1982): Carbamazepine-isoniazid interaction. *Pediatrics*, 69:494–495.

10. Bonduelle, M., Bouygues, P., Sallou, C., and Chemaly, R. (1964): Expérimentation clinique de l'antiépileptique G32.883 (Tegretol): Résultats portant sur 100 cas observés en trois ans. *Rev. Neurol. (Paris)*, 110:209–215.

11. Bonduelle, M., Bouygues, P., Sallou, C., and Chemaly, R. (1962): Bilan de l'expérimentation clinique de l'antiépileptique G32883. In: *3rd Congress of the International Collegium Neuro-psychopharmacologicum*, Munich, Sept. 2–5, 1962.

12. Callaghan, N., Kenny, R. A., O'Neill, B., Crowley, M., and Goggin, T. (19855): A prospective study between carbamazepine, phenytoin and sodium valproate as monotherapy in previously untreated and recently diagnosed patients with epilepsy. *J. Neurol. Neurosurg. Psychiat.*, 48:639–644.

13. Callaghan, N., O'Callaghan, M., Duggan, M., and Feely, M. (1978): Carbamazepine as a single drug in the treatment of epilepsy. A prospective study of serum level and seizure control. *J. Neurol. Neurosurg. Psychiat.*, 41:907–912.

14. Canger, R., Belvedere, D., Cornaggia, C. M., et al. (1987): Studio clinicofarmacocinetica della CBZ convenzionale versus la CBZ a rilascio controllato (CR): trial multicentrico in doppio cieco, cross-over. *Boll. Lega It. Epil.*, 58/59:309–311.

15. Cereghino, J. J. (1975): Serum carbamazepine concentration and clinical control. In: *Advances in Neurology*, Vol. 11, edited by J. K. Penry and D. D. Daly, pp. 309–330. Raven Press, New York.

16. Cereghino, J. J., Brock, J. T., Van Meter, J. C., Penry, J. K., Smith, L. D., and White, B. C. (1974): Carbamazepine for epileptic patients. A controlled prospective evaluation. *Neurology (Minneap)*, 24:401–410.

17. Christiansen, J., and Dam, M. (1973): Influence of phenobarbital and diphenylhdantoin on plasma carbamazepine levels in patients with epilepsy. *Acta Neurol. Scand.*, 49:543–546.

18. Christiansen, J., and Dam, M. (1975): Drug interactions in epileptic patients. In: *Clinical Phar-*

macology of Antiepileptic Drugs, edited by H. Schneider, D. Janz, C. Gardner-Thorpe, H. Meinardi, and A. L. Sherwin, pp. 197–200. Springer-Verlag, Berlin.

19. Dalby, M. A. (1971): Antiepileptic and psychotropic effect of carbamazepine (Tegretol) on psychomotor epilepsy. *Epilepsia* 12:325–334.

20. Dalby, M. A. (1975): Behavioral effects of carbamazepine. In: *Advances in Neurology*, Vol. 11, edited by J. K. Penry and D. D. Dalby, pp. 331–343. Raven Press, New York.

21. Dalton, M. J., Powell, J. R., Messenheimer, Jr. A., and Clark, J. (1986): Cimetidine and carbamazepine: A complex drug interaction. *Epilepsia*, 27:553–558.

22. Dam, M., and Christiansen, J. (1977): Interaction of propoxyfen with carbamazepine. *Lancet*, ii:509.

23. Dam, M., Jensen, A., and Christiansen, J. (1975): Plasma level and effect of carbamazepine in grand mal and psychomotor epilepsy. *Acta Neurol. Scand.*, (suppl) 60:33–38.

24. Dam, M., Kristensen, C. B., Hansen, B. S., and Christiansen, J. (1977): Interaction between carbamazepine and propoxyfene in man. *Acta Neurol. Scand.*, 56:603–607.

25. Dodrill, C. B., and Troupin, A. S. (1977): Psychotropic effects of carbamazepine in epilepsy: A double-blind comparison with phenytoin. *Neurology*, 27:1023–1028.

26. Dodson, W. H., and Trimble, M. R. (1987): Introductory remarks and symposium overview. Carbamazepine's place in antiepileptic therapy. *Epilepsia*, 28 (suppl 3)vii.

27. Dravet, C., Mesdjian, E., Cenraud, B., and Roger, J. (1977): Interaction between carbamazepine and triacetyloleandomycin. *Lancet*, i:810–811.

28. Dreyer, R. (1965). Erfahrungen mit Tegretol. *Nervenarzt*, 36:442–445.

29. Dulac, O., Bouguerra, L., Rey, E., de Lauture, D., and Arthuis, M. (1983): Monothérapie par la carbamazepine dans les épilepsies de l'enfant. *Arch. Fr. Pédiat.*, 40:415–419.

30. Eichelbaum, M., Bertilsson, L., Lund, L., Palmer, L., and Sjoqvist, F. (1976): Plasma levels of carbamazepine and carbamazepine-10,11-epoxide during treatment of epilepsy. *Eur. J. Clin. Pharmacol.*, 9:417–421.

31. Eichelbaum, M., Ekbom, K., Bertilsson, L., Ringberger, V. A., and Rane, A. (1975): Plasma kinetics of carbamazepine and its epoxide metabolite in man after single and multiple doses. *Eur. J. Clin. Pharmacol.*, 8:337–341.

32. Eichelbaum, M., Kothe, K. W., Hoffmann, F., and Von Unruh, G. E. (1979): Kinetics and metabolism of carbamazepine during combined antiepileptic drug therapy. *Clin. Pharmacol. Ther.*, 26:366–371.

33. Evans, R. W., and Gualtieri, C. T. (1985): Carbamazepine: A neuropsychosocial and psychiatric profile. *Clin. Neuropharmacol.*, 8:221–241.

34. Froscher, W., Eichelbaum, M., Hildebrand, G. et al. (1982): Prospective Untersuchungen zur

Epilepsietherapie mit Carbamazepine. *Forstchr. Neurol. Psychiat.,* 50:396–408.

35. Gamstorp, I. (1966): A clinical trial of Tegretol in children with severe epilepsy. *Develop. Med. Child Neurol.,* 8:296–300.

36. Gamstorp, I. (1970): Long-term follow-up of children with severe epilepsy treated with carbamazepine (Tegretol, Geigy). *Acta Paediat. Scand.,* 59, (suppl.) 206:997.

37. Gamstorp, I. (1975): Treatment with carbamazepine: Children. In: *Advances in Neurology,* Vol. 11, edited by J. K. Penry and D. D. Daly, pp. 237–246. Raven Press, New York.

38. Ghose, K., Fry, D. E., and Christfides, J. A. (1983): Effect of dosage frequency of carbamazepine on drug serum levels. *Eur. J. Clin. Pharmacol.,* 24:375–381.

39. Goulden, K. J., Camfield, P., Dooley, J. M., Fraser, A., Meek, D. C., Renton, K. W., and Tibbles, J. A. R. (1986): Severe carbamazepine intoxication after comedication of erythromycin. *J. Pediatrics,* 109:135–138.

40. Guizzaro, A., Tata, M. R., Parisi, A., and Monza, C. G. (1987): Carbamazepine in formulazione a rilascio controllato: Studio clinico e farmacocinetico. *Bull. Lega It. Epil.,* 58/59:313–315.

41. Gupta, A. K., and Jeavons, P. M. (1985): Complex partial seizures: EEG foci and response to carbamazepine and sodium valproate. *J. Neurol. Neurosurg. Psychiat.,* 48:1010–1014.

42. Hakkarainen, H. (1981): Carbamazepine and diphenylhydantoin as monotherapy or in combination in the treatment of adult epilepsy. In: *Epilepsy International Congress* 1981, Abstracts, p. 140. Kyoto, Japan.

43. Hakkarainen, H. (1984): Aspects of carbamazepine treatment. In: *Rational Approaches to Anticonvulsant Drug Therapy,* edited by S. D. Shorvon and G. F. B. Birdwood, pp. 43–52. Hans Huber, Bern.

44. Hassan, R. N., and Parsonage, M. J. (1977): Experience in the long-term use of carbamazepine (Tegretol) in the treatment of epilepsy. In: *Epilepsy: The Eighth International Symposium,* edited by J. K. Penry, pp. 35–44. Raven Press, New York.

45. Hedrick, R., Williams, F., Morin, R., Lamb, W. A., and Cate, I. V. J. C. (1983): Carbamazepine-erythromycin interaction leading to carbamazepine toxicity in four epileptic children. *Ther. Drug Monit.,* 5:405–407.

46. Henriksen, O., Johannessen, S. I., and Munthe-Kaas, A. W. (1983): How to use carbamazepine. In: *Antiepileptic Drug Therapy in Pediatrics,* edited by P. L. Morselli, C. E. Pippenger, and J. K. Penry, pp. 227–243. Raven Press, New York.

47. Holcombe, V., Brandt, J., and Carden, F. (1987): Effects of Tegretol or phenytoin on cognitive function and behavior in epileptic children younger than 6 years. *Neurology,* 37 (suppl. 1):92.

48. Höppener, R. J., Kuyer, A., and Meijer, J. W. A. (1980): Correlations between daily fluctuations of carbamazepine serum levels and intermittent side-effects. *Epilepsia,* 21:341–350.

49. Huf, R., and Schain, R. J. (1980): Long-term experiences with carbamazepine in children with seizures. *J. Pediatr.,* 97:310–312.

50. Jeavons, P. (1983): Monotherapy with sodium valproate and carbamazepine. In: *Research Progress in Epilepsy,* edited by F. Clifford Rose, pp. 406–412. Pitman, Bath.

51. Johannessen, S. I., Barruzzi, A., Gomeni, R., Strandjord, R. E., and Morselli, P. L. (1979): Further observations on carbamazepine and carbamazepine-10,11-epoxide kinetics in epileptic patients. In: *Antiepileptic Drug Monitoring,* edited by C. Gardner-Thorpe, D. Janz, H. Meinardi, and C. E. Pippenger, pp. 110–127. Pitman Press, Avon.

52. Johannessen, S. I., and Henriksen, O. (1987): Comparison of the serum concentration profiles of Tegretol and two new slow-release preparations. In: *Advances in Epileptology,* Vol. 16, edited by P. Wolf, M. Dam, D. Janz, and F. E. Dreifuss, pp. 421–424. Raven Press, New York.

53. Johnsen, S. D., Tarby, T. J., and Sidell, A. D. (1984): Carbamazepine-induced seizures. *Ann. Neurol.,* 16:392–393.

54. Jongmans, J. W. M. (1964): Report on the antiepileptic action of Tegretol. *Epilepsia,* 5:74–82.

55. Keränen, T., Reinikainen, K., and Riekkinen, D. J. (1984): Carbamazepine monotherapy versus polytherapy in chronic epilepsies. *Acta Neurol. Scand.,* 69, suppl. 98:87–88.

56. Klee, J. G., Andersen, E. B., and Philbert, A. (1981): Carbamazepine (Tegretol) monotherapy in epilepsy. A retrospective study in outpatients. In: *Advances in Epileptology,* Vol. 12, edited by M. Dam, and J. K. Penry, pp. 509–514. Raven Press, New York.

57. Kosteljanetz, M., Christiansen, J., Mouritzen Dam, A., Steensgaard Hansen, B., Blatt Lyon, B., Pedersen, M., and Dam, M. (1979): Carbamazepine vs phenytoin. A controlled clinical trial in focal motor and generalized epilepsy. *Arch. Neurol.,* 36:22–24.

58. Kutt, S., Solomon, G., Wasterlain, C., Peterson, H., Louis, S., and Carruthers, R. (1975): Carbamazepine in difficult to control epileptic outpatients. *Acta Neurol. Scand.,* suppl. 60:27–32.

59. Lerman, P., and Kivity-Ephraim, S. (1974): Carbamazepine sole anticonvulsant for focal epilepsy of childhood. *Epilepsia,* 15:229–234.

60. Levy, R. H., Moreland, T. A., Morselli, P. L., Guyot, M., Brachet-Liermain, A., and Loiseau, P. (1984): Carbamazepine/valproic acid interaction in man and in rhesus monkey. *Epilepsia,* 25:338–345.

61. Levy, R. H., Pitlick, W. H., Troupin, A. S., and Green, J. R. (1976): Pharmacokinetic implications of chronic drug treatment in epilepsy: Carbamazepine. In: *The Effects of Disease States on Drug Pharmacokinetics,* edited by L. Z. Benet, pp. 87–95. APLA/Academy of Pharmaceutical Sciences, Washington.

62. Levy, R. H., Rettermeir, A. W., Bailli, T. A.,

Howald, W. N., Wilensky, P. N., and Anderson, G. (1987): Formation of hepatotoxic metabolites of valproate in patients on carbamazepine or phenytoin. *Epilepsia*, 28:627.

63. Livingston, S., Villamater, C., Sakata, Y., and Pauli, L. L. (1967): Use of carbamazepine in epilepsy. *J.A.M.A.*, 200:116–120.

64. Loiseau, P., Guyot, M., Pautrizel, B., Vincon, G., and Albin, H. (1985): Intoxication par la carbamazepine due à l'interaction carbamazepine-erythromycine. *Presse Méd.*, 14:162.

65. Lorge, M. (1963): Klinische Erfahrungen mit einem neuen Antiepilepticum, Tegretol (G 32.883), mit besonderer Wirkung auf die epileptische Wesensveränderung. *Schweiz Med. Wochensch.*, 93:1042–1047.

66. MacKauge, L., Tyrer, J. H., and Eadie, M. J. (1981): Factors influencing simultaneous concentrations of carbamazepine and its epoxide in plasma. *Ther. Drug Monit.*, 3:63–70.

67. MacKichan, J. J., Duffner, P. K., and Cohen, M. E. (1981): Salivary concentrations and plasma protein binding of carbamazepine and carbamazepine-10,11-epoxide in epileptic patients. *Brit. J. Pharmacol.*, 12:31–37.

68. Marjerisson, G., Jedlicki, S. M. Keogh, R. P., Hrychuk, W., and Poulakakis, G. M. (1968). Carbamazepine: Behavioral, anticonvulsant and EEG effects in chronically-hospitalized epileptics. *Dis. Nerv. Syst.*, 29:133–136.

69. Mattson, R. H., Cramer, J. A., Collins, J. F., et al. (1985): Comparison of carbamazepine, phenobarbital, phenytoin, and primidone in partial and secondarily generalized tonic-clonic seizures. *New Engl. J. Med.*, 313:145–151.

70. Meijer, J. W. A., Binnie, C. D., Debets, R. M. C., Van Parys, J. A. P., and De Beer-Pawlikowski, N. K. B. (1984): Possible hazard of valpromide-carbamazepine combination therapy in epilepsy. *Lancet*, i:802.

71. Mesdjian, E., Dravet, C., Cenraud, B., and Roger, J. (1980): Carbamazepine intoxication due to triacetyleandomycin administration in epileptic patients. *Epilepsia*, 21:489–496.

72. Mikkelsen, B., Bergree, P., Joensen, P., Kristensen, O., Kohler, O., and Ohrt Mikkelsen, B. (1981): Clonazepam (Rivotril) and carbamazepine (Tegretol) in psychomotor epilepsy: A randomized multicenter trial. *Epilepsia*, 22:415–420.

73. Mitchell, W. G., and Chavez, J. M. (1987): Carbamazepine versus phenobarbital for partial seizures in children. *Epilepsia*, 28:56–60.

74. Monaco, A., Riccio, A., Benna, P., Covacich, A., Durelli, L., Fantini, M., Furlan, P. M., Gilli, M., Mutani, R., Troni, W., Gerna, M., and Morselli, P. L. (1976): Further observations on carbamazepine plasma levels in epileptic patients. *Neurology*, 26:936–943.

75. Morselli, P. L. (1985): Carbamazepine: Absorption, distribution and excretion. In: *Advances in Neurology*, Vol. 11, edited by J. K. Penry and D. D. Daly, pp. 279–293. Raven Press, New York.

76. Morselli, P. L., and Bossi, L. (1982): Carbamazepine. Absorption, distribution and excretion. In: *Antiepileptic Drugs*, edited by D. M. Woodbury, J. K. Penry, and C. E. Pippenger, pp. 465–482. Raven Press, New York.

77. Morselli, P. L., Monaco, E., Gerna, M., Recchia, M., and Riccio, A. (1975): Bioavailability of two carbamazepine preparations during chronic administration to epileptic patients. *Epilepsia*, 16:759–764.

78. Müller, H. A. (1963): Ein neuartiges Antiepilepticum bei chronisch anstaltsbedürftigen Epileptikern. *Nervenarzt*, 34:463–464.

79. Pakesch, E. (1963): Untersuchungen über ein neuartiges Antiepileptikum. *Wien Med. Wschr.*, 113:794–796.

80. Parsonage, M. (1975): Treatment with carbamazepine:Adults. In: *Advances in Neurology*, Vol. 11, edited by J. K. Penry and D. D. Daly, pp. 221–234. Raven Press, New York.

81. Parsonage, M., Yeung, R., and Laljee, H. C. K. (1980): Clinical experience with carbamazepine in the treatment of grand mal epilepsy. In: *Epilepsy Updated: Causes and Treatment*, edited by Preston Robb, pp. 213–228. Year Book Medical Publisher, Chicago.

82. Pellock, J. M., Carzo, C. G., and Garnett, W. R. (1984): Carbamazepine in children: Clinical and laboratory adverse effects. *Ann. Neurol.*, 16:392.

83. Pisani, F., Fazio, A., Oteri, G., Perruca, E., Russo, A., Trio, R., and Pisani, B. (1986a): Carbamazepine-viloxazine interactions in patients with epilepsy. *J. Neurol. Neurosurg. Psychiat.*, 49:1142–1145.

84. Pisani, F., Fazio, A., Oteri, G., Ruello, C., Gitto, C., Russo, F., and Perruca, E. (1986b): Sodium valproate and valpromide: Differential interactions with carbamazepine in epileptic patients. *Epilepsia*, 27:548–552.

85. Placidi, G. F., Lenzi, A., Lazzerini, F., et al. (1986): The comparative efficacy and safety of carbamazepine versus lithium: A randomized, double-blind 3-year trial in 83 patients. *J. Clin. Psychiatr.*, 47:490–494.

86. Porter, R. J. (1984): Therapy: Partial seizures. In: *Epilepsy: 100 Elementary Principles*, pp. 75–85. W.B. Saunders Co., London.

87. Porter, R. J. (1987): How to initiate and maintain carbamazepine therapy in children and adults. *Epilepsia*, 28 (suppl 3):S59–S63.

88. Pryse-Phillips, W. E. M., and Jeavons, P. M. (1970): Effect of carbamazepine (Tegretol) on the electroencephalograph and ward behavior of patients with chronic epilepsy. *Epilepsia*, 1:263–279.

89. Rajotte, P., Jilek, W., Jilek, L., Perales, A., Giard, N., Bordelan, J. M., and Tetreault, L. (1967): Propriétés antiépileptiques et psychotropes de la carbamazepine (Tegretol). *Union Med. Canada*, 96:1200–1206.

90. Ramsay, R. E., Wilder, B. J., Berger, J. R., and Bruni, J. (1983): A double-blind study comparing carbamazepine with phenytoin as initial seizure therapy in adults. *Neurology*, 33:904–910.

91. Rane, A., Hojer, B., and Wilson, J. T. (1970): Kinetics of carbamazepine and its 10,11-epoxide

metabolite in children. *Clin. Pharmacol. Therap.*, 19:276–283.

92. Rett, A. (1962). Zur Beurteilung der Wirkung von Anticonvulsive im Kindesalter—ein klinisches und entwicklungsphysiologisches Problem. *Neue Öst Z Kinderheilk,* 7:178–191.

93. Reynolds, E. H., and Shorvon, S. D. (1981): Monotherapy or polytherapy for epilepsy? *Epilepsia,* 22:1–10.

94. Riva, R., Albani, F., Ambrosetto, G., Contin, M., Cortelli, P., Perruca, E., and Baruzzi, A. (1984): Diurnal fluctuations in free and total steady-state plasma levels of carbamazepine and correlation with intermittent side-effects. *Epilepsia,* 25:476–481.

95. Rodin, E. A., Rim, C. S., Kitano, H., Lewis, R., and Rennick, P. M. (1976): A comparison of the effectiveness of primidone versus carbamazepine in epileptic out-patients. *J. Nerv. Ment. Dis.,* 163:41–46.

96. Rodin, E. A., Rim, C. S., Rennick, P. M. (1974): Effect of carbamazepine on patients with psychomotor epilepsy: Results of a double-blind study. *Epilepsia,* 15:547–561.

97. Roger, J., Dravet, C., Blanc-Bacci, M. J., and Mesdjian, E. (1980): Monothérapie par la carbamazepine dans les épilepsies partielles avec crises à séméiologie complexe. *Boll. Lega It. Epil.,* 29/30:163–166.

98. Sachdeo, R. C., and Belindiuk, G. (1987): Generic versus branded carbamazepine. *Lancet,* i:1432.

99. Sachdeo, R. C., Chokroverty, S., and Belindiuk, G. (1987): Risk of switching from brand name to generic drugs in seizure disorder. *Epilepsia,* 28:581.

100. Schain, R. J., Ward, J. W., and Guthrie, D. (1977): Carbamazepine as anticonvulsant in children. *Neurology (Minneap),* 27:476–480.

101. Scheffner, D., and Schiefer, I. (1972): The treatment of epileptic children with carbamazepine Follow-up studies of clinical course and EEG. *Epilepsia,* 13:819–829.

102. Schmidt, D., and Richter, K. (1986): Alternative single anticonvulsant drug therapy for refractory epilepsy. *Ann. Neurol.,* 19:85–87.

103. Schneider, H. (1975a): Carbamazepine: An attempt to correlate serum levels with anti-epileptic side-effects. In: *Clinical Pharmacology of Antiepileptic Drugs,* edited by H. Schneider, D. Janz, C. Gardner-Thorpe, H. Meinardi, and A. L. Shervin, pp. 151–158. Springer-Verlag, Berlin.

104. Schneider, H. (1975b): Carbamazepine: The influence of other antiepileptic drugs on its serum levels. In: *Clinical Pharmacology of Antiepileptic Drugs,* edited by H. Schneider, D. Janz, C. Gardner-Thorpe, H. Meinardi, and A. L. Shervin, pp. 189–196. Springer-Verlag, Berlin.

105. Schneider, H. (1977): Long-term treatment in severe epilepsy (institutionalized patients): II: Retrospective evaluation of carbamazepine. In: *Epilepsy: The Eighth International Symposium,* edited by J. K. Penry, pp. 57–62. Raven Press, New York.

106. Shakir, R. A. (1980): Sodium valproate, phenytoin and carbamazepine as sole anticonvulsants. In: *The Place of Sodium Valproate in the Treatment of Epilepsy,* R. Soc. Med. International Congress and Symposium Series, pp. 7–16. Academic Press, London.

107. Shields, W. D., and Saslow, E. (1983): Myoclonic atonic and absence seizures following institution of carbamazepine therapy in children. *Neurology (N.Y.),* 33:1487–1489.

108. Shorvon, S. D., Chadwick, D., Galbraith, A. W., and Reynolds, E. H. (1978): One drug for epilepsy. *Brit. Med. J.,* 1:474–476.

109. Shorvon, S. D., Galbraith, A. W., Laundy, M., Vydelingum, L., and Reynolds, E. H. (1980): Monotherapy for epilepsy. In: *Antiepileptic Drugs: Advances in Drug Monitoring,* edited by S. Johannessen et al., pp. 213–220. Raven Press, New York.

110. Sigwald, J., Bonduelle, M., Sallou, C., Raverdy, P. C., Pito, C., and Van Steenbrugghe, A. (1964): Un nouvel antiepileptique, le carbamyldibenzazepine ou 5-carbamoyl-5-H-dibenzo(b,f)azepine (G 32 883). *Presse Med. (Paris),* 72:2323–2324.

111. Sillanpää, M. (1981): Carbamazepine. Pharmacology and clinical uses. *Acta Neurol. Scand.,* Suppl. 88, 64:1–202.

112. Silverstein, F. S., Parrish, M. A., and Johnston, M. V. (1982): Adverse behavioral reactions in children treated with carbamazepine. *J. Pediatr.,* 101:785–787.

113. Simonsen, N., Olsen, I. Z., Kuhl, V., Lund, M., and Wendelboe, J. (1976): A comparative controlled study between carbamazepine and diphenylhydantoin in psychomotor epilepsy. *Epilepsia,* 17:169–176.

114. Singh, A. N., Saxena, B. M., and Germain, M. (1977): Anticonvulsive and psychotic effects of carbamazepine in hospitalized epileptic patients: A long-term study. In: *Epilepsy: The Eighth International Symposium,* edited by J. K. Penry, pp. 47–56. Raven Press, New York.

115. Smith, D. B., Mattson, R. H., Cramer, J. A., Collins, J. F., Novelly, R. A., Craft, B., and the V.A. Epilepsy Cooperative Study Group (1987): Results of a nationwide Veterans Administration cooperative study comparing the efficacy and toxicity of carbamazepine, phenobarbital, phenytoin and primidone. *Epilepsia,* 28 (suppl. 3):550–558.

116. Snead, O. C., and Hosey, L. C. (1985): Exacerbation of seizures in children by carbamazepine. *New Engl. J. Med.,* 313:916–921.

117. Stefan, H., Schäfer, H., Kreiten, K., and Kuhnen, M. (1987): Once daily evening dose of carbamazepine sustained release: Profiles of 24-hour plasma levels. In: *Advances in Epileptology,* Vol. 16, edited by P. Wolf, M. Dam, D. Janz, and F. E. Dreifus, pp. 425–428. Raven Press, New York.

118. Stefan, H., Schafer, H., and Kuhnen, C. (1986): Abendliche Einnalgabe von carbamazepine slow release (CRS). *Nervenanzt,* 57:415–417.

119. Strandjord, R. E., and Johannessen, S. I. (1980):

Single-drug therapy with carbamazepine in patients with epilepsy: Serum levels and clinical effect. *Epilepsia*, 21:655–662.

120. Thompson, P. J., and Trimble, M. R. (1982): Anticonvulsant drugs and cognitive functions. *Epilepsia*, 23:531–544.

121. Tomson, T. (1984): Interdosage fluctuations in plasma carbamazepine concentration determine intermittent side-effects. *Arch Neurol. (Chi.)*, 41:830–833.

122. Trimble, M. R. (1987): Anticonvulsant drugs and cognitive function: A review of the literature. *Epilepsia*, 28 (suppl. 3):S37–S45.

123. Troupin, A. S., Green, J. R., and Levy, R. H. (1974): Carbamazepine as an anticonvulsant: A pilot study. *Neurology*, 24:863–869.

124. Troupin, A. S., Ojeman, L. M., Halpern, L., Dodrill, C., Wilkus, R., Friel, P., and Feigl, P.

(1977): Carbamazepine—A double blind comparison with phenytoin. *Neurology*, 27:511–519.

125. Valsalan, V. C., and Cooper, G. L. (1982): Carbamazepine intoxication caused by interaction with isoniazid. *Brit. Med. J.*, 285:261–262.

126. Vincon, G., Albin, H., Demotes-Mainard, F., Guyot, M., Bistue, C., and Loiseau, P. (1987): Effects of josamycin on carbamazepine kinetics. *Eur. J. Clin. Pharmacol.*, 32:321–323.

127. Yerby, M. S. (1987): Problems and management of the pregnant woman with epilepsy. *Epilepsia*, 28 (suppl. 3):S29–S38.

128. Yerbi, M. S., Friel, P. N., Miller, D. Q. (1987): Carbamazepine protein binding and disposition in pregnancy. In: *Advances in Epileptology*, Vol. 16, edited by P. Wolf, M. Dam, D. Janz, and F. E. Dreifuss, pp. 547–549. Raven Press, New York.

Antiepileptic Drugs, Third Edition, edited by
R. Levy, R. Mattson, B. Meldrum,
J. K. Penry, and F. E. Dreifuss.
Raven Press, Ltd., New York © 1989.

38

Carbamazepine

Toxicity

Lennart Gram and Peder Klosterskov Jensen

Carbamazepine (CBZ) has become one of the major drugs in the treatment of epilepsy. It exhibits excellent antiepileptic properties, and compared with several of the older antiepileptic drugs, toxicity seems to be less pronounced. Despite this, some kind of adverse effect occurs in as many as one-third to one-half of all patients treated with CBZ (102,120). However, side effects appear more frequently when CBZ is used in combination with other drugs. In large groups of patients, only 5% discontinued CBZ treatment because of side effects (102,120).

Currently, there are more than 1,000 reports of the side effects of CBZ. This chapter reviews CBZ-induced toxicity according to the organ systems involved and emphasizes reviews and recent well-documented case reports of the problem.

NEUROLOGICAL ADVERSE EFFECTS

Although adverse reactions involving the nervous system are probably the most common side effects of CBZ therapy, their estimated incidence varies considerably (from 18% to 56%) (66,111). Nausea, headache, dizziness, and diplopia are the most frequent side effects. They are dose-related and reversible (50). Often they appear early in the course of treatment, but tolerance usually develops rapidly, allowing contin-

uation of the drug (16). To minimize the neurological side effects, the dose should be gradually increased over 10 to 14 days (32). Since these side effects are related to peak plasma levels of the drug (50), use of a controlled-release formulation should be considered (62,69). In countries where such a formulation is not available, division of the daily dose into three to six doses may be as effective (35,143).

Carbamazepine is metabolized through oxidation to the active metabolite, carbamazepine-10,11-epoxide (CBZ-epoxide). A connection between side effects and plasma CBZ-epoxide concentration has been indicated in some studies (91,101,118), but not in others (122,137). Neurological side effects are more frequent in patients treated with a combination of CBZ and other antiepileptic drugs than in those receiving only CBZ. It also appears that elderly patients are more sensitive to neurological side effects than the rest of the population (112).

Different types of involuntary movement have been reported in connection with CBZ treatment (14,21,59,144). This symptom is very rare, however, and is often associated with antiepileptic drug polytherapy (21,59) in patients with brain damage or toxic plasma levels of CBZ (14).

Several antiepileptic drugs may cause at least electromyographic signs of peripheral neuropathy (34). Since the interindividual variation in nerve conduction velocities is much greater than the intraindividual variation (54), any comparison should be made within patients. Lüdorf et al. (85) found no relationship between nerve conduction velocities and CBZ after 3 months of treatment.

Exacerbation of seizures by CBZ has been reported in some patients, mostly in connection with acute drug intoxication and plasma CBZ levels greatly exceeding the therapeutic range (70). A few cases of increased seizure frequency have been reported in children with epilepsy, often associated with known brain damage (63,125,130). The seizures, mainly atypical absences and minor motor seizures, worsened a few days after institution of CBZ therapy and subsided upon discontinuation of the treatment.

Electroencephalographic changes observed during treatment with CBZ were recently reviewed by Besser and Krämer (12). They concluded that CBZ causes slowing of the alpha activity and an increase in theta and delta activity, but found no relation between paroxysmal activity and CBZ.

HYPERSENSITIVITY

Skin rash is a common side effect of CBZ, with a reported incidence of 2.2% to 16.8% (18,127). Most of the cutaneous symptoms are mild and transient, even with continuation of the treatment (71,127). A variety of cutaneous manifestations may be seen, of which the maculopapular, morbilliform, and urticarial types are the most common (71). Serious and potentially life-threatening skin reactions (i.e., exfoliative dermatitis, Steven-Johnson syndrome, and Lyell's syndrome) are very rare and account for less than 10% of all skin reactions to CBZ (127).

Systemic lupus erythematosus (SLE) may be induced by CBZ (7,88). According to information from the main manufacturer of carbamazepine (Ciba-Geigy Ltd., Basel), 41 cases of SLE were reported as of April 1987. A definite connection between CBZ and the development of SLE could be established in only one of these cases. In contrast with many other skin reactions, the symptoms of SLE usually appear 6 to 12 months after the initiation of CBZ therapy (7,88). Discontinuation of the drug always leads to gradual improvement and eventual disappearance of the symptoms. A positive antinuclear-factor titer may still be present long after the disappearance of clinical symptoms (7,88).

In addition to the mild hypersensitivity reactions to CBZ, a more extensive reaction, with fever, skin rashes, and lymphadenopathy, may occur (28,52,79,145). Skin rash accompanied by fever, generalized lymphadenopathy, hepatomegaly, splenomegaly, and pulmonary symptoms has been described (79,145). Various other organ systems may be involved, and vasculitis, myocarditis, interstitial pneumonia, and tubulointerstitial nephritis have sometimes been included in these rare hypersensitivity reactions (28,55,139). After discontinuation of CBZ, all the symptoms gradually disappear. Corticosteroids may have a positive influence on the symptoms (126,139). Although the exact etiology of these multiorgan hypersensitivity reactions is unknown, there is some evidence that they may be Type III or Type IV hypersensitivity reactions. It has been suggested that the involvement of the different organs may be the result of a deposition of immune complexes, with CBZ or its metabolites acting as the antigenic stimulus (43,79).

The diagnosis of drug hypersensitivity to CBZ can be established by either *in vivo* reexposure or *in vitro* stimulation tests. These tests should be performed if there is any doubt about the diagnosis, or if treatment with CBZ is of crucial importance to the patient. A more precise estimation of the incidence of the multisystem hypersensitivity syndrome is still not possible. However, it should be stressed that this syndrome is very rare compared with the usual cutaneous reactions to CBZ.

GASTROINTESTINAL AND HEPATIC SIDE EFFECTS

Gastrointestinal adverse effects of CBZ in the form of vomiting, nausea, and diarrhea have been described anecdotally, but not a single report dealing specifically with these aspects has been published. According to Sillanpää (127), gastrointestinal disturbances accounted for 6.5% of the total number of adverse effects reported to the manufacturer of CBZ. A single case in which CBZ was suspected of causing pancreatitis has been reported (131).

The most frequently observed CBZ-induced hepatic abnormality consists of elevation of the liver enzymes, which occurs in 5% to 10% of patients treated with the drug (102). In a recent series comprising more than 200 children, 5.9% of them showed elevated liver enzymes which were, however, not of any clinical significance (102). Enzyme induction is a well-known effect of treatment with CBZ. The clinical consequences of this phenomenon have been reviewed (103). Studies comparing the enzyme-inducing potential of phenobarbital, phenytoin, and CBZ indicate similar enzyme-inducing potential of these drugs, as measured by antipyrine clearance and urinary excretion of D-glucaric acid (105,124).

The association between hepatic disorders and CBZ has been well reviewed (40,57,61). Although there is some disagreement about the incidence of CBZ hepatotoxicity, about 20 cases were reported by 1980s (56). Hepatitis due to CBZ exposure is a hypersensitivity reaction, presumably mediated by immunological mechanisms (40), sometimes affecting various organ systems. Consequently, symptoms occur shortly after exposure to the drug, usually within weeks. Signs of hypersensitivity such as fever, rash, eosinophilia, and development of granulomas in the liver (78,93) are prominent. In some cases, rechallenge to the drug has resulted in immediate recurrence of the symptoms (68,78,109). The mortality rate seems to be about 25% (40,56). Only a few cases of hepatitis have been described in children (31,147). A single report on CBZ-induced acute cholangitis has appeared (75).

HEMATOLOGICAL TOXICITY

In rare cases, CBZ may cause serious hematological toxicity (i.e., aplastic anemia, persistent leukopenia, and thrombocytopenia). Fewer than 30 cases of aplastic anemia have been associated with CBZ monotherapy or polytherapy, but the outcome of this most feared hematological complication of CBZ therapy is often very severe, with a mortality rate of 33% to 50% (44,72,107). A more precise estimation of the risk of developing aplastic anemia during CBZ treatment is difficult, since multiple-drug therapy and other factors are often involved. However, an incidence of 0.5 cases per 100,000 treatment-years has been reported (44). Neither the duration of treatment nor the age of the patient appears to be a major factor in the development of aplastic anemia (44). In addition, two cases of megaloblastic anemia (107) have been reported.

Transient leukopenia occurs in approximately 10% of patients treated with CBZ (38,67,82). This form of leukopenia resolves despite continuation of treatment and is of no clinical relevance. There seems to be no correlation between the dose of CBZ and the leukocyte count. Transient leukopenia is more common in patients with low white blood cell counts before treatment (67). Persistent leukopenia has been reported in up to 8% of patients treated with CBZ (44). Leukopenia associated with agranulocytosis in 16 patients had a fatal outcome in one of them (108). It is uncertain whether this form of leukopenia is dose related. Although isolated thrombocytopenia occurred during treatment with CBZ (5,117), the fall in platelet count was mostly slight and transient despite continuation of the treatment (44,115).

ENDOCRINOLOGICAL ADVERSE EFFECTS

Antidiuretic Hormone and Water Retention

Hyponatremia and water retention are well-known side effects of CBZ. The risk seems to increase with age and with the serum level of the drug (64,73,104). The reported frequency ranges from 6% to 31%. Hyponatremia does not seem to occur in children (46).

The antidiuretic effect of CBZ was first described in 1966, when it was observed that patients with diabetes insipidus improved during treatment with the drug (15). However, the mechanism of action is still a matter of debate. The two possibilities that have been proposed are (a) a hypothalamic effect on the osmoreceptors mediated via secretion of the antidiuretic hormone (ADH), and (b) a direct influence on the renal tubules. Some investigators have observed increased arginine vasopressin levels (a measure of ADH activity) during CBZ treatment (4,129), suggesting a hypothalamic effect, and others have observed decreased levels, speaking in favor of a renal antidiuretic effect (45,135). Further evidence in favor of a renal effect of CBZ stems from the fact that the antidiuretic effect may be reversed by demeclocycline (6,114). This compound is known to antagonize ADH-sensitive receptors in the kidneys. However, apparently in some cases, hyponatremia may be normalized by concomitant treatment with phenytoin (132), which is known to inhibit the ADH release from the posterior pituitary (27).

Clinical complications of the antidiuretic effect of CBZ in the form of increased seizure frequency have not been reported. However, the relation between water balance and epilepsy is well recognized (89): forced water intake has been used as a diagnostic test to provoke seizures (90), and fluid restriction has been used in the successful treatment of seizures (138). Therefore, since several of the symptoms of hyponatremia, namely, dizziness, headache, drowsiness, and nausea may mimic well-known side effects of CBZ, CBZ-induced hyponatremia should be considered when these symptoms are combined with loss of seizure control.

Thyroid Hormones and Adrenal Cortical Function

Although several studies have examined the effect of CBZ on thyroid hormones, only study designs using the patients as their own controls will be considered here. Such investigations have demonstrated that CBZ causes a significant reduction in total and free thyroxine levels, but total and free triiodothyronine concentrations and TSH levels are unaffected (9,80,84,116,136). Presumably this effect of CBZ is caused by the enzyme-inducing potential of the drug, which seems to cause increased peripheral metabolism of the hormones (1). Overt hypothyroidism has been described in two patients, one treated with CBZ monotherapy and one receiving a combination of CBZ and phenytoin (2). Treating thyroxine-substituted hypothyroid children with CBZ requires an increase in the dose of thyroxine to maintain the euthyroid state (23).

Adrenal Cortical Function

Carbamazepine causes an increase in free cortisol levels (83). In spite of this, cushingoid symptoms have not been observed during treatment with the drug.

Sex Hormones

Although the total concentration of testosterone increases, the biologically active free fraction of the hormone decreases during treatment with CBZ (22). It is not clear whether this effect may play a role in impotence among men with epilepsy. Due to the liver enzyme-inducing potential of CBZ, the drug may augment the degradation of estrogen and progesterone (119). Consequently, the effect of oral contraceptives may be impaired (20,60). Breakthrough bleeding (47) and a number of unintended pregnancies have occurred in patients treated with CBZ (119).

Vitamin D

Biochemical changes in the metabolism of vitamin D may be observed during treatment with CBZ (39,100). However, the question of whether overt osteomalacia may develop during treatment with the drug is a matter of debate (53,142). According to Schmidt and Seldon (120), only a single case of osteomalacia, with clear-cut symptoms, has occurred during treatment with CBZ.

CARDIAC TOXICITY

Experimental studies have demonstrated that CBZ prolongs the atrioventicular conduction time and suppresses ventricular ectopic activity in dogs (134). In humans, cardiac side effects seem to be especially likely to develop in older patients, in whom conduction disturbances are most frequent. The most important toxic effect is the development of conduction distrubances, resulting in bradycardia or Stokes-Adams attacks (8,13,17,42,48), which may develop after several years of CBZ therapy. There is some evidence that this kind of toxicity is dose related (26). It is noteworthy that none of the patients who experienced cardiac toxicity had epilepsy as the indication

for treatment with CBZ. Often treatment of trigeminal neuralgia or other types of pain requires a rapid dose increase, or immediate administration of a maintenance dose of CBZ, but in epilepsy a gradual increase in the dosage is usual. It is possible that these different approaches to treatment play a role in the cardiac toxicity of the drug.

Aggravation of sick sinus syndrome (49) and development of congestive heart failure (141) during CBZ treatment have also been reported.

RENAL ADVERSE EFFECTS

Renal side effects of CBZ therapy are relatively rare. Renal failure, oliguria, hematuria, and proteinuria account for approximately 3% of the side effects of CBZ reported to the manufacturer (127). Reported were two cases of acute renal failure due to presumed CBZ-induced acute tubulointerstitial nephritis (52) and a case of membranous glomerulopathy presumably caused by a Type III allergic reaction to CBZ (55).

PSYCHIC EFFECTS

Carbamazepine may cause a variety of psychic disturbances, including asthenia, restlessness, insomnia, agitation, and anxiety (127). In addition, CBZ has been implicated in sporadic cases of psychosis (33,77,92). Development of an acute state of manic exultation during CBZ treatment has also been described (25).

TERATOGENICITY

Several independent studies have shown that the incidence of malformations in children born to women with epilepsy is about two to three times higher than in the normal population (94,123,133). However, any judgment of the influence of antiepileptic drug treatment on these children is difficult, since the epilepsy itself, the seizure type, and the number of seizures during pregnancy may influence the malformation rate (29,30,65). Lindhout et al. (81) reported congenital anomalies in 2% of the infants born to women treated with CBZ monotherapy compared with 14% for phenobarbital and 9% for phenytoin. Bertollini et al. (11) observed a lower rate of malformation during CBZ monotherapy than should be expected in the investigated population. Although major malformations have not been connected with CBZ monotherapy (96), minor anomalies like fingernail and toenail hypoplasia have been reported (98).

MISCELLANEOUS ADVERSE EFFECTS

Several studies indicate that CBZ may influence the heme biosynthesis (95,110), and reports of CBZ-induced attacks of nonhereditary porphyria exist (113,146). Nevertheless, the use of CBZ is advocated in patients with acute intermittent porphyria (74,106).

There have been only three reports of pulmonary complications of CBZ (24,121,127). Apparently, all three patients developed an allergic interstitial pneumonia, and one of them had a positive lymphocyte transformation test for CBZ. Gilhus et al. (37) found no significant differences in concentrations of immunoglobulins or in frequency of respiratory-tract infections between patients receiving CBZ or phenobarbital and control subjects. This finding is contrary to that observed for phenytoin (36).

A reversible retinotoxic effect of CBZ was suspected in two patients (97). Following several years of treatment with the drug, their vision deteriorated from damage to the retinal epithelium. Discontinuation of the drug led to improvement of the visual function and of the morphological changes. A number of tricyclic psychotropic drugs are known to be retinotoxic (97). Consequently,

the chemical structure of CBZ might be responsible for this side effect.

OVERDOSAGE AND TREATMENT

A total of 311 cases of CBZ overdosage, with nine fatalities, have been reported (10,51,58,70). The lethal dose of CBZ in these cases ranged from 4 to 60 g. However, one patient survived the ingestion of 80 g of the drug (99).

The most prevalent symptoms of CBZ overdosage are nystagmus, ophthalmoplegia, cerebellar and extrapyramidal signs, and impairment of consciousness progressing to a comatose state, possibly accompanied by convulsions and respiratory dysfunction. Cardiac symptoms consist of tachycardia, arrhythmia, conduction disturbances, and low blood pressure. Gastrointestinal and anticholinergic symptoms may also supervene. Coma may develop at blood CBZ levels as low as 80 μmol/liter (76,140).

In CBZ intoxication, the concentration of CBZ epoxide may exceed that of the parent compound (41). It has been suggested that the evolution of the intoxication correlates more closely with the course of the epoxide level than with the concentration of CBZ itself, which declines rapidly (86).

Apart from symptomatic treatment, the recommended measures are gastric lavage, which should be undertaken up to 12 hr after ingestion (87), and hemoperfusion, which may accelerate the elimination of carbamazepine (19,99). Forced diuresis, peritoneal dialysis, and hemodialysis are not recommended (58).

CONCLUSION

Although CBZ may cause a multiplicity of side effects, severe adverse reactions are rather infrequent, and in comparison with many other antiepileptic drugs, it is relatively safe. Nevertheless, several avenues have been pursued with the aim of further minimizing the drug's adverse effects. The pharmacokinetics of CBZ imply significant fluctuations in the 24-hr profile of the plasma concentration, and it is well established that the resulting peak concentrations are responsible for intermittent side effects (50,143). Consequently, the development of a slow-release formulation of the drug should result in a reduction in side effects and permit less frequent dosing. Initial comparative studies of conventional CBZ and slow-release formulations show that both of these advantages may be obtained (3,128). An alternative possibility would be to screen chemical analogs of CBZ in the hope of obtaining a compound with similar or better antiepileptic effect than the parent drug combined with a reduction in adverse effects. The development of oxcarbazepine is the result of such an approach (see Chapter 67).

REFERENCES

1. Aanderud, S., Myking, O. L., and Strandjord, R. E. (1981): The influence of carbamazepine on thyroid hormones and thyroxine-binding globulin in hypothyroid patients substituted with thyroxine. *Clin. Endocrinol.*, 15:247–252.
2. Aanderud, S., and Strandjord, R. E. (1980): Hypothyroidism induced by antiepileptic drugs. *Acta Neurol. Scand.*, 61:330–332.
3. Aldenkamp, A. P., Alpherts, W. C. J., Moerland, M. C., Ottevanger, N., and Van Parys, J. A. P. (1987): Controlled-release carbamazepine: Cognitive side effects in patients with epilepsy. *Epilepsia*, 28:507–514.
4. Ashton, M. G., Ball, S. G., Thomas, T. H., and Lee, M. R. (1977): Water intoxication associated with carbamazepine treatment. *Br. Med. J.*, 1:1134–1135.
5. Baciewicz, G., and Yerevanian, B. I. (1984): Thrombocytopenia associated with carbamazepine. Case report and review. *J. Clin. Psychiat.*, 45:315–316.
6. Ballardie, F. W., and Mucklow, J. C. (1984): Partial reversal of carbamazepine-induced water intolerance by demeclocycline. *Br. J. Clin. Pharmacol.*, 17:763–765.
7. Bateman, D. E. (1985): Carbamazepine induced systemic lupus erythematosus: Case report. *Br. Med. J.*, 291:632–633.
8. Beerman, B., Edhag, O., and Vallin, H. (1975): Advanced heart block aggravated by carbamazepine. *Br. Heart J.*, 37:668–671.
9. Bentsen, K. D., Veje, A. G., and Gram, L. (1983): Serum thyroid hormones and blood folic acid during monotherapy with carbamazepine and valproate. *Acta Neurol. Scand.*, 67:235–241.
10. Berry, D. J., Wiseman, H. M., and Volans, G. N. (1983): A survey of non-barbiturate anticonvulsant drug overdosage. *Human Toxicol.*, 2:357–360.
11. Bertollini, R., Källen, B., Mastroiacovo, P., and Robert, E. (1987): Anticonvulsant drugs in monotherapy. Effect on the fetus. *Eur. J. Epidemiol.*, 3:164–171.
12. Besser, R., and Krämer, G. (1987): Carbamazepin und EEG. In: *Carbamazepin in der Neurologie*, edited by G. Krämer, and H. C. Hopf, pp. 142–146. Georg Thieme Verlag, Stuttgart.
13. Boesen, F., Andersen, E. B., Jensen, E. K., and Ladefoged, S. D. (1983): Cardiac conduction disturbances during carbamazepine therapy. *Acta Neurol. Scand.*, 68:49–52.
14. Bradbury, A. J., Bentick, B., and Todd, P. J. (1982): Dystonia associated with carbamazepine toxicity. *Postgrad. Med. J.*, 58:525–526.
15. Braunhofer, J., and Zicha, L. (1966): Does carbamazepine offer new possibilities for the treatment of certain neurologic and endocrine diseases? A clinical, electroencephalographic and thin-layer chromatographic study. *Med. Welt*, 36:1875–1880.
16. Brodie, M. J. (1985): The optimum use of anticonvulsants. *Practitioner*, 229:921–927.
17. Byrne, E., Wong, H., Chombers, D. G., and Rice, J. P. (1979): Carbamazepine therapy complicated by nodal bradycardia and water intoxication. *Aust. N.Z. J. Med.*, 9:295–296.
18. Chadwick, D., Shaw, M. D. M., Foy, P., Rawlins, M. D., and Turnbull, D. M. (1984): Serum anticonvulsant concentrations and the risk of drug induced skin eruptions. *J. Neurol. Neurosurg. Psychiat.*, 47:642–644.
19. Chan, K. M., Aguanno, J. J., Janssen, R., and Dietzler, D. N. (1981): Charcoal hemoperfusion for treatment of carbamazepine poisoning. *Clin. Chem.*, 27:1300–1302.
20. Coulam, C. B., and Annegers, J. F. (1979): Do anticonvulsants reduce the efficacy of oral contraceptives? *Epilepsia*, 20:519–526.
21. Crosley, C. J., and Swender, P. T. (1979): Dystonia associated with carbamazepine administration: Experience in brain-damaged children. *Pediatrics*, 63:612–615.
22. Dana-Haeri, J., Oxley, J., and Richens, A. (1982): Reduction of free testosterone by antiepileptic drugs. *Br. Med. J.*, 284:85–86.
23. DeLuca, F., Arrigo, T., Pandullo, E., Siracusano, M. F., Benvenga, S., and Trimarchi, F. (1986): Changes in thyroid function tests induced by 2-month carbamazepine treatment in L-thyroxine-substituted hypothyroid children. *Europ. J. Pediat.*, 145:77–79.
24. De Swert, L. F., Ceuppens, J. L., Teuwen, D., Wijndaele, L., Casaer, P., and Casteels van

Daele, M. (1984): Acute interstitial pneumonitis and carbamazepine therapy. *Acta Paediatr. Scand.,* 73:285–288.

25. Drake, M. E., and Peruzzi, W. T. (1986): Manic state with carbamazepine therapy of seizures. *J. Nat. Med. Ass.,* 78:1105–1107.

26. Durelli, L., Mutani, R., Sechi, G. P., Monaco, F., Glorioso, N., and Gusmaroli, G. (1985): Cardiac side effects of phenytoin and carbamazepine. A dose-related phenomenon? *Arch. Neurol.,* 42:1067–1068.

27. Fichman, M. P., Kleeman, C. R., and Bethune, J. E. (1970): Inhibition of antidiuretic hormone secretion by diphenylhydantoin. *Arch. Neurol.,* 22:45–53.

28. Florabel, G. M., McAllister, H. A., Wagner, B. M., and Fenoglia, J. J. (1979): Drug related vasculitis. *Human Pathol.,* 10:313–325.

29. Friis, M. L., Broeng-Wieken, B., Sindrup, E. H., Fogh-Andersen, M., and Hauge, M. (1981): Facial clefts among epileptic patients. *Arch. Neurol.,* 38:227–229.

30. Friis, M. L. (1979): Epilepsy among parents of children with facial clefts. *Epilepsia,* 20:66–76.

31. Galeone, D., Lamontanara, G., and Torelli, D. (1985): Acute hepatitis in a patient treated with carbamazepine. *J. Neurol.,* 232:301–303.

32. Gamstorp, I. (1972): Nine years' experience with Tegretol in epileptic children. In: *Tegretol in Epilepsy,* edited by C. A. S. Wink, pp. 6–11. C. Nichols and Co., Manchester.

33. Gehlen, W., Fröscher, E., and Bron, B. (1978): Nebenwirkungen antiepileptischer Medikamente. *Intern. Prax.,* 18:333–339.

34. Geraldini, C., Faedda, M. T., and Sideri, G. (1984): Anticonvulsant therapy and its possible consequence on the peripheral nervous system. A neurographic study. *Epilepsia,* 25:502–505.

35. Ghose, K., Fry, D. E., and Christfides, J. A. (1983): Effects of dosage frequency of carbamazepine on drug serum levels in epileptic patients. *Eur. J. Clin. Pharmacol.,* 24:375–381.

36. Gilhus, N. E., and Aarli, J. (1981): Respiratory disease and nasal immunoglobulin concentrations in phenytoin-treated epileptic patients. *Acta Neurol. Scand.,* 63:34–43.

37. Gilhus, N. E., Strandjord, R. E., and Aarli, J. (1982): Respiratory disease in patients with epilepsy on single-drug therapy with carbamazepine and phenobarbital. *Europ. Neurol.,* 21:284–288.

38. Gilhus, N. E., and Matre, R. (1986): Carbamazepine effects on mononuclear blood cells in epileptic patients. *Acta Neurol. Scand.,* 74:181–185.

39. Gough, H., Goggins, T., Bissessar, A., Baker, M., Crowley, M., and Callaghan N. (1986): A comparative study of the relative influence of different anticonvulsant drug, UV exposure and diet on vitamin D and calcium metabolism in out-patients with epilepsy. *Quart. J. Med.,* 59:569–577.

40. Gram, L., and Bentsen, K. D. (1983): Hepatic toxicity of antiepileptic drugs: A review. *Acta Neurol. Scand.,* 68 (suppl. 97):81–90.

41. Groot, de G., van Heijst, A. N. P., and Maes, R.

A. A. (1984): Charcoal hemoperfusion in the treatment of two cases of acute carbamazepine poisoning. *Clin. Toxicol.,* 22:349–362.

42. Hamilton, D. V. (1978): Carbamazepine and heart block. *Lancet* 1:1365.

43. Harabs, N., and Shalit, M. (1987): Carbamazepine induced vasculitis. (letter) *J. Neurol. Neurosurg. Psychiat.,* 50:1241–1242.

44. Hart, R. G., and Easton, J. D. (1982): Carbamazepine and hematological monitoring. *Ann. Neurol.,* 11:309–312.

45. Heim, M., Conte-Devoix, B., Bonnefoy, M., and Boyard, P. (1979): Measurements of serum 8-arginine vasopressin level by radioimmunoassay in normal subjects during water loading before and during carbamazepine treatment. *Pathol. Biol.,* 27:95–98.

46. Helin, I., Nilsson, K. O., Bjerre, I., and Vegfors, P. (1977): Serum sodium and osmolality during carbamazepine treatment in children. *Br. Med. J.,* 2:558.

47. Hempel, E., and Klinger, W. (1976): Drug stimulated biotransformation of hormonal steroid contraceptives. Clinical implications. *Drugs,* 12:442–448.

48. Herzberg, L. (1978): Carbamazepine and bradycardia. *Lancet* 1:1097–1098.

49. Hewetson, K. A., Ritch, A. E. S., and Watson, R. D. S. (1986): Sick sinus syndrome aggravated by carbamazepine therapy for epilepsy. *Postgrad. Med. J.,* 62:497–498.

50. Höppener, R. J., Kuyer, A., Meijer, J. W. A., and Hulsman, J. (1980): Correlation between daily fluctuations of carbamazepine serum levels and intermittent side effects. *Epilepsia,* 21:341–350.

51. Hofliger, M. (1987): Vergiftungen mit Carbamazepin. *Schweiz Apoth. Ztg.,* 125:288–293.

52. Hogg, R. J., Sawayer, M., Hecox, K., and Eigenbrodt, E. (1981): Carbamazepine-induced acute tubulointerstitial nephritis. *J. Pediat.,* 98:830–831.

53. Hoikka, V., Alhava, E. M., Karjalainin, P., Keränen, T., Sovalainen, K. E., Reikkinen, P., and Korhonen, R. (1984): Carbamazepine and bone mineral metabolism. *Acta Neurol. Scand.,* 69:77–80.

54. Hopf, H. C. (1968): Ueber die Veränderung der Leitfunktion peripherer motorischer Nervenfasern durch Diphenylhydantoin. *Deutsche Zeitsch. Nervenheil.,* 193:41–56.

55. Hordon, L. D., and Turney, J. H. (1987): Membranous glomerulopathy associated with carbamazepine. *Br. Med. J.,* 294:375.

56. Horowitz, S., Patwarden, R., and Marcus E. (1986): Carbamazepine hepatotoxicity. *Epilepsia,* 27:592.

57. Horowitz, S., Patwardhan, R., and Marcus, E. (1988): Hepatoxic reactions associated with carbamazepine therapy. *Epilepsia,* 29:149–154.

58. Hruby, K., Lenz, K., Druml, W., and Kleinberger, G. (1982): Erfahrungen mit akuten Carbamazepin-Vergiftungen. *Nervenarzt,* 53:414–418.

59. Jacome, D. (1979): Carbamazepine induced dystonia. *J.A.M.A.*, 241:2263.

60. Janz, D., and Schmidt, D. (1974): Anti-epileptic drugs and failure of oral contraceptives. *Lancet*, 1:1113.

61. Jeavons, P. M. (1983): Hepatotoxicity of antiepileptic drugs. In: *Chronic Toxicity of Antiepileptic Drugs*, edited by J. Oxley, D. Janz, and H. Meinardi, pp. 1–45. Raven Press, New York.

62. Johannessen, S. I., and Henriken, O. (1985): A comparison of the serum concentration profiles of Tegretol and two new slow-release preparations. *16th Epilepsy International Symposium*, Hamburg.

63. Johnsen, S. D., Tarby, T. J., and Sidell, D. (1984): Carbamazepine-induced seizures (letter). *Ann. Neurol.*, 16:392–393.

64. Kalff, R., Houtkooper, H. A., Meyer, J. W. A., Goedhart, D. M., Augusteijn, R., and Meinardi, H. (1984): Carbamazepine and sodium levels. *Epilepsia*, 25:390–397.

65. Kelly, Th. E., Rein, M., and Edwards, P. (1984): Teratogenicity of anticonvulsant drugs (1984): The Association of Clefting and Epilepsy. *Am. J. Hum. Genet.*, 19:451–458.

66. Killian, J. M., and From, G. H. (1968): Carbamazepine in treatment of neuralgia. Use and side-effects. *Arch. Neurol.*, 19:129–136.

67. Killian, J. M. (1969): Tegretol in trigeminal neuralgia with special references to hematopoietic side effects. *Headache*, 9:58–63.

68. Knudsen, L., and Jensen, K. B. (1979): Medikamentel hepatitis. *Ugeskr. Laeg.*, 141:3160–3163.

69. Krämer, G., Besser, R., Katzmann, K., and Theisohn, M. (1985): Carbamazepine retard in der Epilepsitherapie. Vergleich der Tagesprofile unter konventionellen Carbamazepin und Carbamazepin retard. *Akt. Neurol.*, 12:70–74.

70. Krämer, G. (1987): Carbamazepine-Intoxikationen. In: *Carbamazepin in der Neurologie*, edited by G. Krämer, and H. C. Hopf, pp. 147–153. Georg Thieme Verlag, Stuttgart.

71. Krämer, G., and Bork, K. (1987): Dermatologische Nebenwirkungen von Carbamazepin. In: *Carbamazepin in der Neurologie*, edited by G. Krämer, and H. C. Hopf, pp. 130–141. Georg Thieme Verlag, Stuttgart.

72. Krämer, G. (1987): Carbamazepin—induzierte Veränderungen von Laborparametern und ihre klinische Relevanz. In: *Carbamazepin in der Neurologie*, edited by G. Krämer, and H. C. Hopf, pp. 107–129. Georg Thieme Verlag, Stuttgart.

73. Lahr, M. B. (1985): Hyponatremia during carbamazepine therapy. *Clin. Pharmacol. Ther.*, 37:693–696.

74. Lai, C. W. (1981): Carbamazepine in seizure management in acute intermittent porphyria. *Neurology*, 31:232.

75. Larray, D., Hadengue, A., Pessayre, D., Choudat, L., Degott, C., and Benhamou, J. P. (1984): Carbamazepine-induced cholangitis. *Dig. Dis. Sci.*, 32:554–557.

76. Lehrmann, S. N., and Bauman, M. L. (1984): Carbamazepine overdose. *Am. J. Dis. Child.*, 135:768–769.

77. Leviatov, V. M., Vselowskaja, T. D., Marienko, G. Ph., and Chtchegoleva, A. P. (1976): Psychoses au Tegretol chez des Epileptiques. *Ann. Med. Psychol.*, 1:473.

78. Levy, M., Goodman, M. W., Van Dyne, B., and Summer, H. W. (1981): Granulomatous hepatitis secondary to carbamazepine. *Ann. Intern. Med.*, 95:64–65.

79. Lewis, I. J., and Rosenbloom, L. (1982): Glandular fever-like syndrome, pulmonary eosinophilia and asthma associated with carbamazepine. *Postgrad. Med. J.*, 58:100–101.

80. Liewendahl, K., Majuri, H., and Helenius, T. (1978): Thyroid function tests in patients on long-term treatment with various anticonvulsant drugs. *Clin. Endocrinol.*, 8:185–191.

81. Lindhout, D., Meinardi, H., and Barth, P. G. (1982): Hazards of fetal exposure to drug combinations. In: *Epilepsy, Pregnancy and the Child*, edited by D. Janz, M. Dam, A. Richens, L. Bossi, H. Helge, and D. Schmidt, pp. 275–282. Raven Press, New York.

82. Livingston, S., Pauli, L. L., and German, W. (1974): Carbamazepine in epilepsy. Nine years' follow-up with special reference on unwanted reactions. *Dis. Nerv. Syst.*, 35:103–107.

83. Lühdorf, K. (1983): Endocrine functions and antiepileptic treatment. *Acta Neurol. Scand.*, 67 (suppl. 94):15–19.

84. Lühdorf, K., Christiansen, C., Hansen, J. M., and Lund, M. (1977): The influence of phenytoin and carbamazepine on endocrine function: Preliminary results. In: *The Eighth International Epilepsy Symposium*, edited by J. K. Penry, pp. 209–213. Raven Press, New York.

85. Lühdorf, K., Nielsen, C. J., Oerbaek, K., and Hammerberg, P. E. (1983): Motor and sensory conduction velocities and electromyographic findings in man before and after carbamazepine treatment. *Acta Neurol. Scand.*, 67:103–107.

86. Luke, D. R., Rocci, M. L., Schaible, D. H., and Ferguson, R. K. (1986): Acute hepatotoxicity after excessive high doses of carbamazepine on two occasions. *Pharmacotherapy*, 6:108–111.

87. Mack, R. B. (1985): Carbamazepine poisoning. *N.C. Med. J.*, 46:41–42.

88. McNicholl, B. (1985): Carbamazepine induced systemic lupus erythematosus (letter). *Br. Med. J.*, 291:1126.

89. McQuarrie, I. (1929): Epilepsy in children. The relationship of water balance to occurrence of fits. *Am. J. Dis. Child.*, 38:451–467.

90. McQuarrie, I., and Peeler, D. B. (1931): The effects of sustained pituitary antidiuresis and forced water drinking in epileptic children. *J. Clin. Invest.*, 10:915–940.

91. Meijer, J. W. A., Binnie, C. D., Deletz, R. M. C., van Parys, J. A. P., and De Beer-Pawlikowski, N. K. B. (1984): Possible hazard of valpromide-carbamazepine combination therapy in epilepsy. *Lancet*, 1:802.

92. Meinardi, H., and Stoel, M. K. (1974): Side effects of antiepileptic drugs. In: *Handbook of Clinical Neurology*, edited by P. J. Vinken and G. W. Bruyn, pp. 705–738, North Holland, Amsterdam.

93. Mitchell, M., Bionett, J., Arregui, A., and Maddrey, W. (1980): Granulomatous hepatitis associated with carbamazepine therapy. *Am. J. Med.*, 71:733–735.

94. Monson, R. R., Rosenberg, L., Hartz, St. C., Shapiro, S., Heinonen, O. P., and Slone, D. (1973): Diphenylhydantoin and selected congenital malformations. *New Engl. J. Med.*, 289:1049–1052.

95. Moore, M. R., McGuire, G., Brodie, M. J., Yeung Laiwah, A. C., Goldenberg, A., Meissmer, P. N., and Kehoe, B. (1983): Carbamazepine and haem biosynthesis. *Lancet*, 2:846.

96. Nakane, Y., Okuma, T., Takahashi, R., Sato, Y., Wada, T., Sato, T., Fukushima, Y., Kumashiro, H., Ono, T., Takahashi, T., Aoki, Y., Kazamatsuri, H., Inami, M., Komai, S., Seino, M., Miyakoshi, M., Tanimura, T., Hazama, H., Kawahara, R., Otsuki, S., Hosokawa, K., Inanaga, K., Nakazawa, Y., and Yamamoto, K. (1980): Multiinstitutional study on the teratogenicity and fetal toxicity of antiepileptic drugs: A report of a Collaborative Study Group in Japan. *Epilepsia*, 21:663–680.

97. Nielsen, N. V., and Syvertsen, K. (1986): Possible retinotoxic effect of carbamazepine. *Acta Ophtalmol.*, 64:287–290.

98. Nilsen, M., and Fröscher, W. (1985): Finger and toenail hypoplasia after carbamazepine monotherapy in late pregnancy. *Neuropediatrics*, 16:167–168.

99. Nilson, C., Sterner, G., and Idvall, J. (1984): Charcoal hemoperfusion for treatment of serious carbamazepine poisoning. *Acta Med. Scand.*, 216:137–140.

100. O'Hare, J. A., Duggan, B., O'Driscoll, B., and Callaghan, N. (1980): Biochemical evidence for osteomalacia with carbamazepine therapy. *Acta Neurol. Scand.*, 62:282–286.

101. Patzalos, P. W., Stephenson, T. J., Korshna, S., Elyas, A. A., Lascelles, P. T., and Wiles, C. M. (1985): Side-effects induced by carbamazepine-10,11-epoxide. *Lancet*, 8:496.

102. Pellock, J. M. (1987): Carbamazepine side effects in children and adults. *Epilepsia*, 28 (suppl. 3):S64–S70.

103. Perucca, E. (1978): Clinical consequences of microsomal enzyme-induction by antiepileptic drugs. *Pharm. Ther.*, 2:285–314.

104. Perucca, E., Garratt, A., Hebdige, S., and Richens, A. (1978): Water intoxication in epileptic patients receiving carbamazepine. *J. Neurol. Neurosurg. Psychiatr.*, 41:713–718.

105. Perucca, E., Hedges, A., Makki, K. A., Ruprah, M., Wilson, J. F., and Richens, A. (1984): A comparative study of the relative enzyme inducing properties of anticonvulsant drugs in epileptic patients. *Br. J. Clin. Pharmacol.*, 18:410–414.

106. Peters, H. A., and Bonkowsky, H. L. (1981): Carbamazepine in seizure management in acute intermittent porphyria. *Neurology*, 31:1579–1580.

107. Pisciotta, A. V. (1975): Hematological toxicity of carbamazepine. *Adv. Neurol.*, 11:355–368.

108. Pisciotta, A. V. (1982): Carbamazepine, hematological toxicity. In: *Antiepileptic Drugs*, 2nd edition, edited by D. M. Woodbury, J. K. Penry, C. E. Pippenger, pp. 538–542. Raven Press, New York.

109. Ramsay, I. D. (1967): Carbamazepine-induced jaundice. *Br. Med. J.*, 4:155.

110. Rapeport, W. G., Thomson, G. G., McInnes, G. T., Moore, M. R., Brodie, M. J., and Goldberg, A. (1982): Carbamazepine and haem biosynthesis in man. *Clin. Sci.*, 63:22P–23P.

111. Redpath, T. H., and Gayford, T. J. (1968): The side effects of carbamazepine therapy. *Oral Surg.*, 26:299–303.

112. Reynolds, E. H. (1975): Neurotoxicity of carbamazepine. *Adv. Neurol.*, 11:345–353.

113. Rideout, J. M., Wright, D. J., Lim, C. K., Rinsler, M. G., and Peters, R. J. (1983): Carbamazepine induced non-hereditary porphyria. *Lancet*, 2:464.

114. Ringel, R. A., and Brick, J. F. (1986): Perspective on carbamazepine-induced water intoxication: Reversal by demeclocycline. *Neurology*, 36:1506–1507.

115. Rodin, E. A., Rim, C. S., and Rennik, P. M. (1974): The effects of carbamazepine on patients with psychomotor epilepsy: Results of a double-blind study. *Epilepsia*, 15:547–561.

116. Rootwelt, K., Ganes, T., and Johannessen, S. I. (1978): Effect of carbamazepine, phenytoin and phenobarbitone on serum levels of thyroid hormones and thyrotropin in humans. *Scand. J. Clin. Lab. Invest.*, 38:731–736.

117. Rutman, J. Y. (1978): Effect of carbamazepine on blood elements. *Ann. Neurol.*, 3:373.

118. Schoeman, J. F., Elyas, A. A., Brett, E. M., and Lascelles, P. T. (1984): Correlation between plasma carbamazepine-10,11-epoxide concentration and drug side effects in children with epilepsy. *Develop. Med. Child. Neurol.*, 26:756–764.

119. Schmidt, D. (1981): Effect of antiepileptic drugs on estrogens and progesterone metabolism and oral contraceptives, In: *Advances in Epileptology: XIIth Epilepsy International Symposium*, edited by M. Dam, L. Gram, and J. K. Penry, pp. 423–431. Raven Press, New York.

120. Schmidt, D., and Seldon, L. (1982): *Adverse Effect of Antiepileptic Drugs.* Raven Press, New York.

121. Schmidt, M., and Brugger, E. (1980): Ein Fall von Carbamazepin-induzierter interstieller Pneumonie. *Med. Klin.*, 75:29–31.

122. Schmidt, D., Corragia, C., and Fabian, A. (1984): Carbamazepine suspension for acute treatment of trigeminal neuralgia: Clinical effects in relation to plasma concentration. In: *Metabolism of Antiepileptic Drugs*, edited by Levy et al., pp. 35–42. Raven Press, New York.

123. Shapiro, S., Hartz, St. C., Siskind, V., Mitchell,

A. A., Söone, D., Rosenberg, L., Monson, R. R., and Heinonen, O. P. (1976): Anticonvulsant and parental epilepsy in the development of birth defects. *Lancet,* I:272–275.

124. Shaw, P. N., Houston, J. B., Rowland, M., Hopkins, K., Thiercelin, J. F., and Morselli, P. L. (1985): Antipyrine metabolite kinetics in healthy human volunteers during multiple dosing of phenytoin and carbamazepine. *Br. J. Clin. Pharmacol.,* 20:611–618.

125. Shields, D., and Saslow, E. (1983): Myoclonic, atonic and absence seizures following institution of carbamazepine therapy in children. *Neurology,* 33:1487–1489.

126. Shuttleworth, D., Graham-Brown, R. A. C., Williams, A. J., Campbell, A. C., and Sewell, H. (1984): Pseudo-lymphoma associated with carbamazepine. *Clin. Exp. Dermatol.,* 9:421–423.

127. Sillanpää, M. (1981): Carbamazepine. Pharmacology and clinical uses. *Acta Neurol. Scand.,* 64 (suppl. 88).

128. Sivenius, J., Heinonen, E., Lehto, H., Järvensivu, P., Anttila, M., Ylinen, A., and Riekkinen, P. (1988): Reduction of dosing frequency of carbamazepine with a slow-release preparation. *Epilepsy Res.,* 2:32–36.

129. Smith, N. J., Espir, M. L. E., and Baylis, P. H. (1977): Raised plasma arginine vasopressin concentration in carbamazepine-induced water intoxication. *Br. Med. J.,* 2:804.

130. Snead, C. O., and Hosey, L. C. (1985): Exacerbation of seizures in children by carbamazepine. *N. Engl. J. Med.,* 15:916–921.

131. Soman, M., and Swenson, C. (1985): A possible case of carbamazepine-induced pancreatitis. *Drug Intell. Clin. Pharm.,* 19:925–927.

132. Sordillo, P., Sagransky, D. M., Mercado, R., and Michelis, M. F. (1977): Carbamazepine-induced syndrome of inappropriate antidiuretic hormone secretion. Reversal by concomitant phenytoin therapy. *Arch. Intern. Med.,* 138:299–301.

133. Speidel, B. D., and Meadow, S. R. (1972): Maternal epilepsy and abnormalities of the fetus and newborn. *Lancet,* II:839–843.

134. Steiner, C., Wit, A. L., Weiss, M. P., and Mamato, A. N. (1970): The anti-arrhythmic action of carbamazepine (Tegretol). *J. Pharmacol. Exp. Ther.,* 173:323–335.

135. Stephens, W. P., Coe, J. Y., and Baylis, P. H. (1978): Plasma arginine vasopressin concentrations and antidiuretic action of carbamazepine. *Br. Med. J.,* 1:1445–1447.

136. Strandjord, R. E., Aanderud, S., Myking, O. L., and Johannessen, S. I. (1981): Influence of carbamazepine on serum thyroid and triiodothyronine in patients with epilepsy. *Acta Neurol. Scand.,* 63:111–121.

137. Strandjord, R. E., and Johannessen, S. I. (1980): Single-drug therapy with carbamazepine in patients with epilepsy: Serum levels and clinical effects. *Epilepsia,* 21:655–662.

138. Stubbe-Teglbjaerg, H. P. (1936): Investigations on epilepsy and water metabolism. *Acta Psychiat. Neurol.,* 9:1–147.

139. Taliercio, C. P., and Olney, B. A. (1985): Myocarditis related to drug hypersensitivity. *Mayo Clin. Proc.,* 60:463–468.

140. Tartara, A., Manni, R., Maurelli, M., Sandrini, M., and Savoldi, F. (1986): Carbamazepine poisoning: A case report. *Ital. J. Neurol. Sci.,* 7:165–166.

141. Terrence, C. F., and Fromm, G. (1980): Congestive heart failure during carbamazepine therapy. *Ann. Neurol.,* 8:200–201.

142. Tjellesen, L., Nilas, L., and Christiansen, C. (1983): Does carbamazepine cause disturbances in calcium metabolism in epileptic patients? *Acta Neurol. Scand.,* 68:13–19.

143. Tomson, T. (1984): Interdosage fluctuations in plasma carbamazepine concentration determine intermittent side-effects. *Arch. Neurol.,* 41:830–834.

144. Wendland, K. I. (1968): Myoclonus following doses of carbamazepine. *Nervenarzt,* 39:231–233.

145. Yates, P., Stockdill, G., and McIntyre, M. (1986): Hypersensitivity to carbamazepine presenting as pseudolymphoma. *J. Clin. Pathol.,* 39:1224–1228.

146. Yeung Laiwh, A. A. C., Rapeport, W. G., and Thompson, G. G. (1983): Carbamazepine-induced non-hereditary acute porphyria. *Lancet,* 1:790–792.

147. Zucker, P., Damm, F., and Cohen, M. I. (1977): Fatal carbamazepine hepatitis. *J. Pediat.,* 91:667–668.

Antiepileptic Drugs, Third Edition, edited by
R. Levy, R. Mattson, B. Meldrum,
J. K. Penry, and F. E. Dreifuss.
Raven Press, Ltd., New York © 1989.

39

Valproate

Mechanisms of Action

Ruggero Fariello and Michael C. Smith

Valproate (VPA) is a unique anticonvulsant. It has a broad spectrum of activity against both the convulsive and nonconvulsive generalized epilepsies. In addition, its simple structure of a branched fatty acid differs markedly from the substituted heterocyclic ring structure common to other anticonvulsants. Despite numerous claims to the contrary, the basis of its anticonvulsant activity remains unknown.

Burton (5) first synthesized this clear, colorless acid in 1882. There was no known clinical use until its anticonvulsant activity was fortuitously discovered in 1963. Meunier, working in the laboratory of G. Carraz, used *N*-dipropylacetic acid (valproic acid) as a vehicle to dissolve the active ingredient in testing anticonvulsant activity of new compounds. The results led to the testing of valproic acid and to the confirmation that it was protective against pentylenetetrazol (PTZ) induced seizures. The first clinical trials of the sodium salt of valproic acid were reported in 1964 by Carraz (7). It was marketed in France in 1967 as Depakine and was released in the United States in 1978 for the treatment of epilepsy.

Valproate was initially used as adjunctive therapy in patients with poorly controlled seizures. It was found to be of most value in the treatment of the primary generalized epilepsies (55,60). Controlled studies have shown that VPA is as effective as ethosuximide in the control of corticoreticular epilepsy (57,63). Although improvement in tonic-clonic seizures was first reported with the use of VPA as adjunctive therapy (29,60), Turnball (67) reported that VPA was as effective as phenytoin when used as monotherapy in adult patients with tonic-clonic seizures. Valproate has also been shown to be effective in the treatment of the myoclonic epilepsies of childhood and adolescence (25). It is as effective as phenobarbital in prophylaxis against febrile seizures (69).

The efficacy of VPA against partial seizures is less well established. Simon and Penry (60) reported that with uncontrolled simple partial seizures there was a positive response (75% reduction in seizures) in 46% of the patients. Only a third of the patients with complex partial seizures had a positive response to VPA adjunctive therapy.

EXPERIMENTAL MODELS

Studies of the mechanisms of action of antiepileptic drugs can be divided into three general types, each with different purposes. Initially, a putative antiepileptic drug undergoes a classic battery of anticonvulsant tests that empirically predict whether generalized tonic-clonic seizures or absence attacks will respond to the drug. The drug is then tested in experimental paradigms that are considered to be models of at least some aspects of human epilepsy. This second type of experimental study also provides information on whether a given compound acts on the epileptiform phenomena at the site of their generation (the focus) or prevents their dissemination or spread (recruitment) throughout the brain. Eventually, when a drug is established as an anticonvulsant, a third type of study is carried out to discover the intimate mechanisms of action of the drug on normal and abnormal (epileptiform) neuronal activity.

Classic Anticonvulsant Tests

The standard tests of an anticonvulsant's effect on tonic-clonic seizures and corticoreticular epilepsy are maximal electroshock threshold (MES) and PTZ-induced seizures, respectively. Although alternative screening tests have been suggested, none have reliably shown better efficacy in predicting the clinical usefulness of antiepileptic drugs. The initial studies by the manufacturing laboratories reported that VPA provided protection from the MES and PTZ seizures in dogs, rabbits, and rats with a therapeutic index (LD_{50}/ED_{50}) of four to eight times. Synergistic anticonvulsant action with phenobarbital, acetylurea, and phenytoin was noted, but there was no synergism with ethosuximide and trimethadione (6).

Swinyard (64) and many other investigators confirmed VPA's usefulness in protecting against PTZ and MES seizures. In general, VPA is more effective against PTZ-induced seizures (a model of corticoreticular epilepsy) than against MES seizures (a model of generalized tonic-clonic seizures). Valproate is also effective in other models of generalized seizures (16,22). For example, at doses of 40 to 400 mg/kg i.p., it protects against seizures induced by bicuculline, glutamic acid, kainic acid,

strychnine, ouabain, and nicotine (8). Pellegrini et al. (53) also found VPA effective in protecting against the feline model of corticoreticular epilepsy induced by intramuscular penicillin.

Thus, these tests suggest that VPA is maximally effective against absence seizures and has good efficacy against tonic-clonic seizures.

Models of Focal and Projected Epileptiform Activity

Cortical cobalt and alumina lesions are models of simple partial seizures. These models of focal seizures are often accompanied by bursts of bilaterally synchronous spikes and waves that represent secondary generalization. In this model, VPA totally supresses the secondary generalized epilepsy, leaving the focal activity unaffected (11). Similarly, in a cortical cobalt-induced epileptogenic focus in cats (68), valproate (200 mg/kg/i.p.) inhibited the spread of seizure activity but did not decrease the focal discharges.

A series of studies (44,45,46) investigated the effects of a single dose of VPA (200 mg/kg/i.p.) on cobalt-induced epileptiform discharges in the cat neocortex and hippocampus and on the threshold, duration, and propagation of the electrical after-discharge (AD) induced in the normal and epileptic hippocampus of cats. Locally induced AD is considered a model equivalent to the maximal electroshock threshold in screening for a drug's antitonic-clonic properties. Valproate was effective in reducing the number and propagation of cobalt-induced seizures. In addition, VPA raised the threshold, reduced the duration, and prevented the spread of the AD from 20 min to 6 hr after the injection. Lockard (32) observed a reduction of the frequency, duration, and severity of seizures in monkeys with an alumina gel focus during constant VPA intravenous infusion. However, focal seizures and focal epileptiform discharges were not suppressed until serum levels greater than 100 μg/ml were reached.

Kindling, another model of focal epileptogenesis and secondary spread, initially induces focal ADs, which then progress to invade distant areas until a generalized AD and clinical seizure follows the originally subthreshold stimulus. In the kindling model, the spread of epileptiform activity in cats was blocked by long-term VPA treatment (31) without affecting local AD or focal seizures.

The majority of these studies, therefore, demonstrate the superior ability of VPA to prevent spread of epileptiform activity versus suppressing it at the site of origin. The systems involved in generalization of seizures seem particularly sensitive to VPA's action.

Intimate Mechanisms of Action

These studies address the fundamental actions of antiepileptic drugs on normal and abnormal epileptiform activity. A hypothesis is usually generated [e.g., VPA's mechanism of action is due to an increase in γ-aminobutyric acid (GABA)] and an experimental paradigm is designed to test the hypothesis. The hypothesis and supporting data must meet two critical criteria. First, the effect of the tested compound must be achieved at a dose and time course analogous to clinical observations. Second, the test system must be relevant to the drug's clinical antiepileptic effect. This is clearly met in VPA's effect on GABA levels, but is not as obvious in VPA's effect on ion conductance in invertebrate neurons. Despite the fact that numerous hypotheses have been generated and tested, the exact mechanisms responsible for VPA's anticonvulsant effect remain unknown.

Increase in GABA Levels

Interference with synaptically available GABA and/or with GABA receptor-me-diated responses are reflected by changes in the convulsant threshold in mammals (12). Thus, decreased GABA function will lower convulsant thresholds, whereas drugs that increase GABA function act as anticonvulsants. GABA levels in the brain increase after VPA, and this fact has been the basis for the earliest and still most cited hypothesis concerning VPA's mechanism of action. However, the available evidence is insufficient to make a final assessment of the validity of this hypothesis.

Evidence in Favor of the GABAergic Hypothesis of VPA

Valproate antagonizes seizures induced by bicuculline and picrotoxin (both potent GABA antagonists (15,70) and seizures induced by 3-mercatopropionic acid, isoniazid, and ally-1-glycine (inhibitors of GABA synthesis [9]).

Godin (21), Loscher (33), Similer (59), and many other investigators (8,39,48) have shown that valproate increases whole brain GABA levels. Godin, from Mendel's laboratory, reported that VPA (400 mg/kg i.p.) increased whole brain GABA 30% to 40% (21). He also reported that VPA inhibits in vitro GABA-transaminase, the first step in GABA degradation. Fowler (13) reported that VPA is only a weak inhibitor of GABA-T in vitro and that high levels, which are clinically unattainable, would be necessary to significantly affect GABA levels. Harvey (23) confirmed that VPA is a more potent inhibitor of in vitro succinic semialdehyde dehydrogenase (SSA-DH), the next enzyme in the GABA degradative pathway.

Regional (54) and whole brain (33,34,35,65) glutaminic acid decarboxylase (GAD) activity is increased after VPA administration. The increased GAD activity, the GABA synthesizing enzyme, results in increased GABA production. GABA in neurons is contained in the synaptosomes of nerve terminals as well as in the neuronal soma and glial cells' metabolic pool. Only the synaptosomal fraction is involved in neurotransmission. Therefore, unless a clear distinction is made between the two pools, it is impossible to establish the effectiveness of increased levels of whole brain GABA in increasing GABA-mediated inhibition (2). Such a distinction can be provided by transecting the striatonigral descending tract, a GABAergic pathway. Eliminating the synaptosomal GABA pool with this procedure prevented the VPA-induced GABA elevation in the substantia nigra (18,19). Furthermore, direct measurement of synaptosomal GABA after VPA confirmed the selective elevation of GABA in this neurotransmission-related subcellular fraction (35). Loscher (37) and Loscher and Siemens (38) reported increased cerebrospinal fluid (CSF) GABA levels in both healthy volunteers and epileptic patients under long-term VPA treatment. Therefore, there is evidence that VPA interferes with GABA-degrading enzymes, that it increases the neurotransmitter-related fraction of GABA's pool, and, at least in one laboratory, CSF GABA was increased after long-term VPA therapy.

Evidence Questioning the Relevance of VPA-Induced GABA Levels to VPA's Effect

Most animal studies of VPA effects on GABA levels and metabolism have used doses 8 to 10-fold higher than the average clinical dose. In one study, a 100% GABA elevation was seen in dogs after 60 mg/kg VPA, a dose not commonly used in humans (36). In VPA trials in Parkinson's disease (51) and schizophrenia (30), CSF GABA levels were not significantly increased. The clinical importance of VPA's effect on SSA-DH was questioned on the basis of the demonstration that even near total blockade of SSA-DH did not raise whole brain GABA levels (59).

In some experimentally induced seizures

(1,9,27), the rise in GABA lags behind the earlier appearance of the anticonvulsant effect (26,28). We are not aware of studies addressing the issue of the time course of GABA elevation versus its antiepileptic action in long-term treatment. Clinically, with VPA treatment, seizure reduction may be delayed and may outlast withdrawal of VPA. Whether or not in such cases the antiepileptic effects follow changes in GABA levels remains to be assessed. Numerous animal studies demonstrate a potentiating role of enhanced GABAergic tone in several models of bilaterally synchronous spike-and-wave discharges (12). Actually, under certain circumstances, GABA agonists may induce such epileptiform paroxysms *ex novo* (12,20). Thus, postulating a GABAergic mechanism as the sole or predominant mechanism of VPA's antiepileptic action against primary generalized epilepsy of the petit mal type contradicts most of the available experimental evidence (10,20).

VPA's Action on Specific Intracerebral Circuitries

Epileptiform activity in the brain appears to be under the regulation of both facilitory and inhibitory influences exerted by neuronal circuitries, of which only a few are known. The caudate nucleus through a VA thalamocortical projection may help control the excitability of the cortex and hippocampus. A single high-intensity pulse to the head of the caudate nucleus elicits cortical caudate spindles believed to be the expression of the state of activation of the caudothalamocortical circuitry. Valproate raises by an average of 75% the electrical threshold necessary to produce caudate spindles (47). When the threshold was lowered by a neocortical focus, VPA raised it above the control (prefocus) values. After administration of VPA, high frequency stimulation of the caudate nucleus failed to elicit the expected ictal discharges in a neocortical cobalt focus (47). In view of the data from Gale's laboratory (18,19,24) showing an increase in the synaptosomal compartment of presynaptic GABA terminal within the substantia nigra, the effect on the caudothalamocortical excitability may be secondary to the biochemical changes in the nigral originating ascending pathways, a recently characterized powerful gating mechanism of cerebral excitability.

Nowack et al. (50) also studied valproate's effect on thalamocortical excitability. They found that both valproate and ethosuximide depressed the average evoked responses seen at the cortex following the second of two stimuli delivered to the ventrolateral thalamus at low stimulus frequencies in the range of 3 Hz. At higher frequency rates, valproate had no significant effect, whereas ethosuximide enhanced evoked potentials at high frequency. This may correlate with ethosuximide's known potential of exacerbating generalized tonic-clonic convulsions. The exact mechanism responsible for the change in thalamocortical excitability remains unknown, but VPA's effect on it may provide the basis to explain its effectiveness against corticoreticular epilepsy.

Utilizing the trigeminal complex in cats as a test system, Fromm and Terrence (17) studied the effects of various antiepileptic drugs on segmental inhibition, descending inhibition, and descending excitation. Segmental inhibition is tested by delivering a conditioning stimulus to the maxillary nerve 100 msec prior to the test stimulus. Descending inhibition is measured by delivering a conditioning stimulus to the periventricular gray matter 100 msec prior to the test stimulus, whereas descending excitation is measured by delivering the conditioning stimulus to the periventricular gray matter 10 msec before the test stimulus to the maxillary nerve. Administration of 20 to 80 mg/kg of VPA depressed the descending and segmental inhibition without affecting the response to the unconditioned maxillary nerve stimulation. In addition, VPA depressed the descending excitation of trigeminal nucleus neurons. In this test model, the results correctly predict VPA's efficacy against both absence and generalized tonic-clonic seizures (17).

Electrophysiological Studies of VPA Action on Neuronal Membrane and Synaptic Transmission

Valproate is similar to the anticonvulsant benzodiazepines and barbiturates in that it selectively potentiates GABA-mediated postsynaptic inhibition *in vitro* (3,26,40,41,66). However, in another *in vitro* preparation, no action of VPA on GABA postsynaptic responses was found (4). On the basis of *in vitro* binding studies, it appears that its action may be exerted at the picrotoxin binding site of the GABA receptor-chloride ionophore complex in the postsynaptic membrane (66). On *Aplysia* neurons, VPA, at concentrations 15 to 50 times higher than clinical levels, directly increases K^+ conductance, a powerful hyperpolarizing mechanism (61).

Several antiepileptic drugs have effects on neuronal conductance when fibers and/or synapses are functioning abnormally. This observation is at the basis of the theory of use- and frequency-dependent pharmacological effect of some anticonvulsants. Valproate at "therapeutic" CSF levels limits the depolarization-induced sustained repetitive firing to a few action potentials (42) through a blockage of voltage-sensitive Na^+ influx. This ability to limit repetitive high-frequency firing may certainly contribute to VPA's efficacy in epilepsy, a condition characterized by excessive high-frequency bursting of neuronal aggregates. Similarly, in studying hippocampal slices, Franceschetti et al. (14) found that VPA markedly depressed frequency potentiation and paired pulse facilitation. It also suppressed spontaneous epileptiform activity and prolonged afterdischarge elicited by antidromic stimulation (14). Their data suggest that VPA does not interfere with Na^+ inward current like phenytoin or carbamazepine, but rather the delayed effect that is seen is best explained by valproate's activation on Ca^{++}-dependent K^+ conductance.

In various models of experimental seizures, VPA has been shown to possess direct membrane effects at clinically obtainable levels. The relationship between these direct membrane effects in these test systems and VPA's anticonvulsant effect, although plausible, remains unproven.

Valproate's effect on whole brain excitatory amino acids has been studied (43). Schechter (58) reported that VPA (400 mg/ kg i.p.) in mice decreased brain aspartate levels and that this decrease correlates temporally with protection against audiogenic seizures. Subcellular studies (56) indicate that the decrease in aspartate is confined to nonsynaptosomal compartments and is thus thought not to be related to a neurotransmitter role of this amino acid. Slevin (62) reported that long-term VPA administration to the rat had no effect on aspartate or glutamic acid uptake or binding activity in cortex and hippocampus. Though there is no consistent evidence that VPA acts as an anticonvulsant through decreasing these excitatory amino acids, further studies examining VPA's effect on regional concentrations of excitatory amino acids are needed.

CONCLUSIONS

Epilepsy is a comprehensive term used clinically for practical purposes, but it is a scientifically vague term. Epilepsy encompasses a wide variety of clinical conditions and a broad spectrum of biochemical and physiological phenomena that occur at various organizational levels of the nervous system, ranging from membrane abnormal-ity to changes in the excitability of the entire brain. Epilepsy is the composite of several electrophysiological abnormalities believed to occur (most of the time) in a stepwise progression from abnormalities underlying the interictal spike through subclinical (electrographic) seizures to the behavioral changes (the actual clinical seizures) that are the essential symptoms for the diagnosis of epilepsy.

Since the exact role of each step in the pathogenesis of seizures is unknown, it would be presumptuous to claim knowledge of the mechanisms of action of any antiepileptic drug. Nevertheless, on the basis of present, limited knowledge, reasonable hypotheses can be proposed to explain the anticonvulsant effect of a drug. For VPA, none of the hypotheses discussed above have satisfactorily explained all of its anticonvulsant activity. It is probable that VPA acts through more than one mechanism in providing its broad anticonvulsant activity. In the classic anticonvulsant tests, VPA protects against PTZ- and MES-induced seizures, consistent with its known effect against both corticoreticular and tonic-clonic epilepsies.

The presently available evidence suggests that VPA may antagonize epileptiform activity at several steps of their organization. Valproate's enhancement of GABAergic tone in the substantia nigra may influence this powerful gating mechanism for generalization of seizures. Related to this may be its inhibiting effect on the caudothalamocortical circuit: excitability of this circuit may be necessary for recruitment of the entire forebrain into generalized tonic-clonic seizures. This anticonvulsant mechanism is supported by (a) the proven increase in nigral levels of GABA and (b) the changes in the excitability threshold of the caudothalamocortical systems seen with VPA administration (47).

Valproate's action on celluar mechanisms is less clear. The most cited hypotheses include the regional and compartmental increase in GABA function supported by multiple investigations, although the relevance of this to its clinical efficacy remains debatable. A second attractive hypothesis is the proven effect of VPA to limit sustained repetitive firing at therapeutically attainable levels. Whether this action is due to interference with the sodium channel (similar to phenytoin and carbamazepine) or to activation of calcium-dependent potassium conductance remains to be determined. Finally, the postulated effect on excitatory amino acid neurotransmission is an attractive hypothesis to explain some of VPA's anticonvulsant effect.

To reach a satisfactory hypothesis of VPA mechanisms of action, we need a better understanding of the pathophysiology of epilepsy. One area of research that may yield useful information is the study of changes in cerebral glucose metabolism after anticonvulsant doses of VPA. This may reveal the loci of action where further neurophysiological and biochemical studies can be targeted to reach a better understanding of their integral relationship. The search for the mechanisms of action of VPA's anticonvulsant activity, though incomplete, has already elucidated important electrophysiologic, anatomic, and biochemical aspects of both focal and generalized epilepsies. Further research into VPA's mechanisms of action should be fruitful in elucidating still further the basic mechanisms of seizure generation and spread.

REFERENCES

1. Anlezark, G., Horton, R. W., Meldrum, B. S., and Sawaya, M. C. B. (1976): Anticonvulsant action of ethanolamine-O-sulphate and di-*n*-propylacetate and the metabolism of GABA in mice with audiogenic seizures. *Biochem. Parmacol.,* 25:413–417.
2. Balazs, R., Machiyama, Y., Hammond, B. J., Julian, T., and Richter, D. (1970): The operation of the GABA bypath tricarboxyclic acid cycle in brain tissue *in vitro. Biochem. J.,* 116:445–467.
3. Baldino, F., and Giller, H. M. (1981): Sodium valproate enhancement of GABA inhibition: Electro-

physiological evidence for anticonvulsant activity. *J. Pharmacol. Exp. Ther.,* 217:445–450.
4. Buchhalter, J. R., and Dichter, M. A. (1986): Effect of valproic acid in cultured mammalian neurons. *Neurology.,* 36:259–262.
5. Burton, B. S. (1882): On the propyl derivatives and decomposition products of ethylacetoacetate. *Am. Chem. J.,* 3:385–395.
6. Carraz, G. (1968): *Pharmacodynamie de l'Acide Dipropylacetique et de ses Amides.* Eymond Ed., Grenoble.
7. Carraz, G., Farr, R., Chateau, R., and Bonnin, J. (1964): First clinical trials of the antiepileptic activity of *n*-dipropylacetic acid. *Ann. Med. Psychol. (Paris),* 122:577–584.
8. Chapman, A., Keane, P. E., Meldrum, B. S., Simiand, J., and Vernieres, J. C. (1982): Mechanism of anticonvulsant action of valproate. *Prog. Neurobiology.,* 19:315–399.
9. Dren, A. T., Giardina, W. J., and Hagen, N. S. (1979): Valproic acid. In: *Pharmacological and Biochemical Properties of Drug Substances,* edited by M. E. Goldberg, APA, Washington.
10. Fariello, R. G., Golden, G. T., and Black, J. A. (1981): Activating effects of homotaurine and taurine in corticoreticular epilepsy. *Epilepsia,* 22:217–224.
11. Fariello, R., and Mutani, R. (1970): Modificazioni dell'attivita del focus epilepttogeno corticomotorio da allumina indotte dal sale disodo dell' acido *N*-diproplacetido (DPA). *Acta Neurol. (Napoli),* 25:116–122.
12. Fariello, R. G., and Ticku, M. K. (1983): Minireview. The perspective of GABA replenishment therapy in the epilepsies: A critical evaluation of hopes and concerns. *Life Sci.,* 33:1629–1640.
13. Fowler, L. J., Beckford, J., and John, R. A. (1975): An analysis of the kinetics of the inhibition of rabbit brain GABA-transaminase by sodium *N*-dipropylacetate and some other simple carboxylic acids. *Biochem. Pharmocol.,* 24:1267–1270.
14. Franceschetti, S., Hamon, B., and Heineman, U. (1986): The action of valproate on spontaneous epileptiform activity in the absence of synaptic transmission and on evoked changes in $[Ca^+]$ and $[K^+]$ in the hippocampal slice. *Brain Res.,* 386:1–11.
15. Frey, H. H., and Loscher, N. (1976): Di-*n*-propylacetic acid profile of anticonvulsant activity in mice. *Arzneimetttelforsch,* 26:299–301.
16. Frey, H. H., Loscher, W., Reiche, R., and Schultz, D. (1983): Anticonvulsant potency of common antiepileptic drugs in the gerbil. *Pharmacology,* 27:330–335.
17. Fromm, G. H., and Terrence, C. F. (1985): Trigeminal nucleus as a model for testing of antiepileptic drugs. LERS Monograph Series, Volume 3, edited by G. Bartholon, L. Bossi, K. G. Lloyd, and P. L. Morselli, pp. 149–157. Raven Press, New York.
18. Gale, K., and Iadorola, M. J. (1980): Seizure protection and increased nerve-terminal GABA: Delayed effects of GABA transaminase inhibition. *Science,* 208:288–291.
19. Gale, K., Iadorala, M. J., Casu, M., and Keating,

R. F. (1982): Relationship between GABA levels *in vivo* and anticonvulsant activity: Importance of cellular compartments and regional localization in brain. In: *Problems in GABA Research From Brain to Bacteria,* edited by Y. Okada and E. Roberts, pp. 159–172. Exerpta Medica, Amsterdam.

20. Gloor, P., and Fariello, R. G. (1987): Generalized epilepsy: Some of its cellular mechanisms differ from those of focal epilepsy. *Trends in NeuroSci.,* 11:63–78.

21. Godin, Y., Heiner, L., Mark, J., and Mandel, P. (1969): Effects of di-*n*-propylacetate, and anticonvulsive compound, on GABA metabolism. *J. Neurochem.,* 16:869–873.

22. Harding, G. F. A., Herrick, G. E., and Jeavons, P. M. (1978): A controlled study of the effects of sodium valproate on photosensitive epilepsy and its prognosis. *Epilepsia,* 19:555–565.

23. Harvey, P. K. B., Bradford, H. F., and Davisson, A. N. (1975): The inhibitory effect of sodium *n*-dipropylacetate on the degradative enzymes of the GABA shunt. *FEBS Lett.,* 52F:251–254.

24. Iadorola, M. J., and Gale, K. (1979): Dissociation between drug-induced increase in nerve terminal and non-nerve terminal pools of GABA *in vivo. Eur. J. Pharmacol.,* 59:125–129.

25. Jeavons, P. M., Clark, J. E., and Maseshwari, M. C. (1977): Treatment of generalized epilepsies of childhood and adolescence with sodium valproate ("Epilim"). *Dev. Med. Child Neurol.,* 19:9–25.

26. Kerwin, R. W., Olpe, H. R., and Schmutz, M. (1980): The effect of sodium-*n*-dipropyl acetate on GABA dependent inhibition in rat cortex *in vivo. Br. J. Pharmac.,* 71:545–551.

27. Kerwin, R. W., and Taberner, P. V. (1981): The mechanism of action of sodium valproate. *Gen. Pharmac.,* 12:71–75.

28. Lacolle, J. Y., Ferrandes, B., and Eymand, P. (1978): Profile of anticonvulsant activity of sodium valproate. Role of GABA. In: *Advances in Epileptology,* edited by H. Meinharde, and A. J. Rowan, pp. 162–167. Swets and Zeitlinger, Amsterdam.

29. Lance, J. W., and Anthony, M. (1977): Sodium valproate and clonazepam in the treatment of intractable epilepsy. *Arch. Neurol.,* 34:14–17.

30. Lautin, A., Angrist, B., Stanley, M., Gershon, S., Heckl, K., and Karobath, M. (1980): Sodium valproate in schizophrenia: Some biochemical correlates. *Br. J. Psychiatr.,* 137:240–244.

31. Leveil, V., and Nanquet, R. (1977): A study of the action of valproic acid on the kindling effect. *Epilepsia,* 18:229–234.

32. Lockard, J., Levy, J. H., Congdon, W. C., DuCharme, L. L., and Patel, I. H. (1977): Efficacy testing of valproic acid to ethosuximide in monkey model: II seizure, EEG, and diurinal variation. *Epilepsia,* 18:205–233.

33. Loscher, W. (1981): Correlation between alterations in brain GABA metabolism and seizure excitability following administration of GABA aminotransferase inhibitors and valproic acid—a Reevaluation. *Neurochem. Int.,* 3:397–404.

34. Loscher, W. (1980): Effects of inhibitors of GABA transaminase on synthesis, binding, uptake, and metabolism of GABA. *J. Neurochem.,* 34:1603–1608.

35. Loscher, W. (1981): Valproate induced changes in GABA metabolism at the subcelluar level. *Biochem. Pharmacol.,* 30:1364–1366.

36. Loscher, W. (1982): GABA in plasma, CSF, and brain of dogs during acute and chronic treatment with acetylenic GABA and valproic acid. In: *Problems in GABA Research From Brain to Bacteria,* edited by Y. Okada and E. Roberts, Exerpta Medica, Amsterdam. pp. 102–109.

37. Loscher, W., and Schmidt, D. (1980): Increase of human plasma GABA by sodium valproate. *Epilepsia,* 21:611–615.

38. Loscher, W., and Siemens, H. (1984): Valproic acid increases GABA in CSF of epileptic children. *Lancet.,* II:225.

39. Lust, W. D., Kupferberg, H. J., Yonekawa, W. D., Penry, J. K., Passoneau, J. V., and Wheaton, A. B. (1978): Changes in brain metabolites induced by convulsants or electroshock: Effect of anticonvulsant agents. *Molec. Pharmacol.,* 14:347–356.

40. MacDonald, R. L. (1986): Mechanisms of anticonvulsant drug action. In: *Recent Advances in Epilepsy,* edited by T. A. Pedley and B. S. Meldrum, pp. 1–23. Churchill Livingstone, Edinburgh.

41. MacDonald, R. L., and Bergey, G. K. (1979): Valproic acid augments GABA mediated post-synaptic inhibition in cultured mammalian neurons. *Brain Res.,* 170:558–562.

42. McClean, M. J., and MacDonald, R. L. (1986): Sodium valproate, but not ethosuximide, produces use and voltage-dependent limitation of high frequency repetitive firing of action potentials of mouse central neurons in cell culture. *J. Pharmacol. Exp. Therap.,* 237:1001–1011.

43. Meldrum, B. S., Anlezark, G. M., Ashton, C. G., Horton, R. W., and Sawaya, C. B. (1979): Neurotransmitters and anticonvulsant drug action. In: *Epilepsy,* edited by J. Majkowski, pp. 139–153. ILEA, Warsaw.

44. Mutani, R., Doriguzzi, T., Fariello, R., and Furlan, P. M. (1968): Azione antiepilettica del sale di sodio dell'acido *N*-dipropilacetico, Studio Sperimentale sul Gatto. *Riv. Patol. Nerv. Ment.,* 89:24.

45. Mutani, R., Doriguzzi, T., Fariello, R., and Furlan, P. M. (1969): Studio dell'azione di alcuni farmaci antiepilettici. *Sistema Nervoso,* 21:160–171.

46. Mutani, R., and Fariello, R. (1969): Effetti dell' acido *N*-dipropilacetico (Depakine) sull'attivita del focus epilettogeno corticale da cobalto. *Riv. Patol. Nerv. Ment.,* 90:40–49.

47. Mutani, R., and Fariello, R. G. (1969): L'azione dell'acido *n*'dipropilacetico (DPA) sulle "caudate spindles" corticali. *Boll. Soc. Ital. Biol. Sper.,* 45:1416–1417.

48. Nau, H., and Loscher, W. (1982): Valproic acid: Brain and plasma levels of the drug and its metabolites, anticonvulsant effects, and GABA metabolism in the mouse. *J. Pharmacol. Exp. Ther.,* 220:654–659.

49. Nosek, T. M. (1985): The effects of valproate and

phenytoin on cAMP and cGMP levels in nervous tissue. *Proc. Soc. Exp. Biol. Med.*, 178:196–199.

50. Nowack, W. J., Johnson, R. N., Englander, R. N., and Hanna, G. R. (1979): Effects of valproate and ethosuximide on thalamocortical excitability. *Neurology*, 29:96–99.

51. Nutt, J., Williams, A., Plotkin, C., Eng, N., Ziegler, M., and Calne, D. B. (1979): Treatment of Parkinson's disease with sodium valproate: Clinical, pharmacologic, and biochemical observations. *Can. J. Neurol. Sci.*, 6:337:343.

52. Patry, G., and Naquet, R. (1971): Action de l'acide dipropylacetique chez le Papio Papio photosensible. *Can. J. Physiol. Pharmacol.*, 49:568–572.

53. Pellegrini A., Gloor, P., and Sherwin, A. L. (1978): Effect of valproate sodium on generalized penicillin in the cat. *Epilepsia*, 19:351–360.

54. Phillips, N. I., and Fowler, L. S. (1982): The effects of sodium valproate on GABA metabolism and behavior in naive and ethanolamine-*O*-sulphate pretreated ras and mice. *Biochem. Pharmacol.*, 31:2257–2261.

55. Richen, A., and Ahmed, S. (1975): Controlled trial of sodium valproate in severe epilepsy. *Br. Med. J.*, 3:255–256.

56. Sarhan, S., and Seiler, N. (1979): Metabolic inhibitors and subcellular distribution of GABA. *J. Neurosci. Res.*, 4:399–421.

57. Sato, S., White, B. G., Penry, J. K., Dreifus, F. E., Sackellares, J. C., and Kupferberg, H. J. (1982): Valproic acid versus ethosuximide in the treatment of absence seizures. *Neurology*, 32:157–163.

58. Schechter, P. J., Trainer, Y., and Grove, J. (1978): Effect of *N*-dipropylacetate on amino acid concentration in mouse brain: Correlations with anticonvulsant activity. *J. Neurochem.*, 3:1325–1327.

59. Simler, S., Ciesielski, L., Klien, M., Gobaille, S., and Mandel, P. (1981): Sur le mechanisme d'action d'un anticonvulsivant, le dipropylacetate de sodium. *C.R. Soc Biol.* (*Paris*), 175:114–119.

60. Simon, D., and Penry, J. K. (1978): Sodium di-*n*-propylacetate (DPA) in the treatment of epilepsy. A review. *Epilepsia*, 19:379–384.

61. Slater, G. E., and Johnston, D. (1978): Sodium valproate increases potassium conductance in *Aplysia* neurons. *Epilepsia*, 19:379–384.

62. Slevin, J. T., and Ferrara, L. P. (1985): Chronic valproic acid therapy and synaptic markers of amino acid neurotransmission. *Neurology*, 35:728–731.

63. Suzuki, M., Maruana, H., Ishibashi, Y., Seki, T., Hoshino, M., Markawa, K., Yogo, T., and Sato, Y. (1982): A doubleblind comparative trial of sodium dipropylacetate and ethosuximide in epilepsy in children with special emphasis on pure petit mal seizures. *Jap. Med. Prog.*, 82:470–488.

64. Swinyard, E. A. (1964): The pharmacology of dipropylacetic acid sodium with special emphasis on its effects on the central nervous system, pp. 1–25. (thesis) University of Utah, College of Pharmacy, Salt Lake City.

65. Taberner, P. V., Charington, C. B., and Unwin, J. W. (1980): Effects of GAD and GABA-T inhibitors on GABA metabolism *in vivo*. *Brain Res. Bull.*, (Suppl 2):621–625.

66. Ticku, M. K., and Davis, W. C. (1981): Effect of valproic acid on H-diazepam and H-dihydropicrotoxin in binding sites at the benzodiazepine-GABA receptor-ionophore complex. *Brain Res.*, 223:218–222.

67. Turnball, D. M., Rawlins, M. D., Weightman, D., and Chadwick, D. W. (1982): A comparison of phenytoin and valporate in previously untreated adult epileptic patients. *J. Neurol. Neurosurg. Psychiat.*, 45:55–59.

68. Van Diujn, H., and Beckman, M. K. F. (1975): Dipropylacetic acid (Depakine) in experimental epilepsy in the alert cat. *Epilepsia*, 16:83–90.

69. Wallace, S. J., and Aldridge-Smith, J. (1980): Successful prophylaxis against febrile convulsions with valproic acid or phenobarbitone. *Br. Med. J.*, 1:353–354.

70. Worms, P., and Lloyd, K. G. (1981): Functional alterations of GABA synapses in relation to seizures. In: *Neurotransmitters, Seizures, and Epilepsy*, edited by P. L. Morselli, K. G. Lloyd, W. Loscher, B. S. Meldnum, and E. H. Reynolds, pp. 37–46. Raven Press, New York.

Antiepileptic Drugs, Third Edition, edited by
R. Levy, R. Mattson, B. Meldrum,
J. K. Penry, and F. E. Dreifuss.
Raven Press, Ltd., New York © 1989.

40

Valproate

Chemistry and Methods of Determination

Harvey J. Kupferberg

Valproate is one of the most widely used agents for the treatment of epilepsy. Once its usefulness was established, numerous methods of analysis were developed, the majority of which used gas-liquid chromatography to separate and quantitate the valproate. Newer analytical methodology for the analysis of valproic acid started to appear in the literature in the late 1970s. The development of immunoassays of the clinically effective antiepileptic agents allowed the clinical laboratory to rapidly integrate their determination into the daily routine. Chromatographic procedures usually entail the extraction of valproic acid from the biological matrix, whereas the immunoassays eliminate this time-consuming step. Clinical and research laboratories have adapted these techniques to their available time, equipment, and personnel. The optimal method depends on the quantity of valproic acid in the matrix. Sensitive methods are needed to measure low concentrations, such as the unbound valproic acid in plasma. Methods of analysis of valproic acid's metabolites usually involve the more specific and sensitive mass spectrometric ion monitoring techniques (see Chapter 42). This chapter presents an overview of the advantages and disadvantages of various methodologies published since the previous review (26).

PHYSICAL AND CHEMICAL PROPERTIES

Valproic acid (2-propylpentanoic acid) is a colorless liquid with a boiling point of 221–222°C at 1 atm (6) (Fig. 1). Its molecular weight is 144.21. It is very slightly soluble in water (1.3 mg/ml) and very soluble in organic solvents. It has an ultraviolet absorption maximum at 213 nm with a molar extinction coefficient of 86. The pK_a of valproic acid is 4.8.

Sodium valproate is a white crystalline material and is highly hygroscopic when relative humidity reaches 50% or more. Its molecular weight is 166.19. It is extremely soluble in water and most polar organic solvents such as methanol and acetone. The calcium and magnesium salts of valproic acid are insoluble in water.

Recently, the stable coordinated complex of equal molar quantities of sodium valproate and valproic acid (sodium hydrogen *bis*-2-propylpentoate of divalproex sodium) has been developed for clinical use.

CHROMATOGRAPHIC METHODS

Gas-Liquid Chromatography

Many of the recent gas-liquid chromatographic (GLC) procedures have not

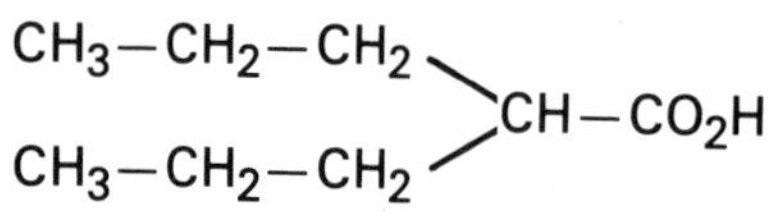

$$CH_3-CH_2-CH_2$$
$$CH-CO_2H$$
$$CH_3-CH_2-CH_2$$

FIG. 1. Structure of valproic acid (2-propyl-pentanoic acid).

changed from the early methods. They require the acidification of plasma and the extraction of valproic acid into a volatile organic solvent. In some cases, the organic solvent is evaporated or concentrated, and in other cases an aliquot of the extracting solvent is injected into the chromatograph. Several methods use derivative formation of valproic acid to produce highly volatile products which chromatograph well (4,5,7,30,35,36,41). In one instance, the extraction of valproic acid is bypassed entirely (9). In all gas chromatographic methods, an internal standard is always added to the biological sample prior to analysis. It is extremely important to emphasize that the internal standard should have physical characteristics similar to valproic acid. Cyclohexane carboxylic acid appears to be the most commonly used internal standard (1,4,7,12,13,16,22,28,31,34,37,38,39), although heptanonic acid (2), caproic (hexanoic) acid (40,41,43,46), caprylic (octanoic) acid (5,23,35,36), 2-ethylbutanoic acid (9), 2-ethyl hexanoic acid (20), 2-methyl-2-ethylcaproic acid (24,29), 2-propylhexanoic acid (33), and sorbic acid (30) have also been used. Two compounds that are not carboxylic acids have been used as internal standards: benzyl alcohol (14) and methyl toluate (49).

Chromatography of underivatized valproic acid requires the use of highly polar stationary phases such as carbowax or diethylene glycol succinate (DEGS). These phases require near maximum operating oven temperatures for the analysis and therefore require monitoring peak shape as a means of evaluating changes in column efficiency. When severe "tailing" of peaks occurs, the column packing should be changed. When a silicone stationary phase (e.g., OV-17) is used, lower oven temperatures are required (8). Care must be taken to assure that the phase exits in a liquid state at these lower temperatures. Hoffman and Porter (20) used a 60 meter OV-351 capillary column for the quantitation of valproic acid. This column was able to resolve valproic acid from hexadeutero and tetradeutero analogs of valproic acid.

Flame ionization detectors have sufficient sensitivity to detect and quantitate therapeutic plasma levels of valproic acid. Some consideration must be given to the organic extracting solvent injected into the chromatograph. Chloroform burns to phosgene and other corrosive products that pit detectors. The more sensitive electron-capture and nitrogen-sensitive detectors can only be used for the quantitation of valproic acid if appropriate derivatives are made.

Nonextractive Methods

Degel et al. (9) developed a method that does not require a prechromatographic separation step. This method uses the "headspace" technique of analysis. When the plasma sample is heated to 90°C in a sealed vial, the volatile valproic acid and internal standard equilibrates between the air and liquid phases. One ml of the atmosphere above the plasma is collected in a gas-tight syringe and injected into the gas chromatograph.

Extractive Methods

Most extractive methods use chloroform as a solvent to remove valproic acid from acidified plasma, although hexane (4,7,35), methylene chloride (13,36,38), carbon tetrachloride (49), diethyl ether (45,46), ethyl acetate (16), toluene (33), and pentane (41) have been used. The amount of organic phase depends on the volume of plasma used. In most cases, the volume of organic solvent is equal to or greater than the volume of plasma. One to two µl of organic phase is injected into the gas chromatograph. Because the concentration of valproic acid in patient plasma is relatively high, it can easily be quantitated in the extract. If the organic phase is removed, evaporated, and the residue reconstituted in small amounts of organic solvent, much lower amounts of valproic acid can be detected. A small amount of isoamylacetate can be added to the extract prior to the evaporation step to overcome the possible evaporation loss of valproic acid.

The use of solid phase extraction has become popular in isolating drugs from plasma. Lin and Kelly (29) used reversed-phase C-18 columns (Bond Elute) and Gast and Thoma (15) used silica columns (Clin Elute) to isolate valproic acid and acetone and hexane to elute the compounds from the C-18 and silica columns, respectively. Andreolini et al. (2) prepared columns containing 0.25 g graphitized carbon black (Carbopack B) to isolate valproic acid and eluted the drugs with a mixture of methanol and water (2).

Derivative Formation

The formation of derivatives of valproic acid produces less polar products with improved chromatographic characteristics and compounds with enhanced detection. Derivatives can be produced either directly within the gas chromatograph injection port (on column) or prior to the chromatographic procedure.

On-column alkylation has been used for many years in the quantitation of anticonvulsants. Morita et al. (33) incorporated on-column propylation in their method, whereas Calendrillo and Reynoso (4) produced methyl derivatives. Propyl derivative is less volatile than the corresponding methyl derivative.

Extractive alkylation methods can be used to produce the methyl ester of valproic acid prior to chromatography. Nishioka et al. (35) used tetrabutylammonium chloride as the counter ion and methyl iodide in methylene chloride as the alkylating agent. Nishioka et al. (36) used hexafluoroisopropanol and trifluorpacetic anydride to produce the hexafluoroisopropyl ester of valproic acid. They hope to produce a derivative with enhanced detectability using electron capture detectors. Unfortunately the sensitivity of the derivative to electron capture was not greater than that using the flame ionization detector.

Rege et al. (41) produced the less volatile phenacylbromide derivative of valproic acid. Valproic acid is extracted into pentane and phenacylbromide and triethylamine is added to the organic solvent. The pentane is rapidly evaporated at 50°C and the residue dissolved in methanol. The commonly used OV-17 columns, operated at 205°C, were used instead of the more polar phases such as SP-1000 or Carbowax.

Other phenacyl derivatives also produce an increase in sensitivity to the detection and quantitation of valproic acid. Cook and Jowett (7) made the p-nitrophenacyl ester of valproic acid. This derivative was produced by adding α-bromo-acetophenone and triethylamine to a hexane extract of patient plasma, whereas Lingeman et al. (30) made amides of valproic acid by adding 2-bromo-1-methylpyridinium iodide and dipropylamine to dichlormethane extracts. Both the nitro group and the amide permit the use of a nitrogen phosphorous detector. Chan (5) modified slightly the method of Cook and Jowett (7) for the more sensitive electron capture detector. This method can measure as little as 100 pg of valproic acid.

High-Performance Liquid Chromatography

High-performance liquid chromatographic (HPLC) methods of valproic acid analysis are similar to those using gas-liquid chromatography. A liquid mobile phase is substituted for the gas phase. Ultraviolet wavelength detectors are used to detect and quantitate valproic acid. Unfortunately, valproic acid does not absorb light very well in this region of the light spectrum, therefore sensitive methods of analysis require the formation of derivatives of valproic acid prior to the chromatographic separation.

A second difference in the methodology is sample preparation. Aqueous extracts can be injected into the chromatograph directly, thus eliminating the use of organic solvents to extract valproic acid from plasma. Many methods use acetonitrile to precipitate plasma proteins and the supernatant is then injected into the chromatograph (1,27,32,34). Any specificity gained in liquid-liquid extraction of the gas chromatographic methods is lost. Specificity within the analysis falls on the resolution characteristics of the chromatographic column. There is always the possibility of interfering materials co-eluting with the analytes, especially when a patient is taking many drugs for other conditions.

Reversed-phase, high-performance columns are used, usually C-18 with mobile phases of either methanol and water or acetonitrile and water mixtures. Derivatives of valproic acid usually have strong ultraviolet absorbances at either 254 nm or 280 nm.

Kline et al. (22) first extracted the plasma samples with methylene chloride prior to the derivatization of the carboxylic to the phenacyl esters. Others have used the acetonitrile supernatant of plasma to form the phenacyl (34), naphthacyl (1), and 4-bromophenacyl (32) esters.

Farinotti and Mahuzier (10) and van der Wal et al. (47) described an HPLC method that did not first form derivatives. The sensitivity of this method is limited because of valproic acid's low molar extinction coefficient, and therefore cannot quantitate valproic acid in small samples or at low concentrations.

ENZYME IMMUNOASSAY METHODS

Immunoassay techniques are now commonly used in therapeutic drug monitoring because of their speed, simplicity, and sensitivity. The technique requires the development of an antibody that recognizes only the molecules to be quantitated. The specific antibodies are then linked to enzymes. Reaction enzyme kinetics for the specific enzyme-substrate are followed for different concentrations of valproic acid. Measurements are made when the reaction kinetics proceed linearly, usually within the first minute. The homogeneous immunoassay or enzyme-multiplied immunoassay technique (EMIT) was the first assay of this type to be developed (21,25). A variety of mechanized and manual enzyme reaction rate analyzers have been adapted using the reagents for this analysis (3,18,19,42). Newer types of immunoassays are commercially available that use fluorescence polarization immunoassay (FPIA) (4,17,47) and substrate-labeled fluorescence immunoassay (SLFIA) (11).

Gas-liquid chromatography was used to validate these immunologic methods of analysis (28). When the values from the two methods were compared, a bias was exhibited by the immunoassay (i.e., the immunoassay tended to give higher values than the chromatographic method). Kumps et al. (25) believe that crossreactivity of some of the valproic acid metabolites occurs with the EMIT antibody. Sedman et al. (44) evaluated the FPIA of valproic acid in patients with chronic renal failure who were not receiving valproic acid. They found that the serum contained material which crossreacted with antibody. The apparent valproic acid concentration never exceeded 1.5 μg/ml.

CONCLUSIONS

The enzyme immunoassay of valproic acid appears to offer the most significant advance in methodology. It is simple and sensitive and can be adapted to measuring both free and total valproic acid. The major drawbacks are the expense of the reagents and that only one drug can be quantitated at a time. Most gas chromatographic methods are similar to the original methods published in the early 1970s. High sensitivity can be obtained with the use of the nitrogen-sensitive and electron-capture detectors and appropriate derivative formation.

CONVERSION

Conversion factor:

$$CF = \frac{1000}{\text{mol. wt.}} = \frac{1000}{144.2} = 6.93$$

Conversion:

$$(\mu g/ml) \times 6.93 = (\mu moles/liter)$$

$$(\mu moles/liter) \div 6.93 = (\mu g/ml)$$

REFERENCES

1. Alric, R., Cociglio, M., Blayac, J. P., and Pluech, R. (1981): Performance evaluation of a reversed-phase, high-performance liquid chromatographic assay of valproic acid involving a "solvent demixing" extraction procedure and pre-column derivatization. *J. Chromatogr.*, 224:289–299.
2. Andreolini, F., Borra, C., Di Corcia, A., and Samperi, R. (1984): Direct determination of valproic acid in minute whole blood samples. *J. Chromatogr.*, 310:208–212.
3. Braun, S. L., Tausch, A., Vogt, W., Jacob, K., and Knedel, M. (1981): Evaluation of a new valproic acid enzyme immunoassay and comparison with capillary gas chromatographic method. *Clin. Chem.*, 27:169–172.
4. Calendrillo, B. A., and Reynoso, G. (1980): A micromethod for the on-column methylation of valproic acid by gas-liquid chromatography. *J. Anal. Toxicol.*, 4:272–274.
5. Chan, S. C. (1980): Monitoring serum valproic acid by gas chromatography with electron capture detection. *Clin. Chem.*, 26:1528–1530.
6. Chang, Z. L. (1979): Sodium valproate and valproic acid. In: *Analytical Profiles of Drug Substances, Vol. 8,* edited by K. Florey, pp. 529–556. Academic Press, New York.
7. Cook, N. J., and Jowett, D. A. (1983): Determination of valproic acid in human serum by gas-

8. Davidson, J. P., and Sinn, J. (1978): Simultaneous quantitative assay of valproate sodium, trimethadione, and ethosuximide by GLC. *Clin. Chem.*, 24:991.
9. Degel, F., Heidrich, R., Schmid, R. D., and Weidemann, G. (1984): Quantitative determination of valproic acid by means of gas chromatographic headspace analysis. *Clin. Chim. Acta,* 139:29–36.
10. Farinotti, R., and Mahuzier, G. (1979): Simultaneous determination of six anticonvulsants in serum by high performance liquid chromatography. *J. Liq. Chromatog.*, 2:345–364.
11. Feinstein, H., Hovav, H., Fridlender, B., Inbar, D. and Buckler, R. T. (1982): Substrate-labeled fluorescent immunoassay (SLFIA) for valproic acid. *Clin. Chem.*, 28:1665.
12. Fredrick, D. L., Kelly, B. R., Fowler, M. W., and Altmiller, D. H. (1979): A rapid gas-liquid chromatographic analysis for valproic acid in serum. *Clin. Chem.*, 25:1118.
13. Freeman, D. J., and Rawal, N. (1980): Extraction of underivatized valproic acid from serum before gas chromatography. *Clin. Chem.*, 26:674–675.
14. Fullinfaw, R. O., and Marty, J. J. (1981): Gas chromatography of valproic acid, with benzyl alcohol as internal standard. *Clin. Chem.*, 27:1176.
15. Gast, B., and Thoma, G. (1979): Glc analysis of valproic acid using an extube extraction and on-column methylation. *Clin. Chem.*, 25:1118.
16. Goudie, J. H., Reed, K., Ayers, G. J., and Burnett, D. (1980): Improved extraction of valproic acid from serum before chromatography. *Clin. Chem.*, 26:1929.
17. Haidukewych, D. (1985): Fluorescence polarization immunoassay and enzyme immunoassay compared for free valproic acid in serum ultrafiltrates from epileptic patients. *Clin. Chem.*, 31:156.
18. Hamlin, C. R., and Sullivan, P. A. (1984): Adaption of EMIT reagents to the Cobas Bio Centrifigal Analyzer. *Clin. Chem.*, 30:314–315.
19. Higgins, T. N., (1983): Enzyme immunoassay of valproic acid using the Abbott ABA 200 analyzer. *Clin. Biochem.*, 16:222–223.
20. Hoffman, D. J., and Porter, W. R. (1983): Resolution of valproic acid from deutrated analogues and their quantitation in plasma using capillary gas chromotography. *J. Chromatog.*, 276:301–309.
21. Izutsu, A., Leung, D., Araps, C., Singh, P., Jaklitsch, A., and Kabakoff, D. S. (1979): Homogeneous enzyme immunoassay for valproic acid in serum. *Clin. Chem.*, 25:1093.
22. Kline, W. F., Enagonio, D. P., Reeder, D. J., and May, W. E. (1982): Liquid chromatographic determination of valproic acid in human serum. *J. Liq. Chromatog.*, 5:1697–1709.
23. Kulpmann, W. R. (1980): Eine gaschromatographische methode zur gleichzeitigen bestimmung von ethosuximid und valproinat im serum. *J. Clin. Chem. Chin. Biochem.*, 18:339–344.
24. Kumps, A., and Mardens, Y. (1980): Simplified simultaneous determination of valproic acid and

liquid chromatography on OV-17 using nitrogen specific detection. *J. Chromatog.*, 272:181–186.

ethosuximide by gas-chromatography. *Clin. Chem.,* 26:1759.

25. Kumps, A. H., Kumps-Grandjean, B., and Mardens, Y. (1981): Enzyme immunoassay and gas-liquid chromatography compared for determination of valproic acid in serum. *Clin. Chem.,* 27:1788–1789.

26. Kupferberg, H. J. (1982): Valproate: Chemistry and methods of determination. In: *Antiepileptic Drugs,* 2nd edition, edited by D. M. Woodbury, J. K. Penry, and C. E. Pippenger, pp. 549–555. Raven Press, New York.

27. Kushida, K., and Ishizaki, T. (1985): Concurrent determination of valproic acid with other antiepileptic drugs by high-performance chromatography. *J. Chromatog.,* 338:131–139.

28. Leroux, M., Budnik, D., Hall, K., Meek, J. I., Otten, N., and Seshia, S. (1981): Comparison of gas-liquid chromatography and EMIT assay for serum valproic acid. *Clin. Biochem.,* 14:87–90.

29. Lin, W., and Kelly, A. R. (1985): Determination of valproic acid in plasma or serum by solid-phase column extraction and gas-liquid chromatography. *Ther. Drug Monitor.,* 7:336–343.

30. Lingeman, H., Haan, H. B. P., and Hulshoff, A. (1984): Rapid and selective derivatization method for the nitrogen-sensitive detection of carboxylic acids in biological fluids prior to gas chromatographic analysis. *J. Chromatog.,* 326:241–248.

31. Manfredi, C., and Zinterhofer, L. (1982): Simplified gas chromatography of valproic acid and ethosuximide. *Clin. Chem.,* 28:246.

32. Moody, J. P., and Allan, S. M. (1983): Measurement of valproic acid in serum as the 4-bromophenacyl ester by high performance liquid chromatography. *Clin. Chim. Acta,* 127:263–269.

33. Morita, Y., Ruo T. I., Lee, M. L., and Atkinson Jr., A. J. (1981): On-column propylation method for measuring plasma valproate concentrations by gas chromatography. *Ther. Drug Monitor.,* 3:193–199.

34. Nakamura, M., Kondo, K., Nishioka, R., and Kawai, S. (1984): Improved procedure for the high performance liquid chromatographic determination of valproic acid in serum as its phenacyl ester. *J. Chromatog.,* 310:450–454.

35. Nishioka, R., Kawai, S., and Toyoda S. (1983): New method for the gas chromatographic determination of valproic acid in serum. *J. Chromatog.,* 277:356–360.

36. Nishioka, R., Takeuchi, M., Kawai, S., Nakamura, M., and Kondo, K. (1985): Improved direct injection method and extractive methylation method for the determination of valproic acid in serum by gas chromatography. *J. Chromatog.,* 342:89–96.

37. Odusote, K. A., and Sherwin, A. L. (1981): A simple, direct extraction method for gas-liquid determination of valproic acid in plasma. *Ther. Drug Monitor.,* 3:103–106.

38. Pena, M. I. A. (1981): Rapid gas chromatographic determination of valproic acid in serum. *J. Chromatog.,* 225:459–462.

39. Petrozolin, A. K., and Ponzo, J. L. (1982): An improved gas-chromatographic determination of valproic acid in serum. *Clin. Chem.,* 28:1588.

40. Puukka, M., and Puukka, R. (1980): A rapid and simple gas-liquid chromatographic determination of valproic acid (α-propyl-valeric acid) in serum. *J. Clin. Chem. Clin. Biochem.,* 18:497–499.

41. Rege, A. B., Lertpra, J. J. L., Whites, L. E., and George, W. J. (1984): Rapid analysis of valproic acid by gas chromatography. *J. Chromatog.,* 309:379–402.

42. Richard, L., Bugugnani, M. J., Fouye, H., and Batten J. (1985): Acide valproique, comparaison entre deux methodes de dosage immunoenzymologie et chromatographie liquide a haute performance. *Ann. Biol. Clin.,* 43:279–284.

43. Riva, R., Albani, F., and Baruzzi, A. (1982): Rapid and simple GLC determination of valproic acid and ethosuximide in plasma of epileptic patients. *J. Pharm. Sci.,* 71:110–111.

44. Sedman, A. J., Molitoris, B. A., Nakata, L. M., and Gal, J. (1986): Therapeutic drug monitoring in patients with chronic renal failures: Evaluation of the Abbott TDx Drug Assay System. *Am. J. Nephrol.,* 6:132–134.

45. Sengupta, A., and Peat, M. A. (1977): Gas-chromatography of eight anticonvulsant drugs in plasma. *J. Chromatog.,* 137:296–309.

46. Tosoni, S., Signorini, C., and Albertini, A. (1983): Gas-chromatographic determination of valproic acid in serum without derivatization. *Clin. Chem.,* 29:990.

47. van der Wal, S. J., Bannister, S. J., Dolan, J. W., and Snyder, L. R. (1980): Co-determination of ethosuximide and valproate in plasma by high performance liquid chromatography on the Technicon Fast-LC system. *Clin. Chem.,* 26:1006.

48. Vincon, G., Demontes-Mainard, F., Bistue, C., Jarry, C., Bracht-Liermain, A., and Albin, H. (1984): Dosages de la theophylline, du phenobarbital et de l'acide valproique par techniques chromatographiques et immunologigues: Comparaison de methodes. *Ann. Biol. Clin.,* 4:427–431.

49. Wu, A., Pearson, M. L., Mertens, S. K., Brett, D. D., and Wolffe, G. S. (1982): Gas chromatography of serum valproic acid, with methy-*m*-toluate as internal standard. *Clin. Chem.,* 28:544.

Antiepileptic Drugs, Third Edition, edited by
R. Levy, R. Mattson, B. Meldrum,
J. K. Penry, and F. E. Dreifuss.
Raven Press, Ltd., New York © 1989.

41

Valproate

Absorption, Distribution, and Excretion

René H. Levy and Danny D. Shen

INTRODUCTION

The branched chain fatty–acid structure of valproic acid (VPA) explains a number of characteristics which dominate its distribution in various body compartments, including the site of action (central nervous system) and organs of elimination (liver, kidney). Valproic acid is highly bound to plasma albumin and this property tends to keep most of the drug within the vascular compartment. As a fatty acid, VPA undergoes beta oxidation to a significant extent and its metabolism through that pathway is affected by the state of endogenous beta oxidation. Early on it was assumed that VPA, being lipophilic like the endogenous long chain fatty acids, readily permeates the blood-brain barrier. However, recent studies suggest that more complex physiologic mechanisms may be involved in the penetration of VPA into brain and cerebrospinal fluid. Those studies are covered in this chapter since they may contribute to an understanding of the neuropharmacologic mechanism of this drug.

Absorption

Early studies on the gastrointestinal absorption of VPA addressed the issue of absolute bioavailability (59,87). Absolute bioavailability was measured using blood-concentration data obtained after intravenous and oral administration. Despite differences in population (healthy volunteers versus epileptic patients) and formulation (oral solution, immediate release tablet, enteric-coated tablet), the absolute bioavailability of sodium VPA was consistently found to be close to unity. These findings can be explained by the fact that it crosses membranes readily and it is not subject to a first-pass effect. Although VPA has no inherent limits with respect to extent of absorption, the rate of absorption is, expectedly, dosage-form–dependent. In general, the rapid–release formulations, i.e., syrup (sodium salt), capsule (acid), and tablet (acid or sodium salt) were absorbed with peak times of less than 2 hr. Enteric-coated tablets that were developed to alleviate gastric discomfort exhibited variable absorption rates (4,10,41,53,57). Peak times ranged between 3 and 8 hr and the extent of absorption were not affected. In many instances, VPA did not appear in circulation until some hours after ingestion of enteric tablets. The delay in onset of absorption is probably due to the variable gastric emptying and dissolution rate of the enteric coating (which is pH dependent). Once absorption begins, the rate of rise of concentration is similar to that observed with rapid–release formulations (41,53,57). This behavior suggests that VPA is absorbed throughout the intestine with no site specificity. Slow–release formulations have also been evaluated in an attempt to reduce fluctuations in plasma valproate concentrations and to lower the frequency of drug intake to twice a day (52).

When gastrointestinal side effects occur, it is generally recommended that VPA be taken with food. The possible effects of food intake on the bioavailability of soft gelatin capsules were examined in healthy subjects, but no significant food effect was found (44).

The bioavailability of VPA administered rectally was examined to determine whether that route can be used in situations where oral administration is not possible (e.g., protracted vomiting, before and after surgery, status epilepticus) (20). In four children on valproate maintenance therapy, the oral capsule of valproic acid was replaced by rectally administered syrup. The steady-state plasma levels achieved by both treatments were comparable and it was concluded that rectal administration of commercially available syrup appears to be a satisfactory alternative to the oral route and that no adjustments in dosage are necessary.

In recent years, newer chemical forms of valproate have been introduced and bioavailability studies were conducted to assess bioequivalence. The calcium salt of valproate was considered because unlike the sodium salt, it is nonhygroscopic and can be dispensed in tablet form without special coatings (36). The bioavailability of calcium valproate tablet in comparison to a free acid capsule and to sodium salt syrup was evaluated in healthy subjects. There were no differences in any of the pharmacokinetic parameters measured. Another new chemical entity is sodium hydrogen divalproate. It quickly dissociates into valproic acid and sodium valproate in water. The bioavailability of sodium hydrogen divalproate enteric-coated tablets was compared to that of sodium valproate enteric-coated tablets in a single-dose, double-blind, crossover study (6). There was no statistically significant difference in area under the plasma concentration time curve or in elimination parameters. Absorption appeared to be slightly more rapid for the sodium hydrogen divalproate tablets.

Several studies have evaluated the amide of valproic acid, valpromide (dipropylacetamide), as a pro-drug for valproate. Valpromide is commercially available in several European countries. The diurnal variations in valproic acid plasma levels were compared in two groups of patients: 47 receiving sodium valproate and 42 receiving valpromide (93). The extent of fluctuations was significantly lower in patients on valpromide. This difference was attributed to slower absorption and slower elimination of valproic acid generated from valpromide. It was concluded that valpromide is a pro-drug or a delayed–release form of valproic acid (data presented in chapters 34 and 35 indicate that valpromide exhibits distinct properties with respect to interactions with carbamazepine-10,11-epoxide). The bioavailability of an enteric-coated valpromide tablet was compared to that of a valpromide oral solution by measuring the valproic acid released. The data were in turn compared to plasma concentrations of acid achieved after a standard valproic acid tablet (10). The fraction of valpromide dose biotransformed to the acid was 0.79 ± 0.24 for the tablet and 0.77 ± 0.12 for the solution. The amide could be detected only in three subjects who received the solution (concentrations in the range 2–14 µg/ml in the period 0.25–3 hr after administration). The fraction of valpromide dose metabolized to the acid was also measured after intravenous administration of single doses of both drugs to healthy subjects (9). This fraction, 0.81 ± 0.10, was comparable to that obtained after oral administration. This study also showed that pharmacokinetic properties of valpromide are quite distinct from those of the acid: valpromide has a much shorter elimination half-life (0.84 ± 0.33 hr), and a larger systemic clearance and volume of distribution. Interestingly, the bioavailability of valproic acid from valpromide appears to be increased by food (92).

DISTRIBUTION

Plasma Protein Binding

The plasma protein binding of valproate has been extensively examined by several investigators. Early studies established the fact that valproate is extensively bound (~90%) in human plasma at therapeutic concentrations (59). Recently several facets of valproate plasma binding have been investigated in more detail.

The recent availability of commercial ultrafiltration devices for routine monitoring of unbound drug concentrations has stimulated research into methodological aspects of valproate unbound fraction determination (58). Incubation of plasma and serum samples at 37° is associated with an increase in free fatty-acid concentration and a concomitant increase in unbound fraction (3). This phenomenon is temperature- and time-dependent and may lead to overestimation of unbound fraction by methods that require long incubations (equilibrium dialysis). Other factors that may affect the determination of unbound fraction include pH, type of buffer (1), and nature of anticoagulant (110).

Earlier estimates of valproate binding parameters to albumin (59) were confirmed by more recent studies. Yu (114) reported the following values from the sera of epileptic children: equilibrium (dissociation) constant = 2.00×10^{-4}M; total concentration of binding sites = 1.45×10^{-3} mole/liter; number of binding sites per mole of albumin = 2.48 (114). Since the therapeutic plasma concentration of VPA approaches the dis-

sociation constant for the valproate/albumin complex, the serum free fraction of VPA is expected to vary with total drug concentration. Several clinical studies have focused on the concentration dependence of valproate binding in serum. In a group of 25 adult patients on valproate monotherapy with normal albumin concentration, Cramer et al. (25) found that the relationship between unbound and total concentration could be fitted to a second-degree polynomial equation. Average unbound fraction ranged between 7% and 9% at total concentrations below 75 mg/ml and increased to 15% at 100 mg/ml, 22% at 125 mg/ml, and 30% at 150 mg/ml. Similar nonlinearity in valproate plasma binding was also documented in several series of studies in epileptic children (101,114).

A number of studies have compared the degree of fluctuation of total and unbound valproate concentrations at steady state (12,13,69,100–102). A consistent finding emerges: fluctuations in unbound concentration were generally twice as large as in total concentrations. Several factors were proposed to explain this phenomenon: concentration-dependence of binding, elevated free fatty–acid levels in early morning samples, and true diurnal differences in unbound and total clearance. The question of whether unbound rather than total valproate concentrations should be monitored was raised by several authors. A definitive assessment of the clinical relevance of monitoring unbound valproate concentration requires prospective clinical trials (61). Since this information is not available, the issue remains unresolved.

The plasma protein binding of valproate explains its distribution in several other body fluids as well as in the fetus during pregnancy. These aspects are considered in the next section.

Central Nervous System

Valproic acid enters the brain and cerebrospinal fluid (CSF) rapidly. Tissue distribution studies in mice and rats (45,63) showed that peak concentration in brain was reached within minutes after either intravenous or intraperitoneal injection of VPA. The subsequent decline of drug concentration in brain paralleled that in plasma, indicating a facile equilibration of VPA between brain and capillary blood. In rhesus monkeys equipped with a chronically implanted ventricular catheter, the upswing and decline of VPA in CSF followed closely the time course of plasma concentration during and after the cessation of intravenous VPA infusion (55,60). A reasonably rapid penetration of VPA into brain also occurs in man as evidenced by the successful treatment of status epilepticus with single-dose oral or rectal administration of VPA (103,109,112).

Much of the existing information on the extent of VPA distribution into the human brain is obtained indirectly through CSF sampling studies. Cerebrospinal fluid data from the various literature sources are presented in Table 1. In general, a good correlation was observed between CSF and total plasma concentration of VPA. The CSF-to-total plasma concentration ratio averaged about 0.1 to 0.15, with notable variation between subjects within any given study. Valproate concentration in CSF also correlated well with free drug concentration in plasma. Except for the one recent report by Löscher et al. (66), in adult patients CSF concentration was found to almost equal the free plasma concentration of VPA. The study of Löscher et al. (66) was conducted in a group of epileptic children ranging in age from 5 months to 11 years. Their data showed that VPA concentration in CSF was consistently lower than the free drug concentration in plasma. The mean CSF-to-free plasma concentration ratio was 0.67 ± 0.20. The reason for the discrepancy between the results of this and the other studies is not clear, although the obvious difference in the age of the subjects may be one explanation. It is interesting to note that in rhesus mon-

keys the CSF concentration of VPA was found to be less than half of plasma free concentration (55).

The only available data on VPA concentration in brain tissue are from the biopsy study of Vajda et al. (111) in a group of neurosurgical patients undergoing brain tumor resection. Prior to surgery, the patients were placed on 1,200 to 1,600 mg of VPA per day for at least 3 days. The brain concentrations were found to be relatively low, varying from 6.8% to 27.8% of total plasma levels and were comparable to levels observed in simultaneously sampled CSF. Thus, unlike many of the aromatic or heterocyclic antiepileptics such as phenytoin and phenobarbital which typically exhibit brain-to-CSF concentration ratios well exceeding unity, VPA does not appear to concentrate in brain tissue. Goldberg and Todoroff (37) have, in fact, reported that VPA does not exhibit binding to rabbit brain homogenates or subcellular fractions of brain tissue.

The transport mechanism of VPA across the blood-brain and blood-CSF barriers has been the subject of a number of recent investigations. It was recognized very early on (31,55) that VPA, being a relatively strong carboxylic acid ($pK_a = 4.56$), is present in predominantly ionized form (>99%) at physiological pH. Therefore, the rather rapid brain uptake of VPA was a surprising observation in view of the classic pH-partition hypothesis, which assumes that only nonionized drugs can diffuse across lipoidal capillary membranes. In fact, Löscher and Frey (64) showed in an anesthetized dog preparation that the penetration of VPA into the CSF is more rapid than other less acidic anticonvulsants with either comparable or slightly higher organic solvent/buffer partition ratios (e.g., phenytoin, phenobarbital, and primidone). To explain these exceptional findings, the existence of a carrier-mediated transport mechanism for VPA was postulated.

The earliest evidence in favor of a carrier

Table 1. *Distribution of valproic acid between plasma and cerebrospinal fluid*

Population	VPA regimen	CSF:plasma total (%)	% Free in plasma	CSF:plasma free	Reference
Adult epileptic patients (N = 22)	long-term	~10	~10	~1	(40)
Adult neurosurgery patients (N = 5)	1,200–1,600 mg/day × 3 + day	17.1 ± 7.9[a]	ND	ND	(111)
Adult nonepileptic patients	Single 1,000 mg	8.9 ± 2.1	8.6 ± 1.8	1.05 ± 0.17	(42)
Adult patients/ myelography or cisternography (N = 17)	30 mg/kg @ 20 and 15 mg/kg @ 2 hr prior	10–22[b]	3.3–25.6(ED)[c] 5.9–2.40(UF)[d]	0.77–1.7(ED) 0.61–2.0(UF)	(97)
Epileptic children/age 5 mo–11 yr (N = 8)	4 days–1 yr	8.9 (5.4–11.4)[b]	14.0 (8.9–22.0)	0.67 (0.45–1.02)	(66)

[a] Mean ± standard deviation.
[b] Range.
[c] ED, equilibrium dialysis.
[d] UF, ultrafiltration.

system mediating the passage of VPA across the blood-brain barrier (BBB) was provided by Frey and Löscher (31). These investigators found that pretreatment with probenecid, which is known to inhibit the active transport of anionic drugs and acidic metabolites of biogenic amines out of the brain, led to an increase in steady-state valproate CSF-to-serum concentration ratio by about 40% during intravenous infusion of VPA in dogs. It has also been reported that in mice and rats VPA treatment elevated cerebral concentration of 5-hydroxyindoleacetic acid (5-HIAA) and homovanillic acid (HVA), probably due to inhibition of their active transport out of brain and CSF (48,67). Therefore, existing evidence suggests that VPA utilizes the same active transport system for the removal of acidic metabolites of monoamines from the central nervous system (CNS).

Although much is known about the brain efflux characteristics of VPA, its exact mode of entry into brain is unclear. There are data suggesting that the uptake rate of VPA into rat brain is saturable. For example, in the early dog experiments of Frey and Löscher (31) a markedly slower rate of entry of VPA into CSF was observed when serum drug concentration was increased from 40–75 µg/ml to over 200 µg/ml. In a recent single-dose–response study in rats, Pollack and Shen (96) found that whole-brain concentration of VPA did not increase proportionately with valproate serum concentration (at 15 min after intravenous drug administration) or dose. Brain-to-serum concentration ratio decreased from about 0.13 to as low as 0.05 when the serum concentration of VPA was increased beyond 300 µg/ml. These observations have given rise to speculation that the uptake of VPA into brain occurs by way of a selective transport system. Using the tissue-sampling, single-injection method (i.e., the Oldendorf technique), Cornford (22) showed that VPA administration did not affect the Brain Uptake Index (BUI) of lactate in rats.

These investigators also failed to observe saturation in valproate uptake at 100 µg/ml injectate concentration. It would appear that the so-called "monocarboxylic acid" carrier system, which is responsible for the uptake of endogenous short-chain fatty acids and ketone bodies, is not involved in the transport of VPA. Future work should be directed toward identification of the putative VPA transporter at the BBB.

One other important aspect of the BBB transport mechanism is the effect of plasma protein binding on the uptake of VPA. The classic notion that drug molecules bound to plasma proteins and blood cells do not diffuse readily across the capillary endothelium appears to hold true in the blood-to-brain distribution behavior of a number of anticonvulsants. This is usually evidenced by equal (nonionized) drug concentration in plasma water and CSF at steady-state. Although the earlier clinical studies reported similar CSF and free plasma concentrations, the realization that VPA is normally present largely in ionized form in body fluids would militate against such a simplistic interpretation of the effect of plasma protein binding on valproate distribution across the BBB. The influence of serum protein binding on the unidirectional blood-to-brain transport of VPA was investigated by Cornford et al. (23). The single-pass extraction of VPA in saline by the adult rat brain was estimated to be 43.4%. Extraction in the presence of 90% human serum was lowered to 18.6%, indicating that serum binding does limit the permeation of VPA across the brain capillary. However, the attenuation in extraction is much less than would be expected if protein-bound drug were completely excluded from the uptake process. Equilibrium dialysis measurement indicated a free fraction of only 9% in the serum injectate, which yields a predicted extraction of 3.9% (i.e., 43.4% × 0.09). Hence, approximately 14.7% (i.e., 18.6% minus 3.9%) of the drug extracted into the brain was derived from serum protein-bound VPA that entered the capillary. It was also shown that although brain extrac-

tion increased with increasing serum concentration of VPA as a result of saturation in serum drug binding, the extraction of the bound moiety remained constant.

The mechanism by which protein-bound drug is released for uptake across the capillary endothelium is not understood (see the review by Cornford and Oldendorf [24] for a discussion of current hypotheses in this area). Furthermore, the dynamics of interaction between the debinding of drug from plasma protein binding sites and drug association with the putative transport carrier need to be delineated. Cornford et al. (23) also observed that the kinetic rate constant for the efflux of VPA from rat brain exceeded the rate constant for uptake into the brain. The asymmetric permeability of VPA across the BBB is consistent with the involvement of separate transport systems for the influx and efflux of VPA in the CNS. It could also explain the earlier observations of a lower CSF valproate concentration relative to plasma free concentration in the monkey (55) and in epileptic children (66).

Aside from the obvious need for studies relating to the brain distribution of VPA, considerable attention has recently been focused on the CNS uptake and accumulation of valproate metabolites, several of which exhibit anticonvulsant activity in rodent seizure models (80). The reason for the interest in valproate metabolites relates to the question of whether the pharmacologically active metabolites contribute significantly to the antiepileptic action of VPA. Much of the work in this area dealt with the CNS kinetics of the mono-unsaturated metabolite Δ^2-VPA. In epileptic patients receiving VPA, the 2-desaturated compound is the predominant oxidative metabolite in circulation. Pharmacokinetic studies in normal volunteers (95) and a pregnant epileptic mother (82) indicated that Δ^2-VPA has a longer plasma half-life than the parent drug. Moreover, Nau and Löscher (79) have shown that in mice the clearance rate of Δ^2-VPA from brain tissue is much slower than that of VPA after single-dose intraperitoneal drug administration. A follow-up sub-chronic VPA treatment study in rats further revealed a slow accumulation of the Δ^2-metabolite in select regions of the brain, namely, in the substantia nigra, superior and inferior colliculus, hippocampus, and medulla (65). The possibility of a protracted build-up of pharmacologically active metabolites in brain is an appealing concept in that it may provide a ready explanation for the well-recognized slow reversibility of the anticonvulsant effect of VPA after prolonged drug treatment (18,62). However, the results of a recent CSF study in epileptic children (66) as well as preliminary findings from a brain biopsy study in neurological patients from the authors' laboratory (*unpublished data*) indicate that Δ^2-VPA is present at exceedingly low concentrations in human brain and CSF. The mean CSF concentration of Δ^2-VPA in epileptic children was reported to be 1.7% that of VPA, ranging from as low as <0.1% to a high of 2.7%. Löscher et al. (66) also noted that the CSF-to-plasma concentration did not vary with the duration of VPA treatment (from 4 days to 1 year). These investigators concluded that the relatively low metabolite concentration reached in CSF casts doubt on the possibility that Δ^2-VPA plays a significant role in the antiepileptic efficacy of VPA. These observations do not, however, rule out the possibility that other unidentified metabolites may be involved or that accumulation of Δ^2-VPA (or other active species) is confined to certain critical human brain areas.

Other Aspects

Whole-body autoradiograms of a pregnant squirrel monkey taken following short intravenous infusions of ^{14}C-VPA showed that the labeled drug crossed the placental barrier freely (107). More recent studies have shown that valproate concentration is 1.5 to 2 times higher in umbilical cord serum than in maternal serum (32,77,81,91). Several investigators examined the possible contribution of protein binding to this phenomenon and consistently found that the unbound fraction of valproate is lower in umbilical cord serum than in maternal serum: 9.1% versus 15% (33), 6% versus 12% (2). A more detailed study of the phenomenon was performed by Nau and Krauer (78). In fetal serum, unbound fractions were 40% to 80% during weeks 13 through 16 of gestation, decreased to 20% around week 20, and continued to decrease to 10% at the end of gestation. This behavior of unbound fraction was explained by the time course of albumin concentrations in fetal serum which increased from 3 to 12 g/liter during early gestation to 30 to 40 g/liter at term. Maternal unbound fractions, on the other hand, increased during pregnancy from 10% to 20%. While the extent of serum protein binding is higher in fetus than in mother at term, the opposite is true during gestation (78). Another study examined the mechanism of impaired serum protein binding in pregnancy and found a significant negative correlation between unbound fraction and albumin level (99).

Consistent with earlier work (29), the concentration of valproate in breast milk was found to be 5% to 10% of the maternal serum concentration (91). The extent of plasma protein binding also explains the relatively low concentrations of valproate in saliva (41,75) and tears (74,75). However, only tears give values which could be used as quantitative indicators of unbound concentration in serum. Expectedly, the plasma protein binding of valproate can be competitively reduced by other drugs bound to albumin. Such is the case for salicylates (30) and naproxen (39). A similar effect is found in the case of endogenous fatty acids (15,86). An elevation in free fatty acid level also explained the decrease in protein binding found in the sera of patients with insulin-dependent diabetes mellitus (35). The extent of plasma protein binding controls partition of valproate in red blood cells. One study has shown that the decrease in plasma protein binding found in patients with renal or hepatic disease is associated with a concomitant increase in red blood cell partitioning (108). Thus red blood cell concentration correlates with unbound concentration in plasma.

ELIMINATION

Clearance

It has long been recognized that the level-dose relationship for VPA is highly variable between patients. Results from therapeutic monitoring studies (11,72,104) have shown that at a given daily dose of VPA the plasma drug level could vary as much as six– to eightfold among individual patients. A recent analysis of the literature (56) indicated that the interpatient variation in valproate level-to-dose ratio largely reflects variability in the clearance characteristics of the drug.

Valproic acid is eliminated almost exclusively by hepatic metabolism (>96% of administered dose). The reported plasma (or metabolic) clearance in healthy volunteers (Table 2) is in the range of 6 to 11 ml/hr/kg. Using a blood-to-plasma VPA concentration ratio of 0.28 (53), the clearance of valproate from whole blood was calculated to range from 25 to 46 ml/min for a 70-kg person. This range of blood clearance represents only a small fraction (≤ 0.03) of the average hepatic blood flow (1,500 ml/min). Thus, VPA may be classified as a low extraction drug with a clearance independent of blood flow (see Chapter 1). Furthermore, since the free fraction of VPA in plasma ($\approx$ 0.05 to 0.1) is larger than the extraction ratio ($E \leq 0.03$), valproate clearance is of the restrictive type and only unbound VPA is cleared (113). Consequently, factors affecting drug plasma protein binding and hepatic drug-metabolizing enzyme activities (presumably those of mitochondrial beta oxidation and microsomal cytochrome P-450 systems) will be important determinants of valproate clearance. A review of the relevant factors is presented in the following sections.

Concomitant Antiepileptic Medications

Valproic acid clearance is typically higher in adult epileptic patients than in healthy volunteers (Table 2). The increase in clearance is generally attributed to induction of liver drug-metabolizing enzymes caused by concurrent antiepileptic medications (11,46,51,71,73,88,98). An approximate 40% to 80% increase in valproate clearance was also observed in epileptic children receiving multiple antiepileptic medications as compared to children on VPA monotherapy (Table 3). The increase in VPA clearance as reflected by a decrease in steady-state plasma drug concentration has been seen in patients on a variety of antiepileptic drugs, including phenobarbital, phenytoin, carbamazepine, or a combination thereof. Thus, higher doses of VPA may be required to maintain therapeutic concentrations in patients receiving polytherapy. Some reports indicate that in some patients these interactions are so pronounced that therapeutic levels of VPA cannot be achieved (46,50).

Development

Physiologic changes occurring during childhood development are known to affect the disposition of many antiepileptic drugs (27,76). A compilation from available literature of data on valproate pharmacokinetics in pediatric patients (Table 3) revealed marked changes in drug clearance throughout the early stages of development.

Valproic acid is not used routinely in the treatment of neonatal seizures, therefore pharmacokinetic data on newborns are scanty. Most of the literature reports were anecdotal observations in infants exposed to VPA *in utero*, which do not provide

Table 2. *Pharmacokinetic parameters of VPA in adult volunteers and epileptic patients*

Populations	Study	VPA regime	AED therapy	(V_d) area[a] liters/kg	T_{1/2β} (hr)	Free fraction[b]	Clearance (ml/hr/kg)[a] Total	Free
Healthy adults (16–60 yr)								
	Various sources[c]	Single dose: 400–800 mg p.o. or i.v.	None	0.12–0.23[d]	12.0–15.8[d]	—	7–11[d]	—
	Perucca et al.[e,f] (89) N = 6	Single dose: 800 mg p.o.	None	0.14 ± 0.02	13.0 ± 2.4	6.6 ± 1.2	7.7 ± 1.5	127 ± 29
	Bialer et al.[e] (7,8) N = 6	Single dose: 1,000 mg p.o.	None	0.14 ± 0.02	14.9 ± 2.4	4.1 ± 1.2	6.7 ± 1.4	170 ± 46
	Gugler et al. (41) N = 6	Steady state: 1,200 mg/day	None	0.15 ± 0.02	15.9 ± 2.6	—	6.4 ± 1.1	—
	Bowdle et al. (14) N = 6	Steady state: 500 mg/day 1,000 mg/day 1,500 mg/day	None	0.13 ± 0.02 0.15 ± 0.04 0.18 ± 0.03	13.6 ± 2.8 13.9 ± 3.4 14.5 ± 4.3	6.4 ± 2.1 9.8 ± 3.1 9.1 ± 0.7	6.7 ± 1.3 6.7 ± 1.5 8.2 ± 1.6	89 ± 71 72 ± 21 91 ± 18
	Bauer et al.[b] (12) N = 6	Steady state 500 mg/day[g]: morning evening	None	— —	— —	6.4 ± 0.8 6.1 ± 1.3	6.7 ± 0.9 7.4 ± 1.0	106 ± 19 123 ± 18
Epileptic adults (16–60 yr)								
	Perucca et al. (88) N = 6	Single dose: 800 mg i.v. 800 mg p.o.	Polytherapy	0.18 ± 0.03 0.18 ± 0.03	9.0 ± 1.4 9.0 ± 1.2	— —	15.1 ± 5.8 17.6 ± 2.8	— —
	Schapel et al. (105) N = 17	Single dose: 600 mg p.o.	Polytherapy	0.19 ± 0.09	9.3 ± 2.0	—	14.8 ± 5.8	—
	Hoffmann et al. (47) N = 6	Steady state	Polytherapy	0.14 ± 0.03	5.2 ± 2.7	—	14.7 ± 8.0	—
	Eadie et al. (28) N = 8	Steady state	Polytherapy	0.19 ± 0.05	8.5 ± 3.3	—	18.1 ± 10.8	—
Healthy elderly (>60 yr)								
	Perucca et al.[f] (89) N = 6	Single dose: 800 mg p.o.	None	0.16 ± 0.02	15.3 ± 1.7	9.5 ± 1.4	7.5 ± 2.2	78 ± 15
	Bauer et al. (13) N = 6	Steady state 500 mg/day[g]: morning evening	None	— —	— —	10.7 ± 1.6 9.7 ± 1.1	6.6 ± 0.5 7.3 ± 0.7	64 ± 12 75 ± 11

[a] In the calculation of (V_d)_area and clearance following oral administration, complete absorption is assumed.
[b] Since plasma protein binding of VPA is saturable, free fraction of VPA varies with the change in total plasma drug concentration over time. Therefore, an average free fraction based on the ratio of free AUC to total AUC is calculated.
[c] Literature reports on single dose pharmacokinetics of VPA in healthy adult volunteers are too numerous to be individually listed in this table (see Levy and Lai, ref. 59, for a summary of much of the early literature). There is generally good agreement between studies, therefore only a summary is presented here. The only references listed individually are those single-dose studies that provide free drug measurements and steady-state studies.
[d] Range of mean estimates.
[e] Free drug concentration measurements were provided in these single-dose studies, thereby allowing the calculation of free drug clearance.
[f] Control data in young adults to be compared with the data in elderly subjects listed below.
[g] Diurnal variation in VPA clearance was examined. Morning and evening doses were administered at 8 a.m. and 8 p.m.

Table 3. Pharmacokinetic parameters for VPA in pediatric patients[a]

Age group	Study	VPA regime	Antiepileptic drug therapy	$(V_d)_{area}$[a] liters/kg	$T_{1/2\beta}$ (hr)	Free fraction %	Clearance (ml/hr/kg) Total	Free
Neonates (0–2 mo)								
	Brachet-Lierman and Demarquez (16); 5 newborns (3 days)	Single dose: 100 mg/kg	None	0.43	40 ± 21	—	18.0	—
	Irvine-Meek et al. (49); 1 neonate (24 days)	Single dose: 7.5 mg/kg	Polytherapy	0.28	17.2	—	10.8	—
	Gal et al. (34); 6 neonates	Steady state	Polytherapy	0.39 ± 0.04	26.4 ± 16.1	13.1 ± 1.9[b]	14.4 ± 9.3	109 ± 96
Infants (2–36 mo)								
	Hall et al. (43)	Steady state	Monotherapy N = 5	0.22 ± 0.05	8.4 ± 2.1	—	19.6 ± 8.2	—
			Polytherapy N = 9	0.28 ± 0.07	5.9 ± 2.1	—	35.6 ± 10.5	—
Children (3–16 yr)								
	Farrell et al. (30) N = 4	Steady state	Monotherapy	—	—	12.0 ± 0.02[c]	17.5 ± 5.4	130 ± 40
	Chiba et al. (19)	Steady state	Monotherapy N = 21	0.22 ± 0.05	12.3 ± 3.1	—	13.0 ± 4.7	—
			Polytherapy N = 16	0.30 ± 0.10	9.4 ± 2.9	—	23.5 ± 6.6	—
	Schobben et al. (106) N = 6	Steady state	Polytherapy	0.25 ± 0.10	9.4 ± 1.4	—	19.1 ± 9.8	—
	Cloyd et al. (21) N = 25	Steady state	Polytherapy	0.26 ± 0.09	7.2 ± 2.3	—	27.2 ± 15.3	—
	Otten et al. (85) N = 4	Steady state	Polytherapy	0.18 ± 0.04	7.2 ± 2.0	9.9 ± 4.8[b]	18.5 ± 4.9	228 ± 151
	Hall et al. (43)	Steady state	Monotherapy N = 8	0.18 ± 0.04	8.6 ± 1.4	—	14.3 ± 4.3	—
			Polytherapy N = 23	0.20 ± 0.05	7.4 ± 2.4	—	20.6 ± 7.8	—

[a] Data are presented as mean ± standard deviation.
[b] Area averaged free fraction.
[c] Plasma free fraction at a total plasma level of 70–85 µg/ml.

clearance estimates (5,16,26,81,94). Gal et al. (34) recently reported a prospective study of valproate efficacy and pharmacokinetics in six neonates with intractable seizures. Valproic acid was added to an existing regimen of anticonvulsants (mainly phenobarbital). Valproate clearance kinetics were studied at steady state. Although highly variable, the steady-state clearance per kilogram of body weight for total drug in serum was within the range of values reported for adult epileptic patients receiving multiple anticonvulsants. The estimates were also consistent with results from two earlier case studies (16,49). The free fractions of VPA in neonatal serum tended to be higher than those reported for adult serum at comparable drug levels (an area average free fraction of 14.4% ± 9.3% in the neonates versus <10% in adults). Consequently, clearance for unbound VPA was in the low range of expected values for adult epileptics, suggesting that the intrinsic metabolic clearance of VPA may be low due to immature drug-metabolizing enzyme activities.

In infants beyond 2 months of age a remarkable increase in valproate clearance, presumably reflecting maturation in drug-metabolizing function, is observed. Data from the study by Hall et al. (43) showed that within the age group of 3 to 36 months, clearance values exceeding 30 ml/min/kg are often observed in polytherapy patients. In such patients, daily dosages much higher than the usually recommended range of 15 to 30 mg/kg/day would be required to achieve plasma VPA levels above the minimum therapeutic concentration of 50 μg/ml.

Ample data are available on valproate clearance in school-age children (3–16 years). Overall, the mean clearance estimates from a number of studies (see Table 3) are in the range of 13 to 18 ml/hr/kg and 19 to 27 ml/hr/kg for monotherapy and polytherapy patients, respectively. These estimates are intermediate between those reported for the infants and young adults. It appears that valproate clearance normalized to per kilogram of body weight begins to decline after infancy and continues on throughout childhood, reaching adult values by adolescence. This pattern of change in clearance relative to body weight over the first decade of life is similar to the general trend observed with other antiepileptic drugs, such as phenytoin and phenobarbital (27). These changes have been attributed to the development of cytochrome P-450–mediated drug metabolism in the liver.

Aging

The pharmacokinetics of VPA in elderly subjects have been studied by several groups of investigators (13,17,89). Both Perucca et al. (89) and Bauer et al. (13) reported that the clearance kinetics of total VPA in serum did not appear to differ between the young and elderly volunteers (Table 2). However, a decrease in serum protein binding of VPA associated with hypoalbuminemia was observed in the elderly group. Consequently, the mean clearance of free drug was 40% lower in the elderly adults than in the young control subjects. This decrease in free drug clearance is consistent with the generally recognized age-related decline in hepatic function, notably with respect to oxidative drug metabolism (38). The results of these studies suggest that monitoring free rather than total serum VPA concentration may be more meaningful in elderly patients.

Pregnancy

A longitudinal study of valproate pharmacokinetics during pregnancy has not been carried out. Anecdotal evidence indicates that alteration in VPA clearance may be observed during pregnancy and after parturition. Plasse et al. (94) reported the level-to-dose ratio of VPA in one pregnant mother. The level-to-dose ratio began to decline in the latter part of the second trimester and continued through the early part of the third trimester, finally reaching nadir within 3 weeks of delivery. Following parturition, valproate level rose rapidly and regained prepregnancy values within 2 to 3 weeks. In a review article, Philbert and Dam (90) cited similar experience in five pregnant patients. At least part of the reason for the apparent increase in clearance during late gestation is a decrease in maternal serum protein binding of VPA as a result of elevated nonesterified fatty acid and hypoalbuminemia (78). The question remains whether there is an actual change in the intrinsic metabolic clearance of VPA during pregnancy.

Disease States

Orr et al. (84) reported the disposition kinetics of VPA in a 9-year-old uremic epileptic child. Total serum clearance was 23.6 ml/hr/kg after the first dose and increased to 40.8 ml/hr/kg after 5 months of therapy. The observed steady-state clearance is higher than reported estimates in polytherapy patients of comparable age (19–28 ml/hr/kg). Serum free fractions were higher than normal, at 22.4% and 27.2%, respectively, for the single-dose and steady-state studies. The corresponding free serum clearances of VPA were calculated to be 149 and 152 ml/hr/kg, which are in line with estimates for children with normal renal function. Thus, the primary effect of uremia is a decrease in serum protein binding resulting in an apparent increase in total drug clearance. Since free drug clearance and, therefore, the average free drug concentration at steady state is not altered, adjustment in valproate dosage may not be necessary in uremic patients. It is also worth noting that only a limited fraction of the valproate dose (<20%) is removed by either hemodialysis (68) or peritoneal dialysis (84).

Therefore, dialysis is not an effective means of detoxification in VPA overdose; neither would there be any need to supplement the valproate dose in renal-failure patients who receive maintenance dialysis treatment.

Valproate pharmacokinetics have also been studied in patients with alcoholic liver cirrhosis and in patients recovering from acute hepatitis (54). Valproate free fraction in serum was increased by more than twofold in patients with liver disease. However, the clearance of VPA was not significantly different from that in healthy volunteers because valproate intrinsic clearance (reflecting drug-metabolizing activity) was also reduced, presumably as a consequence of hepatocellular damage. Thus, hepatic disease causes two opposing effects resulting in no apparent change in total clearance. Accordingly, total serum-valproate levels at steady state would not change, whereas valproate free levels would be increased in such a situation (see Chapter 1).

Dose Dependency

During long-term drug administration a nonlinear relationship between plasma valproate level and dose has been noted in a number of studies (11,26,40,50,79,81,109). Above a daily dose of 500 mg/kg, the steady-state plasma concentration of VPA increased *less* than proportionately with an increase in dose (i.e., a convex plot of concentration versus dose).

The mechanism of nonlinearity in VPA clearance was examined in a multiple-dose study in healthy volunteers (14). Each volunteer received 500, 1,000, and 1,500 mg/day in three consecutive steps. The nonlinearity in clearance was attributed principally to an increase in free fraction (as VPA concentration increases). The hypothesis that increases in free fraction lead to increases in plasma clearance of VPA explains why the nonlinearity in the level-dose relationship is of a convex nature (see Fig. 3 in Chapter 1).

Half-Life

The reported elimination half-life ($T_{1/2\beta}$) of VPA in healthy adult volunteers ranged from 12 to 16 hr (Table 2). The half-life of VPA is typically shorter in epileptic patients, which is attributable to induction of valproate metabolism by other antiepileptic drugs. The mean half-life in epileptic adults is around 9 hr (Table 2). However, elimination half-life as short as 5 hr has been documented (47). The relatively short half-life of VPA explains (at least in part) the frequently observed fluctuation in valproate levels during long-term therapy.

Pronounced changes in valproate half-life were observed during the postnatal period (Table 3). Within the first 10 days after birth, half-lives ranging between 10 and 67 hr have been observed (16). Longer half-lives appeared to be associated with low birth weight (<3,000 g) and prematurity. Between the ages of 10 days and 2 months, the half-life of VPA declines rapidly, reflecting both maturation in drug-metabolizing activity and a decrease in extravascular distribution volume. During middle and late infancy, at a time when serum clearance of VPA exceeds adult capacity, mean elimination half-lives of 8.4 ± 2.1 hr and 5.9 ± 2.1 hr have been reported for monotherapy and polytherapy patients, respectively (43). The elimination half-life of VPA begins to assume adult values during the early years of childhood. The observed half-lives in school-age children and young adolescents are well within the range of adult values (see Table 3).

The elimination half-life of VPA during long-term valproate treatment in one uremic child was reported to be 10.2 hr (84), which agrees with expected values for epileptic children of this age. The rise in serum free fraction induced by uremia had no apparent effect on half-life, since there was a comparable increase in both clearance and apparent volume of distribution.

The half-lives of VPA in patients with liver diseases have also been determined. The mean half-life in seven patients with alcoholic cirrhosis was 18.9 ± 5.1 hr, and in patients recovering from acute hepatitis it was 17.0 ± 3.7 hr (54). Again, the increase in serum valproate free fraction associated with liver dysfunction alone is not expected to have any effect on half-life of the drug. The prolongation in half-life is more a reflection of the decrease in intrinsic metabolic clearance of VPA in hepatic diseases.

Urinary Excretion

Renal clearance represents a very minor route of elimination for VPA. The mean fraction of dose of VPA excreted unchanged in urine was 1.8% after a single dose and 3.2% at steady-state in six healthy volunteers (41). The renal clearance of free VPA (2–4 ml/min) is very small relative to glomerular filtration rate, suggesting that VPA is significantly reabsorbed in the renal tubule.

REFERENCES

1. Albani, F., Riva, R., Contin, M., and Baruzzi, A. (1984): Valproic acid binding to human serum albumin and human plasma: Effects of pH variation and buffer composition in equilibrium dialysis. *Ther. Drug Monit.*, 6:331–333.
2. Albani, R., Riva, R., Contin, M., Baruzzi, A., Altomare, M., Merlini, G. P., and Perucca, E. (1984): Differential transplacental binding of valproic acid: Influence of free fatty acids. *Br. J. Clin. Pharmac.*, 17:759–762.
3. Albani, F., Riva, R., Procaccianti, G., Baruzzi, A., and Perucca, E. (1983): Free fraction of valproic acid: *In vitro* time-dependent increase and correlation with free fatty acid concentration in human plasma and serum. *Epilepsia*, 24:65–73.
4. Albright, P. S., Bruni, J., and Suria, D. (1984): Pharmacokinetics of enteric-coated valproic acid. *Ther. Drug Monit.*, 6:21–23.
5. Alexander, F. W. (1979): Sodium valproate and pregnancy. *Arch. Dis. Child.*, (*Correspondence*) 54:240–245.
6. Anderson, P., and Elwin, C.-E. (1985): Single-dose kinetics and bioavailability of sodium-hydrogen divalproate. *Clin. Neuropharmacol.*, 8:156–164.

7. Bialer, M., Hussein, Z., Dubrovsky, J., Raz, I., and Abramsky, O. (1984): Pharmacokinetics of valproic acid obtained after administration of three oral formulations to humans. *Isr. J. Med. Sci.*, 20:46–49.

8. Bialer, M., Hussein, Z., Raz, I., Abramsky, O., Herishanu, Y., and Pachys, F. (1985): Pharmacokinetics of valproic acid in volunteers after a single dose study. *Biopharm. Drug Disp.*, 6:33–42.

9. Bialer, M., Rubinstein, A., Dubrovsky, J., Raz, I., and Abramsky, O. (1985): A comparative pharmacokinetic study of valpromide and valproic acid after intravenous administration in humans. *Int. J. Pharmaceut.*, 23:25–33.

10. Bialer, M., Rubinstein, A., Raz, I., and Abramsky, O. (1984): Pharmacokinetics of valpromide after oral administration of a solution and a tablet to healthy volunteers. *Eur. J. Clin. Pharmacol.*, 27:501–503.

11. Baruzzi, B., Bondo, B., Bossi, L., Castelli, D., Gerna, M., Tognoni, G., and Zagnoni, P. (1977): Plasma levels of di-*n*-propylacetate and clonazepam in epileptic patients. *Int. J. Clin. Pharmacol.*, 15:403–408.

12. Bauer, L. A., Davis, R., Wilensky, A., Raisys, V., and Levy, R. H. (1984): Diurnal variation in valproic acid clearance. *Clin. Pharmacol. Ther.*, 35:505–509.

13. Bauer, L. A., Davis, R., Wilensky, A., Raisys, V., and Levy, R. H. (1985): Valproic acid clearance: Unbound fraction and diurnal variation in young and elderly adults. *Clin. Pharmacol. Ther.*, 37:697–700.

14. Bowdle, T. A., Patel, I. H., Levy, R. H., and Wilensky, A. J. (1980): Valproic acid dosage and plasma protein binding and clearance. *Clin. Pharmacol. Ther.*, 28:486–492.

15. Bowdle, T. A., Patel, I. H., Levy, R. H., and Wilensky, A. J. (1982): The influence of free fatty acids on valproic acid plasma protein binding during fasting in normal humans. *Eur. J. Clin. Pharmacol.*, 23:343–347.

16. Brachet-Liermain, A., and Demarquez, J. L. (1977): Pharmacokinetics of dipropylacetate in infants and young children. *Pharm. Weekbl.*, 112:293–297.

17. Bryson, S. M., Verma, N., Scott, P. J. W., and Rubin, P. C. (1983): Pharmacokinetics of valproic acid in young and elderly subjects. *Br. J. Clin. Pharmacol.*, 16:104–105.

18. Chapman, A., Keane, P. E., Meldrum, B. S., Simiand, J., and Vernieres, J. C. (1982): Mechanism of anticonvulsant action of valproate. *Prog. Neurobiol.*, 19:315–359.

19. Chiba, K., Suganuma, T., Ishizaki, T., Iriki, T., Shirai, Y., Naitoh, H., and Hori, M. (1985): Comparison of steady-state pharmacokinetics of valproic acid in children between monotherapy and multiple antiepileptic drug treatment. *J. Pediatr.*, 106:653–658.

20. Cloyd, J. C. and Kriel, R. L. (1981): Bioavailability of rectally administered valproic acid syrup. *Neurology*, 31:1348–1352.

21. Cloyd, C. J., Kriel, R. L., Fischer, J. H., Sawchuk, R. J., and Eggerth, R. M., (1983): Pharmacokinetics of valproic acid in children: I. Multiple antiepileptic drug therapy. *Neurology*, 33:185–191.

22. Cornford, E. M. (1983): Blood-brain barrier permeability to valproic acid: Preliminary indications of the independence of lactate and valproate transport. *Epilepsia*, 24:250.

23. Cornford, E. M., Diep, C. P., and Pardridge, W. M. (1985): Blood-brain barrier transport of valproic acid. *J. Neurochem.*, 44:1541–1550.

24. Cornford, E. M. and Oldendorf, W. H. (1986): Epilepsy and the blood-brain barrier. *Advances in Neurology*, 44:787–812.

25. Cramer, J. A., Mattson, R. H., Bennett, D. M., and Swick, C. T. (1986): Variable free and total valproic acid concentrations in sole- and multidrug therapy. *Ther. Drug Monit.*, 8:411–415.

26. Dickinson, R. G., Harland, R. C., Lynn, R. K., Smith, W. B., and Gerber, N. (1979): Transmission of valproic acid (Depakene) across the placenta: Half-life of the drug in mother and baby. *J. Pediatr.*, 94:832–835.

27. Dodson, E. W. (1987): Special pharmacokinetic considerations in children. *Epilepsia*, 28:S56–S70.

28. Eadie, M. J., Heazlewood, V., McKauge, L., and Tyrer, J. H. (1983): Steady-state valproate pharmacokinetics during long term therapy. *Clin. Exp. Neurol.*, 19:183–191.

29. Espin, M. L. E., Benton, P., Will, E., Hayes, M. J., and Walker, G. (1979): Sodium valproate (Epilim)—Some clinical and pharmacological aspects. In: *Clinical and Pharmacological Aspects of Sodium Valproate (Epilim) in the Treatment of Epilepsy*, edited by N. J. Legg, pp. 145–151. MCS Consultants, Tunbridge Wells, Kent.

30. Farrell, K., Orr, J. M., Abbott, F. S., Ferguson, S., Sheppard, I., Godolphin, W., and Bruni, J. (1982): The effect of acetylsalicylic acid on serum free valproate concentrations and valproate clearance in children. *J. Pediatr.*, 101:142–144.

31. Frey, H.-H. and Löscher, W. (1978): Distribution of valproate across the interface between blood and cerebrospinal fluid. *Neuropharmacology*, 17:637–642.

32. Froescher, W., Eichelbaum, M., Neisen, M., Altmann, D., and Von Unruh, G. E. (1981): Antiepileptic therapy with carbamazepine and valproic acid during pregnancy and lactation period. In: *Advances in Epilepsy: the XIIth Epilepsy International Symposium*, edited by M. Dam, L. Gram, and J. K. Penry, pp. 581–588. Raven Press, New York.

33. Froescher, W., Gugler, R., Niesen, M., and Hoffmann, F. (1984): Protein binding of valproic acid in maternal and umbilical cord serum. *Epilepsia*, 25:244–249.

34. Gal, P., Oles, K. S., Gilman, T., and Weaver, R. (1988): Valproic acid efficacy, toxicity, and pharmacokinetics in neonates with intractable seizures. *Neurology*, 38:467–471.

35. Gatti, G., Crema, F., Attardo-Parrinello, G., Fra-

tino, P., Aguzzi, F., and Perucca, E. (1987): Serum protein binding of phenytoin and valproic acid in insulin-dependent diabetes mellitus. *Therapeutic Drug Monitoring,* 9:389–391.

36. Glazko, A. J., Chang, T., Daftsios, A. C., Eiseman, I., Smith, T. C., and Buchanan, R. A. (1983): Bioavailability of calcium valproate in normal men compared with free acid and sodium salt. *Ther. Drug Monit.,* 5:409–417.
37. Goldberg, M. A., and Todoroff, T. (1980): Brain binding of anticonvulsants: Carbamazepine and valproic acid. *Neurology,* 30:826–831.
38. Greenblatt, D. J., Sellers, E. M., and Shader, R. I. (1982): Drug disposition in old age. *N. Engl. J. Med.,* 306:1081–1088.
39. Grimaldi, R., Lecchini, S., Crema, F., and Perucca, E. (1984): *In vivo* plasma protein binding interaction between valproic acid and naproxen. *Eur. J. Drug Metab. Pharmacokinetics,* 9(4):359–363.
40. Guelen, P. J. M., and van der Kleijn, E. (1978): Anti-epileptic drugs in saliva and cerebrospinal fluid. In: *Rational Anti-Epileptic Drug Therapy,* pp. 28–36. Elsevier/North-Holland Biomedical Press, Amsterdam, New York, Oxford.
41. Gugler, R., Schell, A., Eichelbaum, M., Fröscher, W., and Schulz, H. U. (1977): Disposition of valproic acid in man. *Eur. J. Clin. Pharmacol.,* 12:125–132.
42. Guyot, M., Loiseau, P., Brachet-Liermain, A., Levy, R. H., and Morselli, P. L. (1982): The distribution of valproic acid between serum and cerebrospinal fluid. In: *Advances in Epileptology: XIIIth Epilepsy International Symposium,* edited by H. Akimoto, H. Kazamatsuri, M. Seino, and A. Ward, pp. 293–296. Raven Press, New York.
43. Hall, K., Otten, N., Johnston, B., Irvine-Meek, J., Leroux, M., and Seshia, S. (1985): A multivariable analysis of factors governing the steady-state pharmacokinetics of valproic acid in 52 young epileptics. *J. Clin. Pharmacol.,* 25:261–268.
44. Hamilton, R. A., Garnett, W. R., Kline, B. J., and Pellock, J. M. (1981): Effects of food on valproic acid absorption. *Am. J. Hosp. Pharm.,* 38:1490–1493.
45. Hariton, C., Ciesielski, L., Simler, S., Valli, M., Jadot, G., Gobaille, S., Mesdjian, E., and Mandel, P. (1984): Distribution of sodium valproate and GABA metabolism in CNS of the rat. *Biopharm. Drug Disp.,* 5:409–414.
46. Henriksen, O., and Johannessen, S. I., (1980): Clinical observations of sodium valproate in children: An evaluation of therapeutic serum levels. In: *Antiepileptic Therapy: Advances in Drug Monitoring,* edited by S. I. Johannessen, P. L. Morselli, C. E. Pippenger, A. Richens, D. Schmidt, and H. Meinardi, pp. 253–261. Raven Press, New York.
47. Hoffmann, F., von Unruh, G. E., and Jancik, B. C. (1981): Valproic acid disposition in epileptic patients during combined antiepileptic maintenance therapy. *Eur. J. Clin. Pharmacol.,* 19:383–385.
48. Horton, R. W., Anlezark, G. M., Sawaya, M. C. B., and Meldrum, B. S. (1977): Monoamine and GABA metabolism and the anticonvulsant action of di-*n*-propylacetate and ethanolamine-*o*-sulfate. *Eur. J. Pharmacol.,* 41:387–397.
49. Irvine-Meek, J. M., Hall, K. W., Otten, N. H., Leroux, M., Budnik, D., and Seshia, S. S. (1982): Pharmacokinetic study of valproic acid in a neonate. *Pediatr. Pharmacol.,* 2:317–321.
50. Johannessen, S. I., and Henriksen, O. (1980): Pharmacokinetic observations of dipropylacetate in children. In: *Xth International Symposium on Epilepsy,* edited by J. A. Wada and J. K. Penry, p. 353. Raven Press, New York.
51. Johannessen, S. I., and Henriksen, O. (1980): Pharmacokinetic observations of sodium valproate in healthy subjects and in patients with epilepsy. In: *Antiepileptic Therapy: Advances in Drug Monitoring,* edited by S. I. Johannessen, P. L. Morselli, C. E. Pippenger, A. Richens, D. Schmidt, and H. Meinardi, pp. 131–137. Raven Press, New York.
52. Klotz, U. (1982): Bioavailability of a slow release preparation of valproic acid under steady state conditions. *Int. J. Pharmacol. Ther. Toxicol.,* 20(1):24–26.
53. Klotz, U., and Antonin, K. H. (1977): Pharmacokinetics and bioavailability of sodium valproate. *Clin. Pharmacol. Ther.,* 21:736–743.
54. Klotz, U., Rapp, T., and Müller, W. A. (1978): Disposition of valproic acid in patients with liver disease. *Eur. J. Clin. Pharmacol.,* 13:55–60.
55. Levy, R. H. (1980): CSF and plasma pharmacokinetics: Relationship to mechanisms of action as exemplified by valproic acid in monkey. In: *Epilepsy: A Window to Brain Mechanism,* edited by J. S. Lockard and A. A. Ward, Jr., pp. 191–200.
56. Levy, R. H. (1984): Variability in level-dose ratio of valproate: Monotherapy versus polytherapy. *Epilepsia,* 25:S10–S13.
57. Levy, R. H., Cenraud, B., Loiseau, P., Akbaraly, R., Brachet-Liermain, A., Guyot, M., Gomeni, R., and Morselli, P. L. (1980): Meal-dependent absorption of enteric-coated sodium valproate. *Epilepsia,* 21:273–280.
58. Levy, R. H., Friel, P. N., Johno, I., Linthicum, L. M., Colin, L., Koch, K., Raisys, V. A., Wilensky, A. J., and Temkin, N. R. (1984): Filtration for free drug level monitoring: Carbamazepine and valproic acid. *Ther. Drug Monit.,* 6:67–76.
59. Levy, R. H., and Lai, A. A. (1982): Valproate: Absorption, distribution, and excretion. In: *Antiepileptic Drugs,* 2nd edition, edited by D. M. Woodbury, J. K. Penry, and C. E. Pippenger, pp. 555–565. Raven Press, New York.
60. Levy, R. H., Lockard, J. S., and Ludwick, B. T. (1981): Nonlinear plasma protein binding and CSF concentration of valproic acid in monkey. *Epilepsia,* 22:229.
61. Levy, R. H., and Schmidt, D. (1985): Utility of free level monitoring of antiepileptic drugs. *Epilepsia,* 26:199–205.
62. Lockard, J. S., and Levy, R. H. (1976): Valproic

acid: Reversibly acting drug? *Epilepsia,* 17:477–479.

63. Löscher, W., and Esenwein, H. (1978): Pharmacokinetics of sodium valproate in dog and mouse. *Arzneim. Forsch./Drug Res.,* 28:782–787.

64. Löscher, W., and Frey, H.-H. (1984): Kinetics of penetration of common antiepileptic drugs into cerebrospinal fluid. *Epilepsia,* 25:346–352.

65. Löscher, W., and Nau, H. (1983): Distribution of valproic acid and its metabolites in various brain areas of dogs and rats after acute and prolonged treatment. *J. Pharmacol. Exp. Ther.,* 226:845–854.

66. Löscher, W., Nau, H., and Siemes, H. (1988): Penetration of valproate and its active metabolites into cerebrospinal fluid of children with epilepsy. *Epilepsia,* 29:311–316.

67. MacMillan, V. (1979): The effects of the anticonvulsant valproic acid on cerebral indole amine metabolism. *Can. J. Physiol. Pharmacol.,* 57:843–847.

68. Marbury, T. C., Lee, C. S., Bruni, J., and Wilder, B. J. (1980): Hemodialysis of valproic acid in uremic patients. *Dial. and Transpl.,* 9:961–964.

69. Marty, J. J., Kilpatrick, C. J., and Moulds, R. F. W. (1982): Intra-dose variation in plasma protein binding of sodium valproate in epileptic patients. *Br. J. Clin. Pharmac.,* 14:399–404.

70. May, C. A., and Garnett, W. R. (1983): Prediction of steady-state concentrations of valproic acid as determined from single plasma concentrations after the first dose. *Clin. Pharm.,* 2:143–147.

71. May, T., and Rambeck, B. (1985): Serum concentrations of valproic acid: Influence of dose and comedication. *Ther. Drug Monit.,* 7:387–390.

72. McQueen, J. K., Blackwood, D. H. R., Minns, R. A., and Brown, J. K. (1982): Plasma levels of sodium valproate in childhood epilepsy. *Scott. Med. J.,* 27:312–317.

73. Mesdjian, E., Dravet, C., and Roger, J. (1984): Sodium valproate plasma levels (total level and free fraction level) in epileptic patients: Influence of dose, age, and associated therapy. In: *Metabolism of Antiepileptic Drugs,* edited by R. H. Levy, W. H. Pitlick, M. Eichelbaum, and J. Meijer, pp. 115–127. Raven Press, New York.

74. Monaco, F., Mele, G., Milona, T., Franca, V., Sotgia, A., and Mutani, R. (1984): A longitudinal study of valproate free fraction in the specific age group at greatest risk for febrile convulsions (children below 3 years). *Epilepsia,* 25:240–243.

75. Monaco, F., Piredda, S., Mutani, R., Mastropaolo, C., and Tondi, M. (1982): The free fraction of valproic acid in tears, saliva, and cerebrospinal fluid. *Epilepsia,* 23:23–26.

76. Morselli, P. L. (1983): Development of physiological variables important for drug kinetics. In: *Antiepileptic Drug Therapy in Pediatrics,* edited by P. L. Morselli, C. E. Pippenger, and J. K. Penry, pp. 1–12. Raven Press, New York.

77. Nau, H., Helge, H., and Luck, W. (1984): Valproic acid in the perinatal period: Decreased maternal serum protein binding results in fetal accumulation and neonatal displacement of the drug and some metabolites. *J. Pediatr.,* 104:627–634.

78. Nau, H., and Krauer, B. (1986): Serum protein binding of valproic acid in fetus-mother pairs throughout pregnancy: Correlation with oxytocin administration and albumin and free fatty acid concentrations. *J. Clin. Pharmacol.,* 26:215–221.

79. Nau, H. and Löscher, W. (1982): Valproic acid: Brain and plasma levels of the drug and its metabolites, anticonvulsant effects and γ-aminobutyric acid (GABA) metabolism in the mouse. *J. Pharmacol. Exp. Ther.,* 220:654–659.

80. Nau, H., and Löscher, W. (1984): Valproic acid and metabolites: Pharmacological and toxicological studies. *Epilepsia,* 25:S14–S22.

81. Nau, H., Rating, D., Koch, S., Häuser, I., and Helge, H. (1981): Valproic acid and its metabolites: Placental transfer, neonatal pharmacokinetics, transfer *via* mother's milk and clinical status in neonates of epileptic mothers. *J. Pharmacol. Exp. Ther.,* 219:768–777.

82. Nau, H., Wittfoht, W., Rating, D., Jakobs, C., Schäfer, H., and Helge, H. (1982): Pharmacokinetics of valproic acid and its metabolites in a pregnant patient: Stable isotope methodology. In: *Epilepsy, Pregnancy, and the Child,* edited by D. Janz, M. Dam, A. Richens, L. Bossi, H. Helge, and D. Schmidt, pp. 131–139. Raven Press, New York.

83. Nitsche, V., and Mascher, H. (1982): The pharmacokinetics of valproic acid after oral and parenteral administration in healthy volunteers. *Epilepsia,* 23:153–162.

84. Orr, J. M., Farrell, K., Abbott, F. S., Ferguson, S., and Godolphin, W. J. (1983): The effects of peritoneal dialysis on the single dose and steady state pharmacokinetics of valproic acid in a uremic epileptic child. *Eur. J. Clin. Pharmacol.,* 24:387–390.

85. Otten, N., Hall, K., Irvine-Meek, J., Leroux, M., Budnik, D., and Seshia, S. (1984): Free valproic acid: Steady-state pharmacokinetics in patients with intractable epilepsy. *Can. J. Neurol. Sci.,* 11:457–460.

86. Patel, I. H., Levy, R. H., Venkatatamanan, R., Viswanathan, C. T., and Moretti-Ojemann, L. (1980): Diurnal variation in protein binding of valproic acid and phenytoin and the role of free fatty acids. *Clin. Pharmacol. Ther.,* 27:277.

87. Perucca, E., Gatti, G., Frigo, G. M., and Crema, A. (1978): Pharmacokinetics of valproic acid after oral and intravenous administration. *Br. J. Clin. Pharmacol.,* 5:313–318.

88. Perucca, E., Gatti, G., Frigo, G. M., Crema, A., Calzetti, S., and Visintini, D. (1978): Disposition of sodium valproate in epileptic patients. *Br. J. Clin. Pharmacol.,* 5:495–499.

89. Perucca, E., Grimaldi, R., Gatti, G., Pirracchio, S., Crema, F., and Frigo, G. M. (1984): Pharmacokinetics of valproic acid in the elderly. *Br. J. Clin. Pharmacol.,* 17:665–669.

90. Philbert, A., and Dam, M. (1982): The epileptic mother and her child. *Epilepsia,* 23:85–99.

91. Philbert, A., Pedersen, B., and Dam, M. (1985):

Concentration of valproate during pregnancy in the newborn and in breast milk. *Acta Neurol. Scand.,* 72:460–463.

92. Pisani, F., D'Agostino, A. A., Fazio, A., Oteri, G., Primerano, G., and Di Perri, G. (1982): Increased dipropylacetic acid bioavailability from dipropylacetamide by food. *Epilepsia,* 23:115–121.

93. Pisani, F., Fazio, A., Oteri, G., and Di Perri, R. (1981): Dipropylacetic acid plasma levels; Diurnal fluctuations during chronic treatment with dipropylacetamide. *Ther. Drug Monit.,* 3:297–301.

94. Plasse, J. -C., Revol, M., Chabert, G., and Ducerf, F. (1979): Neonatal pharmacokinetics of valproic acid. In: *Progress in Clinical Pharmacy,* edited by D. Schaaf and E. van der Kleijn, pp. 247–252. Elsevier/North-Holland Biomedical Press, Amsterdam, New York.

95. Pollack, G. M., McHugh, W. B., Gengo, F. M., Ermer, J. C., and Shen, D. D. (1986): Accumulation and washout kinetics of valproic acid and its active metabolites. *J. Clin. Pharmacol.,* 26:668–676.

96. Pollack, G. M., and Shen, D. D. (1985): A timed intravenous pentylenetetrazol infusion seizure model for quantitating the anticonvulsant effect of valproic acid in the rat. *J. Pharmacol. Meth.,* 13:135–146.

97. Rapeport, W. G., Mendelow, A. D., French, G., MacPherson, P., Teasdale, E., Agnew, E., Thompson, G. G., and Brodie, M. J. (1983): Plasma protein-binding and CSF concentrations of valproic acid in man following acute oral dosing. *Br. J. Clin. Pharmacol.,* 16:365–369.

98. Richens, S. A., Scoular, I. T., Ahmad, S., and Jordan, B. J. (1976): Pharmacokinetics and efficacy of Epilim in patients receiving long-term therapy with other antiepileptic drugs. In: *Clinical and Pharmacological Treatment of Epilepsy,* edited by N. J. Legg, pp. 78–88. MCS Consultants, Tunbridge Wells, Kent.

99. Riva, R., Albani, F., Contin, M., Baruzzi, A., Altomare, M., Merlini, G. P., and Perucca, E. (1984): Mechanism of altered drug binding to serum proteins in pregnant women: Studies with valproic acid. *Ther. Drug Monit.,* 6:25–30.

100. Riva, R., Albani, F., Cortelle, P., Bobbi, G., Perucca, E., and Baruzzi, A. (1983): Diurnal fluctuations in free and total plasma concentrations of valproic acid at steady state in epileptic patients. *Ther. Drug Monit.,* 5:191–196.

101. Riva, R., Albani, F., Franzoni, E., Perucca, E., Santucci, M., and Baruzzi, A. (1983): Valproic acid free fraction in epileptic children under chronic monotherapy. *Ther. Drug Monit.,* 5:197–200.

102. Roman, E. J., Ponniah, P., Lambert, J. B., and Buchanan, N. (1982): Free sodium valproate monitoring. *Br. J. Clin. Pharmac.,* 13:452–455.

103. Rosenfeld, W. E., Leppik, I. E., Gates, J. R., and Mireles, R. E. (1987): Valproic acid loading during intensive monitoring. *Arch. Neurol.,* 44:709–710.

104. Sackellares, C., Sato, S., Dreifuss, F. E., and Penry, J. K. (1981): Reduction of steady-state valproate levels by other antiepileptic drugs. *Epilepsia,* 22:437–441.

105. Schapel, G. J., Beran, R. G., Doecke, C. J., O'Reilly, W. J., Reece, P. A., Rischbieth, R. H. C., Sansom, L. N., and Stanley, P. E. (1980): Pharmacokinetics of sodium valproate in epileptic patients: Prediction of maintenance dosage by single-dose study. *Eur. J. Clin. Pharmacol.,* 17:71–77.

106. Schobben, F., van der Kleijn, E., and Gabreëls, F. J. M. (1975): Pharmacokinetics of di-*n*-propylacetate in epileptic patients. *Eur. J. Clin. Pharmacol.,* 8:97–105.

107. Schobben, F., Vree, T. B., and van der Kleijn, E. (1978): Pharmacokinetics, metabolism and distribution of 2-*n*-propyl-pentanoate (sodium valproate) and the influence of salicylate co-medication. In: *Advances in Epileptology, 1977,* edited by H. Meinardi and A. J. Rowan, pp. 271–277. Swets & Zeitlinger, Amsterdam.

108. Shirkey, R. J., Jellett, L. B., Kappatos, D. C., Maling, T. J. B., and Macdonald, A. (1985): Distribution of sodium valproate in normal whole blood and in blood from patients with renal or hepatic disease. *Eur. J. Clin. Pharmacol.,* 28:447–452.

109. Snead III, O. C., and Miles, M. V., (1985): Treatment of status epilepticus in children with rectal sodium valproate. *J. Pediatr.,* 106:323–325.

110. Tarasidis, C. G., Garnett, W. R., Kline, B. J., and Pellock, J. M. (1986): Influence of tube type, storage time, and temperature on the total and free concentration of valproic acid. *Ther. Drug Monit.,* 8:373–376.

111. Vajda, F. J. E., Donnan, G. A., Phillips, J., and Bladin, P. F. (1981): Human brain, plasma, and cerebrospinal fluid concentration of sodium valproate after 72 hours of therapy. *Neurology,* 31:486–487.

112. Vajda, F. J. E., Mihaly, G. W., Miles, J. L., Donnan, G. A., and Bladin, P. F. (1978): Rectal administration of sodium valproate in status epilepticus. *Neurology,* 28:897–899.

113. Wilkinson, G. R., and Shand, D. G. (1975): A physiological approach to hepatic drug clearance. *Clin. Pharmacol. Ther.,* 18:377–390.

114. Yu, H. -Y. (1984): Clinical implications of serum protein binding in epileptic children during sodium valproate maintenance therapy. *Ther. Drug Monit.,* 6:414–423.

Antiepileptic Drugs, Third Edition, edited by
R. Levy, R. Mattson, B. Meldrum,
J. K. Penry, and F. E. Dreifuss.
Raven Press, Ltd., New York © 1989.

42

Valproate

Biotransformation

Thomas A. Baillie and Albert W. Rettenmeier

INTRODUCTION

Following the serendipitous discovery of the anticonvulsant properties of valproic acid (VPA) and its subsequent development as an antiepileptic drug in France in the early 1960s (74), a number of preliminary reports appeared on the pharmacokinetics and metabolic disposition of VPA in animal species (for reviews, see 56, 114). Although few metabolites of the drug were identified in these early studies, which relied mainly on the use of [1-^{14}C] VPA as a tracer, measurements of radioactivity in excreta indicated that VPA was well absorbed following oral administration and that it was metabolized extensively to products that appeared in the urine, with only a few percent of the dose (depending on species) being excreted in unchanged form. It was not until the 1970s, when combined gas chromatography-mass spectrometry (GC-MS) systems became commercially available, that significant progress was made on the structural characterization of VPA metabolites. Indeed, by 1978, most of the major products of VPA metabolism in the urine of rats (31,42,48,56,73), rabbits (31), dogs (31,42), mice (42), and humans (31,33,42,48) had been identified on the basis of their respective mass spectral fragmentation patterns.

During the past decade, interest in the metabolic fate of VPA has been stimulated by a growing body of evidence suggesting that metabolites of the drug may contribute significantly to both its anticonvulsant properties and to its serious hepatotoxic side effects (84). Consequently, a relatively large number of studies on VPA biotransformation have been reported in the recent literature, almost all of which have been conducted with the aid of GC-MS methodology. The reason for the dominant position of GC-MS techniques among the analytical methods used in these investigations stems from a consideration of some of the unique physicochemical properties of VPA, which were alluded to by Gugler and von Unruh (37) in their comprehensive review of the literature on VPA metabolism prior to 1980. Thus, metabolites of VPA are structurally similar to endogenous organic acids: they lack a suitable chromophore that can be exploited for detection by high-performance liquid chromatography (HPLC) techniques, they are relatively volatile, and certain members of the family (e.g., 3-oxo-VPA) are chemically and/or thermally unstable (111), thereby necessitating the use of specialized procedures for their isolation in order to avoid the formation of artifacts. Given these analytical difficulties and the associated need for highly specific methods of identification, GC-MS has become an indispensable tool in studies of VPA biotransformation and has been primarily responsible for the increase in number of known VPA metabolites from seven in 1978 to around 50 (not including conjugates or stereoisomers) in 1988. Many of these new metabolites have been synthesized and, in some cases, have been shown to be either pharmacologically active or hepatotoxic in nature. Many others remain to be studied and their metabolic origins and interrelationships established. At this point, it is clear that despite the deceptively simple chemical structure of VPA, its metabolic fate is highly complex and reflects the entry of this unusual fatty acid derivative into pathways (e.g., β-oxidation) normally reserved for endogenous lipids. Indeed, it is this interplay between intermediary and xenobiotic metabolism that makes the study of VPA biotransformation both a fascinating and challenging endeavor, and has led to the adoption of VPA as a model compound for studies on the role of metabolism in mediating the adverse effects of aliphatic acids (19).

METABOLIC PATHWAYS OF VALPROIC ACID

Valproic acid undergoes metabolism by a variety of conjugation and oxidative processes, several of which have been cited in previous reviews (17,19,37,84,114). The discussion that follows attempts to classify many of the seemingly diverse metabolites of VPA according to the biochemical pathways from which they most likely derive.

Conjugation Reactions

Glucuronidation

Conjugation to D-glucuronic acid has been shown to represent the major route of VPA biotransformation in humans and most animals, and results in the corresponding 1-O-acyl-β-linked ester glucuronide (Fig. 1) which is excreted into urine (22,36,53). This

conjugate, which has been characterized directly by GC-MS (73), is also present at high concentrations in the bile of rats given VPA (22). The latter observation is consistent with the finding that VPA undergoes enterohepatic recycling in the rat (21,97). In addition, the marked choleretic activity of VPA in this species appears to be due to the osmotic properties of VPA glucuronide in bile and it is not surprising, therefore, that agents inhibiting glucuronide conjugation in vivo (e.g., borneol and galactosamine) decrease   VPA-induced   choleresis (41,126,127). Interestingly, however, compounds such as phenobarbital that induce glucuronidation of VPA (125) fail to stimulate either the biliary excretion of VPA glucuronide or its choleretic action, indicating that biliary transport of the conjugate is already maximal in the non-induced state (127).

Recently, it has been shown that VPA glucuronide undergoes pH-dependent rearrangement reactions to yield isomeric forms that are resistant to hydrolysis by β-glucuronidase (23). The disposition of these rearranged glucuronides in vivo differs from that of the primary isomer (21,24,26), and it is of some interest that abnormally high concentrations of VPA conjugates, consisting largely of the rearranged glucuronide isomers, were detected in the plasma of a patient diagnosed with VPA-associated hepatobiliary and renal dysfunction (25). The toxicological implications of these findings remain to be established.

Finally, it should be noted that glucuronidation also represents an important pathway of biotransformation for primary metabolites of VPA that have been formed by   initial   oxidative   processes (36,104,105,107,120); in the case of hydroxylated VPA metabolites, both ether and ester glucuronides could result, although no information is available on the preferred sites at which conjugation takes place in these polyfunctional compounds. The kinetics of VPA glucuronidation in vitro have

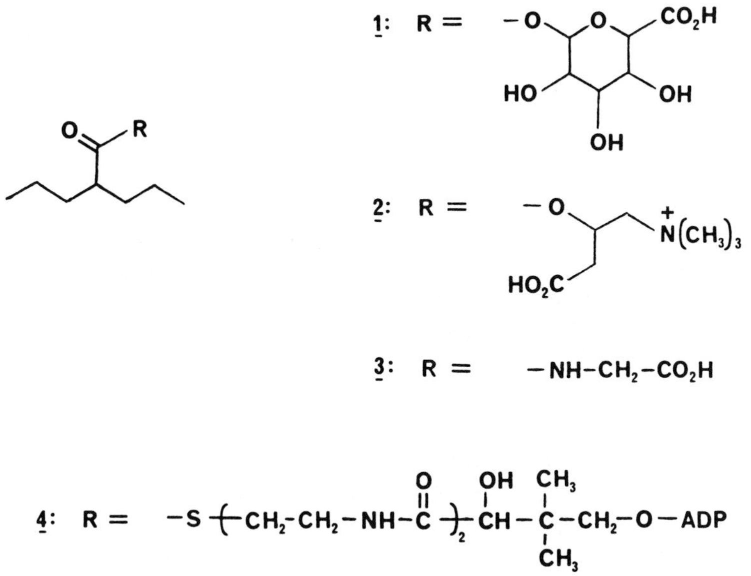

FIG. 1. Structures of conjugates of VPA. **1**: VPA glucuronide; **2**: VPA carnitine; **3**: VPA glycine; **4**: VPA-coenzyme A (ADP, adenosine diphosphate).

been examined using a rat liver microsomal system, and it has been shown that VPA can serve as a competitive inhibitor of the conjugation of other drugs that form glucuronide conjugates (119).

Carnitine Ester Formation

Using a combination of fast atom bombardment mass spectrometry and thermospray liquid chromatography-mass spectrometry, Millington and co-workers identified valproylcarnitine (Fig. 1) as a novel metabolite of VPA in the urine of pediatric patients receiving prolonged administration of the drug (13,61,75). Excretion of this conjugate in urine, where it accounted for less than 10% of the total acylcarnitines (13) and probably less than 1% of the dose of VPA, may nevertheless be significant in that VPA therapy has been associated with a secondary carnitine deficiency and, more rarely, with a Reye-like syndrome (15,18,57), either of which might be precipitated (or ex-

acerbated) by diversion of carnitine to VPA conjugate formation.

Conjugation with Glycine

In early studies of the metabolic fate of VPA in human subjects, Gompertz et al. (33) analyzed the urine from two children with neurological disease for the presence of valproylglycine. Although the authors had available an authentic sample of this compound as reference material, none was detected in the urine specimens and it was concluded that glycine conjugation is not a pathway of metabolism for VPA. In rat urine, however, small amounts of the glycine conjugate have been identified, together with somewhat greater quantities of glycine conjugates of unsaturated VPA metabolites (36). Moreover, when the unsaturated metabolite of valproate, Δ^4-VPA, was administered to rhesus monkeys, the glycine conjugate of (2E)-$\Delta^{2,4}$-VPA was identified in the urine (104). Thus, it appears that glycine conjugation, although normally a very minor biotransformation pathway for the parent drug, assumes greater importance for unsaturated metabolites of VPA.

Conjugation with Coenzyme A

Although the coenzyme A thioester derivative of VPA has been prepared synthetically and used both as a reference compound and as a substrate for metabolic experiments (11,16,121,122), rigorous structural characterization of this conjugate has not been reported. However, persuasive evidence that such a conjugate does exist as a metabolic intermediate in liver tissue has accumulated from animal studies, and it has been proposed that either VPA-CoA itself, or depletion of free coenzyme A pools through VPA-CoA formation, causes inhibition of a variety of key processes of intermediary metabolism (11,121,122). In support of the latter hypothesis, it has been shown that VPA-CoA is a poor substrate for medium-chain acyl-CoA hydrolases (76). The conjugate has not been detected, however, in either brain tissue of adult rats (11) or in rat conceptuses exposed to VPA (16), suggesting that VPA-CoA does not play a role in modulating either the anticonvulsant activity or the teratogenic effects of the parent drug.

Additional (indirect) evidence for the existence of coenzyme A derivatives of VPA and some of its metabolites derives from the fact that both carnitine and glycine conjugates have been detected as urinary metabolites of VPA (see above), the formation of which would be expected to proceed via coenzyme A thioesters. A similar argument can be made on the basis of the participation of VPA in the fatty acid β-oxidation pathway (see below). Xenobiotic carboxylic acids also have been found to be incorporated, via their respective coenzyme A derivatives, into triglycerides and phospholipids, although no evidence that VPA gains entry into such biosynthetic pathways has been obtained to date (9).

β-Oxidation

Products of the "β-oxidation" pathway (Fig. 2) which comprise Δ^2-VPA (formed predominantly as the E-isomer) (53), 3-hydroxy-VPA (73), and 3-oxo-VPA (73), were so termed because of their structural resemblance to intermediates of fatty acid β-oxidation. However, the site of formation of these metabolites at the subcellular level remains to be established unequivocally. On the one hand, it has been claimed that VPA undergoes β-oxidation in peroxisomes (38) with concomitant production of excess hydrogen peroxide, a toxic by-product (98,123). On the other hand, it has been stated that VPA is not a substrate for the hepatic peroxisomal fatty acid β-oxidation system (27), although prolonged administration of VPA to rats does cause proliferation of peroxisomes in a fashion similar to that observed with clofibrate and other hypolipidemic drugs (27,40). Clearly, appropriate *in vitro* studies with isolated organelles are needed in order to resolve which of these discrete β-oxidation systems participates in the biotransformation of VPA.

Regardless of the intracellular origin of the "β-oxidation pathway" metabolites, the available evidence indicates that VPA and endogenous lipids do compete for the enzymes of β-oxidation (12). Thus, co-administration of VPA and isoleucine to rats resulted in marked suppression of the urinary excretion of 3-hydroxy- and 3-oxo-VPA (73), and pretreatment with clofibrate stimulated the excretion of the 3-oxo metabolite (38). These effects were attributed to competitive inhibition and induction, respectively, of β-oxidation activity *in vivo*. Additional experiments in rats showed that both formation and elimination of Δ^2-VPA was sensitive to nutritional status (47) and that injection of fatty acids (in the form of

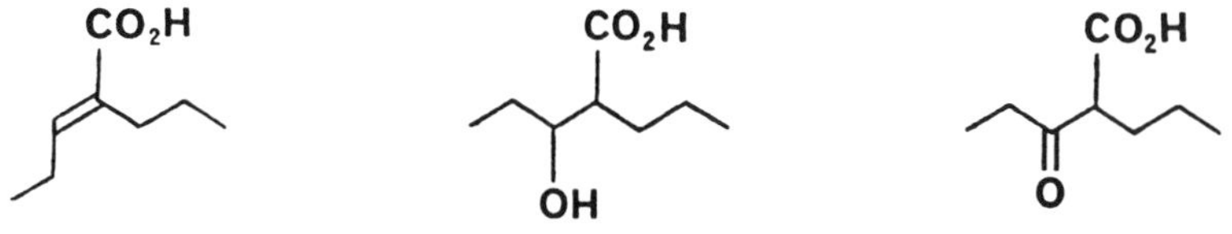

FIG. 2. Structures of metabolites of VPA associated with the β-oxidation pathway. **5**: (E)-Δ^2-VPA; **6**: 3-hydroxy-VPA; **7**: 3-oxo-VPA. As discussed in the text, 3-hydroxy-VPA also derives from a direct hydroxylation pathway.

olive oil) had a marked influence on the urinary excretion of 3-hydroxy- and 3-oxo-VPA (38). More recently, stable isotope labeling techniques have been employed to investigate the β-oxidation pathway of VPA metabolism in the rat, and have demonstrated that 3-hydroxy-VPA is not (as was originally suspected) an exclusive product of β-oxidation, but has a dual origin *in vivo*, being derived in part by direct, cytochrome P-450-dependent hydroxylation of the parent drug (103). This study also confirmed an earlier observation (96) that 3-oxo-VPA appeared to be formed mainly by oxidation of Δ^2-VPA, rather than derived from 3-hydroxy-VPA. Therefore, since the 3-hydroxy compound in urine does not necessarily represent an intermediate in the β-oxidation of VPA, measurement of the combined excretion in urine of the three "β-oxidation" metabolites may give a false estimate of the flux of VPA through this metabolic pathway.

The fact that β-oxidation intermediates are excreted into urine in the case of VPA, a branched-chain fatty acid, but not to any appreciable extent in the case of its endogenous, straight-chain counterparts, implies that the branched structure of VPA renders this compound a poor substrate for β-oxidation enzymes. Consequently, it may be expected that thiolase-mediated cleavage of 3-oxo-VPA to yield propionic and valeric acids, in a reaction corresponding to the final step of β-oxidation, may be similarly inefficient. Interestingly, there have been reports of increased urinary excretion of

propionic acid in patients treated with VPA (55,113), together with elevated plasma concentrations of propionate-derived amino acids, e.g., β-alanine and α-aminobutyric acid (72). Although, cleavage of 3-oxo-VPA would account for these observations and would also explain the increased urinary output of other organic acids that are synthesized from propionate, e.g., methylmalonic acid (48), succinic acid (36), etc., appropriate isotope labeling experiments to confirm the incorporation of elements of the VPA structure into these endogenous metabolites have yet to be reported. In the absence of such data, it becomes difficult to distinguish mechanisms involving degradation of VPA to products that enter biosynthetic pathways versus direct effects of VPA on routes of lipid metabolism. Tracer experiments are needed to resolve these issues, especially in light of the findings of a clinical study designed to assess the influence of VPA therapy on plasma and urinary short-chain fatty acids. The study failed to demonstrate any VPA-induced effects on these compounds (129).

Other Oxygenation Pathways

Hydroxylation

Valproate is hydroxylated mainly at positions 4 and 5, which correspond to the ω- and (ω-1) positions of fatty acids (Fig. 3). As in the case of its endogenous counterparts, VPA undergoes hydroxylation at

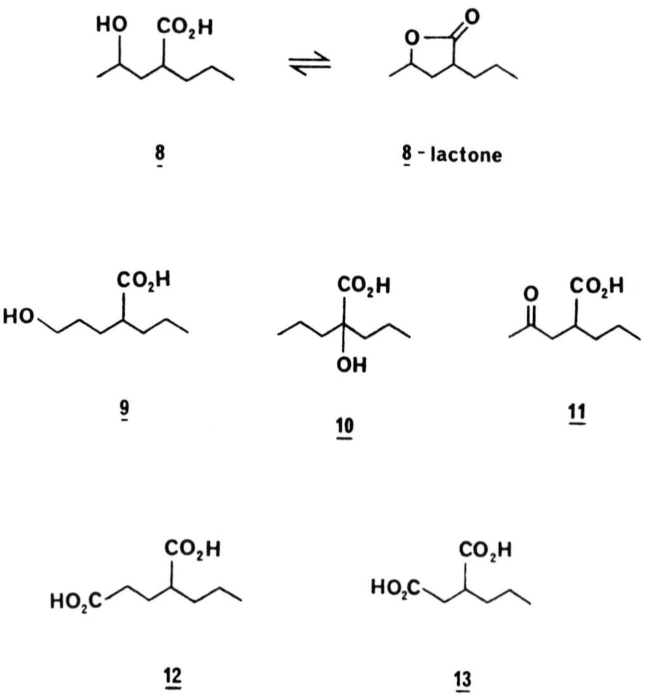

FIG. 3. Structures of oxygenated metabolites of VPA. **8**: 4-Hydroxyl-VPA (and its γ-lactone); **9**: 5-hydroxy-VPA; **10**: 2-hydroxy-VPA; **11**: 4-oxo-VPA; **12**: PGA; **13**: PSA.

these sites by the action of cytochrome P-450 enzymes (101), mainly in liver tissue but also in other organs (4-hydroxylation of VPA in the adrenal gland of human conceptuses has been found to be especially efficient [108]). The 4-hydroxy compound readily forms a γ-lactone, whereas 5-hydroxy-VPA can be transformed to the corresponding δ-lactone when exposed to strong acid (111). As indicated above, 3-hydroxy-VPA was found to derive from both β-oxidation and cytochrome P-450-catalyzed processes (101,103), although the most recently detected metabolite of VPA, 2-hydroxy-VPA (Fig. 3), is of unknown origin (120). Hence, it is evident that VPA undergoes hydroxylation at all of the possible sites on the molecule. It should be pointed out that hydroxylation at positions 3, 4, or 5 generates a chiral center at C-2, and hydroxylation at C-3 and C-4 produces an additional asymmetric center at the ox-idized carbon. Nothing, however, is known about the absolute stereochemistry of chiral metabolites of VPA, although information on this topic may provide a unique insight into the enzymes that participate in VPA biotransformation.

Ketone Formation

From the information currently available, it appears likely that 3-oxo-VPA, a major urinary metabolite of valproate in most species (73), derives largely from (E)-Δ²-VPA via β-oxidation (103), although an alternative route involving oxidation of 3-hydroxy-VPA by cytosolic dehydrogenases cannot be excluded. Of all of the metabolites of VPA hitherto identified, 3-oxo-VPA has probably been the most troublesome from an analytical standpoint in that the compound undergoes spontaneous heat- and acid-catalyzed decarboxylation to produce 3-heptanone. Carefully controlled conditions are essential, therefore, for the successful isolation of intact 3-oxo-VPA from biological fluids, and it is likely that early measurements of this metabolite in blood and urine (33) represent underestimates of the true values.

In contrast to 3-oxo-VPA, the corresponding 4-oxo compound (Fig. 3), which is formed from 4-hydroxy-VPA (36) and which was first identified as a human metabolite of VPA in a stable isotope "pulse dose" experiment (7), presents few difficulties from an analytical standpoint. It should be noted, however, that protocols for the assay of urinary organic acids which entail an aqueous-phase oximation step to derivatize keto functionalities may lead to the generation of artifacts from VPA-derived components; VPA itself is converted, in part, to a hydroxamic acid under such conditions (62).

Dicarboxylic Acid Formation

2-*n*-Propylglutaric acid (PGA) (56) and 2-*n*-propylsuccinic acid (PSA; Fig. 3) (36) are believed to derive from further oxidation of 5-hydroxy- and 4-hydroxy-VPA, respectively (36). As discussed previously, other dicarboxylic acids identified in the urine of VPA-treated humans or animals may, or may not, be genuine metabolites of the drug.

Epoxidation

In principal, any of the unsaturated metabolites of VPA could undergo epoxidation as a second step of biotransformation. Such a process has been documented, however, only in the case of Δ^4-VPA which is converted, in a cytochrome P-450-mediated reaction, to a putative unstable 4,5-epoxide (36,107). Stable isotope labeling experiments using ^{18}O as a metabolic tracer have

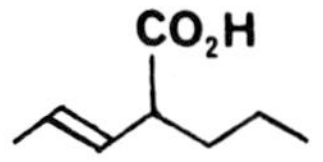

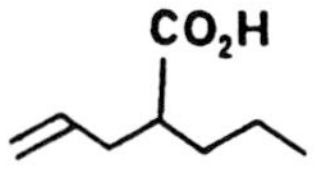

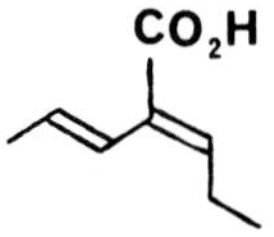

FIG. 4 Unsaturated metabolites of VPA. **14**: Δ^3-VPA; **15**: Δ^4-VPA; **16**: (2E, 3'E)-$\Delta^{2,3'}$-VPA; **17**: (2E)-$\Delta^{2,4}$-VPA.

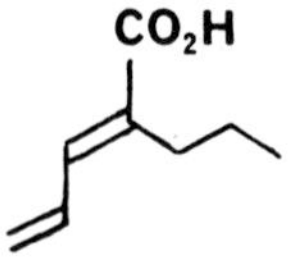

indicated that this epoxide intermediate undergoes facile intramolecular rearrangement to yield the stable, cyclized product, 4,5-dihydroxy-VPA-γ-lactone (102).

Desaturation

Early studies on the metabolism of VPA in human subjects and animals revealed the presence of urine and plasma of mono-unsaturated derivates of the drug (48,53), the first to be positively identified as Δ^2-VPA. As discussed above, this metabolite is generally considered to be a product of VPA β-oxidation, although it is not clear whether this pathway generates both the E (major) and Z (minor) geometric isomers typically found in biological fluids. A survey of metabolites of VPA in serum of epileptic children resulted in the identification of two further positional isomers Δ^3-VPA (present in both E and Z forms) and the terminal olefin, Δ^4-VPA (Fig. 4) (49). All of these mono-unsaturated VPA metabolites have been detected subsequently in body fluids from animal species, e.g., rat (36) and monkey (104), and studies on their respective metabolic relationships *in vivo* have indicated that Δ^3-VPA is formed reversibly from the Δ^2 isomer, whereas Δ^4-VPA has a quite distinct origin (103). Interestingly, recent work has shown that the Δ^4 metabolite is formed by cytochrome P-450-mediated desaturation of VPA in liver microsomes (109), thus confirming the above conclusion that two quite separate desaturation pathways operate for VPA, one in the endoplasmic reticulum (producing Δ^4-VPA) and the other in mitochondria (giving Δ^2- and Δ^3-VPA).

In addition to the above mono-unsaturated metabolites, a series of diene derivatives of VPA has been detected in the plasma and urine of patients receiving VPA therapy (6,51). The major component of this group in both humans and animals has been reported to be the (2E,3'E)-diene (6,36,51,103), although (2E)-$\Delta^{2,4}$-VPA was also identified in these studies (Fig. 4). Evidence has been obtained suggesting that the 2,3'-diene probably is formed by further desaturation of Δ^3-VPA (103), whereas the 2,4-diene is known to be a secondary metabolite of Δ^4-VPA in the rat (36,45,107,117) and monkey (104). Interest in the identities and toxicological properties of these compounds, and the numerous positional and geometric isomers thereof that remain to be fully characterized, stems largely from the observation by Kochen et al. (50) that the concentrations of unsaturated metabolites of VPA were markedly elevated in the plasma of a patient who died from VPA-induced liver failure. Whether this accumulation of unsaturated metabolites represented a cause of the toxicity or was merely a manifestation of an already-damaged liver is not known, although further oxidative metabolism of at least one member of the series, Δ^4-VPA, has been shown to lead to the generation of chemically reactive, potentially hepatotoxic intermediates (102,104,107).

Finally, it may be noted that at least two triene metabolites of VPA have been detected in studies in rats, but these have not yet been characterized (36,45). It is also noteworthy that a number of investigators have verified in control experiments that unsaturated derivatives of VPA are not formed by dehydration of hydroxy-VPA precursors (36,49,51,109). Thus, unsaturated metabolites of VPA isolated from biological sources are considered to be genuine products of biotransformation, and are not artifacts formed during sample work-up.

Miscellaneous Pathways

Investigations of the further biotransformation of primary VPA metabolites in animals have revealed the participation of some rather unusual pathways of drug metabolism. Thus, addition of the elements of water across the double bond of Δ^4-VPA has been proposed to explain the conversion of this olefin to 5-hydroxy-VPA in rats (36,107) and monkeys (104), although a different mechanism involving an oxidation/reduction sequence would be a plausible alternative in this case (107). Reduction of the two other mono-unsaturated metabolites of VPA, Δ^2- and Δ^3-VPA, to yield the parent drug has also been reported to take place in rats, where up to 2% of an administered dose of these compounds was recovered in the urine as VPA (36). As indicated earlier, Δ^2- and Δ^3-VPA appear to be interconverted by an isomerization process (103) which would account satisfactorily for the observation that both olefins are converted in the rat to a common metabolite, 3-oxo-VPA (36).

QUANTITATIVE ASPECTS OF VPA METABOLISM

Assay Methods

Although a variety of assay procedures have been developed for VPA itself (cited in 120), relatively few methods are available for VPA metabolites due to their complexity and generally low concentrations in biological fluids. With the exception of the assay reported by Löscher in 1981 (64), which was based on gas chromatographic analysis of the underivatized metabolites, all of the subsequent methods have employed selected ion monitoring GC-MS techniques with either packed (1,95) or more efficient capillary column separation (2,3,106,117,120). Limits of detection by these highly specific GC-MS assays have been in the order of 20 to 30 ng ml^{-1} plasma (using 100 μl plasma samples) or 20 to 30 ng g^{-1} brain tissue (using 100 mg specimens) when trimethylsilyl or *tert.*-butyldimethylsilyl derivatives were used and ionization was carried out by electron impact (68). Sensitivity can be increased further (by 30 to 50-fold) when negative ion chemical ionization methods are employed with the pentafluorobenzyl ester derivatives (2). Recent developments in automation of GC-MS systems have led to the introduction of a quantitative procedure for the determination of VPA and 14 of its metabolites in plasma or urine, in which sample injection, data acquisition, integration, calibration, and quantitative report functions are carried out during unattended operation under computer control (106).

Numerous applications of the above assay procedures have been made to studies of the pharmacokinetics of VPA itself, such as those involving administration of a "pulse dose" of stable-isotope labeled VPA to individuals receiving unlabeled VPA chronically (8,39,124), although there appear to have been few studies on the kinetics of metabolites of VPA formed from the parent drug (52). Representative values for the concentrations of VPA and its metabolites in plasma of epileptic patients are reproduced in Table 1, and Table 2 summarizes typical urinary recoveries of VPA metabolites, expressed as percentages of the administered dose.

Effect of Dose, Age and Polytherapy on VPA Metabolism

In a detailed study on the influence of dose size on the metabolic fate of VPA in healthy adults, Granneman et al. (34) studied blood levels and urinary excretion patterns of VPA metabolites following single oral doses of 250, 500, or 1,000 mg. While the fraction of the dose excreted in urine as VPA glucuronide increased markedly with increasing dose (from 4.5% at 250 mg to 35.2% at 1,000 mg), the opposite trend was observed with products of the β-oxidation pathway (e.g., 3-oxo-VPA, which fell from 33.7% at 250 mg to 20.7% at 1,000 mg). Cytochrome P-450-dependent pathways (ω- and [ω-1] oxidation), on the other hand, were relatively independent of dose. These findings were interpreted to indicate that at high doses, mitochondrial β-oxidation of VPA becomes saturated due to the limited availability of the necessary cofactor, coenzyme A, and that increased glucuronidation of VPA serves as a compensatory mechanism. Thus, the contribution of mitochondrial versus microsomal processes to VPA metabolism falls appreciably as the dose is increased.

Relatively little attention has been paid to the influence of age on the metabolism of VPA, although the known susceptibility of young children to VPA-induced hepatic injury (29) indicates that age-related changes in VPA biotransformation may be a contributing factor. Shen et al. (116) assessed the effect of age on the pharmacokinetics of VPA metabolites by measuring the time-averaged steady-state serum concentrations of metabolites relative to those of parent drug in 22 infants (4 months–2 years), children (2–15 years), and 12 adult patients. These concentration ratios were found to increase as a function of age for 3-oxo-VPA, to remain constant for Δ^2-VPA, and to decrease for Δ^4-VPA. The latter observation is of interest in that it implies that young infants may be exposed to higher circulating

TABLE 1. *Concentration ranges for VPA and its metabolites in the plasma of epileptic patients*

Compound	Plasma concentration (μg ml^{-1})		
	Children on VPA monotherapy ($N = 34$) (from ref. 3)	Patients (4–19 yr) on monotherapy ($N = 12$) (from ref. 120)	Adults on mono- or polytherapy ($N = 19$) (from ref. 106)
VPA	11.8–105	113.4–146.2	7.1–206
(E)-Δ^2-VPA	0.95–11.3	2.60–6.84	0.55–4.66
(Z)-Δ^2-VPA	0.06–0.40	0.02–0.16	0.04–0.31
Δ^3-VPA	0.25–1.86	0.17–0.68	0.41–1.68
Δ^4-VPA	0.16–1.22	0.05–0.24	Tr[a]–0.64
(2E)-$\Delta^{2,4}$-VPA	0.02–0.58	—[b]	0.07–0.90
(2E, 3'E)-$\Delta^{2,3'}$-VPA	0.50–7.29	—	0.94–4.69
3-OH-VPA	—	0.53–0.88	0.17–1.12
4-OH-VPA	Tr–1.78	0.45–1.05	Tr–2.97
5-OH-VPA	Tr–1.25	0.12–0.55	Tr–1.06
3-oxo-VPA	0.29–15.6	1.02–4.56	2.26–14.7
4-oxo-VPA	0.01–1.29	0.03–0.41	Tr–4.50
PSA	Tr–0.44	—	Tr–0.08
PGA	Tr–1.23	N.D.[c]–0.05	Tr–0.22

[a] Tr, trace; [b] —, not reported; [c] N.D., not detected.

concentrations of the hepatotoxic Δ^4 metabolite than older children or adults.

Effect of Co-Administered Drugs on VPA Metabolism

Since elimination of VPA *in vivo* is highly dependent upon metabolism, it would be predicted that agents modulating the activity of microsomal and/or mitochondrial enzyme systems would alter the pharmacokinetics and biotransformation of this drug. That this is indeed the case was first demonstrated in animal studies, where rats given phenobarbital (a selective inducer of microsomal enzymes) or clofibrate (a selective inducer of mitochondrial and peroxisomal β-oxidation) excreted greater amounts of VPA metabolites in urine than did control animals (38). Phenobarbital pretreatment stimulated glucuronidation of VPA and its diacid metabolite, PGA, and also enhanced cytochrome P-450-dependent hydroxylation reactions. Clofibrate, on the other hand, induced metabolism of VPA to the 3-oxo compound.

The influence of polytherapy on the disposition of VPA in humans has been the subject of recent communications. Abbott et al. (5) showed in a group of pediatric patients that carbamazepine induces the metabolism of VPA by microsomal ω- and (ω-1) oxidation, but that the drug also stimulates, somewhat unexpectedly, the urinary excretion of 3-oxo-VPA. In order to explain the latter finding, the authors speculated that carbamazepine induces the β-oxidation of VPA (which was proposed to occur in peroxisomes), although it is possible that it is actually microsomal (ω-2)-hydroxylation (101) which is stimulated, and that the resultant excess 3-hydroxy-VPA undergoes dehydrogenation to produce the urinary 3-oxo-VPA. A drug interaction that more likely does involve the fatty acid β-oxidation complex occurs between VPA and salicylates. Following antipyretic doses of aspirin to children, urinary excretion of (E)-Δ^2- and 3-oxo-VPA was found to be reduced by 38% and 69%, respectively, presumably due to competitive inhibition of valproyl-CoA formation by aspirin (4). Preliminary studies have also been carried out on the effect of co-therapy with inducers (phenytoin, carbamazepine) and an inhibi-

TABLE 2. *Urinary excretion of VPA and its metabolites in adult epileptic patients treated with prolonged administration of VPA monotherapy*

Compound[a]	Urinary excretion (% dose)[b]
VPA	38 ± 17
(E)-Δ^2-VPA	1.2 ± 0.2
(Z)-Δ^2-VPA	0.33 ± 0.16
Δ^3-VPA	0.02 ± 0.01
Δ^4-VPA	0.05 ± 0.02
(2E)-$\Delta^{2,4}$-VPA	0.13 ± 0.06
(2E, 3'E)-$\Delta^{2,3'}$-VPA	2.3 ± 0.9
3-OH-VPA	1.5 ± 1.0
4-OH-VPA	3.3 ± 1.4
5-OH-VPA	1.5 ± 0.8
3-oxo-VPA	32 ± 21
4-oxo-VPA	1.3 ± 0.6
PSA	0.06 ± 0.03
PGA	2.3 ± 1.0
	Total: 83.6 ± 22.8

[a] Metabolites were quantified following treatment of urine with β-glucuronidase.
[b] Values represent means ± S.D. ($N = 10$) for metabolites excreted during one dosing interval (8 or 12 hr). The mean (± S.D.) daily dose of VPA was 1,392 ± 560 mg.
(Adapted from ref. 59.)

tor (stiripentol) of cytochrome P-450 enzymes on production of the hepatotoxic olefin, Δ^4-VPA (58,59). The formation clearance of this metabolite was respectively increased and decreased by these regimens, as were the clearances of other metabolites generated by cytochrome P-450.

Effect of Altered Physiological States on VPA Metabolism

Pregnancy

In light of the teratogenic potential of VPA, there has been interest in defining the pharmacokinetics and disposition of VPA in human pregnancy. Stable isotope "pulse" dose experiments performed in a pregnant epileptic patient on VPA maintenance therapy showed that kinetic parameters for the parent drug during the first trimester were similar to those of nonpregnant adults (128).

In the later states of pregnancy, hepatic and renal clearances and the volume of distribution of VPA increased, and protein binding decreased (81,94). However, the profile of plasma and urinary metabolites of the drug remained relatively constant (94). Both VPA and its metabolites undergo placental transfer, and it was found that the elimination half-lives of these species were much longer in the fetus than in the mother, resulting in accumulation of VPA and its metabolites in the fetal compartment (81,89,90). Interestingly, the fetus possesses the ability to metabolize VPA, as shown by *in vitro* experiments with human conceptuses (108). Metabolites detected in the serum of newborn infants from mothers receiving VPA therapy comprised 3-oxo- and Δ^2-VPA (major constituents) and 3-, 4-, and 5-hydroxy-VPA and Δ^4-VPA (minor constituents). Although VPA and 3-oxo-VPA were found in breast milk, their concentrations were only 3% to 7% of those in maternal serum, suggesting that breast-feeding would not result in exposure of the neonate to appreciable quantities of these compounds (89).

Liver Disease

Several case reports have appeared describing VPA metabolism in patients with abnormal liver function or VPA-induced hepatic failure (14,15,25,50,54). In all instances, the profile of VPA metabolites was abnormal, although pronounced interpatient differences were evident. In two cases (14,54), ω-oxidation of VPA was markedly enhanced as judged by the urinary excretion of PGA, whereas β-oxidation (judged by 3-oxo-VPA output in urine) was suppressed. Glucuronidation and desaturation of VPA were considered to be normal in these patients, although Dickinson et al. (25) reported unusually high concentrations of rearranged isomers of the glucuronide in plasma and urine of a patient with VPA-related hepatic disease. β-Oxidation was also defective in the cases reported by Böhles et al. (15) and Kochen et al. (50). However, in the latter patient (a child who died from VPA-induced liver failure), extremely high levels of unsaturated, hepatotoxic metabolites of VPA were present in biological fluids immediately before death. Although the current information base is limited, the above findings suggest that different profiles of VPA metabolites in plasma and urine may reflect different types of hepatic dysfunction, and it has been proposed that it may be possible to distinguish VPA-induced versus non-VPA-induced liver damage on this basis (14).

Species Differences

The pharmacokinetics and metabolism of VPA have been examined in a number of animal species and compared to those in humans (84). Although the same pathways of VPA biotransformation appear to be followed in each species (β-oxidation apparently being more pronounced in the dog than in other animals [65,68]), pharmacokinetics differ widely, the plasma half-life of the parent drug being more than an order of magnitude greater in humans than in monkeys, dogs, rats, or mice (84). For this reason, Nau and co-workers have advocated the use of an osmotic delivery system for constant-rate drug administration in animal studies of the toxicity of VPA and its metabolites (88,93,96).

PHARMACOLOGICAL ACTIVITY OF VPA METABOLITES

Evidence that metabolites of VPA may contribute significantly to the therapeutic effects of the parent drug derives from two observations (84,99, and references therein): (a) the anticonvulsant activity of VPA correlates poorly with steady-state VPA serum concentrations; and (b) the time

course of anticonvulsant effect differs from that predicted from the pharmacokinetics of VPA, in that protection against seizures is not maximal until some time after the attainment of steady-state concentrations of VPA in serum or brain tissue, and persists long after the parent drug has been cleared from the systemic circulation.

In an attempt to define the role of active metabolites in the pharmacological actions of VPA, Löscher and colleagues have examined the abilities of all of the major and several of the minor VPA metabolites to increase electro- and chemoconvulsive thresholds in mice (63,70,84) and to elevate GABA levels in mouse brain and in brain synaptosomes *in vitro* (66). These studies demonstrated that the mono-unsaturated metabolites of VPA are the most active, with the (E)-Δ^2 and Δ^4 species having anticonvulsant potencies comparable to that of VPA itself. Furthermore, since (E)-Δ^2-VPA is the only metabolite found in appreciable quantities in mammalian brain following administration of VPA (67,68,83), and since this metabolite is cleared from brain tissue and plasma more slowly than the parent drug (83,96), it has been proposed that Δ^2-VPA accumulates with time in the central nervous system and contributes to the therapeutic effects of the parent drug (68). In addition, the relatively slow washout kinetics of Δ^2-VPA as compared with those of VPA may account for the persistence of antiepileptic activity following discontinuance of VPA administration (83).

Studies in animals given preformed Δ^2-VPA have shown that the metabolite is bound extensively to plasma proteins (typically >90%), resulting in lower concentrations in liver (69,85) and embryonic tissue (88) than would be the case with VPA itself. Indeed, Δ^2-VPA appears to be neither hepatotoxic (45) nor strongly embryotoxic (71,79) and, in view of its favorable anticonvulsant activity, it has been proposed as a potentially valuable alternative to VPA in the treatment of human epilepsy (71,87).

This view has been disputed, however, on the grounds that Δ^2-VPA is a weaker anticonvulsant than VPA with more potent sedative activity (44,77).

TOXICOLOGICAL PROPERTIES OF VPA METABOLITES

VPA-Induced Teratogenesis

Following early clinical reports that therapy with VPA during pregnancy was associated with a significantly higher incidence in offspring of neural tube defects, notably spina bifida, interest has centered on the mechanism of VPA-induced teratogenesis and in the possible role of metabolites of the drug in the process (82). Both parent drug and metabolites have been shown to accumulate to some degree in the early mammalian embryo, probably as a result of the relatively high intracellular pH of this tissue (91,92). Also, several VPA metabolites are embryotoxic in the mouse model, the most potent being Δ^4-VPA whose teratogenicity is similar to that of the parent drug (84,86). However, several lines of evidence suggest that VPA itself, and not one of its known metabolites, is the causative agent *in vivo* (78,82): (a) metabolite levels in the embryo are very low; (b) coadministration of VPA and phenobarbital (an inducer of VPA biotransformation) to either animals or epileptic patients reduces the teratogenic effects of valproate (80); (c) the teratogenicity of VPA in animal models correlates well with circulating levels of the parent drug; and (d) VPA is embryotoxic under *in vitro* conditions where little metabolism takes place, and only hydroxylated (nontoxic) products are formed (108). Despite the negative findings from studies on the embryotoxicity of VPA metabolites and analogs thereof, it should be pointed out that such investigations have provided valuable information on structure-activity relationships for the teratogenicity of branched-chain fatty acids (19,80,86).

VPA-Induced Hepatotoxicity

In contrast to the situation discussed in the preceding section, metabolites of VPA probably do play a significant role in the rare, but potentially fatal, hepatotoxicity associated with VPA therapy. In a case report of a child who developed a Reye-like syndrome while receiving VPA, Gerber et al. (32) were the first to speculate on the involvement of a toxic metabolite of the drug as a mediator of the liver damage. As additional cases of VPA-related hepatic injury came to light, this possibility of toxic metabolite involvement was echoed by others (130,131) who developed further the notion that VPA may undergo biotransformation to a product that resembles, both structurally and functionally, 4-pentenoic acid, a known hepatoxin. With the availability of the rat model for VPA-induced hepatic microvesicular steatosis (43,60), Kesterson, Granneman, and co-workers conducted detailed in *in vivo* toxicological studies with VPA and several of its metabolites (35,45). These experiments, which were supported by independent *in vitro* studies (12,46,110), indicated that the unsaturated metabolites Δ^4- and $\Delta^{2,4}$-VPA were the most potent hepatotoxins *in vivo* where they caused damage to liver mitochondria, inhibition of fatty acid β-oxidation activity, and accumulation of hepatic lipid. Additional studies with Δ^4-VPA (a metabolic precursor of $\Delta^{2,4}$-VPA) served to reinforce the view that this terminal olefin, like 4-pentenoic acid (115), acts as a mechanism-based irreversible inhibitor of enzymes of the fatty acid β-oxidation complex (104,107,112). In addition, it causes autocatalytic destruction of hepatic cytochrome P-450 (102) and generates reactive metabolites, which become covalently linked to cellular macromolecules (100). The recent finding that Δ^4-VPA is formed metabolically by the action of hepatic cytochrome P-450 enzymes that are induced by phenobarbital (109) and other antiepileptic drugs

(59) provides a plausible explanation of the potentiating effect of such agents on VPA-induced hepatotoxicity in rats (60,118) and epileptic patients (28,116).

Although the "Δ⁴" pathway of VPA metabolism seems likely to contribute to VPA-related liver damage (10), other mechanisms, at present poorly defined, are probably also involved, e.g., competitive inhibition of β-ketothiolase by 3-oxo-VPA (20), carnitine deficiency induced by VPA administration (18), depletion of mitochondrial pools of free coenzyme A by VPA (45,76), or interference by VPA with processes of intermediary metabolism in a liver whose function is already compromised by severe illness and exposure to multiple anticonvulsant drugs (28,30). Whatever the precise underlying factors, it is evident that a detailed knowledge of the metabolism of VPA, and of the properties of its biotransformation products, will prove germane to our understanding of VPA-induced hepatotoxicity.

CONCLUSIONS

Judging from the expansive literature published over the past few years dealing with valproate metabolism, it appears that products of VPA biotransformation are attracting increasing attention as mediators of certain serious adverse reactions to the drug, and also as contributors to its beneficial antiepileptic effects. Although the biological activities of several metabolites of VPA have been examined in some detail, those of many others have not, most notably the recently characterized group of doubly-unsaturated compounds which can assume quantitative importance in certain situations and whose metabolic origin remains obscure.

Much remains to be learned about the enzyme systems that participate in the biotransformation of VPA, and about the confluent pathways of intermediary and xenobiotic metabolism reflected in the structures of the diverse array of metabolites of this drug. Moreover, virtually nothing is known about stereochemistry of VPA metabolites, the majority of which, in contrast to the parent drug, are chiral molecules. In this context, it is likely that VPA will find application in more fundamental work as a model compound for the study of metabolic processes involving fatty acids and their derivatives.

A fuller appreciation of VPA metabolism will afford a better understanding of the pharmacological and toxicological properties of this unusual antiepileptic drug. It should also provide new leads for the rational design of novel, safer anticonvulsants of the alkanoic acid class. It is in these areas where progress is likely to be made in the years ahead, and we look forward with keen interest to the next decade of research on VPA biotransformation.

ACKNOWLEDGMENTS

We would like to thank Mr. Robert Gollehon for assistance in manuscript preparation. The authors' work on VPA metabolism has been supported by the Epilepsy Foundation of America, by research grants GM 32165, NS 17111, and DK 30699 from the National Institutes of Health, and by a fellowship (to A. W. Rettenmeier) from the Deutsche Forschungsgemeinschaft, all of which are gratefully acknowledged.

REFERENCES

1. Abbott, F. S., Burton, R., Orr, J., Wladichuk, D., Ferguson, S., and Sun, T.-H. (1982): Valproic acid analysis in saliva and serum using selected ion monitoring (electron ionization) of the *tert*-butyldimethylsilyl derivatives. *J. Chromatogr.*, 227:433–444.
2. Abbott, F. S., Kassahun, K., and Panesar, S. (1987): Negative ion chemical ionization GCMS analysis of valproic acid in saliva and serum and its metabolites in saliva. Presented at the 35th

ASMS Conference on Mass Spectrometry and Allied Topics, Denver, Colorado.

3. Abbott, F. S., Kassam, J., Acheampong, A., Ferguson, S., Panesar, S., Burton, R., Farrell, K., and Orr, J. (1986): Capillary gas chromatography-mass spectrometery of valproic acid metabolites in serum and urine using *tert*-butyldimethylsilyl derivatives. *J. Chromatogr.*, 375:285–298.

4. Abbott, F. S., Kassam, J., Orr, J. M., and Farrell, K. (1986): The effect of aspirin on valproic acid metabolism. *Clin. Pharmacol. Ther.*, 40:94–100.

5. Abbott, F., Panesar, S., Orr, J., Burton, R., and Farrell, K. (1986): Effect of carbamazepine on valproic acid metabolism. *Epilepsia*, 27:591.

6. Acheampong, A., and Abbott, F. S. (1985): Synthesis and stereochemical determination of diunsaturated valproic acid analogs including its major diunsaturated metabolite. *J. Lipid Res.*, 26:1002–1008.

7. Acheampong, A., Abbott, F., and Burton, R. (1983): Identification of valproic acid metabolites in human serum and urine using hexadeuterated valproic acid and gas chromatographic mass spectrometric analysis. *Biomed. Mass Spectrom.*, 10:586–595.

8. Acheampong, A. A., Abbott, F. S., Orr, J. M., Ferguson, S. M., and Burton, R. W. (1984): Use of hexadeuterated valproic acid and gas chromatography-mass spectrometry to determine the pharmacokinetics of valproic acid. *J. Pharm. Sci.*, 73:489–494.

9. Aly, M. I., and Abdel-Latif, A. A. (1980): Studies on distribution and metabolism of valproate in rat brain, liver, and kidney. *Neurochem. Res.*, 5:1231–1242.

10. Baillie, T. A. (1988): Metabolic activation of valproic acid and drug-mediated hepatotoxicity. Role of the terminal olefin, 2-*n*-propyl-4-pentenoic acid. *Chem. Res. Toxicol.*, 1:195–199.

11. Becker, C.-M, and Harris, R. A. (1983): Influence of valproic acid on hepatic carbohydrate and lipid metabolism. *Arch. Biochem. Biophys.*, 223:381–392.

12. Bjorge S, M., and Baillie, T. A. (1985): Inhibition of medium-chain fatty acid β-oxidation *in vitro* by valproic acid and its unsaturated metabolite, 2-*n*-propyl-4-pentenoic acid. *Biochem. Biophys. Res. Commun.*, 132:245–252.

13. Bohan, T. P., Millington, D. S., Roe, C. R., Yergey, A. L., and Liberato, D. J. (1984): Valproylcarnitine: A novel metabolite of valproic acid. *Ann. Neurol.*, 16:394.

14. Bohan, T. P., Tennison, M. B., Rettenmeier, A., and Baillie, T. A. (1987): Valproic acid (VPA) metabolism in a boy with liver failure. *The Pharmacologist*, 29:179.

15. Böhles, H., Richter, K., Wagner-Thiessen, E., and Schäfer, H. (1982): Decreased serum carnitine in valproate induced Reye syndrome. *Eur. J. Pediatr.*, 139:185–186.

16. Brown, N. A., Farmer, P. B., and Coakley, M. (1965): Valproic acid teratogenicity: Demonstration that the biochemical mechanism differs from that of valproate hepatotoxicity. *Biochem. Soc. Trans.*, 13:75–77.

17. Chapman, A., Keane, P. E., Meldrum, B. S., Simiand, J., and Vernieres, J. C. (1982): Mechanism of anticonvulsant action of valproate. *Prog. Neurobiol.*, 19:315–359.

18. Coulter, D. L. (1984): Carnitine deficiency: A possible mechanism for valproate hepatotoxicity. *Lancet*, 689.

19. Di Carlo, F. J., Bickart, P., and Auer, C. M. (1986): Structure-metabolism relationships (SMR) for the prediction of health hazards by the Environmental Protection Agency. II. Application to teratogenicity and other toxic effects caused by aliphatic acids. *Drug Metab. Rev.*, 17:187–220.

20. Dickinson, R. G., Bassett, M. L., Searle, J., Tyler, J. H., and Eadie, M. J. (1985): Valproate hepatotoxicity: A review and report of two instances in adults. *Clin. Exp. Neurol.*, 21:79–91.

21. Dickinson, R. G., Eadie, M. J., and Hooper, W. D. (1985): Glucuronidase-resistant glucuronides of valproic acid: Consequences to enterohepatic recirculation of valproate in the rat. *Biochem. Pharmacol.*, 34:407–408.

22. Dickinson, R. G., Harland, R. C., Ilias, A. M., Rodgers, R. M., Kaufman, S. N., Lynn, R. K., and Gerber, N. (1979): Disposition of valproic acid in the rat: Dose-dependent metabolism, distribution, enterohepatic recirculation and choleretic effect. *J. Pharmacol. Exp. Ther.*, 211:583–595.

23. Dickinson, R. G., Hooper, W. D., and Eadie, M. J. (1984): pH-Dependent rearrangement of the biosynthetic ester glucuronide of valproic acid of β-glucuronidase-resistant forms. *Drug Metab. Dispos.*, 12:247–252.

24. Dickinson, R. G., Kluck, R. M., Eadie, M. J., and Hooper, W. D. (1985): Disposition of β-glucuronidase-resistant "glucuronides" of valproic acid after intrabiliary administration in the rat: Intact absorption, fecal excretion and intestinal hydrolysis. *J. Pharmacol. Exp. Ther.*, 233:214–221.

25. Dickinson, R. G., Kluck, R. M., Hooper, W. D., Patterson, M., Chalk, J. B., and Eadie, M. J. (1985): Rearrangement of valproate glucuronide in a patient with drug-associated hepatobiliary and renal dysfunction. *Epilepsia*, 26:589–593.

26. Dickinson, R. G., Kluck, R. M., Wood, B. T., Eadie, M. J., and Hooper, W. D. (1986): Impaired biliary elimination of β-glucuronidase-resistant "glucuronides" of valproic acid after intravenous administration in the rat. Evidence for oxidative metabolism of the resistant isomers. *Drug Metab. Dispos.*, 14:255–262.

27. Draye, J.-P., and Vamecq, J. (1987): The inhibition by valproic acid of the mitochondrial oxidation of monocarboxylic and ω-hydroxymonocarboxylic acids: Possible implications for the metabolism of gamma-aminobutyric acid. *J. Biochem.*, 102:235–242.

28. Dreifuss, F. E., and Langer, D. H. (1987): He-

patic considerations in the use of antiepileptic drugs. *Epilepsia*, 28(Suppl.2):S23–S29.

29. Dreifuss, F. E., Santilli, N., Langer, D. H., Sweeney, K. P., Moline, K. A., and Menander, K. B. (1987): Valproic acid hepatic fatalities: A retrospective review. *Neurology*, 37:379–385.

30. Eadie, M. J., Hooper, W. D., and Dickinson, R. G. (1988): Valproate-associated hepatotoxicity and its biochemical mechanisms. *Med. Toxicol.*, 3:85–106.

31. Ferrandes, B., and Eymard, P. (1977): Metabolism of valproate sodium in rabbit, rat, dog, and man. *Epilepsia*, 18:169–182.

32. Gerber, N., Dickinson, R. G., Harland, R. C. Lynn, R. K., Houghton, D., Antonias, J. I., and Schimschock, J. C. (1979): Reye-like syndrome associated with valproic acid therapy. *J. Pediatr.*, 95:142–144.

33. Gompertz, D., Tippett, P., Bartlett, K., and Baillie, T. (1977): Identification of urinary metabolites of sodium dipropylacetate in man; potential sources of interference in organic acid screening procedures. *Clin. Chim. Acta*, 74:153–160.

34. Granneman, G. R., Marriott, T. B., Wang, S. I., Sennello, L. T., Hagen, N. S., and Sonders, R. C. (1984): Aspects of the dose-dependent metabolism of valproic acid. In: *Metabolism of Antiepileptic Drugs*, edited by R. H. Levy, W. H. Pitlick, M. Eichelbaum, and J. Meijer, pp. 97–104. Raven Press, New York.

35. Granneman, G. R., Wang, S.-I., Kesterson, J. W., and Machinist, J. M. (1984): The hepatotoxicity of valproic acid and its metabolites in rats. II. Intermediary and valproic acid metabolism. *Hepatology*, 4:1153–1158.

36. Granneman, G. R., Wang, S.-I., Machinist, J. M., and Kesterson, J. W. (1984): Aspects of the metabolism of valproic acid. *Xenobiotica*, 14:375–387.

37. Gugler, R., and von Unruh, G. E. (1980): Clinical pharmacokinetics of valproic acid. *Clin. Pharmacokin.*, 5:67–83.

38. Heinemeyer, G., Nau, H., Hildebrandt, A. G., and Roots, I. (1985): Oxidation and glucuronidation of valproic acid in male rats—influence of phenobarbital, 3-methylcholanthrene, β-naphthoflavone and clofibrate. *Biochem. Pharmacol.*, 34:133–139.

39. Hoffmann, F., von Unruh, G. E., and Janick, B. C. (1981): Valproic acid disposition in epileptic patients during combined antiepileptic maintenance therapy. *Eur. J. Clin. Pharmacol.*, 19:383–385.

40. Horie, S., and Suga, T. (1985): Enhancement of peroxisomal β-oxidation in the livers of rats and mice treated with valproic acid. *Biochem. Pharmacol.*, 34:1357–1362.

41. Howell, S. R., Hazelton, G. A., and Claassen, C. D. (1986): Depletion of hepatic UDP-glucuronic acid by drugs that are glucuronidated. *J. Pharmacol. Exp. Ther.*, 236:610–614.

42. Jakobs, C., and Löscher, W. (1978): Identification of metabolites of valproic acid in serum of humans, dog, rat, and mouse. *Epilepsia*, 19:591–602.

43. Jezequel, A. M., Bonazzi, P., Novelli, G., Venturini, C., and Orlandi, F. (1984): Early structural and functional changes in liver of rats treated with a single dose of valproic acid. *Hepatology*, 4:1159–1166.

44. Keane, P. E., Simiand, J., and Morre, M. (1985): Comparison of the pharmacological and biochemical profiles of valproic acid (VPA) and its cerebral metabolite (2-en-VPA) after oral administration in mice. *Meth. Find. Exptl. Clin. Pharmacol.*, 7:83–86.

45. Kesterson, J. W., Granneman, G. R., and Machinist, J. M. (1984): The hepatotoxicity of valproic acid and its metabolites in rats. I. Toxicologic, biochemical and histopathologic studies. *Hepatology*, 4:1143–1152.

46. Kingsley, E., Gray, P., Tolman, K. G., and Tweedale, R. (1983): The toxicity of metabolites of sodium valproate in cultured hepatocytes. *J. Clin. Pharmacol.*, 23:178–185.

47. Koch, K. M., Baillie, T. A., Prickett, K. S., Rettenmeier, A., and Levy, R. H. (1985): β-Oxidation of valproate in rat: Effects of fasting and glucose. *Epilepsia*, 26:519.

48. Kochen, W., Imbeck, H., and Jakobs, C. (1977): Untersuchungen über die Ausscheidung von Metaboliten der Valproinsäure im Urin der Ratte und des Menschen. *Arzneim.-Forsch.*, 27:1090–1099.

49. Kochen, W., and Scheffner, H. (1980): On unsaturated metabolites of the valproic acid (VPA) in serum of epileptic children. In: *Antiepileptic Therapy: Advances in Drug Monitoring*, edited by S. I. Johannessen, P. L. Morselli, C. E. Pippenger, A. Richens, D. Schmidt, and H. Meinardi, pp. 111–120. Raven Press, New York.

50. Kochen, W., Schneider, A., and Ritz, A. (1983): Abnormal metabolism of valproic acid in fatal hepatic failure. *Eur. J. Pediatr.*, 141:30–35.

51. Kochen, W., Sprunck, H. P., Tauscher, B., and Klemens, M. (1984): Five doubly unsaturated metabolites of valproic acid in urine and plasma of patients on valproic acid therapy. *J. Clin. Chem. Clin. Biochem.*, 22:309–317.

52. Kochen, W., Tauscher, B., Klemens, M., and Depene, E. (1982): The application of deuterated valproic acid (VPA) in chronically treated epileptic patients under monotherapy and polypharmacy. In: *Stable Isotopes*, edited by H.-L. Schmidt, H. Förstel, and K. Heinzinger, pp. 271–276. Elsevier, Amsterdam.

53. Kuhara, T., Hirohata, Y., Yamada, S., and Matsumoto, I. (1978): Metabolism of sodium dipropylacetate in humans. *Eur. J. Drug Metab. Pharmacokin.*, 3:171–177.

54. Kuhara, T., Inoue, Y., Matsumoto, M., Shinka, T., Matsumoto, I., Kitamura, K., Fuji, H., and Sakura, N. (1985): Altered metabolic profiles of valproic acid in a patient with Reye's syndrome. *Clin. Chim. Acta*, 145:135–142.

55. Kuhara, T., Iwai, Y., Haraguchi, S., Shinka, T., and Matsumoto, I. (1978): Metabolic profile of biological constituents: (1) The effects of sodium

dipropylacetate on human urinary acids. In: *Recent Developments in Mass Spectrometry in Biochemistry and Medicine*, edited by A. Frigerio, pp. 191–202. Plenum Press, New York.

56. Kuhara, T., and Matsumoto, I. (1974): Metabolism of branched medium chain length fatty acid. I. ω-Oxidation of sodium dipropylacetate in rats. *Biomed. Mass Spectrom.*, 1:291–294.

57. Laub, M. C., Paetzke-Brunner, I., and Jaeger, G. (1986): Serum carnitine during valproic acid therapy. *Epilepsia*, 27:559–562.

58. Levy, R. H., Loiseau, P., Guyot, M., Acheampong, A., Tor, J., and Rettenmeier, A. W. (1987): Effects of stiripentol on valproate plasma level and metabolism. *Epilepsia*, 28:605.

59. Levy, R. H., Rettenmeier, A. W., Baillie, T. A., Howald, W. N., Wilensky, A. J., Friel, P. N., and Anderson, G. (1987): Formation of hepatotoxic metabolites of valproate in patients on carbamazepine or phenytoin. *Epilepsia*, 28:627.

60. Lewis, J. H., Zimmerman, H. J., Garrett, C. T., and Rosenberg, E. (1982): Valproate-induced hepatic steatogenesis in rats. *Hepatology*, 2:870–873.

61. Liberato, D. J., Millington, D. S., and Yergey, A. L. (1985): Analysis of acylcarnitines in human metabolic disease by thermospray liquid chromatography/mass spectrometry. In: *Mass Spectrometry in the Health and Life Sciences*, edited by A. L. Burlingame and N. Castagnoli, Jr., pp. 333–346. Elsevier, Amsterdam.

62. Libert, R., Van Hoof, F., Schanck, A., and Hoffmann, E. (1986): The hydroxamate of valproic acid, a compound produced by oximation of urine from patients under valproic therapy. *Biomed. Mass Spectrom.*, 13:599–603.

63. Löscher, W. (1981): Anticonvulsant activity of metabolites of valproic acid. *Arch. Int. Pharmacodyn. Ther.*, 249:158–163.

64. Löscher, W. (1981): Concentration of metabolites of valproic acid in plasma of epileptic patients. *Epilepsia*, 22:169–178.

65. Löscher, W. (1981): Plasma levels of valproic acid and its metabolites during continued treatment in dogs. *J. Vet. Pharmacol. Ther.*, 4:111–119.

66. Löscher, W., Böhme, G., Schäfer, H., and Kochen, W. (1981): Effect of metabolites of valproic acid on the metabolism of GABA in brain and brain nerve endings. *Neuropharmacol.*, 20;1187–1192.

67. Löscher, W., and Nau, H. (1982): Valproic acid: Metabolic concentrations in plasma and brain, anticonvulsant activity, and effects on GABA metabolism during subacute treatment in mice. *Arch. Int. Pharmacodyn.*, 257:20–31.

68. Löscher, W., and Nau, H. (1983): Distribution of valproic acid and its metabolites in various brain areas of dogs and rats after acute and prolonged treatment. *J. Pharmacol. Exp. Ther.*, 226:845–854.

69. Löscher, W., and Nau, H. (1984): Comparative transfer of valproic acid and of an active metabolite into brain and liver: Possible pharma-

cological and toxicological consequences. *Arch. Int. Pharmacodyn.*, 270:192–202.

70. Löscher, W., and Nau, H. (1985): Pharmacological evaluation of various metabolites and analogues of valproic acid. Anticonvulsant and toxic potencies in mice. *Neuropharmacol.*, 24:427–435.

71. Löscher, W., Nau, H., Marescaux, C., and Vergnes, M. (1984): Comparative evaluation of anticonvulsant and toxic potencies of valproic acid and 2-en-valproic acid in different animal models of epilepsy. *Eur. J. Pharmacol.*, 99:211–218.

72. Matsumoto, I., Kuhara, T., Shinka, T., Inoue, Y., and Matsumoto, M. (1984): Effect of valproic acid on amino acid and organic acid metabolism. In: *Metabolism of Antiepileptic Drugs*, edited by R. H. Levy, W. H. Pitlick, M. Eichelbaum, and J. Meijer, pp. 169–175. Raven Press, New York.

73. Matsumoto, I., Kuhara, T., and Yoshino, M. (1976): Metabolism of branched medium chain length fatty acid. II. β-Oxidation of sodium dipropylacetate in rats. *Biomed. Mass Spectrom.*, 3:235–240.

74. Meunier, H., Carraz, G., Meunier, Y., Eymard, P., and Aimard, M. (1963): Propriétés pharmacodynamiques de l'acide *n*-dipropylacetique. *Therapie*, 18:435–438.

75. Millington, D. S., Bohan, T. P., Roe, C. R., Yergey, A. L., and Liberato, D. J. (1985): Valproylcarnitine: A novel drug metabolite identified by fast atom bombardment and thermospray liquid chromatography-mass spectrometry. *Clin. Chim. Acta*, 145:69–76.

76. Moore, K. H., Decker, B. P., and Schreefel, F. P. (1988): Hepatic hydrolysis of octanoyl-CoA and valproyl-CoA in control and valproate-fed animals. *Int. J. Biochem.*, 20:175–178.

77. Morre, M., Keane, P. E., Vernières, J. C., Simiand, J., and Roncucci, R. (1984): Valproate: Recent findings and perspectives. *Epilepsia*, 25 (Suppl. 1):S5–S9.

78. Nau, H. (1986): Species differences in pharmacokinetics and drug teratogenesis. *Environ. Health Persp.*, 70:113–129.

79. Nau, H. (1986): Transfer of valproic acid and its main active unsaturated metabolite to the gestational tissue: Correlation with neural tube defect formation in the mouse. *Teratology*, 33:21–27.

80. Nau, H. (1986): Valproic acid teratogenicity in mice after various administration and phenobarbital-pretreatment regimens: The parent drug and not one of the metabolites assayed is implicated as teratogen. *Fund. Appl. Toxicol.*, 6:662–668.

81. Nau, H., Helge, H., and Luck, W. (1984): Valproic acid in the perinatal period: Decreased maternal serum protein binding results in fetal accumulation and neonatal displacement of the drug and some metabolites. *J. Pediatr.*, 104:627–634.

82. Nau, H., and Hendrickx, A. G. (1987): Valproic acid teratogenesis. *ISI Atlas of Science*, 1:52–56.

83. Nau, H., and Löscher, W. (1982): Valproic acid: Brain and plasma levels of the drug and its metabolites, anticonvulsant effects and γ-aminobu-

tyric acid (GABA) metabolism in the mouse. *J. Pharmacol. Exp. Ther.*, 220:654–659.

84. Nau, H., and Löscher, W. (1984): Valproic acid and metabolites: Pharmacological and toxicological studies. *Epilepsia*, 25 (Suppl. 1):S14–S22.

85. Nau, H., and Löscher, W. (1985): Valproic acid and active unsaturated metabolite (2-en): Transfer to mouse liver following human therapeutic doses. *Biopharm. Drug Dispos.*, 6:1–8.

86. Nau, H., and Löscher, W. (1986): Pharmacologic evaluation of various metabolites and analogs of valproic acid: Teratogenic potencies in mice. *Fund. Appl. Toxicol.*, 6:669–676.

87. Nau, H., Löscher, W., and Schäfer, H. (1984): Anticonvulsant activity and embryotoxicity of valproic acid. *Neurology*, 34:400–401.

88. Nau, H., Merker, H.-J., Brendel, K., Gansau, Ch., Häuser, I., and Wittfoht, W. (1984): Disposition, embryotoxicity and teratogenicity of valproic acid in the mouse as related to man. In: *Metabolism of Antiepileptic Drugs*, edited by R. H. Levy, W. H. Pitlick, M. Eichelbaum, and J. Meijer, pp. 85–96. Raven Press, New York.

89. Nau, H., Rating, D., Koch, S., Häuser, I., and Helge, H. (1981): Valproic acid and its metabolites: Placental transfer, neonatal pharmacokinetics, transfer *via* mother's milk and clinical status in neonates of epileptic mothers. *J. Pharmacol. Exp. Ther.*, 219:768–777.

90. Nau, H., Schäfer, H., Rating, D., Jakobs, C., and Helge, H. (1982): Placental transfer and neonatal pharmacokinetics of valproic acid and some of its metabolites. In: *Epilepsy, Pregnancy, and the Child*, edited by D. Janz, M. Dam, A. Richens, L. Bossi, H. Helge, and D. Schmidt, pp. 367–372. Raven Press, New York.

91. Nau, H., and Scott, W. J., Jr. (1986): Weak acids may act as teratogens by accumulating in the basic milieu of the early mammalian embryo. *Nature*, 323:276–278.

92. Nau, H., and Scott, W. J. (1987): Teratogenicity of valproic acid and related substances in the mouse: Drug accumulation and pH_i in the embryo during organogenesis and structure-activity considerations. *Arch. Toxicol.*, Suppl. 11:128–139.

93. Nau, H., and Spielmann, H. (1983): Embryotoxicity testing of valproic acid. *Lancet*, 763–764.

94. Nau, H., Wittfoht, W., Rating, D., Jakobs, C., Schäfer, H., and Helge, H. (1982): Pharmacokinetics of valproic acid in a pregnant patient: Stable isotope methodology. In: *Epilepsy, Pregnancy, and the Child*, edited by D. Janz, M. Dam, A. Richens, L. Bossi, H. Helge, and D. Schmidt, pp. 131–139. Raven Press, New York.

95. Nau, H., Wittfoht, W., Schäfer, H., Jakobs, C., Rating, D., and Helge, H. (1981): Valproic acid and several metabolites: Quantitative determination in serum, urine, breast milk and tissues by gas chromatography-mass spectrometry using selected ion monitoring. *J. Chromatogr.*, 226:69–78.

96. Nau, H., and Zierer, R. (1982); Pharmacokinetics of valproic acid and metabolites in mouse plasma and brain following constant-rate application of the drug and its unsaturated metabolite with an osmotic delivery system. *Biopharm. Drug Dispos.*, 3:317–328.

97. Ogiso, T., Ito, Y., Iwaki, M., and Yamahata, T. (1986): Disposition and pharmacokinetics of valproic acid in rats. *Chem. Pharm. Bull. (Tokyo)*, 34:2950–2956.

98. Olson, M. J., and Thurman, R. G. (1984): Increase in catalase-H_2O_2 and inhibition of ketogenesis by valproate in perfused rat liver. *The Toxicologist*, 4:43.

99. Pollack, G. M., McHugh, W. B., Gengo, F. M., Ermer, J. C., and Shen, D. D. (1986): Accumulation and washout kinetics of valproic acid and its active metabolites. *J. Clin. Pharmacol.*, 26:668–676.

100. Porubek, D. J., Grillo, M. P., and Baillie, T. A. (1989): Covalent binding to protein of valproic acid and its hepatotoxic metabolite, 2-*n*-propyl-4-pentenoic acid, in rats and in isolated rat hepatocytes. *Drug Metab. Dispos. (in press)*.

101. Prickett, K. S., and Baillie, T. A. (1984): Metabolism of valproic acid by hepatic microsomal cytochrome P-450. *Biochem. Biophys. Res. Commun.*, 122:1166–1173.

102. Prickett, K. S., and Baillie, T. A. (1986): Metabolism of unsaturated derivatives of valproic acid in rat liver microsomes and destruction of cytochrome P-450. *Drug Metab. Dispos.*, 14:221–229.

103. Rettenmeier, A. W., Gordon, W. P., Barnes, H., and Baillie, T. A. (1987): Studies on the metabolic fate of valproic acid in the rat using stable isotope techniques. *Xenobiotica*, 17:1147–1157.

104. Rettenmeier, A. W., Gordon, W. P., Prickett, K. S., Levy, R. H., and Baillie, T. A. (1986): Biotransformation and pharmacokinetics in the rhesus monkey of 2-*n*-propyl-4-pentenoic acid, a toxic metabolite of valproic acid. *Drug Metab. Dispos.*, 14:454–464.

105. Rettenmeier, A. W., Gordon, W. P., Prickett, K. S., Levy, R. H., Lockard, J. S., Thummel, K. E., and Baillie, T. A. (1986): Metabolic fate of valproic acid in the rhesus monkey. Formation of a toxic metabolite, 2-*n*-propyl-4-pentenoic acid. *Drug Metab. Dispos.*, 14:443–453.

106. Rettenmeier, A. W., Levy, R. H., Witek, D. J., Baillie, T. A., and Howald, W. N. (1987): Quantitative metabolic profiling of drugs by automated GC/MS. Application to studies on the biodisposition of valproic acid in humans. Presented at the 35th ASMS Conference on Mass Spectrometry and Allied Topics, Denver, Colorado.

107. Rettenmeier, A. W., Prickett, K. S., Gordon, W. P., Bjorge, S. M., Chang, S.-L., Levy, R. H., and Baillie, T. A. (1985): Studies on the biotransformation in the perfused rat liver of 2-*n*-propyl-4-pentenoic acid, a metabolite of the antiepileptic drug valproic acid. Evidence for the formation of chemically reactive intermediates. *Drug Metab. Dispos.*, 13:81–96.

108. Rettie, A. E., Rettenmeier, A. W., Beyer, B. K., Baillie, T. A., and Juchau, M. R. (1986): Valproate hydroxylation by human fetal tissues and

embryotoxicity of metabolites. *Clin. Pharmacol. Ther.*, 40:172–177.

109. Rettie, A. E., Rettenmeier, A. W., Howald, W. N., and Baillie, T. A. (1987): Cytochrome P-450-catalyzed formation of Δ^4-VPA, a toxic metabolite of valproic acid. *Science*, 235:890–893.

110. Rogiers, V., Vandenberghe, Y., and Vercruysse, A. (1985): Inhibition of gluconeogenesis by sodium valproate and its metabolites in isolated rat hepatocytes. *Xenobiotica*, 15:759–765.

111. Schäfer, H., and Lührs, R. (1978): Metabolite pattern of valproic acid. Part I: Gas chromatographic determination of the valproic acid metabolite artifacts, heptanone-3, 4- and 5-hydroxy-valproic acid lactone. *Arzneim.-Forsch.*, 28:657–662.

112. Schäfer, H., and Lührs, R. (1984): Responsibility of the metabolite pattern for potential side-effects in the rat being treated with valproic acid, 2-propylpenten-2-oic acid, and 2-propylpenten-4-oic acid. In: *Metabolism of Antiepileptic Drugs*, edited by R. H. Levy, W. H. Pitlick, M. Eichelbaum, and J. Meijer, pp. 73–83. Raven Press, New York.

113. Schmid, R. D. (1977): Propionic acid and dipropylacetic acid in the urine of patients treated with dipropylacetic acid. *Clin. Chim. Acta*, 74:39–42.

114. Schobben, F., and van der Kleijn, E. (1982): Valproate: Biotransformation. In: *Antiepileptic Drugs*, 2nd edition, edited by D. M. Woodbury, J. K. Penry, and C. E. Pippenger, pp. 567–578, Raven Press, New York.

115. Schulz, H. (1983): Metabolism of 4-pentenoic acid and inhibition of thiolase by metabolites of 4-pentenoic acid. *Biochemistry*, 22:1827–1832.

116. Shen, D. D., Pollack, G. M., Cohen, M. E., Duffner, P., Lacey, D., and Ryan-Dudek, P. (1984): Effect of age on the serum metabolic pattern of valproic acid in epileptic children. *Epilepsia*, 25:674.

117. Singh, K., Abbott, F. S., and Orr, J. M. (1987): Capillary GCMS assay of 2-*n*-propyl-4-pentenoic acid (4-ene VPA) in rat plasma and urine. *Res. Commun. Chem. Pathol. Pharmacol.*, 56:211–223.

118. Sugimoto, T., Woo, M., Nishida, N., Takeuchi, T., Sakane, Y., and Kobayashi, Y. (1987): Hepatotoxicity in rat following administration of valproic acid. *Epilepsia*, 28:142–146.

119. Taburet, A.-M., and Aymard, P. (1983): Valproate glucuronidation by rat liver microsomes. Interaction with parahydroxyphenobarbital. *Biochem. Pharmacol.*, 32:3859–3861.

120. Tatsuhara, T., Muro, H., Matsuda, Y., and Imai, Y. (1987): Determination of valproic acid and its

metabolites by gas chromatography-mass spectrometry with selected ion monitoring. *J. Chromatogr.*, 399:183–195.

121. Thurston, J. H., Carroll, J. E., Hauhart, R. E., and Schiro, J. A. (1985): A single therapeutic dose of valproate affects liver carbohydrate, fat, adenylate, amino acid, coenzyme A, and carnitine metabolism in infant mice: Possible clinical significance. *Life Sci.*, 36:1643–1651.

122. Thurston, J. H., Carroll, J. E., Norris, B. J., Hauhart, R. E., and Schiro, J. A. (1983): Acute *in vivo* and *in vitro* inhibition of palmitic acid and pyruvate oxidation by valproate and valproyl-coenzyme A in livers of infant mice. *Ann. Neurol.*, 14:384–385.

123. Van den Branden, C., and Roels, F. (1985): Peroxisomal β-oxidation and sodium valproate. *Biochem. Pharmacol.*, 34:2147–2149.

124. Von Unruh, G. E., Janick, B. CH., and Hoffmann, F. (1980): Determination of valproic acid kinetics in patients during maintenance therapy using a tetradeuterated form of the drug. *Biomed. Mass Spectrom.*, 7:164–167.

125. Watkins, J. B., Gregus, Z., Thompson, T. N., and Klaassen, C. D. (1982): Induction studies on functional heterogeneity of rat liver UDP-glucuronyl transferases. *Toxicol. Appl. Pharmacol.*, 64:439–446.

126. Watkins, J. B., and Klaassen, C. D. (1981): Choleretic effect of valproic acid in the rat. *Hepatology*, 1:341–347.

127. Watkins, J. B., and Klaassen, C. D. (1982): Effect of inducers and inhibitors of glucuronidation on the biliary excretion and choleretic action of valproic acid in the rat. *J. Pharmacol. Exp. Ther.*, 220:305–310.

128. Wittfoht, W., Nau, H., Rating, D., and Helge, H. (1982): [13]-C-Labelled valproic acid pulse dose during steady-state antiepileptic therapy for pharmacokinetic studies during pregnancy. In: *Stable Isotopes*, edited by H.-L. Schmidt, H. Förstel and K. Heinzinger, pp. 265–270. Elsevier, Amsterdam.

129. Zaccara, G., Boncinelli, L., Paganini, M., Campostrini, R., Arnetoli, G., and Zappoli, R. (1983): Treatment of epileptic patients with valproic acid does not modify plasma and urine short-chain fatty acids. *Acta Neurol. Scand.*, 68:241–247.

130. Zafrani, E. S., and Berthelot, P. (1982): Sodium valproate in the induction of unusual hepatotoxicity. *Hepatology*, 2:648–649.

131. Zimmerman, H. J., and Ishak, K. G. (1982): Valproate-induced hepatic injury: Analyses of 23 fatal cases. *Hepatology*, 2:591–597.

Antiepileptic Drugs, Third Edition, edited by
R. Levy, R. Mattson, B. Meldrum,
J. K. Penry, and F. E. Dreifuss.
Raven Press, Ltd., New York © 1989.

43

Valproate

Interactions with Other Drugs

Richard H. Mattson and Joyce A. Cramer

Valproate (VPA) frequently interacts with other antiepileptic drugs. The extent of such interactions often is sufficient to alter the pharmacokinetics of both VPA and the interacting drug in clinically significant ways. Available evidence not only indicates the probability of an interaction between VPA and phenobarbital as well as between VPA and phenytoin, but also the mechanisms responsible for the interaction (41,75). This understanding has allowed prediction of similar changes in pharmacokinetics when VPA is used in combination with other drugs for which fewer observations and studies are available. Endogenous substances and disease states also may alter VPA pharmacokinetics.

VALPROATE-INDUCED CHANGES IN THE PHARMACOKINETICS OF OTHER DRUGS

Phenobarbital

In many early clinical trials, sedation often appeared when VPA was given to patients already receiving phenobarbital and/or other antiepileptic drugs (5,23,24,29,61,74). An interaction was suspected because sedative side effects eased with a decrease in phenobarbital dosage. Also, sedation was much less, even on higher VPA dosage, when VPA was given as the sole drug. Subsequent clinical trials confirmed that serum phenobarbital levels rose when valproate therapy was initiated. Schobben et al. (69) reported three patients who had increases in phenobarbital levels ranging from 35% to 200%. Later reports confirmed these changes (Table 1). The increases usually have ranged from 15% to 70%, but at times have been much higher.

Although changes in absorption, protein binding, or urinary excretion have been considered as possible mechanisms to explain increased serum phenobarbital concentration when VPA and phenobarbital are co-administered, no studies support these possibilities (9,31,39,51). On the other hand, considerable evidence indicates that VPA may inhibit biotransformation of phenobarbital to oxidized metabolites. Wilson (76) first pointed out that fatty acids bind to hepatic microsomes, including the phenobarbital site. Because VPA is chemically similar to these fatty acids, he suggested that a blockade of phenobarbital metabolism in the liver would cause secondary accumulation of phenobarbital and elevated serum levels.

The possibility that VPA could inhibit phenobarbital metabolism has been studied (Table 2). Loiseau et al. (39) noted elevation of serum phenobarbital levels and an increase in phenobarbital half-life from a

TABLE 1. *Serum phenobarbital increases after initiation of valproate therapy*

No. of patients	Patients affected (%)	Increase in serum PB level (%)	Ref.
3	100	35–200	69
7	100	17–48	62
6	100	34–71	73
—	33	30	23
—	—	66	57
11	87	46[a]	75
5[b]	70	10–25	2
7[c]	50	30–59	78
5	39	34–126	58

[a] Percent that PB dosage had to be decreased to avoid elevation of serum level.
[b] Phenobarbital derived from primidone in four patients.
[c] Phenobarbital derived from primidone in one patient.
PB, phenobarbital.

mean of 83 to 105 hr after administering VPA. At the same time, they observed a decrease in urinary output of hydroxyphenobarbital but no change in phenobarbital excretion. Bruni et al. (9) reported similar results in four patients whose serum phenobarbital levels rose after addition of VPA. The 24-hr urinary output of hydroxyphenobarbital to phenobarbital decreased simultaneously. Patel et al. (51) studied six volunteers given phenobarbital and then both phenobarbital and VPA in a second phase. The phenobarbital half-life increased from 100 to 144 hr. Plasma clearance decreased while renal excretion of phenobarbital remained unchanged. Kapetanovic et al. (31) carried out an especially careful study of VPA-phenobarbital interaction. After giving a single pulse dose of phenobarbital containing a stable isotope, they observed the patient at steady-state for a month and established the drug's elimination half-life to be 126 hr. After addition of VPA, phenobarbital levels rose 25% without change in dosage. A second pulse dose of isotope containing phenobarbital allowed repeated half-life determination that demonstrated increased half-life of the drug from 126 to 181 hr. The daily urinary excretion of phenobarbital actually increased somewhat, whereas output of the metabolite, hydroxyphenobarbital, decreased from 60 to 40 mg/day.

In summary, evidence converging from many studies indicates that the co-administration of VPA and phenobarbital increases the latter's elimination half-life, and ultimately causes elevation of serum phenobarbital levels. The probability of the interaction varies among individuals as a consequence of genetics. Dosage and levels of the drugs also are important factors.

Such an interaction has not occurred in all patients, and evidence is insufficient to allow prediction of who will be affected. High serum levels of phenobarbital before the initiation of VPA may make interaction more probable. We (45) found no significant

TABLE 2. *Changes in half-life and urinary excretion of phenobarbital and p-hydroxyphenobarbital following addition of valproate*

T$_{1/2}$ (hr)		Urinary excretion			
PB	PB + VPA	PB	p-OHPB	Ratio of p-OHPB/PB	Ref.
83	105	[a]	↓	↓	39
		↑	↓	↓	9
100	144	[a]	↓	↓	51
126	181	↑	↓	↓	31

[a] No change.
PB, phenobarbital; p-OHPB, p-hydroxyphenobarbital; VPA, valproate.

changes in serum phenobarbital levels in adult patients on a mean phenobarbital dose of 90 mg/day, whereas Vakil et al. (73) noted increased levels of phenobarbital in six patients, all of whom were receiving a phenobarbital dose of 200 mg/day.

High concentrations of VPA may compete with phenobarbital for microsomal oxidation. At low to moderate levels of VPA, the major metabolite is 3 OXO-VPA oxidized in the mitochondria. Higher levels of VPA saturate this pathway and lead to microsomal smooth endoplasmic reticulum production of metabolites 4-OH-VPA, 5-OH VPA, and conjugates to D-glucuronide (3). These latter actions provide a site of competition for phenobarbital metabolism.

Phenytoin

Early reports provided conflicting evidence of an interaction between VPA and phenytoin. Richens et al. (62) noted no consistent change in phenytoin levels when VPA was begun. Vakil et al. (73) reported an initial fall in phenytoin levels after administration of VPA but a later rise to preadministration of VPA. Bruni et al. (10) observed a decrease in plasma phenytoin levels in seven of eight patients but also noted a return to higher levels after a year of therapy without any change in phenytoin dosage. Bardy et al. (4) found a rise in serum phenytoin levels when VPA was discontinued in six patients and inferred that VPA therapy actually had lowered the phenytoin levels. Subsequent reports have consistently noted a fall in phenytoin levels (2,10,15,20,38,45,49,52,53,67). We (45) found a decrease in mean serum phenytoin levels in 21 patients: the levels dropped from 19.4 μg/ml to 14.6 μg/ml after a week of VPA therapy. After 2 to 3 months and higher dosages of VPA, phenytoin levels declined further to 11.1 μg/ml. The changes were highly significant ($p < 0.001$).

The mechanism by which VPA causes a fall in total plasma phenytoin levels appears to be well established. Valproate is highly protein bound in plasma and displaces phenytoin from binding sites (30). Lascelles, in the discussion of the report by Vakil et al. (72), postulated that such an effect might cause increased free phenytoin levels in blood and produce acute neurotoxicity. Confirming this possibility was the finding of increased phenytoin levels in brains of rats when VPA was administered after pretreatment with phenytoin (52). Evidence of toxicity was observed, which was not seen after giving either drug alone. We (45) reported in a clinical study that a rise in the percentage of free phenytoin accompanied the fall in total serum phenytoin levels when VPA therapy was initiated. Yet, free phenytoin concentrations in blood did not change significantly. When VPA displaces phenytoin from plasma protein, the increased free levels are cleared by the liver.

Valproic acid has a strong affinity for protein and is highly bound to serum albumin (80–95%), with increasing free fraction at higher total concentration (12). Cramer et al. (13) depicted the saturation of VPA binding *in vivo*, showing a nonlinear increase in free VPA: 7% free at 50 μg/ml; 9% free at 75 μg/ml; 15% free at 100 μg/ml; 22% free at 125 μg/ml; and 30% free at 150 μg/ml total VPA (Fig. 1).

When VPA is taken together with phenytoin, the competitive displacement produces an increase in the percentage of free phenytoin. The acute change may produce paradoxical neurotoxicity with redistribution of free drug. Brain levels rise while total plasma levels decrease. After clearance and re-equilibration, total phenytoin concentrations are lowered and free levels remain unchanged. Changes in phenytoin dosage to bring total levels back to the usual therapeutic range (10–20 μg/ml) may raise free phenytoin to toxic levels. In general, changes in total levels induced by binding changes do not affect pharmacologically ac-

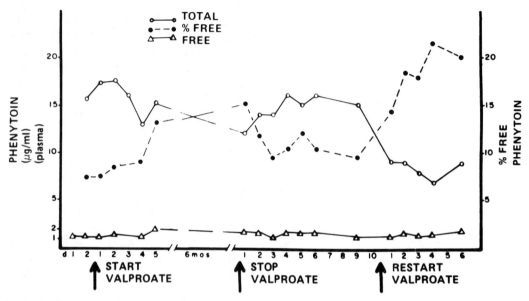

FIG. 1. Characteristic changes in total, percent free, and free phenytoin with initiation and discontinuation of VPA therapy in one patient. (From Mattson et al., ref. 45, with permission.)

tive drug and are not important if understood and anticipated (64). Such effects may be transient but recurrent and easily escape detection if total rather than free drug concentrations are used to assess efficacy and toxicity.

Figure 1 illustrates these changes in one patient. The rise in percentage of free phenytoin was associated with a transient increase in urinary excretion of hydroxyphenylphenylhydantoin (HPPH), the primary phenytoin metabolite. Increased hepatic clearance established a new steady-state with free phenytoin levels unchanged from those present prior to initiation of VPA therapy, even though total serum levels were lower (45). Bruni et al. (10) confirmed these changes in HPPH excretion. They also noted a later rise in total serum phenytoin to levels similar to those present before VPA was given, even though dosage was not changed. Percentage of free phenytoin remained high throughout the observation period. They concluded that a secondary inhibition of hydroxylation of phenytoin had occurred comparable to the

mechanism producing elevated phenobarbital levels. These dual interactions have been confirmed by others (54) and may explain some early reports that failed to note decreased phenytoin levels.

Initial *in vitro* studies of the VPA-phenytoin interaction reported displacement of phenytoin, but only at very high levels of VPA (30). Patsalos and Lascelles (52) found evidence of decreased protein binding of phenytoin when it was combined with VPA in defatted plasma. Our subsequent studies (12) as well as those of others (7,35,48) reported more marked changes at VPA levels well within the therapeutic range (50–150 μg/ml). The percentage of free phenytoin rises increasingly with higher VPA concentration (Table 3).

Phenytoin protein binding varies directly with, and is sensitive to, changes in VPA serum concentration during a dosing interval. Riva et al. (63) demonstrated significant increases in free PHT (20–46%) during a period of rising VPA concentrations. These diurnal changes in free and total phenytoin were significantly greater when VPA was

TABLE 3. *Percent free phenytoin when combined with different concentrations of valproate* in vitro[a]

Valproate (μg/ml)	Percent free phenytoin
0	19.6%
45	21.5%
90	26.1%

[a] Adapted from Cramer and Mattson (ref. 12).

co-administered than when phenytoin was used alone. Thus, sampling time becomes an important consideration for phenytoin, as does direct measurement for free phenytoin concentration (36). Such fluctuations can be expected to produce transient and possibly unrecognized changes in efficacy and toxicity.

Barbiturates

An increase in sedation has been observed when VPA was added to primidone therapy (23,61). Windorfer et al. (77) reported that mean serum primidone levels more than doubled (7.0 to 15.7 μg/ml) in seven patients, but Adams et al. (32) found only a modest 17% increase in five patients after addition of VPA. The variability between peak and predose blood levels of primidone or of other drugs with a relatively short half-life makes interpretation and recognition of interaction difficult unless the time of sampling has been carefully controlled.

Not surprisingly, levels of phenobarbital metabolically derived from primidone have been observed to rise in some patients after administration of VPA (see Table 1). A few patients received mephobarbital when VPA was initiated, but effects have not been reported. Phenobarbital derived from biotransformation of mephobarbital also may be expected to rise with addition of VPA.

Ethosuximide

Despite the frequent combined use of VPA and ethosuximide, few studies have found evidence of an interaction (42). We found that five of six patients had a mean increase of 53% in ethosuximide levels when VPA was added to the regimen. All affected patients were taking multiple drugs, and the mechanism of action was suspected to be an inhibition of oxidation similar to the VPA-phenobarbital interaction (42).

In a study of six volunteers, Pisani et al. (56) also found significant increases in ethosuximide half-life from 44 to 54 hr and decreased clearance from 11.2 to 9.5 ml/min when VPA levels ranged from 67 to 95 μg/ml. Two subjects showed no evidence of interaction, suggesting interindividual variability.

Carbamazepine

Evidence of an effect of VPA on carbamazepine has been reported with increasing frequency. Some patients have developed sedation, nausea, diplopia, and/or a confusional state when VPA was added to carbamazepine therapy. Toxic symptoms cleared only with reduction or discontinuation of carbamazepine (2,24,29,34). These anecdotal case reports suggest an interaction, but none was proved with blood level changes. The considerable variation in carbamazepine levels between doses would make analysis difficult unless determinations were consistently made both predose and at times of clinical toxicity. In addition, clinical effects of carbamazepine probably result from both the parent drug as well as the metabolically derived carbamazepine 10,11-epoxide.

Monkey studies by Levy et al. (37) demonstrated inhibition of CBZ epoxide oxidation by VPA. Assuming the same interaction in humans, the increase in pharmacodynamically active CBZ epoxide (72) might well explain the side effects, which would not be recognized if only plasma carbamazepine levels were measured.

Because carbamazepine is moderately protein bound (75%) (17,26), it may be postulated that displacement by VPA analogous to the VPA-phenytoin interaction could occur clinically. We found that when VPA was added *in vitro* to plasma samples containing carbamazepine in concentrations of 12 μg/ml, the free, pharmacologically active fraction of carbamazepine increased 25% (46). In clinical use, such an increase might produce toxicity without evidence of increased total carbamazepine levels. Höopener et al. (27) have shown that periodic diurnal carbamazepine toxicity does occur. This effect may be compounded with VPA therapy. Carbamazepine toxicity would be likely to occur at times of peak concentrations of both drugs, but would be transient and recurrent. The interaction might easily escape detection by predose determination of total drug levels. Serum samples obtained at times of side effects and analyzed specifically for free carbamazepine levels would be most useful. Further clinical studies are needed to clarify this possible interaction between VPA and carbamazepine.

Levy et al. (37) distinguished between metabolic inhibition and protein binding displacement as the basis for carbamazepine-VPA interactions. They found that carbamazepine levels were reduced in six of seven patients when VPA was added, due to protein binding displacement as verified by *in vitro* tests. Parallel assessments in monkeys also showed carbamazepine displacement by VPA and inhibition of carbamazepine metabolism demonstrated by decreased clearance of free drug. Carbamazepine epoxide free fraction was increased by VPA as was the ratio of free CBZ epoxide to free CBZ.

Inhibition of CBZ epoxide metabolism was demonstrated in the monkey studies and can be assumed to occur in humans. They suggested that decreased elimination clearance and lower formation clearance of CBZ epoxide may be responsible if toxicity

appears. In such a case, it may be advisable to monitor free carbamazepine as well as CBZ epoxide when carbamazepine is used with VPA (36). A more marked inhibition of metabolism and increase in total and free CBZ epoxide have been reported with co-administration of the valpromide formulation (55). Although these interactions may occur, no significant changes in carbamazepine protein binding were observed when VPA was co-administered (51,68).

Benzodiazepines

The combined use of VPA with benzodiazepines (diazepam, nitrazepam, clorazepate, clonazepam) is not unusual because there is considerable overlap in the indication for their use in treatment of seizures. There is no evidence of a change in benzodiazepine serum levels when used in combination with VPA, although Dhillon and Richens (16) found that VPA displaces diazepam from protein binding sites similar to the effect on phenytoin previously described. However, a clinical interaction between clonazepam and VPA was reported by Jeavons and Clark (28). Absence status developed in five of 12 patients placed on the two drugs. Nine of the 12 patients had unwanted side effects leading to discontinuation of the clonazepam. The observation is unexplained, and the mechanism of the suspected interaction is unknown. However, the interaction is uncommon and should not preclude using the drugs together when otherwise indicated.

PHARMACODYNAMIC INTERACTION

Little clinical or animal experimental evidence exists to indicate a supra-additive (synergistic) or infra-additive (antagonistic) pharmacodynamic interaction at the effector site when VPA is co-administered with one or more other drugs (44). A combination of drugs, such as phenytoin or carbamazepine with VPA, might provide additive efficacy with infra-additive toxicity due to different dose limiting neurotoxicity, yielding an improved therapeutic index for the combination. At present, controlled trials have not been completed to test this possibility. Reports have described instances of profound sedation with addition of VPA to a regimen of phenobarbital (31,65). The response was much greater than expected from either drug used alone or the added effect of their sedative properties. The symptoms occurred much too early to be explained by increased phenobarbital levels caused in inhibition of metabolism, and suggested a supra-additive (synergistic) neurotoxic effect. In contrast to the equivocal evidence of any direct pharmacodynamic interactions at the neuronal level, changes in drug efficacy and toxicity are common as indirect effects resulting from very frequent pharmacokinetic interactions.

CHANGES IN VPA PHARMACOKINETICS INDUCED BY OTHER DRUGS

Antiepileptic Drugs

Other drugs have important effects on the pharmacokinetics of VPA. Coulthard (11) noted increasing serum levels of VPA and improved seizure control in one patient only after discontinuation of phenytoin. He postulated that other drugs caused hepatic enzyme induction and increased metabolism of VPA. Subsequent studies lend strong support to this observation. Reunanen et al. (60) reported the serum concentration of VPA found in patients treated with single or combined drugs and found that for those on VPA alone, the concentration in blood was 22.4 μmole/liter per mg/kg, whereas for those on carbamazepine or phenytoin it was 13.8 and 14.4 μmole/liter per mg/kg, respectively. Similarly, Mihaly et al. (47) found that average doses of 25.4 mg/kg of

TABLE 4. *Maximum and minimum VPA concentrations*

	VPA alone (N = 26)	VPA and other drug (N = 32)
Max. total	106.0 ± 39[a]	89.5 ± 35
Min. total	70.5 ± 34[b]	50.2 ± 22
Δ μg/ml	36.3 ± 23	39.3 ± 18
Max. free	18.9 ± 9.3[b]	12.0 ± 6.2
Min. free	9.8 ± 6.3[c]	4.4 ± 2.6
Δ μg/ml	9.1 ± 5.4	7.5 ± 4.7
Max. % free	19.2 ± 6[a]	15.7 ± 7
Min. % free	11.7 ± 4[b]	8.5 ± 3
Δ%	7.5 ± 4	7.2 ± 6

[a] $p < 0.05$
[b] $p < 0.01$
[c] $p < 0.001$
From Cramer et al., ref. 14.

VPA in patients receiving VPA alone produced plasma VPA levels of 90.3 μg/ml, whereas patients concomitantly receiving other antiepileptic drugs took a higher average dose of 41.6 mg/kg of VPA and yet achieved mean VPA levels of only 73.5 μg/ml.

Sackellares et al. (66) noted similar effects in a group of children treated with VPA alone or in combination with phenytoin and/or phenobarbital. Despite a comparable dosage per unit body weight, the mean plasma VPA levels were much higher in the patients receiving VPA alone (99.3 versus 63.0 μg/ml). Richens et al. (62) reported a VPA half-life of 5.88 hr in patients treated with VPA combined with other drugs, whereas the half-life was 9.21 hr in patients receiving only VPA. Other studies have confirmed that report (57).

We studied differences in total and free VPA serum concentrations by analyzing serial blood samples from 26 patients on VPA alone and 32 patients on VPA plus another antiepileptic drug (14) (Table 4). The groups took equivalent daily VPA doses: 32.4 ± 12 mg/kg and 30.5 ± 11 mg/kg, respectively. Mean morning trough and postdose peak levels were significantly higher for the VPA group for both total and free levels. Patients on multiple drugs had almost triple (4.4 to 12.0 μg/ml) the concentration of free VPA while those on VPA alone doubled (9.8 to 18.9 μg/ml) their free levels from predose to peak. Total VPA levels rose 50% (71 to 107 μg/ml) for the VPA group and 78% (50 to 90 μg/ml) for the multidrug group.

These data confirm observations that other drugs influence VPA disposition, probably by enzyme induction, thereby affecting maximum and minimum plasma levels. These mean changes indicate the large doses needed in some patients to achieve therapeutic levels and efficacy with concomitant use of enzyme-inducting drugs. Similarly, children could not be brought to therapeutic levels without very high dosage when VPA was given with enzyme-inducing drugs (25). The timing of induction or disinduction of VPA metabolism by the addition or removal of enzyme-inducing drugs has received little study. We found the rise in VPA levels to begin in some patients while still receiving 100 to 200 mg of phenytoin. In others, no change occurred for 1 to 2 weeks after phenytoin was discontinued (44).

The co-administration of enzyme-inducing drugs not only increases the clearance of VPA but also may change metabolic pathways (3). Increases in the putative hepatotoxic 4-en-VPA and 2-4-en-VPA may be one reason for greater incidence of VPA hepatotoxicity in patients treated with polytherapy (18). The 4-en-VPA metabolite was found in every hepatotoxic death studied by Scheffner et al. (67). Tennison et al. (71) did not consider it a useful screening test because the hepatotoxicity is so rare, and they found that metabolite correlated mainly with polytherapy.

An increase in the VPA elimination rate constant and clearance was found in patients concomitantly receiving other drugs. When administered with VPA, carbamazepine (6,47,60), phenobarbital (66), and phenytoin (47,60,66) each altered VPA pharmacokinetics in the same manner. Sufficient data are not available to know if other drugs have similar effects. The mechanism of action has not been fully studied, but hepatic microsomal enzyme induction and secondary increased clearance are very likely.

Nonantiepileptic Drugs

Occasions are few that allow clinical observations of VPA interactions with nonantiepileptic drugs, but the potential for a competitive effect with other highly protein-bound drugs has been tested *in vitro* (19,48). Salicylic acid displaced VPA from protein, resulting in higher free VPA levels. Schobben et al. (70) noted a significant rise in urinary excretion of VPA after administration of 1 to 2 g of aspirin daily to two human volunteers. They suggested that salicylic acid had displaced VPA from protein, resulting in an increased volume of distribution and subsequent higher hepatic clearance. In addition to changes in binding, aspirin has been found to alter VPA metabolism by competing with VPA for mitochondrial oxidation. This leads to an increase in microsomal metabolism with production of 4-en-VPA (1). With the exception of aspirin, the changes in VPA protein binding caused by exogenous displacers are relatively small compared to endogenous effects. Studies indicate lesser interaction with phenylbutazone and no effect of warfarin on VPA protein binding (19,40). Saturation of binding sites at higher levels of VPA (80–90 μg/ml) (12,50) leads to a rapid increase in free VPA many times greater than that induced by phenytoin or other drugs (Fig. 2). Interaction with endogenous free fatty acids also can produce a marked change in VPA binding (50).

DISEASES ALTERING VPA LEVELS

The extensive binding of VPA to serum albumin can be changed not only by aspirin and endogenous fatty acid displacers but also by disease. *In vitro* studies have shown twice as much free VPA available in low-

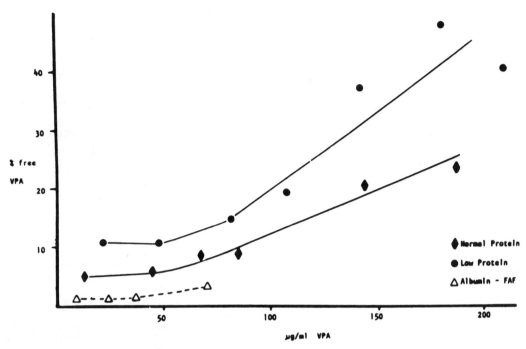

FIG. 2. Variable valproic acid binding to plasma proteins *in vitro*. Binding is maximal with fatty-acid-free (FAF) albumin and least with low concentration of protein. (From Cramer and Mattson, ref. 12, with permission.)

protein plasma (Fig. 2) (12,52). Lower levels of serum albumin may be found in association with malnutrition and impaired synthesis in hepatic disease and malignancy, or associated with protein loss secondary to burns and renal or gastrointestinal disease. In such cases, total VPA concentration will decrease although quantities of free pharmacologically active drug will remain unchanged (8,22,33,59,64).

Decreased binding is found in uremia and can only partly be attributed to decreased protein concentration (64). Allosteric changes in plasma protein have been suggested (54) and may explain increased levels of free VPA. Endogenous "toxic" uremic displacers also may be responsible for the decrease in VPA binding (8). In either case, the result is a lower total serum VPA concentration and an increase in percentage of free VPA without any change in the amount of free drug. Consequently, dosage need not be increased (54,64).

CONCLUSIONS AND CLINICAL IMPLICATIONS

Pharmacokinetic interactions between VPA and other drugs are frequent and potentially important. Accumulating evidence suggests not only the areas of interaction but also the mechanisms responsible for these interactions. VPA is metabolized almost completely in the liver and can interfere with the usual biotransformation of other antiepileptic drugs. Specifically, VPA slows hydroxylation and elimination of some other antiepileptic drugs, causing a rise of serum levels, e.g., CBZ epoxide, phenobarbital, and ethosuximide. Some evidence suggests a similar effect on phenytoin metabolism which is masked by changes in protein binding that produce opposite results. The increase in levels of other drugs may lead to neurotoxicity and require a reduction in their dosage. Valproate does not induce its own metabolism or that of other drugs (30,45). Evidence strongly suggests, however, that many other drugs induce hepatic enzymatic activity to accelerate VPA metabolism and clearance. This results in lower plasma VPA concentrations per dose and a shorter VPA half-life. The high levels achieved with VPA as the sole drug often exceed 80 to 90 μg/ml, at which point a much higher percent of free, pharmacologically active drug becomes available. Conversely, in polytherapy the lower VPA and other antiepileptic drug levels may prevent the patient from obtaining maximal therapeutic effect from the VPA. Although the conversion to valproate monotherapy requires special effort, the benefits from avoiding interactions with other drugs are worthwhile (43). The frequency of VPA interactions calls for clinical awareness and appropriate determinations of blood levels of both VPA and other drugs, at times including free levels.

ACKNOWLEDGMENTS

This work was supported by the Veterans Administration Medical Research Service and NINCDS Grant No. NSO6208-22.

REFERENCES

1. Abbott, F. S., Kassam, J., Orr, J. M., and Farrell, K. (1986): The effect of aspirin on valproic acid metabolism. *Clin. Pharmacol. Therap.*, 40:94–100.
2. Adams, D. J., Luders, H., and Pippenger, C. E. (1978): Sodium valproate in the treatment of intractable seizure disorders: A clinical and electroencephalographic study. *Neurology*, 28:152–157.
3. Baillie, T. A. (1988): Metabolic activation of valproic acid and drug-mediated hepatotoxicity. Role of the terminal olefin, 2-*n*-propyl-4-pentenoic acid. *Chem. Res. Toxicol.*, 1:195–199.
4. Bardy, A., Hari, R., Lehtovaara, R., and Majuri, H. (1977): Valproate may lower serum phenytoin. *Lancet*, 1:1256–1257.
5. Barnes, S. E., and Bower, B. D. (1975): Sodium valproate in the treatment of intractable childhood epilepsy. *Dev. Med. Child. Neurol.*, 17:175–181.
6. Bowdle, T. A., Levy, R. H., and Cutler, R. E. (1979): Effects of carbamazepine on valproic acid

kinetics in normal subjects. *Clin. Pharmacol. Ther.*, 26:629–634.
7. Bruni, J., Gallo, J. M., and Wilder, B. J. (1979): Effect of phenytoin on protein binding of valproic acid. *Can. J. Neurol. Sci.*, 6:433–434.
8. Bruni, J., Wang, L. H., Marburt, T. C., Lee, C. S., and Wilder, B. J. (1980): Protein binding of valproic acid in uremic patients. *Neurology*, 30:557–559.
9. Bruni, J., Wilder, B. J., Perchalski, R. J., Hammond, E. J., and Villareal, H. J. (1980): Valproic acid and plasma levels of phenobarbital. *Neurology*, 30:94–97.
10. Bruni, J., Wilder, B. J., Willmore, L. J., and Barbour, B. (1979): Valproic acid and plasma levels of serum phenytoin. *Neurology*, 29:904–905.
11. Coulthard, M. G. (1975): Sodium valproate in the treatment of intractable childhood epilepsy. *Dev. Med. Child. Neurol.*, 17:534.
12. Cramer, J. A., and Mattson, R. H. (1979): Valproic acid: *In vitro* plasma protein binding and interactions with phenytoin. *Therap. Drug Monit.*, 1:105–116.
13. Cramer, J. A., Mattson, R. H., Bennett, D. M., and Swick, C. T. (1984): Variable free and total valproic acid concentrations in sole and multi drug therapy. In: *Metabolism of Antiepileptic Drugs*, edited by R. H. Levy et al., pp. 105–114. Raven Press, New York.
14. Cramer, J. A., Mattson, R. H., Bennett, D. M., and Swick, C. T. (1986): Variable free and total valproic acid concentrations in sole and multi drug therapy. *Therap. Drug Monit.*, 8:411–416.
15. Dahlqvist, R., Borga, O., Rane, A., Walsh, Z., and Sjoqvist, F. (1979): Decreased plasma protein binding of phenytoin in patients on valproic acid. *Br. J. Clin. Pharmacol.*, 8:547–552.
16. Dhillon, S., and Richens, A. (1982): Valproic acid and diazepam interaction *in vivo*. *Br. J. Clin. Pharmacol.*, 13:553–560.
17. Disalle, E., Pacifici, G. M., and Morselli, P. L. (1974): Studies on plasma protein binding of carbamazepine: Studies on plasma protein binding of carbamazepine. *Pharmacol. Res. Communic.*, 6:193–202.
18. Dreifuss, F. E., Santilli, N., Langer, D. H., Sweeney, K. P., Moline, K. A., and Menander, K. B. (1987): Valproic acid hepatic fatalities: A retrospective review. *Neurology*, 37:379–385.
19. Fleitman, J. S., Bruni, J., Perrin, J. H., and Wilder, B. J. (1980): Albumin binding interactions of sodium valproate. *J. Clin. Pharmacol.*, 20:314–317.
20. Friel, P. N., Leal, K. W., and Wilensky, A. J. (1979): Valproic acid–phenytoin interaction. *Therap. Drug Monit.*, 1:243–248.
21. Frigo, G. M., Lecchini, S., Gatti, G., Perucca, E., and Crema, A. (1979): Modification of phenytoin clearance by valproic acid in normal subjects. *Br. J. Clin. Pharmacol.*, 8:553–556.
22. Gugler, R., and Mueller, G. (1978): Plasma protein binding of valproic acid in healthy patients and in patients with renal disease. *Br. J. Clin. Pharmacol.*, 5:441–446.

23. Harwood, G., and Harvey, P. K. P. (1976): Results of a clinical trial on the use of Epilim in convulsive disorders, with special reference to its efficacy in temporal lobe attacks with focal features. In: *Clinical and Pharmacological Aspects of Sodium Valproate (Epilim)*, edited by N. J. Legg, pp. 40–43. MCS Consultants, Tunbridge Wells, Kent.

24. Hassan, M. N., Laljee, H. C. K., and Parsonage, M. J. (1976): Sodium valproate in the treatment of resistant epilepsy. *Acta Neurol. Scand.*, 54:209–218.

25. Henricksen, O., and Johannessen, S. I. (1982): Clinical and pharmacokinetic observations on sodium valproate—A 5 year followup study in 100 children with epilepsy. *Acta Neurol. Scand.*, 65:504–523.

26. Hooper, W. D., Dubetz, D. K., Bochner, F., Cotter, L. M., Smith, G. A., Eadie, M. J., and Tyrer, J. H. (1976): Plasma protein binding of carbamazepine. *Clin. Pharmacol. Therap.*, 17:433–440.

27. Höopener, R. J., Kuyer, A., Meijer, J. W. A., and Hulsman, J. (1980): Correlation between daily fluctuations of carbamazepine serum levels and intermittent side effects. *Epilepsia*, 21:341–350.

28. Jeavons, P. M., and Clark, J. E. (1974): Sodium valproate in treatment of epilepsy. *Br. Med. J.*, 2:584–586.

29. Jeavons, P. M., Clark, J. E., and Maheswari, M. C. (1977): Treatment of generalized epilepsies of childhood and adolescence with sodium valproate (Epilim). *Dev. Med. Child. Neurol.*, 19:9–25.

30. Jordan, B. J., Shillingford, J. S., and Steed, K. P. (1976): Preliminary observations on the protein binding and enzyme-inducing properties of sodium valproate (Epilim). In: *Clinical and Pharmacological Aspects of Sodium Valproate (Epilim) in the Treatment of Epilepsy*, edited by N. J. Legg, pp. 112–116. Editor: MCS Consultants, Tunbridge Wells, Kent.

31. Kapetanovic, I., Kupferberg, H. J., Porter, R. J., and Penry, J. K. (1980): Valproic acid–phenobarbital interaction: A systematic study using stable isotopically labeled phenobarbital in an epileptic patient. In: *Antiepileptic Therapy: Advances in Drug Monitoring*, edited by P. L. Morselli, C. E. Pippenger, A. Richens et al., pp. 373–380. Raven Press, New York.

32. Kater, R. M. H., Carulli, N., and Iber, F. L. (1969): Differences in the rate of ethanol metabolism in recently drinking alcoholic and nondrinking subjects. *Am. J. Clin. Nutr.*, 22:1608–1617.

33. Klotz, U., Rapp, T., and Mueller, W. A. (1978): Disposition of valproic acid in patients with liver disease. *Eur. J. Clin. Pharmacol.*, 13:55–60.

34. L'Hermitte, F., Marteau, R., and Serdaru, M. (1978): Dipropylacetate (valproate de sodium) et carbamazepine: Une association antiepileptique suspecte. *Presse Med.*, 7:3780.

35. Lecchini, S., Gatti, G., DeBernardi, M., Caravaggi, M., Frigo, G., Galzetti, S., and Visinitini, D. (1978): Serum protein binding of diphenylhydantoin in man: Interaction with sodium valproate. *Farmaco*, 33:80–82.

36. Levy, R. H., and Koch, K. M. (1982): Drug interactions with valproic acid. *Drugs*, 24:543–556.

37. Levy, R. H., Moreland, P. L., Morselli, M., Guyot, A., Brachet-Liermain, A., and Loiseau, P. (1984): Carbamazepine/valproic acid interaction in man and rhesus monkey. *Epilepsia*, 25:338–345.

38. Lines, D. R. (1978): Sodium valproate (Epilim) in the treatment of refractory epilepsy. *N. Z. Med. J.*, 87:9–12.

39. Loiseau, P., Orgogozo, J. M., Centaud, B., and Brachet-Liermain, A. (1980): Further pharmacokinetic observations on the interaction between phenobarbital and valproic acid in epileptic patients. In: *Advances in Epileptology: The Xth Epilepsy International Symposium*, edited by J. A. Wada, and J. K. Penry, pp. 353–354. Raven Press, New York.

40. Lundberg, B., Nergardh, A., Ritzen, E. M., and Samuelsson, K. (1986): Influence of valproic acid on the gonadotropin-releasing hormone test in puberty. *Acta Paediatr. Scand.*, 75:787–792.

41. Mattson, R. H. (1979): Valproate and the management of seizures. In: *Current Neurology*, edited by R. Tyler, and D. Dawson, pp. 233–234. Houghton Mifflin, Boston.

42. Mattson, R. H., and Cramer, J. A. (1980): Valproic acid and ethosuximide interaction. *Ann. Neurol.*, 7:583–584.

43. Mattson, R. H., and Cramer, J. A. (1988): Crossover from polytherapy to monotherapy in primary generalized epilepsy. *Amer. J. Med.*, 84 (Suppl):23–28.

44. Mattson, R. H., Cramer, J. A. (1989): Antiepileptic drug interactions in clinical use: An overview. In: *Drug Interactions*, edited by W. Pitlick, Demos Press, New York, pp. 75–85.

45. Mattson, R. H., Cramer, J. A., Williamson, P. D., and Novelly, R. (1978): Valproic acid in epilepsy: Clinical and pharmacological effects. *Ann. Neurol.*, 3:20–25.

46. Mattson, G. F., Mattson, R. H., and Cramer, J. A. (1982): Interaction between valproic acid and carbamazepine: An *in vitro* study of protein binding. *Therap. Drug Monit.*, 4:181–184.

47. Mihaly, G. W., Vajda, F. J., Miles, J. L., and Louis, W. J. (1979): Single and chronic dose pharmacokinetic studies of sodium valproate in epileptic patients. *Eur. J. Pharmacol.*, 15:23–29.

48. Monks, A., Boobis, S., Wadsworth, J., and Richens, A. (1978): Plasma protein binding interaction between phenytoin and valproic acid *in vitro*. *Br. J. Clin. Pharmacol.*, 6:487–492.

49. Monks, A., and Richens, A. (1980): Effect of single doses of sodium valproate on serum phenytoin concentration and protein binding in epileptic patients. *Clin. Pharmacol. Ther.*, 27:89–95.

50. Patel, I. H., Levy, R. H. (1979): Valproic acid binding to human serum albumin and determination of free fraction in the presence of anticonvulsants and free fatty acids. *Epilepsia*, 20:85–90.

51. Patel, I. H., Levy, R. H., and Cutler, R. E. (1980): Phenobarbital-valproic acid interaction in normal man. *Clin. Pharmacol. Ther.*, 27:515–521.

52. Patsalos, P. N., and Lascelles, P. T. (1977): Effect

of sodium valproate on plasma protein binding of diphenylhydantoin. *J. Neurol. Neurosurg. Psychiat.*, 50:570–574.

53. Penry, J. K., Porter, R. J., Sato, S., Redenbaugh, J., and Dreifuss, F. E. (1976): Effect of sodium valproate on generalized spike-wave paroxysms in the electroencephalogram. In: *Clinical and Pharmacological Aspects of Sodium Valproate (Epilim) in the Treatment of Epilepsy*, edited by N. J. Legg, pp. 158–164. MCS Consultants, Tunbridge Wells, Kent.

54. Perrucca, E., Gatti, G., Frigo, G. M., Crema, A., Calzetti, S., and Visintini, D. (1978): Sodium valproate in epileptic patients. *Br. J. Pharmacol.*, 5:495–499.

55. Pisani, F., Fazio, A., Oteri, G., Ruello, C., Gitto, C., Russo, F., and Perucca, E. (1986): Sodium valproate and valpromide: Differential interactions with carbamazepine in epileptic patients. *Epilepsia*, 27:548–552.

56. Pisani, F., Narbone, M. C., Trunfio, C., Fazio, A., La Rosa, G., Oteri, G., and Di Perri, R. (1984): Valproic acid–ethosuximide interaction: A pharmacokinetic study. *Epilepsia*, 25:229–233.

57. Potolicchio, S. J. (1977): L'Efficacité du di-*n*-propylacetate de sodium (Depakine) en monotherapie dans les absences simples et complexes. Thesis, University de Geneve.

58. Redenbaugh, J. E., Sato, S., Penry, J. K., Dreifuss, F. D., and Kupferberg, H. J. (1980): Sodium valproate: Pharmacokinetics and effectiveness in treating intractable seizures. *Neurology*, 30:1–6.

59. Reidenberg, M. M. (1977): The binding of drugs to plasma proteins and the interpretation of measurements of plasma concentrations of drugs in patients with poor renal function. *Am. J. Med.*, 62:466–470.

60. Reunanen, J. I., Luoma, P., Myllyla, V. V., and Hokkanen, E. (1980): Low serum valproic acid concentrations in epileptic patients on combination therapy. *Curr. Therap. Res.*, 28:455–462.

61. Richens, A., and Ahmad, S. (1975): Controlled trial of sodium valproate in severe epilepsy. *Br. Med. J.*, 4:255–256.

62. Richens, A., Scoular, I. T., Ahmad, S., and Jordan, B. J. (1976): Pharmacokinetics and efficacy of Epilim in patients receiving long-term therapy with other antiepileptic drugs. In: *Clinical and Pharmacological Aspects of Sodium Valproate (Epilim) in the Treatment of Epilepsy*, edited by N. J. Legg, pp. 78–88. MCS Consultants, Tunbridge Wells, Kent.

63. Riva, R., Albani, F., Conten, M., Perucca, E., Ambrosetto, G., Gobbi, G., Santucci, M., and Procaccianti, G. (1985): Time dependent interaction between phenytoin and valproate acid. *Neurology*, 35:510–515.

64. Rowland, M. (1980): Plasma protein binding and therapeutic drug monitoring. *Therap. Drug Monit.*, 2:29–37.

65. Sackellares, J. C., Lee, S. I., and Dreifuss, F. E. (1979): Stupor following administration of valproic acid to patients receiving other antiepileptic drugs. *Epilepsia*, 20:697–703.

66. Sackellares, J. C., Sato, S., Dreifuss, F. E., and Penry, J. K. (1981): Reductions of steady state valproate levels by other antiepileptic drugs. *Epilepsia*, 22:437–441.

67. Sansom, L. N., Beran, R. C., and Schapel, G. J. (1980): Interaction between phenytoin and valproate. *Med. J. Aust.*, 2:212.

68. Scheffner, D., Konig, S. T., Rauterberg-Ruland, I., Kochem, W., Hofmann, W. J., and Unkelbach, S. T. (1988): Fatal liver failure in 16 children with valproate therapy. *Epilepsia*, 29:530–542.

69. Schobben, F., van der Kleijn, D., and Gabreels, F. J. M. (1975): Pharmacokinetics of di-*N*-propylacetate in epileptic patients. *Eur. J. Clin. Pharmacol.*, 8:97–105.

70. Schobben, F., Vree, T. B., and vander Kleijn, D. (1978): Pharmacokinetics, metabolism and distribution of 2-*N*-propyl pentanoate (sodium valproate) and the influence of salicylate comedication. In: *Advances in Epileptology*, edited by H. Meinardi, and A. J. Rowan, pp. 271–277. Swets & Zeitlinger, Amsterdam.

71. Tennison, M. B., Miles, M. V., Pollack, G. M., Thorn, M. D., and Dupuis, R. E. (1988): Valproate metabolites and hepatotoxicity in an epileptic population. *Epilepsia*, 29:543–547.

72. Tomson, T., and Bertilsson, L. (1984): Potent therapeutic effect of carbamazepine-10,11 epoxide in trigeminal neuralgia. *Arch. Neurol.*, 41:598–601.

73. Vakil, S. D., Critchley, E. M. R., Philips, J. C., Haydock, C., Cocks, A., and Dyer, T. (1976): The effect of sodium valproate (Epilim) on phenytoin and phenobarbitone blood levels. In: *Clinical and Pharmacological Aspects of Sodium Valproate (Epilim) in the Treatment of Epilepsy*, edited by N. J. Legg, pp. 75–77. MCS Consultants, Tunbridge Wells, Kent.

74. Voelzke, E., and Doose, H. (1973): Dipropylacetate (Depakine, Ergenyl) in the treatment of epilepsy. *Epilepsia*, 14:185–193.

75. Wilder, B. J., Willmore, L. J., Bruni, J., and Villareal, H. J. (1978): Valproic acid: Interaction with other anticonvulsant drugs. *Neurology*, 28:892–896.

76. Wilson, A. (1976): Discussion of Vakil, S. D., Critchley, E. M. R., Philips, J. C., Haydock, C., Cocks, A., and Dyer, T.: The effect of sodium valproate (Epilim) on phenytoin and phenobarbitone blood levels. In: *Clinical and Pharmacological Aspects of Sodium Valproate (Epilim) in the Treatment of Epilepsy*, edited by N. J. Legg, pp. 77. MCS Consultants, Tunbridge Wells, Kent.

77. Windorfer, A., Sauer, W., and Gadeke, R. (1972): Elevation of diphenylhdantoin and primidone serum concentration by addition of dipropylacetate, a new anticonvulsant drug. *Acta Paediatr. Scand.*, 64:771–772.

78. Varma, R., and Hoshimo, A. (1979): Simultaneous gas-chromatographic measurement of valproic acid in psychiatric patients: Effect on levels of other simultaneously administered anticonvulsants. *Neurosci. Lett.*, 11:353–356.

Antiepileptic Drugs, Third Edition, edited by
R. Levy, R. Mattson, B. Meldrum,
J. K. Penry, and F. E. Dreifuss.
Raven Press, Ltd., New York © 1989.

44

Valproate

Clinical Use

Blaise F. D. Bourgeois

Since its first clinical use in France in 1964 (12) valproate or valproic acid (VPA) has rapidly established itself worldwide as a major antiepileptic drug against several types of seizures. It was soon recognized as a highly effective first line drug against the primary generalized seizures encountered in idiopathic epilepsies: absence, generalized tonic-clonic, and myoclonic seizures. Clinical experience with VPA has continued to grow in recent years and is still the subject of numerous studies and publications. Optimal use, new indications, and new galenic preparations have been the main focus of interest. Antiepileptic therapy with VPA has been the subject of several reviews (8,30,58,66).

ABSENCE SEIZURES

When VPA was released for clinical use in North America in 1978, the primary indication was the treatment of absence seizures. A reduction of spike-and-wave discharges was demonstrated repeatedly when VPA was administered to patients with typical and atypical absences (1,4,49,52). In a group of 25 patients with absence seizures treated with VPA for 10 weeks, 19 patients experienced a reduction in seizure frequency and 21 had a reduction in the total time of spike-and-wave discharge (73). The

reduction was greater than 75% in 11 patients. The efficacy of VPA and ethosuximide in the treatment of absence seizures was compared in a double-blind, crossover study of 16 patients not previously treated for absence seizures and 29 refractory patients. The measure of efficacy was based on the frequency and duration of 3/sec generalized spike-wave bursts on 12-hr telemetered EEG recordings. In the patients who had not previously received antiepileptic therapy, VPA and ethosuximide were equally effective. In various series complete control of simple absence seizures was achieved with VPA monotherapy in 10 of 12 patients (33), 11 of 12 patients (16), 14 of 17 patients (26), and 20 of 21 patients (5). Complete control of absence seizures appears to be more likely when they occur alone than when they occur in combination with another seizure type (5,33). When atypical or "complex" absences are included, results are generally less favorable than for patients with simple absences only (16,24).

GENERALIZED TONIC-CLONIC SEIZURES

Despite its initial use for the treatment of absences, VPA has since been recognized to be effective in convulsive seizures as well

(22,71). Therapy with VPA as the only drug was used in 36 patients with primary tonic-clonic seizures, of whom 24 had been previously treated with other antiepileptic drugs (16). Complete seizure control was achieved in 33 patients. In a series of 100 children with intractable epilepsy, grand mal seizures were completely controlled by the addition of VPA in 14 of 42 patients (33). Wilder et al. (74) compared VPA with phenytoin in 61 previously untreated patients with generalized tonic-clonic, clonic, or tonic seizures in a randomized fashion. No seizures recurred in 73% of patients treated with VPA and in 47% of patients treated with phenytoin. These percentages increased to 82% for VPA and 76% for phenytoin when seizures that had occurred at a time when therapeutic plasma drug levels had not yet been reached were discounted. In another randomized study of the relative efficacy of VPA and phenytoin, a 2-yr remission was used as the endpoint (70). In patients with previously untreated tonic-clonic seizures, this remission was achieved in 27 of 37 cases with VPA and 22 of 39 cases with phenytoin. In two studies of monotherapy for primary (or idiopathic) generalized epilepsies with VPA, complete control of generalized tonic-clonic seizures was achieved in 51 of 60 patients (26) and in 39 of 44 patients (5) in whom only these types of seizures occurred. Excellent results for generalized tonic-clonic seizures were also obtained with VPA monotherapy in children (21).

MYOCLONIC SEIZURES

Myoclonic seizures occurring in patients with primary or idiopathic generalized epilepsies respond particularly well to VPA (5,16,26). Sixteen patients among a group of 23 patients with myoclonic epilepsy of adolescence were completely controlled with VPA monotherapy (16). Among 22 patients with myoclonic epilepsy of adoles-

cence and abnormality on intermittent photic stimulation, 17 were completely controlled, although 17 patients had not responded to previous medications (16). In general, photosensitivity is easily controlled by VPA, whether it is associated with tonic-clonic, absence, or myoclonic seizures (40). A good response to VPA in the treatment of juvenile myoclonic epilepsy was also reported by Delgado-Escueta and Enrile-Bacsal (18). In a study of VPA monotherapy for primary generalized epilepsies, myoclonic seizures were suppressed in 18 of 22 patients (5). Twenty of these 22 patients had another type of seizure (either absence or tonic-clonic) in addition to the myoclonic seizures. Good results with VPA monotherapy were also obtained in children with the so-called benign myoclonic epilepsy of infancy (21). Valproate has also been used successfully against the postanoxic intention myoclonus (9,61) and, in conjunction with clonazepam, against the myoclonic and tonic-clonic seizures occuring with severe progressive myoclonus epilepsy (36).

INFANTILE SPASMS AND LENNOX-GASTAUT SYNDROME

Like all other antiepileptic therapies that have been used so far, therapy with VPA has been less successful for the generalized seizures encountered in the symptomatic generalized epilepsies (e.g., Lennox-Gastaut syndrome) and for the prevention of infantile spasms occurring as part of the West syndrome. There is also much less information available on the use of VPA in these forms of epilepsy than in the treatment of the primary generalized epilepsies. In the series by Covanis et al. (16), three of six patients with myoclonic absence seizures were fully controlled, but none of the patients was treated with VPA alone. Among their 38 patients with myoclonic astatic epilepsy (a term used by the authors synonymously with Lennox syndrome), only seven patients became and remained seizure free with VPA. However, adding VPA was associated with a 50% to 80% improvement in one-third of the patients and other antiepileptic drugs could be withdrawn or reduced after the introduction of VPA. In their series of 100 children treated with VPA, Henriksen and Johannessen (33) report that 12 of 27 children with "absences and other seizures" and 9 of 39 children with atonic seizures became seizure-free.

Several studies on the use of VPA for the prevention of infantile spasms were based either on small numbers of patients (3,56,60) or on a combination of VPA and corticotropin given simultaneously (6,75). In a series of 19 babies with infantile spasms (2), VPA was never used simultaneously with corticotropin. Good control was achieved with VPA as a first drug in eight patients, and these patients therefore did not require corticotropin. The doses of VPA ranged from 20 to 60 mg/kg per day. An analysis of the cases of initial failure with either corticotropin or VPA and subsequent treatment with the other drug revealed a tendency toward a better response to corticotropin. However, treatment with VPA was associated with a lower incidence and severity of side effects. In another study, VPA was given at a dosage of 20 mg/kg per day to 18 infants with infantile spasms who were never treated with corticotropin (57). Short-term results were good to excellent in 12 patients. Follow-up revealed that seven patients still had residual seizures and 16 had either moderate or severe mental retardation. The results were judged to be similar to those obtained with corticotropin or steroids, but VPA was found to have fewer side effects.

PARTIAL SEIZURES

Since the efficacy of VPA has been well established for the treatment of generalized seizures, the emphasis has shifted in recent years toward the study of its use against partial seizures. The number of reports dealing with the specific use of VPA against partial seizures is considerably smaller than for generalized seizures. Difficulties associated with the evaluation of the efficacy of VPA against partial seizures include the fact that VPA was often used initially as an add-on drug, and in patients who had been resistant to therapy for many years. Furthermore, in contrast to the primary generalized seizures, partial seizures are not a homogeneous and easily defined entity, and a more definitive determination of the role of VPA in the treatment of partial seizures might require a distinction between various types of partial seizures according to their functional anatomy.

Information about the effect of VPA against partial seizures is derived in part from small numbers of patients in studies not dealing primarily with partial seizures. In the series by Covanis et al. (16), nine patients with simple partial seizures responded poorly to VPA, and five of 11 patients with complex partial seizures were seizure-free on VPA, mostly in combination with carbamazepine. Among the 100 children with uncontrolled epilepsy reported by Henriksen and Johannessen (33), 13 had simple partial seizures. Of those only one became seizure-free after the addition of VPA, and a seizure reduction of more than 75% and 50% to 75% was observed in three patients each. Among 19 patients with complex partial seizures, four became seizure-free, five experienced a seizure reduction of 75% and 5 experienced a seizure reduction of 50% to 75%. In 24 adults with poorly controlled complex partial seizures, Bruni and Albright (7) added VPA to the pre-existing regimen. A greater than 50% seizure reduction was initially achieved in 12 patients, but in seven patients this improvement was temporary. Thus, a long-term benefit was obtained in only five of 24 patients. Better results were observed when

VPA was compared with carbamazepine in an open study of 31 previously untreated patients with partial seizures (47). Seizures were completely controlled by VPA in 11 patients and by carbamazepine in eight patients. However, only 19 patients were followed for a period of 1 year. Callaghan et al. (11) compared monotherapy with carbamazepine, phenytoin, and VPA in 181 previously untreated patients, with a median follow-up ranging from 14 to 24 months. In the 79 patients with simple or complex partial seizures, there was no significant difference between the three drugs with regard to both seizure reduction and complete control of seizures. In another series of 140 adults with previously untreated seizures, monotherapy with phenytoin and VPA were compared in a randomized design, 76 patients having tonic-clonic seizures only and 64 patients having predominantly complex partial seizures (70). Using time to 2-yr remission and time to first seizure as parameters of efficacy, the authors could find no difference between the two drugs in either group. Among patients with partial seizures, 27% had a 2-yr remission while receiving VPA, and 29% while on phenytoin.

Gupta and Jeavons (32) compared 40 patients with complex partial seizures who responded to carbamazepine monotherapy with 45 patients who were not seizure-free on carbamazepine monotherapy and in whom VPA was added as a second drug. Their response to therapy was analyzed as a function of the side of the interictal EEG abnormality. Carbamazepine alone fully controlled the seizures in 24 of 37 patients who had a left temporal EEG abnormality exclusively, and in only 7 of 33 patients with a right abnormality. Among those who were not controlled by carbamazepine alone, the addition of VPA was associated with full control in 18 of the 26 patients with a right temporal abnormality and in only 1 of the 13 patients with a left temporal abnormality. Although these results suggest a better re-

sponse to carbamazepine alone in patients with a left temporal abnormality and a better response to the addition of VPA to carbamazepine in patients with a right temporal abnormality, a control group with VPA as the only drug was not included in the study. The most recent evaluation of the effect of VPA monotherapy in partial seizures is a retrospective study of 30 patients with simple and complex partial seizures who had not tolerated or not responded to conventional initial drugs (17). Change to VPA monotherapy was associated with surprisingly good results. Twelve patients became seizure-free, 10 experienced reduced seizure frequency by more than 50%, and nine were not improved. All generalized components of partial seizures were controlled in these patients. A prospective controlled multicenter trial of carbamazepine versus VPA in partial seizures is currently underway (51).

FEBRILE SEIZURES

The effectiveness of VPA in the prevention of febrile convulsions has been well documented (13,55). In a group of 196 children with febrile seizures of which 69 received prolonged treatment with phenobarbital, 32 with primidone, and 95 with VPA, Minagawa and Miura (54) found no statistical difference between the recurrence rate in the three groups. At a VPA dose of 20 to 25 mg/kg per day, they found three daily doses to be more effective than two doses. In another series of 90 children with febrile seizures (44), a recurrence occurred in 12 out of 25 untreated children, in eight out of 33 children taking phenobarbital prophylaxis, and in four out of 32 children on VPA therapy. The difference between treatment and no therapy was significant for VPA but not for phenobarbital. The amide of VPA (dipropylacetamide or valpromide) was compared with no treatment, with phenobarbital, and with VPA in four groups of 50 children each (19). Valpromide was as effective as phenobarbital in preventing febrile seizures and was superior to VPA. In a placebo-controlled study (50), the recurrence rate was estimated to be 35% with placebo, 19% with phenobarbital, and 4% with VPA. Herranz et al. (34) conducted a study in which not only the efficacy in preventing febrile seizures but also the incidence of side effects were considered. Recurrences were prevented in 80% of the patients taking phenobarbital, with side effects in 77% of the cases, the corresponding figures being 88% and 53% for primidone, and 92% and 45% for VPA.

Although VPA is effective in the prophylaxis of febrile seizures, it should be emphasized here that the use of prophylactic treatment in patients with febrile seizures has declined markedly in recent years. This has been due mainly to a reassessment of the risk versus benefit ratio and to the increasing use of intermittent rectal diazepam during febrile episodes. The latter approach was found to be as effective as prophylactic treatment with VPA in a group of children with a high risk of recurrence of febrile seizures (45).

NEONATAL SEIZURES AND OTHER USES

Valproate has also been used for the treatment of seizures during the neonatal period. Two newborns whose seizures were not controlled by conventional antiepileptic drugs responded well to a rectal infusion of VPA (68). In a more recent trial, VPA was administered orally as syrup in six neonates who had persistent seizures despite levels of phenobarbital of more than 40 μg/ml, and despite the administration of an additional anticonvulsant in five of the six infants (28). The loading dose was 20 to 25 mg/kg and the initial maintenance dose was 5 to 10 mg/kg every 12 hr. The seizures were controlled in all but one infant, a 30-week gestational age newborn with meningitis. An elevation of serum ammonia was observed in all patients. This elevation was reversible despite continuation of the VPA therapy in three cases. Seizures recurred in two cases after VPA was discontinued because of hyperammonemia. The mean VPA elimination half-life in five of these newborns was 26.4 hr, a value which is considerably higher than in children and adults.

Good results were obtained with VPA in patients with intractable hiccups, which is considered to be a form of myoclonus. Jacobson et al. (39) used VPA in five patients in whom previous therapies failed. Four patients became asymptomatic and one was markedly improved. Similarly good results were obtained when VPA was administered to five patients with Sydenham's chorea (20). The involuntary movements disappeared completely within a week after onset of therapy. Valproate has also been used successfully in primary psychiatric disorders. An acute antimanic effect of VPA was demonstrated and it appears that VPA is particularly effective in bipolar or schizoaffective disorders with no evidence of paroxysmal EEG abnormalities (23,53). Positive results with the use of VPA were also reported for the treatment of the alcohol withdrawal syndrome (43). When tested in a double-blind, placebo-controlled study for the treatment of tardive dyskinesia, VPA could not be shown to be effective (27).

ADMINISTRATION AND CONCENTRATION-EFFECT RELATIONSHIP

In various parts of the world, the drug is marketed as valproic acid, sodium valproate, magnesium valproate, sodium hydrogen divalproate, or valpromide, the amide of VPA. Valproate is available as oral syrup, immediate release formulations, and enteric-coated tablets. Slow release oral preparations have recently become available in certain countries. Valproate has not been marketed for parenteral use. Although valproic acid syrup has been used for rectal administration (15,69), sodium valproate suppositories are available in certain countries. The suppositories were found to be well tolerated, even when administered for several days, and to have the same bioavailability as the oral preparations (38). The question of the appropriate daily dose of valproate has been addressed in numerous reports.

Because of pronounced pharmacokinetic interactions, the dose of VPA will differ markedly between patients on VPA monotherapy and patients on combination therapy, if similar concentrations are to be achieved. Furthermore, the adequate VPA dose or concentration can be a function of the patient's seizure type (48). In patients on VPA monotherapy, doses between 10 and 20 mg/kg/day will usually achieve a good clinical response, and will result in concentrations within the generally accepted therapeutic range (5,26,33,74). Due to age-dependent kinetics, younger children may require higher doses (16,59). Patients on combination therapy will almost invariably need higher doses if the same concentrations are to be obtained, usually between 30 and 60 mg/kg/day. This effect of comedication is particularly pronounced in children in whom VPA concentrations in the accepted therapeutic range can often not be achieved, even with doses above 100 mg/kg/day (33). A curvilinear relationship between VPA dose and concentration was reported by Gram et al. (31), with relatively smaller increases in concentrations at higher doses. Among the different possible explanations, the most likely seems to be a higher free fraction at higher concentrations, resulting in a higher total drug clearance. If therapeutic levels of VPA are to be achieved rapidly, a loading dose of 12.5 mg/kg given orally was shown to be adequate (62). Although it has been a common prac-

tice to divide the daily dose of VPA into two or three single doses beause of the short elimination half-life, several authors have obtained equally good results when VPA was administered as a single daily dose (16,29,67). In patients with primary generalized epilepsy, a mean VPA dose of 15.6 mg/kg per day administered once daily was adequate (67). Despite the fact that maximal concentrations were about two times higher than minimal concentrations, side effects were rare. This leads to the next question, namely the concentration-effect relationship for valproate and the value of determining plasma or serum concentrations.

There are two main reasons for the difficulties associated with interpretation of VPA levels obtained in patients: first, VPA levels fluctuate considerably during a 24-hr period due to the short half-life, and second, no good correlation between VPA levels at a given time and clinical effects at the same time have been demonstrated so far. Studying the photoconvulsive response in man, Rowan et al. (63) found that reduction or abolition of photosensitivity in the EEG occurred on the average 3 hr after peak serum valproate levels had been achieved, and persisted for hours as the levels continued to decrease. Burr et al. (10) measured the course of spike-wave discharge rate in the EEG and analyzed its relationship to fluctuations in VPA levels. They found no significant correlation, whether they analyzed the actual discharge profile or the profile of changes in discharge rate. During long-term VPA therapy, a continued reduction of spike-wave activity or seizure frequency occurred even after a steady state had been reached (5,6,8). This phenomenon is probably not due to delayed brain penetration, selective concentration, or slow elimination of VPA from the brain, since a good correlation between brain and cerebrospinal fluid concentration and free plasma concentrations could be demonstrated in patients undergoing neurosurgery (72). In a group of 25 patients with absence seizures,

Villareal. et al. (73) found no correlation between plasma VPA concentrations and EEG changes, but they observed a clinical response when levels reached 50 to 60 μg/ml (347–417 nmol/l). Among children with absence seizures, those who became seizure-free on VPA monotherapy had a mean plasma concentration of 83.1 μg/ml (VPA as a first drug) and 59.6 μg/ml (patients previously refractory to ethosuximide) (64). In a group of 28 children whose seizures were completely controlled by VPA monotherapy, the mean plasma level was 65.1 μg/ml (452 nmol/l) (42). Farrell et al. (25) found serum levels of 140 to 420 nmol/l (20.2–50.5 μg/ml) by gas chromatography and 210 to 560 nmol/l (30.2–80.6 μg/ml) by EMIT in 80% of children with complete seizure control. Ishikawa et al. (37) reported mean levels of 47.8 μg/ml (332 nmol/l) to 8.52 μg/ml (592 nmol/l) in children whose seizures were well controlled. Younger children had lower average concentrations and half of them were controlled with levels of less than 50 μg/ml (350 nmol/l). In the series by Covanis et al. (16), mean serum levels in seizure-free patients ranged from 82 to 109.5 μg/ml (569–760 nmol/l), and these authors recommend a therapeutic range of 60 to 120 μg/ml (417–833 nmol/l). There is no evidence in any of the studies cited above that VPA was actually titrated to the minimally effective dose or concentration. In the series by Henriksen and Johannessen (33), clinical effect was observed only after the fasting serum VPA levels had reached values of about 300 nmol/l (43.2 μg/ml), and seizure control was frequently achieved only after these levels had persisted for 2 to 4 weeks. Lethargy and drowsiness were noticed at levels above 600 nmol/l in almost all cases. In previously untreated adults, adverse effects were common when plasma VPA levels were above 100 μg/ml (700 nmol/l) on monotherapy and primarily generalized tonic-clonic seizures did not occur at levels of more than 50 μg/ml (350 nmol/l) (71). A lower limit for the prevention of partial seizures could not be determined in this study.

Based on their finding of a good linear correlation between VPA dose and level in patients on monotherapy, Lundberg et al. (48) considered that monitoring VPA levels was not necessary in patients on monotherapy. In a group of 88 children on VPA monotherapy, those presenting certain side effects had received significantly higher doses than patients without side effects (35). However, a relationship between the incidence of side effects and plasma VPA levels could not be established except for children presenting with lassitude and drowsiness, whose levels were significantly higher (mean values of 94.5 and 80.4 μg/ml, respectively). In their study on the prevention of febrile seizures, Herranz et al. (34) found no difference in doses or plasma levels among patients with or without recurrence of seizures or with or without side effects. However, patients with side effects were on a higher VPA dose. Schobben et al. (65) also found that the therapeutic effect correlated better with the VPA dose in mg/kg body weight than with the plasma concentration. Gram et al. (31) concluded that seizure control was better at serum levels of 300 to 350 nmol/l (43–50 μg/ml) than at lower values, but found no correlation between VPA levels and side effects. The value of a single trough level of VPA was questioned by Loiseau et al. (46), based on the observation that the mean fluctuation in concentrations was 113% during a 24-hr period, and that consecutive fasting levels were not reproducible.

In conclusion, although VPA levels can be valuable in selected cases, and particularly during combination therapy, a single measurement is often of limited value and results should be interpreted cautiously (14). Rigid adherence by the physician to the indicated therapeutic range, usually 50 to 100 μg/ml (350–700 nmol/l), is not likely to be beneficial to the patient.

REFERENCES

1. Adams, D. J., Lüders, H., and Pippenger, C. E. (1978): Sodium valproate in the treatment of intractable seizure disorders: A clinical and electroencephalo-graphic study. *Neurology*, 28:152–157.
2. Bachman, D. S. (1982): Use of valproic acid in treatment of infantile spasms. *Arch. Neurol.*, 39:49–52.
3. Barnes, S. E., and Bower, B. D. (1975): Sodium valproate in the treatment of intractable childhood epilepsy. *Dev. Med. Child Neurol.*, 17:175–181.
4. Bergamini, L., Mutani, R., and Fulan, P. M. (1975): The effect of sodium valproate (Epilim) on the EEG. *Electroencephalogr. Clin. Neurophysiol.*, 39:429.
5. Bourgeois, B., Beaumanoir, B., Blajev, B., de la Cruz, N., Despland, P. A., Egli, M., Geudelin, B., Kaspar, U., Ketz, E., Kronauer, Ch., Meyer, Ch., Scollo-Lavizzari, G., Tosi, C., Vassella, F., and Zagury, S. (1987): Monotherapy with valproate in primary generalized epilepsies. *Epilepsia, 28* (Suppl 2):S8–S11.
6. Brachet-Liermain, A., and Demarquez, J. L. (1977): Pharmacokinetics of dipropylacetate in infants and young children. *Pharm. Weekbl.*, 112:293–297.
7. Bruni, J., and Albright, P. (1983): Valproate acid therapy for complex partial seizures. Its efficacy and toxic effects. *Arch. Neurol.*, 40:135–137.
8. Bruni, J., and Wilder, B. J. (1979): Valproic acid. Review of a new antiepileptic drug. *Arch. Neurol.*, 36:393–398.
9. Bruni, J., Willmore, L. J., and Wilder, B. J. (1979): Treatment of postanoxic intention myoclonus with valproic acid. *Can. J. Neurol. Sci.*, 6:39–42.
10. Burr, W., Fröscher, W., Hoffmann, F., and Stefan H. (1984): Lack of significant correlation between circadian profiles of valproic acid serum levels and epileptiform electroencephalographic activity. *Ther. Drug Monit.*, 6:179–181.
11. Callaghan, N., Kenny, R. A., O'Neill, B., Crowley, M., and Groggini, T. (1985): A prospective study between carbamazepine, phenytoin and sodium valproate as monotherapy in previously untreated and recently diagnosed patients with epilepsy. *J. Neurol. Neurosurg. Psychiatr.*, 48:639–720.
12. Carraz, G., Gau, R., Chateau, R., and Bonnin, J. (1964): Communication à propos des premiers essais cliniques sur l'activité anti-epileptique de l'acide *n*-dipropylacetique (sel de Na⁺). *Ann. Med. Psychol.*, 122:577–585.
13. Cavazzutti, G. B. (1975): Prevention of febrile convulsions with dipropylacetate (Depakine). *Epilepsia*, 16:647–648.
14. Chadwick, D. W. (1985): Concentration-effect relationships of valproic acid. *Clin. Pharmacokin.*, 10:155–163.
15. Cloyd, J. C., and Kriel, R. L. (1981): Bioavailability of rectally administered valproic acid syrup. *Neurology*, 31:1348–1352.
16. Covanis, A., Gupta, A. K., and Jeavons, P. M. (1982): Sodium valproate: Monotherapy and polytherapy. *Epilepsia*, 23:693–720.
17. Dean, C., and Penry, J. K. (1987): Valproate monotherapy in 30 patients with partial seizures. *Epilepsia*, 28:605.
18. Delgado-Escueta, A. V., and Enrile-Bacsal, F. (1984): Juvenile myoclonic epilepsy of Janz. *Neurology*, 34:285–294.
19. DeMarco, P. (1981): A new prophylactic treatment of febrile convulsions: Dipropylacetamide (Depamide). Preliminary report. *Eur. Rev. Med. Pharmacol. Sci.*, 3:15–18.
20. Dhanaraj, M., Radhakrishnan, A. R, Srinivas, K., and Sayeed, Z. A. (1985): Sodium valproate in Sydenham's chorea. *Neurology*, 35:114–115.
21. Dulac, O., Steru, D., Rey, E., and Arthuis, M. (1986): Sodium valproate monotherapy in childhood epilepsy. *Brain Dev.*, 8:47–52.
22. Dulac, O., Steru, D., Rey, E., Perret, A., and Arthuis, M. (1982): Monotherapie par le valproate de sodium dans les epilepsies de l'enfant. *Arch. Fr. Pediatr.*, 39:347–352.
23. Emrich, H. M., Dose, M., and von Zerssen, D. (1985): The use of sodium valproate, carbamazepine and oxcarbazepine in patients with affective disorders. *J. Affective Disord.*, 8:243–250.
24. Erenberg, G., Rothner, A. D., Henry, C. E., and Cruse, R. P. (1982): Valproic acid in the treatment of intractable absence seizures in children. A single-blind clinical and quantitative EEG study. *Am. J. Dis. Chil.*, 136:526–529.
25. Farrell, K., Abbott, F. S., Orr, J. M., Applegarth, D. A., Jan, J. E., and Wong, P. K. (1986): Free and total serum valproate concentrations: Their relationship to seizure control, liver enzymes and plasma ammonia in children. *Can. J. Neurol. Sci.*, 13:252–255.
26. Feuerstein, J. (1983): A long-term study of monotherapy with sodium valproate in primary generalized epilepsy. *Br. J. Clin. Practice*, 27:(Suppl 1):17–23 (Third International Symposium on Sodium Valproate).
27. Fisk, G. G., and York, S. M. (1987): The effect of sodium valproate on tardive dyskinesia-revisited. *Br. J. Psychiatry*, 150:542–546.
28. Gal, P., Oles, K. S., Gilman, J. T., and Weaver, R. (1988): Valproic acid efficacy toxicity and pharmacokinetics in neonates with intractable seizures. *Neurology*, 38:467–471.
29. Gjerloff, I., Arentsen, J., Alving, J., and Secher, B. G. (1984): Monodose versus 3 daily doses of sodium valproate: A controlled trial. *Acta Neurol. Scand.*, 69:120–124.
30. Gram, L., and Bentsen, K. D. (1985): Valproate: An updated review. *Acta Neurol. Scand.*, 72:129–139.
31. Gram, L., Flachs, H., Würtz-Jorgensen, A., Parnas, J., and Andersen, R. (1979): Sodium valproate, serum level and clinical effect in epilepsy: A controlled study. *Epilepsia*, 20:303–312.
32. Gupta, A. K., and Jeavons, P. M. (1985): Complex partial seizures: EEG foci and response to car-

bamazepine and sodium valproate. *J. Neurol. Neurosurg. Psychiatry*, 45:131–138.

33. Henriksen, O., and Johannessen, S. I. (1982): Clinical and pharmacokinetic observations on sodium valproate—A 5-year follow-up study in 100 children with epilepsy. *Acta. Neurol. Scandinav.*, 65:504–523.

34. Herranz, J. L., Armijo, J. A., and Arteaga, R. (1984): Effectiveness and toxicity of phenobarbital, primidone and sodium valproate in the prevention of febrile convulsions, controlled by plasma levels. *Epilepsia*, 25:89–95.

35. Herranz, J. L., Arteaga, R., and Armijo, J. A. (1982): Side effects of sodium valproate in monotherapy controlled by plasma levels: A study in 88 pediatric patients. *Epilepsia*, 23:203–214.

36. Iivanainen, M., and Himberg, J. J. (1982): Valproate and clonazepam in the treatment of severe progressive myoclonus epilepsy. *Arch. Neurol.*, 39:236–238.

37. Ishikawa, T., Ogino, C., Furuyama, M., Kauayama, J., Auaya, A., and Yamaguchi, A. (1987): Serum valproate concentrations in epileptic children with favourable responses. *Brain Devel.*, 9:283–287.

38. Issakainen, J., and Bourgeois, B. F. D. (1987): Bioavailability of sodium valproate suppositories during repeated administration of steady-state in epileptic children. *Eur. J. Pediatr.*, 146:404–407.

39. Jacobson, P. L., Messenheimer, J. A., and Farmer, T. W. (1981): Treatment of intractable hiccups with valproic acid. *Neurology*, 31:1458–1460.

40. Jeavons, P. M., Bishop, A., and Harding, G. F. A. (1986): The prognosis of photosensitivity. *Epilepsia*, 27:569–575.

41. Jeavons, P. M., Clark, J. E., and Maheshwari, M. C. (1977): Treatment of generalized epilepsies of childhood and adolescence with sodium valproate (Epilim). *Develop. Med. Child. Neurol.*, 19:9–25.

42. Klotz, V., and Schweizer, C. (1980): Valproic acid in childhood epilepsy: Anticonvulsant efficacy in relation to its plasma levels. *Int. J. Clin. Pharmacol. Ther. Toxicol.*, 18:461–465.

43. Lambie, D. G., Johnson, R. H., Vijayasenan, M. E., and Whiteside, E. A. (1980): Sodium valproate in the treatment of the alcohol withdrawal syndrome. *Aust. N.Z. J. Psychiatry*, 14:213–215.

44. Lee, K., and Melchoir, J. C. (1981): Sodium valproate versus phenobarbital in the prophylactic treatment of febrile convulsions in childhood. *Eur. J. Pediatr.*, 137:151–153.

45. Lee, K., Taudorf, K., and Hvorslev, V. (1986): Prophylactic treatment with valproic acid or diazepam in children with febrile convulsions. *Acta Paediatr. Scand.*, 75:593–597.

46. Loiseau, P., Cenraud, B., Levy, R. H., Akbaraly, R., Brachet-Liermain, A., Guyot, M., and Morselli, P. L. (1982): Diurnal variations in steady-state plasma concentrations of valproic acid in epileptic patients. *Clin. Pharmacokin.*, 7:544–552.

47. Loiseau, P., Cohadon, S., Jogeix, M., Legroux, M., and Artigues, J. (1984): Efficacité du valproate de sodium dans les epilepsies partielles. *Rev. Neurol. (Paris)*, 140:434–437.

48. Lundberg, B., Nergardh, A., and Boreus, L. O. (1982): Plasma concentrations of valproate during maintenance therapy in epileptic children. *J. Neurol.*, 228:133–141.

49. Maheshwari, M. C., and Jeavons, P. M. (1975): The effect of sodium valproate (Epilim) on the EEG. *Electroencephalogr. Clin. Neurophysiol.*, 39:429.

50. Mamelle, N., Mamelle, J. C., Plasse, J. C., Revol, M., and Gilly, R. (1984): Prevention of recurrent febrile convulsions—A randomized therapeutic assay: Sodium valproate, phenobarbital and placebo. *Neuropediatrics*, 15:37–42.

51. Mattson, R. H. (1987): Study design for a multicenter antiepileptic drug trial of carbamazepine versus valproate. *Epilepsia*, 28:605–606.

52. Mattson, R. H., Cramer, J. A., Williamson, P. D, and Novelly, R. (1978): Valproic acid in epilepsy: Clinical and pharmacological effects. *Ann. Neurol.*, 3:20–25.

53. McElroy, S. L., Keck, P. E., and Pope, H. G. (1987): Sodium valproate: Its use in primary psychiatric disorders. *J. Clin. Psychopharmacol.*, 7:16–24.

54. Minagawa, K., and Miura, H. (1981): Phenobarbital, primidone and sodium valproate in the prophylaxis of febrile convulsions. *Brain Dev.*, 3:385–393.

55. Ngwane, E., and Bower, B. (1980): Continuous sodium valproate or phenobarbital in the prevention of "simple" febrile convulsions. *Arch. Dis. Child.*, 55:171–174.

56. Olive, D., Tridon, P., and Weber, M. (1969): Action du dipropylacetate de sodium sur certaines varietés d'encephalopathies epileptogenes du nourrisson. *Schweiz. Med. Wochenschr.*, 99:87–92.

57. Pavone, L., Incorpora, G., LaRosa, M., LiVolti, S., and Mollica, F. (1981): Treatment of infantile spasms with sodium dipropylacetic acid. *Dev. Med. Child Neurol.*, 23:454–461.

58. Pinder, R. M., Brodgen, R. N., and Speight, T. M. (1977): Sodium valproate: A review of its pharmacological properties and therapeutic efficacy in epilepsy. *Drugs*, 13:81–123.

59. Redenbaugh, J. E., Sato, S., Penry, J. K., Dreifuss, F. E., and Kupferberg, H. J. (1980): Sodium valproate: Pharmacokinetics and effectiveness in treating intractable seizures. *Neurology*, 30:1–6.

60. Rohmann, E., and Arndi, R. (1976): The efficacy of Ergenyl (dipropyl acetate) in clonic-, jackknife-, and salaam spasms. *Kinderaertzl Prax.*, 44:109–113.

61. Rollinson, R. D., and Gilligam, B. S. (1979): Postanoxic action myoclonus (Lance-Adams syndrome) responding to valproate. *Arch. Neurol.*, 36:44–45.

62. Rosenfeld, W. E., Leppik, I. E., Gates, J. R., and Mireles, R. E. (1987): Valproic acid loading during intensive monitoring. *Arch. Neurol.*, 44:709–710.

63. Rowan, A. J. Binnie, C. D., Warfield, C. A., Meinardi, H., and Meijer, J. W. A. (1979): The delayed effect of sodium valproate on the photoconvulsive response in man. *Epilepsia*, 20:61–68.

64. Sato, S., White, B. G., Penry, J. K., Dreifuss, F. E., Sackellares, J. C., and Kupferberg, H. J. (1982): Valproic acid versus ethosuximide in the treatment of absence seizures. *Neurology*, 32:157–163.

65. Schobben, F., van der Kleijn, E., and Vree, T. B. (1980): Therapeutic monitoring of valproic acid. *Ther. Drug Monit.*, 2:61–71.

66. Simon, D., and Penry, J. K. (1975): Sodium di-*n*-propylacetate (DPA) in the treatment of epilepsy: A review. *Epilepsia*, 22:1701–1708.

67. Stefan, H., Burr, W., Fichsel, H., Fröscher, W., and Penin, H. (1984): Intensive follow-up monitoring in patients with once daily evening administration of sodium valproate. *Epilepsia*, 25:152–160.

68. Steinberg, A., Shalev, R. S., and Amir, N. (1986): Valproic acid in neonatal status convulsions. *Brain Dev.*, 8:278–279.

69. Thorpy, M. J. (1980): Rectal valproate syrup and status epilepticus. *Neurology*, 30:1113–1114.

70. Turnbull, D. M., Howel, D., Rawlins, M. D., and Chadwick, D. W. (1985): Which drug for the adult epileptic patient: Phenytoin or valproate? *Br. Med. J.*, 290:816–819.

71. Turnbull, D. M., Rawlins, M. D., Weightman, D., and Chadwick, D. W. (1982): A comparison of phenytoin and valproate in previously untreated adult epileptic patients. *J. Neurol. Neurosurg. Psychiatr.*, 45:55–59.

72. Vajda, F. J. E., Donnan, G. A., Phillips, J., and Bladin, P. F. (1981): Human brain, plasma and cerebrospinal fluid concentration of sodium valproate after 72 hours of therapy. *Neurology*, 31:486–487.

73. Villareal, H. J., Wilder, B. J., Willmore, L. J., Bauman, A. W., Hammond, E. J., and Bruni, J. (1978): Effect of valproic acid on spike and wave discharges in patients with absence seizures. *Neurology*, 28:886–891.

74. Wilder, B. J., Ramsey, R. E., Murphy, J. V., Karas, B. J., Marquardt, K., and Hammond, E. J. (1983): Comparison of valproic acid and phenytoin in newly-diagnosed tonic-clonic seizures. *Neurology*, 33:1474–1476.

75. Yokoyama, S., Kodama, S., and Ogini, H. (1976): Study on the treatment of infantile spasms. *Brain Dev.*, 8:447–453.

Antiepileptic Drugs, Third Edition, edited by
R. Levy, R. Mattson, B. Meldrum,
J. K. Penry, and F. E. Dreifuss.
Raven Press, Ltd., New York © 1989.

45

Valproate

Toxicity

Fritz E. Dreifuss

Adverse drug reactions constitute an ever-increasing proportion of hospital admissions, but as noted by Napke (73), it is difficult to distinguish between a drug adverse reaction, a suspected-drug adverse reaction, and a mere accusation of a possible drug adverse reaction. This is because the cause-and-effect relationship is difficult to establish, particularly since the allegation of adverse reaction is frequently made by other than experts in the field under purview. Many such reactions preclude the dechallenge and rechallenge mode of investigation. Although in clearly dose-related adverse reactions the problem is relatively simple, it becomes more challenging in the case of unusual, unexpected, or idiosyncratic side effects or toxic effects that occur after prolonged administration or in the face of intercurrent illness.

Adverse reactions to valproate may be divided into physiological or dose-related side effects, metabolic effects, and peculiar and therefore unusual or rare drug reactions, including idiosyncrasies and effects other than those due to the pharmacology of the drug. Such reactions may be mediated by the formation of unusual or novel metabolites, and altered target organ responses may be the result of genetic abnormalities. Finally, teratogenicity represents an adverse drug reaction which, in the case of valproate, appears to be dose-related, at least in part.

DOSE-RELATED SIDE EFFECTS

Acute Overdosage

Massive overdoses of valproate are usually the result of attempted suicide. Several fatalities have been reported (15,46), but the majority have survived with up to 20 times therapeutic blood levels. An immediate complication appears to be cerebral edema (6,37), but most acute overdosage results in no ill effects (56,77,96,100). One patient achieved a blood level of 1,500 mcg/ml and survived following hemodialysis.

Gastrointestinal Side Effects

Nausea, vomiting, and gastrointestinal distress are among the most common side effects accompanying the initiation of valproate therapy. The symptoms may be appeased by giving the drug after meals or beginning with low doses and gradually increasing the dose until tolerance develops (26). These symptoms may occur in up to 25% of patients, but the majority of discomfort may be avoided by the administration of enteric-coated preparation (102).

Excessive Weight Gain

An excessive increase in body weight of patients taking valproate has been reported frequently (13,22,29,35). This has occasionally been sufficiently severe to require discontinuation of treatment. This is particularly bothersome in young women and appears to be the result of a central effect on the satiety mechanism. Conscious reduction of caloric intake is usually sufficient to counteract this problem.

Hair Changes

Some patients experience hair thinning or alopecia (51,57,74,88). Some authors have reported increased curliness of the regrown hair and Herranz et al. (36) report some change in hair color. It is not clear whether the hair changes are related to dosage or to duration of therapy, though dose reduction may be helpful.

Tremor

Dose-related tremor is seen in long-term valproate therapy in about 10% of patients (41,52). This has the appearance of an adrenergic or essential tremor and may respond to dosage reduction or to the administration of propranalol (52), though the latter is rarely necessary and the tremor is rarely sufficiently severe to limit treatment with valproate. Asterixis has been reported (8).

Other Neurological Side Effects

As in all drugs affecting the central nervous system function, some neurological side effects are to be expected; these include drowsiness, acute confusional states, and irritability. Many of these are seen in relation to polytherapy. Sedation alone occurs in about 2% (48). A reversible dementia was reported by Zaret and Cohen (110): the patient described had a 3-year history of progressive decline in cognitive abilities which reversed within 2 months of discontinuation of valproate. Other studies (94,98,99) indicated that valproate had little effect on psychological performance and cognitive function and that the latter was less effected than with other antiepileptic drugs. This was also the conclusion of the American Academy of Pediatrics Committee on Drugs (1).

Jeavons et al. (50) described an interaction between valproate and clonazepam in which there was the induction of spike-wave stupor. Apart from an occasional anecdotal account, this has not been confirmed as a common complication. In fact, Mireles and Leppik (69) failed to observe a single such case among 55 patients who received combination therapy with valporate and clonazepam.

Stupor or Coma

Changes in alertness amounting to stupor and even coma have been reported both in the presence and in the absence of overt metabolic changes such as hyperammonemia, increased blood phenobarbital levels, and other drug interactions (12,65, 68,85,92,101). Hyperammonemia and drug interactions have been implicated from time to time (107), but the majority of these reported cases is not thus explicable. The stupor is usually associated with bilaterally synchronous high-voltage, slow-wave EEG activity.

Metabolic Disturbances

Various metabolic disorders have been described in patients receiving valproate since this agent was first introduced in the treatment of seizures. However, the clinical significance of the effect of mitochondrial dysfunction and its various biochemical alterations have not been clarified.

Hyperammonemia is a common consequence of valproate administration. It may be seen in the absence of hepatic dysfunction (71,109) and may be the consequence of increased renal production of ammonia (67) or inhibition of nitrogen elimination via inhibition of urea synthesis, or both (38,39). There may be significant nutritional influences (59,60). Hyperammonemia may be enhanced in the presence of polytherapy (79,104,108). Coulter and Allen (18) considered that hyperammonemia might be secondary to increased glycine and propionic acid concentrations and suggested a mechanism similar to that postulated in propionyl CoA carboxylase deficiency. In addition, ornithine transcarbamylase deficiency has been described in a person dying with hyperammonemia who had been given valproate (53). Here the hyperammonemia was probably secondary to the underlying metabolic abnormality (39,95). Other workers (16,75,58,72) postulated carnitine deficiency as a significant factor. Carnitine levels are diminished in patients receiving valproate but whether or not this reaches clinical significance is in doubt (67). It is interesting, however, that in patients on polytherapy with drugs that induce cytochrome P-450, carnitine is depleted to a greater degree.

Valproate induces hyperglycinemia and hyperglycinuria (43,44,70). In most patients these metabolic disturbances have been detected with laboratory screening and were not associated with clinical symptoms. Where it has been tested, valproate-induced hyperglycinemia has not been associated with elevated spinal fluid glycine levels.

Transient amenorrhea has been described in young women following initiation of therapy following valproic acid (66). This may persist for up to a year before regular menstrual cycles recur.

IDIOSYNCRATIC REACTIONS

Hematologic Side Effects

These include neutropenia (45,91) and bone marrow suppression (62,89). The most commonly recognized hematologic side effects are thrombocytopenia and inhibition of platelet aggregation. There have been clinical reports of hematoma, epistaxis, and increased bleeding after surgery (62,81), and fibrinogen depletion may also occur (48,64). The subject has been reviewed by Loiseau (62) who concluded that these side effects have little clinical importance except in patients undergoing surgery.

Hepatotoxicity

Hepatic reactions to antiepileptic drugs range from transient elevations of hepatic enzymes (19,25,28,88,105) without clinical signs or symptoms of hepatic dysfunction to fatal hepatotoxicity.

Drug-induced hepatotoxicity can be categorized into two distinct types, predictable and nonpredictable, according to the pathogenesis or mechanism of toxicity (32,111). Predictable hepatotoxicity is produced by agents known to have direct effects on hepatic cells. Such toxicity has a high incidence among those at risk, is dose-dependent, and is early in onset. Nonpredictable hepatotoxicity is an idiosyncratic reaction and may be due to drug hypersensitivity in which there may be fever, rash, eosinophilia, and a relatively short exposure prior to the onset of symptoms. Nonpredictable hepatotoxicity may also result from aberrant metabolism-producing toxic metabolites. Hepatic injury in this event may not become clinically apparent early in the course of treatment and it is into this group that valproate hepatotoxicity tends to fall.

Although dose-related elevations in liver enzymes may occur in over 40% of patients

(90), these elevations are not generally accompanied by clinical symptoms or by abnormalities in the synthetic function of the liver. To some extent this may be a dose-related phenomenon. Enzyme elevation is usually transient whether the dose is reduced or maintained, and may reflect enzyme induction rather than hepatotoxicity. The subject has been reviewed extensively by Zimmerman and Ishack (111), Gram and Bentsen (32), Powell-Jackson et al. (78), Jeavons (47–49), Dreifuss et al. (28), Berkovic et al. (5), and Dickinson et al. (20).

Because of the apparent high mortality rate and because of the opportunity presented by the collection of data on persons at risk despite the absence of definitive metabolic markers, an analysis of the United States experience with fatal hepatotoxicity was analyzed (28). According to these findings the overall incidence of hepatic failure was approximately 1 in 10,000, but the retrospective review indicated that very young children are disproportionately vulnerable to a fatal hepatic dysfunction, especially when receiving valproate as part of multiple anticonvulsant therapy. The primary risk of fatal hepatic dysfunction was found to be in children under 2 years of age receiving valproate as polytherapy. The rate of hepatic fatality in this high risk group was about 1 in 500. The risk of fatal hepatic toxicity declines with age and in patients above the age of 2 years receiving valproate as polytherapy the rate decreases to 1 in 12,000. When valproate was given as monotherapy the rate of hepatic fatality was about 1 in 37,000 for all monotherapy patients, though it was still 1 in 7,000 in the 0 to 2 year age group. Even monotherapy patients in this age group are more vulnerable than older patients. Patients over the age of 2 years on monotherapy had a fatality rate of 1 in 45,000.

Most polytherapy patients in the 0 to 2 year age group failed on previous anticonvulsants, and these high-risk infants also had severe epilepsy and other medical conditions including mental retardation, developmental delay, congenital anomalies, and other neurological diseases. In this series there were no reports of fatal hepatic dysfunction in patients over the age of 10 years receiving monotherapy.

The key clinical features associated with hepatotoxicity are nausea, vomiting, anorexia, lethargy sometimes accompanied by edema, and jaundice. Abdominal pain, easy bruising, and sudden loss of seizure control may indicate hepatic involvement. On the other hand, liver dysfunction may develop secondarily to status epilepticus-induced shock.

Recent evidence suggests that some cases previously reported as valproate-induced liver failure were misdiagnosed and appeared to have been cases of a familial hepatic dysfunction (9,29). In our series, at least one of the patients who developed hepatic failure while receiving valproate had a sibling who also developed fatal hepatic dysfunction but had never been treated with valproate.

The onset of hepatic illness with valproate usually occurs within the first 90 days of therapy though occasionally it may occur considerably later (97).

Scheffner's series from Germany suggests a less predictable age and polytherapy relationship (55,86,87) and he does not believe the high risk group to be as well delineated by these factors.

On the other hand, in the United States the previous reports have been followed by changes in prescribing patterns, and the incidence of fatal hepatotoxicity in patients over the age of 2 years receiving monotherapy has declined to 1 in 49,000 (16,25). Since the initial report more patients have been receiving valproate as monotherapy, and considerably more low risk patients and fewer high risk patients are being treated with valproate. This change in exposure pattern appears to have had a positive impact on the number of hepatic fatalities (4 among 198,000 patients treated) (27).

Table 1. *Rate of hepatic fatality by age group in patients receiving valproate as monotherapy or polytherapy*

Age group	Monotherapy			Polytherapy[a]		
	Total patients	Deaths	Rate per 10M	Total patients	Deaths	Rate per 10M
0–2	7,025	1	1.42	7,889	15	19.01
3–10	35,593	4	1.12	39,975	7	1.75
11–20	51,951	0	0	58,348	5	0.86
21–40	59,107	0	0	66,386	4	0.60
41 +	34,125	0	0	38,351	1	0.26
Monotherapy total	187,821	5	0.27			
Polytherapy total				210,949	32	1.52
Combined total				398,770	37	0.93

[a] Other anticonvulsants taken with valproate: phenytoin (17 patients); phenobarbital (16); clonazepam (10); carbamazepine (8); primidone (3); diamox, diazepam, and paraldehyde (2 each); ethosuximide and mesantoin (1 each).

From Dreifuss et al., ref. 25, with permission.

Patients who develop fatal hepatic dysfunction have had histological features quite different from those reported with phenytoin and carbamazepine hepatotoxicity in that microvesicular steatosis usually with necrosis is the most prominent finding (111). This finding resembles the histologic picture of Jamaican vomiting sickness and Reye's syndrome which are characterized by a very similar clinical picture. This has led to the suspicion that valproate hepatotoxicity may reflect aberrant metabolism of valproate to a toxic metabolite such as 4-pentonic acid which can produce in animals a condition similar to Reye's syndrome (54). Rettie et al. (80) have shown that 2-*n*-propyl-4-pentonic acid is a metabolite formed via the omega oxidation pathway from valproate. It inhibits both cytochrome P-450 and fatty acid beta oxidation and induces microvesicular steatosis *in vivo*. The production of the 4-ene metabolite is dependent on cytochrome P-450; this in turn is induced by phenobarbital and other enzyme-inducing antiepileptic drugs. This may in part be the explanation why patients on polytherapy are at considerably greater risk of developing fatal hepatic dysfunction than patients receiving valproate monotherapy. It is recommended (24) that valproate not be administered as part of anticonvulsant polytherapy in children under the age of 3 years unless monotherapy has failed or the potential benefit of polypharmacy merits the risks, that valproate administration be avoided in patients with pre-existing liver disease and/or a family history of childhood hepatic disease, that valproate be administered in as low a dose as possible consistent with seizure control, that concomitant administration of salicylates be avoided, and that symptoms such as vomiting, headache, edema, jaundice, or seizure breakthrough, especially after a febrile illness, be regarded as potentially serious.

Not all severe hepatotoxicity is fatal and early discontinuation of the drug and the institution of supportive therapy may result in reversibility (14,20,93).

Pancreatitis

Acute pancreatitis, occasionally fatal, has been reported in patients receiving valproate. This is usually of the acute hemorrhagic variety (11,17,23,76,84,103,106). Complications may include pericardial infusion, laparotomy wound infection, and coagulopathy, and pancreatic pseudocysts may result (4,10). On several occasions rechallenge after recovery led to recurrence of pancreatitis. Although this has been associated with fatal outcome, the condition is usually reversible on withdrawal of valproate. The complication of pancreatitis is a serious one and has to be considered in patients on valproic acid who experience severe abdominal pain and vomiting. The complication may arise at any stage of treatment. The serum amylase level is usually diagnostic.

TERATOGENICITY

The first report of neural tube defect in the offspring of a patient on valproate was published by Gomez in (31). In 1982, Robert and Guibaud (82) showed increased incidence of myelomeningocele in children born to epileptic mothers taking valproate. The frequency of this occurrence is approximately 1% to 2% (7,33,61,83). This is about the same frequency of recurrence as would be expected where there is spina bifida in the sibling. The risk of exposure is during the first trimester of pregnancy. It has been suggested that patients at risk receive prenatal counseling, amniocentesis, alpha-fetoprotein determination, and ultrasonography before the 20th week of gestation in order to detect neural tube defects.

Since the first descriptions of the so-called "fetal hydantoin syndrome" (34), it has become evident that similar anomalies may be seen with other anticonvulsants. A number of anomalies including craniofacial and digital involvement may be seen as a result of in utero exposure to valproate (2,21,40,42). These effects appear to be dose related. Jaeger-Roman et al. (42) monitored 26 pregnancies involving valproate with 12 patients on combination therapy, 14 on monotherapy, and 26 matched-pair controls. Valproate doses and blood levels were higher in the monotherapy group, especially in the first trimester. Four of the infants in this group had major malformations and the median number of minor malformations including craniofacial and digital anomalies as described by DiLiberti et al. (21) exceeded that of controls.

Most maternal exposures to valproate do not appear to have adverse outcomes (83). In fact, for defects other than spina bifida, there is at present insufficient data to demonstrate that alternative agents have any less risk than does valproate (3).

REFERENCES

1. American Academy of Pediatrics' Committee on Drugs. (1985): Behavioral and cognitive effects of anticonvulsant therapy. *Pediatrics,* 76:644–647.
2. Bantz, E. W. (1984): Valproic acid and congenital malformations. A case report. *Clin. Pediatr.,* 23:352–353.
3. Bapst-Reiter, J., Bureau, M., Cenraud, B., Cohadon, S., et al. (1984): Teratogenic risk of antiepileptic drugs with special reference to sodium valproate (valproic acid) therapy. In: *Advances in Epileptology,* edited by R. J. Porter, R. H. Mattson, A. A. Ward, Jr., and M. Dam. Raven Press, New York.
4. Baskies, A. M. (1984): Case report: Pancreatic pseudocyst associated with valproic acid therapy. *J. Med. Soc. N.J.,* 81:399–400.
5. Berkovic, S. F., Bladin, P. F., Jones, D. B., Smallwood, R. A., and Vajda, F. J. (1983): Hepatotoxicity of sodium valproate. *Clin. Exp. Neurol.,* 19:192–197.
6. Bigler, D. (1985): Neurological sequelae after intoxication with sodium valproate. *Acta Neurol. Scan.,* 72:351–352.
7. Bjerkedal, T., Czeizel, A., Goujard, J., et al. (1982): Valproic acid and spina bifida. *Lancet,* 2:1096.
8. Bodensteiner, J. B., Morris, H. H., and Golden, G. S. (1981): Asterixis associated with sodium valproate. *Neurology,* 31:186–190.
9. Bohan, T., *personal communication.*
10. Braun, E., Spannagel, B., and Bundschu, H. D. (1987): Inapparent verlaufende Pankreatitis mit Pseudozystenbildung und cholestatischem Ikterus unter antikonvulsiver Therapie mit Valproinsaure. *Klin. Wochenschr.,* 65:433–436.
11. Camfield, P. R. (1979): Pancreatitis due to valproic acid. *Lancet,* 1:1198–1199.
12. Campostrini, R., Zaccara, G., Rossi, L., Paganini, M., Dorigotti, A., and Zappoli, R. (1985): Valproate-induced hyperammonaemia in two epileptic identical twins. *J. Neurol.,* 232:167–168.
13. Clark, J. E., Covanis, A., Gupta, A. K., and Jeavons, P. M. (1980): Unwanted effects of sodium valproate in children and adolescents. In: *The Place of Sodium Valproate in the Treatment of Epilepsy,* edited by M. J. Parsonage and A. D. S.

Caldwell, pp. 223–233. Royal Society of Medicine, London.

14. Colletti, R. B., Trainer, T. D., and Karwisz, B. R. (1986): Reversible valproate fulminant hepatic failure. *J. Pediatr. Gastroenterol. Nutr.,* 5(6):990–994.

15. Connacher, A. A., Macnab, M. S., Moody, J. P., and Jung, R. T. (1987): Fatality due to massive overdose of sodium valproate. *Scott. Med. J.,* 32:85–86.

16. Coulter, D. L. (1984): Carnitine deficiency: A possible mechanism for valproate hepatotoxicity. *Lancet,* 1:689.

17. Coulter, D. L., and Allen, R. J. (1980): Pancreatitis associated with valproic acid therapy for epilepsy. *Ann. Neurol.,* 7:92.

18. Coulter, D. L., and Allen, R. J. (1980): Secondary hyperammonemia: A possible mechanism for valproate encephalopathy. *Lancet,* 2:1310–1311.

19. Covanis, A., Gupta, A. K., and Jeavons, P. M. (1982): Sodium valproate and polytherapy. *Epilepsia,* 23:693–720.

20. Dickinson, R. G., Bassett, M. L., Searle, J., Tyrer, J. H., and Eadie, M. J. (1985): Valproate hepatotoxicity: A review and report of two instances in adults. *Clin. Exp. Neurol. (Australia),* 21:79–91.

21. DiLiberti, J. H., Farndon, P. A., Dennis, N. R., and Curry, C. J. (1984): The fetal valproate syndrome. *Am. J. Med. Genet.,* 19:473–481.

22. Dinesen, H., Gram, L., Anderson, T., and Dam, M. (1984): Weight gain during treatment with valproate. *Acta Neurol. Scand.,* 70:65–69.

23. Dobrilla, G., Felder, M., and Chilovi, F. (1985): Medikamentos induzierte akute Pankreatits. *Schweiz. Med. Wochenschr.,* 115:850–858.

24. Dreifuss, F. E. (1987): Fatal liver failure in children on valproate. *Lancet,* 1:47–48.

25. Dreifuss, F. E., and Langer, D. H. (1987): Hepatic considerations in the use of antiepileptic drugs. *Epilepsia,* 28 (Suppl. 2):S23–S29.

26. Dreifuss, F. E., Langer, D. H. (1988): Side effects of valproate. *Am. J. Med.,* 84 (Suppl. 1A):39–41.

27. Dreifuss, F. E., Langer, D. H., Moline, K. A., and Maxwell, J. E. (1989): Valproic acid hepatic fatalities II: U.S. experience since 1984. *Neurology,* 39:201–207.

28. Dreifuss, F. E., Santilli, N., Langer, D. H., Sweeney, K. P., Moline, K. A., and Menander, K. B. (1987): Valproic acid hepatic fatalities: A retrospective review. *Neurology,* 37:379–385.

29. Egger, J., Harding, B. N., Boyd, S. G., et al. (1987): Progressive neuronal degeneration of childhood with liver disease. *Clin. Pediatr.,* 26:167–173.

30. Garden, A. S., Benzie, R. J., Hutton, E. M., and Gare, D. J. (1985): Valproic acid therapy and neural tube defects. *Can. Med. Assoc. J.,* 132:933–936.

31. Gomez, M. (1981): Possible teratogenicity of valproic acid. *J. Ped.,* 98:508–509.

32. Gram, L., and Bentsen, K. D. (1983): Hepatic toxicity of antiepileptic drugs: A review. In: *Current Therapy in Epilepsy,* edited by M. V. Iiv-anainen, *Acta Neurol. Scand.* 68 (Suppl. 97):81–90.

33. Guibaud, S., Simplot, A., Boissson, C., and Pison, H. (1987): Depistage prenatal de 4 cas de spina bifida chez de meres traitées par le valproate. *J. Genet. Hum.,* 35:231–235.

34. Hanson, J. W., and Smith, D. W. (1975): The fetal hydantoin syndrome. *J. Pediatr.,* 87:285–290.

35. Hassan, M. N., Laljee, H. K., and Parsonage, M. J. (1976): Sodium valproate in the treatment of resistant epilepsy. *Acta Neurol. Scand.,* 54:209–218.

36. Herranz, J. L., Arteaga, R., and Armijo, J. A. (1981): Change in hair colour induced by valproic acid. *Dev. Child Neurol.,* 23:386–387.

37. Hintze, G., Klein, H. H., Prange, H., and Krequer, H. (1987): A case of valproate intoxication with excessive brain edema. *Klin. Wochenschr.,* 65:424–427.

38. Hjelm, M., Oberholzer, V., Seakins, J., Thomas S., and Kay, J. D. S. (1986): Valproate-induced inhibition of urea synthesis and hyperammonemia in healthy subjects. *Lancet,* 2:859.

39. Hjelm, M., de Silva, L. V., Seakins, J. W., Oberholzer, V. G., and Rolles, C. J. (1986): Evidence of inherited urea cycle defect in a case of fatal valproate toxicity. *Br. Med. Jr.,* 292:23–24.

40. Huot, C., Gauthier, M., Lebel, M., and Larbrisseau, A. (1987): Congenital malformations associated with maternal use of valproic acid. *Can. J. Neurol. Sci.,* 14:290–293.

41. Hyuman, N. M., Dennis, P. D., and Sinclar, K. G. (1979): Tremor due to sodium valproate. *Neurology,* 29:1177–1180.

42. Jaeger-Roman, E., Deichl, A., Jakob, S., et al. (1986): Fetal growth, major malformations, and minor anomalies in infants born to women receiving valproic acid. *J. Peds.,* 108:997–1004.

43. Jaeken, J., Casaer, P., and Corbeel, L. (1980): Valproate, hyperammonaemia and hyperglycinaemia. *Lancet,* 2:260.

44. Jaeken, J., Corbeel, L., Casaer, P., Carchon, H., Eggermont, E., and Eeckels, R. (1977): Dipropylacetate (valproate) and glycine metabolism. *Lancet,* 2:617.

45. Jaeken, J., van Goethem, C., Casaer, P., Devlieger, H., and Eggermont, E. (1979): Neutopenia during sodium valproate treatment. *Arch. Dis. Child,* 54:985–986.

46. Janssen, F., Rambeck, B., and Schnabel, R. (1985): Acute valproate intoxication with fatal outcome in an infant. *Neuropediatrics,* 16:235–238.

47. Jeavons, P. M. (1980): Sodium valproate and acute hepatic failure. *Dev. Med. Child Neurol.,* 22:547–548.

48. Jeavons, P. M. (1982): Valproate toxicity. In: *Antiepileptic Drugs,* 2nd edition, edited by D. M. Woodbury, J. K. Penry, and C. E. Pippenger, pp. 647–653. New York, Raven Press.

49. Jeavons, P. M. (1984): Non–dose-related side effects of valproate. *Epilepsia,* 25 (Suppl. 1):S50–S55.

50. Jeavons, P. M., and Clark, J. E. (1974): Sodium

valproate in treatment of epilepsy. *Br. Med. J.*, 2:584–586.

51. Jeavons, P. M., Clark, J. E., and Harding, G. F. A. (1977): Valproate and curly hair. *Lancet*, 1:359.

52. Karas, B. J., Wilder, B. J., Hammond, E. J., and Bauman, A. W. (1983): Treatment of valproate tremors. *Neurology*, 33:1380–1382.

53. Kay, J. D., Hilton-Jones, D., and Hyman, N. (1986): Valproate toxicity and ornithine carbamoyltransferase deficiency. *Lancet*, 2:1283–1284.

54. Kochen, W., Schneider, A., Ritz, A. (1983): Abnormal metabolism of valproic acid in fatal hepatic failure. *Eur. J. Pediatrics*, 141:30–35.

55. Konig, S., Scheffner, D., Rauterberg-Ruland, I., Kochen, W., Hofmann, W. J., Wokittel, E., and Schick, U. (1987): Todliches Leberversagen bei einem altersgemass entwickelten funf Jahre alten Jungen unter VPA-Monotherapie. *Monatsschr. Kinderheilkd.*, 135:310–313.

56. Lakhani, M., and McMurdo, M. E. (1986): Survival after severe self poisoning with sodium valproate. *Postgrad. Med. J.*, 62(727):310–313.

57. Laljee, H. C. K., and Parsonage, M. J. (1980): Unwanted effects of sodium valproate (Epilim) in the treatment of adult patients with epilepsy. In: *The Place of Sodium Valproate in the Treatment of Epilepsy*, edited by M. J. Parsonage and A. D. S. Caldwell, pp. 234–274. Royal Society of Medicine, London.

58. Lamb, W. C., Paetzke-Brunner, I., and Jaeger, G. (1986): Serum carnitine during valproic acid therapy. *Epilepsia*, 27:559–562.

59. Laub, M. C. (1986): Hyperammonamie wahrend Valproat-Therapie bei Kindern und Jugendlichen. *Nervenarzt*, 57:314–318.

60. Laub, M. C. (1986): Nutritional influence on serum ammonia in young patients receiving sodium valproate. *Epilepsia*, 27:55–59.

61. Lindhout, D., and Meinardi, H. (1984): Spina bifida and *in utero* exposure to valproate. *Lancet*, 2:396.

62. Loiseau, P. (1981): Sodium valproate platelet dysfunction and bleeding. *Epilepsia*, 22:141–146.

63. MacDougall, L. G. (1982): Pure red cell aplasia associated with sodium valproate therapy. *J.A.M.A.*, 247:53–54.

64. Majer, R. V., and Green, P. J. (1987): Neonatal afibrinogenaemia due to sodium valproate. *Lancet*, 2:740–741.

65. Marescaux, C., Micheletti, G., Warter, J. M., Rumbach, L., Inder, M., Koehil, C., and Kuntz, D. (1982): Valprote de sodiu, etats stuporeus et hyperammoniumie. *J. Med. (Strasbourg)*, 13:705–711.

66. Margraf, J. W., and Dreifuss, F. E. (1981): Amenorrhea following initiation of therapy with valproic acid. *Neurology*, 31:159.

67. Matsuda, I., Ohtani, Y., and Ninomiya, N. (1986): Renal handling of carnitine in children with carnitine deficiency and hyperammonemia associated with valproate therapy. *J. Pediatr.*, 109:131–134.

68. Milandre, L., Rey, M., Boudouresques, G., Farnarier, G., and Poncet, M. (1987): Etat stuporeux chez un epileptique traite par le valproate de sodium. Problemes diagnostiques. *Acta Neurol. Belg.*, 87:70–75.

69. Mireles, R., and Leppik, I. E. (1985): Valproate and clonazepam comedication in patients with intractable epilepsy. *Epilepsia*, 26:122–126.

70. Mortensen, P. B., Koluraa, S., and Christensen, E. (1980): Inhibition of the glycine cleavage system: Hyperglycinemia and hyperglycinuria caused by valproic acid. *Epilepsia*, 21:563–569.

71. Murphy, J. V., and Marquard, K. (1982): Asymptomatic hyperammonemia in patients receiving valproic acid. *Arch. Neurol.*, 39:591–592.

72. Murphy, J. V., Marquardt, K. M., and Shug, A. L. (1985): Valproic acid associated abnormalities of carnitine metabolism. *Lancet*, 1:820–821.

73. Napke, E. (1983): Adverse reactions: Some pitfalls and postulates. In: *Side Effects of Drugs Annual 7*, edited by M. N. G. Dukes, pp. xx–xxvi. Amsterdam, Excerpta Medica.

74. Noronha, M. J., and Bevan, P. L. T. (1976): A literature review of unwanted effects of treatment with Epilim. In: *Clinical and Pharmacological Aspects of Sodium Valproate (Epilim) in the Treatment of Epilepsy*, edited by N. J. Legg, pp. 61–67. MCS Consultants, Tunbridge Wells, Kent.

75. Ohtani, Y., Eudo, F., and Matsuda, J. (1982): Carnitine deficiency and hyperammonemia associated with valproic acid therapy. *J. Pediatr.*, 101:782–785.

76. Parker, P. H., Helinek, G. L., et al (1981): Recurrent pancreatitis induced by valproic acid. *Gastroenterology*, 80:825–828.

77. Pedersen, B., and Juul-Jensen, P. (1984): Electroencephalographic alterations during intoxication with sodium valproate: A case report. *Epilepsia*, 25:121–124.

78. Powell-Jackson, P. R., Tredger, J. M., and Williams, R. (1984): Hepatotoxicity to sodium valproate: A review. *Gut*, 25:673–681.

79. Ratnaike, R. N., Schapel, G. J., Purdie, G., Rischbieth, R. H., and Hoffman, S. (1986): Hyperammonaemia and hepatotoxicity during chronic valproate therapy: Enhancement by combination with other antiepileptic drugs. *Br. J. Clin. Pharmacol.*, 22:100–103.

80. Rettie, A. E., Rettenmeier, A. W., Howald, W. N., and Baillie, T. A. (1987): Cytochrome P450-catalyzed formation of VPA, a toxic metabolite of valproic acid. *Science*, 235:890–893.

81. Richardson, S. G. N., Fletcher, D. J., Jeavons, P. H., and Stuart, J. (1976): Sodium valproate and platelet dysfunction. *Brit. Med. J.*, 3:179.

82. Robert, E., and Guibaud, P. (1982): Maternal valproic acid and congenital neural tube defects. *Lancet*, 2:937.

83. Rosa, F. W. (1984): Teratogenesis in epilepsy: Birth defects with maternal valproic acid exposures. In: *Advances in Epileptology*, edited by R. J. Porter, R. J. Mattson, A. A. Ward Jr., and M. Dam. Raven Press, New York.

84. Rosenberg, H. K., and Ortega, W. (1987): Hemorrhagic pancreatitis in a young child following valproic acid therapy. Clinical and ultrasonic assessment. *Clin. Pediatr.,* 26:98–101.

85. Sackellares, J. C., Lee, S. I., and Dreifuss, F. E. (1979): Stupor following administration of valproic acid to patients receiving other antiepileptic drugs. *Epilepsia,* 20:697–703.

86. Scheffner, D. (1986): Fatal liver failure in children on valproate. *Lancet,* 2:511.

87. Scheffner, D., and Konig, S. (1987): Valproate hepatotoxicity. *Lancet,* 2:389–390.

88. Sherard, E. S., Steiman, G. S., and Couri, D. (1980): Treatment of childhood epilepsy with valproic acid: Results of the first 100 patients in a 6-month trial. *Neurology,* 30:31–35.

89. Smith, F. R., and Boots, M. (1980): Sodium valproate and bone marrow suppression. *Ann. Neurol.,* 8:197–199.

90. Sussman, N. M., and McLain, L. W. (1979): A direct hepatotoxic effect of valproic acid. *J.A.M.A.,* 242:1173–1174.

91. Symon, D. N., and Russell, G. (1983): Sodium valproate and neutropenia. *Arch. Dis. Child,* 58:235.

92. Tartara, A., and Manni, R. (1985): Sodium valproate "encephalopathy": Report of three cases with generalised epilepsy. *Ital. J. Neurol. Sci.,* 6:93–95.

93. Thygesen, J., and Boesen, F. (1982): Two cases of reversible liver lesion induced by valproate. *Acta Eurol. Scan.,* 66:396–399.

94. Trimble, M. R., and Thompson, P. J. (1984): Sodium valproate and cognitive function. *Epilepsia,* 25 (Suppl. 1):S60–S64.

95. Tripp, J. H., et al. (1981): Sodium valproate and orinthine carbanyl transferase deficiency. *Lancet,* 1:1165–1166.

96. van der Merwe, A. C., Albrecht, C. F., Brink, M. S., and Coetzee, A. R. (1985): Sodium valproate poisoning. A case report. *S. Afr. Med. J.,* 67:735–736.

97. van Egmond, H., Degomme, P., de Simpel, H., Dierick, A. M., and Roels, H. (1987): A suspected case of late-onset–sodium-valproate-induced hepatic failure. *Neuropediatrics,* 18:96–98.

98. Vining, E. P. G. (1987): Cognitive dysfunction associated with antiepileptic drug therapy. *Epilepsia,* 28 (Suppl 2):S18–S22.

99. Vining, E. P. G., Mellits, E. D., Cataldo, M. F.,

Dorsen, M. M., Spielberg, S. P., and Freeman, J. M. (1983): Effects of phenobarbital and sodium valproate on neuropsychological function and behavior. *Ann. Neurol.* (abstr.), 14:360.

100. Volans, G. N., Berry, D. J., and Wiseman, H. M. (1983): Overdose with valproate. *Brit. J. Clin. Pract.,* (Symp suppl.) 27:58–62.

101. Wason, S., and Savitt, D. (1985): Acute valproic acid toxicity at therapeutic concentrations. *Clin. Pediatr.,* 24:466–467.

102. Wilder, B. J., Ramsay, R. E., Murphy, J. V., Karas, B. J., Marquardt, K., and Hammond, E. J. (1983): Comparison of valproic acid and phenytoin in newly diagnosed tonic-clonic seizures. *Neurology,* 33:1474–1476.

103. Williams, L. H., Reynolds, R. P., and Emery, J. L. (1983): Pancreatitis during sodium valproate treatment. *Arch. Dis. Child,* 58:543–544.

104. Williams, C. A., Tiefenbach, S., and McReynolds, J. W. (1984): Valproic acid-induced hyperammonemia in mentally retarded adults. *Neurology,* 34:550–553.

105. Willmore, L. J., Wilder, B. J., Bruni, J., and Villareal, H. J. (1978): Effect of valproic acid on hepatic function. *Neurology,* 28:961–964.

106. Wyllie, E., Wyllie, R., Cruse, R. P., Erenberg, G., and Rothner, A. D. (1984): Pancreatitis associated with valproic acid therapy. *Am. J. Dis. Child,* 138:912–914.

107. Zaccara, G., Paganini, M., Campostrini, R., Arnetoli, G., Zappoli R., and Moroni, F. (1984): Hyperammonemia and valproate-induced alterations of the state of consciousness. A report of 8 cases. *Eur. Neurol.,* 23(2):104–112.

108. Zaccara, G., Paganini, M., Campostrini, R., Moroni, F., Valenza, T., Messori, A., Bartelli, M., Arnetoli, G., and Zappoli, R. (1985): Effect of associated antiepileptic treatment on valproate-induced hyperammonemia. *Ther. Drug Monit.,* 7(2):185–190.

109. Zaret, B. S., Becker, R. R., Marini, A. M., Wagle, W., and Passarelli, C. (1982): Sodium valproate induced hyperammonemia without clinical hepatic dysfunction. *Neurology,* 32:206–208.

110. Zaret, B. S., and Cohen, R. A. (1986): Reversible valproic acid-induced dementia: A case report. *Epilepsia,* 27:234–240.

111. Zimmerman, H., and Ishak, K., (1982): Valproate-induced hepatic injury: Analyses of 23 fatal cases. *Hepatology,* 2:591–597.

Antiepileptic Drugs, Third Edition, edited by
R. Levy, R. Mattson, B. Meldrum,
J. K. Penry, and F. E. Dreifuss.
Raven Press, Ltd., New York © 1989.

46

Ethosuximide

Mechanisms of Action

James A. Ferrendelli and Katherine D. Holland

Ethosuximide (ESM), α-ethyl-α-methyl-succinimide, has been used extensively for the treatment of absence (petit mal) seizures. Despite its frequent use, the site(s) and mechanism(s) of action of ESM are still poorly defined. In this chapter, the available published data on basic pharmacological actions of ESM is reviewed. To facilitate presentation, this information is divided into the following categories: effects on clinical and experimental seizures, molecular action, cellular actions, and effects on neuronal systems. Finally, an hypothesis attempting to explain the drug's probable mechanism of action is presented.

EFFECTS ON CLINICAL AND EXPERIMENTAL SEIZURES

One of the most intriguing facts about ESM is its highly selective effect on clinical and experimental seizures. It completely, or almost completely, prevents absence seizures in about 50% of patients with petit mal epilepsy and reduces their frequency in another 40% to 45% (3). In contrast, it has no apparent effect against generalized tonic-clonic convulsions or partial seizures.

The high degree of therapeutic specificity of ESM in human seizure disorders is reflected by its selective anticonvulsant action against experimental seizures. It is well known that ESM prevents pentylenetetrazol (PTZ; Metrazol) seizures at nontoxic doses in experimental animals but has no effect on maximal electroshock seizures except at very high, toxic concentrations (5). Ethosuximide has also been reported to have an anticonvulsant action on seizures induced by implantation of cobalt into the cerebral cortex (13,29,50), systemic administration of γ-hydroxybutyrate (24,53,54), application of conjugated estrogen to the brain (28), inhalation of fluorothyl (1) or enflurane (49), barbiturate withdrawal (44), and systemic administration of penicillin (26). However, it seems to be inactive against allylglycine seizures in photosensitive baboons (40), stroboscopic seizures in epileptic fowl (12), and seizures produced by application of aluminum hydroxide (37) to the cerebral cortex.

MOLECULAR ACTIONS

Cerebral Metabolism

Nahorski (43) measured the effects of ESM on brain levels of glycolytic intermediates, adenine nucleotides, phosphocreatine, tricarboxylate cycle intermediates, and some amino acids. He reported that ESM elevated brain glucose levels and increased the brain/blood glucose ratio. In addition, ESM increased brain malate levels and decreased levels of fructose-1,6-biphosphate, pyruvate, aspartate, and α-oxoglutarate, but there were no detectable concentration changes in any of the other substances examined in this study. In a similar study, Gueldry et al. (27) found that single-dose administration of ESM produced no significant change in the adenine nucleotide content in brain but did increase cerebral glucose levels when ESM was given in doses that exceeded therapeutic levels. Finally, ESM reduces the oxygen consumption in brain tissue both *in vitro* and *in vivo* (35). These effects are similar to those seen following the administration of anesthetics and other antiepileptic drugs such as valproate and phenytoin. They probably do not reflect a specific etiology but rather are the result of a general depression of the metabolic rate.

Brain Enzyme Activity

Two laboratories have reported that ESM inhibits (Na$^+$,K$^+$)-ATPase activity but not Mg^{++}-ATPase activity in subcellular fractions of cortical tissue (21,22,23,35). The data of Gilbert and colleagues suggest that the site of (Na$^+$,K$^+$)-ATPase inhibition may be restricted to the nerve terminal plasma membrane (23). Unfortunately, these effects were found at ESM concentrations (2.5 mM and 25 mM) considerably greater than those producing anticonvulsant effects. In addition, although Leznicki and Dymecki (35) reported that ESM inhibits (Na$^+$,K$^+$)-ATPase in brain homogenates, they have also found that long-term treatment of animals resulted in an increase in (Na$^+$,K$^+$)-ATPase activity.

Although ESM has been reported to have little or no direct effect on the γ-aminobutyric acid (GABA) synthesizing enzyme glutaminic acid decarboxylase (GAD) (35), it antagonizes isoniazid-induced inhibition of GAD (38). However, single-dose administration of ESM in anticonvulsant doses has no effect on brain GABA concentrations (36). Thus alterations in brain GABA levels do not contribute to the anticonvulsant effects of ESM. Ethosuximide has no effect on the activities of a variety of enzymes involved in the breakdown of neurotransmitters including GABA transaminase, monoamine oxidase, acetylcholinesterase, and arylsulfatase (35).

Ethosuximide inhibits NADPH-linked aldehyde reductase in bovine brain (16). This enzyme can convert succinic semialdehyde to γ-hydroxybutyrate and may be the mechanism by which long-term ESM treatment decreases brain γ-hydroxybutyrate levels (55,59). In light of the behavioral and EEG similarities between human absence seizures and administration of exogenous γ-hydroxybutyrate alterations, endogenous γ-hydroxybutyrate levels may be relevant to the antiabsence actions of ESM (24,53,65). However, this is unable to account for either the anti-PTZ actions of ESM or the ability of ESM to block seizures caused by exogenous γ-hydroxybutyrate. In addition, it is important to note that single-dose administration of ESM produces an increase in brain γ-hydroxybutyrate, and that this increase is coincident with the onset of anticonvulsant effects (55).

Membrane Transport Processes and Voltage Gated Channels

Gray and Gilbert (25) reported that ESM stimulated the uptake of xylose into brain slices, probably by increasing the affinity of the carrier for xylose. Our laboratory has shown that ESM has no effect on the basal level of Ca^{++} uptake into synaptosomes (58). Unlike phenytoin and carbamazepine, which inhibit Ca^{++} accumulation into veratridine depolarized synaptosomes at therapeutic concentrations, ESM is ineffective except at concentrations exceeding 10 mM. More recently, Crowder and Bradford (10) have confirmed this work and have also found that ESM has no effect on veratridine-stimulated amino acid neurotransmitter release.

Recent experiments by Coulter, Huguenard, and Prince (7,8,9) have shown that therapeutic concentrations of ESM reduce the low-threshold calcium current (LTCC) in thalamic neurons. Ethosuximide's blockade of the LTCC was highly voltage-dependent with larger reductions of LTCC observed at more hyperpolarized membrane potentials. Ethosuximide did not affect the gating properties of the channel; it either reduced the number of LTCC channels or the single channel conductance. Both dimethadione and phenobarbital reduced the LTCC but carbamazepine, phenytoin, and valproate had no effect at clinically relevant concentrations.

Fohlmeister, Aldelman, and Brennan (17) examined the effects of ESM and valproate on excitable Na^+ and K^+ channels in voltage-clamped squid giant axons. They reported that ESM applied to the external surface of the axon reduced Na^+ current in a voltage-independent manner, reduced maximal K^+ conductance, and slowed K^+ channel gating. Internally applied ESM slowed Na^+ and K^+ channel gating and reduced the peak conductance of the Na^+ channel in a voltage-dependent fashion. The significance of these observations in invertebrate neurons as related to the anticonvulsant mechanism of ESM is unclear because of both the species difference and the heroic concentrations of ESM used (60 mM). Others have reported that ESM was unable to inhibit ^2H-batrachotoxinin A 20-α-benzoate binding to sodium channels and batrachotoxinin-induced Na^+ flux in neuroblastoma cells and rat brain synaptosomes at concentrations up to 1 mM (63,64). This data suggests that the sodium channel is not the site of anticonvulsant action.

Neurotransmitter Processes

A relationship between ESM and GABA has been suggested by several studies (31,33). Because anticonvulsants such as valproate, phenobarbital, and benzodiazepines potentiate GABA function, several laboratories have recently examined the possibility that ESM may modify GABAergic neurotransmission. These studies revealed that the anticonvulsant decreased GABA responses in cultured cortical and spinal cord neurons (2,39). Barnes and Dichter (2) report that 500 μM ESM decreased the mean GABA response by 30%. The GABA receptor-chloride ionophore complex contains at least three distinct binding sites: the GABA site, the benzodiazepine site, and the picrotoxin site. In radioligand binding studies, ESM has no effect on diazepam and GABA binding to rat brain membranes at concentrations below 1 mM (52). At higher concentrations ESM substantially inhibited GABA, but not benzodiazepine binding (Holland and Ferrendelli, *unpublished*). In contrast, the binding of ^{35}S-*t*-butylbicyclophosphorothionate (TBPS), the radioligand used to study the picrotoxin receptor, is decreased competively at concentrations comparable to those used by Barnes and Dichter (47, Holland and Ferrendelli, *unpublished*). This suggests that ESM-induced antagonism of GABA responses is due to its action at the picrotoxin site and also implies that the anticonvulsant actions of ESM are not mediated by a postsynaptic enhancement of GABA responses.

Several laboratories have demonstrated that γ-hydroxybutyrate produces seizures in experimental animals. These seizures resemble human absence seizures behaviorally, electrically, and pharmacologically (24,53,54,55). Although the mechanism by which γ-hydroxybutyrate produces seizures remains obscure, specific high affinity γ-hydroxybutyrate binding sites associated with the GABA-mediated chloride ionophore have been identified (56,57) and it has been established that γ-hydroxybutyrate is capable of blocking flow through dopaminergic neurotransmitter systems (48). Ethosuximide is highly effective in preventing γ-hydroxybutyrate–induced seizures. However, ESM is not able to compete with ^{3}H-γ-hydroxybutyrate for binding to rat brain (56). This suggests that the anti–γ-hydroxybutyrate and antiabsence effects of this drug are not due to direct action at the putative γ-hydroxybutyrate binding site. Ethosuximide inhibits depolarization-evoked release of γ-hydroxybutyrate from hippocampal slices (60). Although this may explain the rise in brain γ-hydroxybutyrate concentration following single-dose ESM administration, this cannot account for the ability of ESM to block seizures produced by exogenously supplied γ-hydroxybutyrate.

We have reported that fluphenazine, a dopamine receptor antagonist, or α-methylparatyrosine, an inhibitor of dopamine synthesis, can block the protective effects of ESM in the γ-hydroxybutyrate seizure model (32). This indicates that the anticonvulsant action of ESM, at least in the γ-hydroxybutyrate model, may be related to some effect on dopaminergic neurotransmission, possibly via augmentation of dopamine-mediated inhibition in the central nervous system. The finding that the augmentation of dopaminergic processes prevents three types of seizures that are also blocked by ESM supports this idea. First, L-DOPA, a dopamine precursor, prevents cobalt-induced seizures which are also prevented by ESM (50). Second, cortical spikes produced by the topical application of penicillin are prevented by systemic L-DOPA and by topical dopamine but not by topical norepinephrine (34). As mentioned earlier, ESM prevents seizures produced by systemic administration of penicillin (26). Finally, dopamine receptor agonists decrease the duration of spike-wave discharges in rats with spontaneous absence-like seizures (61). Ethosuximide is also able to abolish seizures in this form of epilepsy (41). However, these results must be interpreted cautiously because at the present time, ESM has not been shown to directly alter dopamine-mediated processes either *in vivo* or *in vitro*.

The role of excitatory amino acids in the pathogenesis of epilepsy is now the subject of intense research. Although the relationship between ESM and excitatory amino acids has yet to be fully investigated, there is some evidence that suggests ESM does not work by a blockade of these processes. Ethosuximide does not prevent seizures induced by either kainic acid or N-methyl-D-aspartate, but nonspecific excitatory amino acid antagonists are very potent blockers of these seizure types (6,11). In addition, the anticonvulsant profiles of ESM and certain excitatory amino acid antagonists differ substantially. This data is certainly not conclusive but does suggest that ESM does not alter excitatory amino acid function, at least via postsynaptic mechanisms.

There is some evidence to suggest that ESM can presynaptically modulate neurotransmitter release. Čapek and Esplin found that ESM accentuated the decline of spinal cord monosynaptic response amplitude evoked by repetitive stimuli, but did not depress synaptic transmission evoked by a single stimulus (4). They suggest that this effect was due to an increased fraction of neurotransmitter release per volley and as a result, ESM partially depletes presynaptic neurotransmitter stores. In addition, Pincus (46) found that ESM augments transmitter release in the frog neuromuscular junction, possibly by increasing Ca^{++} flux into the presynaptic terminal. Unfortunately the molecular mechanisms underlying these observations are unclear. As mentioned earlier, ESM did not affect the release of GABA, aspartate, or glutamate *in vitro*, nor did ESM alter Ca^{++} flux into synaptosomes at concentrations used by Pincus

(10,58). Thus, the relationship between these observations and the antiabsence effects of ESM is unclear.

CELLULAR ACTIONS

The observations of Pincus (46) and Čapek and Esplin (4) show that *in vivo* effects of ESM do not necessarily correspond to what is found *in vitro*. This phenomenon is also apparent in studies of the effect of ESM on repetitive firing of neurons. In cultured neurons ESM has no effect on the repetitive firing of action potentials (39); however, *in vivo* ESM is able to depress specific types of repetitive activation. Ethosuximide significantly reduces PTZ-induced photic recruitment and photic after-discharges and completely suppresses PTZ-induced spindle activity (62). These rhythmic activities are thought to be an expression of synchronous after-discharges of the thalamocortical system.

It was suggested that the effect of ESM was mediated by either direct influences on inhibitory cells in the thalamic relay or by actions on ascending reticular activation. The lateral geniculate body has been discounted as the site of action because injections of ESM into the lateral geniculate could not abolish these photic after-discharges (30). The effects of anticonvulsants on thalamocortical excitability have been examined by recording the cortical response elicited by a pair of stimuli given to the ventral lateral thalamus (14,15,45). These reports show that phenytoin, carbamazepine, and diazepam depressed evoked responses at all frequencies, and ESM and valproate decreased evoked responses at 3 Hz. This provides a basis for the effectiveness of ESM and valproate in controlling absence seizures characterized by 3 Hz spike-and-wave activity.

Fromm and co-workers have shown that antiabsence drugs preferentially depress central nervous system inhibitory pathways that require considerable repetitive stimulation for activation (18,19,20,51). They suggest that this could account for the therapeutic specificity of ESM because they believe absence seizures involve paroxysmal activity in inhibitory pathways (15,20). If this is the case, the observation that GABA responses are reduced by ESM could provide a basis for the antiabsence properties of this drug. However, this theory cannot account for the ability of ESM to protect animals from seizures caused by picrotoxin, whose convulsant actions are thought to be due to its ability to noncompetitively antagonize GABA-mediated inhibition.

NEURAL SYSTEMS EFFECTS

It has become increasingly clear that subcortical brain regions play a crucial role in the propagation of generalized seizures. An important characteristic of anticonvulsant compounds is their ability to depress repetitive impulses in the reticular core. Antiabsence drugs such as ESM have been shown to depress descending reticular inhibitory pathways (20). In addition, we have shown a selective enrichment of ^{14}C-2-deoxyglucose incorporation into the mammillary bodies and their connections during ESM-induced suppression of PTZ seizures (42). This may represent a unique neurosystem of ESM that is important for its anti-PTZ, and perhaps antiabsence activity. However, these observations do not clearly establish the functional anatomy of ESM action and much additional research on this question is needed.

POSSIBLE MECHANISMS OF ACTION OF ESM

Any complete description of the mechanisms of action of an antiepileptic drug would require a full understanding of the pathophysiological mechanisms of epilepsy and an explanation of how the drug modifies these to prevent seizures. Since the patho-physiological mechanisms of epilepsy are still incompletely understood, one can only speculate about the mechanisms of action of most antiepileptic drugs.

We suggest that a drug may produce an anticonvulsant effect by two general mechanisms: (a) direct modification of membrane function in excitable cells, and/or (b) alteration of chemically mediated neurotransmission.

There is no evidence that ESM indirectly and nonspecifically alters membrane structure, thereby disrupting ionic channels. It is highly water soluble, so it is unlikely that much of it inserts into cellular membranes that have a high lipid content. Furthermore, it has none of the properties of general anesthetics which are thought to exert their effects by a direct action on cellular membranes. The observation that ESM inhibits (Na^+, K^+)-ATPase activity in plasma membranes *in vitro* does not explain its antiepileptic effects. On the contrary, inhibition of the sodium pump would cause accumulation of intracellular sodium, make the membrane potential more positive, increase excitability, and thus perhaps produce seizures rather than prevent them. There is also no data indicating that ESM has any effect on Cl^-, K^+, or Na^+ conductances at therapeutic concentrations.

Coulter and his colleagues (7,8,9) have proposed that the antiabsence properties of ESM are a result of its ability to reduce LTCC in thalamic neurons. The observation that ESM depresses thalamocortical excitability supports this hypothesis because LTCC is believed to play an important role in the generation of thalamocortical rhythms. However, several questions remain unanswered. Phenobarbital, which does not consistently prevent absence seizures, also inhibits the thalamic LTCC. Also, valproate which has antiabsence properties, does not significantly inhibit the thalamic LTCC. Finally, LTCC is blocked

by ESM in only a portion of thalamic neurons with this channel. Thus, although these observations are promising, more research on the role of the LTCC in absence seizures and the effect of ESM on this current is necessary.

If further studies indicate that the antiepileptic effect of ESM is not fully explained by its action on the low-threshold calcium current, then its effect may be explained as a result of some effect on neurotransmission. There is indirect evidence to indicate that it may deplete excitatory neurotransmitter stores mediating the spinal monosynaptic reflex. This is thought to occur by an increase in fractional release per stimulus without resultant increase in synthesis. Although a similar effect in brain might selectively depress repetitive impulses, thereby preventing seizures, it is not likely because the increased release of excitatory neurotransmitters on initial impulses might be enough to potentiate seizure activity. In addition, direct measurements of neurotransmitters indicate that in many systems, synthesis can more than compensate for increased release even at the highest firing rates attainable. A more tenable explanation is that ESM may increase the influence of inhibitory neurotransmitters. The fact that ESM causes depression of cerebral metabolic rate is consistent with this idea. Also, the suggested depressant effects of ESM on corticofugal inhibition of the spinal trigeminal nucleus may well be a result of some action on neuronal pathways subserved by inhibitory neurotransmitters. Present evidence suggests that ESM does not significantly effect GABA-mediated inhibitory processes. Possibly the anticonvulsant effect of ESM may involve dopamine-mediated neurotransmission, but this is uncertain. Other still unidentified, inhibitory neurotransmitter systems may also be responsible for or have a role in ESM mechanisms of action.

REFERENCES

1. Adler, M. W. (1972): The effect of single and multiple lesions of limbic system on cerebral excitability. *Psychopharmacologia*, 24:218–230.
2. Barnes, D. M., and Dichter, M. A. (1984): Effects of ethosuximide and tetramethylsuccinimide on cultured cortical neurons. *Neurology*, 34:620–625.
3. Browne, T. R., Dreifuss, F. E., Dyken, P. R., Goode, D. J., Penry, J. K., Porter, R. J., White, B. G., and White, P. T. (1975): Ethosuximide in the treatment of absence (petit mal) seizures. *Neurology*, 25:515–524.
4. Čapek, R., and Esplin, B. (1977): Effects of ethosuximide on transmission of repetitive impulses and apparent rates of transmitter turnover in the spinal cord monosynaptic pathway. *J. Pharmacol. Exp. Ther.*, 201:320–325.
5. Chen, A., Weston, J. K., and Bratton, A. C., Jr. (1963): Anticonvulsant activity and ethosuximide. *Epilepsia*, 4:66–76.
6. Clifford, D. B., Lothman, E. W., Dodson, W. E., and Ferrendelli, J. A. (1982): Effect of anticonvulsant drugs on kainic acid-induced epileptiform activity. *Exp. Neurol.*, 76:156–167.
7. Coulter, D. A., Huguenard, J. R., and Price, D. A. (1988): Anticonvulsants depress calcium spikes and calcium currents of mammalian thalamic neurons *in vitro*. *Soc. Neurosci. Abstr.*, 14:644.
8. Coulter, D. A., Huguenard, J. R., and Price, D. A. (1989): Characterization of ethosuximide reduction of low-threshold calcium current in thalamic neurons. *Ann. Neurol. (in press)*.
9. Coulter, D. A., Huguenard, J. R., and Price, D. A. (1989): Specific petit mal anticonvulsants reduce calcium currents in thalamic neurons. *Neurosci. Lett. (in press)*.
10. Crowder, J. M., and Bradford, H. F. (1987): Common anticonvulsants inhibit Ca^{2+} uptake and amino acid neurotransmitter release *in vitro*. *Epilepsia*, 28:378–382.
11. Czuczwar, S. J., Frey, H.-H., and Löscher, W. (1986): *N*-Methyl-D,L-aspartic acid–induced convulsions in mice and their blockade by antiepileptic drugs and other agents. In: *Neurotransmitters, Seizures, and Epilepsy III*, edited by G. Nishicó, P. L. Morselli, K. G. Lloyd, R. G. Fariello, and J. Engel, Jr., pp. 235–246. Raven Press, New York.
12. Davis, H. L., Johnson, D. D., and Crawford, R. D. (1978): Epileptiform seizures in domestic fowl. IX. Implications of the absence of anticonvulsant activity on ethosuximide in a pharmacological model of epilepsy. *Can. J. Physiol. Pharmacol.*, 56:893–896.
13. Dow, R. C., Forfar, J. C., and McQueen, J. K. (1973): The effects of some anticonvulsant activity on cobalt-induced epilepsy. *Epilepsia*, 14:203–212.
14. Englander, R. N., Johnson, R. N., Brickley, J. J., and Hanna, G. R. (1977): Effects of antiepileptic drugs on thalamocortical excitability. *Neurology*, 27:1134–1139.
15. Englander, R. N., Johnson, R. N., and Hanna, G. R. (1977): Ethosuximide and bicuculline inhibition in petit mal epilepsyy. *Neurol. Neurochir. Psychiatr.*, 18:265–275.
16. Erwin, V. G., and Deitrich, R. A. (1973): Inhibition of bovine brain aldehyde reductase by anticonvulsant compounds. *Biochem. Pharmacol.*, 2:2615–2624.
17. Fohlmeister, J. F., Adelman, W. J., and Brennan, J. J. (1984): Excitable channel currents and gating times in the presence of anticonvulsants ethosuximide and valproate. *J. Pharmacol. Exp. Ther.*, 230:75–81.
18. Fromm, G. H., Glass, J. D., Chattha, A. S., and Martinez, A. J. (1981): Effect of anticonvulsant drugs on inhibitory and excitatory pathways. *Epilepsia*, 22:65–73.
19. Fromm, G. H., Glass, J. D., Chattha, A. S., Martinez, A. J., and Silverman, M. (1980): Antiabsence drugs and inhibitory pathways. *Neurology*, 30:126–131.
20. Fromm, G. H., and Terrence, C. F. (1987): Effect of antiepileptic drugs on the brainstem. In: *Epilepsy and the Reticular Formation: The Role of the Reticular Core in Convulsive Seizures*, edited by G. H. Fromm, D. L. Faingold, R. A. Browning, and W. M. Burnham, pp. 119–136. Alan R. Liss, Inc., New York.
21. Gilbert, J. C., Buchan, P., and Scott, A. K. (1974): Effects of anticonvulsant drugs on monosaccharide transport and membrane ATPase activities of cerebral cortex. In: *Epilepsy*, edited by P. Harris and C. Mawdsley, pp. 98–104. Churchill Livingstone, Edinberg.
22. Gilbert, J. C., Scott, A. K., and Wyllie, M. G. (1974): Effects of ethosuximide on adenosine triphosphatase activities of some subcellular fractions prepared from rat cerebral cortex. *Br. J. Pharmacol.*, 50:452P–453P.
23. Gilbert, J. C., and Wyllie, M. G. (1974): The effects of the anticonvulsant ethosuximide on adenosine triphosphatase activities of synaptosomes prepared from rat cerebral cortex. *Br. J. Pharmacol.*, 52:139P–140P.
24. Godschalk, M., Dzoljíc, M. R., and Bonta, I. L. (1976): Antagonism of gamma-hydroxybutyrate–induced hypersynchronization in the ECoG of the rat by anti-petit mal drugs. *Neurosci. Lett.*, 3:145–150.
25. Gray, P., and Gilbert, J. C. (1970): Anticonvulsant drugs and xylose uptake by cerebral slices. *Biochem. J.*, 120:27P–28P.
26. Guberman, A. G., Gloor, P., and Sherwin, A. L. (1975): Response of generalized penicillin epilepsy in the cat to ethosuximide and diphenylhdantoin. *Neurology*, 25:758–764.
27. Gueldry, S., Rochette, L., and Bralet, J. (1987): Comparison of the effects of valproate, ethosuximide, phenytoin, and pentobarbital on cerebral energy metabolism in the rat. *Epilepsia*, 28:160–168.
28. Julien, R. M., Fowler, G. W., and Danielson, M.

G. (1975): The effect of antiepileptic drugs on estrogen-induced electrographic spike-wave discharges. *J. Pharmacol. Exp. Ther.*, 193:647–656.

29. Kastner, I., Klingberg, F., and Muller, M. (1970): Zur Wirkung des Ethosuximids auf die Kobalt-induzierte "Epilepsie" der Ratte. *Arch. Int. Pharmacodyn. Ther.*, 186:220–226.

30. Kastner, I., and Rougerie, A. (1978): Photisch ausgelöste potentialfolgen nach lokaler applikation von ethosuximid ins corpus geniculatum laterale. *Acta Biol. Med. Germ.*, 37:677–679.

31. Klunk, W. E., Covey, D. F., and Ferrendelli, J. A. (1982): Structure-activity relationships of alkyl substituted γ-butyrolactones and succinimides. *Mol. Pharmacol.*, 22:444–450.

32. Klunk, W. E., and Ferrendelli, J. A. (1980): Reversal of the anticonvulsant action of ethosuximide by drugs that diminish CNS dopaminergic neurotransmission. *Neurology*, 30:421.

33. Klunk, W. E., Kalman, B. L., Ferrendelli, J. A., and Covey, D. F. (1983): Computer-assisted modeling of the picrotoxinin and γ-butyrolactone receptor site. *Mol. Pharmacol.*, 23:511–518.

34. Kobayashi, K., Shirakabe, T., Kishikawa, H., and Mori, K. (1976): Catacholamine levels in penicillin-induced epileptic focus of the cat cerebral cortex. *Acta Neurochir. [Suppl]*, 23:93–100.

35. Leznicki, A., and Dymecki, J. (1974): The effect of certain anticonvulsants *in vitro* and *in vivo* on enzyme activities in rat brain. *Neurol. Neurochir. Pol.*, 24:413–419.

36. Lin-Mitchell, E., Chweh, A. Y., and Swinyard, E. A. (1986): Effect of ethosuximide alone and in combination with γ-aminobutyric acid receptor agonists on brain γ-aminobutyric acid concentration, anticonvulsant activity and neurotoxicity in mice. *J. Pharmacol. Exp. Ther.*, 237:486–489.

37. Lockard, J. S., Levy, R. H., Congdon, W. C., DuCharme, L. L., and Patel, I. H. (1977): Efficacy testing of valproic acid compared to ethosuximide in monkey model: II: Seizure, EEG, and diurnal variation. *Epilepsia*, 18:205–224.

38. Löscher, W., and Frey, H.-H. (1977): Effects of convulsant and anticonvulsant agents on level and metbolism of γ-aminobutyric acid in mouse brain. *Naunyn-Schmiedeberg's Arch. Pharmacol.*, 296:263–269.

39. McLean, M. J., and MacDonald, R. L. (1986): Sodium valproate, but not ethosuximide, produces use- and voltage-dependent limitation of high frequency repetitive firing of action potentials of mouse central neurons in cell culture. *J. Pharmacol. Exp. Ther.*, 237:1001–1011.

40. Meldrum, B. S., Horton, R. W., and Toseland, P. A. (1975): A primate model for testing anticonvulsant agents. *Mol. Pharmacol.*, 14:347–356.

41. Micheletti, G., Vergnes, M., Marescaux, C., Reis, J., Depaulis, A., Rumbach, L., and Wartar, J.-M. (1985): Antiepileptic drug evaluation in a new animal model: Spontaneous *petit mal* epilepsy in the rat. *Arzneimittel-Forsch./Drug Res.*, 35:473–475.

42. Mirski, M. A., and Ferrendelli, J. A. (1986): Selective metabolic activation of the mammillary bodies and their connections during ethosuximide-induced suppression of pentylenetetrazol seizures. *Epilepsia*, 27:194–203.

43. Narhorski, S. R. (1972): Biochemical effects of the anticonvulsants trimethadione, ethosuximide, and chlordiazepoxide in rat brain. *J. Neurochem.*, 19:1937–1946.

44. Norton, P. R. E. (1970): The effects of drugs on barbiturate withdrawal convulsions in the rat. *J. Pharm. Pharmacol.*, 22:763–766.

45. Nowack, W. J., Johnson, R. N., Englander, R. N., and Hanna, G. R. (1979): Effects of valproate and ethosuximide on thalamocortical excitability. *Neurology*, 29:96–99.

46. Pincus, J. H. (1977): Anticonvulsant actions at a neuromuscular synapse. *Neurology*, 27:374–375.

47. Pitkänen, A., Saano, V., Tuomisto, L., and Riekkinen, P. J. (1987): Effect of anticonvulsant drugs on (^{35}S)t-butylbicyclophosphorothionate binding *in vitro* and *ex vivo*. *Pharmacol. Toxicol.*, 61:103–106.

48. Roth, R. H., Walters, J. R., and Aghajanian, G. K. (1973): Effect of impulse flow on the release and synthesis of dopamine in the rat striatum. In: *Frontiers in Catacholamine Research*, edited by E. Udsin and S. H. Snyder, pp. 567–574. Pergamon Press, Oxford.

49. Schettini, A., and Wilder, B. J. (1974): Effects of anticonvulsant drugs on enflurane cortical dysrhythmias. *Anesth. Analg.*, 53:951–962.

50. Scuvee-Moreau, J., Lepot, M., Brotchi, J., Gerebtzott, M., and Dresse, A. (1977): Action of phenytoin, ethosuximide, and of the carbidopa-L-dopa association in semi-chronic cobalt-induced epilepsy in the rat. *Arch. Int. Pharmacodyn. Ther.*, 230:92–99.

51. Shibuya, T., Fromm, G. H., and Terrence, C. F. (1987): Differential effect of ethosuximide and of electrical stimulation on inhibitory and excitatory mechanisms. *Epilepsy Res.*, 1:35–39.

52. Skerritt, J. H., and Johnston, G. A. R. (1983): Interactions of some anesthetic, convulsant, and anticonvulsant drugs at GABA-benzodiazepine receptor-ionophore complexes in rat brain synaptosomal membranes. *Neurochem. Res.*, 8:1351–1362.

53. Snead, O. C. (1978): Gammahydroxybutyrate in the monkey: II. Effect of chronic oral anticonvulsant drugs. *Neurology*, 28:643–648.

54. Snead, O. C. (1978): Gammahydroxybutyrate in the monkey: III. Effect of intravenous anticonvulsant drugs. *Neurology*, 28:1173–1178.

55. Snead, O. C., Bearden, L. J., and Pergram, V. (1980): Effect of acute and chronic anticonvulsant administration on endogenous γ-hydroxybutyrate in rat brain. *Neuropharmacology*, 19:47–52.

56. Snead, O. C. and Liu, C.-C. (1984): Gamma-hydroxybutyric acid binding sites in rat and human brain synaptosomal membranes. *Biochem. Pharmacol.*, 33:2587–2590.

57. Snead, O. C., and Nichols, A. C. (1987): γ-Hydroxybutyric acid binding sites: Evidence for coupling to a chloride anion channel. *Neuropharmacology*, 26:1519–1523.

58. Sohn, R. S., and Ferrendelli, J. A. (1976): Anti-

convulsant drug mechanisms phenytoin, pheno-barbital, and ethosuximide and Ca^{++} flux in iso-lated presynaptic endings. *Arch. Neurol.*, 33:626–629.

59. Tabakoff, B., and von Wartburg, J. P. (1975): Sep-aration of aldehyde reductases and alcohol dehy-drogenase from brain by affinity chromatography: Metabolism of succinic semialdehyde and ethanol. *Biochem. Biophys. Res. Commun.*, 63:957–966.

60. Vayer, P., Charlie, B., Mandel, P., and Maitre, M. (1987): Effect of anticonvulsant drugs on γ-hy-droxybutyrate release from hippocampal slices: Inhibition by valproate and ethosuximide. *J. Neu-rochem.*, 49:1022–1024.

61. Warter, J.-M., Vergnes, M., Depaulis, A., Tran-chant, C., Rumbach, L., Michelletti, G., and Ma-rescaux, C. (1988): Effects of drugs affecting do-paminergic neurotransmission in rats with spontaneous *petit mal*-like seizures. *Neurophar-macology*, 27:269–274.

62. Wenzel, J., Krueger, E., and Mueller, M. (1971): Hemmung pentylenetetrazol-induzierter hyper-synchroner Aktivität im thalamokortikalen system durch ethosuximid. *Acta Biol. Med. Germ.*, 26:567–572.

63. Willow, M., and Catterall, W. A. (1982): Inhibition of binding of [^{3}H]batrachotoxinin A 20-α-benzoate to sodium channels by the anticonvulsant drugs diphenylhydantoin and carbamazepine. *Mol. Pharmacol.*, 22:627–635.

64. Willow, M., Kuenzel, E. A., and Catterall, W. A. (1984): Inhibition of voltage-sensitive sodium channels in neuroblastoma cells and synaptosomes by the anticonvulsant drugs diphenylhydantoin and carbamazepine. *Mol. Pharmacol.*, 25:228–234.

65. Winters, W. D., and Spooner, C. E. (1965): A neu-rophysiological comparison of gamma-hydroxy-butyrate with pentobarbital in cats. *Electroence-phalogr. Clin. Neurophysiol.*, 18:287–296.

Antiepileptic Drugs, Third Edition, edited by
R. Levy, R. Mattson, B. Meldrum,
J. K. Penry, and F. E. Dreifuss.
Raven Press, Ltd., New York © 1989.

47

Ethosuximide

Chemistry and Methods of Determination

Tsun Chang

Ethosuximide (Zarontin) is one of the substituted succinimides discovered in the Parke-Davis Laboratories in the early 1950s. Its clinical antiepileptic properties were first reported by Vossen (49) and Zimmerman and Burgmeister (52). Because of its excellent clinical efficacy and low incidence of side effects, ethosuximide still remains the drug of choice for children with typical absence seizures.

CHEMISTRY

Ethosuximide (Fig. 1), 2-ethyl-2-methyl-succinimide, is a white crystalline compound with an empirical formula $C_7H_{11}NO_2$ and molecular weight of 141.17. It has a melting point of 64° to 65°C, a partition coefficient of 9 (chloroform/water; pH 7), and a water solubility of 190 mg/ml. Owing to its low molecular weight and high volatility, special care must be exercised to prevent drug losses during evaporation of organic extracts for analytical work-up. Methods of chemical synthesis have been described by Miller and Long (29).

METHODS OF DETERMINATION

An ultraviolet spectrophotometric procedure was first used for measuring etho-suximide in biological fluids (14). The method lacked specificity and sensitivity, and was not suitable for clinical therapeutic drug monitoring. Subsequently, a thin-layer chromatographic technique was used in an attempt to impart some degree of specificity (48,51). Both of these methods were tedious and at best semiquantitative. With the advent of gas chromatography, high-performance liquid chromatography, and immunoassays, these early assays are no longer of interest.

Gas chromatography and high-performance liquid chromatography are currently the methods of choice for simultaneous determination and quantitation of several anticonvulsant drugs in a single sample (34), whereas immunoassays are suitable for the analysis of a single drug at a time.

Gas Chromatography

Gas chromatography (GC) has been the most widely used method for the quantitative measurement of ethosuximide in biological fluids. The early phases of GC assay development have been reviewed by Glazko and Dill (12) and Glazko (11). Table 1 summarizes chronologically the GC methods available.

In 1965, Dill et al. (8) described the first gas chromatographic assay, which used a

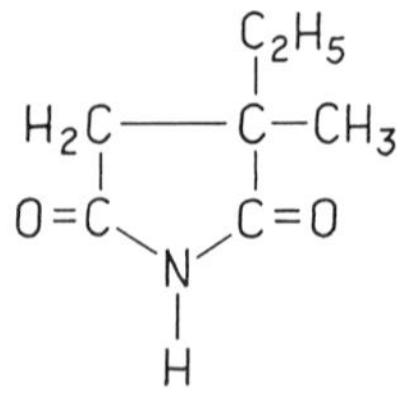

H₂C——C–CH₃ (with C₂H₅ above the central carbon)

O=C, C=O

N

H

FIG. 1. Chemical structure of ethosuximide.

close analog of ethosuximide, 2,2-dimethyl-3-methylsuccinimide, as the internal standard. Ethosuximide and the internal standard were extracted from biological samples by chloroform. A small amount of amyl acetate was added to the chloroform extract to prevent evaporation loss of the drug. A detailed description of the procedure, including a micro-method suitable for analysis of finger tip blood (0.2 ml) from pediatric patients, was given in the first edition of *Antiepileptic Drugs* (12). Development of this assay allowed, for the first time, definitive characterization of the pharmacokinetics of ethosuximide in animals and in man. Several modified versions of the original procedure were subsequently published by other investigators (5,9,15).

In the decade that followed, numerous GC assays were developed for the therapeutic drug monitoring of several anticonvulsant drugs simultaneously (4,26,36,47). Various steps and manipulations were devised to keep the methods simple, rapid, and adaptable to small sample sizes (10–100 μl). A modified extraction procedure used only 0.2 ml of chloroform to eliminate the need for solvent evaporation (46). Temperature programming was used to achieve separation of several underivatized anticonvulsant drugs (4,36). Ethosuximide was successfully assayed on highly polar column packings with excellent peak symmetry (3,16). A nitrogen selective detector was introduced to improve assay sensitivity (45).

Other investigators (7,17,24) developed assays for underivatized ethosuximide fol-

lowed by on-column methylation or silylaction to allow quantitation of other anticonvulsants at elevated column temperatures. The on-column flash methylation technique (40) was combined with temperature programming to determine multiple anticonvulsant drugs, including ethosuximide (41). The use of a new internal standard, 2-methyl-2-propylsuccinimide, was advocated for improved peak separation (42). Other alkylation methods (25,28) were subsequently used to circumvent several disadvantages of the on-column methylation procedure (i.e., need for high injection port temperature), and slow injection was used to reduce pyrolysis of the reagent. Despite these drawbacks, the on-column methylation approach has by far been the most widely used method.

Wallace et al. (50) derivatized ethosuximide and desmethylmethsuximide with pentafluorobenzoyl chloride, making it amendable for electron-capture detection. The internal standard proposed by Solow et al. (42) was used for ethosuximide. Between-day relative standard deviation was less than 4%.

Since 1980 very few new GC methods have been reported. Arranz-Pena (2) described a rapid isothermal GC method for the quantitation of five anticonvulsant drugs, including ethosuximide. Chromatographic separation was achieved on SP 2110/SP 2510 column at 110°C for ethosuximide and at 240°C for the other four drugs. With the introduction of valproate for clinical use, several methods were developed for the determination of ethosuximide and valproic acid. In the method of Kulpmann (22), valproic acid and ethosuximide were extracted from patient serum with chloroform and 2 μl of the extract was injected directly into the column without prior evaporation. Chromatographic separations were performed on a SP 1000 column under isothermal conditions. Between-day precision averaged 2.6% for ethosuximide. Other investigators (13,23,27,37) also reported the

TABLE 1. *Gas chromatographic assays for ethosuximide*

Reference	Year	Column packing	Derivatization	Detector	Internal standard	Other drugs
Dill (8)	1965	XE-60	No	FID[d]	DMS[g]	No
Buchanan (5)	1969	XE-60	No	FID	DMS	No
Solow (40)	1971	OV-17	Flash-methylation	FID	DMS	No
Solow (41)	1972	OV-17	Flash-methylation	FID	DMS	Yes
Van der Kleijn (46)	1973	OV-17	No	FID	Naphthalene	Yes
Harvey (15)	1973	XE-60/OV-17	No	FID	DMS	No
Cremers (7)	1973	OV-225	No	FID	Ethosuximide	Yes
Ritz (36)	1975	OV-225	No	FID	DMS	Yes
Toseland (45)	1975	Carbowax 20/TPA[a]	No	NPD[e]	Heptabarbital	Yes
Bonitati (4)	1976	OV-17	No	FID	Fluorene	Yes
Least (25)	1975	OV-1	N-butyl	FID	DMS	No
Heipertz (16)	1977	SP-1000	No	NPD	Mephenytoin	Yes
Hill (17)	1977	OV-225	No	FID	DMS	No
Menyharth (28)	1977	OV-101	N-butyl	NPD	DMS	No
Berry (3)	1978	OV-225	No	FID	Dimethyl phthalate	No
Solow (42)	1978	OV-17	Flash-methylation	FID	MPS[h]	No
Fellenberg (9)	1978	DGA/phosphoric acid	No	FID	DMS	No
Loscher (26)	1978	OV-17	No	FID	MPS	Yes
Wallace (50)	1979	OV-17	PFB[c]	EC[f]	MPS	Yes
Kumps (23)	1980	SP-1000	No	FID	DMS	Yes
Kulpmann (22)	1980	SP-1000	No	FID	DMS	Yes
Grgurinovich (13)	1980	Carbowax 20M/TPA	No	FID	Methsuximide	Yes
Arranz-Pena (2)	1981	SP 2110/SP 2150	No	FID	DMS	Yes
Manfredi (27)	1982	SP-1000	No	FID	DMS	Yes
Riva (33)	1982	DEGS[b]	No	FID	DMS	Yes

[a] TPA, terephthalic acid
[b] DEGS, diethylene glycol succinate
[c] PFB, pentafluorobenzoyl
[d] FID, flame ionization detector

[e] NPD, nitrogen-phosphorus detector
[f] EC, electron-capture
[g] DMS, 2,2-dimethyl-3-methylsuccinimide
[h] MPS, 2-methyl-2-propyl-succinimide

development of simple and rapid GC procedures for simultaneous determinations of these two drugs.

Gas Chromatography-Mass Spectrometry

Horning et al. (18,19) applied gas chromatography-mass spectrometry (GC-MS) to therapeutic drug monitoring of ethosuximide in patients' serum or saliva. Ethosuximide was converted to the trimethylsilyl derivative prior to analysis on a quadruple mass spectrometer operated in the chemical ionization mode. Quantitation was achieved by the selective ion monitoring technique.

High-Performance Liquid Chromatography

In the last decade, high-performance liquid chromatography (HPLC) has rapidly replaced GC as the preferred technique for anticonvulsant drug determinations in many clinical laboratories. The procedure offers several advantages over GC, including speed and versatility in choice of chromatographic variables, and usually does not require derivative formations. Most of the methods employed reversed-phase column and ultraviolet detection at wavelengths of 195 to 210 nm.

Early work by Adams and Vandemark (1) used an ODS-Sil XL reversed phase column and a solvent mixture of acetonitrile and water (17:83) to measure ethosuximide, phenobarbital, phenytoin, methosuximide, and carbamazepine in a single run. Phenacetin was used as internal standard. Comparison with GC results showed excellent agreement between the two methods. Soldin and Hill (39) described a rapid micromethod for ethosuximide and other anticonvulsant drugs. Serum samples were deproteinized with acetonitrile and an aliquot of the supernatant was injected directly into a μBondapack C_{18}-reversedphase column. Cyheptamide was added as internal standard. Chromatographic separations were achieved using a mobile phase of acetonitrile and pH 8 phosphate buffer (1:1). Kabra et al. (21) modified this procedure by using a pH 4 buffer and acetonitrile as mobile phase. In the method of Freeman and Rawal (10) ethosuximide and other antiepileptic drugs were determined using a methanolic mobile phase.

Christofides and Fry (6) described a reversed-phase ion-pair HPLC method for simultaneous determination of ethosuximide, ethylphenacemide, primidone, phenobarbital, carbamazepine, and phenytoin in serum. The drugs were extracted with ethylacetate at neutral pH. Heptabarbital was used as internal standard. Chromatographic separation was achieved on a SAS Hypersil column with a mobile phase of acetonitrile/tetrabutylammonium phosphate (2:8) at ambient temperature. The interday relative standard of deviation varied from 5.1% and 9.6% for ethosuximide concentrations of 200 to 400 μmole/ml.

Quattrone and Putnam (33) separated theophylline, acetaminophen, or ethosuximide on a μBondapack C_{18} column using mobile phases free of inorganic buffers to prolong the life of valves and fittings of the autoinjector.

Riedmann et al. (36) described a HPLC procedure for optimum resolution and analysis of eight antiepileptic drugs including ethosuximide. The influence of column temperature on resolution and analysis time was studied in detail. By this method 50 samples can be extracted and analyzed in a day.

Kabra et al. (20) reported a fast HPLC method for the analysis of ethosuximide along with four other anticonvulsant drugs using a liquid-solid extraction technique. The drugs in 200 μl of serum were eluted from a Bond-Elut cartridge with 300 μl of methanol. A 5 μl aliquot of the eluate was analyzed on a 3- or 5-micron reversedphase column with a mobile phase of acetonitrile/methanol/phosphate buffer (13.5:35:51.5) at a flow rate of 3 ml/min. The column was maintained at 50°C. The analysis run time was very short ranging from 1.4 min to 2.5 min for the 3- and 5-micron columns, respectively. The sensitivity of the method for all drugs was less than 1 μg/ml.

In another method described by Neels et al. (31) 30 μl of plasma containing ethosuximide and other anticonvulsant drugs was deproteinized with acetonitrile and the supernatant was injected directly onto a 5-micron Lichrosorb RP-18 reversed-phase column maintained at 50°C. The mobile phase consisted of acetonitrile/phosphate buffer, pH 6.9 (40/60). Total separation of five drugs and separation of active metabolites of two drugs was achieved in 12 min without sacrificing sensitivity and column life.

Immunoassays

The immunoassay technique is ideally suited for laboratories lacking expensive chromatographic equipment and the appropriate expertise, as all reagents are supplied in prepackaged kits. However, it should be noted that immunoassays are designed to measure a single drug, whereas chromatographic methods are capable of multiple drug determinations. Three commercially developed, nonisotopic immunoassays are currently available for routine clinical monitoring of blood ethosuximide levels. These include the EMIT system by Syva Company, the *aca* system by DuPont, and a fluorescence polarization immunoassay (FPIA) in the Abbott TDx system.

The EMIT system is currently the most widely used method. Its performance in ethosuximide assays has been extensively evaluated (30,38,43), and the results were found to be in good agreement with those obtained by GC procedures. Although the antibody used in the EMIT ethosuximide kit was been shown to be specific, Pippenger and Kutt (32) reported some crossreactivity with the desmethyl metabolite of methsuximide.

Recently Stewart and Bottorff (44) compared the performance of FPIA (TDx) for ethosuximide with EMIT and *aca*. The TDx assay produced within- and between-day coefficient variations of less than 5% at the low, medium, and high ranges of the calibration curve. Of the 100 ethosuximide serum and plasma samples analyzed, good correlations were found between the TDx and EMIT or *aca* assays. Values obtained by TDx were consistently lower than by *aca* or EMIT methods. The difference was attributed to the fact that antibody used in the TDx method is more specific and less likely to be subject to interference by metabolites. Despite these differences, all three immunoassays are deemed suitable for routine clinical use.

CONVERSION

Conversion factor:

$$CF = \frac{1000}{\text{mol. wt.}} = \frac{1000}{141.2} = 7.08$$

Conversion:

$$(\mu g/ml) \times 7.08 = (\mu moles/liter)$$

$$(\mu moles/liter) \div 7.08 = (\mu g/ml)$$

REFERENCES

1. Adams, R. F., and Vandemark, F. L. (1976): Simultaneous high-performance liquid chromatographic determination of some anticonvulsants in serum. *Clin. Chem.*, 22:25–31.
2. Arranz Pena, M. I. (1981); Rapid determination of anticonvulsant drugs by isothermal gas-liquid chromatography. *J. Chromatogr.*, 222:486–490.
3. Berry, D. J., and Clarke, L. A. (1978): Gas chromatographic analysis of ethosuximide (2-ethyl-2-methyl succinimide) in plasma at therapeutic concentrations. *J. Chromatogr.*, 150:537–541.
4. Bonitati, J. (1976): Gas chromatographic analysis for succinimide anticonvulsants in serum: Macro- and micro-scale methods. *Clin. Chem.*, 22:341–345.
5. Buchanan, R. A., Fernandez, L., and Kinkel, A. W. (1969): Absorption and elimination of ethosuximide in children. *J. Clin. Pharmacol.*, 9:393–398.
6. Christofides, J. A., and Fry, D. E. (1980): Measurement of anticonvulsants in serum by reversed-phase ion-pair liquid chromatography. *Clin. Chem.*, 26:499–501.
7. Cremers, H. M. H. G., and Verheesen, P. E. (1973): A rapid method for the estimation of anti-epileptic drugs in blood serum by gas-liquid chromatography. *Clin. Chim. Acta*, 48:413–420.
8. Dill, W. A., Peterson, L., Chang, T., and Glazko, A. J. (1965): Physiological disposition of a α-methyl-α-ethylsuccinimide (ethosuximide, Zarontin) in animals and in man. Abstract of Papers, 149th National Meeting, American Chemical Society, Detroit, Michigan, p. 30N. American Chemical Society, Washington.
9. Fellenberg, A. J., and Pollard, A. C. (1978): Gas-liquid chromatographic microdetermination of underivatized ethosuximide (alpha-ethyl-alpha-methyl succinimide) in plasma or serum. *Clin. Chem.*, 24:1821–1823.
10. Freeman, D. J., and Rawal, N. (1979): Serum anticonvulsant monitoring by liquid chromatography with a methanolic mobile phase. *Clin. Chem.*, 25:810–811.
11. Glazko, A. J. (1982): Ethosuximide: Chemistry and methods for determinations. In: *Antiepileptic Drugs*, 2nd edition, edited by D. M. Woodbury, J. K. Penry, and C. E. Pippenger, pp. 617–622. Raven Press, New York.
12. Glazko, A. J., and Dill, W. A. (1972): Ethosuximide: Chemistry and methods for determinations. In: *Antiepileptic Drugs*, 1st edition, edited by D. M. Woodbury, J. K. Penry, and R. P. Schmidt, pp. 413–415. Raven Press, New York.

13. Grgurinovich, N., and Miners, J. O. (1980): Simple rapid procedure for the determination of valproate and ethosuximide in plasma by gas-liquid chromatography. *J. Chromatogr.*, 182:237–240.

14. Hansen, S. E. (1963): Quantitative determination of ethosuximide. *Acta Pharmacol. Toxicol. (Kbh).*, 20:286–290.

15. Harvey, C. D., and Sherwin, A. L. (1979): Gas-liquid chromatographic quantitation of ethosuximide. In: *Antiepileptic Drugs: Quantitative Analysis and Interpretation*, edited by C. E. Pippenger, J. K. Penry, and H. Kutt, pp. 87–93, Raven Press, New York.

16. Heipertz, R., Pilz,H., and Eickhoff, K. (1977): Evaluation of a rapid gas-chromatographic method for the simultaneous quantitative determination of ethosuximide, phenylethylmalonediamide, carbamazepine, phenobarbital, primidone and diphenylhydantoin in human serum. *Clin. Chim. Acta*, 77:307–316.

17. Hill, R. E., and Latham, A. N. (1977): Simultaneous determination of anticonvulsant drugs by gas-liquid chromatography. *J. Chromatogr.*, 131:341–346.

18. Horning, M. G., Brown, L., Nowlin, J., Lertratanangkoon, K., Kellaway, P., and Zion, T. E. (1977): Use of saliva in therapeutic drug monitoring. *Clin. Chem.*, 23:157–164.

19. Horning, M. G., Lertratanangkoon, K. Nowlin, J., Stillwell, W. G., Zion, T. E., Kellaway, P., and Hill, R. M. (1974): Anticonvulsant drug monitoring by GC-MS-COM techniques. *J. Chromatogr. Sci.*, 12:630–635.

20. Kabra, P. M., Nelson, M. A., and Marton, L. J. (1983): Simultaneous very fast liquid-chromatographic analysis of ethosuximide, primidone, phenobarbital, phenytoin, and carbamazepine in serum. *Clin. Chem.*, 29:473–476.

21. Kabra, P. M., Stafford, B. E., and Marton, L. J. (1977): Simultaneous measurement of phenobarbital, phenytoin, primidone, ethosuximide and carbamazepine in serum by high-pressure liquid chromatography. *Clin. Chem.*, 23:1284–1288.

22. Kulpmann, W. R. (1980): Eine gaschromatographische methode zur gleichzeitigen bestimmung von ethosuximid und valproinat im serum. *J. Clin. Chem. Clin. Biochem.*, 18:339–344.

23. Kumps, A., and Mardens, Y. (1980): Simplified simultaneous determination of valproic acid and ethosuximide in serum by gas-liquid chromatography. *Clin. Chem.*, 26:1759.

24. Latham, A. N., and Varlow, G. (1976): Simultaneous quantitative gas-chromatographic analysis of ethosuximide, phenobarbitone, primidone and diphenylhydantoin. *Br. J. Clin. Pharmacol.*, 3:145–150.

25. Least, C. J., Johnson, G. F., and Solomon, H. M. (1975): A quantitative gas chromatography determination of ethosuximide based on *N*-butylation. *Clin. Chim. Acta*, 60:285–292.

26. Loscher, W., and Gobel, W. (1978): Consecutive gas chromatographic determination of phenytoin, phenobarbital, primidone, phenylethylmalonediamide, carbamazepine, trimethadione, dimetha-dione, ethosuximide, and valproate from the same serum specimen. *Epilepsia*, 19:463–473.

27. Manfredi, C., and Zinterhofer, L. (1982): Simplified gas chromatography of valproic acid and ethosuximide. *Clin. Chem.*, 28:246.

28. Menyharth, P., Lehane, D. P., and Levy, A. L. (1977): Rapid gas chromatographic method for the determination of ethosuximide in serum. *Clin. Chem.*, 23:1795–1796.

29. Miller, C. A., and Long, L. M. (1953): Anticonvulsants III. A study of *N*,alpha,beta-alkylsuccinimides. *J. Am. Chem. Soc.*, 75:373–375.

30. Mulkus, H., Dicesare, J. L., Meola, J. M., Pippenger, C. E., Ibanex, J., and Castro, A. (1978): Evaluation of EMIT methods for the determination of the five major antiepileptic drugs on an automated kinetic analyzer. *Clin. Biochem.*, 11:139–142.

31. Neels, N. M., Totte, J. A., Verkerk, R. M., Vlietinck, A. J., Scharpe, S. L. (1983): Simultaneous high performance liquid-chromatographic determination of carbamazepine, carbamazepine-10,11-epoxide, ethosuximide, phenobarbital, phenytoin, primidone and phenylethyl-malonediamide in plasma. *J. Clin. Chem. Clin. Biochem.*, 21:295–299.

32. Pippenger, C. E., and Kutt, H. (1978): Common errors in the analysis of antiepileptic drugs. In: *Antiepileptic Drugs: Quantitative Analysis and Interpretation*, edited by C. E. Pippenger, J. K. Penry, and H. Kutt, pp. 199–208. Raven Press, New York.

33. Quattrone, A. J., and Putnam, R. S. (1981): A single liquid-chromatographic procedure for therapeutic monitoring of theophylline, acetaminophen, or ethosuximide. *Clin. Chem.*, 27:129–132.

34. Riedel, E., Klocke, H., and Bayer, H. (1973): Separation of drugs by gas-liquid chromatography (GLC) and high-pressure liquid chromatography (HPLC). In: *Methods of Analysis of Anti-Epileptic Drugs*, edited by J. W. A. Meijer, H. Meinardi, C. Gardner-Thorpe, and E. van der Kleijn, pp. 194–197. Excerpta Medica, Amsterdam.

35. Riedmann, M., Rambeck, B., and Meijer, J. W. (1981): Quantitative simultaneous determination of eight common antiepileptic drugs and metabolites by liquid chromatograph. *Ther. Drug Monit.*, 3:397–413.

36. Ritz, D. P., and Warren, C. G., (1975): Single extraction of six commonly prescribed antiepileptic drugs. *Clin. Toxicol.*, 8:311–324.

37. Riva, R., Albani, F., and Baruzzi, A. (1982): Rapid and simple GLC determination of valproic acid and ethosuximide in plasma of epileptic patients. *J. Pharm. Sci.*, 71:110–111.

38. Schottelium, D. D. (1978): Homogeneous immunoassay system (EMIT) for quantitation of antiepileptic drugs in biological fluids. In: *Antiepileptic Drugs: Quantitative Analysis and Interpretation*, edited by C. E. Pippenger, J. K. Penry, and H. Kutt, pp. 95–108. Raven Press, New York.

39. Soldin, S. J., and Hill, J. G. (1976): Rapid micromethod for measuring anticonvulsant drugs in serum by high-performance liquid chromatography. *Clin. Chem.*, 22:856–859.

40. Solow, E. B., and Green, J. B. (1971): The determination of ethosuximide in serum by gas chromatograph. *Clin. Chem. Acta*, 33:87–90.

41. Solow, E. B., and Green, J. B. (1972): The simultaneous determination of multiple anticonvulsant drug levels by gas-liquid chromatography. *Neurology (Minneap.)*, 22:540–550.

42. Solow, E. B., Tupper, N. L., and Kenfield, C. P. (1978): An alternative internal standard for analysis of ethosuximide by on-column methylation and gas chromatography. *J. Anal. Toxicol.*, 2:39–40.

43. Sun, L., and Szafir, I. (1977): Comparison of enzyme immunoassay and gas chromatography for determination of carbamazepine and ethosuximide in human serum. *Clin. Chem.*, 23:1753–1756.

44. Stewart, C. F., and Bottorff, M. B. (1986): Fluorescence polarization immunoassay for ethosuximide evaluated and compared with two other immunoassay techniques. *Clin. Chem.*, 32:1781–1783.

45. Toseland, P. A., Albani, M., and Gauchei, F. D. (1975): Organic nitrogen-selective detector used in gas-liquid chromatographic determination of some anticonvulsant and barbiturate drugs in plasma and tissues. *Clin. Chem.*, 21:98–103.

46. Van der Kleijn, E., Collste, P., Norlander, B., Agurell, S., and Sjöqvist, F. (1973): Gas chromatographic determination of ethosuximide and phensuximide in plasma and urine of man. *J. Pharm. Pharmacol.*, 25:324–327.

47. Varma, R. (1978): Therapeutic monitoring of anticonvulsant drugs in psychiatric patients: Rapid, simultaneous gas-chromatographic determination of six commonly used anticonvulsants without interference from other drugs. *Biochem. Exp. Biol.*, 14:311–318.

48. Vedso, S., Rud, C., and Place, J. F. (1969): Determination of phenytoin in serum in the presence of barbiturates, sulthiame and ethosuximide by thin layer chromatography. *Scand. J. Clin. Lab Invest.*, 23:175–180.

49. Vossen, R. (1958): On the anticonvulsant effect of succinimides. *Dtsch. Med. Wochenschr.*, 83:1227–1230.

50. Wallace, J. E., Schwertner, H. A., Hamilton, H. E., and Shimek, E. L. (1979): Electron-capture gas-liquid chromatographic determination of ethosuximide and desmethylmethsuximide in plasma and serum. *Clin. Chem.*, 25:252–255.

51. Wechselberg, K., and Hubel, G., (1967): Zur resoption and verteilung von methyl-athyl-succinimid (MAS) im serum und liquor bei kindern. *Z. Kinderheilkd*, 100:10–19.

52. Zimmerman, F. T., and Burgmeister, B. B. (1958): A new drug for petit mal epilepsy, *Neurology (Minneap.)*, 8:769–775.

Antiepileptic Drugs, Third Edition, edited by
R. Levy, R. Mattson, B. Meldrum,
J. K. Penry, and F. E. Dreifuss.
Raven Press, Ltd., New York © 1989.

48

Ethosuximide

Absorption, Distribution, and Excretion

Tsun Chang

Early ethosuximide pharmacokinetic results reported by Hansen and Feldberg (14) and Wechselburg and Hübel (31) were at best tenuous due to the nonspecific nature of the analytical methods used. Development of specific chemical assays such as those described in Chapter 47 made it possible to characterize the pharmacokinetics of ethosuximide and permitted the determination of optimal plasma drug concentrations for seizure control without undue side effects (28,29,30). A complete understanding of the pharmacokinetics of ethosuximide is essential to the proper clinical use of this drug. To that end, the present chapter focuses primarily on the preclinical and clinical pharmacokinetics of ethosuximide based on data obtained from modern chromatographic or radiotracer techniques.

ABSORPTION

Single-Dose Studies

A number of clinical studies have shown that ethosuximide is rapidly absorbed, and is systemically available following oral administration. In the initial study by Dill et al. (8), three volunteers were given a single 1-g oral dose of ethosuximide. Peak plasma ethosuximide concentrations of 18 to 24 µg/ml were reached within 1 to 4 hr after drug

administration. Similar results in four healthy adult subjects receiving 0.5-g of ethosuximide were reported by Eadie et al. (9). The bioavailability and pharmacokinetics of ethosuximide capsules were compared relative to those of a syrup formulation in five institutionalized children (3). The syrup was found to be more rapidly absorbed than the capsule but both formulations demonstrated equivalent total absorption (Fig. 1). Peak plasma concentrations of 38 µg/ml occurred within 3 to 7 hr regardless of the formulations used.

The absolute oral bioavailability of ethosuximide in humans has not been determined because parenteral formulation for human use is not available. However, results in animal studies indicate that oral absorption of ethosuximide is nearly complete. The work by Patel et al. (22) showed that absolute oral bioavailability of ethosuximide syrup in monkeys was 93%, 97.5%, and 96.8% following 30, 50, and 90 mg/kg doses, respectively. Similarly, an oral bioavailability of 88% to 95% was reported in dogs by El Sayed et al. (10).

Multiple-Dose Studies

The first multiple dose clinical pharmacology study of ethosuximide was carried out at the Parke-Davis Laboratories (6).

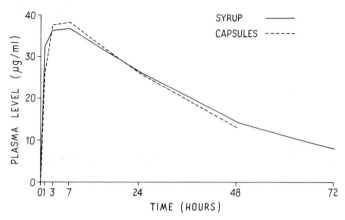

FIG. 1. Plasma ethosuximide levels in children receiving single 0.5-g doses of ethosuximide as capsules (dotted line) or syrup (solid line). (From Buchanan et al., ref. 3.)

Two groups of five healthy subjects each received 0.25-g or 0.5-g of ethosuximide twice daily for 28 days. Plasma concentrations measured 4 hr after the first dose were nearly proportional to dose. Steady-state plasma concentrations of 27 to 29 μg/ml were reached after 8 to 10 days of twice daily doses of 0.25-g. The high dose group (0.5 g BID) showed unacceptable side effects following 10 days of administration and the dose was subsequently reduced to 0.25-g two times daily.

In a subsequent trial, Buchanan et al. (5) administered a 0.5-g oral dose of ethosuximide once daily to healthy volunteers for 21 days, followed by an increased dose of 1-g once daily on days 22 through 28. The resulting mean plasma ethosuximide concentration-time profiles are given in Fig. 2. The 0.5-g once daily dose produced a mean steady-state plasma concentration of 34 μg/ml following approximately 9 days of dosing with a mean maximum-to-nadir variation of 8 μg/ml. The duration of the 1-g daily dose was too short to achieve steady-state levels.

The feasibility of once-daily dose administration was determined in nine children with absence seizures (4). Plasma concentrations resulting from a single daily dose were compared to concentrations after divided daily administration. Plasma concentrations during the single-dose phase peaked more rapidly and fell more quickly than during the divided-dose period, but mean concentrations remained in the therapeutic range. There was no difference in frequency of grand mal seizures between the dosage regimens. Goulet et al. (12) performed a similar study in 10 healthy volunteers with a 500-mg dose of ethosuximide given once daily for 14 days and in 10 additional subjects with a 250-mg dose given twice daily over the same period. Both groups then received a 750-mg daily dose or a 250-mg dose given three times daily. Absorption was rapid in both groups, and plasma ethosuximde concentrations were directly proportional to dose.

Haerer et al. (13) reported plasma concentration in 21 epileptic children and young adults (ages 4 to 27) using divided doses of 250 mg to 1 g of ethosuximide each day over a period of 1 month. The average daily dose was 20.7 ± 5.8 mg/kg and the plasma concentrations averaged 40 ± 14.9 μg/ml. Their data also suggested that once-daily administration should be possible. Browne et al. (2) demonstrated that a statistically significant relationship existed between dosage and plasma ethosuximide

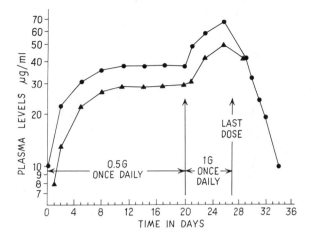

FIG. 2. Plasma ethosuximide levels in normal human subjects receiving 0.5-g doses once daily for 21 days, followed by 1-g once daily for an additional 7 days. Blood samples were taken before the daily morning dose (▲), and again 4 hr after dosing (●). (From Chang et al., ref. 6.)

concentrations in children with absence seizures. The rise in plasma concentrations with increasing dosage was lower in children under 10 years of age than in older children. Sherwin (29) confirmed the observation of Browne et al. (2) regarding the dosage versus plasma concentration relationship in children of different age groups.

DISTRIBUTION

Protein Binding

Ethosuximide is only minimally bound to plasma protein, as determined by chromatography on a Sephadex column (6) and equilibrium dialysis (10,27). El Sayed et al. (10) showed that ethosuximide binding to dog and rat serum proteins was approximately 8% to 9% at concentrations of 10 to 20 μg/ml and decreased to less than 2% at a higher concentration (74 μg/ml). The reported plasma to cerebrospinal fluid (CSF) (10) and plasma to saliva (16) ratio of near unity further suggests that most of the drug present in plasma is in the unbound form.

Tissue Distribution

Ethosuximide is uniformly distributed throughout the body. Dill et al. (8) showed

that ethosuximide was evenly distributed in rat tissues with concentrations nearly identical to those in plasma, except for body fat, which contained lower concentrations (Table 1). Similar results were found by Chang et al. (6) using radio-labeled ethosuximide. The analytical data are given in Table 2. Kidney radioactivity concentrations were highest owing to the presence of high levels of radioactivity in urine. Spleen, lung, and liver ^{14}C concentrations were significantly lower, and other tissues were slightly below this level. Concentrations of ethosuximide in body fat were much lower

TABLE 1. *Plasma and tissue levels of ethosuximide in rats*

| | Ethosuximide levels (μg/g) Time after dosing | |
Tissue	1 hr	2 hr
Plasma	99	65
Liver	99	72
Spleen	81	62
Kidney	100	68
Lung	87	62
Heart	97	68
Muscle	82	62
Brain	94	67
Fat	29	23

100 mg/kg peroral dose; GLC assay.

TABLE 2. *Distribution of ^{14}C-ethosuximide in rat tissues*

Tissue	Control (no drug)	3 days[a]	5 days	7 days	9 days	11 days
Kidney	0	346	34.7	0.9	1.0	0.8
Spleen	0	217	–	0.5	–	0.2
Lung	0	209	–	1.0	–	0.4
Liver	0	197	5.3	1.0	0.6	0.7
Plasma	0	163	3.4	0.4	0.1	0.1
Brain	0	158	–	0.4	–	0.2
Testes	0	142	–	0.4	–	0.1
Heart	0	140	–	0.5	–	0.5
Red cells	0	137	4.5	1.6	1.4	1.7
Pancreas	0	134	–	0.4	–	0.2
Muscle	0	124	–	0.4	–	0.3
Body fat	0	43	–	0.1	–	<0.1

[a] 3 days after start of dosing = 24 hr after last dose.
Animals were dosed perorally with 300 mg/kg ^{14}C-ethosuximide once daily for a total of three doses (0–24–48 hr); single animals were sacrificed at intervals indicated after start of dosing, and tissues were assayed for total ^{14}C activity. Assays reported as μg ethosuximide-equivalents per g tissue or per ml of plasma or red cells.

than in other tissues. It should be noted that radioactivity concentrations reported in this study represented a composite of unchanged drug and its metabolites.

Ethosuximide readily penetrates the blood-brain barrier. El Sayed et al. (10) reported a CSF entry half-life of 4 to 5 min in dogs, and equilibrium was reached in 20 to 30 min, resulting in identical serum and CSF concentrations. Similar findings were also reported in patients following repeated drug administration (27). The mean plasma-to-CSF ratio was 1.01 ± 0.15. Furthermore, CSF concentrations paralleled those in plasma, indicating that plasma concentrations provide a good index of central nervous system drug concentrations.

In the initial study by Dill et al. (8), the whole brain-to-plasma concentration ratio was shown to be near unity. Subsequent investigation by Patel et al. (24) on the distribution of ethosuximide in four discrete areas of rat brain supported the early results. These authors reported that mean brain-to-plasma ratios were 0.917, 0.942, 0.902, and 0.903 for cortex, midbrain, cerebellum, and pons-medulla, respectively.

The distribution ratio was independent of dose and plasma concentration.

Volume of Distribution

In accord with its uniform distribution in body tissues, the apparent volume of distribution of ethosuximide is approximately 70% of body weight, 0.69 liter/kg in children under 10 years of age (3) and 0.62 to 0.67 liter/kg in adults (9). Volume of distribution following intravenous doses ranged from 57% to 71% of body weight in dogs (10). Similarly, values of 0.79 to 0.82 liter/kg were reported in monkeys (22).

Placental Transfer and Secretion into Milk, Saliva, and Tears

Placental transfer of ethosuximide was first demonstrated by Chang et al. (6) in rats fed a drug diet admixture. Concentrations of ethosuximide in fetus and fetal liver and kidney were very close to those found in maternal tissues. Horning et al. (17) provided evidence of placental transfer of unchanged ethosuximide and its metabolites in the urine of a newborn infant. Koup et al. (18) studied ethosuximide concentrations in a pregnant patient near term who was maintained on daily doses of ethosuximide. Plasma concentrations of 40 to 50 μg/ml were measured before delivery and rose to 60 to 70 μg/ml after delivery. The cord blood ethosuximide concentration at birth was 61.9 μg/ml, providing additional evidence for placental transfer. A similar rise in maternal plasma ethosuximide concentration was reported by Rane and Tunell (26).

In the same study by Koup et al. (18), the ethosuximide concentration in breast milk was found to be approximately 94% of plasma concentrations, confirming earlier observations of Hill et al. (15). The authors estimated that the infant would receive a total daily ethosuximide dose of 12.8 to 38.4 mg from the mother's milk. Rane and Tunell (26) and Kuhnz et al. (19) also showed that an average milk-to-plasma concentration ratio of 0.8 to 0.86 persisted in nursing mothers. The nursed infants maintained serum levels between 15 and 40 μg/ml (19).

The concentration of ethosuximide in saliva was found to be equal to that in plasma (16,20,25). Furthermore, in tears collected from epileptic subjects, the tear-to-plasma ethosuximide concentration ratio was not significantly different from the saliva-to-plama ratio (25). Thus, determination of saliva or tear concentrations of ethosuximide provide a convenient, noninvasive method for therapeutic drug monitoring.

ELIMINATION AND EXCRETION

Half-Life

Ethosuximide is cleared slowly from the body, resulting in a long elimination half-life, which is also shown to be age dependent. In healthy adults, an apparent half-life of 60 hr was first reported by Dill et al. (8). This was confirmed later by other investigators who reported mean values of 53 hr (5) to 56 hr (9) in the same population, with wide variability between individual subjects. The elimination half-life of ethosuximide appears to be unaffected by dose size (5), and is constant with repeated dosing (4). Total body clearance in adult subjects averaged 0.01 ± 0.04 liters/kg/hr (9), considerably lower than the hepatic plasma flow of 0.9 liter/kg/hr, indicating that drug clearance is not blood-flow limited. Bachmann et al. (1) devised a method permitting estimation of ethosuximide clearance using a single blood or saliva sample. In healthy adult subjects, the clearance values calculated from single 120-hr serum and saliva samples were 0.0091 and 0.0089 liter/kg/hr, respectively.

In children ethosuximide is eliminated more rapidly than in adults. A mean half-life of 30 hr was found in five children ranging in age from 6 years, 11 months to 8 years, 7 months (3). In a more detailed study of children, aged 5 to 15 years, with absence seizures, ethosuximide half-life ranged from 15 to 68 hr, with a mean of 36 to 39 hr. There was no signficant change in half-life between the first dose and the eighth week of dosing, and there was no difference attributable to age. Koup et al. (18) reported a half-life of 41.3 hr in a neonate, and Kuhnz et al. (19) documented half-life of 32, 37, and 38 hr in three neonates.

The slow rate of elimination of ethosuximide must be taken into consideration in managing acute massive overdose and in cases of dose reduction to alleviate adverse effects. Considerable time is required before the drug is cleared from the body or reaches lower steady-state levels.

In laboratory animals, ethosuximide elimination half-life varies: 1 hr in mice, 10 to 12 hr in rats (6), 11 to 25 hr in dogs (10), and 22 to 30 hr in monkeys (6,22).

Excretion

Ethosuximide is eliminated primarily by metabolism with subsequent excretion of the metabolites in urine. Urinary excretion of unchanged drug in humans accounts for approximately 18% to 19% of the dose (3,5). Using an assay procedure for measuring urinary excretion of the major metabolite of ethosuximide, metabolite II (2-[1-hydroxy ethyl]-2-methyl-succinimidel), Glazko (11) showed that peak excretion rates for unchanged drug occurred in the first 12 hr after dosing, but the excretion rate for the metabolite was greatest in the 24- to 48-hr period (Fig. 3). This is consistent with the slow elimination of ethosuximide and the long elimination half-life. The combined recovery of unchanged ethosuximide and metabolite II accounted for 50% to 76% of the dose. Similar excretion patterns were observed in a study comparing a single dose with a divided daily dose (12). The total recovery, ethosuximide plus metabolite II, accounted for as much as 80% of the dose.

Mass balance studies in laboratory animals with ^{14}C-labeled ethosuximide (6) showed that in rhesus monkeys 77% of a single intraperitoneal dose was recovered as total radioactivity in urine and 1.5% in feces. In rats, 80% to 88% of single oral and intraperitoneal doses was excreted in urine and less than 4% in feces.

PHARMACOKINETIC MODELING

The pharmacokinetics of ethosuximide have been characterized in humans after oral dosing, and in animals following both intravenous and oral routes of administration. The elimination of ethosuximide from systemic circulation follows first order kinetics.

In children, the plasma ethosuximide concentration–time profile of the individual subjects following single oral doses of capsule or syrup formulations was best fitted to a one-compartment model with first-order input (3). The absorption rate constant ranged from 0.73 to 2.85 hr.$^{-1}$ and elimination half-life varied from 24.8 to 41.7 hr. Colburn and Gibaldi (7) computer fitted to a one-compartment model the data from Goulet et al. (12) on repetitive single and divided daily oral doses, and the pharmacokinetic parameters (elimination rate constant, excretion rate constant, and apparent volume of distribution) were similar for the two dosing regimens. The results of the

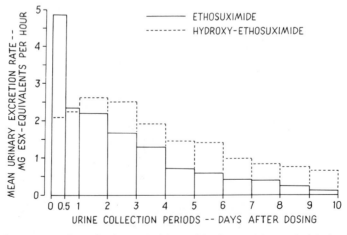

FIG. 3. Mean urinary excretion of ethosuximide and hydroxy-ethosuximide in six normal adult males receiving 1-g oral doses of ethosuximide. (From Glazko, ref. 11.)

study supported the conclusion of Goulet et al. (12) that the use of a single daily dose may be an effective regimen.

After single intravenous and oral doses, the pharmacokinetic profiles of ethosuximide in monkeys and dogs were best described by a one-compartment model with first order elimination for intravenous kinetics and a one-compartment model with first-order absorption for oral kinetics (10,22). In the monkey study (22), a close agreement between experimental data and least squares fitted lines was observed at all three dose levels studied (30, 60, and 90 mg/kg), indicating the appropriateness of the model. Volume of distribution, total body clearance, and elimination half-life were independent of dose.

Patel et al. (21) studied the repetitive dose pharmacokinetics of ethosuximide in monkeys using three dosing regimens: constant rate intravenous infusion, infusion at three consecutive rates with priming doses, and oral multiple dosing at two levels with priming doses. Infusion rates and priming doses were calculated based on single dose pharmacokinetic data. Experimental- and model-predicted plasma and urine data were in good agreement for all three dosing schemes. Total body clearance and elimination half-life were similar for single- and multiple-dose data. The authors concluded that single-dose pharmacokinetic parameters could be used to predict multiple-dosing schedules, suggesting that the pharmacokinetics of ethosuximide are linear. Subsequent work by Patel et al. (23) demonstrated a circadian rhythm in rhesus monkeys with higher steady-state ethosuximide levels in the morning than in the evening.

REFERENCES

1. Bachmann, K., Schwartz, J., Sullivan, T., and Jauregui, L. (1986): Single sample estimates of ethosuximide clearance. *Int. J. Clin. Pharmacol. Ther. Toxicol.*, 24:546–550.
2. Browne, T. R., Dreifuss, F. E., Dyken, P. R.,
   Goode, D. J., Penry, J. K., Porter, R. J., White, B. G., and White, P. T. (1975): Ethosuximide in the treatment of absence (petit mal) seizures. *Neurology (Minneap.)* 25:515–524.
3. Buchanan, R. A., Fernandez, L., and Kinkel, A. W. (1969): Absorption and elimination of ethosuximide in children. *J. Clin. Pharmacol.*, 9:393–398.
4. Buchanan, R. A., Kinkel, A. W., Turner, J. L., and Heffelfinger, J. C. (1976): Ethosuximide dosage regimens. *Clin. Pharmacol. Ther.*, 19:143–147.
5. Buchanan, R. A., Kinkel, A. W., and Smith, T. C. (1973): The absorption and excretion of ethosuximide. *Int. J. Clin. Pharmacol.*, 7:213–218.
6. Chang, T., Dill, W. A., and Glazko, A. J. (1972): Ethosuximide: Absorption, distribution and excretion. In: *Antiepileptic Drugs,* 1st edition, edited by D. M. Woodbury, J. K. Penry, and R. P. Schmidt pp. 417–423. Raven Press, New York.
7. Colburn, W. A., and Gibaldi, M. (1978): Use of MULTDOS for pharmacokinetic analysis of ethosuximide data during repetitive administration of single or divided daily doses. *J. Pharm. Sci.*, 67:574–575.
8. Dill, W. A., Peterson, L., Chang, T., and Glazko, A. J. (1965): Physiologic disposition of α-methyl-α-ethylsuccinimide (ethosuximide; Zarontin) in animals and man. Abstracts, 149th National Meeting American Chemical Society, Detroit, Michigan. American Chemical Society, Washington, p. 30N.
9. Eadie, M. J., Tyrer, J. H., Smith, G. A., and McKauge, L. (1977): Pharmacokinetics of drugs used for petit mal "absence" epilepsy. *Clin. Exp. Neurol.*, 14:172–183.
10. El Sayed, M. A., Löscher, W., and Frey, H.-H. (1978): Pharmacokinetics of ethosuximide in the dog. *Arch. Int. Pharmacodyn.*, 234:180–192.
11. Glazko, A. J. (1975): Antiepileptic drugs: Biotransformation, metabolism and serum half-life. *Epilepsia*, 16:367–391.
12. Goulet, J. R., Kinkel, A. W., and Smith, T. C. (1976): Metabolism of ethosuximide. *Clin. Pharmacol. Ther.*, 20:213–218.
13. Haerer, A. F., Buchanan, R. A., and Wiygul, F. M. (1970): Ethosuximide blood levels in epileptics. *J. Clin. Pharmacol.*, 10:370–374.
14. Hansen, S. E., and Feldberg, L. (1964): Absorption and elimination of Zarontin. *Dan. Med. Bull.*, 11:54–55.
15. Hill, R., Horning, M., and Horning, E. (1973): Identification of transplacentally acquired anticonvulsant agents in the neonate. In: *Methods of Analysis of Antiepileptic Drugs*, edited by J. W. A. Meijer, H. Meinardi, C. Gardner-Thorp, and E. van der Kleijn, pp. 14–147. American Elsevier, New York.
16. Horning, M. G., Brown, L., Nowlin, J., Lertratanangkoon, K., Kellaway, P., and Zion, T. E. (1977): Use of saliva in therapeutic drug monitoring. *Clin. Chem.*, 23:157–164.
17. Horning, M. G., Stratton, C., Nowlin, J., Harvey, D. J., and Hill, R. M. (1973): Metabolism of 2-ethyl-2-methylsuccinimide in the rat and human. *Drug Metab. Dispos.*, 1:569–576.

18. Koup, J. R., Rose, J. Q., and Cohen, M. E. (1978): Ethosuximide pharmacokinetics in a pregnant patient and her newborn. *Epilepsia*, 19:535–539.
19. Kuhnz, W., Koch, S., Jacob, S., Hartman, A., Helge, H., and Nan, H. (1984): Ethosuximide in epileptic women during pregnancy and lactation period. Placental transfer, serum concentrations in nursed infants and clinical status. *Br. J. Clin. Pharmacol.*, 18:671–677.
20. McCauliffe, J. J., Sherwin, A. L., Leppick, I. E., Fayle, S. A., and Pippenger, C. E. (1977): Salivary levels of anticonvulsants: A practical approach to drug monitoring. *Neurology (Minneap.)*, 27:409–413.
21. Patel, I. H., and Levy, R. H. (1975): Pharmacokinetic properties of ethosuximide in monkeys. II. Chronic intravenous and oral administration. *Epilepsia*, 16:717–730.
22. Patel, I. H., Levy, R. H., and Bauer, T. G. (1975): Pharmacokinetic properties of ethosuximide in monkeys. I. Single-dose intravenous and oral administration. *Epilepsia*, 16:705–716.
23. Patel, I. H., Levy, R. H., and Lockard, J. S. (1977): Time-dependent kinetics II: Diurnal oscillations in steady-state plasma ethosuximide levels in rhesus monkeys. *J. Pharm. Sci.*, 66:650–653.
24. Patel, I. H., Levy, R. H., and Rapport, R. L. (1977): Distribution characteristics of ethosuximide in discrete areas of rat brain. *Epilepsia*, 18:533–540.
25. Piredda, S., and Monaco, F. (1981): Ethosuximide in tears, saliva, and cerebral fluid. *Ther. Drug Monit.*, 3:321–323.
26. Rane, A., and Tunell, R. (1981): Ethosuximide in human milk and in plasma of a mother and her nursed infant. *Br. J. Clin. Pharmacol.*, 12:855–858.
27. Sherwin, A. L. (1978): Clinical pharmacology of ethosuximide. In: *Antiepileptic Drugs: Quantitative Analysis and Interpretation*, edited by C. E. Pippenger, J. K. Penry, and H. Kutt, pp. 283–295. Raven Press, New York.
28. Sherwin, A. L., Lechter, M., Marlin, A. E., and Robb, J. P. (1971): Plasma ethosuximide (Zarontin) levels: As new aid in the management of epilepsy. *Ann. R. Coll. Physicians Surg. Can.*, 4:48–49.
29. Sherwin, A. L., and Robb, J. P. (1972): Ethosuximide: Relation of plasma levels to clinical control. In: *Antiepileptic Drugs*, 1st edition, edited by D. M. Woodbury, J. K. Penry, and R. P. Schmidt, pp. 443–448. Raven Press, New York.
30. Sherwin, A. L., Robb, J. P., and Lechter, M. (1973): Improved control of epilepsy by monitoring plasma ethosuximide. *Arch. Neurol.*, 28:178–181.
31. Wechselburg, K., and Hübel, G. (1967): Zur resorption und Verteilung von Methyl-äthyl-succinimid (MAS) in serum und liquor bei kindern. *Z. Kinderheilkd.*, 100:10–19.

Antiepileptic Drugs, Third Edition, edited by
R. Levy, R. Mattson, B. Meldrum,
J. K. Penry, and F. E. Dreifuss.
Raven Press, Ltd., New York © 1989.

49

Ethosuximide

Biotransformation

Tsun Chang

Ethosuximide is eliminated primarily by metabolism with 10% to 20% of the administered dose excreted in urine unchanged. Using a gas chromatographic method (GC), Dill et al. (4) detected several metabolites in animal urine. However, the chemical structures were not elucidated.

Biotransformation studies with ethosuximide were greatly facilitated by the synthesis of [1-^{14}C]ethosuximide (2). This involved the preparation of 2-ethyl-2-methylsuccinic acid (10) and ring closure with ammonia. The resulting product was labeled in the C-1 position of the succinimide ring and had a specific activity of 1.22 μCi/mg (Fig. 1).

Thin-layer chromatography (TLC) of urine specimens from rats dosed with [^{14}C]ethosuximide clearly indicated the presence of unchanged drug plus two major radioactive fractions. A typical TLC chromatogram is shown in Fig. 2. In this system, ethosuximide had the highest R_f value, metabolite II had an intermediate value, and metabolite I was closest to the origin, representing the most polar metabolites or water-soluble conjugates.

ETHOSUXIMIDE FRACTION

Ethosuximide used in clinical practice has one chiral carbon and consists of a ra-

cemic mixture of two enantiomers. If the two enantiomers are metabolized by different pathways at different rates, as occurs with glutethimide (7), the residual ethosuximide excreted in the urine should be optically active.

To examine this possibility, unchanged ethosuximide was isolated from rat urine using solvent extraction and preparative TLC techniques. Urine collected from rats dosed perorally with ethosuximide (100 mg/kg) was adjusted to pH 5 to 6 and extracted twice with chloroform. The combined extracts were evaporated to dryness. The residue was dissolved in a small amount of chloroform and chromatographed on silica gel GF$_{254}$ TLC plates using chloroform:ethyl acetate (2:1) as the developing solvent. The band corresponding to ethosuximide was eluted, and the solution was evaporated to dryness, leaving about 9 mg of a crystalline solid. Subsequent gas-liquid chromatography (GLC) of this material indicated that the retention time was the same as that of ethosuximide and that the preparation was free of impurities. The optical rotation of the purified material was zero, indicating that in the rat the two enantiomers were metabolized at the same rate.

METABOLITE II

Metabolite II, shown in Fig. 2, was isolated from rat urine and identified as 2-(1-

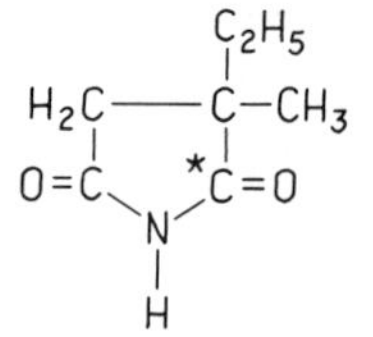

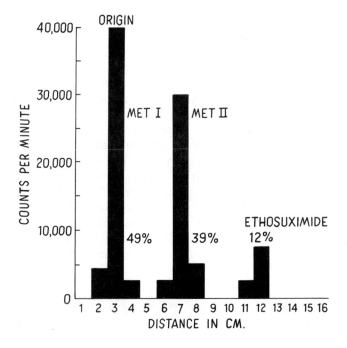

FIG. 1. Structure of ethosuximide showing the location of the ^{14}C label (*asterisk*). This is the C-1 location in the 2-ethyl-2-methylsuccinimide nomenclature.

hydroxyethyl)-2-methylsuccinimide (1). Hydroxylation of the ethyl side chain at the C-1 position results in the formation of a new chiral center. Optical rotation measurements indicated that the isolated material was levorotatory ($[\alpha]_D^{25} = -7.9°$). The diastereoisomers were readily separated by GLC as their trimethylsilyl (TMS) derivatives, and metabolite II was found to be a 40:60 mixture of the diastereoisomers. Oxidation of metabolite II with chromic acid produced the corresponding ketone derivative, 2-acetyl-2-methylsuccinimide.

A small amount of 2-(1-hydroxyethyl)-2-methylsuccinimide (metabolite II) was syn-

thesized for use as reference standard (2). Comparison of the synthetic material with the isolated metabolite showed that the two compounds were identical in their infrared absorbance characteristics and GLC retention times, supporting the proposed structure. The nuclear magnetic resonance (NMR) spectrum of the synthetic compound was slightly different from that of the urinary metabolite because of differences in the proportions of the diastereoisomers in the two preparations. The structure of metabolite II was confirmed later by Horning et al. (6) and Preste et al. (9) using gas chromatography–mass spectrometry (GC-MS).

Urine from a human subject receiving repeated doses of ethosuximide was incubated overnight with β-glucuronidase (Glusulase) to hydrolyze any conjugates. It was then passed through an Amberlite XAD-2 column to retain ethosuximide and its metabolites. These were eluted with methanol, which was then evaporated to dryness. The residue was derivatized with *bis*-(trimethylsilyl)acetamide and subjected to gas chromatography. The chromatographic profile

FIG. 2. Thin-layer chromatogram of rat urine following a 66 mg/kg peroral dose of [1-^{14}C]ethosuximide. Silica gel GF; ethyl acetate:carbon tetrachloride (2:1).

indicated a double peak with retention times of 7.1 min and 8.1 min caused by the diastereoisomers of metabolite II.

The possible presence of a glucuronide conjugate of metabolite II was examined in animals and in man. Rats weighing 250 g were dosed with 10 mg of [^{14}C]ethosuximide, and urine was collected over a 24-hr period. Thin-layer chromatography of the urine on silica gel with chloroform:methanol:water (3:2:1, lower phase) resulted in the appearance of three peaks similar to those seen in Fig. 2. In this case, the radioactivity in the ethosuximide fraction represented about 10% of the total ^{14}C on the plate; the intermediate peak corresponding to metabolite II had 54% of the total radioactivity, and the area near the origin had 36% of the radioactivity. The latter peak was eluted from the silica gel with methanol, evaporated to dryness, and redissolved in 6 ml of pH 5 acetate buffer (0.1 M). Half of this was incubated at 37°C for 24 hr with β-glucuronidase plus one drop of chloroform; the other half served as a control without β-glucuronidase. Thin-layer chromatography of the two preparations resulted in most of the radioactivity (88%) remaining at the origin, with a small amount of activity (12%) appearing in the location of metabolite II. However, the chromatographic patterns were identical in the control and enzyme-treated preparations, indicating that metabolite II probably was not conjugated to any great extent in the rat. Horning et al. (6) later reported the presence of several glucuronides of hydroxyethosuximides in rat urine. When we repeated the same experiment with urine from a monkey dosed with ethosuximide, treatment of the TLC fraction near the origin with β-glucuronidase resulted in the release of material with the same chromatographic characteristics as metabolite II. These observations indicate that significant amounts of a glucuronic acid conjugate of metabolite II are present in monkey urine.

Similar observations were made with

Table 1. *Anticonvulsant effect of ethosuximide and metabolite II against pentylenetetrazol-induced clonic seizures in mice*

Ethosuximide		Metabolite II	
Dose (mg/kg)[a]	Protected/ dose (N)	Dose (mg/kg)[a]	Protected/ dosed (N)
125	5/5	250	2/5
62.5	3/5	125	0/5

[a] Drug was given intraperitoneally 30 min prior to pentylenetetrazol.

human urine specimens obtained from subjects receiving a single 1-g oral dose of ethosuximide. The urine was saturated with sodium chloride and extracted with *n*-butanol, concentrated by evaporation, and chromatographed by GLC. When direct extraction without enzymatic hydrolysis was employed, 14% of the dose was recovered as free metabolite II. Treatment of the urine with β-glucuronidase before extraction resulted in 39% of the dose being recovered in the form of metabolite II, indicating that much of this metabolite was conjugated. Quantitative data obtained in the Parke-Davis laboratories, reported by Glazko (5), indicated that the excretion of metabolite II in human urine accounted for 33% to 41% of the administered dose.

The anticonvulsant effect of metabolite II was tested in mice, using pentylenetetrazol to induce clonic seizures (3). Groups of five mice were predosed with ethosuximide or with metabolite II (isolated from rat urine). These compounds were administered intraperitoneally as aqueous solutions 30 min before the test dose of pentylenetetrazol. The results shown in Table 1 indicate no significant anticonvulsant activity of metabolite II at a dose of 125 mg/kg, whereas ethosuximide gave complete protection at the same dose level.

OTHER METABOLITES

Using GC-MS techniques, Horning et al. (6) identified two minor metabolites, 2-

ethyl-3-hydroxy-2-methylsuccinimide and 2-(2-hydroxyethyl)-2-methylsuccinimide, in rat urine and human urine. Male rats receiving a single intraperitoneal dose (83 mg) of ethosuximide excreted approximately 5.7 mg and 1.9 mg of the 3-hydroxy- and 2-hydroxyethyl metabolites, respectively, in 48-hr urine (6). However, the diastereoisomers of the 1-hydroxyethyl metabolite accounted for a total of 44.2 mg in the same collection period. Assuming an area response factor of unity relative to the internal standard, Horning et al. (6) estimated that as much as 16 mg was excreted as glucuronide conjugates of the hydroxyethosuximides in rat urine. A dihydroxy metabolite of unknown structure was also detected in rat urine. In rat plasma, unchanged ethosuximide was the predominant component, but only trace amounts of the isomeric 1-hydroxyethyl metabolites were found. In human adult and infant plasma, the hydroxyethosuximides were the major products.

Preste et al. (9) confirmed the structure of 2-ethyl-3-hydroxy-2-methylsuccinimide by low- and high-resolution mass spectrometry as well as by NMR spectroscopy. Gas-liquid chromatography of urine from patients receiving ethosuximide suggested that nearly as much of the 3-hydroxy metabolite might be present as the stereoisomeric 1-hydroxyethyl-ethosuximide. However, quantitative data were not obtained (9).

Petterson (8) subsequently reported the identification of 2-carboxymethyl-2-methylsuccinimide from urine of a patient treated with ethosuximide for petit mal epilepsy. This metabolite is likely formed by further oxidation of the primary alcohol function of 2-(2-hydroxyethyl)-2-methylsuccinimide to a carboxy group.

METABOLIC PATHWAYS

Previous work with urine from rats and rhesus monkeys receiving [^{14}C-]-ethosuximide demonstrated the presence of a polar fraction that did not migrate far from the

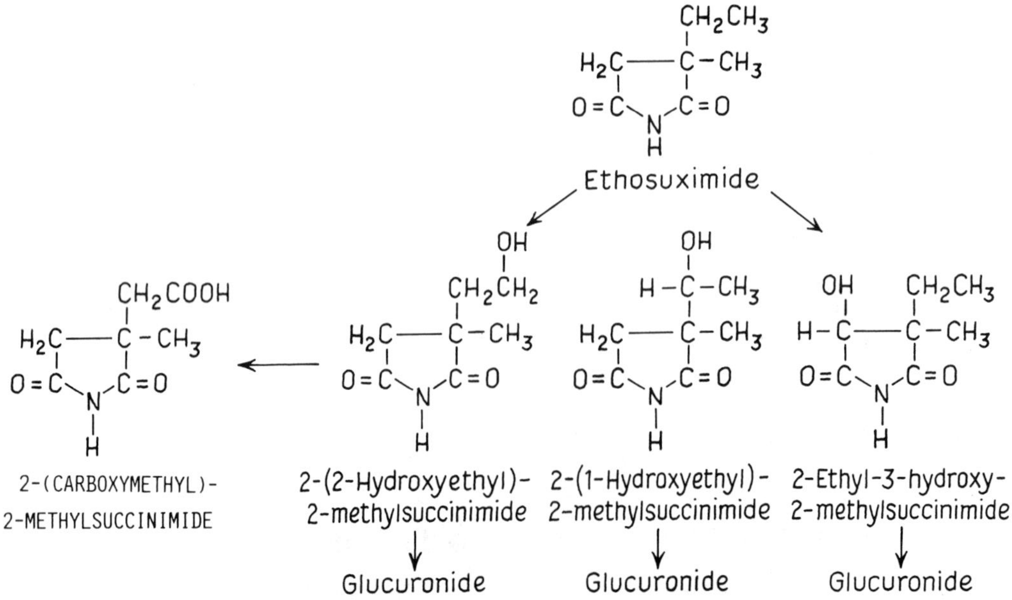

FIG. 3. Metabolic disposition of ethosuximide.

origin of TLC plates (Fig. 2). This appears to be a mixture of metabolites, including the glucuronic acid conjugate of 2-(1-hydroxyethyl)-2-methylsuccinimide. However, after enzymatic hydrolysis, TLC indicated that a polar residue remained at the origin. On heating in strong hydrochloric acid, the succinimide ring appeared to open, forming an insoluble product whose structure has not been established.

On the basis of the information we have on the metabolic disposition of ethosuximide, the biotransformation pathways can be summarized as shown in Fig. 3.

REFERENCES

1. Burkett, A. R., Chang, T., and Glazko, A. J. (1971): A hydroxylated metabolite of ethosuximide (Zarontin®) in rat urine. *Fed. Proc.,* 30:391.
2. Chang, T., Burkett, A. R., and Glazko, A. J. (1972): Ethosuximide: Biotransformation. In: *Antiepileptic Drugs,* 1st edition, edited by D. M. Woodbury, J. K. Penry, and R. P. Schmidt, pp. 425–429. Raven Press, New York.
3. Chen, G., and Portman, R. (1952): Titration of central nervous system depression. *Arch. Neurol. Psychiatry,* 68:498–505.
4. Dill, W. A., Peterson, L., Chang, T., and Glazko, A. J. (1965): Physiologic disposition of α-methyl-α-ethylsuccinimide (ethosuximide; Zarontin) in animals and in man. In: *Abstracts of Papers, 149th National Meeting, American Chemical Society, Detroit, Michigan,* p. 30N. American Chemical Society, Washington.
5. Glazko, A. J. (1975): Antiepileptic drugs: Biotransformation, metabolism, and serum half-life. *Epilepsia,* 16:367–391.
6. Horning, M. G., Stratton, J., Nowlin, D. J., Harvey, D. J., and Hill, R. M. (1973): Metabolism of 2-ethyl-2-methyl succinimide (ethosuximide) in the rat and human. *Drug Metab. Dispos.,* 3:569–576.
7. Kerberle, H., Hoffman, K., and Bernhard, K. (1962): The metabolism of glutethimide (Doriden®). *Experientia,* 18:105–162.
8. Pettersen, J. E. (1978): Urine metabolites of 2-ethyl-2-methyl-succinimide (ethosuximide) studied by combined gas chromatography mass spectrometry. *Biomed. Mass. Spectrom.,* 5:601–603.
9. Preste, P. G., Westerman, C. E., Das, N. P., Wilder, B. J., and Duncan, J. H. (1974): Identification of 2-ethyl-2-methyl-3-hydroxysuccinimide as a major metabolite of ethosuximide in humans. *J. Pharm. Sci.,* 63:467–469.
10. Smith, P. A. S., and Horwitz, J. P. (1949): A synthesis of unsymmetrically substituted succinic acids. *J. Am. Chem. Soc.,* 71:3418–3419.

Antiepileptic Drugs, Third Edition, edited by
R. Levy, R. Mattson, B. Meldrum,
J. K. Penry, and F. E. Dreifuss.
Raven Press, Ltd., New York © 1989.

50

Ethosuximide

Clinical Use

Allan L. Sherwin

Ethosuximide is specifically indicated for the control of absence (petit mal) seizures, an age-related manifestation of generalized epilepsy beginning in childhood or early adolescence (1,63). If absence attacks are the sole seizure pattern, ethosuximide provides a relatively safe and effective form of monotherapy. If tonic-clonic seizures occur, ethosuximide can be readily combined with carbamazepine, phenytoin, or other agents, since clinically significant drug interactions are rare. Valproate monotherapy, which provides protection against both absence and tonic-clonic seizures, should receive serious consideration in such instances (7,56). Ethosuximide remains the contemporary drug of choice for children with typical absence seizures, in whom the potential hepatotoxicity of valproate is an important consideration.

TYPICAL ABSENCE SEIZURES

Typical absence seizures are characterized by brief episodes of transient loss of awareness, responsiveness, and memory without gross convulsive movements. The onset of the attack is sudden, interrupting ongoing activity; the eyes drift upward with slight beating of the eyelids. Absences may be simple or often somewhat more complex, in which case impairment of consciousness is associated with mild clonic movements, loss of postural tone, simple automatisms, or other minor movements (1,5,42). Sweating and changes in color are unusual, and although the body may sway, patients seldom fall. The attacks usually last a few seconds, seldom more than half a minute, and usually terminate abruptly without after effects. Seizures occur daily, especially in the morning, and range in frequency from five to 50 or more a day. The children are usually unaware of them. Absence seizures are relatively uncommon, accounting for 5% to 10% of seizure patterns observed in childhood. Fortunately, in the majority of cases where typical absence is the only seizure pattern, they cease to be a clinical problem by 20 years of age (14,28). The prognosis is less favorable in the presence of tonic-clonic seizures, which occur at some time in one-third to one-half of patients with absence attacks (7,39,49).

The first clinical and electroencephalogram (EEG) manifestations in absence seizures indicate that both cerebral hemispheres are involved; they are accordingly classified as one of the generalized epilepsies (17). This is presumably a reflection of widespread neuronal discharge, usually with impaired consciousness as the initial manifestation. Seizures lasting more than a few seconds are commonly associated with other manifestations, such as mild clonic movements of the eyelids or corners of the mouth or transient alterations of tone in postural muscles, resulting in drooping of the head or some movement of the extremities. Automatism consisting of quasipurposeful movements like licking of the lips, swallowing, or fumbling with clothes may be observed. Involvement of the central noradrenergic and parasympathetic systems results in dilatation of the pupils, brief respiratory arrest, and rarely urinary incontinence. Autonomic features include incontinence, which is fortunately infrequent. The ictal EEG in patients with typical absence seizures reveals regular and symmetrical 2.5 to 3.5 Hz spike-and-wave complexes or multiple spike-and-slow-wave complexes that emerge abruptly from a normal background activity (Fig. 1). The neurological examination results, intelligence, and neuroimaging of the brain are usually normal.

ATYPICAL ABSENCE SEIZURES

Patients with atypical absence seizures have a somewhat similar seizure pattern but the onset and cessation of seizures may be more gradual and they exhibit more pronounced changes in tone, including drop attacks. Both onset and cessation of the seizures may be more gradual. The EEG findings in this group of patients are more heterogeneous, with slow-spike-and-slow-wave complexes that, in this case, arise out of an abnormal background activity which can be asymmetrical. The neurological examination, psychological tests, and neuroimaging usually reveal some degree of ab-

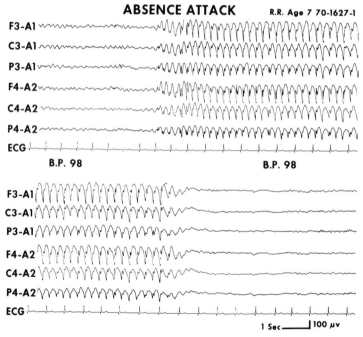

FIG. 1. EEG recorded from a 7-year-old boy before and during an absence seizure that lasted approximately 9 sec. The generalized and bilaterally synchronous spike-and-wave activity at 2.5 to 3 Hz emerges abruptly from a normal background activity. Complete seizure control was achieved with ethosuximide monotherapy (30 mg/kg, plasma concentration 85 μg/ml); seizure-free at 13 years; no history of tonic-clonic seizures.

normality. Although these patients also respond to ethosuximide therapy, they frequently exhibit other types of seizures, including myoclonus, tonic-clonic seizures, and drop attacks. The prognosis for the eventual complete remission of the epilepsy in such patients must be more guarded (14,39,53).

DIAGNOSIS OF ABSENCE SEIZURES

Absence seizures constitute a distinct clinical entity readily diagnosed on the basis of a sound medical history. Attacks can frequently be elicited by 3 to 5 min of forceful voluntary hyperventilation which is a useful and safe clinical test (1). Photic stimulation induces absence attacks in only a minority of patients. This activation procedure was known to the ancient Greeks (40) although good clinical descriptions of absence attacks date from the 18th century (18,36). Modern progress stems from the correlation of typical absence (petit mal) attacks with 3 Hz spike-and-wave discharges, which spring from a normal background (24,25). The wave is considered to be the more consistent feature (36), and modern EEG recordings reveal that the frequency can vary between 2.5 to 3.5 Hz. This was an important discovery in the history of neurology because it showed that absence seizures differ from other types of nonconvulsive attacks, not only in degree but also in kind (24).

Genetic analysis of this pattern in patients and their near relatives indicate that the EEG trait, but not the epilepsy, is inherited in an autosomal dominant pattern with age-related penetrance (35). Absence seizures now appear to fit the genetic model of multifactorial inheritance in which environmental factors are also considered to be important in determining whether clinical seizures occur (2,5).

The differential diagnosis of absence seizures includes brief, complex partial seizures originating in the temporal or frontal lobe. These can usually be distinguished by the presence of an aura, the longer duration of the attacks, and the presence of postictal confusion. Careful analysis of the EEG provides a more precise electroclinical correlation. Nonepileptic states like tics, daydreaming, and psychiatric disorders can usually be readily eliminated by a careful medical history and ancillary data.

ABSENCE STATUS

Absence status refers to an almost continuous state of abnormal behavior and response that ranges from mild confusion to stupor (3). It differs from absence attacks in that patients do not blink or stare but instead appear to be inattentive and disoriented. The EEG abnormalities (44) consist of nearly continuous spike-and-wave discharges, but in some cases the tracing may bear only a faint resemblance to the classic pattern. The episodes usually last just a few minutes but occasionally persist for hours or even days. Absence status is not age-determined and may present at any time in life, often without a previous history of epilepsy. The differential diagnosis includes complex partial status, which can be distinguished by the presence of continuously recurring cycles of the clinical stages of the individual seizures, amnestic states resembling posttraumatic amnesia, hysterical behavior, and schizophrenic reactions. Absence status can be prevented or controlled by ethosuximide, especially if plasma levels greater than 120 µg/ml are achieved (44), or by valproate (18).

PATHOPHYSIOLOGICAL CHARACTERISTICS OF ABSENCE SEIZURES

Absence seizures result from a generalized epileptic disturbance that is somewhat different from the focal epileptic spike discharge characteristic of partial seizures. Generalized and bilaterally synchronous spike-and-wave discharges begin in the cerebral cortex and result from the development of a markedly increased excitation of neurons (25,46). This excitation appears to be the major event and is followed by inhibition, which increases in response to the excitation. The spike-and-wave complex results from a remarkable oscillation between periods of increased excitation of cortical neurons corresponding to the spike, and periods of decreased firing corresponding to the wave. Thalamocortical volleys may help pace and synchronize the bilateral 3 Hz spike-and-wave activity which, however, is generated at the level of the cerebral cortex (47). Ethosuximide acts on low-frequency inhibitory pathways to prevent or reduce the duration of 3 Hz spike-and-wave discharges which are the electrographic manifestation of absence seizures (20,38).

Ethosuximide selectively depresses the synaptic transmission of repetitive stimulation (13,58) such as inhibitory pathways in the reticular formation, unlike drugs effective in complex partial and tonic-clonic seizures, which supress excitatory pathways (22,23). Ethosuximide, in contrast to phenytoin, prevents seizures in an experimental model of absence attacks induced in the cat by intramuscular injection of penicillin (26). Studies of the mechanisms of action of drugs like ethosuximide lend support to the notion that the clinical and electrographic features of absence seizures constitute a distinct nosological entity (18,23,37).

PLASMA ETHOSUXIMIDE LEVELS AND CLINICAL CONTROL OF ABSENCE SEIZURES

Despite their brevity, frequent absence seizures require treatment because of their disruptive effect on the child's normal activities. Often they lead to embarrassment at school or interference with work, and the possibility of accidental injury is always present. There is also evidence that the generalized 3 Hz spike-and-wave epileptic discharge, the hallmark of this seizure pattern, causes impairment in sustained attention (9,42,45). Because absence seizures can usually be precipitated by hyperventilation, the physician is nearly always able to make a direct observation and improve the accuracy of the diagnosis (1). Moreover, absence seizures are accompanied by quantifiable EEG spike-and-wave discharges that can be recorded by prolonged EEG telemetry (41,42). Consequently, this type of epilepsy permits accurate assessment of the relationship of plasma ethosuximide levels to clinical control (10), particularly since ethosuximide has a direct and rather specific action and all its metabolites are inactive (4).

Comparison of plasma ethosuximide levels with clinical control was first reported by Haerer et al. (27) in a study of 21 outpatients. Ten patients were found to be markedly improved, seven moderately improved, and four either slightly or less than 50% improved, but plasma ethosuximide levels were comparatively low. Solow and Green (60) found that ethosuximide levels in 50 patients with controlled absence seizures ranged from 25 to 168 μg/ml, the average plasma level being 63.2 μg/ml, with an average dose of 20.6 mg/kg. Eadie and Tyrer (19) reported that absence attacks were fully controlled with plasma ethosuximide levels ranging between 26 and 180 μg/ml and that these levels were well tolerated by the majority of patients. These early clinical efficacy studies tended to involve refractory cases and addition of the drug to existing polytherapy. A consistent definition of absence seizures was not employed, and determination of seizure control was based exclusively on parental observations.

There is no single satisfactory definition of clinical control; neurologists disagree about the meaning of "satisfactory control" and "complete control," but in general, reduction of seizure frequency is the most useful indicator. When control is incomplete, any change in the character and/or duration of the seizure becomes important. For example, in absence seizures, several isolated brief staring episodes will be less likely to impair performance than a prolonged attack associated with automatisms. General difficulties in defining control and additional nonpharmacological factors that influence the frequency of seizures are discussed in Chapters 6 and 7.

Browne et al. (8) and Penry et al. (42) were the first to carry out a comprehensive prospective study of the efficacy of ethosuximide in controlling absence attacks. Methods to quantitate the degree of seizure control in patients were developed. Moreover, the characteristics of absence seizures were clearly described in general accordance with the International Classification of Epileptic Seizures (17). Each patient was admitted to the study only after an absence seizure, as defined above, was observed by the principal investigator. The frequency of seizures in each patient was measured by (a) observation by a trained observer, (b) observation by the ward staff, (c) mother's observation of seizure frequency before and during ethosuximide administration, (d) examination by a physician, which included hyperventilation, and (e) standardized video tape-EEG recording. The five types of data on the seizure frequency were combined into a "seizure index." Data analysis revealed that seven of 37 patients (19%) had a 100% reduction in seizure index, that is, were seizure-free during the eighth treatment week. Eighteen patients (49%) had a 90% or greater reduction, and 35 (95%) had a 50% or greater reduction in seizures. The antiabsence effect of a given dose of ethosuximide appeared to be almost fully achieved during the first week of oral administration. The doses of ethosuximide ranged from 6.5 to 36.7 mg/kg, and plasma concentrations ranged from 16.6 to 104.0 μg/ml, with a significant relationship between an increased ethosuximide dose and an increased plasma concentration ($r = 0.86$; $p < 0.01$). The mean ratio of plasma ethosuximide concentration (μg/ml) to dose (mg/kg) was 2.95. However, it is important to note that for any given dose, there was such a wide variability in the plasma-to-dose ratio among patients that it was impossible to predict a given patient's plasma concentration from the ethosuximide dose. The optimal range of plasma ethosuximide concentrations as determined with the aid of the seizure index was 40 to 100 μg/ml in this study.

Sherwin et al. (57) carried out a prospective study of 70 patients with absence seizures selected according to clinical and electrographic criteria similar to those of the Collaborative Study of Absence Seizures (8,53). This group of patients had been treated with the aid of therapeutic monitoring of plasma ethosuximide levels for up to 2.5 years, 75% of the group being evaluated for periods greater than 1.5 years. The group comprised 38 females and 32 males aged 4 to 28 years (median, 12 years). Absence attacks were the sole manifestation of epilepsy in 38 (54%) of the patients. Tonic-clonic seizures were also present in 21 patients (30%), and an additional 11 patients (16%) had a history of one or more generalized seizures. The dosage of ethosuximide employed ranged from 0.5 to 1.75 g/day (9.4 to 73.5 mg/kg). Other drugs administered concurrently to some patients included phenytoin (30 patients), phenobarbital (six patients), and various minor psychotropic drugs (five patients). All patients were examined at 6-month intervals, and more frequently if necessary, with detailed recording of seizure frequency and plasma antiepileptic drug levels. In the group of 33 patients with complete seizure control, only 9% had plasma ethosuximide levels below 40 μg/ml, with none below 30 μg/ml. Thus, efforts were directed toward achieving ethosuximide levels greater than

40 μg/ml in patients with uncontrolled seizures.

These efforts resulted in a significant improvement in the clinical control of absence seizures within the first 2.5 years (Fig. 2). Only three of the 70 patients had an increased seizure frequency compared with their status at the onset of the study. Nineteen patients had a significant increase in plasma ethosuximide concentration, resulting from a prescribed dosage increase in seven, from better cooperation in 10, and from both factors in two. Thirteen of these 19 patients improved clinically, with 10 achieving complete seizure control. Patients with absence seizures tend to cease having attacks with advancing age (14,19), although some studies have reported a more guarded prognosis (49). Janz (28) observed that the rate of spontaneous arrest of absence attacks over 2-year periods was approximately 3%. This gradual rate of improvement could not account for the marked increase in the number of controlled

patients (13 of 37 uncontrolled patients) observed during the first 2.5-year period. During this time, the mean plasma ethosuximide levels in the newly controlled patients rose from 57.2 μg/ml to 76.1 μg/ml, a significant increase ($p < 0.05$) that was not observed in those patients who continued to have frequent attacks. This improvement was continued in the second half of the 5-year study. However, patients who continued to have tonic-clonic seizures despite combination therapy with appropriate agents were less likely to have attained control of absence attacks (Fig. 3). Okuma et al. (39) observed a remission rate of 68% in typical absence, but the rate in absence seizures combined with tonic-clonic seizures was 50%. Dalby (14) found that though absence attacks ceased in 79% of patients with no other seizure type, after a period of 5 years or more, tonic-clonic seizures occurred in 46% of patients with absences and seizures ceased in only 33% of this group. This fits with the observation of Rodin (49)

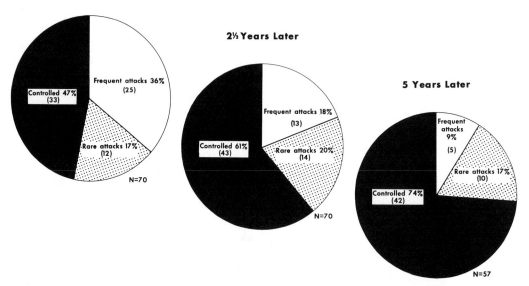

FIG. 2. Control of absence attacks before and after commencing regular plasma concentration monitoring with titration of ethosuximide dosage. There is a highly significant alteration in the distribution of clinical control (Chi-square test, $p < 0.005$). The improvement noted in the first 2.5 years is far greater than would be expected from the natural course of absence seizures. Approximately two-thirds of the patients were managed on ethosuximide monotherapy.

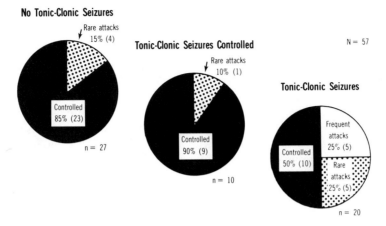

FIG. 3. Correlation between control of absence attacks and control of tonic-clonic seizures after 5 years of ethosuximide therapy. Patients with no tonic-clonic seizures received ethosuximide monotherapy. Phenytoin, phenobarbital, and primidone were used to control tonic-clonic seizures. Six additional patients were fully controlled without medication; one of these had an early history of tonic-clonic seizures. One patient died accidentally, and six patients were lost to follow-up. Ethosuximide was less efficacious in patients who continued to have tonic-clonic seizures.

that the incidence of remission is inversely related to the duration of follow-up. There is no clear evidence that drug therapy influences the remission rate of absence seizures (39).

Ethosuximide and valproate appear to be equally effective in controlling simple absence seizures (61). Table 1 summarizes six studies employing careful clinical observation and/or prolonged telemetered EEG re-

cordings. The investigators compared the number of patients considered to have 100% seizure control as assessed by each technique. Double-blind control studies in which ethosuximide is compared with valproate indicates that both drugs are equally effective in controlling absence seizures (22). In clinical practice individual patients may respond to one or the other drug in monotherapy. Rowan et al. (51) carefully

TABLE 1. *Complete control of absence seizures: Ethosuximide versus valproate*

Refs.	Ethosuximide			Valproate		
	Clinical control[a]	EEG control[b]	Serum level (μg/ml)	Clinical control	EEG control	Serum level (μg/ml)
11	8/11	–	35–53	8/12	–	32–114
12	8/14	6/14	26–88	6/14	4/14	47–121
54	–	6/11	63–97	–	9/12	49–115
52	21/43	–	–	6/7	–	–
32	8/10	8/10	51–114	7/10	7/10	68–131
6	9/11	8/11	25–139	–	–	–
Total	54/89 (61%)	28/46 (61%)	25–139	27/43 (63%)	20/36 (55%)	32–131

[a] 100% control of absence seizures as determined by clinical observation.
[b] Monitored by means of EEG-telemetry.
Modified from Fromm and Crumrine (22), with permission.

studied five patients with absence seizures refractory to treatment with either ethosuximide or valproate. The resultant data confirmed the beneficial clinical and EEG effects of combination therapy in controlling absence seizures. Jeavons et al. (29) observed that patients with a long history of poorly controlled atypical absence seizures or myoclonic absences respond best to these drugs in combination (7,22).

PLASMA ETHOSUXIMIDE LEVEL AND DOSE

The relationship of the plasma ethosuximide level to the dose administered is illustrated in Fig. 4. Plasma ethosuximide levels were determined from single blood samples in patients known to be receiving constant dosages of ethosuximide either alone or in combination with other anticon-

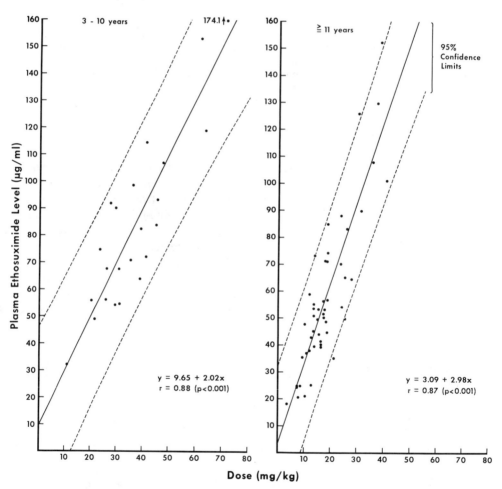

FIG. 4. Relationship of plasma ethosuximide concentration to dosage at steady state. The slope of the regression line for patients aged 3 to 10 years ($N = 23$) is significantly less than that for patients 11 years of age and older ($N = 49$) ($p < 0.01$). These regression lines are useful to select appropriate dosage. Significant differences between male and female children were not observed.

vulsants. In agreement with the data of Browne et al. (8), the slope of the linear regression line of ethosuximide dose to plasma level was significantly less ($p <$ 0.01) in children aged 3 to 10 years than in patients 11 years of age and over. Thus, a daily dose of 20 mg/kg of ethosuximide in children 11 years of age or less will result in mean plasma ethosuximide levels of 50 μg/ml, and in older patients a dose of approximately 15 mg/kg will result in similar levels. The generally accepted maximum daily dose is 30 mg/kg for adults and 40 mg/kg for children. The daily dose may be increased every 4 to 7 days until seizure control and the desired plasma concentration are achieved. In a study of plasma ethosuximide levels examined at 3-month intervals in 245 patients receiving stable doses, there was a highly significant variation in the dose-to-plasma level relationship with increasing age ($p < 0.001$). The mean plasma ethosuximide levels were not significantly different between males and females in any age group, which is in contrast with differences observed by Smith et al. (59) in a group of 36 patients aged 1.5 to 38 years.

Plasma ethosuximide levels remain extremely stable on successive examination of patients when the medication is taken regularly. Although trough levels are theoretically more accurate, it appears that the time of day that the blood sample is obtained is not likely to alter significantly the therapeutic implications of the plasma ethosuximide level. Saliva and plasma ethosuximide levels are very similar, and salivary levels can be used to monitor therapy, providing controls of pooled normal saliva spiked with ethosuximide are utilized to determine the standard curve used in the assay (34).

The pharmacokinetic profile of ethosuximide, including relatively little hepatic microsomal enzyme induction and negligible binding by plasma proteins, enhances its usefulness as a comedication in patients requiring combination therapy for resistant absence seizures, myoclonic absences, or tonic-clonic seizures. Mattson et al. (33) observed sedation accompanied by increased plasma ethosuximide levels in children on multiple drug therapy because the addition of valproate inhibited the metabolism of ethosuximide. Both the toxic symptomatology and elevated drug levels were promptly reversed by a modest reduction in ethosuximide dosage, emphasizing the value of monitoring plasma ethosuximide levels. Subsequently a careful pharmacokinetic study by Pisani et al. (43) showed that valproate decreases total body clearance of ethosuximide; a similar inhibitory interaction has been reported for isoniazid (62). Bachmann et al. (4) showed that following a single test dose of ethosuximide (10 mg/kg), the total body clearance of the drug can be estimated from a single plasma sample at 96 hr or a salivary level at 120 hr later. Ethosuximide's potential value as a single sample probe of host factor influences on hepatic mixed-function oxidase activity derives from its first-order kinetics and its extensive oxidative metabolism. With the ready availability of accurate plasma drug levels, clinicians could employ this method of probing host factor influences on drug metabolism whenever unusual dose-to-plasma drug level responses are encountered.

Acute behavioral disturbances are occasionally observed within days to weeks following the initiation of ethosuximide therapy. Anxiety, depression, and frank psychosis with visual and auditory hallucinations along with paranoid ideation have been reported (50,64). Symptoms usually resolve with discontinuation of the drug and its gradual elimination and in one case returned when the drug was reintroduced (21). This adverse effect is uncommon in children and most of the reported cases involved adolescents or young adults with a history of significant emotional problems or overt psychiatric disease.

Fortunately typical absence seizures have often ceased to be a major problem by the time many patients reach childbearing age. If so it may be possible to discontinue therapy before conception, though if tonic-clonic seizures are also present therapy with carbamazepine or other agents must be maintained (55). Plasma ethosuximide levels usually remain fairly constant during pregnancy with a modest increase in maternal levels reported after delivery (16,30,31). The mean fetal-to-maternal plasma concentration ratio was 0.97 at birth, indicating that the fetus is exposed to similar drug concentrations as the mother (31). Ethosuximide therapy during pregnancy, usually in combination with other antiepileptics, has been associated with congenital malformations. Dansky et al. (16) monitored ethosuximide in five patients, one of whom had a malformed child. Her mean dosage (17.3 mg/kg) and mean plasma ethosuximide level (42.2 μg/ml), though within the therapeutic range, were about twice the corresponding mean values for the four mothers with normal children (10 mg/kg, 27 μg/ml). There are insufficient data on ethosuximide monotherapy in pregnancy to predict the precise risk of fetal malformations, but because effective free drug plasma levels of this nonprotein bound drug are 20-fold greater than carbamazepine levels, the fetus will be exposed to higher concentrations of a foreign chemical. Dansky et al. (15) also demonstrated a positive correlation between mean maternal phenytoin concentrations and the risk of malformed offspring.

Though pharmacogenetic, metabolic, and genetic factors are the prime determinants of teratogenicity, it would seem prudent to minimize fetal exposure to ethosuximide by keeping maternal plasma drug levels as low as possible. Breast milk ethosuximide concentrations are approximately 90% of the mother's steady-state plasma levels, which is likely due in part to the drug's negligible binding by plasma proteins. Kuhnz et al. (31) noted neonatal behavioral toxicity in seven of 10 breast-fed infants in whom plasma ethosuximide levels ranged between 15 and 40 μg/ml. Corresponding maternal steady-state plasma ethosuximide concentrations ranged between 28 and 84 μg/ml. Rane et al. (48) in reporting a single case observed significant amounts of ethosuximide in the baby's plasma during nursing without adverse behavioral effects. Both authors recommend monitoring of plasma and if possible breast milk ethosuximide concentrations. The major problem in the management of mothers with either nonconvulsive or convulsive epilepsies is the risk of dropping the infant from a height or while in a bath during an absence seizure. Regular therapeutic drug monitoring and frequent visits are essential to maintain optimal antiepileptic drug therapy for each clinical seizure type. If one entertains the notion that exposure to CNS-active drugs *in utero* or early life may result in subtle adverse effects later in life, the recent study of Mirsky et al. (37) on the mechanisms of action of ethosuximide (see Chapter 47) is of great importance. They observed that this drug enhanced metabolic activity in key brain stem structures, including the thalamic midbrain pathway, which plays an important inhibitory role in the pathogenesis of corticoreticular (generalized) epilepsy.

PROGNOSTIC FACTORS IN ABSENCE SEIZURES

The relationship of plasma ethosuximide levels to clinical seizure control is profoundly influenced by the natural history observed in children with absence seizures. Sato et al. (53) reported a longitudinal, long-term, prospective follow-up study of patients selected solely on the basis of clinical observations but all meeting the clinical and EEG classification of epileptic seizures.

The data strongly illustrated the point that patients presenting initially with absence seizures alone have a significantly better outcome for the eventual cessation of seizures than do patients presenting with both absence and generalized tonic-clonic seizures. The two most important factors favoring natural cessation of absence attacks were the presence of normal EEG background activity and a normal or above normal intelligence quotient. There was also a more favorable prognosis for seizure cessation in males. The authors suggested that effective treatment should be instituted early in the course of the illness. Normal neurological examination results and a shorter duration of illness tended to favor cessation of seizures. For any seizure type, significant prognostic factors were a negative history of generalized tonic-clonic seizures, normal or above normal intelligence, and a negative family history of seizure disorders. Nearly 90% of the patients with all significant prognostic factors for both absence seizures and seizures of all types became seizure-free. In contrast, the patients who lacked all significant prognostic factors had a poor outlook for seizure relief.

SUMMARY AND CONCLUSIONS

The guidelines for ethosuximide therapy in typical and atypical absence seizures are summarized as follows:

Maintenance dosage: 15–40 mg/kg/day, once daily or with meals
Peak levels: children, 3–7 hr; adults, 2–4 hr
Dose-related effects: gastric distress, nausea, vomiting, anorexia, fatigue, lethargy, headache, dizziness, hiccups, behavioral changes
Plasma concentrations: effective levels 40–100 μg/ml (285–710 nmole/liter), but levels of up to 150 μg/ml (1,000 nmole/liter) may be required and well tolerated.
Time to reach steady state: children, 6 days; adults, 12 days

Absorption: 100%, capsules or syrup
Half-life: children, 30 hr; older children and adults, 60 hr
Major route of elimination: hepatic; no active metabolites
Interactions: minimal with other antiepileptic drugs; negligible binding by plasma proteins; levels increased by valproate alone or in combination with other drugs
Indications for therapeutic drug monitoring: poor response, noncompliance, suboptimal dosage, and to maintain optimal concentration
Maintenance of therapeutic drug monitoring: 4–6 month intervals if good response; trough specimens preferable but not essential; salivary levels similar
Monitoring of adverse effects: Complete blood cell counts and liver function tests monthly for 6 months and periodically thereafter

Monitoring of plasma ethosuximide levels is helpful in individualizing drug regimens and identifying noncompliant patients. Maintenance of plasma ethosuximide at levels of 40 to 100 μg/ml will be associated with practical control in 80% of patients, 60% becoming seizure-free. The starting dosage should be 20 mg/kg per day to anticipate a plasma level of 50 to 60 μg/ml, which can be adjusted after repeated plasma level monitoring. Plasma ethosuximide levels ranging from 40 to 100 μg/ml are considered optimal for effective seizure control but concentrations up to 150 μg/ml may be efficacious and well tolerated (19,44,60). Ethosuximide is particularly indicated as monotherapy in patients with absence seizures as the sole seizure type when both the IQ and EEG background activity are within the normal range. However, ethosuximide is also highly effective in atypical absence seizures. If seizure control is not attained with ethosuximide, valproate monotherapy should be gradually introduced. If seizure control is not obtained with valproate alone, then comedication with valproate and ethosuximide is frequently successful, especially in patients with myoclonic absences (5,17,29). Patients with a history of tonic-clonic seizures must also be maintained on combination therapy, preferably with carbamazepine. Valproate monotherapy is an attractive alternative in this situation.

When absence seizures have been controlled for 2 years, consideration may be given to the discontinuation of ethosuximide therapy, particularly if EEG examination, including 3 min of forceful hyperventilation, fails to reveal evidence of 3 Hz spike-and-wave discharges. Ethosuximide therapy can be discontinued but the patient should be re-examined 1 month later and the EEG with hyperventilation repeated (18). If clinical seizures and/or epileptogenic discharges are recorded, continuation of drug therapy should be seriously considered.

ACKNOWLEDGMENTS

This work was supported by a grant from the Medical Research Council of Canada. The author wishes to acknowledge the expert assistance of Roberta Todd in preparing the manuscript.

REFERENCES

1. Aicardi, J. (1986) *Epilepsy in Children*, pp. 97–99. Raven Press, New York.
2. Andermann, E. (1980): Multifactorial inheritance in the epilepsies. In: *Advances in Epileptology: XIth Epilepsy International Symposium*, edited by R. Canger, F. Angeleri, and J. K. Penry, pp. 297–309. Raven Press, New York.
3. Andermann, F., and Robb, J. P. (1972): Absence status: A reappraisal following a review of 38 patients. *Epilepsia*, 13:177–187.
4. Bachmann, K., Schwartz, J., Sullivan, T., and Jauregui, L. (1986): Single sample estimate of ethosuximide clearance. *Int. J. Clin. Pharmacol. Ther. Toxicol.*, 24:546–550.
5. Bercovic, S. F., Andermann, F., Andermann, E., and Gloor, P. (1987): Concepts of absence epilepsies: Discrete syndromes or biological continuum. *Neurology (Cleveland)*, 37:993–1000.
6. Blomquist, H. K., and Zetterlund, B. (1985): Evaluation of treatment in typical absence seizures.

The roles of long-term EEG monitoring and ethosuximide. *Acta Paediatr. Scand.*, 74:409–415.
7. Browne, T. R. (1983): Ethosuximide (Zarontin) and other succinimides. In: *Epilepsy, Diagnosis and Management*, edited by T. R. Browne and R. G. Feldman, ch. 19, pp. 215–224. Little Brown, Boston.
8. Browne, T. R., Dreifuss, F. E., Dyken, P. R., Goode, D. J., Penry, J. K., Porter, R. J., White, B. G., and White, P. T. (1975): Ethosuximide in the treatment of absence (petit mal) seizures. *Neurology (Minneap.)*, 25:515–524.
9. Browne, T. R., Penry, J. K., Porter, R. J., and Dreifuss, F. E. (1974): Responsiveness before, during and after spike-wave paroxysms. *Neurology (Minneap.)*, 24:659–665.
10. Buchanan, R. A., Kinkel, A. W., and Smith, T. C. (1976): Ethosuximide dosage regimens. *Clin. Pharmacol. Ther.*, 20:213–218.
11. Callaghan, N., O'Driscoll, D., and Daley, M. (1980): A comparative study between ethosuximide and sodium valproate in the treatment of petit mal epilepsy. In: *Royal Society of Medicine International Congress and Symposium, No. 30: The place of sodium valproate in the treatment of epilepsy*, pp. 47–52. Academic Press, London.
12. Callaghan, N., O'Hara, J., O'Driscoll, D., O'Neill, B., and Daly, M. (1982): Comparative study of ethosuximide and sodium valproate in the treatment of typical absence seizures (petit mal). *Dev. Med. Child Neurol.*, 24:830–836.
13. Capek, R., and Esplin, B. (1977): Effects of ethosuximide on transmission of repetitive impulses and apparent rates of transmitter turnover in the spinal monosynaptic pathway. *J. Pharmacol. Exp. Ther.*, 201:320–325.
14. Dalby, M. A. (1969): Epilepsy and 3 per second spike-and-wave rhythms. *Acta Neurol. Scand.*, 45 (Suppl. 40):1–83.
15. Dansky, L., Andermann, E., Andermann, F., Sherwin, A. L., and Kinch, R. A. (1982): Maternal epilepsy and congenital malformations: Correlation with maternal plasma anticonvulsant levels during pregnancy. In: *Epilepsy, Pregnancy and the Child*, edited by D. Janz, M. Dam, A. Richens, L. Bossi, H. Helge, and D. Schmidt, pp. 251–258. Raven Press, New York.
16. Dansky, L., Andermann, E., and Sherwin, A. L. (1981): Maternal epilepsy and birth defects: A prospective study with monitoring of plasma anticonvulsant levels during pregnancy. In: *Advances in Epileptology: XIIth Epilepsy International Symposium*, edited by M. Dam, L. Gram, and J. K. Penry, pp. 607–612. Raven Press, New York.
17. Dreifuss, F. E. (1981): Proposals for revised clinical and electroencephalographic classification of epileptic seizures. *Epilepsia*, 22:489–501.
18. Dreifuss, F. E. (1983): Treatment of the nonconvulsive epilepsies. *Epilepsia*, 24 (Suppl. 1):S45–S54.
19. Eadie, M. J., and Tyrer, J. H. (1980): *Anticonvulsant Therapy. Pharmacological Basis and Practice,* 2nd edition, pp. 211–223. Churchill Livingstone, Edinburgh.

20. Englander, R. N., Johnson, R. N., Brickley, J. J., and Hanna, G. R. (1979): Effects of antiepileptic drugs on thalamocortical excitability. *Neurology,* 29:96–99.

21. Fischer, M., Korskjaer, G., and Pederson, E. (1965): Psychotic episodes in Zarontin treatment. *Epilepsia,* 6:325–334.

22. Fromm, G., and Crumrine, P. (1986): Ethosuximide: An update. In: *Recent Advances in Epilepsy,* edited by A. Pedley and B. S. Meldrum, pp. 279–294. Churchill Livingstone, Edinburgh.

23. Fromm, G. H., Glass, J. F., Chattha, A. S., and Martinez, A. J. (1981): Effect of anticonvulsant drugs on inhibitory and excitatory pathways. *Epilepsia,* 22:65–73.

24. Gibbs, F., Davis, H., and Lennox, W. (1935): The electroencephalogram in epilepsy and in conditions of impaired consciousness. *Arch. Neurol. Psychiatry,* 3:1133–1148.

25. Gloor, P. (1979): Generalized epilepsy with spike-and-wave discharge: A reinterpretation of its electrographic and clinical manifestations. *Epilepsia,* 20:571–588.

26. Guberman, A., Gloor, P., and Sherwin, A. L. (1975): Response of generalized penicillin epilepsy in the cat to ethosuximide and diphenylhydantoin. *Neurology (Minneap.),* 25:758–764.

27. Haerer, A. F., Buchanan, R. A., and Wiygul, F. M. (1970): Ethosuximide blood levels in epileptics. *J. Clin. Pharmacol.,* 10:370–374.

28. Janz, D. (1969): *Die Epilepsien-Spezielle Pathologie und Therapie,* p. 94. Georg Thieme, Stuttgart.

29. Jeavons, P. M., Covanis, A., and Gupta, A. H. (1980): Monotherapy with sodium valproate. *Advances in Epileptology, XI Epilepsy International Symposium,* edited by R. Canger, F. Angeleri, and J. K. Penry, pp. 415–418. Raven Press, New York.

30. Koup, J. R., Rose, J. Q., and Cohen, M. E. (1978): Ethosuximide pharmacokinetics in a pregnant patient and her newborn. *Epilepsia,* 19:535–539.

31. Kuhnz, W., Koch, S., Jakob, S., Hartmann, A., Helge, H., and Nau, H. (1984): Ethosuximide in epileptic women during pregnancy and lactation period. Placental transfer, serum concentrations in nursed infants and clinical status. *Br. J. Clin. Pharmacol.,* 18:671–677.

32. Martinovic, Z. (1983): Comparison of ethosuximide with sodium Valproate. In: *Advances in Epileptology, XIVth Epilepsy International Symposium,* edited by M. Parsonage, R. H. E. Grant, A. G. Craig, and A. A. Ward, Jr., pp. 301–305. Raven Press, New York.

33. Mattson, R. H., and Cramer, J. A. (1980): Valproic acid and ethosuximide interaction. *Ann. Neurol.,* 7:583–584.

34. McAuliff, J. J., Sherwin, A. L., Leppik, I. E., Fayle, S. A., and Pippenger, C. E. (1970): Salivary levels of anticonvulsants: A practical approach to drug monitoring. *Neurology (Minneap.),* 27:409–413.

35. Metrakos, K., and Metrakos, J. D. (1961): Genetic and electroencephalographic studies in centrencephalic epilepsy. *Neurology (Minneap.),* 11:474–483.

36. Mirsky, A. F., Duncan, C. C., and Myslobodsky, M. S. (1986): Petit mal epilepsy: A review and integration of recent information. *J. Clin. Neurophysiol.,* 3:179–208.

37. Mirski, M. A., and Ferrendelli, J. A. (1986): Selective metabolic activation of the mammillary bodies and their connections during ethosuximide-induced suppression of pentylenetetrazol seizures. *Epilepsia,* 27:194–203.

38. Nowack, W. J., Johnson, R. N., Englander, R. N., and Hanna, G. R. (1979): Effects of valproate and ethosuximide on thalamocortical excitability. *Neurology (Minneap.),* 29:96–99.

39. Okuma, T., and Kumashiro, H. (1981): Natural history and prognosis of epilepsy: Report of a multi-institutional study in Japan. *Epilepsia,* 22:35–53.

40. Penfield, W., and Jasper, H. (1954): *Epilepsy and the Functional Anatomy of the Human Brain,* pp. 3–19, Little Brown, Boston.

41. Penry, J. K., Porter, R. J., and Dreifuss, F. E. (1971): Quantitation of paroxysmal abnormal discharge in the EEG's of patients with absence (petit mal) seizures for evaluation of antiepileptic drugs. *Epilepsia,* 12:278–279.

42. Penry, J. K., Porter, R. J., and Dreifuss, F. E. (1975): Simultaneous recording of absence seizures with video tape and electroencephalography: A study of 374 seizures in 48 patients. *Brain,* 98:427–440.

43. Pisani, F., Narbone, M. C., Trunfio, C., Fazio, A., La Rosa, G., Oteri, G., and Di Perri, R. (1984): Valproic acid—ethosuximide interaction—A pharmacokinetic study. *Epilepsia,* 25:229–233.

44. Porter, R. J., and Penry, J. K. (1983) Petit mal status. In: *Advances in Neurology; Vol 34: Status Epilepticus: Mechanisms of Brain Damage and Treatment,* edited by A. V. Delgado-Escueta, C. G. Wasterlain, D. M. Trieman, and R. J. Porter, pp. 61–67. Raven Press, New York.

45. Porter, R. J., Penry, J. K., and Dreifuss, F. E. (1973): Responsiveness at the onset of spike-wave bursts. *Eletroencephalogr. Clin. Neurophysiol.,* 34:239–245.

46. Quesney, L. F. (1977): *Pathophysiology of Generalized Penicillin Epilepsy in the Cat: The Role of Cortical and Subcortical Structures.* Ph.D. Thesis, McGill University, Montreal.

47. Quesney, L. F., and Gloor, P. (1978): Generalized penicillin epilepsy in the cat: Correlation between electrophysiological data and distribution of ^{14}C-penicillin in the brain. *Epilepsia,* 19:35–45.

48. Rane, A., and Tunell, R. (1981): Ethosuximide in human milk and in the plasma of a mother and her nursed infant. *Br. J. Clin. Pharmacol.,* 12:855–858.

49. Rodin, E. A. (1968): *The Prognosis of Patients with Epilepsy.* Charles C Thomas, Springfield, Illinois.

50. Roger, J., Grangeon, H., Guey, J., and Lob, H. (1968): Psychiatric and physiological effects of ethosuximide treatment in epileptics. *Encephale,* 57:407–438.

51. Rowan, A. J., Meijer, J. W., de Beer-Pawlikowski,

N., van der Geest, P., and Meinardi, H. (1983): Valproate–ethosuximide combination therapy for refractory absence seizures. *Arch. Neurol.,* 40:797–802.

52. Santavuori, P. (1983): Absence seizures: Valproate or ethosuximide? *Acta Neurol. Scand.,* 69 (Suppl. 97):41–48.

53. Sato, S., Dreifuss, F. E., and Penry, J. K. (1976): Prognostic factors in absence seizures. *Neurology (Minneap.),* 26:788–796.

54. Sato, S., White, B. G., and Penry, J. K. (1982): Valproic acid versis ethosuximide in the treatment of absence seizures. *Neurology,* 32:157–163.

55. Schmidt, D., Beck-Mannagetta, G., Janz, D., and Koch, S. (1982): The effect of pregnancy on the course of epilepsy: A prospective study. In: *Epilepsy, Pregnancy and the Child,* edited by D. Janz, M. Dam, A. Richens, L. Bossi, H. Helge, and D. Schmidt, pp. 39–49. Raven Press, New York.

56. Sherwin, A. L. (1983): Absence Seizures. In: *Antiepileptic Drug Therapy in Pediatrics,* edited by P. L. Morselli, C. E. Pippenger, and J. K. Penry, pp. 153–161. Raven Press, New York.

57. Sherwin, A. L., Robb, J. P., and Lechter, M. (1973): Improved control of epilepsy by monitoring plasma ethosuximide. *Arch. Neurol.,* 28:178–181.

58. Shibuya, T., Fromm, G. H., and Terrence, C. F. (1987): Differential effects of ethosuximide and of

electrical stimulation inhibitory and excitatory mechanisms. *Epilepsy Res.,* 1:35–39.

59. Smith, G. A., McKauge, L., Dubetz, D., Tyrer, J. H., and Eadie, M. J. (1979): Factors influencing plasma concentrations of ethosuximide. *Clin. Pharmacokinet.,* 4:38–52.

60. Solow, E. B., and Green, J. B. (1972): The simultaneous determination of multiple anticonvulsant drug levels by gas-liquid chromatography. *Neurology (Minneap.),* 22:540–550.

61. Suzuki, M., Maruyama, H., Ishibashi, Y., Ogawa, S., Seki, T., Hoshino, M., Mackawa, K., Yo, T., and Sato, Y. (1972): A double-blind comparative trial of sodium dipropylacetate and ethosuximide in children, with special emphasis on pure petit mal seizures. *Med. Prog. (Jpn),* 82:470–488.

62. Van Wieringen, A., and Vrijlandt, C. M. (1983): Ethosuximide intoxication caused by interaction with isoniazid. *Neurology,* 33:1227–1228.

63. Wallace, S. J. (1986): Use of ethosuximide and valproate in the treatment of epilepsy. In: *Neurology Clinics,* edited by R. J. Porter and W. H. Theodore, pp. 601–616. W.B. Saunders, Philadelphia.

64. Wolfe, P., Inone, Y., Roder-Wanner, U. U., and Tsai, J. J. (1984): Psychiatric complications of absence therapy and their relation to alteration of sleep. *Epilepsia,* 25(Suppl. 1):556–559.

Antiepileptic Drugs, Third Edition, edited by
R. Levy, R. Mattson, B. Meldrum,
J. K. Penry, and F. E. Dreifuss.
Raven Press, Ltd., New York © 1989.

51

Ethosuximide

Toxicity

Fritz E. Dreifuss

All drugs are toxic in overdose, and there is great variation in sensitivity to drugs from person to person, so that a safe dose for one person may be an excessive dose for another. Even a therapeutic dose may have unavoidable side effects.

Adverse effects of ethosuximide may be divided into (a) toxic effects that are the result of overdose or unwanted reactions that may accompany a dose in the therapeutic range—these effects usually occur soon after administration of the drug and fall into the general category of acute toxicity; (b) specific organ effects, including dermatological and most hematological complications, and alterations of the immune system with the appearance of immunologic disturbances such as systemic lupus erythematosus and drug allergies; (c) drug interactions; and (d) teratogenic effects. The latter three reactions may be considered long-term drug toxicity in that they rarely occur with single-dose administration but may be observed after weeks, months, or even years of use.

The incidence of adverse drug effects varies greatly, ranging in different studies from 1% (18,30) to 9% (56), 31% (16), 33% (4), and 44% (55). Most of these are associated with direct dose-related problems.

ACUTE TOXICITY

Dose Related Side Effects

The majority of toxic effects of ethosuximide as reported in different series are accounted for by relatively few symptoms, including nausea, abdominal discomfort, drowsiness, anorexia, hiccups, and headache. Nausea, the most common side effect, usually occurs within the first few days of ethosuximide administration and is frequently alleviated by reduction of the dose. Drowsiness and anorexia likewise respond to dosage reduction. Headache often proves rather more persistent and falls into the category of unwanted accompanying reactions rather than being strictly dose related and therefore amenable to dose reduction. In the study by Browne et al. (4), 13 of 39 patients experienced side effects of ethosuximide. Nausea was described in nine instances and drowsiness five times, indicating that most of the side effects were of a benign, dose-related nature. This was also the experience in other reports (5,10,16,21,55,56).

Side Effects Unrelated to Dose

Ethosuximide has been reported to cause the exacerbation of various types of seizures. DeHaas and Kuilman, in a study of 107 patients, noted exacerbation of seizures, except for absence attacks, in seven patients (9). Gordon (18) reported that of four patients with myoclonus, two became worse after ethosuximide administration, and Friedel and Lempp (14) described the transformation of absence seizures into "grand mal" during the course of treatment with trimethadione, methsuximide, and ethosuximide in 22 of 85 patients. Todorov et al. (51) reported that exacerbation of absence seizures in a patient undergoing treatment with ethosuximide was ameliorated with phenobarbital. Most authors, however, specifically noted no instances of exacerbation of any seizure type during administration of ethosuximide (4,5,21,53,56). In view of the occurrence of generalized tonic-clonic seizures at some time during the course of absence seizures in some 25% of patients, it would not be surprising to find the emergence of generalized tonic-clonic seizures coincidentally with ethosuximide therapy in a certain number of patients, and this is the probable explanation for some, if not most, of the reported events.

Behavioral changes have been reported in persons taking ethosuximide. The psychopharmacology of antiepileptic drugs is in an unsatisfactory state because of inadequate and unsophisticated behavior evaluation. Most reports deal with persons who are taking several drugs, and most contain no mention of monitoring antiepileptic drug levels. Many of the reports do not adequately distinguish between mental or behavioral changes that may result from seizures and those that may be related to drug effects.

One of the first reports came from Fischer et al. (13) who reported on five psychotic episodes in three adult patients occurring within a few days of starting treatment with ethosuximide. The report dealt with a total of 105 patients, and the seizure types were not clearly distinguished. The psychotic episodes consisted of intermittent impairment of consciousness, anxiety, depression, and visual and auditory hallucinations, which improved following cessation of treatment with ethosuximide. All patients had a history of mental disorder. Individual cases of psychotic behavior were noted by Cohadon et al. (6), Lairy (27), and Sato et al. (41). Roger et al. (40) and Soulayrol and Roger (46) described the falling off of school performance and efficiency and, on occasion, the appearance of hallucinations and ideas of persecution. The symptoms remitted when ethosuximide was discontinued and recurred on reinstitution of treatment.

There appeared to be a reciprocal relationship between the epilepsy and the psychosis in that when seizures were controlled the psychosis remitted and vice versa. A similar phenomenon in complex partial seizures was described by Landolt (29). Guey et al. (19) reported on 25 children with absence attacks who were assessed before and after the administration of ethosuximide. They found memory and speech disturbances, particularly in the older patients and those who were receiving large doses of the drug. Fifteen of the patients were mentally retarded, no control group was included in the study, and antiepileptic drug levels were not monitored. As pointed out by Trimble and Reynolds (52), such studies should have control groups for comparison, as the EEG spike-and-wave activity of absence seizures may be related to impaired visual-motor performance (17,38).

Smith et al. (45) described a double-blind study in which verbal and full-scale IQ scores improved in nonepileptic children given ethosuximide. Browne et al. (4) studied psychometric performance in 39 children, using matched controls, and found that performance improved significantly in 17 patients treated with ethosuximide. Only one showed diminished ability because of a decrease in alertness. This group was more homogeneous than that reported by Guey et al. (19), mental retardation was less prevalent, and barbiturate administration was less pervasive. Also, the blood levels of ethosuximide were within the therapeutic range. None of the other studies included data on blood ethosuximide levels, and some of the mental symptoms may have stemmed from drug intoxication.

DELAYED SPECIFIC ORGAN EFFECTS

An idiosyncratic reaction has been defined as a peculiar and therefore unusual or rare drug reaction (3). Reasons for the reaction may be multifactorial. Strictly speaking, pharmacologists tend to regard an idiosyncratic reaction as a genetically determined abnormal reactivity to drugs, and a complete understanding of such a reaction requires knowledge of the mechanisms by which the usual drug effect is altered in the genetically variant person, of the biochemical abnormality involved, and of the pattern of inheritance. For example, prolonged apnea occurring after induced hemolytic anemia, and acute intermittent porphyria enhanced by drugs are true genetically determined idiosyncrasies on the basis of individual genotypes. In this context, the reactions to antiepileptic drugs, including ethosuximide, described below are not truly idiosyncratic, although further study may show them to be related to a genetic trait, at least as one of a number of factors.

Skin rashes have been frequently described, as have erythema multiforme and the Stevens-Johnson syndrome (36,49), in the course of treatment with ethosuximide. The dermatological complications usually remit after withdrawal of the drug, but steroid therapy is sometimes indicated, especially in the more severe cases. Teoh and Chan (50) reported that lupus erythematosus and scleroderma were reversed after withdrawal of medication. Readministration of ethosuximide for the treatment of persistent seizures resulted in a relapse with predominant sclerodermatous features that

again resolved after ethosuximide withdrawal.

Systemic lupus erythematosus (SLE) or a lupus-like syndrome as an adverse reaction to antiepileptic drugs has been the subject of many reports (1,2,5,8,22,31,35, 44,45,50). It is likely that the SLE-activating properties of anticonvulsant drugs reside in their potential to induce antinuclear antibodies. Drugs that activate SLE may do so by pharmacological properties of their own or by causing allergic reactions, which in turn bring about SLE (1). Many persons develop antinuclear antibodies without developing SLE, and it may be that only predisposed individuals among those with antinuclear antibodies will become symptomatic. Most anticonvulsants elicit antibodies primarily directed to soluble nucleoprotein, but each may do so by altering different sites in the nucleoprotein molecule. Development of DNA antibodies may result from action of the drugs on an antigenic site of nucleoprotein closely related to the nucleic acid or from the fact that patients who develop anti-DNA antibodies have underlying SLE as a basis for their seizures (1). The lupus-like illness consists of fever, malar rash, arthritis, lymphadenopathy, and, on occasion, pleural effusions, myocarditis, and pericarditis. Most patients developing a lupus-like syndrome have a relatively benign, albeit prolonged, course after cessation of the medication. Singsen et al. (44) reported no improvement in one of five affected children after withdrawal of ethosuximide, and this patient had renal involvement, which is an unusual organ involvement in drug-induced lupus.

Three types of lupus-like reactions have been described. In one type, the patients develop only antinuclear antibodies. Asymptomatic children with antinuclear antibodies should be carefully observed, but they do not usually develop evidence of lupus. In the second type, a classic lupus-like illness develops. Silverman et al. (43) described a third type in which clinical and chemical evidence of an immunologic disorder, including a nephrotic syndrome, occurs. Results of lupus preparations are negative and antinuclear antibodies are absent, and the apparent immunologic disorder abates on cessation of ethosuximide.

Nishiyama et al. (37) described two cases of autoimmune thyroiditis in patients receiving antiepileptic therapy, including one taking ethosuximide.

There is one report of adverse effects of anticonvulsant therapy, including ethosuximide, on renal allograft survival (54). This may occur through interference with the immune system or alteration of metabolism of administered corticosteroids, leading to less effective immunosuppression and hence a higher incidence of graft failure.

Basal ganglia involvement has been reported several times. Some of these have been acute reactions to ethosuximide similar to those seen after administration of some phenothiazines (12,25). The symptoms respond to withdrawal of the drug or the administration of diphenhydramine hydrochloride. More severe bradykinesia, as a manifestation of ethosuximide toxicity (among other drugs administered) and occurring after several years of treatment, has been described (38), as has parkinsonian syndrome (16).

Blood dyscrasias are among the most serious side effects of treatment with antiepileptic drugs (4,5,7,11,24,26,33,47,55). Mature cell lines may be damaged, in which case often only one element is involved, resulting in a disorder such as thrombocytopenia. In more severe cases of bone marrow hypoplasia with involvement of less differentiated cell types, pancytopenia or aplastic anemia is the result. Bone marrow depression may be the result of an allergic phenomenon or of a toxic effect. In the former, the platelets have been implicated as targets of allergic drug reactions, and antibodies to the drug have been demonstrated in the serum of patients developing thrombocytopenic purpura. In chloramphenicol toxicity and in the case of the anticonvulsant drugs, it would appear that bone marrow toxicity is a more likely explanation than an allergic phenomenon.

Depression of blood-forming elements has been mentioned sporadically in many of the larger studies of patients treated with ethosuximide (4,5,24,55). Further, specific cases were reported by Koutsoulieris (26), who reported a case of fatal bone marrow aplasia, and by Spittler (47), who reported a fatal case of agranulocytosis in a 7-year-old patient who had been treated for 9 weeks when the condition was diagnosed and who subsequently succumbed to complications. Cohn (7) reported a child who died approximately 6 months after the institution of ethosuximide therapy. Buchanan (5) noted two fatal cases, one an 11-year-old child who developed pancytopenia some 7 months after beginning treatment and another a 6-year-old who developed aplastic bone marrow some 6 weeks after the addition of ethosuximide to the regimen.

In the hope of detecting bone marrow depression early, it is generally recommended that periodic blood counts be performed at no greater than monthly intervals for the duration of treatment with ethosuximide and that the dosage be reduced or the drug discontinued if the total white blood cell count falls below 3,500 or the proportion of granulocytes falls below 25% of the total white blood cell count. Prescribing physicians are advised to observe patients for the development of fever, sore throat, or cutaneous and other hemorrhages, in addition to periodic hematological monitoring.

In the author's experience, ethosuximide-related granulocytopenia frequently responds to reduction of the dose and does not always require cessation of therapy, indicating that to some extent at least, this may be a dose-related phenomenon.

DRUG INTERACTIONS

No significant interactions between ethosuximide and other antiepileptic drugs have been reported. Enzyme induction does not appear to occur to any significant degree (15). There is no significant increase in the plasma concentration of phenobarbital derived from primidone with the addition of ethosuximide as there is with phenytoin (38), but one report suggests that some increase does occur (42). Another report suggests that the plasma phenytoin concentration increases with the administration of ethosuximide (28).

TERATOGENIC EFFECTS

It is generally accepted that birth defects occur with increased frequency in children born of mothers with epilepsy who were exposed to anticonvulsant drugs in pregnancy and that this frequency exceeds that occurring in children born of mothers with epilepsy who did not take drugs during pregnancy (23,32,34). The drugs most often implicated are phenytoin and phenobarbital, and these are, of course, the most commonly used drugs. Trimethadione, although now rarely used, carries by far the greatest risk of teratogenicity.

Little information is available concerning the risk to the fetus exposed to ethosuximide. The primary indication for the administration of ethosuximide is absence seizures, and these rarely persist into the childbearing years. Absence seizures appear to be largely age-limited; they tend to abate in the teenage years and no longer require treatment with the drug. Experimental data (48), however, suggest that ethosuximide is considerably less teratogenic than phenytoin, carbamazepine, phenobarbital, or primidone.

Teratogenic effects must be distinguished from mutagenic or genetic effects. The former are more likely to result from toxic affliction or organogenesis, either directly or through metabolic changes (folic acid metabolism abnormalities have come under scrutiny). Certain agents, of course, have mutagenic and carcinogenic effects as well as teratogenic activity, but most teratogens are neither mutagenic nor carcinogenic. The latter actions require heritable alteration in a cell line, such as cytogenetic abnormalities of the translocation type.

In general, it is recommended that the medication regimen be kept as simple as possible during pregnancy, with administration of the smallest possible number of agents. Only rarely will it be necessary to continue antiabsence drugs in the childbearing age group.

SUMMARY

The side effects associated with ethosuximide include dose-related reactions such as nausea, gastrointestinal discomfort, drowsiness, and anorexia. These are common, relatively trivial in the context of overall patient management, and usually respond to dosage reduction.

Side effects not related to the dose include exacerbation of various types of seizures. This is a rare complication and more likely represents the natural history of epilepsy than a cause-and-effect relationship. Behavioral changes, including transient psychoses, and interference with cognitive function, apart from some idiosyncratic phenomena, may be related to drug intoxication, as they are not prominent when blood ethosuximide levels are within the therapeutic range.

Delayed specific organ sensitivities, including hematological, dermatological, and immunologic disorders, represent the most serious and potentially lethal complications. These are rare and, in some degree, avoidable by careful monitoring and ameliorable by early intervention.

Neither drug interactions nor teratogenicity is believed to play a significant role in ethosuximide pharmacotherapy.

REFERENCES

1. Alarcon-Seqovia, D., Fishbein, E., Reyes, P. A., Dies, H., and Shwadsky, S. (1972): Antinuclear antibodies in patients on anticonvulsant therapy. *Clin. Exp. Immunol.*, 12:39–47.
2. Beernink, D., and Miller, J. J. (1973): Anticonvulsant induced antinuclear antibodies and lupus like disease in children. *J. Pediatr.*, 82:113–117.
3. Booker, H. E. (1975): Idiosyncratic reactions to the antiepileptic drugs. *Epilepsia*, 16:171–181.
4. Browne, T. R., Dreifuss, F. E., Dyken, P. R., Goode, D. J., Penry, J. K., Porter, R. J., White, P. T., and White, B. G. (1975): Ethosuximide in the treatment of absence (petit mal) epilepsy. *Neurology (Minneap.)*, 25:515–525.
5. Buchanan, R. A. (1972): Ethosuximide: Toxicity. In: *Antiepileptic Drugs*, 1st edition, edited by D. M. Woodbury, J. K. Penry, and R. P. Schmidt, pp. 449–454. Raven Press, New York.
6. Cohadon, F., Loiseau, P., and Cohadon S. (1964): Results of treatment of certain forms of epilepsy of the petit mal type by ethosuximide. *Rev. Neurol.*, 110:201–207.
7. Cohn, R. (1968): A neuropathological study of a case of petit mal epilepsy. *Electroencephalogr. Clin. Neurophysiol.*, 24:282.
8. Dabbous, I. A., and Idriss, H. M. (1970): Occurrence of systemic lupus erythematosus in association with ethosuximide therapy. *J. Pediatr.*, 76:617–620.
9. deHaas, A. M. L., and Kuilman, M. (1964): Ethosuximide (α-ethyl-α-methylsuccinimide) and grand mal. *Epilepsia*, 5:90–96.
10. deHaas, A. M. L., and Stoel, L. M. K. (1959): Experiences with α-ethyl-α-methylsuccinimide in the treatment of epilepsy. *Epilepsia*, 1:501–511.
11. DeVries, S. I. (1965): Haematological aspects during treatment with anticonvulsant drugs. *Epilepsia*, 7:1–15.
12. Ehyai, A., Kilroy, A. W., and Fenicheal, G. M. (1978): Dyskinesia and akathisia induced by ethosuximide. *Am. J. Dis. Child*, 132:527–528.
13. Fischer, M., Korskjeer, G., and Pederson, E. (1965): Psychotic episodes in Zarondan treatment. *Epilepsia*, 6:325–334.
14. Friedel, B., and Lempp, R. (1962): Grand-mal Provokation bei der Behandlung Kindlicher petit-mal mit Oxazolidinen oder Succinimiden und ihre therapeutischen Konsequenzen. *Z. Kinderheilkd.*, 87:42–51.
15. Gilbert, J. C., Scott, A. K., Galloway, D. B., and Petrie, J. C. (1974): Ethosuximide: Liver enzyme induction and D-glucaric acid excretion. *Br. J. Clin. Pharmacol.*, 1:249–252.
16. Goldensohn, E. S., Hardie, J., and Borea, E.

(1962): Ethosuximide in the treatment of epilepsy. *J.A.M.A.*, 180:840–842.
17. Goode, D. J., Penry, J. K., and Dreifuss, F. E. (1970): Effects of paroxysmal spike-wave on continuous motor performance. *Epilepsia*, 11:241–254.
18. Gordon, N. (1961): Treatment of epilepsy with α-ethyl-α-methylsuccinimide. (P.M. 671). *Neurology (Minneap.)*, 11:266–268.
19. Guey, J., Charles, C., Coquery, C., Roger, J., and Soulayrol, R. (1967): Study of psychological effects of ethosuximide (Zarontin) on 25 children suffering from petit mal epilepsy. *Epilepsia*, 8:129–141.
20. Hammond, W. A. (1874): *Clinical Lectures on Diseases of the Nervous System.* T. M. B. Cross, New York.
21. Heathfield, K. W. G., and Jewesbury, E. C. O. (1964): Treatment of petit mal with ethosuximide: Follow-up report. *Br. Med. J.*, 3:616.
22. Jacobs, J. C. (1963): Systemic lupus erythematosus in childhood. Report of 35 cases, with discussion of seven apparently induced by anticonvulsant medication, and of prognosis and treatment. *Pediatrics*, 32:257.
23. Janz, D. (1975): The teratogenic risk of antiepileptic drugs. *Epilepsia*, 16:159–169.
24. Kiorboe, E., Paludan, J., Trolle, E., and Overvad, E. (1964): Zarontin (ethosuximide) in the treatment of petit mal and related disorders. *Epilepsia*, 5:83–89.
25. Kirschberg, G. J. (1975): Dyskinesia—An unusual reaction to ethosuximide. *Arch. Neurol.*, 32:137–138.
26. Koutsoulieris, E. (1967): Granulopenia and thrombocytopenia after ethosuximide. *Lancet*, 2:310–311.
27. Lairy, C. C. (1964): Psychotic signs in epileptics during treatment with ethosuximide. *Rev. Neurol.*, 110:225–226.
28. Lander, C. M., Eadie, M. J., and Tyrer, J. (1975): Interactions between anticonvulsants. *Proc. Aust. Assoc. Neurol.*, 12:111–116.
29. Landolt, H. (1958): Serial electroencephalographic investigations during psychotic episodes in epileptic patients and during schizophrenic attacks. In: *Lectures on Epilepsy*, edited by A. M. L. deHaas. Elsevier, Amsterdam.
30. Livingstone, S., Pauli, L., and Najimabadi, A. (1952): Ethosuximide in the treatment of epilepsy. *J.A.M.A.*, 180:104–107.
31. Livingstone, S., Rodriguez, H., Greene, C. A., and Pauli, L. (1968): Systemic lupus erythematous. Occurrence in association with ethosuximide therapy. *J.A.M.A.*, 203:731–732.
32. Lowe, C. R. (1973): Congenital malformations among infants born to epileptic women. *Obstet. Gynecol. Surv.*, 28:493–494.
33. Mann, L. B., and Habenicht, H. A. (1962): Fatal bone marrow aplasia associated with administration of ethosuximide (Zarontin) for petit mal epilepsy. *Bull. Los Angeles Neurol. Soc.*, 27:173–176.
34. Meyer, J. G. (1973): Teratological effects of anti-

convulsants and the effects on pregnancy and birth. *Eur. Neurol.,* 10:179–190.

35. Monnet, P., Salle, B., Poncet, J., Gauthier, J., Philippe, N., and Germain, D. (1967): Disseminated lupus erythematosus induced by ethosuximide in a girl aged 6. *Rev. Med. Dijon.,* 2:319–330.

36. Mueller, K. (1963): Erythema exudativum multiforme majus (Stevens-Johnson syndrome) infolge Suxinutin-Uberempfindlichkeit. *Z. Kinderheilkd.,* 88:548–563.

37. Nishiyama, J., Matsukura, M., Fugimoto, S., and Matsuda, I. (1983): Reports of 2 cases of antoimmune thyroiditis while receiving anticonvulsant therapy. *Europ. J. Pediatr.,* 140:116–117.

38. Porter, R. J., Penry, J. K., and Dreifuss, F. E. (1973): Responsiveness at the onset of spike-wave bursts. *Electroencephalogr. Clin. Neurophysiol.,* 34:239–245.

39. Prensky, A. L., DeVivo, D. C., and Palkes, H. (1971): Severe bradykinesia as a manifestation of toxicity in antiepileptic medications. *J. Pediatr.,* 78:700–704.

40. Roger, J., Grangeon, H., Guey, J., and Lob, H. (1968): Psychiatric and psychological complications of ethosuximide treatment in epileptics. *Encephale,* 57:407–438.

41. Sato, T., Kondo, Y., Matsuo, T., Iwata, H., Okuyama, Y., and Aoki, Y. (1965): Clinical experiences of ethosuximide (Zarontin) in therapy-resistent epileptics. *Brain Nerve (Tokyo),* 17:958–964.

42. Schmidt, D. (1975): The effect of phenytoin and ethosuximide on primidone metabolism in patients with epilepsy. *J. Neurol.,* 209:115–123.

43. Silverman, S. H., Gribetz, D., and Rausen, A. R. (1978): Nephrotic syndrome associated with ethosuccimide. *Am. J. Dis. Child,* 132:99.

44. Singsen, B. H., Fishman, L., and Hanson, V. (1976): Antinuclear antibodies and lupus-like syndromes in children receiving anticonvulsants. *Pediatrics,* 57:529–534.

45. Smith, L. W., Phillips, M. J., and Guard, H. L. (1968): Psychometric study of children with learning problems and 14-6 positive spike EEG patterns, treated with ethosuximide (Zarontin) and placebo. *Arch. Dis. Child.,* 43:616–619.

46. Soulayrol, R., and Roger, J. (1970): Adverse psychiatric effects of antiepileptic drugs. *Rev. Neuropsychiatr. Infant,* 18:591.

47. Spittler, J. F. (1974): Agranulocytosis due to ethosuximide with a fatal outcome. *Klin. Paediatr.,* 186:364–366.

48. Sullivan, F. M., and McElhatton, P. R. (1977): A comparison of the teratogenic activity of the antiepileptic drugs carbamazepine, clonazepam, ethosuximide, phenobarbital, phenytoin and primidone in mice. *Toxicol. Appl. Pharmacol.,* 40:365–378.

49. Taaffe, A., and O'Brien, C. (1975): A case of Stevens-Johnson syndrome associated with the anticonvulsants sulthiame and ethosuximide. *Br. Dent. J.,* 138:172–174.

50. Teoh, P. C., and Chan, H. L. (1975): Lupus-scleroderma syndrome induced by ethosuximide. *Arch. Dis. Child,* 50:658–661.

51. Todorov, A. B., Lenn, N. J., and Gabor, A. J. (1978): Exacerbation of generalized non-convulsive seizures with ethosuximide therapy. *Arch. Neurol.,* 35:389–391.

52. Trimble, M. R., and Reynolds, E. H. (1976): Anticonvulsant drugs and mental symptoms. *Psychol. Med.,* 6:169–178.

53. Vossen, R. (1958): The anticonvulsive effect of succinimides. *Dtsch. Med. Wochenschr.,* 83:1227–1230.

54. Wassner, S. J., Pennisi, A. J., Malekzadeh, M. H., and Fine, R. N. (1976): The adverse effect of anticonvulsant therapy on renal allograft survival. A preliminary report. *J. Pediatr.,* 88:134–137.

55. Weinstein, A. W., and Allen, R. J. (1966): Ethosuximide treatment of petit mal seizures. A study of 87 pediatric patients. *Am. J. Dis. Child,* 111:63–67.

56. Zimmerman, F. T., and Burgemeister, B. B. (1958): A new drug for petit mal epilepsy. *Neurologr (Minneap.),* 8:769–776.

Antiepileptic Drugs, Third Edition, edited by
R. Levy, R. Mattson, B. Meldrum,
J. K. Penry, and F. E. Dreifuss.
Raven Press, Ltd., New York © 1989.

52

Other Succinimides

Methsuximide

Thomas R. Browne

Methsuximide (N,2-dimethyl-2-phenyl-succinimide, Celontin) and the other succinimide antiepileptic drugs, ethosuximide (Zarontin) and phensuximide (Milontin), are all derivatives of a five-membered succinimide ring. Animal screening tests of numerous succinimide derivatives for antiepileptic activity (9,10,24) show that (a) methyl and ethyl substitutions at the 2 and 3 positions produce drugs that are more effective against seizures induced by pentylenetetrazol (PTZ) than against maximal electroshock (MES) seizures, (b) methylation at the 5 position increases activity against PTZ seizures, (c) activity against PTZ seizures decreases with increasing length of alkyl chain substitutions at the 2, 3, and 5 positions, and (d) phenyl substitution at the 2 and 3 positions decreases activity against PTZ seizures and increases activity against MES seizures.

A drug's effectiveness against seizures induced by PTZ in animals is thought to correlate with clinical efficacy against absence seizures, and activity against MES seizures in animals is thought to correlate with clinical activity against tonic-clonic and complex partial seizures (see Chapter 5). The rank order of the therapeutic index of the succinimides against PTZ seizures in animals is from most to least effective: (a) ethosuximide, (b) methsuximide and (c) phensuximide, and against MES seizures in animals is from most to least effective: (a) methsuximide, (b) phensuximide and (c) ethosuximide (10). Clinically, ethosuximide is more effective than methsuximide against absence seizures, and methsuximide has some efficacy against complex partial seizures, whereas ethosuximide has almost none.

CHEMISTRY AND METHODS OF DETERMINATION

Methsuximide (Fig. 1) has a molecular weight of 203.23 and a melting point of 52°C. The solubility in water at pH 7.0 (25°C) is 2.8 mg/ml (17). Methsuximide is prepared by the action of methylamine on methylphenylsuccinic acid (25). The drug is marketed in the United States as 150-mg and 300-mg capsules.

Methsuximide is rapidly demethylated to form 2-methyl-2-phenylsuccinimide (*N*-desmethylmethsuximide), (Fig. 2). Only *N*-desmethylmethsuximide accumulates in the plasma in detectable quantities during long-term methsuximide administration (6,12,16,17,25,26,32,33). Gibbs et al. (16) reported no plasma methsuximide concentrations above 1 μg/ml in more than 100 patients on long-term methsuximide therapy.

Colorimetric and gas-liquid chromatographic methods have been used for the de-

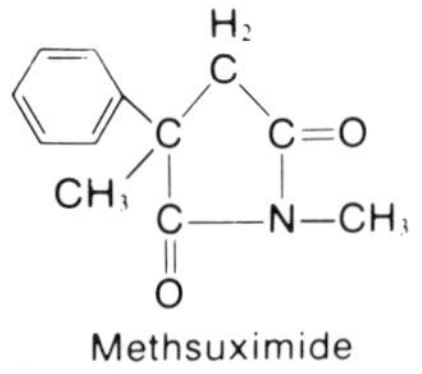

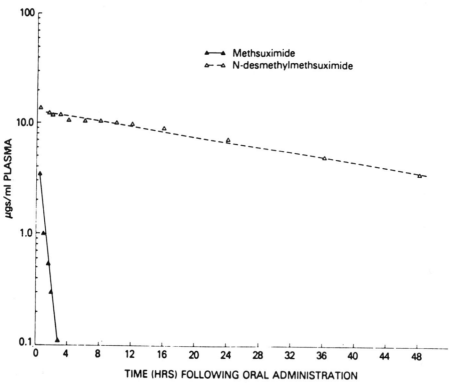

FIG. 1. Structure of methsuximide.

termination of methsuximide in biological fluids (12,17,35), but their sensitivity is not sufficient to detect the low concentrations of methsuximide present in plasma after administration of the drug at typical dosing rates (26,32) (see Fig. 2). There are, however, two gas chromatographic-mass spectrometric (GC-MS) methods with sufficient sensitivity (0.1 μg/ml) to detect the usual plasma concentrations of methsuximide and N-desmethylmethsuximide (26,32).

For routine therapeutic drug monitoring, only the plasma concentration of N-desmethylmethsuximide needs to be determined (6,16,26,32). Szabo and Browne (33) reported a simple isocratic high-performance liquid chromatographic method for simultaneous determination of N-desmethylmethsuximide along with phenytoin, phenobarbital, primidone, carbamazepine, and ethosuximide in plasma (Fig. 3).

ABSORPTION, DISTRIBUTION, AND EXCRETION

In humans, maximum plasma concentration of methsuximide occurs 1 to 4 hr after an oral dose (17). Peak plasma levels of methsuximide (may actually have been N-desmethylmethsuximide) occurred 4 hr after oral administration to two dogs (17).

FIG. 2. Plasma concentration time course for methsuximide and N-desmethylmethsuximide after a single 1,200-mg dose of methsuximide. From Porter et al., ref. 26, with permission.

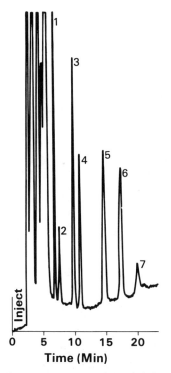

FIG. 3. Chromatogram of 5-µl injection of serum sample supplemented to give the following concentrations of drugs: (**1**) ethosuximide 20 µg/ml, (**2**) primidone 5 µg/ml, (**3**) phenobarbital 15 µg/ml, (**4**) *N*-desmethylmethsuximide 10 µg/ml, (**5**) tolybarb 10 µg/ml (internal standard), (**6**) phenytoin 10 µg/ml, (**7**) carbamazepine 4 µg/ml. From Szabo and Browne, ref. 33, with permission.

The disappearance of [^{14}C]methsuximide from the stomach and small intestine of the rat was found to be first-order, with an elimination half-life of 52 min from the stomach and 17 min from the small intestine (25). After 6 hr 87% was absorbed from the rat gastrointestinal tract (25).

Methsuximide is a lipid-soluble compound and rapidly distributes to lipid-containing tissues of animals, including fat, kidney, liver, and adrenal glands (17,25). Methsuximide crosses the blood-brain barrier (17,25).

Little, if any, methsuximide is excreted unchanged in humans (17) or dogs (25). In dogs, methsuximide is excreted primarily as conjugated metabolites, especially α-(*p*-hydroxyphenyl)-α-methylsuccinimide and *N*-methyl-α-(*p*-hydroxyphenyl)-α-methylsuccinimide (25). The metabolites of methsuximide in humans are discussed in the following section.

BIOTRANSFORMATION AND CLINICAL PHARMACOKINETICS

Methsuximide is rapidly converted to *N*-desmethylmethsuximide with an elimination half-life of 1 to 2.6 hr (17,26,32). *N*-Desmethylmethsuximide is then slowly metabolized, with an apparent elimination half-life of 34 to 80 hr (6,16,26). The metabolite accumulates to steady-state serum concentrations that are, on the average, about 600 to 800 times higher than the concentration of the parent drug methsuximide (25,26,32). The following observations indicate that the metabolite is probably the effective agent in patients receiving methsuximide: (a) plasma *N*-desmethylmethsuximide levels are much higher than methsuximide levels, (b) methsuximide and *N*-desmethylmethsuximide are similarly efficacious against PTZ and MES seizures in animals (9), and (c) in a small clinical trial, the efficacy of methsuximide and *N*-desmethylmethsuximide against absence seizures was similar (37).

The major urinary metabolites of methsuximide were hydroxylated at the 3 and 4 positions of the phenyl ring by an epoxide-diol pathway (19), but because the analytical method involved methylation, the relative proportions of hydroxylated methsuximide and hydroxylated *N*-desmethylmethsuximide in the urine were not determined. The following substances are lesser urinary metabolites of methsuximide: unmetabolized methsuximide, *N*-desmethyl-2 - hydroxy - methyl - 2 - phenylsuccinimide, *N*,2-dimethyl-3-hydroxy-2-phenylsuccinimide, and a dihydrodiol derivative (17, 19,25).

N-Desmethylmethsuximide and pheny-toin share a common arene oxidase step in their major route of metabolism (19) (see Chapter 12). This is the presumed site of major interactions between these two drugs (see below). The arene oxidase pathway exhibits nonlinear (dose-dependent) pharmacokinetics for phenytoin at therapeutic plasma concentrations in humans (see Chapter 12); This raises the possibility that N-desmethylmethsuximide may also exhibit the same pharmacokinetic profile, and Browne et al. (6) have presented indirect evidence for this possibility. If N-desmethylmethsuximide has nonlinear pharmacokinetics, its elimination half-life would be longer at steady-state serum concentrations than in single-dose studies (5,6,7).

The package insert states that increases in the methsuximide dosing rate may be made at weekly intervals. However, the dosing rate should only be increased at intervals of 14 days or longer because (a) a drug's accumulation half-life should be similar to its elimination half-life, and five half-lives are required to attain a steady-state plasma concentration of N-desmethylmethsuximide (6), and (b) the elimination half-life of N-desmethylmethsuximide at low plasma concentrations is 34 to 80 hr and may be longer at steady-state concentrations (see above). If the methsuximide dosing rate is increased at weekly intervals, the plasma concentration of N-desmethyl-methsuximide will rise rapidly because of the combined effects of the continuing rise in plasma concentration from the previous dosing rate which had not risen to a steady-state level, and the new increase in dosing rate. This rise may lead to toxic plasma concentrations of N-desmethyl-methsuximide (6).

RELATIONSHIP OF PLASMA CONCENTRATION TO SEIZURE CONTROL

The plasma concentration of methsuximide in patients taking the usual doses of the drug is so small that it can be measured accurately only by GC-MS (6,26,32). There is no apparent correlation between the dose of methsuximide and its antiepileptic effect or plasma concentration, presumably because methsuximide is so rapidly converted to N-desmethylmethsuximide (6).

There is a significant correlation between the methsuximide dose and the plasma concentration of N-desmethylmethsuximide (6,32). On average, the plasma concentration of N-desmethylmethsuximide (in μg/ml) is 1.6 to 2.0 times the daily dose of methsuximide (in mg/kg) (6,32). Several studies indicate that the therapeutic plasma concentration of N-desmethylmethsuximide ranges from 10 to 40 μg/ml (6,11,26,32,36).

DRUG INTERACTIONS

Patients taking methsuximide in addition to phenytoin and/or phenobarbital have higher plasma N-desmethylmethsuximide concentrations than patients taking methsuximide alone (27). The addition of methsuximide to a regimen of phenytoin or phenobarbital results in an appreciable increase in the plasma concentrations of the latter two drugs in many patients (6,27,31). These observed interactions among phenytoin, phenobarbital, and N-desmethyl-methsuximide probably occur as a result of competition for the arene oxidase metabolic pathway shared by all three drugs.

Browne et al. (6) reported that the addition of methsuximide to primidone was accompanied by a significant 17% increase ($p < 0.05$) in the serum concentration of phenobarbital derived from primidone. The addition of methsuximide to carbamazepine was accompanied by a 23% decrease in the plasma carbamazepine concentration in six patients ($p = 0.08$) (6).

DOSE-RELATED SIDE EFFECTS

Large series report side effects from methsuximide in 11% to 57% (median, 35%)

of patients taking the drug (Table 1). The side effects usually do not abate or disappear with continued drug administration, and methsuximide often has to be discontinued. Some of the drowsiness, irritability, and ataxia associated with methsuximide therapy may be due to the drug's interference with the elimination of phenobarbital or phenytoin rather than to a direct toxic effect of methsuximide or its metabolites.

Four patients experiencing methsuximide overdose all recovered without sequelae (2,15,21,30). Methsuximide overdose is characterized by stupor and coma, which may develop slowly or may have a biphasic (coma–more alert–coma) course. The late worsening may be due to conversion of methsuximide to *N*-desmethylmethsuximide or to methsuximide's interference with metabolism of other antiepileptic drugs. Other clinical features of methsuximide overdosage include respiratory depression, central neurogenic hyperventilation, increased reflexes, decreased reflexes, myoclonus, and second-degree heart block. Charcoal hemoperfusion was employed in one case and resulted in a high rate of *N*-desmethylmethsuximide clearance and rapid clinical improvement (22). A single case of massive combined overdosage of methsuximide and primidone resulted in flaccid coma, respiratory arrest, hypotension, and death (20).

IDIOSYNCRATIC SIDE EFFECTS

Extensive toxicity testing of methsuximide in animals showed no abnormalities on hematologic and chemical tests of blood (10). Autopsy studies of mice, rats, dogs, and monkeys showed no abnormalities except for "mild centrilobular hepatic necrosis" in rats receiving 600 mg/kg of methsuximide daily (10). These changes were thought to be reversible and of no functional consequence.

No serious hepatic damage has ever been reported in humans taking methsuximide. Dow et al. (13) found an increase in cephalin flocculation in 2 of 62 patients taking methsuximide, as well as other antiepileptic drugs.

Trolle et al. (34) reported a case of transient leukopenia in which blood cell counts returned to normal while the patient was still taking methsuximide, and described a patient with multiple small bruises in which a platelet count was not performed. Stenzel et al. (31) observed another case of appar-

TABLE 1. *Incidence of side effects of ethosuximide and methsuximide in series with 50 or more patients*

Side effects	Ethosuximide[a]		Methsuximide[b]	
	Range (%)	Median (%)	Range (%)	Median (%)
Drowsiness	0–16	7	0–28	16
Gastrointestinal disturbances (anorexia, nausea, vomiting, or abdominal pain)	4–29	13	2–30	6
Hiccups	0–5	0	0–6	0
Ataxia	0–1	0	0–13	6
Dizziness	0–4	1	0–13	0
Irritability	0	0	0–6	0
Rash	0–6	0	0–17	6
Leukopenia	0–7	0	0–2	0
Any side effect	26–46	37	11–57	35

[a] Based on 12 published reports.
[b] Based on 8 published reports.
From Browne, ref. 4, with permission.

ently transient leukopenia. The only reported fatal blood dyscrasia associated with methsuximide was a case of pancytopenia occurring in a middle-aged woman 3 months after beginning methsuximide (18). It is not certain that methsuximide was the cause of the pancytopenia because the woman had breast carcinoma and was taking four other medications.

Neonatal hemorrhage has occurred after combined maternal therapy with methsuximide and metharbital (3). Reversible osteomalacia was found in a patient on methsuximide monotherapy (1). Other rare complications of methsuximide therapy are behavioral changes, confusion, diplopia, headache, periorbital edema, extrapyramidal reactions, and Stevens-Johnson syndrome (11,17,25). Methsuximide may precipitate attacks of hepatic porphyria in susceptible persons (28). Rashes can occur with methsuximide therapy (see Table 1).

MECHANISM OF ACTION

The mechanism of action of methsuximide is unknown and possibly multiple. Methsuximide has a heterocyclic ring with alkyl substitutions and exhibits activity against PTZ seizures in animals and absence seizures in humans. This suggests that it may have a mechanism of action similar to that of ethosuximide (see Chapter 46). Methsuximide also has a phenyl substituent and exhibits activity against MES seizures in animals and complex partial seizures in humans. Thus, it may have a mechanism of action similar to that of phenytoin (see Chapter 9).

THERAPEUTIC USE

Absence Seizures

The treatment of absence seizures is the only indication for methsuximide approved by the FDA. In four series with 20 or more

patients in which methsuximide was used as an adjunctive drug for absence seizures, the seizures were completely controlled in 0% to 31% of patients, and the frequency of absence seizures was reduced by 50% or more in 13% to 66% of patients (13,14,23,38). In the one study in which methsuximide was used in previously untreated absence seizures, only 20% of the patients had a 50% or greater reduction in frequency of seizures, and in none were the seizures completely controlled (23).

Ethosuximide has many advantages over methsuximide for the treatment of absence seizures. With ethosuximide, absence seizures are controlled in a higher percentage of cases (see Chapter 50), and the common side effects of succinimides (drowsiness, gastrointestinal disturbances) are less severe and less persistent (see Table 1). Furthermore, methods for determination of plasma ethosuximide concentrations are more generally available, and ethosuximide has fewer interactions with other antiepileptic drugs (see Chapter 50).

Methsuximide is indicated for the treatment of absence seizures only when less toxic drugs fail to produce adequate control.

Complex Partial Seizures

In seven series with 18 or more patients in which methsuximide was used as an adjunctive drug for complex partial seizures, complete seizure control was obtained in 4% to 30% of patients, and a 50% or greater reduction in seizure frequency was obtained in 25% to 80% of patients (6,8,11,14,29,36,39). Three recent series (6,11,36), which are more applicable to contemporary practice, indicate that many patients who have failed a trial of phenytoin and phenobarbital will have a 50% or greater reduction in seizure frequency immediately after the addition of methsuximide, but that a majority of patients who have failed a trial of phenytoin, phenobarbital, and carbamazepine will not have the same response to the addition of methsuximide. These studies also indicate that some patients will become tolerant to the antiepileptic effect of methsuximide after 4 to 7 months of maximal therapy and that the response rate may be higher in patients with focal spike-and-wave EEG patterns (complexes consisting of a spike, often blunt, followed by a slow wave at a frequency of 1 to 2 Hz occurring predominantly in one temporal region).

In the one study in which methsuximide was used in previously untreated complex partial seizures, a 50% or greater reduction in seizure frequency occurred in 27% of patients, and 18% of patients experienced complete seizure control (23).

Other Seizure Types

Stenzel et al. (31) reported some success with methsuximide in patients with "complex atypical absences" and "slow spike-wave, or sharp and slow". Trials of methsuximide for tonic-clonic and simple partial seizures generally have been discouraging.

Dosage and Administration

The usual starting dose of methsuximide is 300 mg per day. The daily dose may be increased in increments of 150 mg or 300 mg per day at intervals of at least 2 weeks (see above). The smaller increment is preferred in small children and persons of any age taking other antiepileptic drugs because of the longer elimination half-life and therefore reduced clearance of *N*-desmethylmethsuximide. Dosage is increased until seizures are controlled, toxicity develops, or a maximum daily dosing rate of 1,200 mg is reached.

CONVERSION

Conversion factor:

$$CF = \frac{1000}{\text{mol. wt.}} = \frac{1000}{203.23} = 4.92$$

Conversion:

$$(\mu g/ml) \times 4.92 = (\mu moles/liter)$$

$$(\mu moles/liter) \div 4.92 = (\mu g/ml)$$

ACKNOWLEDGMENT

This work was supported in part by the Veterans Administration.

REFERENCES

1. Aponte, C. J., and Petrelli, M. P. (1973): Anticonvulsants and vitamin D metabolism. *J.A.M.A.*, 225:1248.
2. Baehler, R. W., Work, J., Smith, W., and Dominic, J. A. (1980): Charcoal hemoperfusion in therapy of methsuximide and phenytoin overdose. *Arch. Int. Med.*, 140:1466–1468.
3. Bleyer, W. A., and Skinner, A. L. (1976): Fatal neonatal hemorrhage after maternal anticonvulsant therapy. *J.A.M.A.*, 235:626–627.
4. Browne, T. R. (1983): Ethosuximide and other succinimides. In: *Epilepsy: Diagnosis and Management*, edited by T. R. Browne and R. G. Feldman, pp. 215–224. Little Brown, Boston.
5. Browne, T. R., Evans, J. E., Szabo, G. K., Evans, B. A., Greenblatt, D. J., and Schumacher, G. E. (1985): Studies with stable isotopes I: Changes in phenytoin pharmacokinetics and biotransformation during monotherapy. *J. Clin. Pharmacol.*, 25:43–50.
6. Browne, T. R., Feldman, R. G., Buchanan, R. A., Allen, N. C., Fawcett-Vickers, L., Szabo, G. K., Mattson, G. F., Norman, S. E., and Greenblatt, D. J. (1983): Methsuximide for complex partial seizures: Efficacy, toxicity, clinical pharmacology, and drug interactions. *Neurology*, 33:414–418.
7. Browne, T. R., Greenblatt, D. J., Evans, J. E., Evans, B. A., Szabo, G. K., and Schumacher, G. E. (1987): Estimation of a drug's elimination half-life at any serum concentration when the drug's K_m and V_{max} are known: Calculations and validation with phenytoin. *J. Clin. Pharmacol.*, 27:318–320.
8. Cardoba, E. F., and Strobos, R. R. J. (1956): *N*-methyl-alpha-alpha-methylphenyl-succinimide in psychomotor epilepsy. *Dis. Nerv. Syst.*, 17:383–385.
9. Chen, G., Portman, R., Ensor, C. R., and Bratton,

A. C., Jr. (1951): The anticonvulsant activity of alpha-phenyl succinimides. *J. Pharmacol. Exp. Ther.,* 103:54–61.

10. Chen, G., Weston, J. K., and Bratton, A. C., Jr. (1963): Anticonvulsant activity and toxicity of phensuximide, methsuximide and ethosuximide. *Epilepsia,* 4:66–76.

11. Dasheiff, R. M., McNamara, D., and Dickson, L. V. (1986): Efficacy of second line antiepileptic drugs in the treatment of patients with medically refractive complex partial seizures. *Epilepsia,* 27:124–127.

12. Dobrinska, M. R., and Welling, P. G. (1977): Pharmacokinetics of methsuximide and a major metabolite in dog. *J. Pharm. Sci.,* 66:688–692.

13. Dow, R. S., Macfarlane, J. P., and Stevens, J. R. (1958): Celontin in patients with refractory epilepsy. *Neurology,* 8:201–207.

14. French, E. G., Rey-Bellet, J., and Lennox, W. G. (1958): Methsuximide in psychomotor and petit-mal seizures. *N. Engl. J. Med.,* 258:892–894.

15. Gellman, V. (1956): A case of accidental methsuximide (Celontin) ingestion. *Manitoba Med. Rev.,* 45:141–143.

16. Gibbs, E. L., Gibbs, T. J., and Appell, M. R. (1974): Subtle side effects caused by Dilantin and Celontin: A report of two pilot volunteer studies. *Clin. Electroencephalogr.,* 5:192–198.

17. Glazko, A. J., and Dill, W. A. (1972): Other succinimides. Methsuximide and phensuximide. In: *Antiepileptic Drugs,* 1st edition, edited by D. M. Woodbury, J. K. Penry, and R. P. Schmidt, pp. 455–464. Raven Press, New York.

18. Green, R. A., and Gilbert, M. G. (1959): Fatal bone marrow aplasia associated with Celontin therapy. *Minn. Med.,* 42:130.

19. Horning, M. G. (1973): Metabolism of N,2-dimethyl-2-phenylsuccinimide (methsuximide) by epoxide-diol pathway in rat, guinea pig, and human. *Res. Commun. Chem. Pathol. Pharmacol.,* 6:565–578.

20. Johnson, G. F., Least, C. J., Jr., Serum, J. W., Solow, E. B., and Soloman, H. M. (1976): Monitoring drug concentration in a case of combined overdosage with primidone and methsuximide. *Clin. Chem.,* 22:915–921.

21. Karch, S. B. (1973): Methsuximide overdose. Delayed onset of profound coma. *J.A.M.A.,* 223:1463–1465.

22. Kupferberg, H. J., Yonekawa, W. D., Lacy, J. R., Porter, R. J., and Penry, J. K. (1977): Comparison of methsuximide and phensuximide metabolism in epileptic patients. In: *Antiepileptic Drug Monitoring,* edited by C. Gardner-Thorpe, D. Janz, H. Meinardi, and C. E. Pippenger, pp. 173–180. Pitman Medical, Tunbridge Wells, Kent.

23. Livingston, S., and Pauli, L. (1957): Celontin in the treatment of epilepsy. *Pediatrics,* 19:614–617.

24. Miller, C. A., and Long, L. M. (1951): Anticon-

vulsants. An investigation of N-R-alpha-R₁-alpha-phenylsuccinimides. *J. Am. Chem. Soc.,* 73:4895–4898.

25. Porter, R. J., and Kupferberg, H. J. (1982): Other succinimides: Methsuximide and phensuximide. In: *Antiepileptic Drugs,* 2nd edition, edited by D. M. Woodbury, J. K. Penry, and C. E. Pippenger, pp. 663–671. Raven Press, New York.

26. Porter, R. J., Penry, J. K., Lacy, J. R., Newmark, M. E., and Kupferberg, H. J. (1979): Plasma concentrations of phensuximide, methsuximide, and their metabolites in relation to clinical efficacy. *Neurology,* 29:1509–1513.

27. Rambeck, B. (1979): Pharmacological interactions of methsuximide with phenobarbital and phenytoin in hospitalized epileptic patients. *Epilepsia,* 20:147–156.

28. Reynolds, N. C., and Miska, R. M. (1981): Safety of anticonvulsants in hepatic porphyrias. *Neurology,* 31:480–484.

29. Scholl, M. L., Abbot, J. A., and Schwab, R. S. (1959): Celontin: A new anticonvulsant. *Epilepsia,* 1:105–109.

30. Schulte, C. J. A., and Good, T. A. (1966): Acute intoxication due to methsuximide and diphenylhydantoin. *J. Pediatr.,* 68:635–637.

31. Stenzel, E., Boenigk, H. E., and Rambeck, B. (1977): Methsuximide in der Epilepsiebehandlung. *Nerveharzt,* 48:377–384.

32. Strong, J. M., Abe, T., Gibbs, E. L., and Atkinson, J. A., Jr. (1974): Plasma levels of methsuximide and N-desmethylmethsuximide during methsuximide therapy. *Neurology,* 24:250–255.

33. Szabo, G. K., and Browne, T. R. (1982): Improved isocratic liquid-chromatographic stimultaneous measurement of phenytoin, phenobarbital, primidone, carbamazepine, ethosuximide, and N-desmethylsuximide in serum. *Clin. Chem.,* 28:100–104.

34. Trolle, E., and Kiorboe, E., (1960): Treatment of petit mal epilepsy with new succinimides: PM60 and Celontin (a clinical comparative study). *Epilepsia,* 1:587–597.

35. Watson, Jr., Lawrence, R. C., and Lovering, E. B. (1978): Simple GLC analysis of anticonvulsant drugs in commercial dosage forms. *J. Pharm. Sci.,* 67:950–953.

36. Wilder, B. J., and Buchanan, R. B. (1981): Methsuximide for refractory complex partial seizures. *Neurology,* 31:741–744.

37. Zimmerman, F. T. (1953): New drugs in the treatment of petit mal epilepsy. *Am. J. Psychiatry,* 109:767–773.

38. Zimmerman, F. T. (1955): Milontin in the treatment of epilepsy. *N.Y. State J. Med.,* 56:1460–1465.

39. Zimmerman, F. T. (1956): N-methyl-alpha-alpha-methylphenylsuccinimide in psychomotor epilepsy therapy. *Arch. Neurol. Psychiat.,* 76:65–71.

Antiepileptic Drugs, Third Edition, edited by
R. Levy, R. Mattson, B. Meldrum,
J. K. Penry, and F. E. Dreifuss.
Raven Press, Ltd., New York © 1989.

53

Trimethadione

Harold E. Booker

Trimethadione (Tridione) is the most important of several antiepileptic oxazolidinediones. Once it was the drug of choice, if not the only truly effective drug for treatment of absence seizures, but interest in trimethadione (TMO) has declined since the introduction of ethosuximide and valproic acid. Consequently, little new information on the pharmacologic and clinical features of TMO has appeared since the extensive reviews in the second edition of *Antiepileptic Drugs* (3,4,12,47,48,49). Nevertheless, TMO remains of interest both for basic studies of convulsant and anticonvulsant mechanisms and for clinical application in areas unrelated to epilepsy (18,21,26,27, 30,37,53). Trimethadione is also of great interest historically as it holds a unique and pivotal position in the development of the pharmacology of epilepsy. Its selective efficacy against absence seizures in man and its profile of efficacy in experimental animal models were quickly recognized to be the inverse of those for phenytoin. This raised the possibility that different seizure types or even epileptic syndromes might have differing molecular pathologies, and initiated a search for other new drugs with more specific or selective antiepileptic efficacy.

Trimethadione probably also holds the record for the rate of drug development, as its clinical utility was clearly established (22,28) within months of its synthesis. This is all the more remarkable as it was synthesized as part of a systematic search for drugs with analgesic properties (35). The critical intermediary step was the demonstration (14,18) of its ability to protect experimental animals from seizures induced by pentylenetetrazol (PTZ). The demonstration that the therapeutic effect of long-term TMO therapy is due to its rapid and almost complete biotransformation to dimethadione (DMO) makes TMO one of the first pro-drugs recognized (6,7,8,20).

CHEMISTRY AND METHODS OF DETERMINATION

Oxazolidine-2,4-dione is a five membered heterocyclic ring whose structure is remarkably similar to the hydantoin, succinimide, and barbiturate rings. The structures of TMO (3,5,5-trimethyloxazolidine-2,4-dione) and DMO (5,5-dimethyloxazolidine-2,4-dione) are shown in Fig. 1.

Trimethadione and dimethadione are bitter white crystalline solids whose molecular weights are 143.15 and 129.12, respectively. Trimethadione melts at 40°C and boils at 79°C; DMO melts at 78°C. Water solubility of TMO is approximately 5% (W/V) and greater than 50% for DMO. Both drugs are moderately soluble in common organic solvents. Both form stable salts with metal ions. Trimethadione is moderately stable in dilute mineral acids but is rapidly degraded by aqueous alkali. Dimethadione is stable in boiling water or dilute mineral acids but the sodium salt is degraded by prolonged boiling. Because of the unsubstituted imide

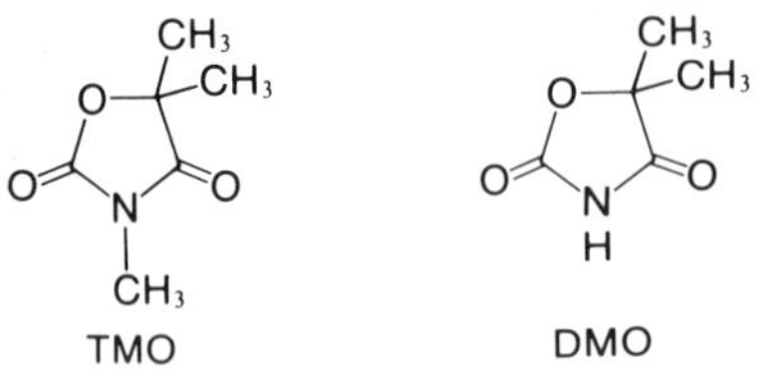

FIG. 1. Structures of trimethadione (TMO) and dimethadione (DMO).

group in DMO, it is a weak monobasic acid with a pK_α of 6.13. Consequently, it is largely ionized at a physiologic pH of 7.4.

Several methods are available for the synthesis of TMO and DMO including preparation of a ^{14}C derivative with the label in the 2 position (12). More recently, an ^{11}C derivative of DMO suitable for use in positron emission tomography has been synthesized (21,30).

A large number of analytical techniques are available for the determination of TMO and DMO concentrations in tissue and biologic fluids. Most clinical laboratories have used one of the several gas-liquid chromatography (GLC) methods available. Inherent problems with GLC, however, include the poor recovery of DMO unless salting out steps are taken, and the potential loss of TMO or DMO with solvent evaporation techniques. Dudley et al. (12) have provided an excellent critical review of these problems and stress the need for internal standards. Tanaka et al. (36) developed a high-performance liquid chromatography technique that should circumvent these problems since direct injection of nonextracted serum is employed. However, the method was not standardized for the high range of DMO levels present following prolonged TMO therapy. Two new GLC methods (16,40) and one utilizing infrared spectrometry (53) have recently been described.

MECHANISM OF ACTION

Clinically the oxazolidinediones are effective in the control of absence and related seizure types but not partial or generalized tonic-clonic seizures. In the laboratory, they antagonize all of the excitatory effects of PTZ in brain and spinal cord but are far less effective in modifying maximal electroshock seizures. This profile of efficacy in experimental models is the inverse of that for drugs (e.g., phenytoin) which have clinical efficacy against partial and generalized tonic-clonic but not absence seizures, and tend to predict drugs (e.g., ethosuximide) whose clinical efficacy will parallel TMO's. Although the mechanism by which PTZ induces seizures in experimental animals and man is not necessarily related to the mechanism(s) underlying absence seizures in human petit mal epilepsy, the anti-PTZ effect of TMO has been extensively studied.

Trimethadione and DMO prevent or reverse a number of metabolic changes in brain induced by PTZ but have little effect on these systems in absence of PTZ stimulation (49,51). They have variable and less potent effects in modifying seizures induced by picrotoxin and strychnine (18), local anesthetics (31), thiosemicarbazide (1), hyperbaric oxygen (23), high doses of methadone (33), and CO_2 withdrawal (50). As with PTZ, several metabolic changes induced by these agents are blocked or reversed by TMO but these effects may result from rather than be the cause of TMO's anticonvulsant effect. Because DMO is a weak acid largely ionized at physiologic pH it produces an extracellular acidosis. It is unlikely this plays a significant role in DMO's mechanism of action as TMO is neutral yet has a stronger anti-PTZ effect.

Little is known of the effects of TMO and DMO on individual neurons and subcellular systems. Trimethadione decreases intracellular Na^{++} in lobster nerve (29) but does not affect synaptic protein phosphorylation or release of acetylcholine or norepinephrine stimulated by Ca^{++}-calmodulin (11). It has little effect on the properties of peripheral nerve or the excitation produced by excessive stimulation or calcium deficit

(42,43). No significant direct effects have been demonstrated on any neurotransmitter system, including GABA (50). Benzodiazepine binding is not altered by TMO (2).

More positive findings emerge when transmission through neuronal networks is considered. Trimethadione enhances presynaptic inhibition in the spinal cord (24) but unlike phenytoin, does not depress posttetanic potentiation (13). The threshold for repetitive discharge is not altered but the polysynaptic transmission of such discharges is inhibited (13). The threshold for cortical after-discharge is lowered by TMO (10) but transmission of cortical seizure discharges to the thalamus is inhibited (25). The threshold for seizure discharges to repetitive stimulation in the thalamus, however, is raised by TMO (32). Thus the main action of TMO and DMO which may have direct relevance for their clinical efficacy appears to be an ability to raise the threshold for repetitive activity in the thalamus and to inhibit corticothalamic transmission. The molecular basis for these effects, however, is uncertain.

PHARMACOKINETICS

Trimethadione is rapidly absorbed after oral, subcutaneous, or intraperitoneal administration in animals (47). Less is known about DMO but it is rapidly absorbed after intraperitoneal injection (50). Absorption of TMO after oral administration in man is apparently complete with peak plasma levels at 30 to 60 min (3,36). Orally administered DMO is absorbed in man (8) but the rate is unknown.

Biotransformation of TMO is limited to demethylation to DMO. No further biotransformations are known for either TMO or DMO. The reaction is essentially complete (6) and less than 5% of oral doses of TMO are excreted unchanged in the urine of man (3). Although the reaction can occur in several tissues, the primary site of metabolism is the liver (41). Appreciable amounts of DMO are present in human plasma within 2 hr of an oral dose of TMO (37). The reaction is inhibited by DMO and by high concentrations of TMO itself (9). The reaction is also inhibited by age (38), hepatic disease (37), and dehydration (39).

Neither TMO or DMO are appreciably bound to serum or tissue proteins. The volume of distribution for TMO ranges from 60% to 90% of total body weight in experimental animals (47) and is estimated to be approximately 60% in man (3,37,38). Tissue-to-blood concentration ratios average around 0.65 for most tissues in animals but were 0.9 for muscle with no apparent selective concentration in different brain regions (41). Somewhat lower ratios (0.4–0.6) were found for DMO in rats (21). After i.v. administration of DMO, equilibrium was attained in 5 min for most vascular tissues (e.g., heart, thyroid), but required 30 to 60 min for brain. Ratios approaching 1 were found in the wall and contents of the gastrointestinal tract at 1 to 2 hr. Since DMO is a weak acid its distribution to tissue will be proportional to intracellular pH, and this phenomenon has frequently been used to measure intracellular pH. More recently Rottenberg et al. (30) exploited this effect, using [^{11}C] DMO and positron emission tomography to diagnose human brain tumors. Dimethadione entered brain rapidly (<5 min) and brain/tumor equilibrium was attained in 30 to 60 min.

Trimethadione is eliminated from the body almost exclusively by metabolism to DMO. The plasma half-life of TMO in normal volunteers after single oral doses ranges from 11 to 16 hr (3,36) but is prolonged in older subjects (38) and in patients with hepatic disease (37). Dimethadione is very slowly excreted in the urine (20,45) and in the bile and pancreatic juice (26,27). Urinary excretion is enhanced by alkalinization. The plasma half-life of DMO is not accurately known but is estimated to be around 10 days (20,26).

RELATION OF PLASMA CONCENTRATION TO SEIZURE CONTROL

Jensen (20) measured DMO plasma levels in subjects treated with TMO and found control of absence seizures associated with DMO levels in excess of 700 μg/ml. Chamberlin et al. (8) repeated the study, but also crossed subjects from TMO therapy to treatment with DMO, adjusting doses to maintain equivalent plasma DMO levels. Control of seizures was unchanged and correlated with DMO levels in the range of 700 μg/ml. Our own data (3) are in good agreement, as DMO levels in controlled subjects ranged from 470 to 1,200 with an average of 765 μg/ml. Plasma DMO levels in uncontrolled subjects (less than 75% reduction in seizures) averaged 465 μg/ml (range, 130 to 690 μg/ml). The average TMO level was higher in the uncontrolled subjects (40 μg/ml) than the controlled subjects (20 μg/ml).

In institutionalized subjects with steady-state plasma drug levels, each mg per kg of a daily TMO dose gave a plasma TMO level of 0.6 μg/ml and DMO level of 12 μg/ml (3). Thus, daily TMO doses of 50 to 60 mg/Kg would be required to maintain therapeutic DMO levels. Because of its long plasma half-life, DMO will accumulate slowly in plasma after treatment with TMO is begun. Thus, therapeutic effects are often delayed for 2 weeks or more after treatment is begun, and persist for similar periods after TMO is discontinued.

TOXICITY

Dose-dependent, reversible adverse effects primarily involve the central nervous system (4). Hemeralopia (night blindness) and photophobia occur in approximately 30% of subjects. Adaptation occurs and the problem can usually be managed by avoiding sunlight and using dark glasses. Sedation, fatigue, and loss of concentration are the next most frequent side effects followed by dizziness and ataxia. Insomnia, restlessness, confusion and hallucinations are rare but have been reported (46). Most of these reactions can be managed by lowering the dose, although there are no data relating them to plasma drug levels.

Skin reactions are common but usually benign (acneform or morbilliform), although erythema multiforme and exfoliative dermatitis have been reported. Bone marrow depression, ranging from a benign, non-progressive depression of the absolute neutrophil count to a fulminant pancytopenia, can occur. A nephrotic syndrome occurs but is usually reversible (46). A myasthenic syndrome has been reported rarely (5). Hemorrhagic disease of the newborn has not been reported in offspring of mothers taking TMO.

Antiepileptic drugs, including TMO, can cause teratogenesis. Although epidemiologic evidence in man implicating the drugs is not strong (19,34), TMO is teratogenic in rodents and can even produce behavioral abnormalities in the absence of physical malformations (44). A somewhat unique combination of physical anomalies, growth retardation, and mental retardation in children whose mothers took TMO during the pregnancy (the fetal TMO syndrome) has been described (15,17,52). The current consensus is that TMO is contraindicated during pregnancy.

CONVERSION

Trimethadione

Conversion factor:

CF = 1000/mol. wt. = 1000/143.1 = 6.99

Conversion:

$$(\mu g/ml) \times 6.99 = (\mu moles/liter)$$

$$(\mu moles/liter)/6.99 = (\mu g/ml)$$

Dimethadione

Conversion factor:

CF = 1000/mol. wt. = 1000/129.1 = 7.75

Conversion:

(μg/ml) × 7.75 = (μmoles/liter)

(μmoles/liter)/7.75 = (μg/ml)

REFERENCES

1. Baniger, R., and Hane, D. (1967): Evaluation of a new convulsant for anticonvulsant screening. *Arch. Int. Pharmacodyn.,* 167:245–249.
2. Bennett, D. A., Geyer, H., Dotta, P., Brogger, S., Fielding, S., and Lal, H. (1982): Comparison of the actions of trimethadione and chlordiazepoxide in animal models of anxiety and benzodiazepine receptor binding. *Neuropharmacology,* 21:1175–1179.
3. Booker, H. E. (1982): Trimethadione: Relation of plasma concentation to seizure control. In: *Antiepileptic Drugs,* 2nd edition, edited by D. M. Woodbury, J. K. Penry, and C. E. Pippenger, pp. 697–699. Raven Press, New York.
4. Booker, H. E. (1982): Trimethadione: Toxicity. In: *Antiepileptic Drugs,* 2nd edition, edited by D. M. Woodbury, J. K. Penry, and C. E. Pippenger, pp. 701–703, Raven Press, New York.
5. Booker, H. E., Chun, R., and Sanguino, M. (1970): Myasthenia Gravis syndrome associated with trimethadione. *J.A.M.A.,* 212:2262–2263.
6. Butler, T. C. (1953): Quantitative studies of the demethylation of trimethadione (Tridione). *J. Pharmacol. Exp. Ther.,* 108:11–17.
7. Butler, T. C., and Waddell, W. (1958): *N*-Methylated derivatives of barbituric acid, hydantoin and oxazolidinedione used in the treatment of epilepsy. *Neurology (Minneap.),* 8:106–112.
8. Chamberlin, H., Waddell, W., and Butler, T. (1965): A study of the product of demethylation of trimethadione in the control of petit mal epilepsy. *Neurology (Minneap.),* 15:499–454.
9. Conney, A. H. (1967): Pharmacologic implications of microsomal enzyme induction. *Pharmacol. Rev.,* 19:317–366.
10. Delgado, J. M. R., and Milailovic, L. (1956): Use of intracerebral electrodes to evaluate drugs that act on the central nervous system. *Ann, N.Y. Acad. Sci.,* 64:644–666.
11. DeLorenzo, R. J. (1986): A molecular approach to the calcium signal in brain: Relationship to synaptic modulation and seizure discharge. In: *Advances in Neurology 44. Basic Mechanisms of the Epilepsies: Molecular and Cellular Approaches,* edited by A. V. Delgado-Escueta, A. A. Ward, Jr., D. M. Woodbury, and R. J. Porter, pp. 435–464. Raven Press, New York.
12. Dudley, K. H., Dios, D. L., and King B. T. (1982): Trimethadione: Chemistry and methods of determination. In: *Antiepileptic Drugs,* 2nd edition, edited by D. M. Woodbury, J. K. Penry, and C. E. Pippenger, pp. 673–679. Raven Press, New York.
13. Esplin, D. W., and Carto, E. W. (1957): Effect of trimethadione on synaptic transmission in the spinal cord: Antagonism of trimethadione and pentylene-tetrazole. *J. Pharmacol. Exp. Ther.,* 121:457–467.
14. Everett, G. M., and Richards, R. K. (1944): Comparative anticonvulsive action of 3,5,5,-trimethyloxazolidine-2,4-dione (Tridione), Dilantin, and phenobarbital. *J. Pharmacol. Exp. Ther.,* 81:402–407.
15. Feldman, G., Weaver D., and Lorrien, E. (1977): The fetal trimethadione syndrome: Report of an additional family and further delineation of their syndrome. *Am. J. Dis. Child.,* 131:1389–1392.
16. Gazdzik, W., and Kwiotek, W. (1986): Rapid and simple gas-liquid chromatographic method for the determination of 5,5-dimethyl-2,4-oxazolidinedione. *J. Chromatog.,* 378:482–485.
17. German, J., Kowal, A., and Ehlers, K. (1970): Trimethadione and human teratogenesis. *Teratology,* 3:349–361.
18. Goodman, L., Toman, J., and Swinyard, E. (1946): The anticonvulsant properties of Tridione: Laboratory and clinical investigations. *Am. J. Med.,* 1:213–228.
19. Janz, D. (1982): Antiepileptic drugs and pregnancy: Altered utilization patterns and teratogenesis. *Epilepsia,* 23(Suppl. 1):53–63.
20. Jensen, B. (1962): Trimethadione in the serum of patients with petit mal. *Dan. Med. Bull.,* 1:213–228.
21. Kearfott, K. J., Junck, L., and Rottenberg, D. A. (1983): C-11 dimethyloxazolidione (DMO): Biodistribution, radiation absorbed dose, and potential for PET measurement of regional brain pH. *J. Nucl. Med.,* 24:805–811.
22. Lennox, W. (1945): The petit mal epilepsies. Their treatment with Tridione. *J.A.M.A.,* 129:1069–1075.
23. Mayevsky, A. (1975): The effects of trimethadione on brain energy metabolism and EEG activity of the conscious rat exposed to HBO. *J. Neurosci. Res.,* 1:131–142.
24. Miyahara, J. T., Esplin, D. W., and Zablocka, B. (1966): Differential effects of depressant drugs on presynaptic inhibition. *J. Pharmacol. Exp. Ther.,* 154:118–127.
25. Morrell, F., Bradley, W., and Ptashne, M. (1959): Effect of drugs on discharge characteristics of chronic epileptogenic lesions. *Neurology (Minneap.),* 9:492–498.
26. Noda, A., Hayakawa, T., Mizuno, R., Hamano, H., Murase, T., and Shibata, T. (1984): The excretion of dimethadione in pure pancreatic juice and bile in postoperative patients. *Gastroenterologica Japonica,* 19:121–126.
27. Noda, A., Shibata, T., Hamano, H., Murase, T., Hayakawa, T., Horiguchi, Y., and Takayama, T.

(1984): Trimethadione (Troxidone) dissolves pancreatic stones. *Lancet,* Aug. 11:351–353.

28. Perlstein, M., and Andelman, M. (1946): Tridione: Its use in convulsive and related disorders. *J. Pediatr.,* 29:20–40.

29. Pincus, J. H., Grove, I., Marino, B. B., and Glaser, G. E. (1970): Studies on the mechanism of action of diphenylhydantoin. *Arch. Neurol. (Chic.),* 22:566–571.

30. Rottenberg, D. A., Ginos, J. Z., Kearfott, K. J., Junck, L., Dhawan, V., and Jarden, J. D. (1985): *In vivo* measurement of brain tumor pH using [^{11}C]DMO and positron emission tomography. *Ann. Neurol.,* 17:70–79.

31. Sanders, H. O. (1967): A comparison of the convulsant activity of procaine and pentylenetetrazol. *Arch. Int. Pharmacodyn.,* 170:165–177.

32. Schallek, W., and Kuehn, A. (1963): Effects of trimethadione, diphenylhydantoin and chlordiazepoxide on after-discharges in brain of cat. *Proc. Soc. Exp. Biol. N.Y.,* 112:813–817.

33. Shannon, H. E., and Holtzman, S. G. (1976): Blockade of the specific lethal effects of narcotic analgesics in the mouse. *Eur. J. Pharmacol.,* 39:295–303.

34. Shapiro, S., Slone, D., Hartz, S. C., Rosenberg, L., Siskind, V., Manson, R. R., Mitchell, A. A., Heinanen, O. P., Idanpaan-Heikkila, J., Haro, S., and Saxen, L. (1976): Anticonvulsants and paternal epilepsy in the development of birth defects. *Lancet,* 1:272–275.

35. Spielman, M. A. (1944): Some analgesic agents derived from oxazolidine-2,4-dione. *J. Am. Chem. Soc.,* 66:1244–1245.

36. Tanaka, E., Hagino, S., Yoshida, I., and Kuroiwa, Y. (1984): Simultaneous determination of trimethadione and its metabolite in rat and human serum by high-performance liquid chromatography. *J. Chromatog.,* 308:393–397.

37. Tanaka, E., Ishikawa, A., Ono, A., Okamura, T., Kobayashi, S., Yashura, H., and Misawa, S. (1986): Trimethadione tolerance test for evaluation of functional reserve of the liver in patients with liver cirrhosis and esophageal varices. *J. Pharmacobio. Dyn.,* 9:297–302.

38. Tanaka, E., Ishikawa, A., Ono, A., Okamura, T., and Misawa, S. (1987): Age-related changes in trimethadione oxidizing capacity. *Br. J. Clin. Pharmacol.,* 23:355–357.

39. Tanaka, E., Kurata, N., Kuriowa, Y., and Misawa, S. (1986): Influence of short-term water deprivation in kinetics of trimethadione and its metabolite in rats. *Japan J. Pharmacol.,* 42:269–274.

40. Tanaka, E., and Misawa, S. (1987): Simultaneous determination of serum trimethadione and its metabolite by gas chromatography. *J. Chromatography,* 413:376–378.

41. Taylor, J. D., and Bertcher, E. L. (1952): The determination and distribution of trimethadione (Tridione) in animal tissues. *J. Pharmacol. Exp. Ther.,* 106:277–285.

42. Toman, J. E. P. (1952): Neuropharmacology of peripheral nerve. *Pharmacol. Rev.,* 4:168–218.

43. Toman, J. E. P. (1969): Discussion. Further observations on diphenylhydantoin. In: *Basic Mechanisms of the Epilepsies,* edited by H. H. Jasper, A. A. Ward, and A. Pope, pp. 682–688. Little, Brown and Co. Boston.

44. Vorhees, C. V. (1983). Fetal anticonvulsant syndrome in rats: Dose and period response relationships of prenatal diphenylhydantoin, trimethadione and phenobarbital exposure on the structural and functional development of the offspring. *J. Pharmacol. Exp. Ther.,* 227:274–287.

45. Waddell, W. J., and Butler, T. C. (1957): Renal excretion of 5,5-dimethyl-2,4-oxazolidinedione (product of demethylation of trimethadione). *Proc. Soc. Exp. Biol. Med.,* 96:563–565.

46. Wells, C. (1957): Trimethadione: Its dosage and toxicity. *Arch. Neurol. Psychiatry,* 77:140–145.

47. Withrow, C. D. (1982): Trimethadione. Absorption, distribution and excretion. In: *Antiepileptic Drugs,* 2nd edition, edited by D. M. Woodbury, J. K. Penry, and C. E. Pippenger, pp. 681–687. Raven Press, New York.

48. Withrow, C. D. (1982). Trimethadione: Biotransformation. In: *Antiepileptic Drugs,* 2nd edition, edited by D. M. Woodbury, J. K. Penry, and C. E. Pippenger, pp. 689–692. Raven Press, New York.

49. Withrow, C. D. (1982): Trimethadione: Mechanisms of action. In: *Antiepileptic Drugs,* 2nd edition, edited by D. M. Woodbury, J. K. Penry, and C. E. Pippenger, pp. 705–709. Raven Press, New York.

50. Withrow, C. D., Stout, R. J., Barton, L. J., Beacham, W. S., and Woodbury, D. M. (1968). Anticonvulsant effects of 5,5-dimethyl-2,4-oxazoli-dinedione (DMO). *J. Pharmacol. Exp. Ther.,* 161:335–341.

51. Woodbury, D. M. (1977). Pharmacology and mechanisms of anti-epileptic drugs. In: *Scientific Approaches to Clinical Neurology,* edited by E. S. Goldensohn and S. J. Appel, pp. 693–727. Lea and Febiger, Philadelphia.

52. Zackai, E., Mellman, W., Neiderer, B., and Hanson, J. (1975). The fetal trimethadione syndrome. *J. Pediatr.,* 87:280–284.

53. Zweens, J., and Franena, H. (1984). Simultaneous determination of dimethadione and trimethadione by infrared-spectrometry: Application for mean intracellular pH measurement. *J. Clin. Chem. Clin. Biochem.,* 22:641–645.

Antiepileptic Drugs, Third Edition, edited by
R. Levy, R. Mattson, B. Meldrum,
J. K. Penry, and F. E. Dreifuss.
Raven Press, Ltd., New York © 1989.

54

Benzodiazepines

Mechanisms of Action

Willy Haefely

The benzodiazepines constitute a class of drugs that contains mostly the benzo-1,4-diazepine nucleus—exceptionally the benzo-1,5-diazepine or the thieno-1,4-diazepine nucleus (18)—and shares a characteristic profile of activity and a main common mechanism of action. They interact specifically with a receptor molecule, called the benzodiazepine receptor (BZR), to modulate the efficiency of the inhibitory neurotransmitter γ-aminobutyric acid (GABA) at the $GABA_A$ receptor. Over 50 new chemical entities of the benzodiazepine class are marketed worldwide. Drugs not belonging to the chemical class of diazepines have been developed (and recently marketed, such as zopiclone and zolpidem) that also produce benzodiazepine-like effects through interaction with the BZR. Moreover, many agents of benzodiazepine and non-benzodiazepine structure have been found to interact with the BZR in such a way as to produce activities antagonistic and even opposite to those of classic benzodiazepines. It is, therefore, more appropriate to use the term BZR ligands for all compounds displaying high affinity for the BZR, and the terms BZR agonists, partial agonists, antagonists, and partial and full inverse agonists for the BZR ligands exerting positive (full or partial), no, or negative (partial or full) modulatory activity on the $GABA_A$ receptor. The term BZR ligands considers only the affinity for the BZR, whereas the other terms specify the positive, absent, or negative intrinsic efficacy. A number of recent reviews and books on BZR and BZR ligands are available for more detailed information (1,2,5,7,9,10,14, 15,18,19,20,30,37,39,42,43).

The classic benzodiazepine tranquilizers were found in the mid-1970s to facilitate GABAergic synaptic transmission in the central nervous system (CNS) (17,11). Shortly afterward, specific high-affinity binding sites for these drugs were identified using the radioligand technique (4,29,40). Around 1980 two classes of BZR ligands were discovered, one class acting as specific antagonists (22), the other producing effects opposite to the classic BZR full agonists (7). This brought into the focus of interest the broad spectrum of intrinsic efficacies displayed by BZR ligands and was the first demonstration of a drug receptor that is able to mediate two opposite effects, both of which can be competitively blocked. This complex operation of a drug receptor had considerable impact on basic aspects of ligand-receptor interaction, but the existence of partial and full inverse BZR agonists also opened new concepts and provided new tools in the exploration of the cellular mechanisms of anxiety and epilepsy. Progress in the purification of the BZR and the use of methods of molecular genetics culminated in a preliminary insight into the primary structure of the molecular complex of the $GABA_A$ receptor-gated chloride channel containing the BZR as an allosteric modulatory unit (34,24). This chapter is a brief account of the present knowledge of the operation of the BZR. Putative mechanisms of action of BZR ligands unrelated to the BZR and of theoretical interest for their anticonvulsant activity are also reviewed.

$GABA_A$-RECEPTOR–CHLORIDE CHANNEL COMPLEX

GABA produces its effects at the subsynaptic membrane by interacting with at least two classes of receptors, called $GABA_A$ and $GABA_B$ receptors, which are characterized by their preferential affinities for agonists and antagonists, by the different signal transduction devices to which they are coupled, and by the modulatory sites with which they are associated (Fig. 1). Their distribution within the CNS also differs in part. The structure of the $GABA_B$

receptor is at present unknown. Benzodiazepine receptor ligands do not affect the function of this class of GABA receptors.

Structure of the Complex

Conventional techniques used for the detergent solubilization of the BZR from neuronal membranes and subsequent purification, greatly facilitated by the photoaffinity labeling of the BZ binding site by radioactive flunitrazepam (28), suggested that the BZR was an integral part of a supramolecular glycoprotein complex consisting of two different subunits. The smaller protein (approximately 53 kD), the α-subunit, is easily photoaffinity-labeled with flunitrazepam and, therefore, appears to bear the binding site of the BZR. The larger protein (approximately 57 kD), called β-subunit, can be photo-labeled with the specific $GABA_A$ agonist muscimol and, hence, contains GABA binding site(s) (35). Monoclonal antibodies raised against the affinity-purified BZR were found to coprecipitate the native membrane receptor complex

	$GABA_A$-RECEPTORS	$GABA_B$-RECEPTORS
COMMON AGONIST	GABA	GABA
SELECTIVE AGONIST	MUSCIMOL	BACLOFEN
SELECTIVE ANTAGONIST	BICUCCULLINE	(δ-AMINO-VALERIC ACID)
EFFECTOR	Cl^- CHANNEL	Ca^{2+}-CHANNEL$\downarrow$ AC$\downarrow$ K^+ CHANNEL$\uparrow$
ALLOSTERIC MODULATION	"BENZODIAZEPINES" BARBITURATES SOME CONVULSANTS	?

FIG. 1. Classification of GABA receptors.

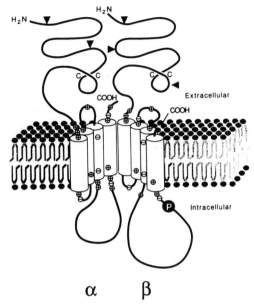

α   β

FIG. 2. Tentative topology of the GABA$_A$ receptor complex derived from its primary structure and the knowledge of other receptor-regulated ion channels. (From Schofield et al., ref. 34, with permission.)

(33). Schofield et al. (34) screened cDNA libraries from bovine brain and calf cortex with synthetic oligodeoxyribonucleotide probes designed after sequenced, cleaved peptide fragments of the native complex. DNA sequencing of hybridizing cDNA clones predicted an α-subunit of 456 amino acids and a β-subunit of 474 amino acids. Both peptides were found to contain N-terminal sequences of 20 to 30 residues typical of N-terminal signal sequences, suggesting mature peptide sizes of 430 and 450 amino acids. Sequence analysis suggested the presence in both subunits of four putative α-helical hydrophobic stretches (M$_1$ to M$_4$) that might act as transmembrane segments, anchoring the peptide complex in the neuronal membrane. A tentative topology of the complex was proposed (Fig. 2). The model shows the four membrane spanning helices, the large N-terminal exobilayer part presumably containing a β-loop formed by a disulphide bridge and two (α-subunit)

to three (β-subunit) potential N-glycosylation sites, as well as the smaller cytoplasmic domains formed by the peptide segments connecting the M$_3$ and M$_4$ helices. The cytoplasmic domain of the β-subunit contains a potential serine phosphorylation consensus sequence.

The remarkable similarities of the deduced primary structure of the GABA$_A$ receptor with the nicotinic cholinoceptor (nAChR) and with the partially sequenced glycine-receptor–gated chloride channel led Schofield et al. (34) to propose that these and probably still other receptor-operated ion channels may be members of a superfamily of receptor-operated ion channels (ROCs), characterized by similar structural and functional features such as partial sequence homologies, presence of four hydrophobic transmembrane helices in each subunit, binding domains for primary signals and secondary allosteric modulatory signals on the ectodomains, as well as phosphorylation sites on the cytoplasmic domains allowing for intracellular covalent modulation. Further similarities between the members of this superfamily may include the richness in threonine and serine residues in the M$_2$ transmembrane helix, providing a lining of the channel with hydrophilic hydroxy groups required for forming a water-filled channel lumen, and the presence of clusters of charged side groups on both ends of the presumed transmembrane domains possibly forming the channel mouth and providing a selectivity filter for cations or anions. The striking, conserved proline residue in M$_1$, possibly resulting in a bend in the helix and a protrusion into the channel, may be crucial for the channel gating triggered by GABA$_A$ receptor activation.

Schofield et al. (34) tested the hypothesis that the two sequenced subunits may form the presumed complete GABA$_A$ receptor by injecting *Xenopus* oocytes with pure mRNAs transcribed *in vitro* from their cloned cDNAs. Although the mRNAs encoding α- and β-subunits alone did not induce a GABA-responsiveness in the oocytes, the injection of the two mRNAs resulted in the translation and membrane incorporation of a complex mediating a chloride conductance on exposure to GABA (blocked by bicuculline and picrotoxin) and being facilitated by pentobarbital and the benzodiazepine chlorazepate. Similar results had been obtained earlier by injection of total mRNA from chick and rat brain (38). Recent and still ongoing studies in several laboratories on GABA$_A$ receptor cloning and *in vitro* expression suggest a more complex situation than emerged from the paper of Schofield et al. (34). Indeed, the structure proposed by these authors appears to be just one of several variants of native receptor types.

A structural heterogeneity of the GABA$_A$-BZR complex, already indicated by the analysis of the native receptor, is likely to exist in bovine, rat, and human brains. Levitan et al. (24) have recently reported the isolation of additional cDNA clones for the α-subunit in the bovine brain and provide evidence that the three α-subunit variants presently characterized arise from different genes. A high degree of homology is observed in the four putative membrane spanning domains and in the ectodomain. A poor sequence conservation is seen in the extreme *N*-terminal region and in the cytoplasmic domain connecting M$_3$ and M$_4$. Heterologous expression in *Xenopus* oocytes showed that any α-subunit variant (α$_1$, α$_2$, α$_3$) injected together with the β-subunit resulted in a functional GABA$_A$ receptor. However, the (α$_1$β), (α$_2$β), and (α$_3$β) receptors showed markedly different sensitivities to GABA, indicating a surprising influence of the α-subunit structure on the affinity of the GABA binding sites on the β-subunit. The heterologously expressed receptor-channel complexes differed from those obtained by injection of native mRNA and from the native neuronal membrane receptor by different cooperative effects of GABA-stimulation and by the absence of modulation by BZR ligands. Whether these studies reflect truly BZR-ligand insensitive GABA$_A$ receptors, as they might exist in the brain, or whether the oocytes fail to perform the correct posttranslational modification, or whether additional components not yet identified are necessary to provide the properties of native BZR-modulated receptors remains to be shown.

Keeping in mind the unsettled problem of GABA$_A$ receptor structural heterogeneity and, in particular, its relevance for the pharmacology of BZR ligands, the following simplified hypothetical model (Fig. 3) of the GABA$_A$-BZR complex is a useful guide to the discussion of the effects of BZR ligands.

The model assumes a tetrameric quaternary (2α, 2β) composition of the receptor-channel complex. The stoichiometry of binding sites is not definitely known. Evidence exists for two GABA binding sites and four benzodiazepine binding sites per receptor-channel complex. Whereas activation of the GABA receptor results in the conversion of the resting, closed channel into the open conformation (large arrow), activation of the BZR mediates allosteric modulation of this gating process (change in the affinity state or accessibility of GABA binding sites or modification of the GABA-induced conformational transition of the channel). Other allosteric sites on the complex are indicated on the β-subunit (although this location is by no way certain); barbiturates, steroids, some convulsants and a heterogeneous group of agents act on this or these sites.

BZR

The BZR, identified by radioligand studies, is an integral part of most or all GABA$_A$ receptors, mediating allosteric modulation of the channel gating function of the GABA$_A$ receptor. The uniqueness of the BZR is to mediate two opposite modulatory

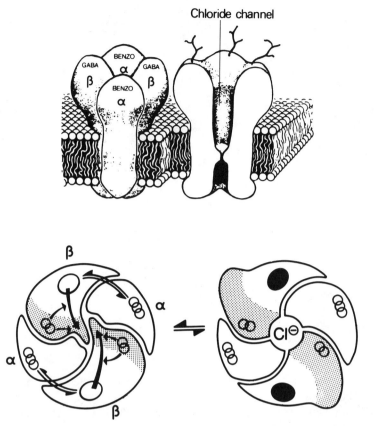

FIG. 3. Hypothetical model of the GABA$_A$-BZR-chloride channel function.

effects, one facilitating, the other depressing the channel gating function. Benzodiazepine receptor ligands with the former action are called BZR agonists and those with the latter action are called inverse BZR agonists (32). A class of BZR ligands exists which produces no modulatory effect on the channel gating function but competitively blocks the effects of both agonists and inverse agonists. As Fig. 4 shows, in reality a full spectrum of BZR ligands exists, from agents exerting full positive intrinsic efficacy, all degrees of partial positive intrinsic efficacies (partial BZR agonists), zero intrinsic efficacy, and various degrees of partial negative intrinsic efficacies (partial or low efficacy BZR inverse agonists), to full negative intrinsic efficacy.

Benzodiazepine receptor ligands, like ligands of any receptor, are characterized by two inherent properties: affinity and intrinsic efficacy. Affinity is the structural property (size, three-dimensional shape, and spatial orientation of functional groups) that determines the relation between ligand concentration and fractional receptor occupancy (number of receptor-ligand complexes) at equilibrium; it is expressed by the dissociation rate constant of the receptor-ligand complex determined by the ligand concentration required for half-maximal occupation of binding sites (K_D) in equilibrium binding studies, or by the ratio of association and dissociation rate constants determined in kinetic binding studies. Intrinsic efficacy is the property (also dependent on

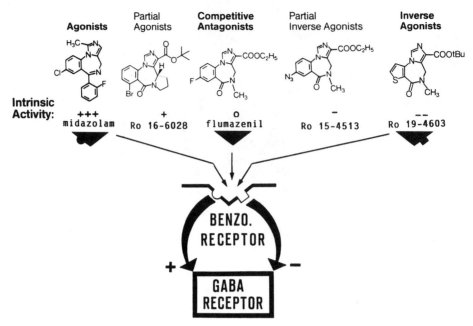

FIG. 4. Spectrum of BZR ligands, exemplified with derivatives of benzodiazepines.

structure) that relates fractional receptor occupancy to the amplitude of effect (in percent of the maximal effect which can be produced through the given receptor). Intrinsic efficacy reflects the fact that formation of a receptor-ligand complex by itself needs not to result in activation of the receptor, i.e., in the conformational change of the receptor which is required to activate the transduction process.

Full agonists may produce maximal effects in a target cell with a high receptor density while occupying only a fraction of the available receptors (Fig. 5); such cells have a receptor reserve or spare receptors for agonists. Partial agonists require a higher fractional receptor occupancy for a maximal effect than full agonists and, depending on the intrinsic efficacy and receptor density, may be unable to produce a full effect even at receptor saturation. In the presence of a full agonist, partial agonists reduce their effect, thus acting as mixed agonists-antagonists. Competitive antagonists bind to a receptor but lack intrinsic efficacy;

their antagonistic effect increases with progressive fractional receptor occupancy. Although the existence of full and low efficacy agonists as well as of antagonists at the BZR is not surprising as it is subject to the basic rules governing receptor-ligand interactions, the discovery of full and partial inverse agonists emerged as a completely novel principle, initially met with great scepticism. Yet, the existence of ligands with negative intrinsic efficacy was predicted long before on purely theoretical grounds (41). These theoretical considerations assumed that a receptor could oscillate spontaneously between two energetically favorable conformational states, representing the active and inactive forms, the equilibrium for different receptors being at any point between highest probability for the active or inactive state. Ligands are proposed to differ in their affinity for the two states (Fig. 6). Full agonists would bind preferably or exclusively to the active conformation, stabilize it and, hence, shift the equilibrium toward the active state. Partial

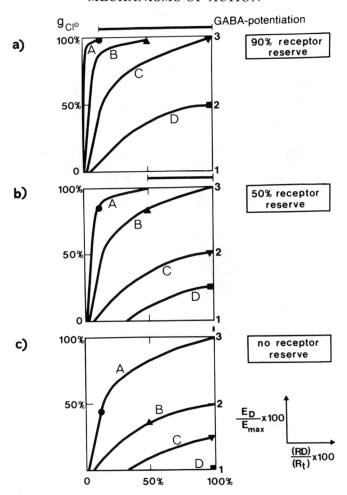

FIG. 5. Schematic diagram illustrating the influence of intrinsic efficacy of ligands and receptor density of target cells on the effect of drugs.

agonists would have a less marked preference for the active state. Inverse agonists are assumed to prefer the inactive state and, hence, shift the receptor toward this conformation. Pure competitive antagonists, by not distinguishing the two conformations, would bind to both conformations equally well and fail to affect the resting equilibrium, but compete with the binding of both agonists and inverse agonists.

This "two-state" hypothesis emphasizes the selection by ligands of two spontaneously occurring conformations, but an alternative "three-state" hypothesis (32) assumes the existence of a functional neutral inactive state and two different states with opposite consequences on the transduction mechanisms, and postulates the need of a ligand to induce the two opposite states. The reasons why a receptor reacting to ligands with positive, zero, and negative intrinsic efficacies have not yet been found aside from the BZR is simple. For most receptors the equilibrium between the two states would logically be close to the inactive state since their role is to activate a resting, inactive receptor-transduction mechanism. Hence, inverse agonists would

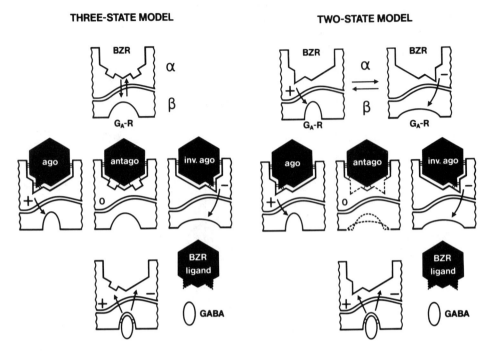

FIG. 6. Two- and three-state model to explain the existence of agonists and inverse agonists.

hardly be able to shift the equilibrium to further inactivity and would appear as pure competitive antagonists when tested in the presence of an agonist. This is likely to be the situation with the $GABA_A$ receptor, as its coupled channel is continuously closed in the absence of GABA. The BZR has a different function; it does not act as channel operator but as modulator of the channel gating process. We may reasonably assume that at rest (in the absence of a ligand) the equilibrium between the positive and the negative modulatory states of the BZR is somewhere in the middle and that, therefore, inverse agonists produce a detectable functional change and can be distinguished from functionally inert competitive antagonists.

Pharmacology of BZR Ligands

The basic changes by BZR ligands in the $GABA_A$ receptor-mediated chloride flux in neuronal membranes is illustrated schematically in Fig. 7. It shows a control dose-response curve for the chloride conductance increase of GABA in a neuron, e.g., a single neuron in cell culture and the changes induced in this curve by prototypes of BZR.

Full BZR Agonists

Full BZR agonists produce a concentration-dependent parallel shift to the left of the GABA dose-response curve without altering its maximum; in other terms, they increase the apparent affinity of GABA or its potency. Curve B (Fig. 7) depicts the effect of a submaximal agonist dose and curve A shows the effect of a maximally active dose. This maximal shift is about two- to threefold. A consequence of this leftward shift is that BZR agonists produce a relevant increase of the effect of GABA at GABAergic

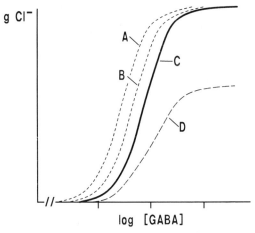

g Cl⁻

log [GABA]

FIG. 7. Theoretical changes induced by BZR ligands on the dose-response curve of GABA for chloride conductance induction. **A,** effect of a maximal dose of full agonist. **B,** leftward shift by a submaximal dose of a full agonist or by a maximal dose of a partial agonist. **C,** control curve in the absence of BZR ligands (or in the presence of a pure competitive BZR antagonist). **D,** effect of a full inverse agonist.

synapses when the synaptic concentrations of GABA are submaximal, they have no effect in the absence of activity in the GABAergic afferent, and they do not increase the effect of maximal concentrations of GABA. Accordingly, varying degrees of facilitation by agonists have been found in different central nervous system (CNS) neurons with spontaneous or electrically stimulated GABAergic inputs, and the ongoing activities of different neurons in the intact CNS show depressions of greatly varying intensity in response to agonists. The facilitation of GABAergic synaptic transmission by BZR agonists readily explains their characteristic and broad profile of pharmacological activity (anxiolytic, anticonvulsant, sedative, and muscle relaxant), although we can only guess as to the CNS structures and neuronal circuits that are involved in the individual effects. Most BZR ligands available in therapy today are full agonists.

Partial BZR Agonists

Partial BZR agonists produce a smaller maximal leftward shift of the GABA dose-response curve than full agonists. Their maximal effect corresponds to the effect of a submaximally effective dose of full agonist (curve B in Fig. 7). The important consequence of the submaximal GABA potentiation is a dramatic change in their pharmacological profile (16): they retain full anxiolytic and anticonvulsant efficiency but the intensity of their sedative and muscle relaxant-ataxic effects is greatly reduced and, in fact, they act as antagonists of full agonists for these effects. Other remarkable consequences of weak intrinsic efficacy are the greatly reduced liability for inducing tolerance and physical dependence. This interesting profile can be explained by the situation theoretically illustrated in Fig. 5, assuming that neurons critically involved in the anxiolytic and anticonvulsant effects have a higher receptor density than those mediating sedative and muscle relaxant effects. Clonazepam, known to have particularly advantageous properties in the antiepileptic therapy, has a submaximal intrinsic efficacy (3). Attempts at designing tailor-made partial BZR agonists as superior antiepileptics appear to be very promising.

Competitive BZR Antagonists

Competitive BZR antagonists have, ideally, zero intrinsic efficacy. The first antagonist available for therapy, flumazenil (22,13) has a very weak intrinsic efficacy, not enough to produce any sedative and anxiolytic effects but sufficient to produce weak antiepileptic effects in mild forms of experimental epileptiform models in animals. Flumazenil, whose established indications are in BZR agonist overdosing and in reversal of agonist-induced sedation in anesthesiology and intensive care medicine, is currently being investigated for potential usefulness in antiepileptic treatment. It is noteworthy that flumazenil is less potent in antagonizing the anticonvulsant effect of BZR agonists than their sedative-muscle relaxant effects. In clinical use, the antagonist has only very rarely been found to induce seizures in agonist-treated epileptics.

Partial and Full Inverse BZR Agonists

Partial and full inverse BZR agonists depress the dose-response curve of GABA, as shown by curve D in Fig. 7. They act as noncompetitive, allosteric GABA antagonists. Accordingly, full inverse agonists are anxiogenic, convulsant, arousing, and spasmogenic. Partial inverse agonists often lack convulsant activity when given alone, but facilitate the effect of convulsants not acting through the BZR (so-called proconvulsant activity). Repeated administration of partial inverse BZR agonists can lead to sensitization (kindling epilepsy).

FACILITATION OF GABAERGIC SYNAPTIC TRANSMISSION AND ANTIEPILEPTIC ACTIVITY

Reduction of the efficiency of GABAergic neurotransmission very consistently induces epileptiform activities. The antiepileptic activity of BZR agonists and partial agonists is, therefore, easily explained by their facilitation of GABAergic transmission. These drugs have been shown to augment all types of synaptic inhibition mediated by GABAergic neurons schematically depicted in Fig. 8. Of particular relevance is the potentiation of recurrent inhibition by BZR agonists on hippocampal and cortical pyramidal cells (20), neurons that are notorious for exhibiting high-frequency bursting activity and that are candidates for epileptic pacemaker cells.

Positive allosteric modulation of the $GABA_A$ receptor function by BZR agonists and partial agonists makes neurons more sensitive to their GABAergic inhibitory synaptic input. Thus, these drugs act simply by reinforcing intrinsic synaptic inhibition mediated by the $GABA_A$ receptor-triggered

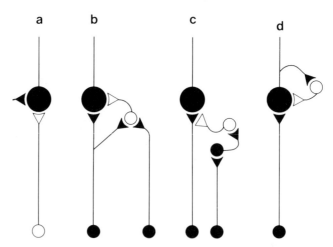

FIG. 8. Prototypes of neuronal circuits containing a GABAergic neuron. Excitatory neurons indicated by filled symbols, GABAergic neurons by open symbols. **a,** direct inhibition by a GABAergic projection neuron (e.g., striatal or nigral efferent neurons). **b,** indirect forward inhibition through a local interneuron. **c,** presynaptic inhibition of primary afferent neurons (axo-axonal GABAergic synapse). **d,** recurrent inhibition.

increase of chloride conductance. The latter induces hyperpolarization in the majority of neurons, in particular when these are highly active and, thereby, reduces their excitability by shifting the membrane potential away from the threshold potential for spike generation. But even in those neurons which have a less pronounced chloride concentration gradient and in which GABA induces depolarization, the chloride conductance shunts the depolarizing effect of the sodium influx that underlies the excitatory synaptic potentials and the rising part of action potentials. Thus, the $GABA_A$ receptor-mediated antiepileptic effect of BZR agonists and partial agonists mainly reflects a reduced synaptic excitability, resulting in prevention or blockade of interictal paroxysmal activity and of the transition into ictal activity in pacemaker neurons, as well as of the propagation and generalization of paroxysmal activity.

EFFECTS OF BZR LIGANDS UNRELATED TO BZR

Although the anticonvulsant effect of BZR agonists and partial agonists in animals, in particular against experimentally induced pentylenetetrazol seizures, shows a clear relationship to fractional BZR occupancy, actions unrelated to the BZR may have an additive or synergistic effect on GABAergic facilitation. Several such actions have been proposed.

Adenosine Potentiation

Several BZR ligands have been reported to potentiate the depressant effect of adenosine on neuronal excitability and activity. This effect has been explained by inhibition of a nucleoside transporter operating in the membrane of a variety of cells (31). Adenosine may be released as neurotransmitter from specific neurons or, nonspecifically, from any metabolically highly active cells

as a breakdown product of the energy-rich adenosine triphosphate. The inhibitory effect on adenosine uptake of BZR ligands at relevant concentrations is rather small and not correlated with the anticonvulsant potency of the ligands studied. Adenosine uptake inhibition is, therefore, unlikely to play a major role in the antiepileptic activity of BZR agonists and partial agonists, but may provide an additional mechanism of action for some of these drugs under special conditions.

Inhibition of Calcium Influx

Bowling and De Lorenzo (6) reported a saturable binding of ^3H-diazepam to brain membrane at micromolar concentrations. Half-maximal saturation of these low-affinity binding sites required about 30,000 times higher concentration than the K_D for the high-affinity BZR. The affinity for micromolar binding sites did not correlate with that for the nanomolar binding site in a small series of compounds tested and there was also no correlation between the affinities for the micromolar binding site and the anticonvulsant potency. The authors claimed that the affinity for the micromolar site correlated with potency in the electroshock seizure model. This is an interesting hypothesis because there are marked discrepancies between antipentylenetetrazol and antielectroshock potencies among BZR agonists; some very potent drugs in the former test are virtually or completely inactive in the latter, e.g., thieno diazepines, triazolo- and imidazobenzodiazepines. Moreover, the concentrations of benzodiazepine-agonists achieved in the brain after doses used to abolish status epilepticus are in a range that could interact with low-affinity binding sites. Unfortunately, the low-affinity binding has not been reproduced in other laboratories and the significance of these binding sites, therefore, remains highly speculative. The micromolar benzodiazepine binding site has been hypothesized to mediate an inhibition of voltage-dependent calcium current (36,23). Although calcium transients have been shown to be depressed by micromolar concentrations also in non-neuronal cells, at present it is not clear whether this mechanism has any relevance for the therapeutic effects of benzodiazepines.

INCREASE OF POTASSIUM CONDUCTANCE

Carlen et al. (8) proposed that BZR agonists increase calcium-induced potassium conductance based on studies in hippocampal slices. Although the induction of potassium conductance could explain part of the stabilizing effect of BZR agonists on neuronal cell activity, the fact that the potassium current activation occurred at subnanomolar and disappeared at low nanomolar concentrations and the failure of other investigations to find consistent changes of the membrane conductance, raise serious doubts as to the validity of this hypothesis.

USE-DEPENDENT BLOCKADE OF FAST SODIUM CHANNELS

Sustained repetitive firing occurs in cultured spinal cord neurons depolarized by constant current injection. Several BZR agonists of the benzodiazepine class, but not of the β-carboline class, were found by McLean and Macdonald (25) to markedly reduce this repetitive firing at high nanomolar concentrations. This effect was ascribed to a use- and voltage-dependent blockade of fast sodium channels, i.e., to a slowing of recovery of these channels from inactivation. BZR antagonist did not reduce the benzodiazepine effects, suggesting that the high-affinity BZR was not involved. Since other anticonvulsants such as diphenylhydantoin, carbamazepine, and valproate produce a similar limitation of re-

petitive firing, the authors proposed that all these drugs share a common mechanism of action. The contribution of this effect to the anticonvulsant action of BZR agonists is at present not clear, as BZR antagonists block their anticonvulsant effects *in vivo*. Moreover, the (convulsant) p-chloroderivative of diazepam also limited repetitive firing. It is imperative to confirm the limiting effect of benzodiazepines on repetitive firing under less artificial conditions before this mechanism can be accepted as relevant for therapeutic antiepileptic activity.

ENDOGENOUS LIGANDS OF THE BZR

The problem of endogenous ligands of the BZR has been reviewed recently (15). None of the candidates with either positive or negative intrinsic efficacy has yet been shown to interact with the BZR *in vivo* under physiological or pathological conditions.

TOLERANCE TO THE ANTIEPILEPTIC ACTION OF BZR AGONISTS

Development of tolerance to the antiepileptic action of BZR agonists is a handicap in the therapeutic use of these drugs. The mechanisms underlying this tolerance are not yet fully elucidated. Experimental evidence suggests that a down-regulation of BZR occurs with repeated exposure (26,27). A desensitization of the $GABA_A$ receptor has also been observed (12). Since GABA induces desensitization of its receptor very quickly, the GABA potentiation achieved with BZR agonists may facilitate this process. Most interestingly, partial BZR agonists have been found to lack the tolerance-inducing liability in animals (21). This property of partial agonists, together with their lower sedative activity, may have great relevance for the treatment of epilepsy.

CONCLUSIONS

Exploration of the mechanism of action of the classic benzodiazepines resulted in the identification of specific high-affinity receptors in neuronal membranes. This BZR is an allosteric modulatory site present on most or all GABA$_A$ receptor-chloride channel complexes. The BZR recognizes ligands of various chemical classes, both benzodiazepines and non-benzodiazepines. These BZR ligands cover a continuum of intrinsic efficacies from full positive over zero to full negative intrinsic efficacy. BZR agonists and partial agonists are ligands which facilitate the chloride channel-gating function of GABA, resulting in an enhancement of GABAergic synaptic transmission. Full and partial BZR inverse agonists depress the gating function and non-competitively reduce GABAergic transmission. Benzodiazepine receptor antagonists bind to the BZR without affecting the gating function but block the effects of both agonists and inverse agonists. A concept of the structure of the GABA$_A$-BZR is beginning to emerge. The enhancement of GABAergic neurotransmission provides different sites of attack for BZR agonists to reduce the excitability of neurons and, thereby, to limit epileptiform activities.

Several direct actions of benzodiazepines on the neuronal membrane unrelated to the GABA$_A$ receptor have been found, such as inhibition of the cellular uptake of adenosine and interaction with potassium, sodium, and calcium channels. The relevance of these effects as secondary components of the antiepileptic activity of benzodiazepines is not yet clear.

REFERENCES

1. Biggio, G., and Costa, E. (eds.) (1983): *Benzodiazepine Recognition Site Ligands: Biochemistry and Pharmacology*. Raven Press, New York.
2. Biggio, G., and Costa, E. (eds.) (1986): *GABAergic Transmission and Anxiety*. Raven Press, New York.
3. Bonetti, E. P., Polc, P., Laurent, J.-P., Schoch, P., and Haefely, W. (1987): Clonazepam is a partial agonist at the benzodiazepine receptor. *Neuroscience,* 22 (Suppl.) S82.
4. Bosman, H. B., Case, K. R., Di Stefano, P. (1977): Diazepam receptor characterization: Specific binding of a benzodiazepine to macromolecules in various areas of rat brain. *TEBS Letters,* 82:368–372.
5. Bowery, N. G. (ed.) (1984): *Actions and Interactions of GABA and Benzodiazepines*. Raven Press, New York.
6. Bowling, A. G., and De Lorenzo, R. J. (1982): Micromolar affinity benzodiazepine receptors: Identification and characterization in central nervous system. *Science,* 216:1247–1250.
7. Braestrup, C., and Nielsen, M. (1983): Benzodiazepine receptors. In: *Handbook of Psychopharmacology*, Vol. 17, edited by L. L. Iversen, S. D. Iversen, and S. H. Snyder, pp. 285–384. Plenum Press, New York.
8. Carlen, P. L., Gurevich, N., Davies, M. F., Blaxter, T. J., O'Beirne, M. (1985): Enhanced neuronal K^+ conductance: A possible common mechanism for sedative-hypnotic drug action. *Canad. J. Physiol. Pharmacol.,* 63:831–837.
9. Costa, E. (1983): *The Benzodiazepines: From Molecular Biology to Clinical Practice*. Raven Press, New York.
10. Costa, E., and Barnard, E. (eds.) (1988): *The Allosteric Modulation of Amino Acid Receptors and Its Therapeutic Implication*. Raven Press, New York.
11. Costa, E., Guidotti, A., and Mao, C. C. (1975): Evidence for involvement of GABA in the action of benzodiazepines: Studies on rat cerebellum. *Advances Biochem. Psychopharmacol.,* 14:113–130.
12. Gallager, D. W., Malcolm, A. B., Anderson, S. A., and Gonsalves, S. F. (1985): Continuous release of diazepam: Electrophysiological and behavioral consequences. *Brain Research,* 342:26–36.
13. Geller, E., and Thomson, D. (eds.) (1988): Proceedings of the International Symposium on flumazenil—The first benzodiazepine antagonist. *Eur. J. Anaesthesiol.* Suppl. 2:1–332.
14. Haefely, W. E. (1987): Structure and function of the benzodiazepine receptor. *Chimia,* 41:389–396.
15. Haefely, W. (1988): Endogenous ligands of the benzodiazepine receptor. *Pharmacopsychiatry,* 21:43–46.
16. Haefely, W. (1988): Pharmacology of the allosteric modulation of GABA$_A$-receptors by benzodiazepine receptor ligands. In: *The Allosteric Modulation of Amino Acid Receptors and Its Therapeutic Implication,* edited by E. Costa and E. Barnard. Raven Press, New York.
17. Haefely, W., Kulcsar, A., Möhler, H., Pieri, L., Polc, P., and Schaffner, R. (1975): Possible involvement of GABA in the central actions of benzodiazepines. *Advances in Biochemical Psychopharmacology,* 14:131–151.
18. Haefely, W., Kyburz, E., Gerecke, M., and Möhler, H. (1985): Recent advances in the molecular

pharmacology of benzodiazepine receptors and in the structure-activity relationships of their agonists and antagonists. *Advances in Drug Research,* 14:165–322.

19. Haefely, W., Pieri, L., Polc, P., and Schaffner, R. (1981): General pharmacology and neuropharmacology of benzodiazepine derivatives. In: *Handbook of Experimental Pharmacology,* Vol. 55/II, edited by F. Hoffmeister and G. Stille, pp. 13–262. Springer Verlag, Berlin.

20. Haefely, W., and Polc, P. (1986): Physiology of GABA enhancement by benzodiazepine and barbiturates. In: *Benzodiazepine/GABA Receptors and Chloride Channels: Structural and Functional Properties,* edited by R. W. Olsen and J. C. Venter, pp. 97–133. Alan R. Liss, New York.

21. Haigh, J. R. M., and Feely, M. (1988): Ro 16-6028, a benzodiazepine receptor partial agonist, does not exhibit anticonvulsant tolerance in mice. *Eur. J. Pharmacol.,* 147:283–285.

22. Hunkeler, W., Möhler, H., Pieri, L., Polc, P., Bonetti, E. P., Cumin, R., Schaffner, R., and Haefely, W. (1981): Selective antagonists of benzodiazepines. *Nature,* 290:514–516.

23. Johansen, J., Taft, W. C., Yang, J., Kleinhans, A. L., and De Lorenzo, R. J. (1985): Inhibition of Ca^{2+} conductance in identified leech neurons by benzodiazepines. *Proc. Natl. Acad. Sci. USA,* 82:3935–3939.

24. Levitan, E. S., Schofield, P. R., Burt, D. R., Rhee, L. M., Wisden, W., Köhler, M., Fujita, N., Rodriguez, H. F., Stephenson, A., Darlison, M. G., Barnard, E. A., and Seeburg, P. H. (1988): Structural and functional basis for GABA$_A$ receptor heterogeneity. *Nature,* 335:76–79.

25. McLean, M. J., and Macdonald, R. L. (1988): Benzodiazepines, but not beta carbolines, limit high frequency repetitive firing of action potentials of spinal cord neurons in cell culture. *J. Pharmacol. Exp. Ther.,* 244:789–795.

26. Miller, L. G., Greenblatt, D. J., Barnhill, J. G., and Shader, R. I. (1988): Chronic benzodiazepine administration. I. Tolerance is associated with benzodiazepine receptor down regulation and decreased gamma-aminobutyric acid A receptor function. *J. Pharmacol. Exp. Ther.,* 246:170–176.

27. Miller, L. G., Greenblatt, D. J., Roy, R. B., Summer, W. R., and Shader, R. I. (1988): Chronic benzodiazepine administration. II. Discontinuation syndrome is associated with upregulation of gamma-aminobutyric acid$_A$ receptor complex binding and function. *J. Pharmacol. Exp. Ther.,* 246:177–182.

28. Möhler, H., Battersby, M. K., and Richards, J. G. (1980): Benzodiazepine receptor protein identified and visualized in brain tissue by a photoaffinity label. *Proc. Natl. Acad. Sci., USA,* 77:1666–1670.

29. Möhler, H., and Okada, T. (1977): Benzodiazepine receptor: Demonstration in the central nervous system. *Science,* 198:849–851.

30. Olsen, R. W. (1982): Drug interactions at the GABA-receptor-ionophore complex. *Ann. Rev. Pharmacol. Toxicol.,* 22:245–277.

31. Phillis, J. W. (1984): Adenosine's role in the central actions of the benzodiazepines. *Progr. Neuropsychopharmacol. Biol. Psychiat.,* 8:495–502.

32. Polc, P., Bonetti, E. P., Schaffner, R., and Haefely, W. (1982): A three-state model of the benzodiazepine receptor explains the interactions between the benzodiazepine antagonist Ro 15-1788, benzodiazepine tranquilizers, β-carbolines and phenobarbitone. *Arch. Pharmacol.,* 321:260–264.

33. Schoch, P., Richards, J. G., Häring, P., Takacs, B., Stähli, C., Staehelin, T., Haefely, W., and Möhler, H. (1985): Co-localization of GABA$_A$ receptors and benzodiazepine receptors in the brain shown by monoclonal antibodies. *Nature,* 314:168–171.

34. Schofield, P. R., Darlison, M. G., Fujita, N., Burt, D. R., Stephenson, F. A., Rodriguez, H., Rhee, L. M., Ramachandran, J., Reale, V., Glencorse, T. A., Seeburg, P. H., and Barnard, E. A. (1987): Sequence and functional expression of the GABA$_A$ receptor shows a ligand-gated receptor super-family. *Nature,* 328:221–227.

35. Sigel, E., Stephenson, F. A., Mamalaki, C., and Barnard, E. A. (1984): The purified GABA$_A$/benzodiazepine barbiturate receptor complex: Four types of ligand binding sites and the interactions between them are preserved in a single isolated protein complex. *J. Recept. Res.,* 4:175–188.

36. Skerrit, J. H., Were, M. A., McLean, M. J., and Macdonald, R. L. (1984): Diazepam and its anomalous *p*-chloro-derivative Ro 5-4864: Comparative effects on mouse neurons in cell culture. *Brain Research,* 310:99–105.

37. Skolnick, P., and Paul, S. M. (1982): Benzodiazepine receptors in the central nervous system. *Internat. Rev. Neurobiol.,* 23:103–140.

38. Smart, T. G., Constanti, A., Bilbe, G., Brown, D. A., and Barnard, E. A. (1983): Synthesis of functional chick brain GABA-benzodiazepine-barbiturate/receptor complex in mRNA-injected Xenopus oocytes. *Neuroscience Letters,* 40:55–59.

39. Smith, D. E., and Wesson, D. R. (eds.) (1985): *The Benzodiazepines, Current Standards for Medical Practice.* MTP Press Ltd., Lancaster.

40. Squires, R. F., and Braestrup, C. (1977): Benzodiazepine receptors in rat brain. *Nature,* 266:732–734.

41. Thron, C. D. (1973): On the analysis of pharmacological experiments in terms of an allosteric receptor model. *Mol. Pharmacol.,* 9:1–9.

42. Trimble, M. R. (ed.) (1983): *Benzodiazepine Divided.* John Wiley & Sons, Chichester.

43. Usdin, E., Skolnick, P., Tallman, J. F., Greenblatt, D., and Paul, S. M. (eds.) (1982): *Pharmacology of Benzodiazepines.* Macmillan, London.

Antiepileptic Drugs, Third Edition, edited by
R. Levy, R. Mattson, B. Meldrum,
J. K. Penry, and F. E. Dreifuss.
Raven Press, Ltd., New York © 1989.

55

Benzodiazepines

Diazepam

Dieter Schmidt

The clinical use of diazepam as an antiepileptic agent has grown in recent years. Diazepam remains the drug of first choice for the treatment of status epilepticus (190). In addition, diazepam has effectively been employed in the acute treatment of ongoing seizures. The introduction of the rectal administration of diazepam has further expanded its use for the prevention of febrile seizures or serial seizures. The potential of newly available benzodiazepine antagonists merits attention. The pharmacokinetics and clinical use of diazepam have been reviewed by Caccia and Garattini (26) and Schmidt (189,191). This chapter reviews selected aspects of the clinical pharmacology of diazepam as related to its therapeutic use and toxic effects in the treatment of epilepsy.

CHEMISTRY AND METHODS OF DETERMINATION

Diazepam is a yellowish crystalline substance with a melting point of 125° to 126°C and a bitter taste. Its chemical name is 7-chloro-1,3-dihydro-1-methyl-5-phenyl-2H-1, 4-benzodiazepin-2-one with a sum formula of $C_{16}H_{13}ClN_2O$. The structural formula is shown in Fig. 3. The molecular weight is 284.8. The pK_a is 3.4. Diazepam is soluble in chloroform, ethanol, dioxane, and dilute hydrochloric acid. It is not sol-uble in water (18). The parenteral solution (Valium[2]) is therefore dissolved in 40% propylene glycol, 10% ethyl alcohol, and a sodium benzoate/benzoic acid buffer or in cremophor EL (Stesolid[R]). The synthesis of the substance was described by Sternbach and Reeder (208). A study of the structure-activity relationship indicates that substitutions on position 7 in the six-membered A ring influence antiepileptic activity and selectivity (210).

The current gas chromatographic (GC) procedures with electron capture detector have a sensitivity of 1 to 10 ng of the compound per ml of plasma and require only 100 μl to 2 ml of plasma (188). The combination of GC with sophisticated mass spectrometer systems is most suitable for metabolic studies and other research purposes (93). Gas-liquid chromatography with flame ionization detectors and enzyme-immunoassay techniques are mainly employed for toxicology and drug abuse detection (78).

ABSORPTION, DISTRIBUTION, AND EXCRETION

Absorption

Oral Administration

Following a single oral dose of 5, 10, or 20 mg of diazepam, mean peak plasma concentrations of 145 ng/ml (110–180 ng/ml),

216 ng/ml (130–300 ng/ml), and 370 ng/ml (300–500 ng/ml), respectively, were obtained, mostly within 30 to 90 min, indicating a rather rapid absorption (Fig. 1) (11,40,60,89,101,126).

Ingestion of metoclopramide (161) and possibly alcohol (83,136) may enhance the absorption. An earlier peak (30 min) is observed in children, as compared with adults and the elderly (63).

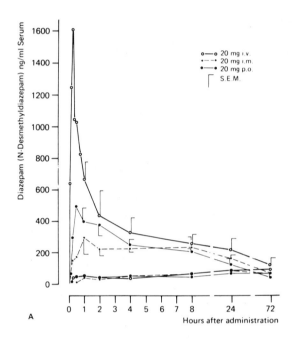

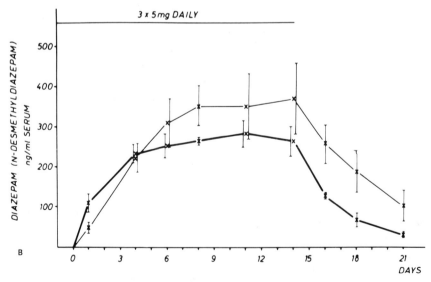

FIG. 1. Serum concentrations of diazepam and *N*-desmethyldiazepam following a single intravenous, intramuscular, or oral dose (**A**), a multiple oral dose (**B**), a single rectal dose (**C**), and a single intramuscular dose (**D**). (**A** and **B** from Hillestad et al., refs. 88, 89, and **C** and **D** from Meberg et al., ref. 151, with permission.)

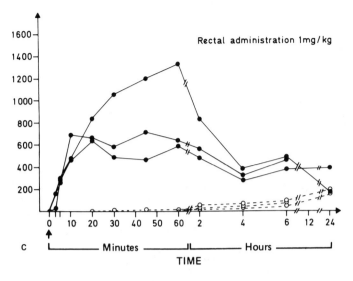

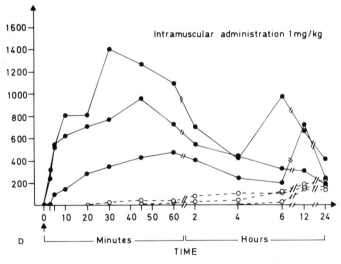

FIG. 1. (*continued*)

Intravenous Administration

Following an intravenous dose of 10 or 20 mg of diazepam, peak plasma concentrations of about 700 to 800 ng/ml and 1,100 to 1,607 ng/ml, respectively, are reached within 3 to 15 min in volunteers (Fig. 1) (11,89). Haram et al. (80) studied the plasma concentration shortly after intravenous administration of 30 mg of diazepam during labor. After 55 sec, a plasma concentration

of 1,047 ng/ml was recorded; at 135 sec after injection, a mean plasma concentration of 991 ng/ml was reached. These data indicate a most rapid increase in plasma concentration, surpassing the 500 ng/ml level that is minimally required for seizure control in less than 1 min. At doses of about 0.2 mg/kg, peak concentrations of approximately 500 ng/ml can be expected in children (4,105). In two newborns, peak concentrations of 5,775 to 10,800 ng/ml and 2,750 to

6,450 ng/ml were recorded 5 min after administration of 1 mg/kg or 0.5 mg/kg, respectively (133). Precipitation may occur when the intravenous diazepam solution is mixed with saline solutions (98). Adsorption of diazepam to the plastic tubing during infusion is possible (142).

Intramuscular Administration

After the intramuscular administration of 10 or 20 mg of diazepam, peak plasma concentrations of 35 to 300 ng/ml and 300 ng/ml, respectively, can be expected in adults within 30 to 60 min (Fig. 1) (12,13,89,128). The wide variation of plasma concentrations quite possible below 500 ng/ml and the late peak do not encourage the use of intramuscular administration in adults. The sources of variation include the site and the depth of the injection, the need to avoid injection into adipose tissue, the needle size, and the expertise of the person who performs the injection (60). In newborns and children up to 12 years, the intramuscular administration gave less erratic results and produced plasma concentrations above 500 ng/ml within the first 10 min. Peak concentrations of 206 to 1,400 ng/ml were recorded at 10 to 60 min after administration of 0.24 to 1 mg/kg (Fig. 1) (4,133,151).

Rectal Administration

Administration of 0.5 mg/kg or 1 mg/kg of diazepam solution in rectioles (rectal tube) resulted in peak plasma concentrations of 300 to 800 ng/ml within 4 to 45 min or of 600 to 1,400 ng/ml within 10 to 60 min. Plasma concentrations of 500 ng/ml required for acute seizure control are reached in infants and children under 11 years within 2 to 6 min (Fig. 1) (4,46,120,133,151). Rectal administration of several preparations of diazepam to six adult patients with epilepsy achieved peak serum concentrations of 375 $\pm$ 77 (S.D.) ng/ml between 10 and 120 min

with a mean of 65 $\pm$ 47 min (154). In contrast, suppositories are not suitable for acute treatment of seizures in children (4,120) or in adults (128,195) because of delayed peaks and low plasma concentrations.

Distribution

After the peak concentration has been reached, a mostly biexponential decline of the plasma concentration can be observed; correspondingly, an open two-compartment model is usually employed. A short distribution half-life ($t_{1/2}\alpha$) of about 1 hr determines the rapid initial decline. Correspondingly, the plasma concentration may drop below therapeutic values (200 ng/ml) within 15 to 20 min after intravenous injection, depending on the initial peak concentration (Fig. 1). The subsequent slower decline results mainly from the elimination of the drug; its slope determines the apparent plasma elimination half-life ($t_{1/2}\beta$) (Table 1). A second smaller peak of the plasma concentration may occur after a meal. The mechanism of the redistribution is unclear: a change in plasma protein binding by food intake (125) and an enterohepatic circulation have been excluded.

Tissue Distribution

As a result of its low pK_a and its lipophilic character, diazepam distributes quickly in lipoid tissues and rapidly crosses the blood-brain barrier. After intravenous administration in mice, N^{14}-CH$_3$-diazepam is seen in brain within 18 sec by whole-body autoradiography (220). Extrapolating to an average body composition for a 70 kg man with 16% body fat, the largest fractions of total body stores of diazepam would be found in muscle (42%), fat (35%), and liver (12%), with smaller stores in brain (4–3%), lung, heart, kidney, and adrenal gland (57). Based on its most rapid antiepileptic effect, sometimes observed within seconds after intravenous administration (Fig. 2), a very rapid penetration of diazepam into the human brain may be assumed. The subsequent decline and selective binding in different brain regions are rather difficult to predict from animal data. The decline probably begins within minutes after administration and is likely to differ for various brain regions. In addition, redistribution into the brain may also occur.

Plasma and Tissue Protein Binding

The apparent volume of distribution of diazepam in volunteers ranges from 1 to 2 liter/kg (Table 1). It is higher in children or the elderly and increases in liver cirrhosis or hepatitis because of a lower protein binding (Table 1). Simultaneous ingestion of ethanol may decrease the volume of distribution (143), which is not affected by alcohol withdrawal (174).

Diazepam and *N*-desmethyldiazepam are both strongly bound to plasma proteins, mainly albumin, over the therapeutic range (Table 1). The apparent association constant K_{app} is $1.3 \text{ M}^{-1}10^{-4}$ for normal serum (123). The high protein binding is responsible for the fact that diazepam distributes only very little into red blood cells, resulting in a blood-to-plasma concentration ratio of 0.58 ± 0.15 (116), or into saliva (2%–3.5%) and cerebrospinal fluid (CSF), representing the free fraction of diazepam (44,84,105).

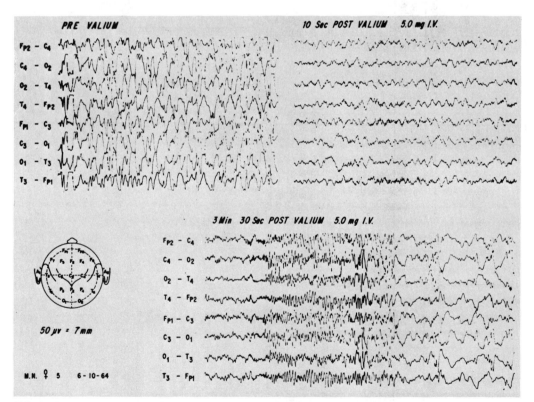

FIG. 2. Ten seconds after intravenous administration of 5 mg diazepam, the electroencephalogram of a 5-year-old girl in status epilepticus is completely free of polyspikes, which return 3½ min later, although there are no clinical signs. (From Lombroso, ref. 137, with permission.)

TABLE 1. *Pharmacokinetics of diazepam, N-desmethyldiazepam, and oxazepam[a]*

	Diazepam	Ref.	N-Desmethyl-diazepam	Ref.	Oxazepam	Ref.
Apparent volume of distribution (liter/kg)						
Volunteers	0.95–2.0	8, 21, 96, 107, 113, 116	0.64–1.11	114, 217	0.7 (47.7–61.2 liters)	110, 203
Epileptic patients			1.58[b], 1.63[c]	225		
Premature newborns	1.8 ± 0.3	159				
Infants	1.3 ± 0.2	159				
Children	2.6 ± 0.5	159				
Elderly (over 60 yr)	0.8–2.2	116	0.85 ± 0.14	117		
Liver disease	0.59–1.74	21, 116	0.63 ± 0.12	114	(52–61 liters)	203
Species differences						
Dog	5.6	113				
Rabbit	5.5	113				
Guinea pig	2.5	113				
Rat	4.5	113				
Plasma protein binding (%)						
Volunteers	96–97	113, 220	96.6	110	87–89	203
Fetus, newborn	84	102				
Liver disease	95.3 ± 1.8	116				
Renal insufficiency	92.0 ± 7.7	100	94.5 ± 2.8	100	86–87	203
Chronic alcoholism	97.8 ± 1.2	214				
Species differences						
Dog	96.0	113	95.9	113		
Rabbit	89.9	113	94.7	113		
Guinea pig	91.3	113	78.6	113		
Rat	86.3	113	90.5	113		
Distribution half-life ($t_{1/2\alpha}$, hr)						
Volunteers	0.96–2.2	107, 113	0.17–0.78	72, 114		
	1.1 ± 0.3[b]	112				
	4.2 ± 2.3[c]	112				
Epileptic patients			1.28 ± 0.44	225		

Apparent elimination half-life ($t_{1/2}\beta$, hr)

Volunteers or psychiatric patients	32–36[b]; 28–54[c]	8, 112; 10, 17, 21, 88, 107, 112, 220	51 ± 6.2; 48–55[b]; 92; 51 ± 7[c]	114, 117; 88, 217	5.1–5.6[b]	203
Epileptic patients	36.4 ± 4.9	85	39.2 ± 14.3[b]; 40.4 ± 6.0[c]	225; 225		
Premature newborns	75 ± 35	159				
Full-term newborns	31 ± 2	159				
Diazepam pretreated	18 ± 1	159				
Barbiturate, pretreated	29 ± 1	159				
Infants	10 ± 2	159				
Children	17 ± 3[b]	159				
Elderly (over 60–65 yr)	80–100	110	151 ± 60	117	5.3–5.8	203
Liver disease	59–116	21, 85, 114, 116	108.2 ± 40.3	114		
Pregnancy	65 ± 29	157				
Species differences						
Dog	7.6	112	9	220		
Rabbit	2.7	112				
Guinea pig	2.4	112				
Rat	1.1	112	4	220		
Mouse						

Plasma clearance (ml/min)

Volunteers or psychiatric patients	15–35; 26.0 ± 10.8[b]; 18.2 ± 7.0[c]; 18.7 ± 2.3[e]	8, 85, 112, 220; 111; 111; 85	7.4–11.3; 16.73 ± 2[d]	114, 117; 217	113–136	203
Epileptic patients			35.8 ± 7.4[b]; 34.6 ± 8.1[c]	225; 225		
Liver disease	8–24	85, 114, 116	4.6	114	137–155	203
Elderly (over 60 yr)	10–32	116	4.3 ± 1.5	117		
Pregnancy	28 ± 10	157				

[a] Data are given as mean ± S.D. or the range of values.
[b] Single dose.
[c] Multiple dose.
[d] Total body clearance.
[e] Metabolic clearance rate.

Protein binding is unaffected by age or food intake (113) but is impaired *in vitro* by oleic acid (206), in liver disease, or in uremia, resulting in lower K_{app} of 0.9 and 0.2 $M^{-1}10^{-4}$, respectively, probably because of inhibitors of binding in serum (123,124). A lower protein binding increases the plasma clearance in man as only the free fraction is extracted by the liver independent of liver blood flow, but significant species differences are obvious, both in percentage of bound diazepam and in the fact that metabolism in dog, rabbit, and rat is affected by liver blood flow (112).

Excretion

Elimination Half-Life

In volunteers, the apparent elimination half-life of diazepam is about 1 to 2 days (Table 1). In patients with epilepsy treated with prolonged use of enzyme-inducing antiepileptic drugs, the elimination half-life is about 30% shorter, corresponding to a higher metabolic clearance rate (Table 1) (85). The elimination is age dependent (Table 1) but independent of the dose, with no evidence for zero-order kinetics (111), and is unaffected by the route of administration (89). Plasma concentrations of 100 to 500 ng/ml were determined in patients with epilepsy who were receiving additional antiepileptic drugs (19,42).

N-Desmethyldiazepam is formed as long as diazepam is returning from the peripheral to the central compartment, which explains why the *N*-desmethyldiazepam elimination half-life tends to be longer when diazepam is given instead of *N*-desmethyldiazepam itself or clorazepate, its pro-drug (Table 1). *N*-Desmethyldiazepam has a longer elimination half-life than diazepam (Table 1). With long-term treatment, *N*-desmethyldiazepam will accumulate more than diazepam in plasma and CSF, resulting in two to five times higher plasma concentrations

when compared with single-dose administration (Fig. 1) (61,88,111). In patients with liver disease, the plasma clearance of *N*-desmethyldiazepam is decreased (Table 1).

Routes of Excretion

Man excretes 62% to 73% of the administered dose of diazepam in the urine and approximately 10% in the feces (196). The main urinary metabolites of diazepam are conjugated oxazepam and conjugated *N*-desmethyldiazepam, whereas conjugated *N*-methyloxazepam and free *N*-desmethyldiazepam or diazepam are of minor significance. During the first 24 hr, about 7% to 11% of the dose is excreted in the urine. With higher doses, e.g., in intoxication, a higher relative amount of the hydroxylated metabolites is excreted (106).

Diazepam or a diazepam metabolite may pass through the intestinal wall into the gut lumen, as about 5% to 18% of the administered [^{14}C] diazepam appears in stool despite the absence of significant biliary excretion of diazepam, which is less than 0.1% of the dose excreted (85,116). Consequently, there is no sound evidence for a significant enterohepatic circulation in man despite earlier suggestions (198,199). There are species differences in the relative amounts excreted in urine and in the feces (196).

BIOTRANSFORMATION

Demethylation of diazepam at N-1 to *N*-desmethyldiazepam, which is further metabolized by oxidation at C-3 to oxazepam, and direct oxidation of diazepam at C-3 to N-methyloxazepam are the major steps in the biotransformation of diazepam in man (Fig. 3). Oxidation of diazepam and *N*-desmethyldiazepam, *N*-methyloxazepam, and oxazepam at C-4 were described in different animal species (see Fig. 3) (6,196). The principal site of biotransformation is in the liver

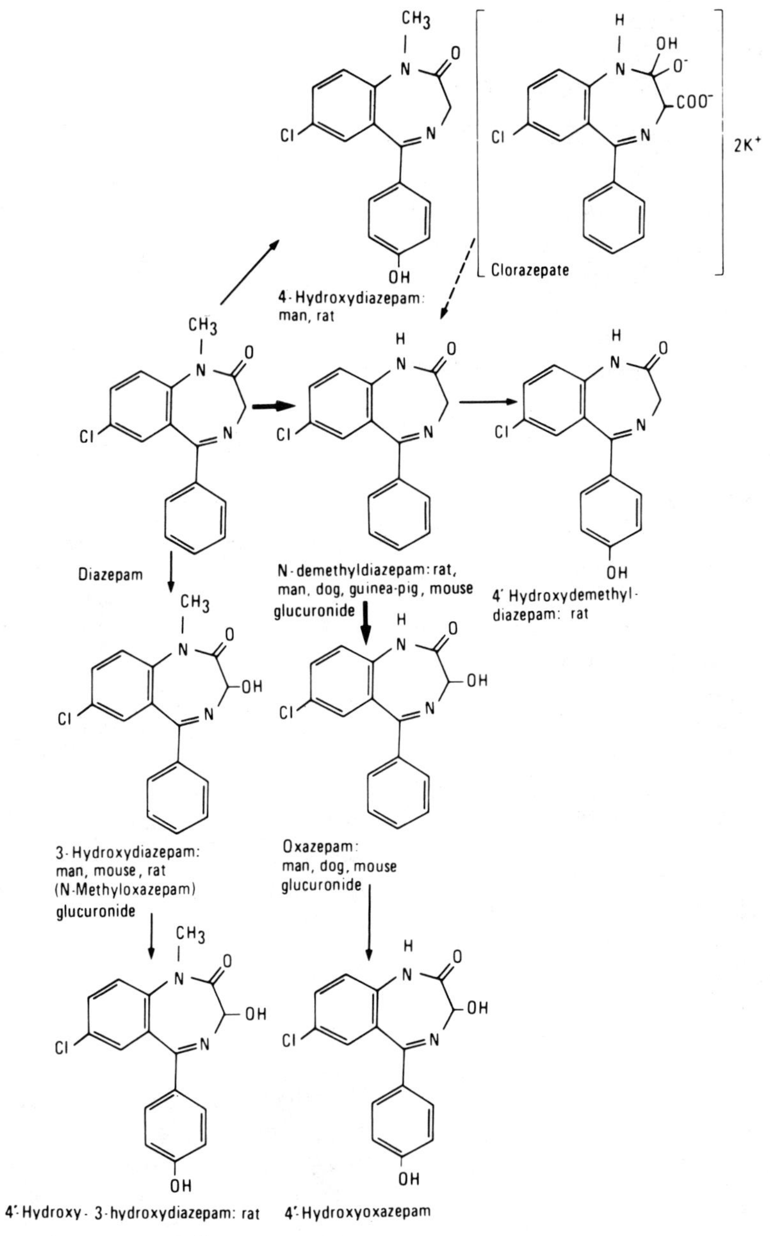

FIG. 3. Biotransformation of diazepam. Major steps are indicated by **thick arrows.** Note that the C1 at the 7 position remains intact. Clorazepate is decarboxylated to *N*-desmethyldiaze-pam. (Modified from Alvin and Bush, ref. 6, with permission.)

microsomes (2). Although the *N*-demethylation is rather rapid, as indicated by the appearance of *N*-desmethyldiazepam about 20 min after a single dose, the oxidation steps are slower (109).

The rapid antiepileptic effect shortly after intravenous administration and before *N*-desmethyldiazepam concentrations are reached indicates that diazepam per se possesses antiepileptic activity. From experimental data a potency ratio of 1.0 : 0.37 can be calculated for diazepam and desmethyldiazepam when the concentration in brain at 50% protection against pentylenetetrazol was determined in mice (56). *N*-Desmethyldiazepam possesses significant antiepileptic and sedative properties (37,217) and can reduce the elimination of diazepam by product inhibition (118). Because of their low plasma concentrations, oxazepam and *N*-methyloxazepam do not significantly contribute to the antiepileptic effect of diazepam treatment.

The biotransformation of diazepam is age dependent. It is metabolized *in vitro* as early as the 13th week of pregnancy by human fetal liver microsomes to *N*-desmethyldiazepam and *N*-methyloxazepam but at a lower rate than by adult liver microsomes (2). In the first days after delivery, a limited *in vivo* capacity to form hydroxylated and demethylated metabolites and a lower glucoronizing capacity have been revealed (159,160). During the first years of life, the relative share of hydroxylated metabolites will continue to increase (159). Phenobarbital treatment during intrauterine life or after delivery will lead to increased biotransformation, resulting in more hydroxylated metabolites in the newborn (159).

There are significant species differences in biotransformation as reviewed earlier (188). It led to more hydroxylated metabolites in mice and to more hydroxylated, *N*-demethylated, and polar metabolites in rats, whereas in guinea pigs, only *N*-demethylated metabolites were increased (188).

INTERACTIONS WITH OTHER DRUGS

Effect of Diazepam on Other Drugs

Diazepam rarely influences the pharmacokinetics of other drugs. It does not increase the urinary excretion of 6-β-hydroxycortisol, indicating that it is not, if at all, a potent enzyme inducer in man, nor does it influence the plasma levels of warfarin (169), ethanol, tricyclic antidepressants (204), or the beta-blocking agent metoprolol (119). It does not displace phenytoin from its plasma protein binding sites (90). Whether it has an effect on the bilirubin-binding capacity of serum in newborns is controversial (3,227). Diazepam does not interfere with measurements of adrenal hormones in urine (33), nor does it affect the metabolic clearance rate of methylprednisolone and its sodium succinate (209). The influence of diazepam on the plasma concentration of phenytoin is controversial; both lower and higher plasma phenytoin levels have been reported after addition of diazepam (94,179,205,219). Diazepam may accelerate the elimination of phenobarbital in man and in the rat (87).

Effect of Other Drugs on Diazepam

Diazepam pharmacokinetics are not significantly influenced by oral steroids (207). Whether phenobarbital or phenytoin influences the plasma concentration of diazepam is controversial (120,223). Disulfiram reduces the plasma clearance of diazepam and *N*-desmethyldiazepam, whereas oxazepam is not affected (144). Cimetidine lowers both the plasma clearance of diazepam and the apparent volume of distribution, which may lead to higher plasma diazepam levels (115). Severe hypothermia has been described in one case of combined treatment with lithium carbonate and diazepam, but neither drug alone (162). The mechanism of the interaction remains unclear.

Aminophylline reverses the protective action of diazepam against electroconvulsions in mice (36) and antagonizes diazepam-induced anesthesia and EEG changes in humans (149). Even though the exact nature of this interaction is unclear, it suggests the participation of a purinergic component in the anticonvulsant action of diazepam. The anticonvulsant effects of diazepam were potentiated by administration of the cannabinoid derivative levonantradol in the amygdaloid-kindled rats (48). Facilitation of the anticonvulsant action of diazepam occurs following the addition of sodium valproate (130). Displacement of protein binding of diazepam through valproate results in an increased free concentration of diazepam (43). This interaction may provide an explanation for the increased anticonvulsant efficacy of diazepam and the observation that the CNS-depressant effects of diazepam are potentiated by the concurrent intake of valproate (192). Obviously, addition of sedative effects is seen when diazepam is combined with sedative or hypnotic drugs or alcohol (158).

Benzodiazepine Antagonists

Flumazeil, an imidazobenzodiazepine, is a benzodiazepine antagonist that specifically blocks by competitive inhibition the central effects of agents acting through the benzodiazepine receptor. The bioavailability of diazepam is not affected by flumazenil (166). Animal experiments suggest that flumazeil competes directly with diazepam for a binding site involved in producing anticonvulsant activity (173). At doses of 1.0 mg/kg and higher flumazeil attenuated the anticonvulsant action of diazepam (1.0 mg/kg) in epileptic chickens (173). In this model flumazeil alone had no anticonvulsant activity even in doses as high as 10 mg/kg. However, when flumazeil was tested together with low doses of diazepam (0.25 mg/kg) in amygdaloid-kindled rats, it appeared

to have moderate anticonvulsant properties, apart from its antagonist effects attenuating the anticonvulsant action of higher doses of diazepam (2 mg/kg) (5). These results and similar data indicate that flumazeil is a benzodiazepine partial agonist with low efficacy as well as a potent antagonist (30,76). Flumazeil precipitates mild and intermediate withdrawal signs when given in baboons after 7 days of diazepam exposure (141). When given to patients with epilepsy, flumazeil caused the disappearance or marked reduction of epileptic potentials in the EEG. Only one of the four patients studied was pretreated with diazepam, the others had no recent exposure to benzodiazepines. Results of this pilot study would suggest further investigation of flumazeil in patients with epilepsy to clarify its potential as an antiepileptic agent. Side effects were not observed (197). Flumazeil may also be useful for the acute treatment of sedative side effects of benzodiazepines with anticonvulsant properties.

Other benzodiazepine antagonists belonging to the group of β-carbolines also antagonize diazepam activity in cats and mice (167,212). The imidazodiazepine Ro 15-4513 completely reversed the anticonvulsant effects of diazepam in mice, suggesting that it is a competitive ligand for benzodiazepine receptors (165). Additional studies are required to evaluate the impact of benzodiazepine antagonists on the treatment of epilepsy and their role as instruments to explore the contribution of benzodiazepine receptor ligands to the regulation of seizure mechanisms in epilepsy.

RELATION OF PLASMA CONCENTRATION TO SEIZURE CONTROL

Relation of Dose to Plasma Concentration

The available clinical evidence suggests that diazepam plasma concentrations differ widely, up to 10-fold after a single oral dose (41,60,147,177,228), and up to threefold with prolonged treatment (17,61,220). Intramuscular injection leads to as much as 10-fold differences in plasma diazepam concentrations and to as much as fourfold differences in the CSF concentrations of diazepam and N-desmethyldiazepam (11,60,84,104,128). Severalfold differences in plasma diazepam concentrations were reported following intravenous (19,21,66) and rectal (4) administration. Experimentally, over 10-fold differences in whole-brain concentration have been shown after intravenous administration of oxazepam (148). In conclusion, the poor correlation between dose and concentration in plasma and CSF (and probably in brain) makes it very difficult to predict correctly the actual concentration from the administered dose, regardless of the mode of administration.

Therapeutic Plasma Concentration

Sound clinical evidence for a relationship between plasma concentration and seizure control is based on prospective trials in which the plasma concentration is monitored before and during seizure control or at recurrence of a seizure. Unfortunately, only a few such studies are available (155). One report indicated that plasma concentrations of 300 to 700 ng/ml were needed for initial control of focal seizures after intravenous administration of 0.14 to 0.34 mg/kg of diazepam in three children aged 4, 5, and 15 years. Seizure control could be maintained with plasma diazepam concentrations of more than 130 to 180 ng/ml (52). In a second study, the individual therapeutic plasma concentrations were not given, but rectal administration (0.12–0.45 mg/kg) produced seizure control 10 min after administration in two children with plasma concentrations of 183 to 1,135 ng/ml (4). Two other children required 330 ng/ml and 250 ng/ml, respectively, for seizure control

(4,223). Knudsen (120) noted that one child had febrile convulsions despite a plasma diazepam level of 1,185 ng/ml after rectal administration of 0.7 mg/kg of the drug.

Relation of Plasma Concentration to EEG Suppression

The clinical evidence in adults is limited to plasma concentrations of diazepam associated with the suppression of EEG discharges. Mattson (150) noted persistent spiking in the EEG of a 52-year-old confused man despite plasma diazepam concentrations of 220 ng/ml. In another case, paroxysmal spiking with photic stimulation disappeared after 10 mg of diazepam was given intravenously and remained controlled at 110 ng/ml. Booker and Celesia (19) found a significant correlation between the suppression of interictal specific paroxysmal discharges in the EEG and the serum concentration of diazepam (Fig. 4). A plasma concentration of 1,300 ng/ml (600–2,000 ng/ml) was necessary in photosensitive patients for protection against stroboscopic stimulation. The suppression was maintained by plasma concentrations of about 500 ng/ml (100–500 ng/ml). In nonphotosensitive patients, the initial concentration for suppression of specific paroxysmal discharges was 1,800 ng/ml (600–1,800 ng/ml). Discharges returned at 800 ng/ml (500–1,400 ng/ml). No suppression effect was observed in either group below 430 ng/ml (300–700 ng/ml).

Dasberg et al. (37) found that a minimal steady-state plasma concentration of 400 ng/ml was necessary for the anxiolytic effect of diazepam. A combination of the anxiolytic and antiepileptic effects of diazepam has been elegantly demonstrated by Mattson (150) who described a 40-year-old man with anxiety-provoked hyperventilation which led to myoclonic seizures. Diazepam at plasma concentrations of 270 ng/ml relieved the anxiety, the emotional stimulus

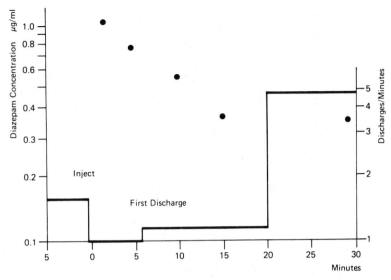

FIG. 4. The effect of intravenous administration of diazepam on 3 to 4 Hz spike-and-wave complexes. Discharges are suppressed at peak concentrations of about 1,000 ng/ml; suppression is maintained for 6 min until the plasma concentration falls below 700 ng/ml. Discharge frequency is indicated by a **bar graph**, scale on right. Diazepam concentrations are indicated by **filled circles**, scale on left. (From Booker and Celesia, ref. 19, with permission.)

apparently was suppressed, and the spiking of the EEG and the seizures improved. Blood levels of more than 100 ng/ml were associated with an increase in β activity and a decrease in α activity in the EEGs of volunteers, as frequently seen with diazepam treatment (24,108,188).

Variation of Therapeutic Concentrations

When diazepam is given to a patient for acute seizure control, clinical and electroencephalographic evidence (reviewed above) indicates that the concentration required for initial control of the seizure or suppression of the EEG discharge is higher than the concentration needed to maintain the desired therapeutic effect. It is tempting to assume that a rapidly occuring change in the "severity" from the ictal to the postictal state is responsible for the lower plasma concentration requirements (194). Age or additional disease, as in hepatic encepha-

lopathy, increases the sensitivity to the muscle-relaxant and depressant effects of diazepam (21,67,95,177).

The severalfold difference in therapeutic concentrations among patients may be the result of differences in the type or "severity" of the epilepsy, or both. In experimental seizures in cats, pentylenetetrazol-induced seizures were controlled by diazepam at concentrations ineffective against focal seizures. Focal seizures were controlled by 4 μg/g or more in brain and 2 μg/ml or more in serum (28). This study suggests that the type of seizure is an important variable accounting for differences of therapeutic plasma concentrations of diazepam. Similar data were recently reported for phenytoin, carbamazepine, and phenobarbital in patients with epilepsy (193). For the treatment of status epilepticus, a long duration of the status and acute underlying brain disease are significantly related to poor prognosis of treatment, which may be expected to require higher therapeutic concentrations if control can be achieved at all. Maintaining suppression of specific focal or generalized discharges requires higher concentrations than does suppression of photosensitivity (19). Generalized EEG discharges are more readily suppressed by diazepam than are focal abnormalities (131,164). This suggests, if extrapolation from EEG data to clinical seizures is allowed, that primary generalized and focal epilepsies may possibly require different therapeutic concentrations for acute or long-term treatment.

Toxic Effects Related to Plasma Concentration

Side effects such as drowsiness, ataxia, and dizziness occur mostly at the beginning of treatment in up to an estimated 10% to 40% of patients (24) and disappear with dose reduction. Irritability, inattention, sedation, and hypotonia are more common in children (4) and may partly be related to the accumulation of N-desmethyldiazepam (120). Diazepam produced little change in REM sleep, but a marked decrease in stage 4 sleep during short-term and subchronic oral administration, and during withdrawal (99). The dose-related side effects tend to lessen or disappear with the duration of treatment because of developing tolerance.

There seems to be a good correlation between the plasma concentration of diazepam and sedative effects after single-dose studies (89,101). At about 200 ng/ml, subjects tended to become slightly tired and drowsy (126). Most subjects were fast asleep at plasma concentrations of 1,600 ng/ml within 15 min after the intravenous administration. A transient deficiency in mental arithmetic, blurred vision, and amnesia persisted during the first 2 hr until the plasma concentration returned below 450 ng/ml (89,126). After intramuscular administration of 10 mg of diazepam, coordinative

and reactive skills were impaired for as long as 5 hr at plasma concentrations exceeding 180 ng/ml (127). In other studies of mood ratings, mental and psychomotor tests, or measures of clinical sedation, the correlation to the plasma concentration was weak (66,103). According to Morselli (159), the appearance of disturbing side effects such as marked drowsiness, vertigo, ataxia, and impaired performance is usually associated with plasma concentrations over 900 to 1,000 ng/ml. With prolonged treatment, the correlation becomes more difficult because of the development of tolerance (88).

The most serious side effects after intravenous administration are the rare development of apnea, hypotension, cardiac arrest, or obtundation. After intravenous administration for status epilepticus and additional sedative drug treatment, mild to severe hypotension or respiratory depression occurred in 5.2% of 246 patients, including one fatal case (0.4%) (163). In otherwise apparently healthy patients with epilepsy, slow intravenous administration usually produces no clinically significant hypotension or hypoventilation (164). As a precaution, however, equipment and personnel trained in cardiopulmonary resuscitation should be available when diazepam is administered intravenously.

The reason for the hypotensive and respiratory depressant action of diazepam is not clear and may involve the propylene glycol solvent (150). Risk factors leading to these rare life-threatening side effects include combination with sedative drugs such as barbiturates (175,185), lidocaine/epinephrine (202), methaqualone (45), chlordiazepoxide, or amobarbital (73), and use of a rapid (bolus) injection of even as little as 2.5 or 5 mg (23,79). Additional risk factors include higher age (67,177) and decompensated liver disease; both increase the sensitivity to diazepam and slow the elimination half-life (21,74,95). A low serum albumin possibly with a higher free fraction, advanced heart or lung disease, or any other severe disease are additional risks (20).

Newborns, especially premature newborns, may develop transient side effects after the transplacental transfer of maternal diazepam. Transient respiratory depression, muscular hypotonia, and absence of primitive reflex action up to several days were seen when more than 175 mg of diazepam was administered to the mother in the 24 hr prior to delivery (7). A transient floppy infant syndrome (68), poor sucking, transient hypothermia (170), loss of beat-to-beat variation in the fetal heart immediately following the intravenous administration (187), occasional slight hyperbilirubinemia (180), and slightly lower Apgar scores in some (49,180) but not all studies (62,81) have been reported.

An apparently rare lethal intoxication by diazepam in combination with other drugs has been described in an addict (27). Massive oral overdose may lead to cardiac arrest (16), hypotension, apnea, and coma (75). Patients intoxicated with plasma concentrations of 20,000 ng/ml of diazepam and 5,000 ng/ml of *N*-desmethyldiazepam and concentrations of oxazepam and *N*-methyloxazepam above 1,000 ng/ml have survived. Rapid clinical recovery from diazepam overdose does not result from rapid elimination, as both *N*-desmethyldiazepam and *N*-methyloxazepam have a long elimination half-life, but is more likely the result of tolerance to the depressant effect of the drug. Patients were fully alert at plasma concentrations of 1,800 to 7,000 ng/ml of diazepam and 600 to 5,000 ng/ml of *N*-desmethyldiazepam 1 or 2 days after a massive overdose (16). In a diazepam-induced coma, bullous skin lesions and exocrine sweat gland necrosis may occur (221). Apart from standard intensive care treatment, exchange transfusion (213) and physostigmine (134) have been employed in diazepam intoxications.

Tolerance

The development of tolerance may be the result of CNS adaptation to the effect of diazepam or a decline in plasma concentration, or both. Experimental evidence suggests that long-term exposure to diazepam diminishes its ability to protect against seizures induced by pentylenetetrazol in rats (69), mice (53), and in amygdaloid-kindled rats (97,139,140). Recent results indicate that tolerance to anticonvulsant activity against bicuculline seizures is temporally related to the onset of reduced γ-aminobutyric acid (GABA) sensitivity on dorsal raphe neurons during prolonged exposure to diazepam (69). Electrophysiological evidence has been presented for decreased postsynaptic sensitivity to GABA following long-term diazepam administration (59). Prolonged exposure of spinal cord cultures to diazepam resulted in a reversible downregulation of diazepam binding and function (201). The development of tolerance was functional, not metabolic, in nature as suggested by data that the plasma concentration of diazepam did not decrease during prolonged treatment (55,140). Long-term treatment in the baboon, *Papio papio*, suggested a possibly dose-dependent development of tolerance to the effect of diazepam on epileptic seizures and measures of electrical activity of the brain (108). The evidence is not conclusive, but several clinical reports suggest that diazepam may lose some of its antiepileptic effect in about 40% of all cases within 4 to 6 months of treatment; plasma concentrations were not recorded, and fluctuation of disease may have occurred independently of drug intake (24,65,218). Diazepam has been shown to be less effective in acute treatment of a recurrent seizure than in the initial seizure (52). In cats, acute tolerance develops to inhibitory effects of diazepam (14). There is suggestive evidence in man that a degree of tolerance to the sedative effects of diazepam during multiple administration or during intoxication develops (75,88).

Habituation

It is not known whether habituation or dependence develops among patients with epilepsy treated with long-term administration of diazepam. The addiction potential of diazepam in the general population is beyond the scope of this chapter (see 145). In newborns exposed to mostly long-term intrauterine diazepam, tremor, irritability and hypertonicity, poor weight gain, and vigorous sucking may occur after delivery and are considered a neonatal withdrawal syndrome (178). Single case reports indicate that in adults, agitation, anxiety, insomnia, tremor, hallucinosis, and generalized tonic-clonic seizures have been seen in relation to the withdrawal of diazepam (145).

Pharmacological Aspects of Clinical Use

Emergency Treatment

Our knowledge of therapeutic plasma concentrations of diazepam is based on rather few data with considerable individual variation. These preliminary data indicate that 500 to 700 ng/ml are a minimum needed rapidly for single-dose seizure control and that more than 150 to 200 ng/ml are necessary for maintenance of seizure control. If the plasma concentrations following different routes of administration are compared with these requirements in mind (Fig. 1), the intravenous administration is preferable to other routes as it produces therapeutic plasma concentrations most rapidly. An initial dose of 0.2 to 0.3 mg/kg i.v. is slowly (2 mg/min) injected in children and adults until the seizure stops or serious side effects occur. Administration of 0.5 to 1 mg/kg of diazepam solution inserted rectally results in therapeutic concentrations within minutes which are maintained for about 1

hr. The rectiole, a rectal tube containing a solution of the drug for application through a 4-cm tube inserted in the rectum, can be used quickly by informed parents. When it is squeezed until it is withdrawn, backflow of the solution into the container can be avoided. Intramuscular administration (0.5–1 mg/kg) is about as effective as rectal administration in children; in adults, however, it cannot be recommended because of erratic and often subtherapeutic concentrations with delayed peaks. Suppositories or oral treatment with diazepam are not suitable for acute treatment of a seizure because of late peaks and inadequately low concentrations in plasma.

Oral Treatment

Oral diazepam therapy is used mainly for associated psychiatric disease in epileptic patients and only rarely as an antiepileptic adjunct in patients with persistent seizures. The recommended therapeutic dose is 0.2 to 0.4 mg/kg for adults. Steady-state plasma concentrations of diazepam and N-desmethyldiazepam are reached within 5 to 10 days and 10 to 15 days after treatment, respectively. This interval will pass before the full therapeutic or toxic response of a dosage change can be anticipated. During prolonged administration of diazepam, plasma N-desmethyldiazepam concentrations will be at least similar to or even higher than the plasma diazepam concentrations. For each 1 mg/kg per day, steady-state concentrations of about 100 ng/ml of diazepam and 200 ng/ml of N-desmethyldiazepam may be expected.

Premature newborns, patients with advanced liver disease, and the elderly have a longer elimination half-life, requiring a lower dose not only for pharmacokinetic reasons but also because the sensitivity to diazepam may be higher in all three patient groups. In contrast, infants or children have a shorter elimination half-life than full-term newborns or adults, who have a similar elimination half-life. The relative ineffectiveness of oral diazepam treatment may reflect the development of tolerance within the first months or subtherapeutic plasma concentrations of less than 500 ng/ml, or both. This suggests that therapeutic drug monitoring is helpful when the desired therapeutic effect is not obtained during long-term treatment or when side effects occur. The toxic plasma concentration ranges above 1,000 ng/ml of diazepam and 2,000 ng/ml of N-desmethyldiazepam, even though only preliminary data are available.

Pregnancy

Pregnancy prolongs the elimination half-life to about 2 to 3 days because of a change in the volume of distribution (Table 1). Cord blood concentrations are similar to or even higher than maternal blood concentrations (51). After repeated administration, accumulation of diazepam and N-desmethyldiazepam occurs in the fetus (81,146). After delivery, diazepam and N-desmethyldiazepam will remain in neonatal plasma for several days, causing mostly sedative side effects, especially in premature newborns, and possibly a neonatal withdrawal syndrome. Diazepam and N-desmethyldiazepam are found in breast milk in a concentration 4 to 10 times lower than in plasma (22,32,50) but may result in neonatal plasma concentrations in the range of 30% to 75% of the maternal concentration. The possible teratogenic effect and the development of side effects in the neonate suggest a critical benefit/risk evaluation prior to the use of diazepam during pregnancy or in nursing mothers.

Teratogenesis

The possible teratogenic effect of diazepam is difficult to assess because of change correlations and confounding factors, e.g.,

maternal illness, familial association with cleft lip and cleft palate (58), and consumption of other drugs (186). No definite causal relationship has been established, even though suggestive retrospective evidence on the association between the first trimester intake of benzodiazepines and oral clefts has been presented (1,182,183,186) but not always confirmed (35). If a teratogenic effect of diazepam exists in fact, it may induce a fourfold increase in relative risk; this implies an actual risk of 0.4% for having a child with cleft lip and cleft palate (183).

TOXICITY

Diazepam-induced disease seems to be exceptionally rare. Apart from transient and mostly mild dose-related neurological side effects, an aggravation of tonic or tonic-clonic seizures may rarely occur, especially in secondary generalized epilepsy (176,211). There is no sound evidence for hematological, hepatic, or renal toxicity. There are two reports of leucopenia (25,77) and one case of acute hepatic necrosis (34) in doubtful relation to diazepam in combination with antibiotics or amitriptyline. The drug is not an enzyme inducer of significance in man (169) but increases the smooth endoplasmic reticulum in human hepatocytes (168). In volunteers, a transient decrease in renal para-aminohippuric acid (PAH) and insulin clearance without clinical symptoms has been reported after its intravenous administration (215). Furthermore, diazepam does not significantly alter thyroid function (184) or tests of thyroid function (31), pituitary function, urinary excretion of catecholamines (82), prolactin levels, or blood sugar levels (152,226). It may increase growth hormone (129) and testosterone levels (9) and may have a varying influence on appetite and weight (24). After intramuscular injection, a transient rise of the serum creatine phosphokinase can be expected (13). Diazepam induces a number of electromyographic changes of no clinical relevance on motor nerves and skeletal muscle (91). Hypersensitivity reactions to diazepam are exceptionally rare (156). Allergic interstitial nephritis has occurred in one patient receiving oral diazepam (181). Hypersensitivity may result from the lipid vehicle of the diazepam preparation Diazemul (38). Whether diazepam inflicts damage to chromosomes is controversial (224). Diazepam may induce a brown coloration of the ocular lens after prolonged intake (172). Usually mild thrombophlebitis occurs in about 3% to 7% of all patients after intravenous administration, especially when diazepam is rapidly administered or injected in a small vein or precipitates develop because of mixture with saline solution (132). Accidental intraarterial administration may lead to painful extensive limb tissue necrosis (71).

PHARMACODYNAMICS

The mechanisms of action of benzodiazepines are reviewed in Chapter 54. In addition to its well known action on postsynaptic GABA function, diazepam may exert effects on endogenous GABA concentrations and GABA release in the human cen-

tral nervous system (CNS) as reflected by elevations of GABA levels in human CSF (Fig. 5) (138).

THERAPEUTIC USE

Emergency Treatment

Bolus Injection

Diazepam is a drug of first choice for the treatment of status epilepticus (Table 2), serial seizures, and ongoing acute seizures. Seizures were controlled in 76% of the episodes treated with 10 mg diazepam i.v. and in 89% treated with 4 mg lorazepam i.v. in a double-blind study of status epilepticus (135). Both drugs were injected over a period of 2 min. Adverse effects occurred in 12.5% of the diazepam-treated patients. Diazepam-related respiratory arrest was observed in one patient, three patients had mild to moderate respiratory depression which was drug related in two cases. In one other patient diazepam-related sedation was observed. None of the patients with adverse effects suffered from concurrent medical problems. Lorazepam was more effective than diazepam in other epileptic seizures excluding generalized tonic-clonic

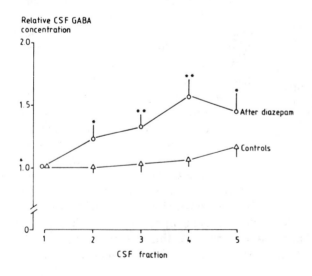

FIG. 5. GABA levels in serial 1.5 ml specimens of lumbar CSF from patients with and without intravenous injection of 5 mg of diazepam. Data are expressed as -fold increase over the GABA level determined in the initial 1.5 ml (CSF fraction 1) in each subject and are given as means $\pm$SEM of 10 patients per group. Significance of differences between controls and data obtained after diazepam: $^*p < 0.05$; $^{**}p < 0.02$. In controls, the absolute GABA level in fraction 1 was 175 (154–200) pmol/ml (geometric mean and range for 1 SEM). (From Löscher and Schmidt, ref. 138, with permission.)

TABLE 2. *Therapeutic effect of diazepam in various types of status epilepticus*[a]

Type of status epilepticus	Seizure-free patients		Number of studies
	N	%	
Grand mal status	177/224	79	10
Petit mal status			
Infantile spasms	6/13	46	3
Myoclonic-astatic seizures	26/43	60	3
Absence seizures	12/16	75	4
Status of partial seizures	59/67	88	6

[a] In many cases, multiple injections were required for lasting seizure control, and most patients received additional sedative or antiepileptic drugs (190).

seizures. Twelve percent of these seizure types were not controlled by lorazepam and 32% of the episodes were not controlled by diazepam. More clinical experience is needed to determine if lorazepam can replace diazepam or phenytoin in the treatment of status epilepticus, but results from this study indicate that lorazepam is at least as effective as diazepam in the initial treatment of status epilepticus.

A single intravenous bolus dose of diazepam in a dosage of 5 to 10 mg at a rate of 1 to 5 mg/min has been reported to stop initial seizure activity in 88% of patients with various seizure types in status epilepticus (see review 24,188,191). The clinical responses to intravenous diazepam given as a bolus of 2 mg/min were studied in detail by Delgado-Escueta and Enrile-Bacsal (39). Convulsions stopped in 32% of patients after 3 min, in 68% of patients after 5 min and in 80% of patients after 10 min. Patients with primarily generalized seizures responded quickly to bolus injections. When bolus injections failed in patients with primarily generalized seizures, metabolic encephalopathies were often found. The most common reasons for failure were rapid progressive CNS diseases, e.g., acute infectious encephalopathies, several cerebral anoxia, and acute cerebral infarction. The

regimen of initial bolus injection of diazepam 2 mg/min combined with intravenous phenytoin and followed, if neccessary, by diazepam infusion was successful in 88% of the cases, even in 7 of 13 patients with progressing neurological lesions. The moderately slow rate of initial injection of 2 mg/min did not lead to hypotension. Respiratory depression could not be studied as the authors elected to artificially ventilate the patients at the start of the treatment. The combination of the fast acting diazepam with phenytoin, which has a longer duration of action, has been recommended by Delgado-Escueta and Enrile-Bacsal (39).

A recent prospective comparison of diazepam i.v. and phenytoin i.v. versus phenobarbital i.v. in the treatment of status epilepticus found both regimens similarly effective and comparable in safety (200). Patients treated with diazepam and phenytoin needed two separate i.v. lines, whereas patients treated with phenobarbital required a second i.v. line only if additional phenytoin was needed. Such a need arose in less than one-half of the patients treated initially with phenobarbital (200). However, the combination of diazepam with phenobarbital is not recommended. These drugs potentiate sedative effects and have caused respiratory depression and hypotension. Contraindications for diazepam include patients who have received high doses of barbiturates or other sedative drugs.

A substantial number of responsive patients experience seizure recurrences 10 to 20 min later, with only 50% seizure-free 2 hr after a single injection (175). The favorable response and the subsequent relapse is thought to be caused by diazepam's rapid redistribution pattern resulting in an abrupt fall of its concentration in the brain, with a significant loss of anticonvulsant effect. After an intravenous bolus of diazepam has been administered to achieve initial control of seizures, additional treatment usually is given. A number of proposals have been made including the use of intravenous phenytoin, phenobarbital, lidocaine, and clonazepam, or a constant infusion of diazepam (15).

Continuous Infusion

The continuous infusion of diazepam has not been studied in randomized controlled clinical trials. To date, the majority of data is retrospective case reports and uncontrolled clinical observations. Single case reports of refractory status epilepticus reported control of seizures without side effects with continuous diazepam infusions of 75 to 100 mg/day (64,163). The first prospective study of six patients reported four patients with complete or satisfactory control, one with temporary control and one who failed. The duration of treatment was 2 to 7 days with 140 to 200 mg diazepam per day. Development of tolerance was noted with infusions lasting longer than one day (171). In a retrospective study of five patients, good seizure control, one breakthrough seizure, and one failure were reported with infusions of 10 to 48 mg per day for 12 to 24 hr (175). A well documented observation of five infants (newborns to age 13 months) with refractory seizures showed adequate seizure control and no adverse effects when 3 to 12 mg diazepam per kg and day were administered for 21 hr to 8 days (216).

Most recently, Delgado-Escueta and Enrile-Bacsal (39) promoted the use of continuous diazepam infusion in patients with refractory status epilepticus. They suggest that patients in status epilepticus first be given a trial of bolus diazepam injections of 10 to 20 mg at a rate of 2 mg/min while simultaneously receiving an intravenous loading of 15 mg/kg phenytoin in the opposite arm. If seizures persist, a continuous infusion of diazepam 4 to 8 mg/hr with 50 mg of diazepam in 500 ml dextrose/water is recommended for 3 hr after an initial loading dose of 20 mg diazepam as a bolus injection. When diazepam is used as an infusion, a maximum of 20 mg should be dissolved and thoroughly mixed in a minimum of 250 ml of solvent. This solution will not precipitate in a 5% to 10% glucose solution or in a 0.9 saline solution. The infusion should be used immediately after mixing, using a large caliber vein. Their report on 18 patients in a review article did not state the exact duration of treatment. The proposed regimen led to seizure control in 12 patients and failed in six. Significantly, in contrast to intravenous bolus injection, diazepam by continuous infusions results in a lower incidence of respiratory depression and hypotension. Continuous electroencephalographic monitoring has been used to evaluate drug efficiency. Delgado-Escueta et al. also recommended following serum diazepam concentrations and suggested that diazepam serum concentrations should exceed 3 μg/ml.

The clinical pharmacokinetics and the preliminary clinical experience would suggest that an initial loading dose of 20 mg should be administered to temporarily control the seizures in a patient in an intensive care unit, followed by a continuous intravenous infusion of diazepam 2 mg/kg/day. The rate of infusion should be clinical, and drug-related changes (e.g., respiratory depression and hypotension), plasma concentration measurement of diazepam and N-desmethyldiazepam, and intensive video-electroencephalographic monitoring is recommended.

Although published data indicate that continuous intravenous infusions of diazepam are safe and effective, more rigorous clinical trials are needed to clarify optimal dosage and administration. Diazepam given as an infusion will effectively control another 25% of patients with refractory status epilepticus (39). If this regimen is not effective and status has continued for an hour, general anesthesia and muscle relaxants should be given (190).

Rectal Solution

The rectal solution of diazepam has been effectively used for the emergency treatment of ongoing seizures. Diazepam rectal solution was given at home to 17 epileptic children with prolonged convulsions (92). An initial dose of 0.5 mg/kg was employed with a maximum of 20 mg per single dose. The drug was used 65 times and given within 5 min of the start of a convulsion in 85% of the episodes. A convulsion lasting longer than 15 min after the drug had been given was classified as an insufficiently slow response and persistence of the seizure for 30 min or longer was classified as a failure. Ten children used rectal diazepam solution that was applied using a disposable plastic syringe attached to a plastic catheter 6 cm long, inserted rectally. The convulsions were stopped within 15 min in 80% of the episodes. Seizure duration was longer than 15 min in 12.3% and longer than 30 min in 7.7% (92). Side effects included temporary respiration difficulties in one patient aged 16 following a rectal application of diazepam (0.5 mg/kg). Concomitant phenobarbital therapy may have contributed. Two children had skin reactions with urticaria and pruritus. Dizziness occurred in one 13-year-old boy. No other side effects were observed.

In a prospective study, 44 children aged 6 months to 5 years were treated with a rectal solution of diazepam during 59 generalized attacks in a hospital. Diazepam i.v. solution was administered rectally with a disposable plastic syringe and a 6 cm long plastic tube with a blunt tip. Children aged less than 3 years received 5 to 7.5 mg diazepam rectally (0.5–0.9 mg/kg per dose); children older than age 3 were given 7.5 to 10 mg diazepam rectally (0.6–0.8 mg/kg per dose). The duration of the convulsion after administration of the drug was registered with a stop watch. When the convulsion had not stopped within 5 min, rectal treatment was repeated or the child was given diazepam intravenously. A total of 44 children received rectal diazepam during 59 convulsions. Rectal diazepam was effective in 80% of the episodes. In 10% rectal diazepam failed although intravenous diazepam was effective, and in 10% diazepam failed after rectal and intravenous administration. No significant respiration depression or other serious side effects were observed (121). The rapid and reliable anticonvulsant effect of diazepam given rectally makes this regimen a valuable alternative when intravenous administration is not feasible.

Diazepam Prophylaxis

The usefulness of the rectal administration of diazepam for the prevention of febrile convulsions has been studied by several authors in recent years. A prospective controlled study evaluated the efficacy of short-term diazepam prophylaxis. A total of 289 children admitted consecutively to the hospital with their first febrile seizure were randomized in two groups. In one group diazepam solution was administered rectally whenever the temperature was 38.5°C or more. The control group received diazepam rectally only for the acute treatment of an ongoing seizure. The rectal administration was effective in the prevention of recurrent febrile seizures. The total number of recurrences was reduced from 77 to 23, and the recurrence rate from 39% to 12%. The risk of subsequent epilepsy was not lowered, however. It was zero in 230 children with simple febrile seizures, 20% after complex febrile seizures, or 50% after seizures associated with several interictal EEG abnormalities (122). No significant side effects were observed in this study.

Treatment of febrile seizures at home with the use of rectal diazepam administration was evaluated in a large cooperative study in Italy (222). Parents of 601 children admitted to a hospital for a febrile seizure were informed how to use a syringe with a plastic tube for rectal application of diazepam solution. Diazepam was administered correctly in 70 episodes of 50 children. Prolonged seizures of more than 15 min occurred six times in the control group and twice in the treated group. In the latter two cases diazepam was expelled immediately. This result shows that rectal administration is useful provided the parents have a full understanding of the procedure (47). Some parents preferred to bring the child to the nearest hospital.

Diazepam has also been used effectively to prevent serial seizures in adult patients with drug-resistant epilepsy. When diazepam was administered rectally immediately after a seizure, it was highly effective in preventing recurrent seizures within a 24-hr observation period. Pharmacokinetic studies showed a mean serum diazepam concentration of 190 ± 73 (SD ng/ml) 60 min after the rectal administration. This study shows that a single-dose rectal administration is useful for the prevention of further seizures in patients known to have serial seizures (153).

Diazepam reduces spike frequency within 10 to 20 min after rectal administration, corresponding with a mean serum concentration of .210 ± 125 ng/ml (154). Within 1 and 9.3 min after the administration of rectal diazepam, fast activities appear in the EEG (54).

Diazepam normally produces an increase in beta activity in the EEG; a poor increase indicates an abnormal region. In 12 of 21 patients with epilepsy, the area of poorest response to diazepam was identical to that of seizure onset (70). Based on pharmacokinetic considerations and the clinical evidence presented above, intravenous diazepam is effective and safe for the emergency treatment of status epilepticus (Table 2). When injected slowly at a rate of 2 mg/min, side effects are rare in patients without risk factors. Resuscitation because of respiratory or cardiovascular depression may rarely become necessary, but it should be available when risk factors are present.

These factors include rapid bolus injection; pretreatment with sedative drugs (e.g., phenobarbital); advanced heart, lung, or liver disease; and status epilepticus secondary to acute brain disease. Infusions of diazepam are effective and safe for patients with refractory status epilepticus. When the intravenous administration cannot be administered without delay, the rectal administration of diazepam solution is the procedure of choice. Rectal diazepam is effective and safe for the immediate home treatment of prolonged seizures and serial seizures and the initial treatment of status epilepticus. Furthermore, rectal diazepam is effective and safe for prophylaxis of febrile seizures and serial seizures.

Diazepam suppositories, and intramuscular and oral diazepam are not suited for emergency treatment.

Oral Treatment

As reviewed earlier (188), oral diazepam is rarely used for treatment of epilepsy. Controlled trials show that diazepam is less effective than phenytoin or phenobarbital for treatment of generalized tonic-clonic seizures (29) and about as effective as pheneturide, a now absolute agent, in control of partial seizures (86). In a recent double-blind, placebo-controlled trial in drug-resistant epilepsy, a single 20 mg dose of oral diazepam significantly reduced the incidence of serial seizures at plasma concentrations of 273 ± 190 (SD) ng/ml (153). The poor efficacy of long-term oral diazepam treatment may be related to the development of tolerance or the difficulty to maintain effective plasma concentrations. Prolonged oral diazepam exposure is fraught with the risk of overdose, dependence, and withdrawal, and is therefore not safe for the treatment of chronic epilepsy.

SUMMARY AND OUTLOOK

Diazepam is a safe and effective drug of first choice for the emergency treatment of status epilepticus, serial seizures, prolonged seizures, and the prophylaxis of febrile seizures. The intravenous route, if immediately available, is preferable for emergency treatment. For immediate treatment at home, administration of rectal solutions of diazepam are safe and effective for the treatment of prolonged seizures, serial seizures, and the initial treatment of status epilepticus. Rectal diazepam also is recommended for the prophylaxis of febrile seizures. Suppositories, intramuscular, or oral administration of diazepam are not suited for emergency treatment. Oral diazepam cannot be recommended for long-term treatment of epilepsy because of poor efficacy, development of tolerance, and associated risks. Areas of future interest are the potential use of partial benzodiazepine agonists with antiepileptic efficacy without sedation and without the development of tolerance, or as yet unforeseeable useful selective modifications of the benzodiazepine GABA receptor in patients with epilepsy.

CONVERSION

Conversion factor:

$$CF = \frac{1000}{\text{mol. wt.}} = \frac{1000}{284.8} = 3.51$$

Conversion:

$$(\mu g/ml) \times 3.51 = (\mu \text{moles/liter})$$

$$(\mu \text{moles/liter}) \div 3.51 = (\mu g/ml)$$

REFERENCES

1. Aarskog, D. (1975): Association between maternal intake of diazepam and oral clefts. *Lancet,* 2:921.
2. Ackermann, E., and Richter, K. (1979): Diazepam metabolism in human foetal and adult liver. *Eur. J. Clin. Pharmacol.,* 11:43–49.
3. Adoni, A., Kapitulnik, J., Kaufmann, N. A., Ron, M., and Blondheim, S. H. (1973): Effect of maternal administration of diazepam on the bilirubin-binding capacity of cord blood serum. *Am. J. Obstet. Gynecol.,* 115:577–579.
4. Agurell, S., Berlin, A., Ferngren, H., and Hellström, B. (1975): Plasma levels of diazepam after paternal and rectal administration in children. *Epilepsia,* 16:277–283.
5. Albertson, T. E., Bowyer, J. F., and Paule, M. G. (1982): Modification of the anticonvulsant efficacy of diazepam by Ro 15-1788 in the kindled amygdaloid seizure model. *Life Sci.,* 31:1597–1601.
6. Alvin, J. D., and Bush, M. T. (1977): Physiological disposition of anticonvulsants. The benzodiazepines. In: *Anticonvulsants,* edited by J. A. Vida, pp. 140–144. Academic Press, New York.
7. Andre, M., Sibout, M., Petry, J. M., and Vert, P. (1973): Dépression respiratoire et neurologique chez le premature nouveau-né de mère traitée par Diazepam. *J. Gynecol. Obstet. Biol. Reprod. (Paris),* 2:357–366.
8. Andreasen, P. B., Hendel, J., Greisen, G., and Hvidberg, E. F. (1976): Pharmacokinetics of diazepam in disorders of liver function. *Eur. J. Clin. Pharmacol.,* 10:115–120.
9. Argüelles, A. E., and Rosner, J. (175): Diazepam and plasma testosterone levels. *Lancet,* 2:607.
10. Arnold, E. (1975): A simple method for determining diazepam and its major metabolites in biological fluids: Application in bioavailability studies. *Acta Pharmacol. Toxicol. (KbH.),* 36:335–352.
11. Baird, E. S., and Hailey, D. M. (1972): Delayed recovery from a sedative: Correlation of the plasma levels of diazepam with clinical effects after oral and intravenous administration. *Br. J. Anaesthesiol.,* 44:803–808.
12. Baird, E. S., and Hailey, D. M. (1973): Plasma levels of diazepam and its major metabolite following intramuscular administration. *Br. J. Anaesthesiol.,* 45:546–548.
13. Bank-Mikkelsen, O. K., Steiness, E., Arnold, E., Hansen, T., Sobye, M., and Lunding, M. (1978): Serum diazepam and serum creatine kinase after intra-muscular injection of diazepam in two different vehicles. *Acta Anaesthesiol. Scand.* (Suppl.), 67:91–95.
14. Barnett, A., and Fiore, J. W. (1983): Acute tolerance to diazepam in cats. In: *The Benzodiazepines,* edited by S. Garattini, E. Mussini, and L. O. Randall, pp. 545–557. Raven Press, New York.
15. Bell, H. E., and Bertino, Jr. J. S. (1984): Constant diazepam infusion in the treatment of continuous seizure activity. *Drug Intell. Clin. Pharm.,* 18:965–970.
16. Berger, R., Green, G., and Melnick, A. (1975): Cardiac arrest caused by oral diazepam intoxication. *Clin. Pediatr.,* 14:842–844.
17. Berlin, A., Siwers, B., Agurell, S., Hiort, A., Sjöqvist, F., and Ström, S. (1972): Determination of bioavailability of diazepam in various formulations from steady state plasma concentration data. *Clin. Pharmacol. Ther.,* 13:733–744.
18. Beyer, K.-H., and Sadée, W. (1969): Analytische Daten von vier 5-Phenyl-1,4-benzodiazepinderivaten in Monographien. 6. Mitteilung zur Chemie

und Analytik von Benzodiazepinderivaten. *Dtsch. Apoth. Z.*, 109:312–314.

19. Booker, H. E., and Celesia, G. G. (1973): Serum concentrations of diazepam in subjects with epilepsy. *Arch. Neurol.*, 29:191–194.

20. Boston Collaborative Drug Surveillance Program (1973): Clinical depression of the central nervous system due to diazepam and chlordiazepoxide in relation to cigarette smoking and age. *N. Engl. J. Med.*, 288:277–280.

21. Branch, R. A., Morgan, M. H., James, J., and Read, A. E. (1976): Intravenous administration of diazepam in patients with chronic liver disease. *Gut*, 17:975–983.

22. Brandt, R. (1976): Passage of diazepam and desmethyldiazepam into breast milk. *Arzneim. Forsch.*, 26:454–457.

23. Brauninger, G., and Ravin, M. (1974): Respiratory arrest following intravenous Valium. *Ann. Ophthalmol.*, 6:805–806.

24. Browne, T. R., and Penry, J. K. (1973): Benzodiazepines in the treatment of epilepsy. *Epilepsia*, 14:277–310.

25. Bussien, R. (1974): Granulocytopénie aigue après administration simultanée de gentamicine et diazépam. *Nouv. Presse Md.*, 3:123.

26. Caccia, S. S., Garattini (1985): Benzodiazepine. In: *Handbook of Experimental Pharmacology. Vol. 74*, edited by H. H. Frey, and D. Janz, pp. 575–593. Springer, Heidelberg, New York.

27. Cardauns, H., and Iffland, R. (1973): Über eine tödliche Diazepam (Valium) Vergiftung bei einem drogenabhängigen Jugendlichen. *Arch. Toxikol.*, 31:147–151.

28. Celesia, G. G., Booker, H. E., and Sato, S. (1974): Brain and serum concentrations of diazepam in experimental epilepsy. *Epilepsia*, 15:417–425.

29. Chien, C., and Keegan, D. (1972): Diazepam as an oral long-term anticonvulsant for epileptic mental patients. *Dis. Nerv. Syst.*, 33:100–104.

30. Chwew, A. Y., Ulloque, R. A., and Swinyard, E. A. (1986): Benzodiazepine inhibition of (H) Flunitrazepam binding and caffeine-induced seizures in mice. *Europ. J. Pharmacol.*, 122:161–165.

31. Clark, F., Hall, R., and Ormston, B. J. (1971): Diazepam and tests of thyroid function. *Br. Med. J.*, 1:585–586.

32. Cole, A. P., and Hailey, D. M. (1975): Diazepam and active metabolite in breast milk and their transfer to the neonate. *Arch. Dis. Child.*, 50:741–742.

33. Cryer, P. E., and Sode, J. (1971): Drug interference with measurement of adrenal hormones in urine: Analgesics and tranquilizer-sedatives. *Ann. Intern Med.*, 75:697–702.

34. Cunningham, M. L. (1965): Acute hepatic necrosis following treatment with amitriptyline and diazepam. *Br. J. Psychiatry*, 111:1107–1109.

35. Czeizel, A. (1976): Diazepam, phenytoin, and aetiology of cleft lip and/or cleft palate. *Lancet*, 1:810.

36. Czuczwar, S. J., Turski, W. A., Ikonomidou, C., and Turski, L. (1985): Aminophylline and CGS 8216 reverse the protective action of diazepam against electroconvulsions in mice. *Epilepsia*, 26(6):693–696.

37. Dasberg, H. H., Van der Kleijn, E., Guelen, P. J. R., and Van Praag, H. M. (1974): Plasma concentrations of diazepam and of its metabolite N-desmethyldiazepam in relation to anxiolytic effect. *Clin. Pharmacol. Ther.*, 15:473–483.

38. Deardon, D. J., and Bird, G. L. A. (1987): Acute (type 1) hypersensitivity to i.v. Diazemuls. *Brit. J. Anaesthes.*, 59:391.

39. Delgado-Escueta, A. V., and Enrile-Bacsal, F., (1983): Combination therapy for status epilepticus: Intravenous diazepam and phenytoin. In: *Advances in Neurology, Vol. 34*, pp. 477–485. Raven Press, New York.

40. De Silva, J. A. F. (1978): Electron capture-GLC in the quantitation of 1.4-benzodiazepines. In: *Antiepileptic Drugs: Quantitative Analysis and Interpretation*, edited by C. E. Pippenger, J. K. Penry, and H. Kutt, pp. 111–138. Raven Press, New York.

41. De Silva, J. A. F., Bekersky, I., Puglisi, C. V., Brooks, M. A., and Weinfeld, R. E. (1976): Determination of 1.4-benzodiazepines and -diazepin-2-ones in blood by electroncapture gas-liquid chromatography. *Anal. Chem.*, 48:10–19.

42. Dhar, A. K., and Kutt, H. (1979): Monitoring diazepam and desmethyldiazepam concentrations in plasma by gas-liquid chromatography, with use of a nitrogen-sensitive detector. *Clin. Chem.*, 25:137–140.

43. Dhillon, S., and Richens, A. (1982): Valproic acid and diazepam interaction *in vivo*. *Br. J. Clin. Pharmacol.*, 13:553–560.

44. DiGregorio, G. J., Piraino, A. J., and Ruch, E. (1978): Diazepam concentrations in parotid saliva, mixed saliva, and plasma. *Clin. Pharmacol. Ther.*, 24:720–725.

45. Doughty, A. (1970): Unexpected danger of diazepam. *Br. Med. J.*, 2:239.

46. Dulac, O., Aicardi, J., Rey, E., and Olive, G. (1978): Blood levels of diazepam after single rectal administration in infants and children. *J. Pediatr.*, 93:1039–1041.

47. Echenne, B., Cheminal, R., Martin, P., Peskine, F., Rodière, M., Astruc, J., and Brunel, D. (1983): Utilisation du diazépam dans le traitement préventif à domicile des récidives de convulsions fébriles. *Arch. F. Pediatr.*, 40:499–501.

48. Ehlers, C. L., Henriksen, S. J., and Bloom, F. E. (1981): Levonantradol potentiates the anticonvulsant effects of diazepam and valproic acid in the kindling model of epilepsy. *J. Clin. Pharmacol.*, 21:4065–4125.

49. Erkkola, R., Kangas, L., and Pekkarinen, A. (1973): The transfer of diazepam across the placenta during labour. *Acta Obstet. Gynaecol. Scand.*, 52:167–170.

50. Erkkola, R., and Kanto, J. (1972): Diazepam and breast-feeding. *Lancet*, 1:1235–1236.

51. Erkkola, R., Kanto, J., and Sellman, R. (1974):

Diazepam in early human pregnancy. *Acta Obstet. Gynaecol. Scand.*, 53:135–138.

52. Ferngren, H. G. (1974): Diazepam treatment for acute convulsions in children. *Epilepsia*, 15:27–37.
53. File, S. E. (1983): Strain differences in mice in the development of tolerance to the anti-pentylenetetrazole effects of diazepam. *Neuroscience Let.*, 42:95–98.
54. Franzoni, E., Carboni, C., and Lambertini, A. (1983): Rectal diazepam: A clinical and EEG study after a single dose in children. *Epilepsia*, 24:35–41.
55. Frey, H. H. (1985): Tolerance and dependence. In: *Handbook of Experimental Pharmacology, Vol. 74* edited by H. H. Frey and D. Janz, pp. 449–477. Springer, Heidelberg, New York.
56. Frey, H. H., and Löscher, W. (1982): Anticonvulsant potency of unmetabolized diazepam. *Pharmacol.*, 25:154–159.
57. Friedmann, H., Ochs, H. R., Greenblatt, D. J., and Shader, R. I. (1985): Tissue distribution of diazepam and its metabolite desmethyldiazepam: A human autopsy study. *J. Clin. Pharmacol.*, 25:613–615.
58. Friis, M. L. (1979): Epilepsy among parents of children with facial clefts. *Epilepsia*, 20:69–76.
59. Gallager, D. W., Lakoski, J. M., Gonsalves, S. F., and Rauch, S. L. (1984): Chronic benzodiazepine treatment decreases postsynaptic GABA sensitivity. *Nature*, 308:74–77.
60. Gamble, J. A. S., Dundee, J. W., and Assaf, R. A. E. (1975): Plasma diazepam levels after single dose oral and intramuscular administration. *Anaesthesia*, 30:164–169.
61. Gamble, J. A. S., Dundee, J. W., and Gray, R. C. (1976): Plasma diazepam concentrations following prolonged administration. *Br. J. Anaesth.*, 48:1087–1090.
62. Gamble, J. A. S., Moore, J., Lamki, H., and Howard, P. J. (1977): A study of plasma diazepam levels in mother and infant. *Br. J. Obstet. Gynaecol.*, 84:588–591.
63. Garattini, S., Marcucci, F., Morselli, P. L., and Mussini, E. (1973): The significance of measuring blood levels of benzodiazepines. In: *Biological Effects of Drugs in Relation to their Plasma Concentrations*, edited by D. S. Davies and B. N. C. Prichard, pp. 211–226. Macmillan, London.
64. Gastaut, H., Naquet, R., Poire, R., and Tassinari, C. A. (1985): Treatment of status epilepticus with diazepam (Valium). *Epilepsia*, 6:167–182.
65. Gastaut, H., Roger, J., and Lob, H. (1973): Medical treatment of epilepsy. In: *Anticonvulsant Drugs. Vol. II*, edited by J. Mercier, pp. 535–598. Pergamon Press, Oxford.
66. Ghoneim, M. M., Mewaldt, S. P., and Ambre, J. (1975): Plasma levels of diazepam and mood ratings. *Anesth. Analg. (Cleve.)*, 54:173–177.
67. Giles, H. G., MacLeod, S. M., Wright, J. R., and Sellers, E. M. (1978): Influence of age and previous use on diazepam dosage required for endoscopy. *Can. Med. Assoc. J.*, 118:513–514.
68. Gillberg, C. (1977): "Floppy infant syndrome" and maternal diazepam. *Lancet*, 2:244.
69. Gonsalves, S. F., and Gallager, D. W. (1987): Time course for development of anticonvulsant tolerance and GABAergic subsensitivity after chronic diazepam. *Brain Res.*, 405:94–99.
70. Gotman, J., Gloor, P., Quesney, L. F., and Olivier, A. (1982): Correlations between EEG changes induced by diazepam and the localization of epileptic spikes and seizures. *EEG Clin. Neurophysiol.*, 54:614–621.
71. Gould, J. D. M., and Lingam, S. (1977): Hazards of intraarterial diazepam. *Br. Med. J.*, 2:298–299.
72. Greenblatt, D. J. (1978): Determination of desmethyldiazepam in plasma by electron-capture GLC: Application to pharmacokinetic studies of clorazepate. *J. Pharm. Sci.*, 67:427–429.
73. Greenblatt, D. J., and Koch-Weser, J. (1973): Adverse reactions to intravenous diazepam: A report from the Boston Collaborative Drug Surveillance Program. *Am. J. Med. Sci.*, 266:261–266.
74. Greenblatt, D. J., and Koch-Weser, J. (1974): Clinical toxicity of chlordiazepoxide and diazepam in relation to serum albumin concentration: A report from the Boston Collaborative Drug Surveillance Program. *Eur. J. Clin. Pharmacol.*, 7:259–262.
75. Greenblatt, D. J., Woo, E., Allen, M. D., Orsulak, P. J., and Shader, R. I. (1978): Rapid recovery from massive diazepam overdose. *J.A.M.A.*, 240:1872–1874.
76. Greksch, G., Prado de Carvalho, L., Venault, P., Chapouthier, G., and Rossier, J. (1983): Convulsions induced by submaximal dose of pentylenetetrazol in mice are antagonized by the benzodiazepine antagonist RO 15-1788. *Life Sci.*, 32:2579–2584.
77. Haerten, K., and Pöttgen, W. (1975): Leukopenie nach Benzodiazepin-Derivaten. *Med. Welt.*, 26:1712–1714.
78. Hailey, D. M. (1974): Chromatography of the 1.4-benzodiazepines. *J. Chromatogr.*, 98:527–568.
79. Hall, S. C., and Ovassapian, A. (1977): Apnea after intravenous diazepam therapy. *J.A.M.A.*, 238:1052.
80. Haram, K., Bakke, O. M., Johannessen, K. H., and Lund, T. (1978): Transplacental passage of diazepam during labor: Influence of uterine concentrations. *Clin. Pharmacol. Ther.*, 24:590–599.
81. Haram, K., Sagen, N., and Brandt, R. D. (1976): Transplacental passage of diazepam following intravenous injection immediately prior to operative vaginal delivery. *Int. J. Gynaecol. Obstet.*, 14:545–549.
82. Havard, C. W. H., Saldanha, V. F., Bird, R., and Gardner, R. (1972): The effect of diazepam on pituitary function in man. *J. Endocrinol.*, 52:79–85.
83. Hayes, S. L., Pablo, G., Radomski, T., and Palmer, R. F. (1977): Ethanol and oral diazepam absorption. *N. Engl. J. Med.*, 296:186–189.
84. Hendel, J. (1975): Cumulation in cerebrospinal fluid of the *N*-desmethyl metabolite after long-

term treatment with diazepam in man. *Acta Pharmacol. Toxicol. (KbH.),* 37:17–22.

85. Hepner, G. W., Vesell, E. S., Lipton, A., Harvey, H. A., Wilkinson, G. R., and Schenker, S. (1977): Disposition of aminopyrine, antipyrine diazepam, and indocyanine green in patients with liver disease or on anticonvulsant drug therapy: Diazepam breath test and correlations in drug elimination. *J. Lab. Clin. Med.,* 90:440–456.

86. Hershon, H. I., and Parsonage, M. (1969): Comparative trial of diazepam and pheneturide in treatment of epilepsy. *Lancet,* 2:859–862.

87. Heubel, F., and Frank, R. (1970): Zur induktiven Wirkung von Diazepam. *Arzneim. Forsch.,* 20:1706–1708.

88. Hillestad, L., Hansen, T., and Melsom, H. (1974): Diazepam metabolism in normal man. II. Serum concentration and clinical effect after oral administration and cumulation. *Clin. Pharmacol. Ther.,* 16:485–489.

89. Hillestad, L., Hansen, T., Melsom, H., and Drivenes, A. (1974): Diazepam metabolism in normal man. I. Serum concentrations and clinical effects after intravenous, intramuscular, and oral administration. *Clin. Pharmacol. Ther.,* 16:479–484.

90. Hooper, W. D., Sutherland, J. M., Bochner, F., Tyrer, J. H., and Eadie, M. J. (1973): The effect of certain drugs on the plasma protein binding of phenytoin. *Aust. N.Z. J. Med.,* 3:377–381.

91. Hopf, H. C., and Billmann, F. (1973): The effect of diazepam on motor nerves and skeletal muscle. *J. Neurol.,* 204:255–262.

92. Hoppu, K., and Santavuori, P. (1981): Diazepam rectal solution for home treatment of acute seizures in children. *Acta Pediatr. Scand.,* 70:369–372.

93. Horning, M. G., Nowlin, J., Butler, C. M., Lertratanangkoon, K., Sommer, K., and Hill, R. M. (1975): Clinical applications of gas chromatography/mass spectrometer/computer systems. *Clin. Chem.,* 21:1282–1287.

94. Houghton, G. W., and Richens, A. (1974): The effect of benzodiazepines and pheneturide on phenytoin metabolism in man. *Br. J. Clin. Pharmacol.,* 1:344–345.

95. Hoyumpa, A. M., Jr. (1978): Disposition and elimination of minor tranquilizers in the aged and in patients with liver disease. *South. Med. J.,* 71 (Suppl.2):23–28.

96. Hvidberg, E. F., and Dam, M. (1976): Clinical pharmacokinetics of anticonvulsants. *Clin. Pharmacokinet.,* 1:161–188.

97. Ichimaru, Y., Gomita, Y., and Moriyama, M. (1987): Effects of clobazam on amygdaloid and hippocampal kindled seizures in rats. *J. Pharmacobiodyn.,* 10:189–194.

98. Jusko, W. J., Gretsch, M., and Gassett, R. (1973): Precipitation of diazepam from intravenous preparations. *J.A.M.A.,* 225:176.

99. Kales, A., and Scharf, M. B. (1973): Sleep laboratory and clinical studies of the effects of benzodiazepines on sleep: Flurazepam, diazepam, chlordiazepoxide, and RO 5-4200. In: *The Benzodiazepines,* edited by S. Garattini, E. Mussini,

and L. O. Randall, pp. 577–598. Raven Press, New York.

100. Kangas, L., Kanto, J., Forsström, J., and Iisalo, E. (1976): The protein binding of diazepam and N-desmethyldiazepam in patients with poor renal function. *Clin. Nephrol.,* 5:114–118.

101. Kanto, J. (1975): Plasma concentrations of diazepam and its metabolites after peroral, intramuscular, and rectal administration. *Int. J. Clin. Pharmacol.,* 12:427–432.

102. Kanto, J., Erkkola, R., and Sellman, R. (1973): Accumulation of diazepam and N-desmethyldiazepam in the fetal blood during the labour. *Ann. Clin. Res.,* 5:375–379.

103. Kanto, J., Iisalo, E. U. M., Hovi-Viander, M., and Kangas, L. (1979): A comparative study on the clinical effects of oxazepam and diazepam. Relationship between plasma level and effect. *Int. J. Clin. Pharmacol. Biopharm.,* 17:26–31.

104. Kanto, J., Kangas, L., and Siirtola, T. (1975): Cerebrospinal-fluid concentrations of diazepam and its metabolites in man. *Acta Pharmacol. Toxicol. (KbH.),* 36:328–334.

105. Kanto, J. H., Pihlajamaki, K. K., and Iisalo, E. U. M. (1974): Concentrations of diazepam in adipose tissue of children. *Br. J. Anaesth.,* 46:168.

106. Kanto, J., Sellman, R., Haataja, M., and Hurme, P. (1978): Plasma and urine concentrations of diazepam and its metabolites in children, adults and in diazepam-intoxicated patients. *Int. J. Clin. Pharmacol.,* 16:258–264.

107. Kaplan, S. A., Jack, M. L., Alexander, K., and Weinfeld, R. E. (1973): Pharmacokinetic profile of diazepam in man following single intravenous and oral and chronic oral administrations. *J. Pharm. Sci.,* 62:1789–1796.

108. Killam, E. K., Matsuzaki, M., and Killam, K. F. (1973): Effects of chronic administration of benzodiazepines on epileptic seizures and brain electrical activity in *Papio papio.* In: *The Benzodiazepines,* edited by S. Garattini, E. Mussini, and L. O. Randall, pp. 443–460. Raven Press, New York.

109. Klotz, U. (1977): Wichtige Faktoren, die beim Menschen die Verteilung und Elimination von Diazepam beeinflussen. *Fortschr. Med.,* 95:1958–1964.

110. Klotz, U. (1978): Klinische Pharmakokinetik von Diazepam und seinen biologisch aktiven Metaboliten. *Klin. Wochenschr.,* 56:895–904.

111. Klotz, U., Antonin, K. H., and Bieck, P. R. (1976): Comparison of the pharmacokinetics of diazepam after single and subchronic doses. *Eur. J. Clin. Pharmacol.,* 10:121–126.

112. Klotz, U., Antonin, K. H., and Bieck, P. R. (1976): Pharmacokinetics and plasma binding of diazepam in man, dog, rabbit, guinea pig and rat. *J. Pharmacol. Exp. Ther.,* 199:67–73.

113. Klotz, U., Antonin, K. H., and Bieck, P. (1977): Food intake and plasma binding of diazepam. *Br. J. Clin. Pharmacol.,* 4:85–86.

114. Klotz, U., Antonin, K. H., Brügel, H., and Bieck, P. R. (1977): Disposition of diazepam and its major metabolite desmethyldiazepam in pa-

tients with liver disease. *Clin. Pharmacol. Ther.,* 21:430–436.

115. Klotz, U., Anttila, V. J., and Reimann, I. (1979): Cimetidine/diazepam interaction. *Lancet,* 2:699.

116. Klotz, U., Avant, G. R., Hoyumpa, A., Schenker, S., and Wilkinson, G. R. (1975): The effects of age and liver disease on the disposition and elimination of diazepam in adult man. *J. Clin. Invest.,* 55:347–359.

117. Klotz, U., and Müller-Seydlitz, P. (1979): Altered elimination of desmethyldiazepam in the elderly. *Br. J. Clin. Pharmacol.,* 7:119–120.

118. Klotz, U., and Reimann, I. (1981): Clearance of diazepam can be impaired by its major metabolite desmethyldiazepam. *Eur. J. Clin. Pharmacol.,* 21:161–163.

119. Klotz, U., and Reimann, I. W. (1984): Pharmacokinetic and pharmacodynamic interaction study of diazepam and metoprolol. *Eur. J. Clin. Pharmacol.,* 26:223–226.

120. Knudsen, F. U. (1977): Plasma-diazepam in infants after rectal administration in solution and by suppository. *Acta Paediatr. Scand.,* 66:563–567.

121. Knudsen, F. U. (1979): Rectal administration of diazepam in solution in the acute treatment of convulsions in infants and children. *Arch. Dis. Child.,* 54:855–857.

122. Knudsen, F. U. (1985): Effective short-term diazepam prophylaxis in febrile convulsions. *J. Pediatr.,* 106:487–490.

123. Kober, A., Jenner, A., Sjöholm, I., Borga, O., and Odar-Cederlöf, I. (1978): Differentiated effects of liver cirrhosis on the albumin binding sites for diazepam, salicylic acid and warfarin. *Biochem. Pharmacol.,* 27:2729–2735.

124. Kober, A., Sjöholm, I., Borga, O., and Odar-Cederlöf, I. (1979): Protein binding of diazepam and digitoxin in uremic and normal serum. *Biochem. Pharmacol.,* 28:1037–1042.

125. Korttila, K., and Kangas, L. (1977): Unchanged protein binding and the increase of serum diazepam levels after food intake. *Acta Pharmacol. Toxicol. (Kbh.),* 40:241–246.

126. Korttila, K., and Linnoila, M. (1975): Absorption and sedative effects of diazepam after oral administration and intramuscular administration into the vastus lateralis muscle and the deltoid muscle. *Br. J. Anaesth.,* 47:857–862.

127. Korttila, K., and Linnoila, M. (1975): Psychomotor skills related to driving after intramuscular administration of diazepam and meperidine. *Anesthesiology,* 42:685–691.

128. Korttila, K., Sothman, A., and Andersson, P. (1976): Polyethylene glycol as a solvent for diazepam: Bioavailability and clinical effects after intramuscular administration, comparison of oral, intramuscular and rectal administration, and precipitation from intravenous solutions. *Acta Pharmacol. Toxicol. (Kbh.),* 39:104–117.

129. Koulu, M., Lammintausta, R., Kangas, L., and Dahlström, S. (1979): The effect of methysergide, pimozide, and sodium valproate on the diazepam-stimulated growth hormone secretion in man. *J. Clin. Endocrinol. Metab.,* 48:119–122.

130. Kulkarni, S. K., and Jog, M. V. (1983): Facilitation of diazepam action by anticonvulsant agents against picrotoxin induced convulsions. *Psychopharmacol.,* 81:332–334.

131. Laguna, J. F., and Korein, J. (1972): Diagnostic value of diazepam in electroencephalography. *Arch. Neurol.,* 26:265–272.

132. Langdon, D. E., Harlan, J. R., and Bailey, R. L. (1973): Thrombophlebitis with diazepam used intravenously. *J.A.M.A.,* 223:184–185.

133. Langslet, A., Meberg, A., Bredesen, J. E., and Lunde, P. K. M. (1978): Plasma concentrations of diazepam and N-desmethyldiazepam in newborn infants after intravenous, intramuscular, rectal and oral administration. *Acta Paediatr. Scand.,* 67:699–704.

134. Larson, G. F., Hurlbert, B. J., and Wingard, D. W. (1977): Physostigmine reversal of diazepam-induced depression. *Anesth. Analg. (Cleve.),* 56:348–351.

135. Leppik, I. E., Derivan, A. T., Homan, R. W., Walker, J., Ramsay, R. E., and Patrick, B. (1983): Double-blind study of lorazepam and diazepam in status epilepticus. *J.A.M.A.,* 249:1452–1454.

136. Linnoila, M., Otterström, S., and Anttila, M. (1974): Serum chlordiazepoxide, diazepam and thioridazine concentrations after the simultaneous ingestion of alcohol or placebo drink. *Ann. Clin. Res.,* 6:4–6.

137. Lombroso, C. T. (1966): Treatment of status epilepticus with diazepam. *Neurology (Minneap.),* 16:629–634.

138. Löscher, W., and Schmidt, D. (1987): Diazepam increases aminobutyric acid in human cerebrospinal fluid. *J. Neurochem.* 49:152–157.

139. Löscher, W., Schmidt, D. (1988): Which animal models should be used in the search for new antiepileptic drugs? A proposal based on experimental and clinical considerations. *Epilepsy Res.,* 2:145–181.

140. Löscher, W., and Schwark, W. S. (1985): Development of tolerance to the anticonvulsant effect of diazepam in amygdala-kindled rats. *Exper. Neurol.,* 90:373–384.

141. Lukas, S. E., and Griffiths, R. R. (1982): Precipitated withdrawal by a benzodiazepine receptor antagonist (Ro 15-1788) after 7 days of diazepam. *Science,* 217:1161–1163.

142. MacKichan, J., Duffner, P. K., and Cohen, M. E. (1979): Absorption of diazepam to plastic tubing. *N. Engl. J. Med.,* 301:332–333.

143. MacLeod, S. M., Giles, H. G., Patzalek, G., Thiessen, J. J., and Sellers, E. M. (1977): Diazepam actions and plasma concentrations following ethanol ingestion. *Eur. J. Clin. Pharmacol.,* 11:345–349.

144. MacLeod, S. M., Sellers, E. M., Giles, H. G., Billings, B. J., Martin, P. R., Greenblatt, D. J., and Marshman, J. A. (1978): Interaction of disulfiram with benzodiazepines. *Clin. Pharmacol. Ther.,* 24:583–589.

145. Maletzky, B. M., and Klotter, J. (1976): Addiction to diazepam. *Int. J. Addict.*, 11:95–115.

146. Mandelli, M., Morselli, P. L., Nordio, S., Pardi, G., Principi, N., Sereni, F., and Tognoni, G. (1975): Placental transfer of diazepam and its disposition in the newborn. *Clin. Pharmacol. Ther.*, 17:564–572.

147. Mandelli, M., Tognoni, G., and Garattini, S. (1978): Clinical pharmacokinetics of diazepam. *Clin. Pharmacokinet.*, 3:72–91.

148. Marcucci, F., Mussini, E., Guaitani, A., Fanelli, R., and Garattini, S. (1971): Anticonvulsant activity and brain levels of diazepam and its metabolites in mice. *Eur. J. Pharmacol.* 16:311–314.

149. Marrosu, F., Marchi, A., De Martino, M. R., Saba, G., and Gessa, G. L. (1985): Aminophylline antagonizes diazepam-induced anesthesia and EEG changes in humans. *Psychopharmacol.*, 85:69–70.

150. Mattson, R. H. (1972): The benzodiazepines. In: *Antiepileptic Drugs,* 1st edition, edited by D. M. Woodbury, J. K. Penry, and R. P. Schmidt, pp. 497–516. Raven Press, New York.

151. Meberg, A., Langslet, A., Bredesen, J. E., and Lunde, P. K. M. (1978): Plasma concentration of diazepam and N-desmethyldiazepam in children after a single rectal or intramuscular dose of diazepam. *Eur. J. Clin. Pharmacol.*, 14:273–276.

152. Mehta, S. (1971): The influence of premedication with diazepam on the blood sugar level. *Anaesthesia,* 26:468–472.

153. Milligan, N. M., Dhillon, S., Griffiths, A., Oxley, J., and Richens, A. (1984): A clinical trial of single dose rectal and oral administration of diazepam for the prevention of serial seizures in adult epileptic patients. *J. Neurol. Neurosurg. Psychiatr.*, 47:235–240.

154. Milligan, N., Dhillon, S., Oxley, J., and Richens, A. (1982): Absorption of diazepam from the rectum and its effects on interictal spikes in the EEG. *Epilepsia,* 23:323–331.

155. Milligan, N., Dhillon, S., Richens, A., and Oxley, J. (1981): Rectal diazepam in the treatment of absence status: A pharmacodynamic study. *J. Neurol. Neurosurg. Psychiatry,* 44:914–917.

156. Milner, L. (1977): Allergy to diazepam. *Br. Med. J.* 1:144.

157. Moore, R. G., and McBride, W. G. (1978): The disposition kinetics of diazepam in pregnant women at parturition. *Eur. J. Clin. Pharmacol.*, 13:275–284.

158. Morland, J., Seteklciv, J., Haffner, J. F. W., Stromsaether, C. E., Danielsen, A., and Wethe, G. G. (1974): Combined effects of diazepam and ethanol on mental and psychomotor functions. *Acta Pharmacol. Toxicol. (Kbh.),* 34:5–15.

159. Morselli, P. L. (1977): Psychotropic drugs—benzodiazepines. In: *Drug Disposition During Development,* edited by P. L. Morselli, pp. 449–459. Spectrum Publications, New York.

160. Morselli, P. L., Principi, N., Tognoni, G., Reali, E., Belvedere, G., Standen, S. M., and Sereni, F. (1973): Diazepam elimination in premature and full term infants, and children. *J. Perinat. Med.,* 1:133–141.

161. Nair, S. G., Gamble, J. A. S., Dundee, J. W., and Howard, P. J. (1976): The influence of three antacids on the absorption and clinical action of oral diazepam. *Br. J. Anaesth.*, 48:1175–1180.

162. Naylor, G. J., and McHarg, A. (1977): Profound hypothermia on combined lithium carbonate and diazepam treatment. *Br. Med. J.*, 2:22.

163. Nicol, C., Tutton, I. C., and Smith, B. H. (1969): Parenteral diazepam in status epilepticus. *Neurology,* 19:332–34.

164. Niedermeyer, E. (1970): Intravenous diazepam and its anticonvulsive action. *Johns Hopkins Med. J.,* 127:79–96.

165. Nutt, D. J., and Lister, R. G. (1987): The effect of the imidazodiazepine Ro 15-4513 on the anticonvulsant effects of diazepam, sodium pentobarbital and ethanol. *Brain Res.,* 413:193–196.

166. O'Boyle, C., Lambe, R., Darragh, A., Taffe, W., Brick, I., and Kenny, M. (1983): RO15-1788 antagonizes the effects of diazepam in man without affecting its bioavailability. *Br. J. Anaesth.*, 55:349–356.

167. Ongini, E., Marzanatti, M., Bamonte, F., Monopoli, A., and Guzzon, V. (1985): A beta-carboline antagonizes benzodiazepine actions but does not precipitate the abstinence syndrome in cats. *Psychopharmacology,* 86:132–134.

168. Orlandi, F., Bamonti, F., Dini, M., Koch, M., and Jezequel, A. (1975): Hepatic cholesterol synthesis in man: Effect of diazepam and other drugs. *Eur. J. Clin. Invest.,* 5:139–146.

169. Orme, M., Breckenridge, A., and Brooks, R. V. (1972): Interactions on benzodiazepines with warfarin. *Br. Med. J.,* 3:611–614.

170. Owen, J. R., Irani, S. F., and Blair, A. W. (1972): Effects of diazepam administered to mothers during labour on temperature regulation of neonate. *Arch. Dis. Child.,* 47:107–110.

171. Parsonage, M. J., and Norris, J. W. (1967): Use of diazepam in treatment of severe convulsive status epilepticus. *Br. Med. J.,* 3:85–88.

172. Pau, H. (1985): Brown disk-shaped deposits in the lens following long-term intake of diazepam (Valium). *Klin. Mbl. Augenheilk.,* 187:219–220.

173. Pedder, S. C. J., Wilcox, R., Tuchek, J. M., Crawford, R. D., and Johnson, D. D. (1987): Benzodiazepine antagonist Ro 15-1788 (flumazeil) attenuates the anticonvulsant activity of diazepam in epileptic fowl. *Brain Res.,* 424:139–143.

174. Pond, S. M., Phillips, M., Benowitz, N. L., Galinsky, R. E., Tong, T. G., and Becker, C. E. (1979): Diazepam kinetics in acute alcohol withdrawal. *Clin. Pharmacol. Ther.,* 25:832–836.

175. Prensky, A. L., Raff, M. C., Moore, M. J., and Schwab, R. S. (1967): Intravenous diazepam in the treatment of prolonged seizure activity. *N. Engl. J. Med.,* 276:779–784.

176. Prior, P. F., MacLaine, G. N., Scott, D. F., and Laurance, B. M. (1971): Intravenous diazepam. *Lancet,* 2:434–435.

177. Reidenberg, M. M., Levy, M., Warner, H., Coutinho, C. B., Schwartz, M. A., Yu, G., and Cher-

ipko, J. (1978): Relationship between diazepam dose, plasma level, age, and central nervous system depression. *Clin. Pharmacol. Ther.*, 23:371–374.

178. Rementeria, J. L., and Bhatt, K. (1977): Withdrawal symptoms in neonates from intrauterine exposure to diazepam. *J. Pediatr.*, 90:123–126.

179. Rogers, H. J., Haslam, R. A., Longstreth, J., and Lietman, P. S. (1979): Phenytoin intoxication during concurrent diazepam therapy. *J. Neurol. Neurosurg, Psychiatry*, 40:890–895.

180. Rosanelli, K. (1970): Über die Wirkung von pränatal verabreichtem Diazepam auf das Frühgeborene. *Geburtshilfe Frauenheilk.*, 30:713–724.

181. Sadjadi, S. A., McLaughlin, K., Shah, R. M. (1987): Allergic interstitial nephritis due to diazepam. *Arch. Intern. Med.*, 147:579.

182. Safra, M. J., and Oakley, G. P., Jr. (1975): Association between cleft lip with or without cleft palate and prenatal exposure to diazepam. *Lancet*, 2:478–480.

183. Safra, M. J., and Oakley, G. P. Jr. (1976): Valium: An oral cleft teratogen? *Cleft Palate J.*, 13:198–200.

184. Saldanha, V. F., Bird, R., and Havard, C. W. H. (1971): Effect of diazepam (Valium) on dialysable thyroxine. *Postgrad. Med. J.*, 47:326–328.

185. Sawyer, G. T., Webster, D. D., and Schut, L. J. (1968): Treatment of uncontrolled seizure activity with diazepam. *J.A.M.A.*, 203:913–918.

186. Saxen, I., and Saxen, L. (1975): Association between maternal intake of diazepam and oral clefts. *Lancet*, 2:498.

187. Scher, J., Hailey, D. M., and Beard, R. W. (1972): The effects of diazepam on the fetus. *J. Obstet. Gynaecol. Brit. Commonw.*, 79:635–638.

188. Schmidt, D. (1982): Benzodiazepines—Diazepam. In: *Antiepileptic Drugs*, 2nd edition, edited by D. M. Woodbury, J. K. Penry, and C. E. Pippenger, pp. 711–735. Raven Press, New York.

189. Schmidt, D. (1983): How to use benzodiazepines. In: *Antiepileptic Drug Therapy in Pediatry*, edited by P. L. Morselli, C. E. Pippenger, J. K. Penry, pp. 269–278. Raven Press, New York.

190. Schmidt, D. (1984): Behandlung der Epilepsien, 2nd edition. Georg Thieme Verlag, Stuttgart.

191. Schmidt, D. (1985): Benzodiazepines—an update. In: *Recent Advances in Epilepsy, No. 2*, edited by T. A. Pedley and B. S. Meldrum, pp. 125–136. Churchill Livingstone, Edinburgh.

192. Schmidt, D. (1989): Adverse effects of antiepileptic drugs in children: The relevance of drug interactions. *Cleveland J. of Med. (in press)*.

193. Schmidt, D., Einicke, I., and Haenel, F. (1986): The influence of seizure type on the efficacy of plasma concentrations of phenytoin, phenobarbital and carbamazepine. *Arch. Neurol.*, 43:263–265.

194. Schmidt, D., and Janz, D. (1977): Therapeutic plasma concentrations of phenytoin and phenobarbitone. In: *Antiepileptic Drug Monitoring*, edited by C. Gardner-Thorpe, D. Janz, H. Meinardi, and C. E. Pippenger, pp. 214–225. Pitman Medical, Tunbridge Wells, Kent.

195. Schwartz, D. E., Vecchi, M., Ronco, A., and Kaiser, K. (1966): Blood levels after administration of 7-chloro-1,3-dihydro-1-methyl-5-phenyl-2H-1,4-benzodiazepine-2-one (Diazepam) in various forms. *Arzneim. Forsch.*, 16:1109–1110.

196. Schwartz, M. A., Koechlin, B. A., Postma, E., Palmer, S., and Krol, G. (1965): Metabolism of diazepam in rat, dog, and man. *J. Pharmacol. Exp. Ther.*, 149:423–435.

197. Scollo-Lavizzari, G. (1984): The anticonvulsant effect of the benzodiazepine antagonist Ro 15-1788: An EEG study in four cases. *Eur. Neurol.*, 23:1–6.

198. Sellman, R., Hurme, M., and Kanto, J. (1977): Biliary excretion of diazepam and its metabolites in man after repeated oral doses. *Eur. J. Clin. Pharmacol.*, 12:209–213.

199. Sellman, R., Kanto, J., and Pekkarinen, J. (1975): Biliary excretion of diazepam and its metabolites in man. *Acta Pharmacol. Toxicol. (Kbh.)*, 37:242–249.

200. Shaner, D. M., McCurdy, S. A., Herring, M. O., and Gabor, A. J. (1988): Treatment of status epilepticus: A prospective comparison of diazepam and phenytoin versus phenobarbital and optional phenytoin. *Neurology*, 38:202–207.

201. Sher, P. K., Study, R. E., Mazzetta, J., Barker, J. L., and Nelson, P. G. (1983): Depression of benzodiazepine binding and diazepam potentiation of GABA-mediated inhibition after chronic exposure of spinal cord cultures to diazepam. *Brain Res.*, 268:171–176.

202. Sherman, P. M. (1974): Cardiac arrest with diazepam. *J. Oral Surg.*, 32:567.

203. Shull, H. J., Wilkinson, G. R., Johnson, R., and Schenker, S. (1976): Normal disposition of oxazepam in acute viral hepatitis and cirrhosis. *Ann. Intern. Med.*, 84:420–425.

204. Silverman, G., and Braithwaite, R. A. (1973): Benzodiazepines and tricyclic antidepressant plasma levels. *Br. Med. J.*, 3:18–20.

205. Siris, J. H., Pippenger, C. E., Werner, W. L., and Masland, R. L. (1974): Anticonvulsant drug-serum levels in psychiatric patients with seizure disorders. *N.Y. State J. Med.*, 74:1554–1556.

206. Sjödin, T. (1977): Circular dichroism studies on the inhibiting effect of oleic acid on the binding of diazepam to human serum albumin. *Biochem. Pharmacol.*, 26:2157–2161.

207. Sonnenberg, A., Koelz, H. R., Herz, R., Benes, I., and Blum, A. L. (1978): Der Einfluss oraler Kontrazeptiva auf die Demethylierung von Diazepam und Dimethyl-N-Aminoantipyrin. *Verh. Deutsch. Ges. Inn. Med.*, 84:1485–1488.

208. Sternbach, L. H., and Reeder, E. (1961): Quinazolines and 1,4-benzodiazepines. IV. Transformations of 7-chloro-2-methylamino-5-phenyl-3H-1,4-benzodiazepine-4-oxide. *J. Org. Chem.*, 26:4936–4941.

209. Stjernholm, M. R., and Katz, F. H. (1975): Effects of diphenylhydantoin, phenobarital, and diazepam on the metabolism of methylprednisolone and its sodium succinate. *J. Clin. Endocrinol. Metab.*, 41:887–893.

210. Swinyard, E. A. (1969): Laboratory evaluation of antiepileptic drugs. Review of laboratory methods. *Epilepsia,* 10:107–119.

211. Tassinari, C. A., Gastaut, H., Dravet, C., and Roger, J. (1971): A paradoxical effect: Status epilepticus induced by benzodiazepines. *Electroencephalogr. Clin. Neurophysiol.,* 31:182.

212. Tenen, S. S., and Hirsch, J. D. (1980): β-Carboline-3-carboxylic acid ethyl ester antagonizes diazepam activity. *Nature,* 288:609–610.

213. Thearle, M. J., Dunn, P. M., and Hailey, D. M. (1973): Exchange transfusion for diazepam intoxication at birth followed by jejunal stenosis. *Proc. R. Soc. Med.,* 66:349–350.

214. Thiessen, J. J., Sellers, E. M., Denbeigh, P., and Dolman, L. (1976): Plasma protein binding of diazepam and tolbutamide in chronic alcoholics. *J. Clin. Pharmacol.,* 16:345–351.

215. Thompson, W. L. (1978): Management of alcohol withdrawal syndromes. *Arch. Intern. Med.,* 138:278–283.

216. Thong, Y. H., and Abramson, D. C. (1974): Continous infusion of diazepam in infants with severe recurrent convulsions. *Med. Ann. Dist. Columbia,* 43:63–65.

217. Tognoni, G., Gomeni, R., De Majo, D., Alberti, G. G., Franciosi, P., and Scieghi, G. (1975): Pharmacokinetics of *N*-demethyldiazepam in patients suffering from insomnia and treated with nortriptyline. *Br. J. Clin. Pharmacol.,* 2:227–232.

218. Trolle, E. (1965): Diazepam (Valium) in the treatment of epilepsy. *Acta Neurol. Scand.,* (Suppl.), 13:535–539.

219. Vajda, F. J. E., Princas, R. J., and Lovell, R. R. H. (1971): Interaction between phenytoin and the benzodiazepines. *Br. Med. J.,* 1:346.

220. Van der Kleijn, E., Van Rossum, J. M., Muskens, E. T. J. M., and Rijntjes, N. V. M. (1971): Pharmacokinetics of diazepam in dogs, mice and humans. *Acta Pharmacol. Toxicol. (Suppl.) (Kbh.),* 3:109–127.

221. Varma, A.-J., Fisher, B. K., and Sarin, M. K. (1977): Diazepam-induced coma with bullae and eccrine sweat gland necrosis. *Arch. Intern. Med.,* 137:1207–1210.

222. Ventura, A., Basso, T., Bortolan, G., Gardini, A., Guidobaldi, G., Lorusso, G., Marinoni, S., Merli, A., Messi, G., Mussi, G., Muner, M., Patamia, F., Rabusin, P., Sacher, B., and Ulliana, A. (1982): Home treatment of seizures as a strategy for the long-term management of febrile convulsions in children. *Helv. Paediatr. Acta,* 37:581–587.

223. Viala, A., Cano, J. P., Dravet, C., Tassinari, C. A., and Roger, J. (1971): Blood levels of diazepam (Valium) and *N*-desmethyldiazepam in the epileptic child. *Psychiatr. Neurol. Neurochir.,* 74:153–158.

224. White, B. J., Driscoll, E. J., Tjio, J. H., and Similack, Z. H. (1974): Chromosomal aberration rates and intravenously given diazepam. A negative study. *J.A.M.A.,* 230:414–417.

225. Wilensky, A. J., Levy, R. H., Troupin, A. S., Moretti-Ojemann, L., and Friel, P. (1978): Clorazepate kinetics in treated epileptics. *Clin. Pharmacol. Ther.,* 24:22–30.

226. Wilson, J. D., King, D. J., and Sheridan, B. (1979): Tranquilisers and plasma prolactin. *Br. Med. J.,* 1:123–124.

227. Windorfer, A., Jr. (1973): Untersuchungen über die Steigerung der Albumin-Bilirubin-Dissoziation durch Medikamente *in vitro* und *in vivo. Monatsschr. Kinderheilkd.,* 121:469–470.

228. Zingales, I. A. (1973): Diazepam metabolism during chronic medication. Unbound fraction in plasma, erythrocytes and urine. *J. Chromatogr.,* 75:55–78.

Antiepileptic Drugs, Third Edition, edited by
R. Levy, R. Mattson, B. Meldrum,
J. K. Penry, and F. E. Dreifuss.
Raven Press, Ltd., New York © 1989.

56

Benzodiazepines

Clonazepam

Susumu Sato

Clonazepam, 5-(2-chlorophenol)-1,3-di-hydro-7-nitro-2H-1,4-benzodiazepin-2-one, a chlorinated derivative of nitrazepam, was approved for use as an antiepileptic drug by the United States Food and Drug Administration in 1975. Benzodiazepines were first synthesized by Dziewónski and Sternbach in 1933 (206), and in 1966 clonazepam was evaluated as one of the antiepileptic benzodiazepines (203). The recent contribution of the benzodiazepines to the management of epilepsy has been reviewed (213).

The clinical application of clonazepam was not undertaken until the early 1970s. Although clonazepam (Clonopin) is used primarily in the treatment of epilepsy (31,33,179,180) there is a recent trend for its use in panic disorders (12,13, 48,74,98,118,181,210) and movement disorders (30,75,111). Clonazepam has the chemical structure shown in Fig. 1.

CHEMISTRY

Benzodiazepines are a class of heterocyclic six-membered ring compounds transformed into novel hetero-ring compounds with a seven-membered ring. Substituents in the 7 position of ring A with the electron-withdrawing properties of heavier halogens, particularly with some nitro and trifluoro-

methyl groups, increase biological potency, e.g., activity against pentylenetetrazol-induced seizures. It has also been found that fluorine, chlorine, or two halogens at the *ortho* position of ring C have potent effects. Clonazepam has a nitro substitution at the 7 position of ring A and a chlorine at the *ortho* position of ring C.

Clonazepam is a light yellow crystalline powder with a molecular weight of 315.7 and pK_a values of 1.5 and 10.5. The pK_a of 1.5 corresponds to the removal of the proton of the protonated nitrogen in the 4 position of the molecule, and the pK_a of 10.5 corresponds to the deprotonation of the nitrogen in the 1 position. Thus, the compound is virtually undissociated throughout the physiological pH range (121).

METHODS OF DETERMINATION

The original method of electron capture gas-liquid chromatographic (GLC) assay for the determination of clonazepam (54,56) required repeated extraction procedures and acid hydrolysis prior to analysis, a time-consuming technique. Since then, the extraction procedure has been improved with the omission of acid hydrolysis (83,167,175). A gas chromatographic-mass spectrometric assay for clonazepam, using positive ion chemical ionization with am-

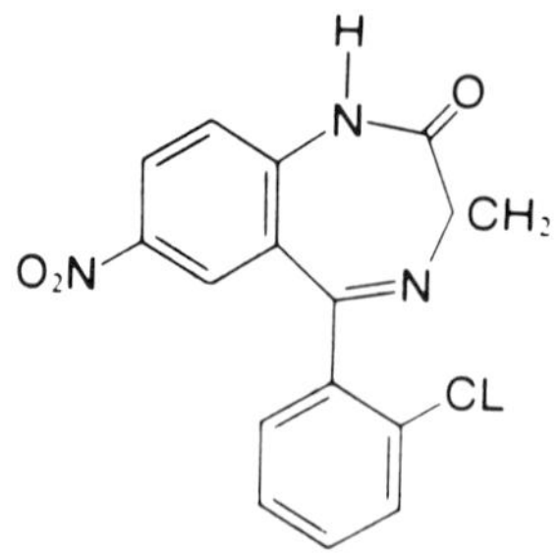

FIG. 1. Structure of clonazepam.

monia, was described in 1977 and 1978 (159,160) and was subsequently modified to employ negative chemical ionization, in which methane was used as both the gas chromatographic carrier gas and the chemical ionization reagent gas (79). The sensitivity of this technique is considerably greater than that of the original method (80). Other modifications of GLC techniques have been reported (37,38,53,63,72,203). High-performance liquid chromatography (HPLC) (178,216) and thin-layer chromatography (211,223) have also been used. Gas and liquid chromatographic methods for the determination of clonazepam and other drugs have been reviewed (35,55), and simple and sensitive HPLC methods have been described (97,120,145,158,235). A simple and specific radioimmunoassay technique for detection of clonazepam in plasma without extraction can be used with antibodies to clonazepam produced in rabbits and exhibiting a high degree of specificity for clonazepam (57,58). When [3H]iodine is used as a tracer, the radioimmunoassay has a limited sensitivity of 5 ng/ml. A more rapid and less costly technique utilizes a radioimmunoassay with [125I] (57).

ABSORPTION, DISTRIBUTION, AND EXCRETION

The pharmacokinetics of clonazepam have been recently reviewed (90). Clona-

zepam is well absorbed, and the peak plasma level occurs within 1 to 4 hr after oral administration, but it may occur as late as 8 hr (20,62,105,121). Benzodiazepines cross the blood-brain barrier easily and distribute rapidly in the brain (77). Clonazepam administered orally in a solution of propylene glycol was absorbed completely, and micronization of clonazepam overcame the dissolution rate-limiting characteristics of the compound in the overall absorption of the drug (121). After a dose of 1.5 mg of [2-14C]clonazepam (68), the absorption rate ranged from 81.2% to 98.1% of the dose, calculated from total radioactivity and concentration mean values of the radioactive compound from the plasma. The distribution is rapid because of its high lipid solubility (130). Clonazepam is $86 \pm 0.5\%$ protein bound (16). The volume of distribution (V_d) ranged from 1.5 to 4.4 liter/kg in eight healthy adult volunteers (22). Following intravenous administration of clonazepam to sheep, there was rapid equilibration of cerebral spinal fluid concentrations and unbound serum concentrations of the drug, and the large V_d suggested tissue binding (174).

Less than 0.5% of clonazepam was recovered unchanged in the urine in a 24-hr period (121,200), indicating extensive biotransformation and/or an alternative route of excretion. Total excretion of clonazepam and unconjugated 7-amino-clonazepam and 7-acetamino-clonazepam amounted to 5% to 20% of the dose given. The 3-hydroxy derivatives of all three compounds were detected only in trace amounts in the urine (200).

METABOLISM AND BIOTRANSFORMATION

Clonazepam is metabolized principally by reduction of the nitro group to produce inactive 7-amino derivatives (184). The following metabolic products of clonazepam have been demonstrated in man (68): free compounds, including unaltered clonazepam; 7-amino derivative as the principal metabolite; 7-acetamido derivative; 3-hydroxy-7-amino derivative; and 3-hydroxy-7-acetamido derivative in small quantities. Conjugate compounds include the 7-amino derivative and the 7-amino-phenol derivative (134). In 27 patients, a daily dose of 6 mg of clonazepam yielded plasma levels of both clonazepam and its principal metabolite, the 7-amino derivative, in the range of 30 to 80 ng/ml (mean, 50 ng/ml). The pharmacokinetic behavior of the 7-amino metabolite of clonazepam adminstered exogenously and formed endogenously from the parent drug was studied in a group of Rhesus monkeys, with constant-rate venous infusions. The biological half-life of the 7-amino metabolite was shorter than that of clonazepam (138). The average peak concentration of the metabolite occurred at approximately the same time as that of the parent compound, and the ratio between them varied from 1 to 3 and 3 to 1 (200). The nitro compounds are pharmacologically active, whereas the amino compounds are not. However, the plasma level of the 3-hydroxy-7-nitro metabolite appears to contribute insignificantly to the pharmacological effect of clonazepam itself (76,129).

PLASMA CLONAZEPAM LEVEL, HALF-LIFE, AND SEIZURE CONTROL

The mean plasma concentration of clonazepam after intravenous and oral administration of 1.5 mg of the drug to four male patients was 5.0 to 7.8 ng/ml and 3.7 to 5.9 ng/ml, respectively (68). The half-life ranged from 30.5 to 40.3 hr after 1.5 mg given intravenously and from 26.5 to 49.2 hr after 1.5 mg given orally. Oral administration of 9 mg gave a similar half-life of 26.8 to 32.5 hr in four patients. Ten adult males given a single 2-mg oral dose of clonazepam showed blood clonazepam levels of 6.5 to

13 ng/ml, and the corresponding half-life ranged from 18.7 to 39.0 hr (mean, 26.4 hr) (121). Five patients received 0.5 mg of clonazepam twice a day for 15 days and had steady-state plasma clonazepam levels of 4.6 to 12.0 ng/ml, with a plasma half-life of 31 to 42 hr (121). These findings were similar to those of single-dose studies, implying an absence of liver enzyme induction (20).

Ten children with absence seizures received clonazepam in daily doses ranging from 0.029 to 0.111 mg/kg for 8 weeks and reached steady-state plasma drug levels of 13 to 72 ng/ml (Fig. 2) and plasma half-lives between 22 and 33 hr (Fig. 3) (59). The relationship between serum clonazepam levels and dosage is more (59,168,200) or less (11) linear (Fig. 2). Children have a considerably lower mean ratio of plasma level to oral dose (11) and a higher relative clearance value (129) than adults, implying that they require a higher dose to reach and maintain the same concentration. In children, who rapidly absorb and eliminate the drug, the daily oral dose should be divided into thirds. Clonazepam appears to be effective in reducing the frequency of absence seizures at serum levels of 13 to 72 ng/ml (11,59,129). Clonazepam administered rectally to 11 children was rapidly absorbed, with a peak plasma concentration of 2.8 to 12.0 ng/ml 20 to 60 min following a dose of 0.05 mg/kg and 18.4 to 40.5 ng/ml 10 min to 2 hr following a dose of 0.1 mg/kg (189). In 18 newborns with convulsions, slow intravenous infusion of clonazepam produced plasma drug levels of 28 to 117 ng/ml in eight patients who received 0.1 mg/kg and 99 to 380 ng/ml in 10 patients who received 0.2 mg/kg, and the plasma half-life ranged from 20 to 43 hr (5). Interestingly, clonazepam was more efficacious in the group receiving the lower dose.

There is no correlation between antiepileptic efficacy and plasma clonazepam levels (169; S. Sato et al., *unpublished data*), although the range of plasma clonazepam levels coinciding with excellent seizure con-

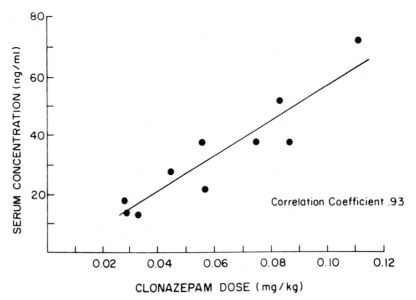

FIG. 2. Relationship of serum clonazepam concentration (ng/ml) to dose (mg/kg) in 10 children. (From Dreifuss et al., ref. 59, with permission.)

trol was similar in several studies (11,59,129). Patients with absence seizures who showed no generalized spike-and-wave discharges on the 12-hr telemetered EEG had clonazepam levels of 8.6 to 19.4 ng/ml during the first week of treatment and 18.4 to 42.5 ng/ml during the eighth and 17th treatment weeks (S. Sato et al., *unpublished data*). Patients with high levels of phenobarbital and clonazepam levels of less than 10 ng/ml responded poorly to the addition of clonazepam (170).

MECHANISMS OF ACTION

Although clonazepam induces a moderate elevation of whole brain serotonin, its effect on the physiological activity of serotonin is uncertain (227). In mice, the increase in serotonin and 5-hydroxyindole-acetic acid observed with single-dose administration of clonazepam was not seen following prolonged administration of high doses for 8 days (114,115). In the mouse, clonazepam elevates brain tryptophan lev-

els (although not because of altered serotonin synthesis), decreases serotonin utilization, and blocks the egress of 5-hydroxyindoleactic acid from the brain (116). Some suggest that clonazepam influences central dopaminergic systems through a direct effect on dopaminergic presynaptic mechanisms (226). The observation that benzodiazepines potentiated the dopamine–GABA-dependent stereotyped gnawing behavior in mice suggested that the benzodiazepines may act by sensitizing γ-aminobutyric acid (GABA) receptors to the action of GABA (6). Stimulation of benzodiazepine receptor binding may involve a novel type of GABA receptor (123). In monkeys, clonazepam abolished γ-hydroxybutyrate–induced EEG changes but exacerbated myoclonic jerks (202).

The discovery of specific benzodiazepine receptors in rat brain (29,163,164) led to the description of [^{3}H]diazepam binding sites in human brain. In the human brain, the cerebral and cerebellar cortical regions contain the highest densities of [^{3}H]diazepam binding sites. Clonazepam and diazepam have

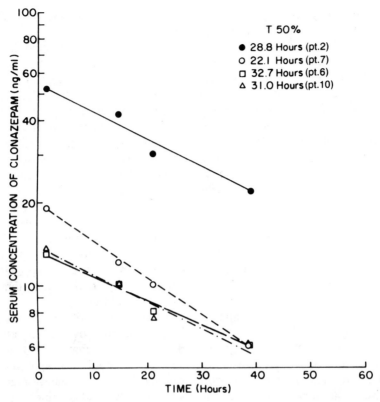

FIG. 3. Serum half-life (hr) of clonazepam in four children. Four serum clonazepam concentrations were determined for each patient within a 40-hr period while the dosage of clonazepam was delayed. (From Dreifuss et al., ref. 59, with permission.)

higher affinities for these binding sites in all human brain regions than do other benzodiazepines. The ability of benzodiazepines to displace [³H]diazepam from the receptors is thought to correlate with the recommended daily clinical doses and clinical effects (28,163,164). The use of [³H]fluoronitrazepam showed specific benzodiazepine binding sites in mouse and human brain identical to those found with [³H]diazepam (46,205). There is substantial agreement between binding affinity and relative potency to block pentylenetetrazol-induced convulsions for a large series of benzodiazepines (184). Benzodiazepines appear to modify neuronal excitability by acting on three different affinity receptor sites: high affinity central receptor, linked

to the inhibitory action of GABA; low affinity membrane site, limiting repetitive firing; and lower affinity site in the presynaptic terminals, decreasing Ca^{++} conductance and neurotransmitter release. The action on the high affinity central benzodiazepine binding sites correlates with anticonvulsant and antimyoclonic action as well as with anxiolytic activity. The two lower affinity systems may be responsible for therapeutic action in status epilepticus and for sedative side effects (153). Benzodiazepine-induced hyperphagia may also be mediated by central-type benzodiazepine binding sites (50). An autoradiographic technique using [³H]flunitrazepam in living cultures of fetal mouse cerebral cortex suggested that multiple cell types (neurons and background cells) may participate in the neuropharmacologic actions of the benzodiazepines (199). Reduced drug efficacy may be due to reduction of benzodiazepine binding, which was found following long-term exposure of cortical cell cultures to clonazepam (198), therefore alternate-day clonazepam treatment was proposed to minimize receptor alterations (197). Benzodiazepine receptors are not involved in either the anticonvulsant action of phenytoin against seizures induced by electroshock or the neurotoxicity of phenytoin (47).

The actions of benzodiazepines have been linked to the functions of receptor-chloride ionophore systems that are regulated by GABA (173). Both presynaptic and postsynaptic GABA-mediated inhibition and the effects of exogenous GABA appear to be facilitated by benzodiazepines. Clonazepam may potentiate the inhibitory effects of GABA but produces no consistent inhibitory effect by itself in in vitro midbrain slices containing the dorsal raphe nucleus (201).

Recent studies suggest that the anticonvulsant effects of the benzodiazepine may not depend entirely upon action on GABAergic neurotransmission or on chloride ion channels. It has also been suggested that the benzodiazepines may exert their pharmacologic effects by mimicking the effects of glycine at its central nervous system receptor sites (234). Clonazepam is effective against generalized tonic-clonic seizures induced in rats by ouabain (52) and in mice and rats by pentylenetetrazol (207,232). It has a very potent inhibitory effect on convulsions induced by maximal electroshock, strychnine, and picrotoxin (232), and little action on seizures induced by maximal electroshock (207). Clonazepam protects dogs (225) and rats (3) against tonic-clonic seizures induced by amygdala kindling. However, it has little effect on afterdischarges induced by stimulation of the cerebral cortex in cats (232). It is very effective against

photically induced epilepsy in *Papio papio* (152) but is ineffective against febrile covulsions in mice subjected to microwave diathermy (119). The anticonvulsant activity of clonazepam experimentally appears to be at least partially mediated by inhibition of synaptic recovery and the enhancement of presynaptic inhibition (232). Clonazepam shortens the duration of primary epileptiform discharge and prolongs the intermittent interval in cortical, amygdaloid, and intralaminar thalamic epileptic foci induced by a high concentration of penicillin G in cats. The anticonvulsant effects of clonazepam may result from blockade of neuronal pathways that spread the discharge from the site of origin to the effector organ and from the elevation of seizure threshold (214).

Microinjection of clonazepam bilaterally into substantia nigra pars reticulata produced a 75% elevation of the generalized seizure threshold in the kindling model, suggesting that the substantia nigra is the one site where benzodiazepines may act to suppress seizures (128). Electroencephalographic studies have shown that clonazepam is particularly effective in suppressing generalized discharge such as the 3 per sec spike-and-wave discharge of absence seizures, the slow spike-and-wave discharge of atypical absence, and the generalized polyspike-and-wave discharge frequently associated with generalized tonic-clonic seizures or myoclonic seizures. It also appears to be effective in suppressing the discharges of reflex epilepsies, particularly photic-induced seizures (18,26,33,44,59,80,81,103,148). The effect on hypsarrhythmia is less striking, but may be quite marked (61,148,220,228). Focal epileptic discharge is less consistently abolished; it may be decreased (2,70,94,106), unchanged (172), or increased (103). However, clonazepam does appear to prevent the propagation of seizures. Both intravenously and orally administered clonazepam may produce rapid beta rhythms (16 to 30 Hz) (33,103).

The degradation of clonazepam in serum during exposure to light (artificial ultraviolet light, sunlight, and room light) can markedly decrease the concentration of the drug (222). This may also contribute to the loss of drug efficacy. Tolerance to the drug's effect can develop without significant changes in plasma clonazepam concentrations (93). Tolerance developed in dogs after 1 to 2 weeks of clonazepam treatment (193), in mice over a 72-hr period (82), and in kindled rats after 5 days (217).

EFFECT OF CLONAZEPAM ON SPECIFIC SEIZURE TYPES

Most therapeutic trials of new anticonvulsant drugs involve the addition of the new drug to the existing regimen of patients with refractory seizures. "Add-on" studies have two major drawbacks. One is the bias introduced by the placebo effect of a new drug. The second is that the most refractory patients may give no indication of how effective the drug will be in previously untreated patients. Controlled clinical trials of the new drug render the most objective, rapid, and definitive answers to questions of the drug's efficacy.

Absence Seizures

Reports on the effectiveness of clonazepam in absence seizures have described open trials (19,26,71,109,140,141,147, 172,215) and controlled trials (44,59,156, 170,215). In all studies, clonazepam was extremely effective in the control of absence seizures. Clonazepam was found to be superior to ethosuximide in the normalization of the EEG (59), but adverse side effects and the development of tolerance to the drug's effect greatly reduced this advantage (S. Sato et al., *unpublished data*). Valproate and clonazepam comedication improved absence seizures in seven of eight

patients with intractable absence seizures (162).

Tonic-Clonic Seizures

In general, phenytoin, phenobarbital, primidone, and carbamazepine are drugs of choice in the treatment of generalized tonic-clonic seizures. However, clonazepam may completely control these seizures in some 10% to 70% of patients (10,19,21,23,41, 65,104,133,143,155,166,185), and even in more than 80% (169). Comedication with valproate and clonazepam improved seizures in 3 of 14 patients with intractable primary generalized tonic-clonic seizures (162). When given intravenously, clonazepam suppresses the EEG abnormality and abolishes generalized tonic-clonic status epilepticus. In some series (133,172), however, the drug has been found to be ineffective in this seizure type, and many reports have indicated that generalized tonic-clonic seizures are exacerbated by the addition of clonazepam to the regimen (26,147,166,183,186).

Complex Partial Seizures

Although phenytoin, carbamazepine, primidone, and phenobarbital are all more effective in protecting experimental animals against maximal electroshock seizures than is clonazepam, this drug has been found effective in several trials, both controlled (22,103,147) and uncontrolled (19,71,104, 124,125,127,141–143,147,155,172,194). The development of tolerance, or decreasing efficacy with long-term administration, has been noted several times (1,71,147,149, 155). Some reports, however, have specifically stated that efficacy was not decreased over time (44,194). Valproate and clonazepam comedication improved seizures in 19 of 39 patients with intractable complex partial seizures (162).

Simple Partial Seizures

In general, clonazepam is less effective than phenytoin, primidone, or carbamazepine in simple partial seizures, but it has been shown to be effective in controlled trials (65,157) and in some uncontrolled studies (1,92,147,169,172,194). The latter studies suggest that the drug is effective even in epilepsia partialis continua. Clonazepam seems to be more effective in partial seizures than in generalized tonic-clonic seizures, and it has been noted that secondary generalization has not been facilitated by the administration of clonazepam (80). The drug's effectiveness in epilepsia partialis continua (104,194) is achieved despite persistence of the electroencephalographic focus.

Atypical Absence (Lennox-Gastaut Syndrome)

The Lennox-Gastaut syndrome is one of the most severe forms of childhood epilepsy. It is a chronic encephalopathy characterized electroencephalographically by slow spikes and waves and often by focal abnormalities with a shifting hemisphere emphasis. It is manifested in a variety of seizures, the most severe of which is the drop attack, in which injuries frequently occur. The benzodiazepines, and particularly clonazepam, have been found to have beneficial effects in many children with this syndrome, and these have been observed in both controlled (164,225) and uncontrolled (10,19,26,61,92,95,103,112,131,134,171, 172,187,188,191,220) studies. The results were frequently better at the beginning of treatment than later, and this may have been because of the development of tolerance to the drug's effect or the rather variable natural history of the condition. On occasion, treatment failures may respond when corticotropin (ACTH) or hydrocortisone (61) is added to the regimen. Valproic

acid has virtually superseded clonazepam in the treatment of Lennox-Gastaut syndrome and is considerably more effective. Valproate and clonazepam comedication improved atonic seizures in three of 14 patients (162).

Massive Infantile Spasms

Infantile spasms consist of a heterogeneous group of seizure disorders usually characterized by massive flexion myoclonic spasms, at times by extensor spasms, and frequently associated with a hypsarrhythmic EEG pattern, intractability to treatment, and mental retardation. Others are phenotypically similar but date from birth and are associated with severe neurological abnormalities. Treatment of choice has been corticosteroids. The effects of benozdiazepines are highlighted by the good results obtained with nitrazepam. The results with clonazepam appear to be disappointing, but they vary widely; some authors have found that the drug is ineffective (92,95,103,132,166), whereas others have met with more success (61,80,148,220,228). Vassella et al. (220) reported control of infantile spasms in about one-third of the patients treated. The limiting factor appeared to be increased bronchial secretions.

Myoclonic Seizures

There are several syndromes described under the rubric of myoclonic epilepsy. These include bilateral massive epileptic myoclonus (juvenile myoclonic epilepsy), a relatively benign seizure form frequently accompanied by generalized tonic-clonic seizures. In this condition, clonazepam has been found to be quite effective in both controlled and uncontrolled studies (15,71,81,156,166,172,179). Other forms of myoclonic epilepsy have also benefited significantly (9,65,95,103,134,140,161). In progressive hereditary myoclonic epilepsy and the Ramsay-Hunt syndrome, clonazepam has been of significant benefit (19,80,139). The intention myoclonus seen in postencephalitic and postanoxic states has been successfully treated with clonazepam (27,39,43,69,86,101,161). Chadwick et al. (42,43) suggested that the protective effect of clonazepam in myoclonic seizures may be the result of increased cerebral serotonin concentrations; it is not surprising, therefore, that the myoclonic seizures responding to clonazepam are those that benefit from 5-hydroxytryptophan. Myoclonus associated with methyl bromide poisoning has been successfully treated with clonazepam (88,212). Valproate and clonazepam comedication improved seizures in eight of nine patients with myoclonic seizures (162) or in some patients with severe progressive myoclonic epilepsy (108).

Photosensitive Seizures

Clonazepam is a potent anticonvulsant in *Papio papio*, a model of light-sensitive epilepsy. Of all medications tested in this model, clonazepam has the greatest protective effect. Photosensitive seizures are of great interest as a form of reflex epilepsy. A large portion of the population is affected by the photomyoclonic and photoconvulsive epilepsies, as well as a variety of self-induced photosensitive seizures. Clonazepam is effective not only in reducing the response to photic stimulation but also in alleviating the desire for self-induction of seizures (4,26,92,104,125,183).

Miscellaneous Paroxysmal Conditions

Clonazepam has been used with some success in a large number of paroxysmal disorders. Successes have been claimed for it in eclamptic convulsive attacks (15), Gilles de la Tourette syndrome (87), trigeminal neuralgia (36,45,51), the stiff man syndrome (220,230), chorea (176), blepharo-spasm (154), restless legs (151), tardive dyskinesia (195), hemifacial spasm (99), paroxysmal awakenings (177), and segmental and essential myoclonus (30,111).

Status Epilepticus

Clonazepam is effective in controlling various forms of status epilepticus involving generalized tonic-clonic seizures, absence seizures, partial seizures with complex symptomatology, simple partial seizures, clonic seizures, tonic seizures, myoclonic seizures, Jacksonian seizures, hemiconvulsions, and epilepsia partialis continua (34,60,78,92,122,126,165,219). A single dose of 1 to 4 mg of clonazepam is usually sufficient to abolish status epilepticus and to ameliorate paroxysmal activity in the EEG. In this use, clonazepam is usually more effective and long-lasting than diazepam (49). However, there was no significant difference between diazepam and clonazepam in the control of status epilepticus in patients with Lennox-Gastaut syndrome (208). The failure of an intravenous benzodiazepine to control nonconvulsive status epilepticus in patients with the Lennox-Gastaut syndrome has been reported (146). In some patients repeated injections may be necessary, up to a total dose of 13 to 18 mg, with poor results in patients with acute brain lesions (208). Both clonazepam (24) and intravenous diazepam (182,209) have been associated with the precipitation of a tonic status episode. A transitory increase in myoclonic jerks and in EEG paroxysmal activity has been described in a case of status epilepticus with the Ramsay-Hunt syndrome (19). Clonazepam is not available for intravenous use in the United States, where diazepam is still the drug of choice for status epilepticus.

CLINICAL TOXICITY

In seven controlled studies (17,22,44, 65,149,156,215), side effects of clonazepam were observed in 16% to 90% (median, 67%) of patients, and led to eventual discontinuation of the drug in 10% to 36%. In other series, side effects in 30% to 82% of patients caused eventual termination of the drug in 12% to 18% of them (104,139,170). Table 1 shows the side effects of clonazepam in a double-blind study of clonazepam versus ethosuximide (S. Sato et al., *unpublished data*). Side effects in 34 (92%) of 37 children with absence seizures required eventual discontinuation of clonazepam in 27% of the patients. The common side effects of clonazepam include drowsiness, ataxia, and behavioral and personality changes. Drowsiness and ataxia usually appear a few hours after the first days of clonazepam therapy and improve with dosage adjustment. Drowsiness occurs in 10% to 85% (median, 62%) of patients and incoordination and ataxia in 7% to 43% (median, 12%). Significant behavioral and personality changes, such as hyperactivity, restlessness, short attention span, irritability, disruptiveness, and aggressiveness, are seen commonly in children and occasionally in adults and occur in 2% to 51% (median, 12%) of patients. Other neurological side effects of clonazepam include, rather commonly, nystagmus, dizziness, dysarthria, and hypotonia and, less commonly, blurred vision, diplopia (18,64), and psychotic reactions (8,140,149).

Increased frequency of various types of seizures has been reported (7,32,166,191). Different varieties of seizures may emerge (7,96,110,148,149,233). Slight weight gain (less than 10% within 17 weeks) was a fairly common problem in our series (S. Sato et al., *unpublished data*). Occasionally, nausea has been reported (18,44). Hypersecretion and hypersalivation may be troublesome in children and infants (180,228). Hematological side effects are rare. Leukopenia has occasionally occurred (25), and thrombocytopenic purpura has been documented (149,221). Dermatological side effects include skin pigmentation (104), transient hair loss (170), and an extensive rash (91). Hepatic or renal complications have

not been observed. Reasons for withdrawing clonazepam include freedom from seizures, lack of clinical effect, intolerable behavior, personality changes, psychotic reactions, persistent drowsiness, leukopenia, increased seizure frequency, and the development of other types of seizures.

There is no correlation between the dose of clonazepam and the occurrence of side effects (143), but this has been disputed (102). The rate of dosage increase is thought to be significant in the development of side effects (67). There is no relationship between side effects and plasma concentration of the drug (11,200). However, drowsiness, dysarthria, irritability, and hypotonia may occurr when plasma clonazepam concentrations range between 22 and 81 ng/ml. In four patients, seizures became more frequent when plasma levels of the drug exceeded 100 ng/ml, and in two patients, status epilepticus was observed when the concentration exceeded 180 ng/ml (11). Serious dysphoria appeared to be associated with an elevated level of clonazepam in some cases, and the upper limit of drug level was thought to be about 70 ng/ml before this toxic effect appeared (200). The main metabolite, 7-amino clonazepam, was found in much higher concentration in patients suffering from withdrawal symptoms (pronounced dysphoria, irritability, restlessness, sleeplessness, and tremor of the hands) than in those who had no such reactions (200).

Convulsion (84) or status epilepticus (184) may be precipitated if the drug is discontinued abruptly (33). A febrile reaction in a severely retarded 18-year-old man who had been taking clonazepam for some 6 months abated within 2 days of discontinuing the drug (89). Anticonvulsant drugs may depress cellular immunity regardless of the drug, the dose, the duration of treatment, or the age when treatment was started (150). A 4-year-old child who ingested a large amount of clonazepam had a plasma level of 69 ng/ml and experienced seven episodes of coma interspersed with alert agitation during the first 24 hr; during the coma

Table 1. *Side effects of clonazepam in 37 children with absence seizures*

Patients			Side effects										Other drugs					
No.	Age	Sex	Drowsiness	Ataxia	Nystagmus	Hyperactivity	Personality change	Increased seizures	Change in seizure type	Weight gain $>10\%$	Leukopenia	Did not complete trial	None	Phenobarbital	Metharbital	Primidone	Phenytoin	Acetazolamide
Untreated																		
1	12	M	x	x	x									x				
2	9	F											x					
3	12	F	x		x								x					
4	13	M			x	x				x						x		
5	6	F		x		x				x			x					
6	12	F	x			x						x	x					
7	9	F	x	x	x					x				x				
8	7	M	x	x		x		x				x	x					
9	8	M	x			x						x	x					
10	9	M				x	x			x			x					
11	5	M		x		x	x					x	x					
12	15	M	x						x					x			x	
13	7	F	x					x				x					x	
14	9	M	x	x				x				x		x				
15	13	F	x						x							x	x	
16	7	M	x	x		x	x						x					
17	11	M											x					
18	8	F												x				
19	6	F				x				x			x					
20	12	F	x											x			x	
Refractory																		
21	5	F	x															
22	9	F			x												x	x
23	11	F	x		x	x				x			x					
24	11	F	x	x	x	x												
25	12	F		x										x				
26	14	F		x	x									x				
27	13	M		x							x	x						
28	10	M	x	x														x
29	9	M	x	x	x					x							x	
30	9	M	x	x			x			x				x				
31	13	F	x											x			x	
32	6	F	x	x						x							x	
33	14	F				x	x	x				x					x	
34	8	F					x	x				x			x			
35	12	F					x			x				x				
36	9	M							x	x				x				
37	7	M	x	x				x				x						
Total			21	16	9	12	7	6	3	11	1	10						

his pupils were pinpoint (229). Intravenous administration of clonazepam for treating status epilepticus may cause cardiovascular and respiratory depression, particularly when it is used after or in combination with phenobarbital (218). Neonatal apnea may be associated with maternal clonazepam therapy (73) Clonazepam does not exacerbate porphyria and has been used to treat seizures in this condition (142). In dogs, slight physical dependence on clonazepam developed after only 1 week of treatment (192). A Tourette-like syndrome may be associated with the use of clonazepam (85).

INTERACTIONS WITH OTHER DRUGS

The potential problem of drug interactions occurs whenever multiple drugs are administered. Clonazepam appears to be relatively inert in this regard. It has been given together with most other antiepileptic drugs, usually without untoward effects. The drug interactions that have been observed appear to be inconstant; thus, serum phenytoin levels after the administration of clonazepam have been noted either to rise (66,104,107) or to fall (17,190). With a fall in the phenytoin levels, there was a concomitant increase in phenytoin metabolites, suggesting an increase in metabolism. The administration of phenytoin has led to a diminution in blood clonazepam levels and levels of its 7-amino clonazepam metabolite (197); similar effects have been observed with other antiepileptic drugs (196).

In other cases, the addition of clonazepam has no effect on blood levels of phenytoin or carbamazepine (144). Lai et al. (135–137) noted that carbamazepine infusion led to diminution in clonazepam levels. They attributed this finding to enzyme induction with an increase in D-glucaric acid, which characterizes such activity. Benetello et al. (17) reported diminished phenobarbital levels, Bekersky et al. (14) found an increased plasma clearance of clonazepam with the addition of phenobarbital, and Nanda et al. (170) observed lower blood

clonazepam levels with the addition of phenobarbital. These reports noted no interaction between clonazepam and the other antiepileptic drugs. Windorfer and Sauer (231) found that serum levels of phenytoin and primidone increased on administration of clonazepam, but Johannessen et al. (117) could find no effect on the levels of phenytoin, phenobarbital, or carbamazepine. It is generally recommended that amphetamines or methylphenidate not be administered together with clonazepam because of the danger of producing nervous system depression and respiratory irregularities (40). The simultaneous administration of clonazepam and valproate carries the danger of exacerbating absence attacks with the possibility of continuous absence seizures (petit mal status) (100,113,204,224). Although some patients tolerate and benefit from this combination of drugs, this hazard must be borne in mind when its use is considered. It also must be remembered that benzodiazepines are known to potentiate the action of central nervous system depressant drugs, such as ethanol and barbiturates (184).

TERATOGENICITY

The anticonvulsant drugs most often implicated in teratogenicity are phenytoin, phenobarbital, and trimethadione. Although now rarely used, trimethadione carries the greatest risk of teratogenicity. There is at the present time no evidence that clonazepam is significantly teratogenic.

SUMMARY

Clonazepam is a potent benzodiazepine anticonvulsant with activity against various types of seizures. It is generally most effective in the treatment of absence seizures, Lennox-Gastaut syndrome, and the myoclonic epilepsies. It is less useful in infantile spasms and partial seizures, although complex partial seizures may be alleviated to some extent. Reflex epilepsies, including photosensitive epilepsy, respond well to clonazepam. Administration of the drug may lead to the emergence of other seizure types. Initial success may be followed by the development of tolerance to the drug's effects. Side effects are common, and most patients experience drowsiness and some ataxia and changes in mood. Severe toxicity is rare, and apart from possible adverse reaction to simultaneous administration of clonazepam and valproate, there is little evidence for clinically significant drug interaction. The drug may exert its effect, at least in part, through modification of GABA-mediated synaptic systems and has an effect on serotonin metabolism. It is well absorbed after oral administration; blood concentration is usually maximal within 2 to 4 hr. Metabolism occurs principally by formation of an inactive 7-amino derivative, and less than 5% of the drug is recovered in the urine unchanged. In recent years, clonazepam has been extensively utilized in the treatment of psychiatric and movement disorders rather than in epilepsy.

CONVERSION

Conversion factor:

$$CF = \frac{1000}{\text{mol. wt.}} = \frac{1000}{315.5} = 3.17$$

Conversion:

$$(\mu g/ml) \times 3.17 = (\mu moles/liter)$$

$$(\mu moles/liter) \div 3.17 = (\mu g/ml)$$

REFERENCES

1. Aarli, J. A. (1973): Effect of clonazepam (Ro 5-4023) on epileptic seizures. *Acta Neurol. Scand.,* 49:11–17.
2. Ahmad, S., Perucca, E., and Richens, A. (1977): Effect of frusemide, mexiletine, (+)-propranolol and three benzodiazepine drugs on interictal spike discharges in the electroencephalogram. *Br. J. Clin. Pharmacol.,* 4:683–688.
3. Albright, P. S., and Burnham, W. M. (1980): Development of a new pharmacological seizure model; Effect of anticonvulsants on cortical- and

amygdala-kindled seizures in the rat. *Epilepsia,* 21:681–689.
4. Ames, F. F., and Enderstein, O. (1976): Clinical and EEG response to clonazepam in four patients with self induced phtosensitive epilepsy. *S. Afr. Med. J.,* 50:1432–1434.
5. Andre, M., Boutroy, M. J., Dubruc, C., Thenot, J. P., Bianchetti, G., Sola, L., Vert, P., and Morselli, P. L. (1986): Clonazepam pharmacokinetics and therapeutic efficacy in neonatal seizures. *Eur. J. Clin. Pharmacol.,* 30:585–589.
6. Arnt, J., Christensen, A. V., and Scheel-Krueger, J. (1979): Benzodiazepines potentiate GABA–dopamine-dependent stereotyped gnawing in mice. *J. Pharm. Pharmacol.,* 31:56–58.
7. Bang, F., Birket-Smith, E., and Mikkelsen, B. (1976): Clonazepam in the treatment of epilepsy. A clinical long-term follow-up study. *Epilepsia,* 17:323–324.
8. Barfod, S., and Wendelboe, J. (1977): Severe psychiatric side effects of clonazepam treatment. 2 cases. *Ugeskr. Laeger,* 139:2450.
9. Bark, N. (1977): Clonazepam in the treatment of epilepsy in handicapped patients. *Br. J. Ment. Subnorm.,* 23:84–87.
10. Barnett, A. M. (1973): Treatment of epilepsy with clonazepam (Ro 5-4023). *S. Afr. Med. J.,* 47:1683–1686.
11. Baruzzi, A., Bordo, B., Bossi, L., Castelli, D., Gerna, M., Tognoni, G., and Zagnoni, P. (1977): Plasma levels of di-*n*-propylacetate and clonazepam in epilepsy patients. *Int. J. Clin. Pharmacol. Biopharm.,* 15:403–408.
12. Beaudry, P., Fontaine, R., Chouinard, G., and Annable, L. (1983): An open clinical trial of clonazepam in treatment of patients with recurrent panic attacks. *Prog. Neuropsychopharmacol. Biol. Psychiatry,* 9:589–592.
13. Beaudry, P., Fontaine, R., Chouinard, G., and Annable, L. (1986): Clonazepam in the treatment of patients with recurrent panic attacks. *J. Clin. Psychiatry,* 47:83–85.
14. Bekersky, I., Maggio, A. C., Mattaliano, V. J., Boxenbaum, H. G., Maynard, D. C., Cohen, P. D., and Kaplan, S. A. (1977): Influence of phenobarbital on the disposition of clonazepam and antipyrine in the dog. *J. Pharmacokinet. Biopharm.,* 5:507–512.
15. Beltrami, M., Mangaldo, R., and Frassinetic, E. (1978): Clonazepam in the treatment of eclampic convulsive attacks. *Minerva Anestesiol.,* 44:257–261.
16. Benet, L. Z., and Sheiner, L. B. (1985): Appendix II. Design and optimization of dosage regimens: Pharmacokinetic data. In: *The Pharmacological Basis of Therapeutics,* 7th edition, edited by A. G. Gilman, L. S. Goodman, T. W. Rall, and F. Murad, pp. 1663–1733. Macmillan, New York.
17. Benetello, P., Furlanut, M., Testa, G., and Santi, R. (1977): Effect of benzodiazepines on serum levels of phenobarbital and diphenylhydantoin. *Riv. Farmacol. Ter.,* 8:109–112.
18. Bensch, J., Blennow, G., Ferngren, H., Gamstorp, I., Herrlin, K. M., Kubista, J., Arvidsson, A., and Dahlstrom, H. (1977): A double-blind

study of clonazepam in the treatment of therapy resistant epilepsy in children. *Dev. Med. Child Neurol.,* 19:355–342.

19. Bergamini, L., Mutani, R., and Liboni, W. (1970): Eleckroenczephalographische under klinische Bewertung des neuen Benzodiazepin Ro 5/4023. *Electroencephalogr. Electromyogr.,* 1:182–188.

20. Berlin, A., and Dahlstrom, H. (1975): Pharmacokinetics of the anticonvulsant drug clonazepam evaluated from single oral and intravenous doses and by repeated oral administration. *Eur. J. Clin. Pharmacol.,* 9:155–159.

21. Bielman, P., Levoc, T., and Gagnon, M. A. (1978): Clonazepam: Its efficacy in association with phenytoin and phenobarbital in mental patients with generalized major motor seizures. *Int. J. Clin. Pharmacol. Biopharm.,* 16:268–273.

22. Birket-Smith, E., Lund, M., Mikkelsen, B., Vestermark, D., Zander Olsen, P., and Holm, P. (1973): A controlled trial on Ro 5-4023 (clonazepam) in the treatment of psychomotor epilepsy. *Acta Neurol. Scand.,* 49:18–25.

23. Birket-Smith, E., and Mikkelsen, B. (1972): Preliminary observations on the effect of a new benzodiazepine (Ro 5-4023) in epilepsy. *Acta Neurol. Scand.,* 48:385–389.

24. Bittencourt, P. R. M., and Richens, A. (1981): Anticonvulsant-induced status epilepticus in Lennox-Gastaut syndrome. *Epilepsia,* 22:129–134.

25. Bittner-Manicka, M., and Wasilewski, R. (1976): Preliminary clinical evaluation of Rivotril in epilepsy. *Neurol. Neurochir. Pol.,* 26:519–525.

26. Bladin, P. F. (1973): The use of clonazepam as an anticonvulsant—Clinical evaluation. *Med. J. Aust.,* 1:683–688.

27. Boudouresques, J., Roger, J., Khalil, R., Vigouroux, R. A., Grossett, A., Pellisier, J. F., and Tassinari, C. A. (1971): A propos de deux observationes de syndrome de Lance et Adams: Effet therapeutique de Ro5-4023. *Rev. Neurol.,* 125:306–309.

28. Braestrup, C., Albrechtsen, R., and Squires, R. F. (1977): High densities of benzodiazepine receptors in human cortical areas. *Nature,* 269:702–704.

29. Braestrup, C., and Squires, R. F. (1977): Specific benzodiazepine receptors in rat brain characterized by high-affinity ^{3}H-diazepam binding. *Proc. Natl. Acad. Sci. U.S.A.,* 74:3805–3809.

30. Bressman, S., and Fahn, S. (1986): Essential myoclonus. *Adv. Neurol.,* 43:287–294.

31. Browne, R. R. (1976): Clonazepam: A review of a new anticonvulsant drug. *Arch. Neurol.,* 33:326–332.

32. Browne, T. R. (1978): Clonazepam. *N. Engl. J. Med.,* 299:812–816.

33. Browne, T. R., and Penry, J. K. (1973): Benzodiazepines in the treatment of epilepsy. *Epilepsia,* 15:277–310.

34. Bückling, P. H. (1977): Electroclinical correlations during anticonvulsive therapy of status epilepticus and chronic focal epilepsies using clo-

nazepam. *Schweiz. Arch. Neurol. Neurochir. Psychiatr.,* 121:187–205.

35. Burke, J. T., and Thenot, J. P. (1985): Review: Determination of antiepileptic drugs. *J. Chromatogr.,* 340:199–241.

36. Caccia, M. R. (1975): Clonazepam in facial neuralgia and cluster headache. *Eur. Neurol.,* 13:560–563.

37. Cano, J. P., Catalin, J., Viala, A., Roger, J., Tassinari, C. A., Dravet, C., and Gastaut, H. (1976): Determination of clonazepam ("Rivotril" or "Ro 5-4023") in plasma by gas chromatography using an internal standard. *Eur. J. Toxicol. Environ. Hyg.,* 9:213–225.

38. Cano, J. P., Guintrand, J., Aubert, C., Viala, A., and Covo, J. (1977): Determination of flunitrazepam, desmethylflunitrazepam and clonazepam in plasma by gas liquid chromatography with an internal standard. *Arzneim. Forsch.,* 27:338–342.

39. Carroll, W. M., and Walsh, P. J. (1978): Functional independence in postanoxic myoclonus: Contribution of L-5-HTP, sodium valproate and clonazepam. *Br. Med. J.,* 2:1612.

40. Carson, J., Jr., and Gilden, C. (1975): Treatment of minor motor seizures with clonazepam. *Dev. Med. Child Neurol.,* 17:306–310.

41. Caso, A., Raphael-Fernandez, G., Romo, A., Martinex, C., Garibay, E., and Padilla, J. (1973): Evaluation neuropsiquiatrica del clonazepam (Ro 5-4023) en pacientes epilepticos. *Gac. Med. Mex.,* 106:385–392.

42. Chadwick, D., and French, A. T. (1979): Uremic myoclonus: An example of reticular reflex myoclonus? *J. Neurol. Neurosurg. Psychiatry,* 42:52–55.

43. Chadwick, D., Hallett, M., Harris, R., Jenner, P., Reynolds, E. H., and Marsden, C. D. (1977): Clinical, biochemical and physiological features distinguishing myoclonus responsive to 5-hydroxytryptophan, tryptophan with a monoamine oxidase inhibitor, and clonazepam. *Brain,* 100:455–487.

44. Chandra, B. (1973): Clonazepam in the treatment of petit mal. *Asian J. Med.,* 9:433–436.

45. Chandra, B. (1976): The use of clonazepam in the treatment of tic douloureux (a preliminary report). *Proc. Aust. Assoc. Neurol.,* 13:119–122.

46. Chang, R. S. L., and Snyder, S. H. (1978): Benzodiazepine receptors: Labeling in intact animals with ^{3}H-flunitrazepam. *Eur. J. Pharmacol.,* 48:213–218.

47. Chweh, A. Y., Swinyard, E. A., and Wolf, H. H. (1985): Benzodiazepine receptors are not involved in the neurotoxicity and anti-electroshock activity of phenytoin in mice. *Neurosci. Lett.,* 24:57(3):279–82.

48. Cohen, L. S., and Rosenbaum, J. F. (1987): Clonazepam: New uses and potential problems. *J. Clin. Psychiatry,* 48 Suppl: 50–56.

49. Congdon, P. J., and Forsythe, W. I. (1980): Intravenous clonazepam in the treatment of status epilepticus in children. *Epilepsia,* 21:97–102.

50. Cooper, S. J., and Gilbert, D. B. (1985): Clonazepam-induced hyperphagia in nondeprived

rats: Tests of pharmacological specificity with Ro5-3663, Ro5-4864, Ro15-1788 and CGS 9896. *Pharmacol. Biochem. Behav.,* 22(5):753–760.

51. Court, J. E., and Kase, C. S. (1976): Treatment of tic douloureux with a new anticonvulsant (clonazepam). *J. Neurol. Neurosurg. Psychiatry,* 39:297–299.

52. Davidson, D. L., Tsukada, Y., and Barbeau, A. (1978): Ouabain induced seizures: Site of production and response to anticonvulsants. *Can. J. Neurol. Sci.,* 5:405–411.

53. De Boer, A. B., Roest-Kaiser, J., Bracht, H., and Breimer, D. D. (1978): Assay of underivated nitrazepam and clonazepam in plasma by capillary gas chromatography applied to pharmacokinetic and bioavailability studies in humans. *J. Chromatogr.,* 145:105–114.

54. de Silva, J. A. F., Bekersky, I., Puglisi, C. V., Brooks, M. A., and Weinfeld, R. E. (1976): Determination of 1,4-benzodiazepines and -diazepine-2-ones in blood by electron-capture gas-liquid chromatography. *Anal. Chem.,* 48:10–19.

55. de Silva, J. A. F., and Pulglisi, C. V. (1983): Electron capture GAS-liquid chromatography in drug analysis. In: *Drug Fate and Metabolism—Methods and Techniques,* edited by E. R. Garrett and J. L. Hirtz, pp. 245–333. Marcel Dekker, New York.

56. de Silva, J. A., Puglisi, C. V., and Munno, N. (1974): Determination of clonazepam and flunitrazepam in blood and urine by electron-capture GLC. *J. Pharm. Sci.,* 63:520–527.

57. Dixon, R., and Crews, T. (1977): An iodine-125 radioimmune assay for the determination of the anticonvulsant agent clonazepam directly in plasma. *Res. Commun. Chem. Pathol. Pharmacol.,* 18:477–486.

58. Dixon, W. R., Young, R. L., Ning, R., and Liebman, A. (1977): Radioimmunoassay of the anticonvulsant agent clonazepam. *J. Pharm. Sci.,* 66:235–237.

59. Dreifuss, E. F., Penry, J. K., Rose, S. W., Kupferberg, H. J., Dyken, P., and Sato, S. (1975): Serum clonazepam concentrations in children with absence seizures. *Neurology (Minneap.),* 23:255–258.

60. Drug and Therapeutics Bulletin (1976): Drugs for status epilepticus. *Drug Ther. Bull.,* 14:89–91.

61. Dumermuth, G., and Kovacs, E. (1973): The effect of clonazepam (Ro 5-4023) in the syndrome of infantile spasms with hypsarrhythmias and in petit mal variant or Lennox syndrome. *Acta Neurol. Scand.,* 49:26–28.

62. Eadie, M. J., Tyrer, J. H., Smith, G. A., and McKauge, L. (1977): Pharmacokinetics of drugs used for petit mal absence epilepsy. *Proc. Aust. Assoc. Neurol.,* 14:172–183.

63. Edlbrook, P. M., and De Wolff, F. A. (1978): Improved micromethod for determination of underivatized clonazepam in serum by gas chromatography. *Clin. Chem.,* 24:774–777.

64. Edwards, V. E. (1974): Side effects of clonazepam therapy. *Proc. Aust. Assoc. Neurol.,* 11:199–202.

65. Edwards, V. E., and Eadie, M. J. (1973): Clonazepam—A clinical study of its effectiveness as an anticonvulsant. *Proc. Aust. Assoc. Neurol.,* 10:61–66.

66. Eeg-Olofsson, O. (1973): Experiences with Rivotril in treatment with epilepsy—particularly minor motor epilepsy—in mentally retarded children. *Acta Neurol. Scand.,* 49:29–31.

67. Elian, M., Lund, M., and Melsen, S. (1973): The rate of dosage increase of clonazepam. *Acta Neurol. Scand.,* 49:32–35.

68. Eschenhof, E. (1973): Untersuchung uber das Schicksal des Antikonvulsivums Clonazepam in Organismus der Ratte, des Hundes und des Menschen. *Arzneim. Forsch.,* 23:390–400.

69. Fahn, S. (1978): Postanoxic action myoclonus: Improvement with valproic acid. *N. Engl. J. Med.,* 299:313–314.

70. Fariello, R., and Mutani, R. (1970): Valutazione sperimentale dell'efficacia del nuovo farmaco anticomiziale Ro 5-4023. *Riv. Neurol. Clin.,* 40:174–183.

71. Fazio, C., Manfredi, M., and Piccinelli, A. (1975): Treatment of epileptic seizures with clonazepam. *Arch. Neurol.,* 32:304–307.

72. Ferguson, J. L., and Couri, D. (1977): Electron capture gas chromatography determination of benzodiazepines and metabolites. *J. Anal. Toxicol.,* 1:171–174.

73. Fisher, J. B., Edgren, B. E., Mammel, M. C., and Coleman, M. (1985): Neonatal apnea associated with maternal clonazepam therapy: A case report: *Obstet. Gynecol.,* 66(3 Suppl):34S–35S.

74. Freinhar, J. P., and Alvarez, W. A. (1985–86): Clonazepam: A novel therapeutic adjunct. *Int. J. Psychiatry Med.,* 15(4):321–328.

75. Fukazawa, T., Tashiro, K., Hamada, T., and Kase, M. (1986): Multisystem degeneration: Drugs and square wave jerks. *Neurology,* 36(9):1230–1233.

76. Fukushima, H., Nakamura, M., and Matsumoto, T. (1977): Pharmacological studies of clonazepam and its metabolites in mice. *Oyo Yakuri,* 14:357–361.

77. Garantti, S., Mussini, E., Marcucci, F., and Gauitam, A. (1973): Metabolic studies on benzodiazepines in various animal species. In: *The Benzodiazepines,* edited by S. Garantti, E. Mussini, and L. O., Randall, pp. 75–128. Raven Press, New York.

78. Garcia, D. A., Malagon, V. J., Franco, D. J., and Ramos, P. J. (1987): Status epilepticus within the Lennox-Gastaut syndrome: Clinical characteristics and management. *Clin. Electroencephalogr.,* 18(2):89–92.

79. Garland, W. A., and Min, B. H. (1979) Determination of clonazepam in human plasma by gas chromatography—Negative ion chemical ionization mass spectrometry. *J. Chromatogr.,* 172:279–286.

80. Gastaut, H. (1970): Properiétés anti-epileptiques exceptionneles d'une benzodiazepine nouvelle le Ro 05-4023. *Vie Med.,* 51:517.

81. Gastaut, H., Courjon, J., Poire, R., and Weber,

M. (1971): Treatment of status epilepticus with a new benzodiazepine more active than diazepam. *Epilepsia,* 12:197–214.

82. Gent, J. P., Feely, M. P., and Haigh, J. R. (1985): Differences between the tolerance characteristics of two anticonvulsant benzodiazepines. *Life Sci.,* 37(9):849–856.

83. Gerna, M., and Morselli, P. L. (1976): A simple and sensitive gas chromatographic method for the determination of clonazepam in human plasma. *J. Chromatogr.,* 115:445–450.

84. Gharirian, A. M., Gauthier, S., and Wong, T. (1987): Convulsions in patients abruptly withdrawn from clonazepam while receiving neuroleptic medication. *Am. J. Psychiatry,* 144(5):686.

85. Gillman, M. A., and Sandyk, R. (1987): Clonazepam-induced Tourette syndrome in a subject with hyperexplexia. *Postgrad. Med. J.,* 63(738):311–1.

86. Goldber, M. A., and Dorman, J. D. (1976): Intention myoclonus: Successful treatment with clonazepam. *Neurology (Minneap.),* 26:24–26.

87. Gonce, M., and Barbeau, A. (1977): Seven cases of Gilles de la Tourett's syndrome: Partial relief with clonazepam: A pilot study. *Can. J. Neurol. Sci.,* 4:279–283.

88. Goulon, M., Nouaihat, F., Escourolle, R., and Zarranz-Imirizaldu, J. J. (1975): Methyl bromide poisoning. Report of 3 cases with one death. Anatomical study in one case of stupor and myoclonus with a 5 year's survey. *Rev. Neurol.,* 131:445–468.

89. Gray, R., and Folkerts, L. N. (1977): Drug fever due to clonazepam. *Drug Intell. Clin. Pharm.,* 11:367.

90. Greenblatt, D. J., Miller, L. G., and Shader, R. I. (1987): Clonazepam pharmacokinetics, brain uptake, and receptor interactions. *J. Clin. Psychiatry,* 48 Suppl:4–11.

91. Gregoriades, A. D., and Franges, E. G. (1977): Clinical observation on clonazepam in intractable epilepsy. In: *Epilepsy: The Eighth International Symposium,* edited by J. K. Penry, pp. 169–175. Raven Press, New York.

92. Groh, C., and Rosenmayr, F. W. (1973): Orale Dauertherapie mit Clonazepam (Ro 05-4023) bei Epilepsien des Kindes und Jugendalters. *Acta Neurol. Scand.,* 49:36–43.

93. Haigh, J. R., Feely, M., and Gent, J. P. (1986): Tolerance to the anticonvulsant effect of clonazepam in mice: No concurrent change in plasma concentration. *J. Pharm. Pharmacol.,* 38(12):931–934.

94. Hakkine, V. (1973): Effect of clonazepam (Ro 5-44023) on interictal EEG abnormalities. *Acta Neurol. Scand.,* 49:44.

95. Hanson, R. A., and Menkes, J. M. (1972): A new anticonvulsant in the management of minor motor seizures. *Dev. Med. Child Neurol.,* 14:3–114.

96. Hansson, O., and Tonnby, B. (1976): Serious psychological symptoms caused by clonazepam. *Lakartidningen,* 73:1209–1210.

97. Haver, V. M., Parter, W. H., Dorie, L. D., and Lea. J. R. (1986): Simplified high performance liquid chromatographic method for the determination of clonazepam and other benzodiazepine in serum. *Ther. Drug Monit.,* 8(3):352–357.

98. Herman, J. B., Rosenbaum, J. F., and Brotman, A. W. (1987): The alprazolam to clonazepam switch for the treatment of panic disorder. *J. Clin Psychopharmacol.,* 7(3):175–178.

99. Herzberg, L. (1985): Management of hemifacial spasm with clonazepam. *Neurology,* 35(11):1676–1677.

100. Hildebrandt, W. K. (1979): Concomitant use of clonazepam and valproic acid in treatment of epileptic seizures (letter). *Am. J. Hosp. Pharm.,* 36:22.

101. Hoehn, M. M., and Cherington, M. (1977): Spinal myoclonus. *Neurology (Minneap.),* 27:942–946.

102. Hollister, L. E. (1975): Dose-ranging studies of clonazepam in man. *Psychopharmacol. Commun.,* 1:89–92.

103. Hooshmand, H. (1972): Intractable seizures. Treatment with a new benzodiazepine anticonvulsant. *Arch. Neurol.,* 27:205–208.

104. Huang, C. Y., McLeod, J. G., Sampson, D., and Hensley, W. J. (1974): Clonazepam in the treatment of epilepsy. *Med. J. Aust.,* 2:5–8.

105. Hvidberg, E. F., and Sjo, O. (1975): Clinical pharmacokinetic experiences with clonazepam. In: *Clinical Pharmacology of Anti-Epileptic Drugs,* edited by H. Schneider, D. Janz, C. Gardner-Thorpe, H. Meinardi, and A. L. Sherwin, pp. 242–246. Springer-Verlag, Berlin.

106. Iinuma, K., Tamahashi, S., Otomo, H., Onuma, A., and Takamatsu, N. (1978): Immediate changes of the electroencephalograms after intravenous injection of clonazepam and their relation to its effect on clinical fits in children with minor seizures. *Tohoku J. Exp. Med.,* 125:223–231.

107. Inami, M., and Hara, T. (1977): The effects of clonazepam on the plasma diphenylhydantoin level in epileptic patients. *Electroencephalogr. Clin. Neurophysiol.,* 43:497.

108. Iivanainen, M., and Himberg, J. J. (1982): Valproate and clonazepam in the treatment of severe progressive myoclonus epilepsy, *Arch Neurol.,* 39:236.

109. Ishikawa, A., Sakuma, N., Nagashima, T., Kohsaka, and Kajii N. (1985): Clonazepam monotherapy for epilepsy in childhood. *Brain Dev.,* 7(6):610–613.

110. Iwakawa, Y., Niwa, T., and Suzuki, H. (1986): Clonazepam-induced tonic seizure. *No To Hattatsu,* 18(5):347–363.

111. Jankovic, J., and Pardo, R. (1986): Segmental myoclonus. *Arch. Neurol.,* 43(10):1025–1031.

112. Jeavons, P. (1977): Management of childhood epilepsy. *Br. Med. J.,* 1:986.

113. Jeavons, R. M., Clark, J. E., and Maheshwari, M. C. (1977): Treatment of generalized epilepsies of childhood and adolescence with sodium valproate ("Epilim"). *Dev. Med. Child Neurol.,* 19:9–25.

114. Jenner, P., Chadwick, D., Reyholds, E. H., and Marsden, C. D. (1975): Altered 5-HT metabolism

with clonazepam, diazepam and diphenylhydantoin. *J. Pharm. Pharmacol.,* 27:707–710.

115. Jenner, P., Chadwick, D., Reynolds, E. H., and Marsden, C. D. (1975): Clonazepam-induced changes in 5-hydroxytryptamine metabolism in animals and man. *J. Pharm. Pharmacol.,* 27:38P.

116. Jenner, P., Marsden, C. D., Pratt, J., and Reynolds, E. H. (1978): Altered serotoninergic activity in mouse brain induced by clonazepam. *Br. J. Pharmacol.,* 64:432.

117. Johannessen, S. I., Strandjord, R. E., and Munthe-Kaas, A. W. (1977): Lack of effort of clonazepam on serum levels of diphenylhydantoin, phenobarbital, and carbamazepine. *Acta Neurol. Scand.,* 55:506–512.

118. Jones, B. D., and Chouinard, G. (1985): Clonazepam in the treatment of recurrent symptoms of depression and anxiety in a patient with systematic lupus erythematosus. *Am. J. Psychiatry,* 142(3):354–355.

119. Julien, R. M., and Fowler, G. W. (1977): A comparative study of the efficacy of newer antiepileptic drugs on experimentally-induced febrile convulsions. *Neuropharmacology,* 16:719–724.

120. Kabra, P. M., and Nzekwe, E. U. (1985): Liquid chromatographic analysis of clonazepam in human serum with solid-phase (Bonet-Elut) extraction. *J. Chromatogr.,* 341(2):383–390.

121. Kaplan, S. A., Alexander, K., Jack, M. L., Puglisi, C. V., deSilva, J. A. F., Lee, T. L., and Weinfeld, R. E. (1974): Pharmacokinetic profiles of clonazepam in dog and humans and of flunitrazepam in dog. *J. Pharm. Sci.,* 63:527–532.

122. Karbowski, K. (1976): Der Petit-mal Status. *Schweis. Med. Wochenschr.,* 29:973–981.

123. Karobath, M., and Sperk, B. (1979): Stimulation of benzodiazepine receptor binding of gamma-aminobutyric acid. *Proc. Natl. Acad. Sci. U.S.A.,* 76:1004–1006.

124. Kato, H., and Mori, T. (1977): A clinical and electroencephalographic study on antiepileptic activity of clonazepam. Relationship between clinical effects of oral administration and electroencephalographic effects of intravenous administration. *Folia Psychiatr. Neurol. Jpn.,* 31:183–194.

125. Kato, H., Mori, T., Moriuchi, I., Yoshimura, T., and Iwata, T. (1976): Antiepileptic activity of clonazepam—An antiepileptic benzodiazepine derivative. *Brain Nerve (Tokyo),* 28:565–577.

126. Ketz, E., Bernomiti, C., and Siegfried, J. (1973): Clinical and EEG study of clonazepam (Ro 5-4023) with particular reference to status epilepticus. *Acta Neurol. Scand.,* 49:47–53.

127. Kick, H., and Dreyer, R. (1973): Klinische Erfahrungen mit Clonazepam unter besonderer Berucksightigung psychomotorische Anfalle, *Acta Neurol. Scand.,* 49:54–59.

128. King, P. H., Shin, C., Mansbach, H. H., Chen, L. S., and McNamara, J. O. (1987): Microinjection of a benzodiazepine into substantia nigra elevates kindled seizures threshold. *Brain Res.,* 423(1–2):261–268.

129. Knop, J. J., Edmunds, L. C., Blom, G. F., Bruens, J. H., Bongers, E., Meinardi, H., Meijer, J. W. A., Guelen, P. J. M., and van der Kleijn, E. (1977): Clonazepam: A clinical trial. Pharmacokinetic and clinical aspects. In: *Antiepileptic Drug Monitoring,* edited by C. Gardner-Thorpe, D. Janz, H. Meinardi, and C. E. Pippenger, pp. 226–263. Pitman Medical, Tunbridge Wells, Kent.

130. Knopp, H. J., van der Kleijn, E., and Edmunds, L. C. (1975): Pharmacokinetics of clonazepam in man and laboratory animals. In: *Clinical Pharmacology of Antiepileptic Drugs,* edited by H. Schneider, D. Janz, C. Gardner-Thorpe, H. Meinardi, and A. L. Sherwin, pp. 247–260. Springer-Verlag, Berlin.

131. Kohler, C., Clere, J., and Girtanner, B. (1975): Interet du clonazepam dans le traitement des manifestations convulsives avec encephalopathic chez l'enfant. *Rev. Neuropsychiatr. Infant,* 23:381–387.

132. Kotlarek, F., Deselares, M., and Hotes, G. (1985): How effective is the treatment schedule in children with infantile spasms? *Lin. Padiatr.,* 197(1):21–24.

133. Krue, P., and Blankenhorn, V. (1973): Zusammenfassender Erfahrungsbericht uber die klinische Anwendung und Wirksamkeit von Ro 5-4023 (Clonazepam) auf verschiedene Formen epilptischer Anfalle. *Acta Neurol. Scand.,* 49:60–71.

134. Krugers Dagneaux, P. G. L., and Klein Elhorst, J. T. (1975): Qualitative analysis of clonazepam and its metabolites in urine and plasma. *Pharm. Weekbl.,* 110:1137–1142.

135. Lai, A. A. (1978): Investigations of the pharmacokinetics of clonazepam and its interaction with carbamazepine in monkeys and humans. *Diss. Abstr. Int. B. 1978,* 39:669.

136. Lai, A. A., and Levy, R. H. (1979): Pharmacokinetic description of drug interactions by induction: Carbamazepine-clonazepam in monkeys. *J. Pharm. Sci.,* 68:416–421.

137. Lai, A., Levy, R. H., and Cutler, R. E. (1978): Time-course of interaction between carbamazepine and clonazepam in normal man. *Clin. Pharmacol. Ther.,* 24:316–323.

138. Lai, A. A., Min, B. H., Garland, W. A., and Levy, R. H. (1979): Kinetics of biotransformation of clonazepam to its 7-amino metabolite in monkey. *J. Pharmacokinet. Biopharm.,* 7:87–95.

139. Laitinen, L., and Toivakka, E. (1973): Clonazepam (Ro 5-4023) in the treatment of myoclonus epilepsy. *Acta Neurol. Scand.,* 49:72–76.

140. Lance, J. W., and Anthony, M. (1977): Sodium valproate and clonazepam in the treatment of intractable epilepsy. *Arch. Neurol.,* 34:14–17.

141. Lance, J. W., and Anthony, M. (1977): Sodium valproate and clonazepam in the treatment of intractable epilepsy. *Proc. Aust. Assoc. Neurol.,* 12:55–60.

142. Larson, A. W., Wasserstrom, W. R., Felsher, B. F., and Chih, J. C. (1978): Posttraumatic epilepsy and acute intermittent porphyria: Effects of phenytoin, carbamazepine and clonazepam. *Neurology (Minneap.),* 28:824–828.

143. Lehtovaara, R. (1973): A clinical trial with clonazepam. *Acta Neurol. Scand.*, 49:77–81.
144. Lehtovaara, R., Bardy, A., Hari, R., and Majuri, H. (1978): Sodium valproate and clonazepam interactions with phenytoin and carbamazepine. In: *Advances in Epileptology, 1977: Psychology, Pharmacotherapy, and New Diagnostic Approaches*, edited by H. Meinardi and A. J. Rowan, pp. 269–270. Swets and Zeitlinger, Amsterdam.
145. Lin, W. N. (1987): Determination of clonazepam in serum by high performance liquid chromatography. *Ther. Drug Monit.*, 9(3):337–342.
146. Livingston, J. H., and Brown, J. K. (1987): Nonconvulsive status epilepticus resistant to benzodiazepines. *Arch. Dis. Child.*, 62(1):41–44.
147. Lund, M., and Trolle, E. (1973): Clonazepam in the treatment of epilepsy. *Acta Neurol. Scand.*, 49:82–90.
148. Martin, D., and Hirt, H. R. (1973): Klinische Erfahrungen mit Clonazepam (Rivotril) in der Epilepsiebehandlung bei Kindem. *Neuropaediatrie*, 4:245–266.
149. Masland, R. L. (1975): A controlled trial of clonazepam in temporal lobe epilepsy. *Acta Neurol. Scand.*, 51:49–54.
150. Massino, L., Pasino, M., Rosanda-Vadala, C., Tonini, G. P., De Negri, M., and Saccomani, L. (1976): Immunological side effects of anticonvulsants. *Lancet*, 1:860.
151. Matthews, E. B. (1979): Treatment of the restless leg syndrome with clonazepam (letter). *Br. Med. J.*, 1:751.
152. Meldrum, B. S., Anlezrk, G., Balzamo, E., Horton, R. W., and Trimble, M. (1975): Photically induced epilepsy in *Papio papio* as a model for drug studies. *Adv. Neurol.*, 10:119–132.
153. Meldrum, B. S., and Chapman, A. G. (1986): Benzodiazepine receptors and their relationship to the treatment of epilepsy. *Epilepsia*, 27(Suppl. 1):S3–S13.
154. Merkikangas, J. R., and Reynolds, C. F. (1979): Blepharospasm: Successful treatment with clonazepam. *Ann. Neurol.*, 5:401–402.
155. Mikkelsen, B., and Birket-Smith, E. (1973): A clinical study of the benzodiazepine Ro 5-4023 (clonazepam) in the treatment of epilepsy. *Acta Neurol. Scand.*, 49:91–96.
156. Mikkelsen, B., Birket-Smith, E., Brandt, S., Holm, P., Lund, M., Thorn, I., Vestermark, S., and Zander Olsen, P. (1976): Clonazepam in the treatment of epilepsy. A controlled clinical trial in simple absences, bilateral massive epileptic myoclonus, and atonic seizures. *Arch. Neurol.*, 33:322–325.
157. Mikkelsen, B., Birket-Smith, E., Holm, P., Lund, M., Vestermark, S., and Zander Olsen, P. (1975): A controlled trial on clonazepam (Ro 5-4023, Rivotril) in the treatment of focal epilepsy and secondary generalized grand mal epilepsy. *Acta Neurol. Scand.*, 51:55–61.
158. Miller, L. G., Friedman, H., and Greenblatt, D. J. (1987): Measurement of clonazepam by electron-capture gas-liquid chromatography with application to single-dose pharmacokinetcs. *J. Anal. Toxicol.*, 11(2):55–57.
159. Min, B. H., and Garland, W. A. (1977): Determination of clonazepam and its 7-amino metabolite in plasma and blood by gas chromatographic-chemical ionization mass spectrometry. *J. Chromatogr.*, 139:121–133.
160. Min, B. H., Garland, W. A., Khoo, K., C., and Torres, G. S. (1978): Determination of clonazepam and its amino and actamido metabolites in human plasma by combined gas chromatography chemical ionization mass spectrometry and selected ion monitoring. *Biomed. Mass Spectrom.*, 5:692–698.
161. Minoli, G., and Tredici, G. (1974): Levodopa in treatment of myoclonus. *Lancet*, 2:472.
162. Mireles, R., and Leppik, I. L. (1985): Valproate and clonazepam comedication in patients with intractable epilepsy. *Epilepsia*, 26(2):122–126.
163. Moehler, H., and Okada, T. (1977): Benzodiazepine receptor: Demonstration in the central nervous system. *Science*, 198:849–851.
164. Moehler, H., Okada, T., Heitz, P., and Ulrich, J. (1978): Biochemical identification of the site of action of benzodiazepines in human brain by ^{3}H-diazepam binding. *Life Sci.*, 22:985–995.
165. Mori, T., Kato, H., Ikeda, S., and Morizaki, I. (1977): Antiepileptic activity of clonazepam: A benzodiazepine antiepileptic. II. Effects of intravenous injection of clonazepam. *Brain Nerve (Tokyo)*, 29:171–180.
166. Munthe-Kaas, A. W., and Strandjord, R. E. (1973): Clonazepam in the treatment of epileptic seizures. *Acta Neurol. Scand.*, 49:97–102.
167. Naestoft, J. J., Larsen, N. E. (1974): Quantitative determination of clonazepam and its metabolites in human plasma by gas chromatography. *J. Chromatogr.*, 93:113–122.
168. Naestoft, J., Lund, M., Larsen, N. E., and Hvidberg, E. (1973): Assay and pharmacokinetics of clonazepam in humans. *Acta Neurol. Scand.*, 49:103–108.
169. Naito, H., Wachi, M., and Nishida, M. (1987): Clinical effects and plasma concentrations of long-term clonazepam monotherapy in previously untreated epilepticus. *Acta Neurol. Scand.*, 76(1):58–63.
170. Nanda, R. N., Johnson, R. H., Keogh, H. J., Lambie, D. G., and Melville, I. D. (1977): Treatment of epilepsy with clonazepam and its effect on other anticonvulsants. *J. Neurol. Neurosurg. Psychiatry*, 40:538–543.
171. Nogen, A. B. (1978): The utility of clonazepam in epilepsy of various types. Observations with 22 childhood cases. *Clin. Pediatr.*, 17:71–74.
172. Oller-Daurella, L. (1969): Resultados obtenidos conmuevos derivados benzodiazepinicos en el tratamiento la epilepsia. *Ciencias Neurol.*, 3:3.
173. Olsen, R. W. (1982): Drug interactions at the GABA receptor-ionophore complex. *Annu. Rev. Pharmacol. Toxicol.*, 22:245–277.
174. Parry, G. G. (1977): Concentration of clonazepam in serum and cerebrospinal fluid of the sheep. *Pharmacology*, 15:318–323.

175. Parry, G. G., and Ferry, D. B. (1976): Rapid gas chromatographic method for the determination of clonazepam in serum and cerebrospinal fluid. *J. Chromatogr.,* 128:166–168.

176. Peiris, J. B., Boralessa, H., and Lionel, N. D. W. (1976): Clonazepam in the treatment of choreiform activity. *Med. J. Aust.,* 1:225–227.

177. Peled, R., and Lavie, P. (1986): Paroxysmal awakenings from sleep associated with excessive daytime somnolence: A form of nocturnal epilepsy. *Neurology,* 36(1):95–98.

178. Perchalski, R. J., and Wildre, B. J. (1978): Determination of benzodiazepine anticonvulsants in plasma by high performance liquid chromatography. *Anal. Chem.,* 59:554–557.

179. Pinder, R. M., Brogden, R. N., Speight, T. M., and Avery, G. S. (1976): Clonazepam: A review of its pharmacological properties and therapeutic efficacy in epilepsy. *Drugs,* 12:321–361.

180. Pinder, R. M., Brogden, R. N., Speight, T. M., and Avery, G. S. (1977): Clonazepam (Rivotril-Roche): An independent report. *Curr. Ther. Res.,* 18:25–32.

181. Pollack, M. H., Rosenbau, J. F., Tesar, G. E., Herman, J. B., and Sachs, G. S. (1987): Clonazepam in the treatment of panic disorder and agoraphobia. *Psychopharmacol. Bull.,* 23(1): 141–144.

182. Prior, P. E., MacLaine, G. N., Scott, D. F., and Laurance, B. M. (1972): Tonic status epilepticus precipitated by intravenous diazepam in a child with petit mal status. *Epilepsia,* 13:467–472.

183. Rail, L. R. (1973): The treatment of self-induced photic epilepsy. *Proc. Aust. Assoc. Neurol.,* 9:121–123.

184. Rall, T. W., and Schleifer, L. S. (1985): Drugs effective in the therapy of the epilepsies. In: *The Pharmacological Basis of Therapeutics,* 7th edition, edited by A. G. Gilman, L. S. Goodman, T. W. Rall, and F. Murad, pp. 446–472. Macmillan, New York.

185. Rett, A. (1973): Zwei Jahre Erfahrungen mit Clonazepam bei zerebralen Krampfanfallen im Kindesalter. *Acta Neurol. Scand.,* 49:109–116.

186. Rosenmayr, F. W., and Groh, C. (1973): Wirkung von Clonazepam auf das EEG von Kindern und Jugendlichen. *Acta Neurol. Scand.,* 49:117–123.

187. Roussounis, S. H., and Rudolf, N. M. (1977): A long term electroclinical study of clonazepam in children with intractable seizures. *Electroencephalogr. Clin. Neurophysiol.,* 43:528–529.

188. Roussounis, S. H., and Rudolf, N. (1977): Clonazepam in the treatment of children with intractable seizures. *Dev. Med. Child Neurol.,* 19:326–334.

189. Rylance, G. W., Poulton, J., Cherry, R. C., and Cullen, R. E. (1986): Plasma concentrations of clonazepam after single rectal administration. *Arch. Dis. Child.,* 61(2):186–188.

190. Saavedra, I. N., Aquilera, L. I., Faure, E., and Galdames, D. G. (1985): Phenytoin/clonazepam interaction. *Ther. Drug Monit.,* 7(4)481–484.

191. Sato, S., Penry, J. K., Dreifuss, F. E., and Dyken, P. R. (1977): Clonazepam in the treatment of absence seizures. *Neurology (Minneap.),* 27:371.

192. Scherkl, R., and Frey, H. H. (1986): Physical dependence on clonazepam in dogs. *Pharmacology,* 32(1):18–24.

193. Scherkl, R., Scheuler, W., and Frey, H. H. (1985): Anticonvulsant effect of clonazepam in the dog: Development of tolerance and physical dependence. *Arch. Int. Pharmacodyn. Ther.,* 278(2):249–260.

194. Scollo-Lavizzari, G., Pralle, W., and dela Cruz, N. (1974): Clinical experience with clonazepam (Rivotril) in the treatment of epilepsy in adults. *Eur. Neurol.,* 11:340–344.

195. Sedman, G. (1976): Clonazepam in treatment of tardive oral dyskinesia. *Br. Med. J.,* 2:583.

196. Shakir, R., Nanda, R. N., Lambie, D. G., and Johnson, R. H. (1979): Comparative trial of valproate and clonazepam in chronic epilepsy. *Arch. Neurol.,* 36:301–304.

197. Sher, P. K. (1985): Alternate-day clonazepam treatment of intractable seizures. *Arch. Neurol.,* 42(8):787–788.

198. Sher, P. K. (1986): Long-term exposure of cortical cell cultures to clonazepam reduces benzodiazepine receptor binding. *Exp. Neurol.,* 92(2):360–368.

199. Sher, P. K., Neale, E. A., and Machen, V. L. (1986): Autoradiographic localization of benzodiazepine receptor binding in dissociated cultures of fetal mouse cerebral cortex. *J. Neurochem.,* 46(3):899–904.

200. Sjo, O., Hvidber, E. F., Naestoft, J., and Lund, M. (1975): Pharmacokinetics and side effects of clonazepam and its 7-amino-metabolite in man. *Eur. J. Clin. Pharmacol.,* 8:249–254.

201. Smith, D., and Gallager, D. (1987): GABA, benzodiazepine and serotonergic receptor development in the dorsal raphe nucleus: Electrophysiological studies. *Brain Res.,* 432(2):191–198.

202. Snead, O. C., III. (1978): Gamma hydroxybutyrate in the monkey. III. Effect of intravenous drugs. *Neurology (Minneap.),* 28:1173–1178.

203. Solow, E. B., and Kenfield, C. D. (1977): A micromethod for the determination of clonazepam in serum by electron-capture gas-liquid chromatography. *J. Anal. Toxicol.,* 1:155–157.

204. Sommerbeck, K. W., Theilgaard, A., and Rasmussen, K. E. (1977): Valproate sodium: Evaluation of so called psychotropic effect. A controlled study. *Epilepsia,* 18:159–167.

205. Speth, R. C., Wastek, G. J., Johnson, P. G., and Yamamura, H. I. (1978): Benzodiazepine binding in human brain: Characterization using ³H-flunitrazepam. *Life Sci.,* 22:859–866.

206. Sternback, L. H. (1973): Chemistry of 1,4-benzodiazepines and some aspects of the structure-activity relationship. In: *The Benzodiazepines,* edited by S. Garattini, E. Mussini, and L. O. Randall, pp. 1–26. Raven Press, New York.

207. Swinyard, E. A., and Castellion, A. W. (1966): Anticonvulsant properties of some benzodiazepines. *J. Pharmacol. Exp. Ther.,* 151:369–375.

208. Tassinari, C. A., Daniele, O., Michelucci, R., Bu-

reau, M., Dravet, C., and Roger, J. (1983): Benzodiazepines: Efficacy in status epilepticus. In: *Advances in Neurology, vol. 34: Status Epilepticus,* edited by A. V. Delgado-Escueta, C. G. Wasterlain, D. M. Treiman, and R. J. Porter, pp. 465–475. Raven Press, New York.

209. Tassinari, C. A., Dravet, C., Roger, J., Cano, J. P., and Gastaut, H. (1972): Tonic status epilepticus precipitated by intravenous benzodiazepine in five patients with Lennox-Gastaut syndrome. *Epilepsia,* 13:421–435.

210. Tesar, G. E., and Rosenbaum, J. F. (1986): Successful use of clonazepam in patients with treatment-resistant panic disorder. *J. Nerv. Ment. Dis.,* 174(8):477–482.

211. Tewari, S. N., and Shukla, S. K. (1977): Separation and indentification of 1,4-benzodiazepine drugs present in the biological fluids by two dimensional TLC. *Pharmazie,* 32:536.

212. Toyonaga, K., and Tokuda, D. (1976): Physiological examination and treatment by clonazepam of action myoclonus due to methyl bromide intoxication. *Clin. Neurol. (Tokyo),* 16:830–831.

213. Trimble, M. R. (1986): Recent contributions of benzodiazepines to the management of epilepsy. *Epilepsia,* 27 (Suppl 1.):S1–S52.

214. Tsuchiya, T., Fukushima, H., and Kitagawa, S. (1976): Effects of benzodiazepines on penicillin-induced epileptic discharges. *Nippon Acta Radiol.,* 72:861–877.

215. Turner, M., Cordero Funes, J. R., Aspinwall, R., Cantlon, B., Fejerman, N., and Lon, J. C. (1970): Ensayo de valoracion clinicoelectroen—Cefalographica de un nuevo derivado benzodiazepinico (Ro 05-4023) por administracion oral en pacientes epilepticos con tecnica de doble ceguera. *Acta Neurol. Lat. Am.,* 16:158–163.

216. Uges, D. R. A., and Bouma, P. (1978): An improved determination of clonazepam in serum by HPLC. *Pharm. Weekbl.,* 113:1156–1158.

217. Vajda, F. J., Lewis, S. J., Harris, Q. L., Jarrott, B., and Yound, N. A. (1987): Tolerance to the anticonvulsant effects of clonazepam and clobazam in the amygdaloid kindled rat. *Clin. Exp. Neurol.,* 23:155–164.

218. van der Kleijn, E., Baars, A. M., Vree, T. B., and van der Dries. A. (1983): Clinical pharmacokinetics of drugs used in the treatment of status epilepticus. In: *Status Epilepticus, Advances in Neurology, vol. 34,* edited by A. V. Delgado-Escueta, C. G. Wasterlain, D. M. Treiman, and R. J. Porter, pp. 421–440. Raven Press, New York.

219. Van Huffelen, A. C., and Magnus, O. (1976): The treatment of status epilepticus with clonazepam. *Ned. Tijdschr. Geneeskd.,* 120:1734–1738.

220. Vassella, F., Pavlincova, E., Schneider, H. J., Rudin, H. J., and Karbowski, K. (1973): Treatment of infantile spasms and Lennox-Gastaut syndrome with clonazepam. *Epilepsia,* 14:165–175.

221. Veall, R. M., and Hogarth, H. C. (1975): Thrombocytopenia during treatment with clonazepam. *Br. Med. J.,* 4:462.

222. Wad, N. (1986): Degradation of clonazepam in serum by light confirmed by means of a high performance liquid chromatographic method. *Ther. Drug Monit.,* 8(3):358–360.

223. Wad, N. T., and Hanfli, E. J. (1977): Simplified thin layer chromatographic method for the simultaneous determination of clonazepam, diazepam and their metabolites in serum. *J. Chromatogr.,* 143:214–218.

224. Watson, W. A. (1979): Interaction between clonazepam and sodium valproate. *N. Engl. J. Med.,* 300:678–679.

225. Wauquier, A., Ashton, D., and Melis, W. (1979): Behavioral analysis of amygdaloid kindling in beagle dogs and effects of clonazepam, diazepam, phenobarbital, diphenylhydantoin, and flunarizine on seizure manifestation. *Exp. Neurol.,* 64:579–586.

226. Weiner, W. J., Goetz, C., Nausieda, P. A., and Klawans, H. L. (1977): Clonazepam and dopamine-related stereotyped behavior. *Life Sci.,* 21:901–905.

227. Weiner, W. J., Goetz, C., Nausieda, P. A., and Kalwans, H. L. (1977): Clonazepam and 5-hydroxytryptophan-induced myoclonic stereotypy. *Eur. J. Pharmacol.,* 46:21–24.

228. Weinmann, H. M., and Willms, E. (1973): Kurzer Erfahrungsbericht uber die Wirksamkeit des antikonvulsivums Ro 5-4023 (Clonazepam) auf verschiedene Epilepsieforme. *Acta Neurol. Scand.,* 49:124–132.

229. Welch, T. E., Rumack, B. H., and Hammond, K. (1977): Clonazepam overdose resulting in cyclic coma. *Clin. Toxicol.,* 10:433–436.

230. Westblom, U. (1977): Stiff man syndrome and clonazepam. *J.A.M.A.,* 237:1930.

231. Windorfer, A., Jr., and Sauer, W. (1977): Drug interactions during anticonvulsant therapy in childhood: Diphenylhydantoin, primidone, phenobarbitone, clonazepam, nitrazepam, carbamazepine and dipropylacetate. *Neuropaediatrie,* 8:29–41.

232. Yajima, T., Uritani, K., Aoki, R., Suzuki, T., and Nakamura, K. (1976): Anticonvulsant activity of clonazepam in experimental animals. *Nippon Acta Radiol.,* 72:763–794.

233. Yamauchi, T., Hirabayashi, Y., and Kataoka, N. (1978): A clinical study of clonazepam in the treatment of epilepsy. *Brain Nerve (Tokyo),* 30:107–116.

234. Young, A., Zukin, S. R., and Syder, S. H. (1974): Interaction of benzodiazepines with central nervous glycine receptors: Possible mechanism of action. *Proc. Natl. Acad. Sci. U.S.A.,* 71:2246–2250.

235. Zill, M. A., and Nisi, G. (1986): Simple and sensitive method for the determination of clobazam, clonazepam and nitrazepam in human serum by high performance liquid chromatography. *J. Chromatogr.,* 378(2):492–497.

Antiepileptic Drugs, Third Edition, edited by
R. Levy, R. Mattson, B. Meldrum,
J. K. Penry, and F. E. Dreifuss.
Raven Press, Ltd., New York © 1989.

57

Benzodiazepines

Nitrazepam

Agostino Baruzzi, Roberto Michelucci, and Carlo Alberto Tassinari

Nitrazepam (1,3-dihydro-7-nitro-5-phenyl-2H-1,4-benzodiazepine-2-one) is a benzodiazepine derivative synthesized by Sternbach et al. (144). It is mainly used as a sleep-inducing agent but, in some countries, it is also utilized in the treatment of selected forms of epilepsy.

CHEMISTRY AND METHODS OF DETERMINATION

Chemistry

Nitrazepam is a yellow, odorless, tasteless crystalline powder with a melting point of 226° to 229°C and a molecular weight of 281.3. The structural formula is shown in Fig. 1. Nitrazepam shows pK_a values of 3.2 and 10.8; the drug is practically insoluble in water but soluble in chloroform, ethanol, ether, and diluted inorganic acids.

The most important structure-activity relationship for the 1,4-benzodiazepines involves the character of the substituent at position 7 in the *a* ring. Electron withdrawing substituents generally increase the activity, with Cl, as in diazepam, imparting broad anticonvulsant efficacy, and NO_2, as in nitrazepam, being more selective for antipentylenetetrazol activity (149).

Methods of Determination

The quantitative determination of nitrazepam in biological fluids can be performed with various methods. Gas-liquid chromatographic (GLC), spectrophotometric, thin-layer chromatographic (TLC), and ^{14}C-labeling techniques developed before 1973 were reviewed by Browne and Penry (17). The TLC and photometric methods were not sufficiently specific or sensitive for clinical monitoring or pharmacokinetic studies, and the ^{14}C-labeling method is not applicable to the detection of plasma nitrazepam concentrations after administration of commercial nitrazepam preparations.

Since 1973, fluorometric, radioimmunoassay, radioreceptor, TLC, GLC, and high-pressure liquid chromatographic (HPLC) techniques have been developed. The fluorometric technique is able to detect nitrazepam and the sum of 7-amino and 7-acetamido metabolites at plasma concentrations over 10 ng/ml after selective extractions of the compounds (129,130). The radioimmunoassay has a sensitivity limit of 4 ng/ml of nitrazepam using 10 μl of plasma. Because of its rapidity and simplicity, it is suitable for clinical monitoring in epileptic patients and for pharmacokinetics and bioavailability studies that require small-volume samples; the limit is represented by

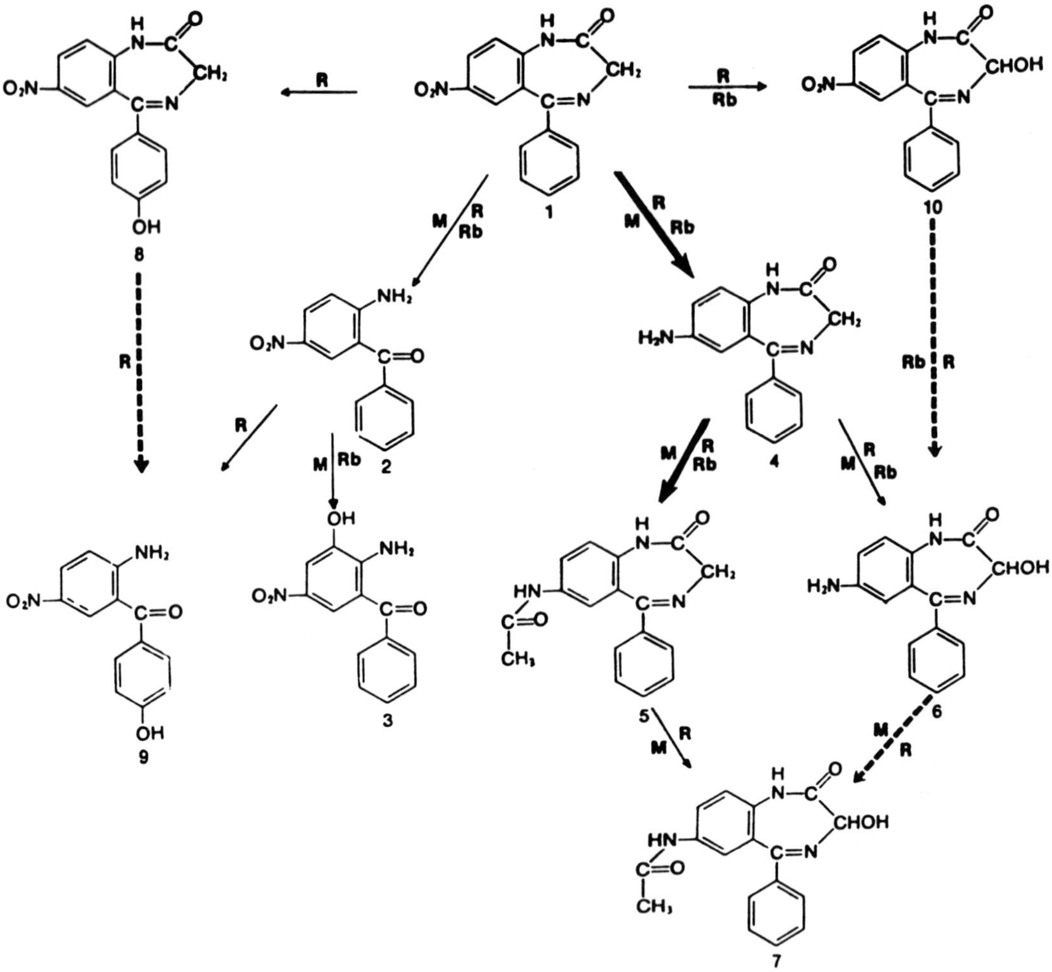

FIG. 1. Proposed metabolic pathways of nitrazepam in man, rat, and rabbit (131,135,162). **1,** nitrazepam; **2,** 2-amino-5-nitrobenzophenone; **3,** 2-amino-3-hydroxy-5-nitrobenzophenone; **4,** 7-aminonitrazepam; **5,** 7-acetamidonitrazepam; **6,** 3-hydroxy-7-aminonitrazepam; **7,** 3-hydroxy-7-acetamidonitrazepam; **8,** 4'-hydroxynitrazepam; **9,** 2-amino-4'-hydroxy-5-nitrobenzophenone; **10,** 3-hydroxynitrazepam; **M,** takes place in man; **R,** takes place in rat; **Rb,** takes place in rabbit. Major metabolic steps are indicated by thick arrows; dashed arrows represent uncertain pathways.

a crossreactivity with some other benzodiazepines (29).

The high affinity that benzodiazepines show for the receptor and the specificity of binding have been utilized for radioreceptor assays (57,63). The inability of radioreceptor assays to differentiate between nitrazepam and other benzodiazepines or benzodiazepine metabolites is a major limitation to the use of these methods in a clinical setting.

Thin-layer chromatography with direct densitometry has been used to determine concentration of nitrazepam and its metabolites in urine with a sensitivity limit (10 ng/ml) suitable for clinical purposes (59).

Gas-liquid chromatography is one of the most widely used procedures. Nitrazepam can be measured with good sensitivity by a direct method (27,69,70,94) or after acid hydrolysis (69,111) utilizing electron capture detectors (ECD); after derivatization (methyl derivative), it has been measured either by ECD or nitrogen-selective detectors (9,28,31).

In the clinical monitoring of nitrazepam in plasma, the direct method is preferred because it is fairly rapid and simple, even though it requires thorough inactivation of the column. The acid hydrolysis and derivatization techniques require more complex extraction and purification procedures (69).

The GLC methods described, which differ in their internal standards and stationary phases, have a sensitivity of 0.2 to 5 ng/ml of plasma and require 0.5 to 1 ml of plasma.

In the main metabolic step nitrazepam loses the electrophilic 7-nitro group, yielding compounds not detectable using an ECD. The 7-amino and 7-acetamido metabolites, however, can be measured in the urine, with a detection limit of 50 ng/ml, utilizing a nitrogen-selective detector (70).

Determination of nitrazepam concentrations in biological fluids in also possible by HPLC. In 1977, Moore et al. (114) analyzed nitrazepam and metabolites in urine by using an anion exchange column and ultraviolet detection. More recently HPLC has been successfully applied to the determination of plasma (serum) concentrations of nitrazepam (54,163) or nitrazepam and metabolites (81,151). These procedures differ in the chromatographic conditions and columns used and in the ability to separate nitrazepam from other benzodiazepines or co-administered drugs. They require 0.5 to 1.0 ml of sample and attain sensitivity limits comparable to those of GLC methods.

A further HPLC procedure for the analysis of nitrazepam and metabolites in urine has also been published (86).

ABSORPTION, DISTRIBUTION, AND EXCRETION

Absorption

After a single oral dose of 5 or 10 mg of nitrazepam, mean peak plasma concentrations of 35 to 47 ng/ml and 83 to 84 ng/ml, respectively, were found in different studies, mostly in young, healthy volunteers (15,16,27,54,55,72,73,75,79,111,131). In some recent studies, relatively higher peak concentrations were found: 65 to 85 ng/ml after 5 mg (62,65) and 119 to 164 ng/ml after 10 mg (1,42). In elderly patients suffering from various debilitating diseases, a mean peak plasma concentration of 22 ng/ml was observed after a single oral dose of 5 mg of nitrazepam (75); in healthy elderly subjects, however, peak concentrations were similar to those in young controls (42,55). Two studies (42,65) reported a slightly lower mean peak concentration in healthy women as compared to men.

Generally, peak absorption after oral administration occurred within 1 hr, but in some cases relatively slow absorption (as much as 4 hr) was reported (1,16,27,42, 55,62,65). When administered rectally as a solution, nitrazepam is absorbed faster than orally (median peak time 18 versus 38 min) with similar peak concentrations (62).

The absolute oral bioavailability of this drug was determined in six healthy adult volunteers who first received an i.v. injection of 10 mg of nitrazepam and, 2 weeks later, an equal oral dose of a brand preparation (131). Despite considerable interindividual variation, ranging from 53% to 94% of the dose, an average of 78% of the unchanged drug was absorbed. In a subsequent study (62), bioavailability after oral and rectal administration was determined in seven healthy volunteers. Oral bioavailability was complete; when nitrazepam was given rectally as a solution, the availability was 20% lower. The rate and degree of rectal absorption appeared to be markedly influenced by the solvent composition.

A few studies have compared the relative bioavailability of different oral preparations. Moller Jensen (111) observed identical serum curves for two brands of nitrazepam, and De Boer et al. (27) showed evidence of significant differences with respect to peak level times. The wide variability in mean peak concentrations observed in different studies is a further indication that some biopharmaceutical difference among the various preparations may exist.

Distribution

The disposition of nitrazepam may be described in terms of a two-compartment open model. In fact, a biexponential decline of the plasma concentration is observed either after i.v. administration or after the peak concentration for oral administration has been reached. The initial rapid decrease of plasma nitrazepam concentration is determined by a short distribution half-life ($T\frac{1}{2}_\alpha$ about 17 min) (62); in some cases the slow absorption and the presence of a second peak concentration at 4 to 8 hr may produce an estimate of larger values for $T\frac{1}{2}_\alpha$ (about 2 hr) (16,73). The subsequent slower decrease, mainly reflecting the elimination of the drug, is consistent with the apparent elimination half-life ($T\frac{1}{2}_\beta$).

The second small increase in plasma concentration observed between 4 and 8 hr after nitrazepam administration appears to be related to food intake (16,27,62). This latter hypothesis could not be confirmed by Kangas et al. (73) who failed to find a second peak concentration in serum following oral administration, but most of his patients had not eaten or had taken only a small amount of food.

The mean apparent volume of distribution in healthy volunteers, calculated during the β elimination phase after i.v. adminis-

tration was about 2.0 liter/kg (62,130). After oral administration, Kangas et al. (75) reported mean volumes of distribution (calculated on the assumption that bioavailability was complete) of 2.4 ± 0.8 and 4.8 ± 1.7 liter/kg, respectively, in groups of 25 young volunteers and of 12 old patients; total clearance was not significantly different in the two groups (68 ± 33 and 78 ± 25 ml/min). The authors suggested that at steady state a greater amount of the administered dose will be present in aged subjects at receptor sites in the central nervous system (CNS) and that the increased sensitivity to nitrazepam in the elderly could possibly result from the increased volume of distribution. In healthy elderly subjects, however, the difference in volume of distribution was less important, though statistically significant: 1.96 (elderly) versus 1.63 liter/kg (young) after oral administration (42), and 2.93 versus 1.93 liter/kg after i.v. administration (64). In this latter study the total nitrazepam clearance was the same in young and elderly subjects, leading the authors to conclude that after a single dose, nitrazepam action may be more persistent in the elderly, whereas similar steady-state levels should be expected during long-term administration in young and old subjects.

The effect of gender on nitrazepam distribution has been examined by Jochemsen et al. (65) who found no difference in volume of distribution and plasma binding between males and females, and by Greenblatt et al. (42) who found a larger volume of distribution in women (an average of 2.56 versus 1.82 liter/kg).

In obese subjects (weighing 121% to 234% of their ideal body weight), volume of distribution (in liter/kg) was only slightly increased as compared to normal controls (mean 2.62 versus 2.27) (1).

Generally, a good correlation between volume of distribution and elimination half-life was observed in all groups studied. The differences observed in volume of distribution related to sex, age, and weight seem to be dependent on the relative proportion of body adipose tissue.

The percentage of the non-protein-bound fraction of nitrazepam at different concentrations has been shown *in vitro* to range from 13.2% to 14.2% (131). Similar findings of 11% to 14% in healthy volunteers (62,65,73), of 9.6% to 15.6% (mean 11.9 ± 2.1%) in 10 women at the end of pregnancy, and of 8.6% to 14.1% (mean 12.0 ± 1.8%) in their 10 newborns (76) were reported. Somewhat higher figures (18–19%) were found by Greenblatt et al. (42). Healthy elderly subjects show the same unbound fraction as young subjects (42,64).

The effect of diseased states on nitrazepam distribution was examined in cirrhotic patients, who showed an increased unbound fraction (18.9% versus 13.8% in controls) but a similar volume of distribution (64).

The high protein binding and the liposolubility of nitrazepam are responsible for the fact that the drug distributes with only a small fraction in liquid body compartments. After i.p. administration of [^{14}C]nitrazepam (40 mg/kg) to "young" and "old" rats, the tissue distribution of radioactivity was found to be higher in kidney and liver, followed by spleen, heart, and lung, than in plasma between 2 and 6 hr after injection (52). The brain-to-plasma ratio was consistently lower in "young" rats than in "old" rats, suggesting a different distribution pattern (52). After i.v. injection of [^{14}C]nitrazepam (5 mg/kg) in rats, a brain-to-plasma concentration ratio of 0.60 was observed between 15 and 30 min after administration (152). After a 5-mg single oral dose in 38 patients with neurological disorders, the percentage ratio between the mean cerebrospinal fluid (CSF) and plasma concentrations increased from 8% at 2 hr to 15.6% at 36 hr (78). Although it was suggested that the CSF concentration can reflect the non-protein-bound fraction in plasma, the time dependence of the CSF-to-plasma ratio indicates that factors other than simple protein binding determine equilibrium of nitrazepam between CSF and plasma. Moreover, these observations suggest a slow equilibration of nitrazepam between plasma and the CSF (78).

A similar time-dependent ratio between saliva and serum concentration was observed (73). Nitrazepam concentration in saliva does not reflect the free plasma concentration (51,73).

Transfer of nitrazepam across the human placenta has been documented both at the beginning of the second trimester and during the last weeks of pregnancy (76). In early pregnancy, the concentration of nitrazepam in umbilical circulation and amniotic fluid was significantly lower than that in maternal plasma (76), but in late pregnancy an equilibrium between fetal and maternal tissues was observed (76,131). Nitrazepam is poorly excreted in the milk of lactating mothers (131); in a few cases, however, the amount of drug was apparently sufficient to produce side effects in the feeding infants (141).

Excretion

Total nitrazepam clearance determined in healthy young volunteers (males and females) was about 1.0 ml/kg/min (42,62,130). When free plasma concentrations were considered, mean unbound clearance (intrinsic clearance) was about 6 to 7 ml/kg/min (42,62). Age seems to have little or no effect on nitrazepam total or unbound clearance: values found in healthy elderly subjects were comparable to those of controls (42,64,75). Clearance values were similar in men and women of similar age (42,65). In cirrhotic patients unbound clearance is reduced (64), but due to increased unbound plasma fraction, total plasma clearance is unaltered. A case report (82) suggests that elimination of nitrazepam might be significantly impaired in hypothyroidism.

In young healthy volunteers the $T\frac{1}{2}_\beta$ of

nitrazepam ranged from 24 to 31 hr after a single oral dose (1,16,27,62,64,65,73,75, 79,111,131) and from 18 to 31 hr after i.v. administration (62,64,131). When elimination was examined separately in males and females some conflicting results were obtained: Jochemsen et al. (65) observed no difference in $T\frac{1}{2}_\beta$ in young men and women (average of 27.3 versus 28.6 hr, respectively), whereas Greenblatt et al. (42) found larger values for women in the young groups (27 hr in women versus 20 hr in men) but not in older subjects (26 versus 28 hr). In a group of 12 geriatric patients (66–89 years old) affected by various disabling diseases and on multidrug therapy, a $T\frac{1}{2}_\beta$ of 40.4 ± 16.2 hr was reported (75). Similarly prolonged $T\frac{1}{2}_\beta$ was found in healthy elderly subjects by Jochemsen et al. (64) (38 hr versus 26 hr in young controls) and Greenblatt et al. (42) (28 hr versus 20 hr in young controls). Considering that no differences in total or unbound nitrazepam clearance was observed between young and elderly subjects, the increase in $T\frac{1}{2}_\beta$ was ascribed to the larger volume of distribution. Elimination half-life was also prolonged in obese subjects as a consequence of the increased volume of distribution (1).

At the end of 2 weeks of continuous nitrazepam treatment in a group of 11 young volunteers and 2 months in a group of 10 old patients, apparent plasma half-lives were 24.2 ± 4.9 and 39.6 ± 13.8 hr, respectively (75). There was no significant change in the elimination half-life of the drug after 24 days of treatment in four healthy subjects (131). In subjects who ingested large amounts of the drug (75–200 mg), the half-life was similar to that found after therapeutic doses (range, 21–35 hr) (74).

The present findings suggest that the elimination of nitrazepam is independent of the dose and route of administration. The unchanged half-life of nitrazepam in the single-dose and long-term studies in both young and old subjects suggests that nitrazepam does not induce its own metabolism. According to published results, the disposition of nitrazepam appears to be modified by age only through changes in body composition (with consequent modification of volume of distribution) or as a consequence of concomitant diseases.

Routes of Excretion

Nitrazepam and its metabolites are mainly excreted in the urine in humans. In six healthy adults, following a single oral administration of 5 mg of nitrazepam labeled with ^{14}C, urinary excretion 144 hr after dosage varied from 45% to 65% of the total radioactivity introduced with the dose (131). In another subject who had received a single oral dose of 10 mg of ^{14}C-labeled nitrazepam and, 3 months later, an equal dose of the same preparation by i.v. injection, the total renal excretion determined during the first 120 hr was 71% and 93%, respectively (131). It was suggested that the lower percentage after oral administration can be explained by incomplete absorption.

Similar results were obtained in 15 healthy volunteers after a single 5-mg tablet of nitrazepam. The mean total 7-day excretion of nitrazepam and its main metabolites in the urine was approximately 50% of the administered dose (71), with a large interindividual variation. With regard to the proportions of the various excretion products appearing in the urine, it was found that unchanged nitrazepam is excreted in small amounts via the kidneys (1%), whereas its main metabolites (7-acetamido- and 7-amino nitrazepam) are excreted to a larger extent (21% and 31%, respectively, as the sum of free and conjugated metabolites) (71).

Fecal excretion of nitrazepam was studied in four healthy adults following the oral or i.v. administration of a 30-mg dose of [2-^{14}C]nitrazepam. At 144 hr after administration, the cumulative fecal excretion of nitrazepam or its metabolites varied from 8% to 13% of the dose when the drug was injected intravenously and 14% to 20% when it was given orally (131).

The rest of the dose, not accounted for by urinary and fecal excretion, may be bound to tissues or to deep compartments from where it is very slowly eliminated, or it may be excreted as metabolites not measurable by available methods (e.g., 3-hydroxynitrazepam, benzophenones [71]).

The possibility of biliary excretion of nitrazepam has been mentioned (71).

Some species variations do exist in the excretory route of most of the benzodiazepines. In rats, fecal excretion is the major route of elimination of nitrazepam, and an enterohepatic cycling of the biliary metabolites of nitrazepam has been established following [^{14}C]nitrazepam intravenous injection (152).

BIOTRANSFORMATION

Rieder and Wendt (131) reviewed the metabolism of nitrazepam in humans and rats in 1973. Since then, not much additional information has been obtained. The main line of metabolism begins with the reduction of the nitro group to the corresponding amine (7-aminonitrazepam); this latter compound is then acetylated to the 7-acetamido derivative (see Fig. 1). A small proportion of these two metabolites is then hydroxylated in position 3, yielding the 3-OH derivatives. Intestinal microflora and/or intestinal tissue enzymes as well as hepatic enzymes play an important role in the first of these metabolic steps (nitroreduction) (53), whereas the acetylation and hydroxylation are performed in the liver (6,7,80). Nitroreduction may involve formation of free radicals and superoxide (132). It has been found that the acetylation of 7-aminonitrazepam is achieved by genetically controlled polymorphic acetylation (33,80), but generally there is no evidence that acetylation phenotype may be important in connection with nitrazepam therapy (96).

A secondary line of metabolism involves the formation of benzophenones: 2-amino-5-nitrobenzophenone and relative hydroxylated compounds (2-amino-3-hydroxy-5-nitrobenzophenone in human and 2-amino-4'-hydroxy-5-nitrobenzophenone in rats) (131). There are significant species differences in biotransformation. Sawada and Hara (135) have shown that 2-amino-3-hydroxy-5-nitrobenzophenone was the major metabolite excreted, mainly in the conjugated form, in the urine of rabbits fed nitrazepam. Additional pathways of nitrazepam metabolism in rats, consisting of 3-hydroxylation and 4'-hydroxylation, have also been described (38,131,162).

INTERACTION WITH OTHER DRUGS

Nitrazepam is probably ineffective in altering the rate of metabolism of concomitantly administered drugs. Stevenson (145) and Stevenson et al. (146) observed no significant change in plasma test drug (antipyrine and phenylbutazone) half-lives or in the urinary output of 6β-hydroxycortisol after nitrazepam treatment. Consistent with these results, nitrazepam does not influence the plasma levels and effects of warfarin (121), phenprocoumon (10), or tricyclic antidepressants (113,138) in humans. Nevertheless, a possible interference of nitrazepam with the anticoagulant effects of phenprocoumon was shown in rats (85), and Ballinger et al. (4) observed a mild and insignificant influence of nitrazepam on plasma imipramine levels in humans.

Adverse drug interaction due to slow acetylation was reported in a patient who had taken phenelzine for 12 years and developed typical symptoms of monoamine oxidase inhibitor toxicity when he took nitrazepam (50).

Benzodiazepines are known to potentiate the action of CNS depressant drugs but specific data for nitrazepam are scarce. In mice, i.p. nitrazepam increases the duration of pentobarbital sodium-induced sleeping times (21). Taberner et al. (150), however, demonstrated that ethanol, at doses corresponding to moderate social drinking, do not potentiate or prolong the depressant effects of nitrazepam and temazepam.

Interaction of clinical significance between nitrazepam and other antiepileptic drugs has not been reported in the literature. Only Jeavons (61) has reported a potentiation of nitrazepam effects induced by sodium valproate.

Oral contraceptive steroids and cimetidine have been shown to reduce nitrazepam clearance (65,118); the clinical implications of these interactions, however, are not established.

RELATION OF PLASMA CONCENTRATION TO CLINICAL EFFECTS

Kangas et al. (75) studied plasma nitrazepam levels in a group of 44 children affected by different types of epilepsy. All subjects were on long-term treatment at a daily oral dose of 280 ± 110 μg/kg. Blood samples were taken 8 to 14 hr after the pre-ceding dose. In 95% of the plasma samples studied, the concentrations of nitrazepam were between 40 and 180 ng/ml (mean, 114 ng/ml); a significant correlation was found between the daily dose and the plasma concentration (Fig. 2). Most children had a successful clinical response, but because all of the patients were on combined anticonvulsant therapy, no desirable "therapeutic" plasma drug level could be defined. However, the authors suggested an upper "therapeutic" level of about 200 to 220 ng/ml, because when higher plasma concentrations were reached, toxic effects (e.g., sedation) developed (Fig. 3).

Kangas et al. (77) observed in 61 patients receiving a single oral 5-mg dose of nitrazepam for premedication in minor surgery, a significant correlation between the subjective sedative effect and plasma concentration of the drug during the period of increasing plasma concentrations. Similar results have been obtained by Kangas et al. (79) in 10 healthy volunteers after a single 10-mg dose. Grundstrom et al. (46), using the critical flicker fusion method, estimated the sedative-hypnotic effects of diazepam and nitrazepam in eight healthy volunteers. The peak effects of sedation occurred 1.5 hr after nitrazepam intake, whereas the peak plasma concentration usually oc-

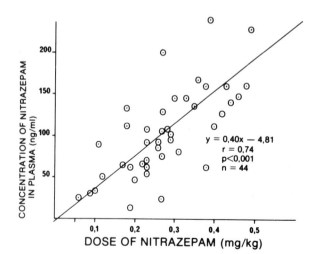

$$y = 0.40x - 4.81$$
$$r = 0.74$$
$$p < 0.001$$
$$n = 44$$

FIG. 2. Correlation between the daily dose and plasma concentration of nitrazepam in epileptic children during continuous treatment with nitrazepam. (From Kangas et al., ref. 75, with permission).

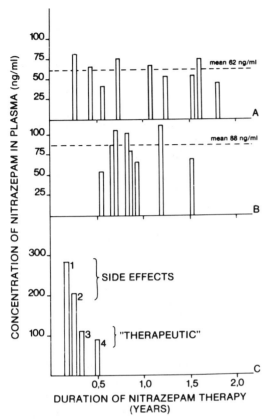

FIG. 3. Plasma concentration of nitrazepam in three epileptic children during continuous therapy. No evidence of enzyme induction causing a decrease in the concentration during long-term treatment was found (note the unchanged daily dose in growing children). **A:** 6- to 8-year-old boy receiving nitrazepam, 3.75 mg/day; mean steady-state concentration, 62 ng/ml. **B:** 8- to 9-year-old girl given nitrazepam, 12.5 mg/day; mean steady-state concentration, 88 ng/ml. **C:** an example of titration of nitrazepam from "toxic" to "therapeutic" level in a 1- to 1.5-year-old boy. The doses of nitrazepam were: **1,** 4.5 mg/day; **2,** 3.75 mg/day; **3,** 3.0 mg/day (2.5 hr after the preceding dose); and **4,** 3.0 mg/day (8.5 hr after the preceding dose). (From Kangas et al. ref. 75, with permission).

curred after 3 to 4 hr. Utilizing a more sensitive neurophysiological test, Bittencourt et al. (11) demonstrated a clear correlation between nitrazepam concentrations and its effect on the peak velocity of saccadic eye movements (which is a measure of brainstem reticular formation function). On the other hand, a lack of correlation between the residual effects (studied by means of psychological tests) of nitrazepam and the corresponding plasma levels has been stressed in several works (41,46,79).

Tolerance

The development of tolerance to the sedative action (156) and to the anticonvulsant effects (39,47–49,108) of nitrazepam has been reported. It is probably caused by a decreased response of the CNS to a constant plasma nitrazepam concentration, since there is no evidence that nitrazepam induces liver microsomal enzymes (120,121,146) and thereby stimulates its own metabolism during long-term treatment (75,131) (see Fig. 3).

Dependence

The development of dependence of the barbiturate-alcohol type after prolonged use of nitrazepam is possible but rare. Darcy (26) described a delirium-tremens–like syndrome after discontinuation of nitrazepam in a 51-year-old man who had been taking the drug (20 mg) nightly for years. In a 92-year-old woman taking nitrazepam 10 mg at night for 17 years, severe muscular spasms and opisthotonos occurred following nitrazepam withdrawal (142). Rebound insomnia is a more important effect after discontinuation of the drug. Adam et al. (2) and Kales et al. (67,68) observed a significant worsening of sleep on withdrawal from nitrazepam. Kales et al. (67) hypothesize that the abrupt withdrawal of benzodiazepine drugs with a short to intermediate duration of action, such as nitrazepam, results in an intensive form of rebound insomnia because of a lag in the production and replacement of endogenous benzodiazepine-like substances whose production decreases if active benzodiazepine drugs are introduced exogenously.

TOXICITY

The most common side effects related to long-term nitrazepam administration include symptoms of CNS depression (drowsiness, ataxia, incoordination) which may be minimized by beginning with a low dose of nitrazepam and slowly increasing the dose (17). These adverse reactions are probably more frequent in the elderly (43) and are dose-related in frequency. On the other hand, symptoms of CNS stimulation such as nightmares, insomnia, and agitation have been reported, but to a lesser extent (40,43,154). Other relatively common side effects are dizziness, inattention, hypotonia, and muscle weakness.

In children, increased salivation and hypersecretion of the tracheobronchial tree have been noted by several investigators (47,48,108,159); in adults, such effects were less frequent or negligible (95). Cases of nitrazepam-induced drooling (47,48,108,159), eating difficulty (159), and aspiration pneumonia (48,60,108,159) have been reported in children. These effects have usually been attributed to salivary and bronchial hypersecretion (47,48,60,159). However, Wyllie et al. (161) performed manometric examinations in two children with nitrazepam-induced drooling and aspiration and demonstrated a delay of the cricopharyngeal relaxation during swallowing. They suggested that nitrazepam-induced drooling and aspiration was caused by impaired swallowing. In light of these results, swallowing disturbance was theoretically postulated as possible cause of death in six children with intractable epilepsy receiving nitrazepam at daily doses ranging from 0.9 to 2.5 mg/kg (117). It was not clear whether nitrazepam played a role in these deaths, but the authors recommended using a dose of nitrazepam below 0.8 mg/kg/day in children.

There is some evidence that nitrazepam may produce respiratory depression and subsequent CO_2 increase in chronic smokers with obstructive bronchitis and ventilatory failure (22,37,109,126,133) and a slight drop in blood pressure in healthy subjects (56).

Several studies have shown that the administration of nitrazepam may impair human performance on the subsequent day (12,98,123,124). Of particular interest are the data concerning the residual effects of nitrazepam on the performance of skills related to driving or other daily activities (91,134). Lahtinen et al. (89) observed in 32 healthy young volunteers 8 hr after 5- or 10-mg oral doses of nitrazepam an impairment of psychomotor skills that was dose-related. It was suggested that precautions must be taken when prescribing large doses (over 5 mg) of nitrazepam as a hypnotic to subjects needing their normal skills in daily work.

Nitrazepam has rarely been shown to increase seizure frequency. Martin (100) reported the occurrence of tonic seizures after an i.v. injection of nitrazepam in a patient with petit mal status, and, as described by Peterson (125), six out of 108 epileptic patients treated with oral nitrazepam had an exacerbation of seizures. Gibbs and Anderson (39) observed 14 patients who experienced increased frequency and severity of grand mal seizures. In a 12-year-old boy affected by Lennox-Gastaut syndrome, parenteral administration of 15 mg of nitrazepam caused tonic status epilepticus 11 min after injection (153).

Miscellaneous Side Effects

MacLean (97) described the case of a 55-year-old woman who developed acroparesthesias after receiving 10-mg doses of nitrazepam as long-term therapy. Hypothermia occurred in an elderly patient following the administration of 5 mg of nitrazepam (58), and a 40-year-old man with a history of gout had acute attacks after taking 10 mg of nitrazepam (90).

A case of leukopenia has been reported to be caused by nitrazepam (125), and of interest are some cutaneous reactions attributed to nitrazepam in the studies of Greenblatt and Allen (43) and Arndt and Jick (3). Generalized urticaria (99), opisthotonos with dystonia (99), headache (125), and anorexia (39) have been reported in single cases.

Nitrazepam and the Elderly

Nitrazepam may be dangerous to the elderly. Evans and Jarvis (32) reported a syndrome characterized by mental confusion, disorientation, ataxia, postural hypotension, and incontinence occurring in old people taking 5 mg of nitrazepam at night. During long-term use in psychogeriatric inpatients, nitrazepam (10 mg) produced impairment of many functions such as ability to move and memory, and caused fecal and urinary incontinence, excessive muscle relaxation, and persistent sedation and drowsiness (92). A deterioration in daytime performance was observed after seven consecutive doses of nitrazepam (5 mg) in elderly patients, an effect consistent with drug accumulation (24,115). Castelden et al. (20) observed an increased sensitivity to a dose of 10 mg of nitrazepam in old age. Since elderly patients are readily susceptible to excessive CNS depression at high drug doses, Greenblatt and Allen (43) suggest that for hypnotic use there is little reason to exceed 5-mg doses of nitrazepam for most older patients.

Overdose

Nitrazepam is a relatively safe drug in overdosage. Out of 1,176 hypnotic drug overdosages, 102 involved nitrazepam; only six patients were deeply comatose, and these recovered uneventfully in 12 hr

(103,104). Bardhan (5) described a case of a 23-year-old man who developed a cerebellar syndrome (nystagmus, ataxia, dysarthria) after taking 180 mg of nitrazepam. Ridley (128) reported the occurrence of bullous lesions of the type sometimes seen with barbiturate overdosage in a 24-year-old woman who was comatose for 36 hr after ingesting 100 tablets of nitrazepam.

Nitrazepam overdosage has been implicated in a comatose patient whose EEG was composed of activity in the alpha frequency range (18,19). The point of major practical importance is that "alpha coma" has been seen mainly in cases of pontomesencephalic infarction or diffuse posthypoxic cerebral cortical necrosis, and in such cases it has usually carried a poor prognosis. It is suggested that when patients in coma exhibit generalized nonreactive alpha activity, a pharmacological intoxication should be considered and if this is confirmed, a complete recovery should be expected.

Teratogenicity

We have been unable to find any published data concerning a possible teratogenic effect of nitrazepam. Only Saxen and Saxen (136) suggested evidence of a correlation between the first-trimester maternal intake of benzodiazepines (diazepam, oxazepam, nitrazepam, chlordiazepoxide) and the occurrence of oral clefts (especially cleft palate) in newborns.

PHARMACODYNAMICS

Anticonvulsant activity of nitrazepam has been evaluated against a wide variety of experimental seizure models. Benzodiazepines, notably nitrazepam, have been shown to be most effective in preventing pentylenetetrazol-induced seizures in both mice and rats (14,87,107,149). A much greater dose is needed to raise the threshold at which maximal electroshock induces seizures in the same animals (107,149). Nitrazepam appeared to be between diazepam and clonazepam in potency and duration of action in the maximal electroshock seizure test (107,149).

In a study carried out to determine whether benzodiazepines preferentially antagonize seizures induced by chemical convulsants acting on the GABA system, such as 3-mercaptopropionic acid (3-MP), biculline, and picrotoxin, nitrazepam seemed to be more effective against pentylenetetrazol than against 3-MP (147). Furthermore, nitrazepam prevents, as do other benzodiazepines, photically induced seizures in the baboon *Papio papio* (83), which may correlate well with the effectiveness of this drug in reducing photosensitivity in humans (35).

With respect to models of partial epilepsy, many studies have detailed the action of benzodiazepines on experimentally induced cortical foci. Benzodiazepines prevent the motor manifestations of focal seizure discharges and depress the spread of abnormal electrical activity from the site of the lesion (17).

Electroencephalographic studies in humans have shown that nitrazepam may produce an increase in low-voltage fast activity and a decrease of alpha frequency, especially in frontal areas (102,112). It has been shown that nitrazepam has a suppressive effect in humans with regard to the photosensitive response in the EEG (35).

Nitrazepam has characteristic effects on sleep stages. As do other benzodiazepines, it reduces the time spent in drowsiness during the night (stage 1), increases the total time in stage 2 sleep, and decreases the time spent in slow-wave sleep (stages 3 and 4); also, the time spent in the paradoxical or rapid eye movement phase is usually shortened (122).

Responses evoked in cortical and subcortical areas by local or sensory inputs have been shown to be altered by benzodiazepines. In the baboon, evoked potential studies showed nitrazepam-induced changes in evoked responses in the occipital regions that paralleled seizure control (83).

In experimental animals, benzodiazepines have various pharmacological effects on limbic system structures. In cats (137) nitrazepam increases the after-discharge threshold of the amygdala and inhibits the response of the hippocampus to stimulation of the ipsilateral amygdala (116).

Data documenting significant participation of the ubiquitous inhibitory neurotransmitter, GABA, in the action of benzodiazepines have been extensively reviewed elsewhere in this book (see Chapter 54). The benzodiazepines potentiate the actions of GABA at both presynaptic and postsynaptic sites (84). Benzodiazepine binding to specific receptors in the brain modulates GABA effects (106). Several recent papers describe in detail the known structure of these receptors and the mechanisms of modulation (101,110,119).

In addition to the modulation of GABA action, the function of several monoamines in the brain may be altered by benzodiazepines (23,36,143). These drugs, notably nitrazepam, may decrease the turnover rate of catecholamines (25,155), acetylcholine (23), and serotonin (143,148). It has been suggested that the impairment of serotonin turnover rate may explain the anxyolitic effects of benzodiazepines (143) and underlie nitrazepam-induced sleep in mice (160).

Nitrazepam, as well as diazepam and other benzodiazepines, shows a high affinity for the brain receptors of glycine, a prominent inhibitory transmitter in the brainstem and spinal cord (140). A glycine-mimetic action would account for the antianxiety and muscle relaxant effects of benzodiazepines (140).

THERAPEUTIC USE

Reports on the efficacy of nitrazepam in long-term oral treatment of epilepsy start in

1963, peak in the 1967–1968 period, and then progressively decrease.

Effective daily doses of nitrazepam range from 0.25 mg/kg to 3 mg/kg, the highest being used in children suffering mainly from hypsarrhythmia. Mean daily doses vary from 0.5 mg/kg in adults to 1 mg/kg in children. Therapeutic plasma levels are quite variable and consequently are considered of little relevance in clinical practice (61).

Nitrazepam has been found effective in a variety of seizures occurring in different forms of epilepsy (17). Most reports, however, seem to indicate that nitrazepam is chiefly useful in the treatment of infantile spasms with hypsarrhythmia (or West syndrome) and in the so-called infantile myoclonic seizures (the two conditions often being reported under the same heading of myoclonic seizures) (105). In 1963 Liske and Forster (93) first used nitrazepam in the treatment of infantile spasms; since then, many other reports showing the efficacy of nitrazepam on this condition have been published. We have reviewed 137 cases of West syndrome (infantile spasms with hypsarrhythmic records occurring mainly in the first 2 years of life), and 93 of these (68%) responded satisfactorily to nitrazepam treatment (8,13,30,34,39,44,66,99,139, 157,159). Gibbs and Anderson (39), however, included under the heading of infantile spasms with hypsarrhythmia subjects up to 12 years of age who could be considered as having a Lennox-Gastaut syndrome. Curiously, Jong (66) considered nitrazepam effective in all cases of epilepsy except hypsarrhythmia, since he did not observe significant effects in his four cases. From the study of Borselli et al. (13) it would seem that patients with symptomatic West syndrome (11 cases) are less likely to respond well (3 out of 11) to nitrazepam treatment, and understandably so. These findings, however, must be considered from the viewpoint of the great heterogeneity of the reported cases, probably related to such significant factors as the age of the patients,

the etiology of the syndrome, the duration of the follow-up, and criteria for the definition of improvement.

In some studies, an attempt has been made to compare the efficacy of nitrazepam and ACTH in the treatment of infantile spasms (17,45). In their review monograph, Lacy and Penry (88) reported excellent seizure response to nitrazepam and ACTH in 30% to 77% and 18% to 60% of patients, respectively. The studies in which these results were achieved, however, varied regarding the patient selection criteria, dosing regimen, and treatment duration. Recently, a 4-week randomized, controlled study comparing the efficacy and safety of nitrazepam and ACTH in the treatment of infantile spasms has been published (30). In this study, 52% of patients in the nitrazepam group (27 cases) and 57% of the ACTH group (21 cases) achieved excellent spasm control (75–100% reduction in seizure frequency). The number of patients who experienced side effects was similar in the two treatment groups, but the adverse effects encountered among the patients treated with ACTH were qualitatively more severe.

In myoclonic seizures occurring mainly in children later in life, as compared to hypsarrhythmia, nitrazepam was also found effective (8,95,108,139). According to Jeavons (61), nitrazepam is likely to be one of the most effective benzodiazepines for the control of myoclonic seizures.

More than 50 cases have been reported under the specific heading of "myoclonic seizures" or "myoclonic epilepsy" but it is quite difficult to determine from these reports precisely if and what kind of "myoclonic seizures" responded best to nitrazepam and for how long the improvement was maintained. Patients with myoclonic or absence seizures, or both, are particularly likely to display photosensitivity, and there is evidence that benzodiazepines, notably nitrazepam, can block paroxysmal responses in both types of seizures (35,127). Nitrazepam was also found effective in some patients with "minor motor seizures" (125), a term that unfortunately covers a wide range of different seizures and forms of epilepsy. Similarly, "astatic seizures" benefited from therapy with nitrazepam.

A number of cases of what could be referred to as Lennox-Gastaut syndrome were classified under different labels in the literature. We found reports of approximately 60 patients affected by such a syndrome (39,44,66,157) who benefited to some extent from treatment with nitrazepam. In an unpublished study, nitrazepam was added to previous treatment in 50 children aged 2 to 12 years with a Lennox-Gastaut syndrome (C. Dravet, J. Roger, C. A. Tassinari, *unpublished data,* 1968). Dosages varied from 15 to 30 mg, with a maximum daily dose of 50 to 75 mg. A very significant clinical and EEG improvement was observed in 27 children. It was noted that nitrazepam could significantly control the atypical absences and that tonic seizures persisted as the sole symptomatology. The positive effects, however, disappeared or significantly decreased over a follow-up period ranging from 8 days to 3 months in 13 patients. The treatment was stopped in five patients because of side effects. Good results persisted for up to 3 months in seven patients and up to 2 years in two others. Nineteen children had only a mild clinical improvement, and four were unhelped by nitrazepam. Interestingly, 25 out of the 27 patients who showed good improvement with nitrazepam therapy had previously been treated with diazepam; 10 of them had more or less transitory good results, and nine did not respond at all. The conclusions were that in the Lennox-Gastaut syndrome nitrazepam was more useful than diazepam, particularly in the control of atypical absences.

With regard to primary generalized epilepsy (typical absences of petit mal and tonic-clonic seizures), we found reports of 48 patients mainly affected by typical absences, of whom 18 significantly improved after nitrazepam treatment (44,66,95, 99,125). Of 27 patients suffering only or mainly from tonic-clonic seizures, nine had a significant improvement following nitrazepam therapy (13,66,99). Vanasse and Geoffroy (157) used nitrazepam as add-on therapy in 62 patients with generalized seizures, either petit mal, grand mal, or both. The addition of nitrazepam was followed by a 50% or greater reduction in seizure frequency in 64.4% of patients. This group was subdivided into grand mal or petit mal attacks or both and the results were essentially the same for each of these subgroups.

Nitrazepam has also been found effective in partial seizures. Clinically significant improvement or, rarely, complete seizure control was observed in 19 out of 35 patients with various partial seizures and in 17 out of 62 patients with psychomotor seizures. (8,66,99). To the previously reported cases we should add those of Lundberg and Stalberg (95), who observed in 21 adult patients (15 with psychomotor epilepsy and six with partial attacks of other types) in whom other therapy had been unsuccessful, that nitrazepam effected excellent control of the seizures in 20 cases with a follow-up of 3 years. In another study the addition of nitrazepam resulted in a significant clinical benefit in 23 out of 43 patients with a diagnosis of "focal and complex partial epilepsy" and in 15 out of 28 patients with "multifocal epilepsy" (157).

Intermittent oral administration of nitrazepam has also been used for the prophylactic treatment of febrile convulsions (158). Thirty-one children with a high risk of recurrence received nitrazepam. The rate of recurrence in this group was 19.3% after a follow-up period of 16 months, compared to 45.8% in 24 children who also had a high risk of recurrence but whose parents refused the medication.

Parenteral Nitrazepam in Treatment of Status Epilepticus

From the reports of Martin (100), Oller-Daurella (*personal communication,* 1968:

14 cases), and Lison and Fassoni (*personal communication*, 1968: 20 cases), as well as from unpublished data from the Center St. Paul, Marseilles, it was concluded that nitrazepam by slow injection is as effective as clonazepam in the control of status epilepticus (unilateral, partial, and generalized, with or without convulsions). However, Martin (100) and Tassinari et al. (153) have observed, as with other benzodiazepines, instances of status epilepticus paradoxically induced by i.v. injection of nitrazepam in cases of Lennox-Gastaut syndrome.

SUMMARY

Nitrazepam is a widely used and safe hypnotic drug. The compound is effective in the treatment of various types of epilepsy, primarily infantile spasms, myoclonic seizures, and Lennox-Gastaut syndrome. Reflex epilepsies, including photosensitive epilepsy, respond well to nitrazepam. Initial success, however, may be followed by the development of tolerance.

Side effects are common but mild: most patients experience drowsiness, ataxia, and, for hypnotic use, impairment of psychomotor skills the morning following oral administration. Also, after prolonged treatment in children, hypotonia and increased salivary and bronchial secretion may often occur. The drug is safe in overdosage.

Nitrazepam probably does not alter the rate of metabolism of concomitantly administered drugs.

Some neurotransmitters, GABA in particular, play an important role in the action of nitrazepam.

The compound is well absorbed after oral administration, and peak plasma concentrations occur within 1 to 4 hr. The main metabolic pathway leads, by reduction of the nitro group, to the corresponding amine and, by acetylation of the latter, to the 7-acetamido derivative.

CONVERSION

Conversion factor:

$$CF = \frac{1000}{mol.\ wt.} = \frac{1000}{281.26} = 3.56$$

Conversion:

$$(\mu g/ml) \times 3.56 = (\mu moles/liter)$$

$$(\mu moles/liter) + 3.56 = (\mu g/ml)$$

REFERENCES

1. Abernethy, D. R., Greenblatt, D. J., Locniskar, A., Ochs, H. R., Harmatz, J. S., and Shader, R. I. (1986): Obesity effects on nitrazepam disposition. *Br. J. Clin. Pharmacol.*, 22:551–557.
2. Adam, K., Adamson, L., Brezinov, V., Hunter, W. M., and Oswald, I. (1976): Nitrazepam: Lastingly effective but trouble on withdrawal. *Br. Med. J.*, 1:1558–1560.
3. Arndt, K. A., and Jick, H. (1976): Rates of cutaneous reactions to drugs: A report from the Boston Collaborative Drug Surveillance Program. *Drug Intell. Clin. Pharm.*, 9:648–654.
4. Ballinger, B. R., Presly, A., Raid, A. H., and Stevenson, I. H. (1974): The effects of hypnotics on imipramine treatment. *Psychopharmacologia*, 39:267–274.
5. Bardhan, K. D. (1969): Cerebellar syndrome after nitrazepam overdosage. *Lancet*, 1:1319–1320.
6. Bartosek, I., Kvetina, J., Guaitani, A., and Garattini, S. (1970): Comparative study of nitrazepam metabolism in perfused isolated liver laboratory animals. *Eur. J. Pharmacol.*, 11:378–382.
7. Bartosek, I., Mussini, E., Saronio, C., and Garattini, S. (1970): Studies on nitrazepam reduction *in vitro*. *Eur. J. Pharmacol.*, 11:249–253.
8. Benedetti, P., Ammaniti, M., and Cogliati Dezza, G. (1967): L'impiego del Ro-4-5360 nell'epilessia infantile, contributo clinico. *Infanzia Anormale (Roma)*, 75:287–296.
9. Bente, H. B. (1978): Nitrogen-selective detectors: Application to quantitation of antiepileptic drugs. In: *Antiepileptic Drugs: Quantitative Analysis and Interpretation*, edited by C. E. Pippenger, J. K. Penry, and H. Kutt, pp. 139–145. Raven Press, New York.
10. Bieger, R., de Jonge, H., and Loeliger, E. A. (1972): Influence of nitrazepam on oral anticoagulation with phenprocoumon. *Clin. Pharmacol. Ther.*, 13:361–365.
11. Bittencourt, P. R. M., Wade, P., Smith, A. T., and Richens, A. (1981): The relationship between peak velocity of saccadic eye movements and serum benzodiazepine concentration. *Br. J. Clin. Pharmacol.*, 12:523–533.
12. Borland, R. G., and Nicholson, A. N. (1975): Comparison of the residual effects of two benzodiazepines (nitrazepam and flurazepam hydro-

chloride) and pentobarbitone sodium on human performance. *Br. J. Clin. Pharmacol.*, 2:9–17.

13. Borselli, L., Corvaglia, E., and Falchi, G. (1967): L'impiego di un nuovo nitroderivato del clordiazepossido (1,3 diidro-7-nitro-5-fenil-2H-1,4-benzodiazepin-2-one o Mogadon) nella terapia dell'epilessia infantile. *Riv. Clin. Pediatr.*, 2:450–456.

14. Boyer, P. A. (1966): Anticonvulsant properties of benzodiazepines. *Dis. Nerv. Syst.*, 27:35–42.

15. Breimer, D. D. (1977): Clinical pharmacokinetics of hypnotics. *Clin. Pharmacokinet.*, 2:93–109.

16. Breimer, D. D., Bracht, H., and De Boer, A. G. (1977): Plasma level profile of nitrazepam (Mogadon) following oral administration. *Br. J. Clin. Pharmacol.*, 4:709–711.

17. Browne, I. R., and Penry, J. K. (1973): Benzodiazepines in the treatment of epilepsy. *Epilepsia*, 14:277–310.

18. Carrol, W. M., and Mastaglia, F. L. (1977): Alpha and beta coma in drug intoxication. *Br. Med. J.*, 2:1518–1519.

19. Carrol, W. M., and Mastaglia, F. L. (1979): Alpha and beta coma in drug intoxication uncomplicated by cerebral hypoxia. *Electroencephalogr. Clin. Neurophysiol.*, 46:95–105.

20. Castelden, C. M., George, C. F., Marcer, D., and Hallet, C. (1977): Increased sensitivity to nitrazepam in old age. *Br. Med. J.*, 1:10–12.

21. Chambers, D. M., and Jefferson, G. C. (1977): Some observations of the mechanism of benzodiazepine-barbiturate interactions in the mouse. *Br. J. Pharmacol.*, 60:393–399.

22. Clark, T. J. H., Collins, J. V., and Tong, D. (1971): Respiratory depression caused by nitrazepam in patients with respiratory failure. *Lancet*, 2:737–738.

23. Consolo, S., Garattini, S., and Ladinsky, H. (1975): Action of the benzodiazepines on the cholinergic system. *Adv. Biochem. Psychopharmacol.*, 14:63–80.

24. Cook, P. J., Huggett, A., Graham-Pole, R., Savage, I. T., and James, I. M. (1983): Hypnotic accumulation and hangover in elderly inpatients: A controlled double-blind study of temazepam and nitrazepam. *Br. Med. J.*, 286:100–102.

25. Corrodi, H., Fuxe, K., Lidbrink, P., and Olson, L. (1971): Minor tranquillizers, stress and central catecholamine neurons. *Brain Res.*, 29:1–16.

26. Darcy, L. (1972): Delirium tremens following withdrawal of nitrazepam. *Med. J. Aust.*, 2:450.

27. De Boer, A. G., Rost-Kaiser, J., Bracht, H., and Breimer, D. D. (1978): Assay of underivatized nitrazepam and clonazepam in plasma by capillary gas chromatography applied to pharmacokinetic and bioavailability studies in humans. *J. Chromatogr.*, 145:105–114.

28. De Silva, J. A. F. (1978): Electron capture-GLC in the quantitation of 1,4-benzodiazepines. In: *Antiepileptic Drugs: Quantitative Analysis and Interpretation*, edited by C. E. Pippenger, J. K. Penry, and H. Kutt, pp. 111–138. Raven Press, New York.

29. Dixon, R., Lucek, R., Yong, R., Ning, R., and Darragh, A. (1979): Radioimmunoassay for nitrazepam in plasma. *Life Sci.*, 25:311–316.

30. Dreifuss, F., Farwell, J., Holmes, G., Joseph, C., Lackman, L., Madsen, J. A., Minarcik, C. J., Rothner, A. D., and Shewmon, D. A. (1986): Infantile spasms: Comparative trial of nitrazepam and corticotropin. *Arch. Neurol.*, 43:1107–1110.

31. Ehrsson, M., and Tilly, A. (1973): Electron capture gas chromatography of nitrazepam in human plasma as methyl derivatives. *Anal. Lett.*, 6:197–210.

32. Evans, J. G., and Jarvis, E. H. (1972): Nitrazepam and the elderly. *Br. Med. J.*, 4:487.

33. Eze, L. C. (1987): High incidence of the slow nitrazepam acetylator phenotype in a Nigerian population. *Biochem. Genet.*, 25:225–229.

34. Feng, Y., Zhang, Z., and Xu, J. (1980): Infantile spasms: A clinicoelectroencephalographic report of 41 cases. *Chin. Med. J.*, 93:439–450.

35. Friedel, B., and Kunath, J. (1970): Anderung der photosensiblen Reizschwelle in EEG durch Nitrazepam. *Arzneim. Forsch.*, 6:168–188.

36. Fuxe, K., Agnati, L. F., Bolme, P., Hokfelt, T., Lidbrink, P., Ljungdahl, A., de la Mora, M. P., and Ogren, S. (1975): The possible involvement of GABA mechanisms in the action of benzodiazepines on central catecholamine neurons. *Adv. Biochem. Psychopharmacol.*, 14:45–61.

37. Gaddie, J., Legge, J. S., Palmer, K. N. V., Petrie, J. C., and Wood, R. A. (1972): Effect of nitrazepam in chronic obstructive bronchitis. *Br. Med. J.*, 2:688–689.

38. Garattini, S., Marcucci, F., and Mussini, E. (1977): The metabolism and pharmacokinetics of selected benzodiazepines. In: *Psychotherapeutic Drugs*, edited by E. Usdin and I. S. Forrest, pp. 1039–1087. Marcel Dekker, Basel, New York.

39. Gibbs, F. A., and Anderson, E. M. (1965): Treatment of hypsarrhythmia and infantile spasms with a Librium analogue. *Neurology*, 15:1173–1176.

40. Girdwood, R. H. (1973): Nitrazepam nightmares. *Br. Med. J.*, 1:353.

41. Godtlibsen, O. B., Jerk, D., Gordeladze, J. O., Bredesen, J. E., and Matheson, I. (1986): Residual effect of single and repeated doses of midazolam and nitrazepam in relation to their plasma concentrations. *Eur. J. Clin. Pharmacol.*, 29:595–600.

42. Greenblatt, D. J., Abernethy, D. R., Locniskar, A., Ochs, H. R., Harmatz, J. S., and Shader, R. I. (1985): Age, sex, and nitrazepam kinetics: Relation to antipyrine disposition. *Clin. Pharmacol. Ther.*, 38:697–703.

43. Greenblatt, D. J., and Allen, M. D. (1978): Toxicity of nitrazepam in the elderly: A report from the Boston collaborative drug surveillance program. *Br. J. Clin. Pharmacol.*, 5:407–413.

44. Grossi-Bianchi, M. L., and Pistone, F. M. (1967): Effetto ipnogeno ed effetto anticomiziale del nitrazepam nei bambini. *Minerva Pediatr.*, 19:1073–1082.

45. Grossi-Bianchi, M. L., and Pistone, F. M. (1968): Comparison of treatment with ACTH and ni-

trazepam in some forms of infantile convulsive syndromes. *Riv. Clin. Pediatr.*, 81:233–234.

46. Grundstrom, R., Holmberg, G., and Hansen, T. (1978): Degree of sedation obtained with various doses of diazepam and nitrazepam. *Acta Pharmacol. Toxicol.*, 43:13–18.

47. Hagberg, B. (1967): The librium-analogue Mogadon in the treatment of epilepsy in children. *Acta Neurol. Scand.*, 31:167.

48. Hagberg, B. (1968): The chlordiazepoxide HCl (Librium) analogue nitrazepam (Mogadon) in the treatment of epilepsy in children. *Dev. Med. Child Neurol.*, 10:302–308.

49. Hambert, O., and Petersen, J. W. (1970): Clinical, electroencephalographical and neuropharmacological studies in syndromes of progressive myoclonus epilepsy. *Acta Neurol. Scand.*, 46:149–186.

50. Harris, A. L., and McIntyre, N. (1981): Interaction of phenelzine and nitrazepam in a slow acetylator. *Br. J. Clin. Pharmacol.*, 12:254–255.

51. Hart, B. J., Wilting, J., and de Gier, J. J. (1987): Complications in correlation studies between serum, free serum and saliva concentrations of nitrazepam. *Meth. Find. Exp. Clin. Pharmacol.*, 9:127–131.

52. Hewick, D. S., and Shaw, V. (1978): Tissue distribution of radioactivity after injection of C^{14}-nitrazepam in young and old rats. *J. Pharm. Pharmacol.*, 30:318–319.

53. Hewick, D. S., and Shaw, V. (1978): The importance of the intestinal microflora in nitrazepam metabolism in the rat. *Br. J. Pharmacol.*, 62:427.

54. Ho, P. C., Triggs, E. J., Heazlewood, V., and Bourne, D. W. A. (1983): Determination of nitrazepam and temazepam in plasma by high-performance liquid chromatography. *Ther. Drug Monit.*, 5:303–307.

55. Holm, V., Melander, A., and Wahlin-boll, E. (1982): Influence of food and of age on nitrazepam kinetics. *Drug-Nut. Int.*, 1:307–311.

56. Hossmann, V., Maling, T. J. B., Hamilton, C. A., Reid, J. L., and Dollery, C. T. (1980): Sedative and cardiovascular effects of clonidine and nitrazepam. *Clin. Pharmacol. Ther.*, 28:167–176.

57. Hunt, P., Husson, J. M., and Raynaud, J. P. (1979): A radioreceptor assay for benzodiazepines. *J. Pharm. Pharmacol.*, 31:448–451.

58. Impallomeni, M., and Ezzat, R. (1976): Hypothermia associated with nitrazepam administration. *Br. Med. J.*, 1:223–224.

59. Inoue, T., and Niwaguchi, T. (1985): Determination of nitrazepam and its main metabolites in urine by thin-layer chromatography and direct densitometry. *J. Chromatogr.*, 339:163–169.

60. Jan, J. E., and Riegl, J. A. (1970): Nitrazepam in the treatment of convulsive disorders. *Clin. Res.*, 18:220.

61. Jeavons, P. M. (1977): Choice of drug therapy in epilepsy. *Practitioner*, 219:542–556.

62. Jochemsen, R., Hogendoorn, J. J. H., Dingemanse, J., Hermans, J., Boeijinga, J. K., and Breimer, D. D. (1982): Pharmacokinetics and bioavailability of intravenous, oral and rectal ni-

trazepam in humans. *J. Pharmacokinet. Biopharm.*, 10:231–245.

63. Jochemsen, R., Horbach, G. J. M. J., and Breimer, D. D. (1982): Assay of nitrazepam and triazolam in plasma by a radioreceptor technique and comparison with a gas chromatographic method. *Res. Commun. Chem. Pathol. Pharmacol.*, 35:259–273.

64. Jochemsen, R., Van Beusekom, B. R., Spoelstra, P., Janssens, A. R., and Breimer, D. D. (1983): Effect of age and liver cirrhosis on the pharmacokinetics of nitrazepam. *Br. J. Clin. Pharmacol.*, 15:295–302.

65. Jochemsen, R., Van der Graaff, M., Boeijinga, J. K., and Breimer, D. D. (1982): Influence of sex, menstrual cycle and oral contraception on the disposition of nitrazepam. *Br. J. Clin. Pharmacol.*, 13:319–324.

66. Jong, T. H. (1964): Klinische erfahrungen mit dem Benzodiazepinderivat Ro-4-5360 bei der Behandlung der epilepsie. *Schweiz. Med. Wochenschr.*, 94:730–733.

67. Kales, A., Scharf, M. B., and Kales, J. D. (1978): Rebound insomnia: A new clinical syndrome. *Science*, 201:1039–1041.

68. Kales, A., Scharf, M. B., Kales, J. D., and Soldatos, C. R. (1979): Rebound insomnia. A potential hazard following withdrawal of certain benzodiazepines. *J.A.M.A.*, 241:1692–1695.

69. Kangas, L. (1977): Comparison of two gas-liquid chromatographic methods for the determination of nitrazepam in plasma. *J. Chromatogr.*, 136:259–270.

70. Kangas, L. (1979): Determination of nitrazepam and its main metabolites in urine by gas-liquid chromatography: Use of electron capture and nitrogen-selective detectors. *J. Chromatogr.*, 172:273–278.

71. Kangas, L. (1979): Urinary elimination of nitrazepam and its main metabolites. *Acta Pharmacol. Toxicol.*, 45:16–19.

72. Kangas, L., Allonen, H., Lammintausta, R., Pynnonen, S., and Salonen, M. (1977): Pharmacokinetics of nitrazepam in human plasma and saliva. *Acta Pharmacol. Toxicol.*, 41:56.

73. Kangas, L., Allonen, H., Lammintausta, R., Salonen, M., and Pekkarinen, A. (1979): Pharmacokinetics of nitrazepam in saliva and serum after a single oral dose. *Acta Pharmacol. Toxicol.*, 45:20–24.

74. Kangas, L., and Breimer, D. D. (1981): Clinical pharmacokinetics of nitrazepam. *Clin. Pharmacokinet.*, 6:346–366.

75. Kangas, L., Iisalo, E., Kanto, J., Lehtinen, V., Pynnonen, S., Ruikka, I., Salminen, J., Sillanpaa, M., and Syvalahti, E. (1979): Human pharmacokinetics of nitrazepam: Effect of age and diseases. *Eur. J. Clin. Pharmacol.*, 15:163–170.

76. Kangas, L., Kanto, J., and Erkkola, R. (1977): Transfer of nitrazepam across the human placenta. *Eur. J. Clin. Pharmacol.*, 12:355–357.

77. Kangas, L., Kanto, J., and Mansikka, M. (1977): Nitrazepam premedication for minor surgery. *Br. J. Anaesth.*, 49:1153–1157.

78. Kangas, L., Kanto, J., Siirtola, T., and Pekkarinen, A. (1977): Cerebrospinal-fluid concentrations of nitrazepam in man. *Acta Pharmacol. Toxicol.,* 41:74–79.

79. Kangas, L., Kanto, J., and Syvalahti, E. (1977): Plasma nitrazepam concentrations after an acute intake and their correlation to sedation and serum growth hormone levels. *Acta Pharmacol. Toxicol.,* 41:65–73.

80. Karim, A. K. M. B., and Price Evans, D. A. (1976): Polymorphic acetylation of nitrazepam. *J. Med. Genet.,* 13:17–19.

81. Kelly, H., Huggett, A., and Dawling, S. (1982): Liquid-chromatographic measurement of nitrazepam in plasma. *Clin. Chem.,* 28:1478–1481.

82. Kenny, R. A., Kafetz, K., Cox, M., and Timmers, J. (1984): Impaired nitrazepam metabolism in hypothyroidism. *Postgrad. Med. J.,* 60:296–297.

83. Killam, E. K., Matsuzaki, M., and Killam, K. F. (1973): Effects of chronic administration of benzodiazepines on epileptic seizures and brain electrical activity in *Papio papio.* In: *The Benzodiazepines,* edited by S. Garattini, E. Mussini, and L. O. Randall, pp. 443–460. Raven Press, New York.

84. Killam, E. K., and Suria, A. (1980): Antiepileptic drugs: Benzodiazepines. In: *Antiepileptic Drugs: Mechanisms of Action,* edited by G. H. Glaser, J. K. Penry, and D. M. Woodbury, pp. 597–615. Raven Press, New York.

85. Kinawi, A., and Teller, C. (1978): Zur interaktion von phenprocoumon mit Diazepam und Nitrazepam. *J. Clin. Chem. Clin. Biochem.,* 16:313–314.

86. Kozu, T. (1984): High-performance liquid chromatographic determination of nitrazepam and its metabolites in human urine. *J. Chromatogr.,* 310:213–218.

87. Krall, R. L., Penry, J. K., White, B. G., Kupferberg, H. J., and Swinyard, E. A. (1978): Antiepileptic drug development: II. Anticonvulsant drug screening. *Epilepsia,* 19:409–428.

88. Lacy, J. R., and Penry, J. K. (1976): *Infantile Spasms.* Raven Press, New York.

89. Lahtinen, U., Lahtinen, A., and Pekkola, P. (1978): The effect of nitrazepam on manual skill, grip strength, and reaction time with special reference to subjective evaluation of effects on sleep. *Acta Pharmacol. Toxicol.,* 42:130–134.

90. Leng, C. O. (1975): Drug-precipitated acute attacks of gout. *Br. Med. J.,* 2:561.

91. Linnoila, M. (1973): Drug interaction on psychomotor skills related to driving: Hypnotics and alcohol. *Ann. Med. Exp. Biol. Fenn.,* 51:118–124.

92. Linnoila, M., and Viukari, M. (1976): Efficacy and side effects of nitrazepam and thioridazine as sleeping aids in psychogeriatric inpatients. *Br. J. Psychiatry,* 128:566–569.

93. Liske, E., and Forster, F. M. (1963): Clinical study of a new benzodiazepine as an anticonvulsant agent. *J. N. Drugs,* 3:241–244.

94. Locniskar, A., and Greenblatt, D. J. (1985): Simplified gas chromatographic assay of underivatized nitrazepam in plasma. *J. Chromatogr.,* 337:131–135.

95. Lundberg, P. O., and Stalberg, E. (1971): Mogadon in der behamdlung von epilepsie bei erwachsenen. *Arch. Psychiatr. Nervenkr.,* 214:46–55.

96. Lunde, P. K. M., Frislid, K., and Hansteen, V. (1977): Disease and acetylation polymorphism. *Clin. Pharmacokinet.,* 2:182–197.

97. MacLean, H. (1973): Nitrazepam: Another interesting syndrome. *Br. Med. J.,* 1:488.

98. Malpas, A., Rowan, A. J., Joyce, C. R. B., and Scott, D. F. (1970): Persistent behavioural and encephalographic changes after single doses of nitrazepam and amylobarbitone sodium. *Br. Med. J.,* 2:762–764.

99. Markham, C. H. (1964): The treatment of myoclonic seizures of infancy and childhood with LA-I. *Pediatrics,* 34:511–518.

100. Martin, D. (1970): Intravenous nitrazepam in the treatment of epilepsy. *Neuropaediatrie,* 2:27–37.

101. Martin, I. L., Brown, C. L., and Doble, A. (1983): Multiple benzodiazepine receptors: Structures in the brain or structures in the mind? A critical review. *Life Sci.,* 32:1925–1933.

102. Matthes, A. (1965): 1,3-Dihydro-7-nitro-5-phenyl-2H-1,4-benzodiazepin-2-on als schlafmittel im kindesalter. *Arzneim. Forsch.,* 15:1157–1158.

103. Matthew, H., Proudfoot, A. T., Aitken, R. C. B., Raeburn, J. A., and Wright, N. (1969): Nitrazepam—A safe hypnotic. *Br. Med. J.,* 3:23–25.

104. Matthew, H., Roscoe, P., and Wright, N. (1972): Acute poisoning. A comparison of hypnotic drugs. *Practitioner,* 208:254–258.

105. Mattson, R. M. (1972): The benzodiazepines. In: *Antiepileptic Drugs,* 1st edition, edited by D. M. Woodbury, J. K. Penry, and R. P. Schmidt, pp. 497–518. Raven Press, New York.

106. Miller, L. G., Greenblatt, D. J., and Shader, R. I. (1987): Benzodiazepine receptor binding: Influence of physiologic and pharmacologic factors. *Biopharm. Drug Disp.,* 8:103–114.

107. Millichap, J. G. (1969): Relation of laboratory evaluation to clinical effectiveness of antiepileptic drugs. *Epilepsia,* 10:315–328.

108. Millichap, J. G., and Ortiz, W. R. (1966): Nitrazepam in myoclonic epilepsies. *Am. J. Dis. Child,* 112:242–248.

109. Model, D. G. (1973): Nitrazepam induced respiratory depression in chronic obstructive lung disease. *Br. J. Dis. Chest,* 67:128–130.

110. Mohler, H., and Richards, J. G. (1983): Benzodiazepine receptors in the central nervous system. In: *The Benzodiazepines: From Molecular Biology to Clinical Practice,* edited by E. Costa, pp. 93–116. Raven Press, New York.

111. Moller Jensen, K. (1975): Determination of nitrazepam in serum by gas-liquid chromatography. *J. Chromatogr.,* 111:389–396.

112. Montagu, J. D. (1971): Effects of quinalbarbitone (secobarbital) and nitrazepam on the EEG in man. Quantitative investigations. *Eur. J. Pharmacol.,* 14:238–249.

113. Moody, J. P., Whyte, S. F., Mac Donald, A. J., and Naylor, G. J. (1977): Pharmacokinetic aspects of protriptyline plasma levels. *Eur. J. Clin. Pharmacol.,* 11:51–56.

114. Moore, B., Nickless, G., Hallet, C., and Howard, A. G. (1977): Analysis of nitrazepam and its metabolites by high-pressure liquid chromatography. *J. Chromatogr.,* 137:215–217.

115. Morgan, E. (1985): Effects or repeated dose of nitrazepam and lormetazepam on psychomotor performance in the elderly. *Psychopharmacology,* 86:209–211.

116. Morillo, A. (1962): Effects of benzodiazepines upon amygdala and hippocampus of the cat. *Int. J. Neuropharmacol.,* 1:353–359.

117. Murphy, J. V., Sawasky, F., Marquardt, K. M., and Harris, D. J. (1987): Deaths in young children receiving nitrazepam. *J. Pediatr.,* 111:145–147.

118. Ochs, H. R., Greenblatt, D. J., Gugler, R., Muntefering, G., Locniskar, A., and Abernethy, D. R. (1983): Cimetidine impairs nitrazepam clearance. *Clin. Pharmacol. Ther.,* 34:227–230.

119. Ogawa, N., Mizuno, S., Tsukamoto, S., and Mori, A. (1984): Relationships of structure to binding of gamma-aminobutyric acid (GABA) and related compounds with the GABA and benzodiazepine receptors. *Res. Commun. Chem. Pathol. Pharmacol.,* 43:355–368.

120. O'Malley, K. (1971): Safety of hypnotics. *Br. Med. J.,* 1:729.

121. Orme, M., Breckenridge, A., and Brooks, R. V. (1972): Interactions of benzodiazepines with warfarin. *Br. Med. J.,* 3:611–614.

122. Oswald, I., Lewis, S. A., Tagney, J., Firth, H., and Haider, I. (1973): Benzodiazepines and human sleep. In: *The Benzodiazepines,* edited by S. Garattini, E. Mussini, and L. O. Randall, pp. 613–625. Raven Press, New York.

123. Peck, A. W., Adams, R., Bye, C., and Wilkinson, R. T. (1976): Residual effects of hypnotic drugs: Evidence for individual differences on vigilance. *Psychopharmacology,* 47:213–216.

124. Peck, A. W., Bye, C. E., and Claridge, R. (1977): Differences between light and sound sleepers in the residual effects of nitrazepam. *Br. J. Clin. Pharmacol.,* 4:101–108.

125. Peterson, W. G. (1967): Clinical study of Mogadon, a new anticonvulsant. *Neurology,* 17:878–880.

126. Pines, A. (1972): Nitrazepam in chronic obstructive bronchitis. *Br. Med. J.,* 3:352.

127. Poiré, R., and Royer, J. (1968): Comparative experimental electrographic study of anticonvulsant properties of a new derivative of the benzodiazepines Ro 5-4023. *Electroencephalogr. Clin. Neurophysiol.,* 27:106.

128. Ridley, C. M. (1971): Bullous lesions in nitrazepam overdosage. *Br. Med. J.,* 3:28.

129. Rieder, J. (1973): A fluorimetric method for determining nitrazepam and the sum of its main metabolites in plasma and urine. *Arzneim. Forsch.,* 23:207–211.

130. Rieder, J. (1973): Plasma levels and derived pharmacokinetic characteristics of unchanged nitrazepam in man. *Arzneim. Forsch.,* 23:212–218.

131. Rieder, J., and Wendt, G. (1973): Pharmacokinetics and metabolism of the hypnotic nitrazepam. In: *The Benzodiazepines,* edited by S. Garattini, E. Mussini, and L. Randall, pp. 99–127. Raven Press, New York.

132. Rosen, G. M., Rauckman, E. J., Wilson, R. L., and Tschanz, C. (1984): Production of superoxide during the metabolism of nitrazepam. *Xenobiotica,* 14:785–794.

133. Rudolf, M., Geddes, D. M., Turner, J. A., and Saunders, K. B. (1978): Depression of central respiratory drive by nitrazepam. *Thorax,* 33:97–100.

134. Saario, I., Linnoila, M., and Maki, M. (1975): Interaction of drugs with alcohol on human psychomotor skills related to driving: Effect of sleep deprivation or two weeks' treatment with hypnotics. *J. Clin. Pharmacol.,* 15:52–59.

135. Sawada, H., and Hara, A. (1976): Novel metabolite of nitrazepam in the rabbit urine. *Experientia,* 32:987–988.

136. Saxen, I., and Saxen, L. (1975): Association between maternal intake of diazepam and oral clefts. *Lancet,* 2:498.

137. Shalleck, W., Thomas, J., Kuehn, A., and Zabransky, F. (1965): Effects of Mogadon on responses to stimulation of sciatic nerve, amygdala and hypothalamus of cat. *Int. J. Neuropharmacol.,* 4:317–326.

138. Silverman, G., and Braithwaite, R. A. (1973): Benzodiazepines and tricyclic antidepressant plasma levels. *Br. Med. J.,* 3:18–20.

139. Snyder, C. H. (1968): Myoclonic epilepsy in children: Short-term comparative study of two benzodiazepine derivatives in treatment. *South Med. J.,* 61:17–20.

140. Snyder, S. H., and Enna, S. J. (1975): The role of central glycine receptors in the pharmacologic actions of benzodiazepines. *Adv. Biochem. Psychopharmacol.,* 14:81–91.

141. Speight, A. N. P. (1977): Floppy infant syndrome and maternal diazepam and/or nitrazepam. *Lancet,* 2:878.

142. Speirs, C. J., Wavey, F. L., Brooks, D. J., and Impallomeni, M. G. (1986): Opisthotonos and benzodiazepine withdrawal in the elderly. *Lancet,* 2:1101.

143. Stein, L., Wise, C. D., and Belluzzi, J. D. (1975): Effects of benzodiazepines on central serotonergic mechanisms. *Adv. Biochem. Psychopharmacol.,* 14:29–44.

144. Sternbach, L. H., Fryer, R. I., Keller, O., Metlesics, W., Sach, G., and Steiger, N. (1963): Quinazolines and 1-4 benzodiazepines. X. Nitro-substituted 5-phenyl-1,4-benzodiazepine derivatives. *J. Med. Pharm. Chem.,* 6:261–265.

145. Stevenson, I. H. (1977): Factors influencing antipyrine elimination. *Br. J. Clin. Pharmacol.,* 4:261–265.

146. Stevenson, I. H., Browning, M., Crooks, J., and O'Malley, K. (1972): Changes in human drug metabolism after long-term exposure to hypnotics. *Br. Med. J.,* 4:322–324.

147. Stone, W. E., and Javid, M. J. (1978): Benzodiazepines and phenobarbital as antagonists of dissimilar chemical convulsants. *Epilepsia,* 19:361–368.

148. Swade, C., Milln, P., and Coppen, A. (1981): The effect of nitrazepam and other hypnotics on platelet 5-HT uptake. *Br. J. Clin. Pharmacol.,* 12:588–590.

149. Swinyard, A., and Castellion, A. W. (1966): Anticonvulsant properties of some benzodiazepines. *J. Pharmacol. Exp. Ther.,* 151:369–375.

150. Taberner, P. V., Roberts, C. J. C., Shrosbree, E., Pycock, C. J., and English, L. (1983): An investigation into the interaction between ethanol at low doses and the benzodiazepines nitrazepam and temazepam on psychomotor performance in normal subjects. *Psychopharmacology,* 81:321–326.

151. Tada, K., Miyahira, A., and Moroji, T. (1987): Liquid chromatographic assay of nitrazepam and its main metabolites in serum, and its application to pharmacokinetic study in the elderly. *J. Liq. Chromatogr.,* 10:465–476.

152. Tanayama, S., Momose, S., and Kanai, Y. (1974): Comparative studies on the metabolic disposition of 8-chloro-6-phenyl-4H-S-triazolo[4,3-α][1,4] benzodiazepine (D-40TA) and nitrazepam after single and repeated administration in rats. *Xenobiotica,* 4:229–236.

153. Tassinari, C. A., Dravet, C., Roger, J., Cano, J. P., and Gastaut, H. (1972): Tonic status epilepticus precipitated by intravenous benzodiazepine in five patients with Lennox-Gastaut syndrome. *Epilepsia,* 13:421–435.

154. Taylor, F. (1973): Nitrazepam and the elderly. *Br. Med. J.,* 1:113–114.

155. Taylor, K. M., and Laverty, R. (1969): The effect of chlordiazepoxide, diazepam and nitrazepam on catecholamine metabolism in regions of the rat brain. *Eur. J. Pharmacol.,* 8:296–301.

156. Tedeschi, G., Griffiths, A. N., Smith, A. T., and Richens, A. (1985): The effect of repeated doses of temazepam and nitrazepam on human psychomotor performance. *Br. J. Clin. Pharmacol.,* 20:361–367.

157. Vanasse, M., and Geoffroy, G. (1980): Treatment of epilepsy with nitrazepam. In: *Advances in Epilepsy: Xth Epilepsy International Symposium,* edited by J. A. Wada and J. K. Penry, p. 503. Raven Press, New York.

158. Vanasse, M., Masson, P., Geoffroy, G., Larbrisseau, A., and Favid, P. C. (1984): Intermittent treatment of febrile convulsions with nitrazepam. *Can. J. Neurol. Sci.,* 11:377–379.

159. Volzke, E., Doose, H., and Stephan, E. (1967): The treatment of infantile spasms and hypsarrhythmia with Mogadon. *Epilepsia,* 8:64–70.

160. Wambebe, C. (1985): Influence of some agents that affect 5-hydroxytryptamine metabolism and receptors on nitrazepam induced sleep in mice. *Br. J. Pharmacol.,* 84:185–191.

161. Wyllie, E., Wyllie, R., Cruse, R. P., Rothner, A. D., and Eremberg, G. (1986): The mechanism of nitrazepam-induced drooling and aspiration. *N. Engl. J. Med.,* 314:35–38.

162. Yanagi, Y., Haga, F., Endo, M., and Kitagawa, S. (1975): Comparative metabolic study of nimetazepam and its desmethyl derivative (nitrazepam) in rats. *Xenobiotica,* 5:245–257.

163. Zilli, M. A., and Nisi, G. (1986): Simple and sensitive method for the determination of clobazam, clonazepam and nitrazepam in human serum by high-performance liquid chromatography. *J. Chromatogr.,* 378:492–497.

Antiepileptic Drugs, Third Edition, edited by
R. Levy, R. Mattson, B. Meldrum,
J. K. Penry, and F. E. Dreifuss.
Raven Press, Ltd., New York © 1989.

58

Benzodiazepines

Clorazepate

Alan J. Wilensky and Patrick N. Friel

Clorazepate dipotassium (Tranxene) is a pro-drug which is converted to the active antiepileptic drug *N*-desmethyldiazepam (DMD). Clorazepate, in acid solution, is rapidly decarboxylated to form DMD (2,64). In man, although not in some other species, this reaction is usually rapid and complete so that after oral administration of clorazepate to man, mainly DMD is found in serum (2,3,5,10,13). *N*-desmethyldiazepam is also a major metabolite of several benzodiazepines, including diazepam. Although diazepam given intravenously is effective against status epilepticus, it is not very useful for the long-term treatment of seizure disorders. The ineffectiveness of diazepam may be secondary to its rapid distribution phase and the delayed appearance, in relatively low levels, of its primary metabolite, DMD. *N*-desmethyldiazepam provides a major portion of the pharmacologic activity when diazepam is given for a prolonged period (37,44). However, attempts to achieve adequate serum levels of DMD with orally administered diazepam are complicated by the rapid peak and short distribution times of diazepam. These attempts produce episodes of acute toxicity if a few large doses are given daily, or an overly demanding medication schedule if multiple small doses are given (75). In contrast, clorazepate provides a means of producing high and stable levels of DMD in the body. Clorazepate has been used since the mid 1960s as an antianxiety agent (75). In addition, it is approved for use in the symptomatic relief of acute alcohol withdrawal and as adjunctive therapy for management of partial seizures.

CHEMISTRY

Clorazepate dipotassium, 7-chloro-1,3-dihydro-2-oxo-5-phenyl-1H-1,4-benzodiazepine-3-carboxylic acid, monopotassium salt, monopotassium hydroxide (Fig. 1), is an off-white to pale yellow, fine, crystalline powder with a molecular weight of 408.93. It does not have a definite melting range but discolors at about 215°C, shrinks between 225° and 235°C, and decomposes between 235° and 295°C (62). The ultraviolet absorption spectrum of clorazepate in aqueous solution has been studied extensively and shows the characteristic benzodiazepine peaks at 230 and 250 nm (78). In contrast to both diazepam and DMD, which are essentially insoluble in water, the solubility of clorazepate is between 100 and 200 mg/ml. Solubilities in ethanol and isopropanol are 0.6 and 0.7 mg/ml, respectively, and in organic solvents solubility is less than 0.5 mg/ml (62).

Schmitt et al. (72) originally synthesized clorazepate in 1955. At pH levels of 4 or

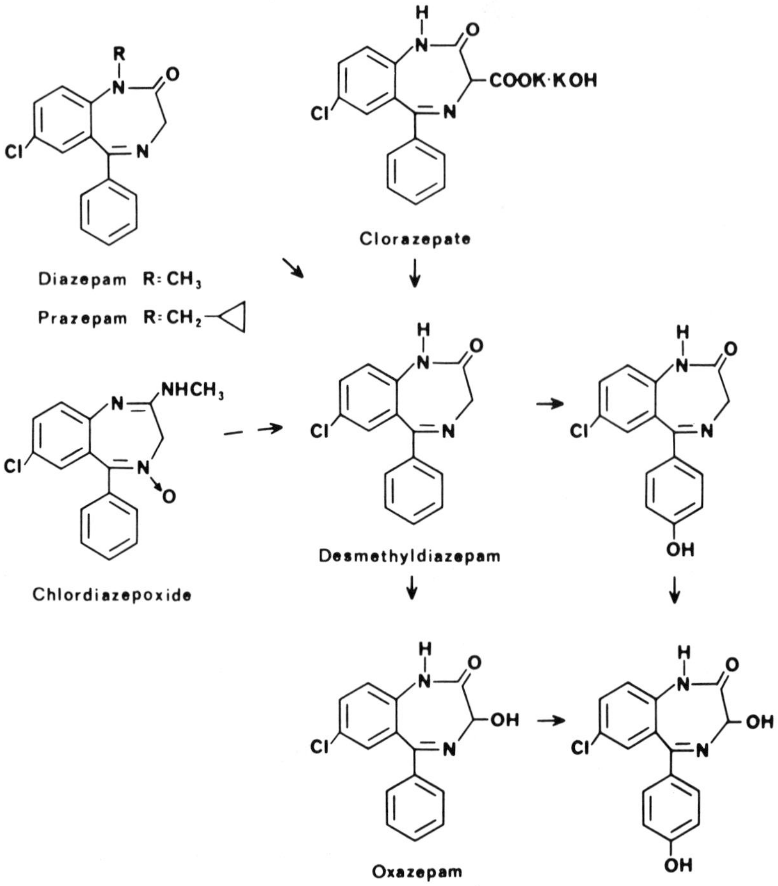

FIG. 1. Metabolic pathways involving clorazepate and *N*-desmethyldiazepam. All three hydroxylated compounds are excreted as conjugates, primarily glucuronides.

less more than 90% is converted to DMD within 10 min. The rate of degradation decreases with increasing pH. At pH 5, 20 min is required for 90% conversion and at pH 6, 50% is converted to DMD in an hour. Clorazepate is more stable in blood at physiological pH, with approximately 33% hydrolyzed to DMD in 24 hours (2,64).

METHODS OF DETERMINATION

Because clorazepate is converted rapidly in the stomach to DMD, the active medication in the blood, most analytical methods are for DMD. The methods of determination involve thin-layer chromatography (TLC), electron capture gas chromatography (GLC/EC), and high-performance liquid chromatography (HPLC). In addition, polaragraphic methodologies have been used in *in vitro* studies of stability (2,78), and a radioimmune assay has been described (19). Initial studies of clorazepate utilized a colorimetric analysis using the Bratton-Marshall reaction following hydrolysis of clorazepate and/or DMD to 2-amino-5-chlorobenzophenone (28). Both clorazepate and DMD can be identified using various mobile phases on TLC either as themselves or after hydrolysis to 2-amino-5-chlorobenzophenone. Care must be taken if clorazepate and DMD are to be separated in these procedures because clorazepate may be degraded to DMD (19,62,64).

More useful and sensitive are the subsequently developed GLC methodologies. The original methodology of De Silva, which was subsequently modified by Hoffman and Chun (34), involves hydrolysis of clorazepate and/or DMD to 2-amino-5-chlorobenzophenone. Later, many procedures were developed utilizing direct assay of DMD and much simpler extraction procedures (10,13,24,31,63). The majority of these procedures have used GLC/EC because of increased sensitivity, but GLC using a nitrogen detector has been described (17). Although relatively simple and precise, GLC assays may be associated with problems with peak symmetry and tailing as well as interferences by other drugs and endogenous substances. Many of these problems can be avoided by precise attention to detail and elaborate preconditioning of the columns, but these standards are difficult to maintain except in research facilities.

The more recently described HPLC methodologies with ultraviolet detection are easier to perform (14,35,58,63). Peaks tend to be more symmetrical and there are fewer interferences. These assays also offer the ability to simultaneously analyze other benzodiazepines such as diazepam, oxazepam, nitrazepam, and chlordiazepoxide without interference or decomposition. Because of these advantages the HPLC assays appear to be somewhat more sensitive than GLC assays, one report quoting analytical sensitivity to 1 ng/ml (14).

These methods measure total clorazepate plus DMD concentrations because clorazepate is converted to DMD during analysis. Special extraction procedures are required to quantitate the compounds separately (10,13,14,34,67).

PHARMACOKINETICS AND METABOLISM

The kinetics of clorazepate have been studied in normal subjects after parenteral and oral administration. The time of peak concentration is approximately 1 hr (T_{max}) after oral administration and 1.4 hr after intramuscular administration. Elimination half-life is approximately 2 hr. The apparent volume of distribution (V_d) is 0.33 liter/kg, significantly less than the value for DMD, a much less polar compound. Total clearance of clorazepate ranges from 1 to 1.8 ml/hr/kg (10,67,80). Clearance is almost doubled in women approaching the end of pregnancy (67).

The pharmacokinetics of DMD derived from both diazepam and clorazepate have been extensively investigated. Table 1 summarizes the pharmacokinetic parameters of DMD derived from orally administered clorazepate.

Biotransformation

Clorazepate is decarboxylated in the acid of the stomach to DMD (2,3,5,10,13). In other species, particularly the dog where the gastric pH is more neutral, appreciable plasma levels of the parent drug can be detected (34). In any case, decarboxylation continues in the blood so that almost all administered drug is eventually converted to DMD even if clorazepate is given parenterally, bypassing the acid of the stomach (3,67). *N*-Desmethyldiazepam is central to the metabolism of many benzodiazepines (Fig. 1). It is the major metabolite of diazepam and one of the metabolites of chlordiazepoxide (19,75). *N*-Desmethyldiazepam is further metabolized by hydroxylation either in the C-3 position, forming oxazepam, or in the *para* position of the C-5 phenyl group. Both these compounds may be further hydroxylated to the

TABLE 1. N-Desmethyldiazepam kinetics after clorazepate administration

Subjects	Age (yr)	Sex	Dose[a] (mg)	Lag time (hr)	T_{max} (hr)	$T_{1/2abs}$ (hr)	V_d (L/kg)	$t_{1/2\beta}$ (hr)	Cl (ml/min/kg)	Ref.
Control	24–74	M, F	15	0.40	1.5	0.94	0.94	57	0.20	1
Obese	23–61	M, F	15	0.20	1.3	0.48	1.52	154	0.14	
Control	27–55	M	15	0.31	1.02	0.07	1.06	65	0.19	13
Control	24–39	—	15	—	—	—	0.75	48	0.18	18
	61–78	—	15	—	—	—	1.29	96	0.17	
Control	23–28	M	20	—	—	—	1.17	55	0.27	52
Smokers	22–79	M	20	—	—	—	1.38	30	0.73	
Control	21–66	M, F	20 IV	0.21	0.9	0.31	1.24	65	0.24	54
			20 IM	0.03	2.7	0.68	—	67	—	
			20	—	—	—	—	62	—	
Control	22–38	M, F	20 IM	—	—	—	1.13	53	—	60
		F	20 × 14 days	—	—	—	1.45	66	—	
		M		—	—	—	0.97	46	—	
Control	21–31	F	20 IM	0.25	11	—	1.8	60	0.43	67
Pregnancy	19–38	F	20 IM	—	11	—	3.1	180	0.37	
Control	23–70	M, F	15	Average for all	1.8	0.25	1.05	64	—	74
Control	23–39	M	15	0.23	1.42	0.41	1.28	83	0.22	76
	26–38	F	15	—	0.88	0.41	1.24	120	0.21	
	64–76	M	15	—	2.14	0.49	1.54	72	0.15	
	56–85	F	15	—	1.48	0.38	—	—	0.27	
Patients	21–41	M, F	0.3 mg/kg	0.25	0.75	—	1.58	39	0.49	86
	21–41	M, F	0.6 mg/kg × 6 days	—	1.0	—	1.63	40	0.48	•
Control	22–47	M, F	10	0.37	1.33	0.21	1.05	57	0.22	88

a Doses are single oral doses unless otherwise indicated.

dihydroxy compound and all of these last three appear in the urine as conjugates (65,66).

Absorption

Clorazepate is available as tablets and capsules with rapid dissolution times, and as a slow release preparation. T_{max} of DMD ranges from 0.5 to 2 hr after ingestion of clorazepate by persons with normal gastric pH (1,3,13,53,74,76,86,88). In contrast, peak time for the slow release tablet, designed for once a day administration, is approximately 12 hr (12). After ingestion there is a lag of 15 to 25 min before DMD appears in the serum and is then rapidly absorbed with a first-order absorption half-life of approximately 20 min (13,74,86,88). This is most likely due to the time required for release and dispersion of clorazepate from the ingested preparation, its decarboxylation, and the subsequent absorption of DMD. Small quantities of clorazepate are absorbed directly from the stomach even at low pH. Peak levels of clorazepate are reached 0.5 to 2 hr after its ingestion and are approximately 15% to 25% those of DMD at the same time postingestion (1,10,13).

The effective dose (ED_{50}) of clorazepate given intravenously in terms of anti-pentylenetetrazol activity in mice is approximately 100 times as great as that of DMD (3). Thus, it is essential that clorazepate be converted to DMD to provide significant therapeutic effect. Since low gastric pH is required for rapid conversion of clorazepate to DMD, any condition that maintains gastric pH at high levels could alter the therapeutic efficacy of clorazepate. Thus, the decreased absorption of DMD by patients who had received abdominal and/or pelvic radiation therapy was possibly due to reduced gastric acidity (79). Abruzzo et al. (3) determined serum clorazepate and DMD levels after single doses in normal subjects

at normal gastric pH and after increasing the pH to greater than 6 with sodium bicarbonate. At the high pH, the peak time for DMD levels increased to between 2 and 24 hr. The maximum serum level decreased by 14% to 46% as compared to control circumstances. The area under the curve over 72 hr was reduced by 5% to 75%. Similar but somewhat less marked changes in the rate of DMD absorption have been shown by two groups using magnesium-aluminum hydroxide to raise gastric pH (13,74). The extent of the effects seems to be related to the dose of antacid used. Neither of the latter two studies measured gastric pH, and the greater effect with sodium bicarbonate may relate to the higher pH maintained during that study.

These findings suggest that the clinical effect of clorazepate might be significantly altered in situations of reduced gastric acidity. Indeed, Shader et al. (74) showed that after a single dose of clorazepate there were changes in self-rated clinical effects in healthy volunteers when clorazepate was administered with antacids. However, after long-term administration of clorazepate, DMD levels in subjects treated with antacids did not differ from those in controls (73). The absorption phase was not evaluated in these subjects but the data suggest that with long-term treatment the extent of conversion of clorazepate to DMD may be similar in the presence or absence of antacids. Ochs et al. (53) also found that low gastric pH is not essential to the appearance of DMD in the serum after ingestion of clorazepate. After single doses of clorazepate in patients following Billroth gastrectomies, plasma concentrations did not differ from those in age-matched controls without gastrointestinal disease. However, age had a significant effect on absorption. Peak DMD concentrations and area under the curve were significantly lower in elderly patients and elderly controls than in young controls, and time to peak concentration was somewhat prolonged, although not significantly so. These data suggest that in the absence of gastric acid DMD levels after clorazepate administration peak more slowly, but that systemic availability is not impaired. Presumably, conversion of clorazepate to DMD occurs in sites other than the stomach, possibly in other portions of the gastrointestinal tract, in the serum, or in the hepatic portal circulation.

The extent of the bioavailability of DMD after oral administration of clorazepate has been studied by comparing concentrations and area under the curve after oral, intravenous, and intramuscular administration of clorazepate (54). Conversion to DMD is essentially complete. As expected, side effects occurred more rapidly and were more intense after oral than after intravenous administration, because DMD is formed more rapidly in the stomach after oral administration of clorazepate than it is in the blood after intravenous administration of clorazepate.

Distribution

Spontaneous hydrolysis of clorazepate to DMD makes it difficult to assess unchanged clorazepate distribution in body tissues. Thus, the available data relate primarily to the distribution of DMD, which is known in some detail.

Following absorption, DMD has a distribution phase with a half-life of 0.7 to 2.2 hr (13,76,86,88). N-Desmethyldiazepam is extensively bound to plasma protein. In healthy adults the free fraction ranges from about 1.7% to 5.3%, with a mean of about 3.0% (4,36,39,69,76). Since binding is largely to serum albumin, the percent bound is directly related to serum albumin concentration and therefore free fraction declines with age (4,76). As with many other drugs, salivary concentrations of DMD reflect the serum free fraction with a mean saliva-to-serum ratio of 0.027 and a range of 0.014 to 0.047 [unpublished data from Wilensky et al. (87)].

In animals DMD rapidly crosses the blood-brain barrier and equilibrates in cerebrospinal fluid (CSF) with free serum concentration (25). Clinical data are limited because of the time lag between drug administration and time of lumbar puncture. However, by 2 hr after an intramuscular injection of diazepam, CSF and free plasma concentrations of DMD are equal (36). With prolonged exposure to DMD, it may accumulate in the CSF. Various studies of DMD distribution in experimental animals suggest that this may reflect increased binding of DMD to myelin lipids (32,59).

Although DMD tissue distribution in experimental animals is well described, there is only one study of its tissue distribution in humans. Friedman et al. (22) studied diazepam and DMD distribution at autopsy in 14 patients who had been treated with either diazepam or CZP. The highest DMD concentrations were found in the adrenal gland, liver, and heart with ratios relative to concentrations in skeletal muscle of 14.4, 6.9, and 3.8, respectively. Intermediate concentrations were found in the kidney, brain, and lung, the brain having a ratio of 1.8. Lowest concentrations were found in skeletal muscle and fat, with fat concentrations being approximately 0.9 relative to muscle. The low concentration in adipose tissue is to be expected given the relative polarity of DMD. Because skeletal muscle and fat make up a major percentage of body mass, one can calculate that in spite of low concentrations, approximately 53% of the tissue stores of DMD in a healthy man are in the skeletal muscle and 18% in fat. Another 17% is in the liver and 5% in the brain.

The V_d of DMD in most subjects varies from about 1 to 1.8 liter/kg (Table 1) (1,18,52,60,67,76,86,88). The single most important factor altering V_d is the degree of body fat. In obese individuals, V_d, on a liter per kilogram basis, is approximately 1.6 times that in normal controls, probably secondary to the increased storage of DMD in body fat. Although there is no change in clearance, this results in a prolongation of the apparent half-life of elimination from 57 to 154 hr (1). Thus, loading doses of clorazepate should take into account the degree of obesity of the patient being treated. Late in pregnancy there is a similar increase in V_d of DMD to approximately 1.6 times the value in nonpregnant women. This too is associated with prolongation of the elimination half-life with no change in clearance values (67). Age and sex also alter the V_d; it increases with age and is greater in women at all ages than in men (60,76). These findings probably reflect the greater percentage of fat to lean body mass in women.

In pregnant women, DMD is transported rapidly across the placenta to the fetus. Clorazepate crosses more slowly and requires 4 hr to equilibrate because of its more polar nature (29,68). Amniotic fluid concentrations of DMD are low and reflect the free serum level (68). DMD also enters breast milk and reaches a concentration approximately 15% to 30% of the maternal level. Despite the newborn's low ability to eliminate DMD, serum concentrations in the newborn are minimal and of no clinical importance unless the mother is receiving very high doses of a DMD precursor (9,68).

Food intake also affects the distribution of DMD. Serum concentration of DMD rises after each meal. With clorazepate administration to epileptic patients, serum DMD concentration increased after meals following a single dose and during prolonged dosing (86). Similar postprandial increases in serum concentrations occur for both diazepam and DMD derived from diazepam (42,51). This increase is clinically important since it can result in a sufficient increase in DMD levels after a meal to produce somnolence. Both enterohepatic cycling and altered protein binding secondary to increased free fatty acids have been suggested to explain this phenomenon, but neither seems to satisfactorily account for the changes (86). Redistribution from the large

tissue-bound pool of drug may be responsible but there is no satisfactory explanation for such a redistribution.

A recent report describes the presence of endogenous DMD in brains of animals and humans who had never received benzodiazepines. The concentrations were sufficient to be pharmacologically active (70). Further research is needed in this area.

Elimination

The conversion of clorazepate to DMD and subsequent metabolism of DMD have been described above (see Fig. 1). After a single dose of clorazepate its biotransformation products are slowly excreted. Approximately 10 days after dosing, metabolites accounting for approximately 1% of the administered dose can still be recovered from the urine over a 24-hr period. Approximately 5% to 9% of the dose is recovered as unchanged DMD. Over half of the remainder is conjugated oxazepam and another quarter is conjugated parahydroxy DMD. Between 15% and 20% of the orally administered dose can be recovered in the feces over the same 10 days (5,65,80). In view of data demonstrating virtually total bioavailability of DMD after oral administration of clorazepate the fecal metabolites probably are due to biliary secretion rather than incomplete absorption. After oral administration of clorazepate less than 1% of the recovered dose in the urine is in the form of clorazepate. In contrast, when clorazepate is given either intravenously or intramuscularly, approximately 7% of the dose is recovered as the parent compound (80).

N-Desmethyldiazepam has a long elimination half-life, which in normal controls varies from 55 to 100 hr (1,18,52,60,76,88). Because of the long elimination half-life, it appears that clorazepate could be administered once a day without an excessive fall in serum levels. However, because of the rapid absorption, relatively high peak concentrations occur after each dose, and toxicity may result if a whole day's dose is given at once. Therefore, the daily dose should be divided or a slow release preparation utilized.

A number of physiological and pathological conditions alter the elimination half-life. As discussed above, half-life is prolonged in late pregnancy and obesity secondary to the increased V_d. There is no significant change in clearance (1,67). In elderly men, but not older women, the elimination half-life is prolonged and clearance reduced. Apparently, there is a decrease in the ability of older men to oxidize DMD to oxazepam (76).

The elimination half-life for neonates ranges from 73 to 132 hr. Here too the long half-life is probably due to a poor ability to oxidize DMD (68). A similar prolongation of DMD half-life is seen in patients with liver disease (40). In situations where DMD elimination half-life is prolonged, the most important clinical effects are increased time to steady state and protracted washout after cessation of drug intake. Also, when clearance is reduced, lower doses are required to achieve a given serum level.

In contrast to the situation where elimination half-life is prolonged, any clinical state that results in enzyme induction in the liver, especially of the mixed-function oxidases, may increase clearance. Thus, smokers have an elimination half-life of 30 versus 55 hr in controls and clearance increases from 0.27 to 0.73 ml/min/kg. Peak serum concentrations are lower in smokers and there is less of a sedative effect (52). Similarly, DMD metabolism is increased in patients taking for prolonged periods antiepileptic drugs that induce microsomal enzymes. In epileptic patients, there is a trend toward shorter half-life and increased clearance compared to normal subjects. Patients receiving clorazepate for the treatment of epilepsy, especially in conjunction with other antiepileptic drugs, require higher doses of clorazepate than normal subjects to achieve a given serum level (86).

INTERACTIONS WITH OTHER DRUGS

As described above, several studies have evaluated the influence of concomitant antacid administration on DMD absorption following administration of clorazepate. Although the rate of absorption is slower and the peak concentrations of DMD are lower after a single dose of clorazepate administered with antacid, there does not seem to be any change in steady-state DMD levels when clorazepate is given for prolonged periods with antacid (2,13,73,74).

The presence of heparin affects DMD distribution. Free fraction and free concentration increase without a change in total drug levels. The mechanisms of this redistribution are complex and involve more than just displacement (69).

Although liver disease alters DMD kinetics, single doses of alcohol taken with clorazepate do not alter clorazepate levels. There is, however, a pharmacodynamic effect. The typical alcohol euphoric effect is enhanced by clorazepate approximately 90 min after ingestion of the two drugs. In contrast, taking clorazepate with alcohol prevents the dysphoric symptoms induced by alcohol the following morning. Thus, clorazepate seems to enhance, through its anxiolytic effect, disinhibition produced by alcohol while at the same time reducing the subsequent hangover (81).

Induction of DMD metabolism by smoking and antiepileptic drugs is discussed above (52). No reciprocal effect on the metabolism of other antiepileptic drugs has been described. Also, any compound inhibiting the mixed-function oxidases will slow the hydroxylation of DMD. Thus, cimetidine significantly increases DMD half-life while decreasing metabolic clearance in both young and old subjects. It also delays the appearance of DMD in the blood, possibly secondary to its reduction of gastric acidity (18,41). These effects must be taken into account whenever cimetidine is given to a patient receiving clorazepate.

If possible, the combination of clorazepate plus barbiturate should be avoided. Feldman (20) described personality changes characterized by depression, irritability, and aggressive behavior in 8 of 17 patients treated with more than 22.5 mg per day of clorazepate. Four of these eight became very hostile and "difficult to live with." Six of the eight were being treated with primidone in combination with clorazepate. One of the other two was receiving phenobarbital and phenytoin and the other methsuximide. Only one of the nine patients who did not exhibit these symptoms was receiving primidone. The mechanism for this effect is unknown but it may be related to excessive sedation or disinhibition by the combination of barbiturate and benzodiazepine.

MECHANISMS OF ACTION

The mechanisms of action of benzodiazepines in general are discussed in detail in Chapter 54. The following discussion is limited to issues related specifically to DMD. Like other benzodiazepines, DMD binds to brain benzodiazepine receptors. Binding to the high affinity (nanomolar) receptor described by Möhler and Okada (49) increases the inhibitory action of γ-aminobutyric acid (GABA) by increasing the number of chloride channels which are opened in response to any given concentration of GABA. This action is correlated with antimyoclonic and antianxiety effects in humans as well as activity against pentylenetetrazol-induced seizures in experimental animals (46). The affinity of DMD for this receptor is approximately an order of magnitude less than that of diazepam and 30 times less than that for clonazepam. Thus, relatively higher doses of DMD than diazepam are required to produce antianxiety effects, and DMD is clearly less potent than clonazepam in controlling myoclonic movements or absence seizures in patients.

N-Desmethyldiazepam shows a relatively higher affinity for the micromolar benzodiazepine binding site described by Bowling and DeLorenzo (8). Binding to this low affinity site seems to correlate with antimaximal electroshock seizure activity, which in turn predicts for activity against generalized tonic-clonic and partial seizures. The recent study of Stéru et al. (82) in mice is consistent with these findings, indicating that the ED_{50} of DMD in the maximal electroshock test is much lower than that seen when it is tested in models of sedation, muscle relaxant, and anxiolytic effects. In fact, DMD seems to be the most specific of the 1,4-benzodiazepines in protection against maximal electroshock seizures (82). Similarly, DMD is effective in blocking kindled seizures in various animal models, a property which suggests activity against partial seizures (84). All these findings are consistent with the clinical reports of effectiveness against generalized tonic-clonic and partial seizures. Affinity to the nanomolar as opposed to micromolar receptor seems also to predict for the development of tolerance to benzodiazepines (46) and, in mice and dogs, tolerance is slower to develop for clorazepate than for other benzodiazepines (21,71). This relative resistance to development of tolerance has also been seen in some clinical studies with clorazepate (47).

CLINICAL USE

Clorazepate was initially introduced in the mid 1960s as an antianxiety agent. Several double-blind studies compared the antianxiety effect of clorazepate with that of diazepam. In general, when large enough doses were given, the antianxiety effect of clorazepate was as good as, and in some cases better than, diazepam's, with fewer side effects. In addition, clorazepate is effective when used as an antispasmodic agent in cases of tetanus and reduces spasticity in patients with chronic neurological diseases such as multiple sclerosis (5).

The first trial of clorazepate in epilepsy was published in the 1960s (48), followed by numerous case reports, several open add-on trials, and one large double-blind study with clorazepate. Evaluation of clorazepate efficacy has been difficult for several reasons. Classification of seizures varies among the studies, especially in the earlier trials. Some studies report each seizure type separately for the same patient so that the number of responses equals the number of seizure types for all the patients. Also, the description of the responses is usually qualitative and in some studies quite vague. Table 2 summarizes the results of most of the published studies of clorazepate in epilepsy.

Miribel and Marinier (48) added four different benzodiazepines to the drug regimens of 61 children aged 6 to 14 years with severe generalized seizures; 11 received

clorazepate. The authors concluded that clorazepate had little anticonvulsant effect. Booker (7) used clorazepate in 59 patients with various seizure types. Best results were obtained in patients with generalized seizures, especially seizure types other than generalized tonic-clonic seizures. Although two patients with simple partial seizures showed marked improvement, none of the 14 with complex partial seizures was considered improved. Initial control was obtained in 6 of these 14 patients, but seizures recurred in 3 to 6 months. Feldman (20) reported a "definite decrease in seizure frequency" in an unknown percentage of 17 patients with temporal lobe seizures who received clorazepate. However, Livingston et al. (43) had disappointing results with the drug in 65 patients with various seizure types, including complex partial seizures. In an open pilot study of eight patients with intractable epilepsy, three of seven with complex partial seizures taking phenytoin

TABLE 2. *Clinical trials of clorazepate in epilepsy*

Seizure type	Response to clorazepate (# of patients)			Reference
	None/ worse	Partial response	Marked improvement	
Generalized	28	7	20	6
Tonic-clonic	12	1	3	7
	4	11	4	47
Total (percent)	44 (49)	19 (21)	27 (30)	
Other generalized seizure	34	9	5	6
types	19	3	16	7
	4	10	9	23[a]
	10	9	6	47
	0	1	0	83
Total (percent)	67 (50)	32 (23)	36 (27)	
Partial seizures	13	6	4	6
	14	0	2	7
	22	6	3	16
	0	1	3	27
	1	1	1	47
	4	3	0	83
	20	18	2	87
Total (percent)	74 (60)	35 (28)	15 (12)	

[a] Data for 23 patients are from unpublished communication. Data in the reference describes 18 patients; 13 improved, 5 markedly.

Note also reference 30. Forty-two of 75 patients with partial seizures had marked improvement and 7 of 23 with generalized seizures had marked improvement.

and phenobarbital improved when clorazepate was substituted for the phenobarbital (83). When Berchou et al. (6) added clorazepate to the regimens of 61 patients with various seizure types, 23% of the patients improved, but improvement was not related to seizure type. Similar results were reported by Dasheiff et al. (16), who found that 29% of subjects with intractable complex partial seizures responded to clorazepate but that the result was not long-lasting. Griffith and Murray (27) described four patients with complex partial seizures with psychic symptomatology who were completely controlled when relatively low doses of clorazepate were added to their regimens.

In contrast with the pessimistic original report of the effect of clorazepate in children with intractable seizures (48), three recent papers have reported excellent results. In two studies (23,47), patients with generalized seizures had improved seizure control in 85% and 75% of cases, respectively. The third study (30) found excellent results in 85% of patients with partial epilepsy and in only 15% of those with generalized epilepsy. Fifteen patients achieved excellent seizure control with clorazepate as monotherapy; three of these had generalized epilepsy and 12 partial epilepsy. Of seven patients with Lennox-Gastaut syndrome, five had a transient initial benefit without long-term improvement.

All the above studies were open add-on trials. Only one double-blind study has been performed (87). The antiepileptic effect of clorazepate plus phenytoin was compared with the effect of phenobarbital plus phenytoin in patients with partial seizures. Thirty of 42 subjects preferred the clorazepate plus phenytoin regimen. There was no statistically significant difference in seizure control between the two drug regimens, but the data are consistent with a clinical decrease in total, simple, and complete partial seizures with clorazepate. With secondarily generalized seizures, the trend was toward more seizures with clorazepate. Subjects with many seizures (more than 20 per month) had significantly fewer seizures with clorazepate. Of the 29 patients who remained on clorazepate after the study, 25 were still taking it 6 months later, and at last contact, 6 to 28 months after the study, 22 remained on the drug. Seizure incidence was unchanged in 18 of the 22 patients and decreased in four with adjustment of the clorazepate dose. Six of the seven patients who had discontinued the drug were having more seizures.

The nature of the available data makes it difficult to assess the place of clorazepate in the treatment of specific seizure types. For every study demonstrating a positive effect, an example of a study which does not show any effect can be cited. It is clear that clorazepate, as an add-on drug and as monotherapy, is effective in some patients with partial seizures. However, it appears to be slightly more effective in patients with generalized seizure types, especially primary generalized tonic-clonic attacks. These equivocal results are not unexpected given the intractable nature of the patients in whom clorazepate was tested and the fact that, except in one study, it was used exclusively as an add-on medication.

The tentative conclusions drawn from these studies is that clorazepate is useful in treating patients with complex partial seizures, especially those with high seizure frequencies and psychic disturbances. There is some evidence that it may be more effective in children than in adults.

The starting dose of clorazepate is usually 0.3 mg/kg per day, and subsequent doses range from 0.4 to 3 mg/kg per day. The higher doses, as for most drugs, are used in children, with the average adult dose being 0.5 to 1 mg/kg per day. Doses substantially lower than this were used in some of the studies that found the drug apparently ineffective. Serum clorazepate levels between 0.5 and 2.0 µg/ml are associated with the best responses, but the therapeutic range is not well defined (7,83,87).

ADVERSE EFFECTS

The most common side effects of clorazepate therapy for epilepsy are sedation, lethargy, ataxia, and, in children, drooling (7,16,23,30,83,87). However, clorazepate appears to be less sedating than diazepam and other benzodiazepines used to treat epilepsy. These effects, especially sedation and lethargy, tend to clear after treatment with clorazepate for 1 to 2 weeks (6,26,47). In normal volunteers, clorazepate impairs measures of attention and reaction time (50). Patients may complain of memory problems, nervousness, depression, irritability, and concentration difficulties. Adverse personality changes, especially irritability, can occur, particularly when clorazepate is combined with primidone and may require stopping the drug (20,30). In nonepileptic patients treated with clorazepate, rage reactions have been reported (38). All these reactions appear to be dose-related and are characteristic of the benzodiazepines.

Patients receiving long-term administration of clorazepate may tolerate large overdoses without loss of consciousness. We have observed DMD levels of 10 μg/ml in patients who have overdosed but remained conscious with ataxia. Treatment of an overdose consists of general supportive care and close observation. On occasion, treatment of hypotension may be required. Recent reports indicate that benzodiazepine antagonists may be useful in treating acute benzodiazepine overdosage (55).

Idiosyncratic and allergic reactions rarely occur with benzodiazepines. There has been one report of hepatic necrosis (56) and one of an esophageal burn associated with clorazepate therapy (45). There also has been a single case of skin blistering and sweat gland necrosis in a patient who overdosed with amitriptyline and clorazepate (33).

Benzodiazepines may be mildly teratogenic (85). If clorazepate has the same teratogenic potential as other benzodiazepines, there may be a slight increased risk of cleft lip and/or cleft palate. A study in mice suggested an increased risk of cleft palate, but studies in rats did not find clorazepate to be teratogenic (15). One newborn child who died at 24 hr of age had multiple limb anomalies; the mother had taken a total of 23 clorazepate capsules during her first trimester (57). Newborns having prolonged exposure to clorazepate *in utero* may exhibit a floppy infant syndrome consisting of floppy movements, hypotonia, hypothermia, poor reflexes, low Apgar scores, and apnea (85). Benzodiazepine withdrawal has also been observed in newborns (85). It has been suggested that since the mother's breast milk contains substantial quantities of DMD, breast feeding could be used as a way to wean an infant gradually from the drug, assuming that the infant is not experiencing toxicity at the time of birth.

TOLERANCE AND WITHDRAWAL

Tolerance to the antiepileptic effects of benzodiazepines is a common problem. Animal models demonstrate that in situations where tolerance develops to diazepam and clonazepam, it is not apparent with long-term clorazepate therapy (21,71). These findings are consistent with results of some clorazepate clinical trials which suggest that tolerance may be less common than for other benzodiazepines, or that it develops very slowly. Patients have been treated successfully for over 2 years with no loss of drug effectiveness (87). However, a number of the clinical studies have reported early successful treatment with clorazepate with later recurrence of the seizures (7,16).

Consistent with the development of tolerance to benzodiazepines is the existence of a withdrawal syndrome that may involve development of psychosis (11,61). In addition, withdrawal seizures may occur. In nonepileptic patients who stop clorazepate abruptly this is rare (77). More commonly, exacerbation of seizures when it is reduced or withdrawn may occur in 5% to 10% of patients with epilepsy taking clorazepate. In the double-blind study of clorazepate withdrawal seizures occurred during the crossover from clorazepate to phenobarbital in two of the 42 patients.

SUMMARY

Clorazepate is a pro-drug which is decarboxylated by acid in the stomach to DMD, an active metabolite of diazepam. It is effective in selected patients with generalized or partial seizures. In patients with partial seizures it appears to be most effective in those with psychic symptomatology as well as those with very frequent seizures (>20/month).

N-Desmethyldiazepam derived from clorazepate is well absorbed after oral administration, with maximal levels within 0.5 to 2 hr. N-Desmethyldiazepam has a long half-life but because of its rapid absorption the daily dose should be divided to prevent absorption peaks, which can result in toxicity.

The primary adverse reaction is lethargy, to which tolerance frequently develops. Occasionally, adverse behavioral changes occur, especially in children. Life-threatening idiosyncratic and allergic reactions are rare. Abrupt decrease in dose or withdrawal of clorazepate should be avoided because of the possibility of withdrawal psychosis and/or seizures.

ACKNOWLEDGMENTS

This work was supported by grant #NS 17111 from the National Institute of Neurological and Communicative Disorders and Stroke. The contributions of all of those who have worked with clorazepate at the University of Washington Epilepsy Center, especially Drs. Allen S. Troupin, Linda M. Ojemann, Carl B. Dodrill, and René H. Levy are gratefully acknowledged.

CONVERSION

Conversion factor:

$$CF = \frac{1000}{\text{mol. wt.}} = \frac{1000}{408.93} = 2.45$$

Conversion:

$$(\mu g/ml) \times 2.45 = (\mu moles/liter)$$

$$(\mu moles/liter) \div 2.45 = (\mu g/ml)$$

REFERENCES

1. Abernethy, D. R., Greenblatt, D. J., Divoll, M., and Shader, R. I. (1982): Prolongation of drug half-life due to obesity: Studies of desmethyldiazepam (Clorazepate). *J. Pharm. Sci.,* 71:942–944.
2. Abruzzo, C. W., Brooks, M. A., Cotler, S., and Kaplan, S. A. (1976): Differential pulse polarographic assay procedure and *in vitro* biopharmaceutical properties of dipotassium clorazepate. *J. Pharmacokinet. Biopharm.,* 4:29–41.
3. Abruzzo, C. W., Macasieb, T., Weinfeld, R., Rider, J. A., and Kaplan, S. A. (1977): Changes in the oral absorption characteristics in man of dipotassium clorazepate at normal and elevated gastric pH. *J. Pharmacokinet. Biopharm.,* 5:377–390.
4. Allen, M. D., and Greenblatt, D. J. (1981): Comparative protein binding of diazepam and desmethyldiazepam. *J. Clin. Pharmacol.,* 21:219–223.
5. Bauer, F. B., Johnson, P. A., and Chebuhar, T. M. (1973): *Tranxene®* (*Clorazepate Dipotassium*) *Drug Monograph.* Abbott Laboratories, North Chicago.
6. Berchou, R. C., Rodin, E. A., and Russell, M. E. (1981): Clorazepate therapy for refractory seizures. *Neurology,* 31:1483–1485.
7. Booker, H. E. (1974): Clorazepate dipotassium in the treatment of intractable epilepsy. *J.A.M.A.,* 229:552–555.
8. Bowling, A. C., and DeLorenzo, R. J. (1982): Micromolar affinity benzodiazepine receptors: Identification and characterization in central nervous system. *Science,* 216:1247–1250.
9. Brandt, R. (1976): Passage of diazepam and desmethyldiazepam into breast milk. *Arzneim-Forsch.,* 26:454–457.
10. Brooks, M. A., Hackman, M. R., Weinfeld, R. E., and Macasieb, T. (1977): Determination of clorazepate and its major metabolites in blood and urine by electron capture gas-liquid chromatography. *J. Chromatogr.,* 135:123–131.
11. Busto, U., Sellers, E. M., Naranjo, C. A., Cappell,

H., Sanchez-Criag, M., and Sykora, K. (1986): Withdrawal reaction after long-term therapeutic use of benzodiazepines. *N. Engl. J. Med.,* 315:854–859.

12. Carrigan, P. J., Chao, G. C., Barker, W. M., Hoffman, D. J., and Chun, A. H. C. (1977): Steadystate bioavailability of two clorazepate dipotassium dosage forms. *J. Clin. Pharmacol.,* 17:18–28.

13. Chun, A. H. C., Carrigan, P. J., Hoffman, D. J., Kershner, R. P., and Stuart, J. D. (1977): Effect of antacids on absorption of clorazepate. *Clin. Pharmacol. Ther.,* 22:329–335.

14. Colin, P., Sirois, G., and Lelorier, J., (1983): High-performance liquid chromatography determination of dipotassium clorazepate and its major metabolite nordiazepam in plasma. *J. Chromatogr.,* 273:367–377.

15. Corwin, H., and DeMyer, W. (1980): Failure of clorazepate to cause malformations or fetal wastage in the rat. *Arch. Neurol.,* 37:347–349.

16. Dasheiff, R. M., McNamara, D., and Dickinson, L. (1986): Efficacy of second line antiepileptic drugs in the treatment of patients with medically refractive complex partial seizures. *Epilepsia,* 27:124–127.

17. Dhar, A. K., and Kutt, H. (1979): Monitoring diazepam and desmethyldiazepam concentrations in plasma by gas-liquid chromatography, with use of a nitrogen-sensitive detector. *Clin. Chem.,* 25:137–140.

18. Divoll, M., Greenblatt, D. J., Abernethy, D. R., and Shader, R. I. (1982): Cimetidine impairs clearance of antipyrine and desmethyldiazepam in the elderly. *J. Am. Geriat. Soc.,* 30:684–689.

19. Dixon, R., Brooks, M. A., Postma, E., Hackman, M. R., Spector, S., Moore, J. D., and Schwartz, M. A. (1976): *N*-Desmethyldiazepam: A new metabolite of chlordiazepoxide in man. *Clin. Pharmacol. Ther.,* 20:450–457.

20. Feldman, R. G. (1976): Clorazepate in temporal lobe epilepsy. *J.A.M.A.,* 236:2603.

21. Frey H.-H., Philippin, H.-P., and Scherkl, R. (1986): Development of tolerance to the anticonvulsant effect of benzodiazepines in dogs. In: *Tolerance to Beneficial and Adverse Effects of Antiepileptic Drugs,* edited by W. P. Koella, H.-H. Frey, D. W. Froscher, and H. Meinardi, pp. 71–79. Raven Press, New York.

22. Friedman, H., Ochs, H. R., Greenblatt, D. J., and Shader, R. I., (1985): Tissue distribution of diazepam and its metabolite desmethyldiazepam: A human autopsy study. *J. Clin. Pharmacol.,* 25:613–615.

23. Graf, W. D., and Rothman, S. J. (1987): Clorazepate therapy in children with refractory seizures. *Epilepsia,* 28:606.

24. Greenblatt, D. J. (1978): Determination of desmethyldiazepam in plasma by electron-capture GLC: Application to pharmacokinetic studies of clorazepate. *J. Pharm. Sci.,* 67:427–429.

25. Greenblatt, D. J., Ochs, H. R., and Lloyd, B. L. (1980): Entry of diazepam and its major metabolite into cerebrospinal fluid. *Psychopharmacology,* 70:89–93.

26. Greenblatt, D. J., Shader, R. I., Harmatz, J. S., and Georgotas, A. (1979): Self-related sedation and plasma concentrations of desmethyldiazepam following single doses of clorazepate. *Psychopharmacology,* 66:289–290.

27. Griffith, J. L., and Murray, G. B., (1985): Clorazepate in the treatment of complex partial seizures with psychic symptomatology. *J. Nerv. Ment. Dis.,* 173:185–186.

28. Gros, P., and Raveux, R. (1969): Étude de l'excrétion du clorazépate dipotassique et de ses métabolites urinaires. I. Fractionnement, identification et dosage des metabolites urinaires. *Chim. Thér.,* 4:312–322.

29. Guerre-Millo, M., Rey, E., Challier, J-C., Turquais, J-M., d'Athis, Ph., and Olive, G. (1979): Transfer *in vitro* of three benzodiazepines across the human placenta. *Eur. J. Clin. Pharmacol.,* 15:171–173.

30. Guggenheim, M. A., Donaldson, J., and Hotvedt, C. (1987): Clinical evaluation of clorazepate. *Ann. Neurol.,* 22:412–413.

31. Haidukewych, D., Rodin, E. A., and Davenport, R. (1980): Monitoring clorazepate dipotassium as desmethyldiazepam in plasma by electron-capture gas-liquid chromatography. *Clin. Chem.,* 26:142–144.

32. Hendel, J. (1975): Cumulation in cerebrospinal fluid of the *N*-desmethyl metabolite after long-term treatment with diazepam in man. *Acta. Pharmacol. Toxicol.,* 37:17–22.

33. Herschthal, D., and Robinson, M. J. (1979): Blisters of the skin in coma induced by amitriptyline and clorazepate dipotassium. *Arch. Dermatol.,* 115:499.

34. Hoffman, D. J., and Chun, A. H. C. (1975): GLC determination of plasma drug levels after oral administration of clorazepate potassium salts. *J. Pharm. Sci.,* 64:1668–1671.

35. Kabra, P. M., Stevens, G. L., and Marton, L. J. (1978): High-pressure liquid chromatographic analysis of diazepam, oxazepam and *N*-desmethyldiazepam in human blood. *J. Chromatogr.,* 150:355–360.

36. Kanto, J., Kangas, L., and Siirtola, T. (1975): Cerebrospinal-fluid concentrations of diazepam and its metabolites in man. *Acta. Pharmacol. Toxicol.,* 36:328–334.

37. Kaplan, S. A., Jack, M. L., Alexander, K., and Weinfeld, R. E. (1973): Pharmacokinetic profile of diazepam in man following single intravenous and oral and chronic oral administration. *J. Pharm. Sci.,* 62:1789–1796.

38. Karch, F. E. (1979): Rage reaction associated with clorazepate dipotassium. *Ann. Int. Med.,* 91:61–62.

39. Klotz, U., Antonin, K-H., and Bieck, P. R. (1976): Pharmacokinetics and plasma binding of diazepam in man, dog, rabbit, guinea pig and rat. *J. Pharmacol. Exp. Ther.,* 199:67–73.

40. Klotz, U., Antonin, K. H., Brügel, H., and Bieck, P. R. (1977): Disposition of diazepam and its major

metabolite desmethyldiazepam in patients with liver disease. *Clin. Pharmacol. Ther.,* 21:430–436.

41. Klotz, U., and Reimann, I. (1980): Influence of cimetidine on the pharmacokinetics of desmethyldiazepam and oxazepam. *Eur. J. Clin. Pharmacol.,* 18:517–520.

42. Korttila, K., and Kangas, L. (1977): Unchanged protein binding and the increase of serum diazepam levels after food intake. *Acta. Pharmacol. Toxicol.,* 40:241–246.

43. Livingston, S., Pauli, L. L., and Pruce, I. (1977): Clorazepate in epilepsy. *J.A.M.A.,* 237:1561.

44. Mandelli, M., Tognoni, G., and Garattini, S. (1978): Clinical pharmacokinetics of diazepam. *Clin. Pharmacokinet.,* 3:72–91.

45. Maroy, B., and Moullot, Ph. (1986): Esophageal burn due to clorazepate dipotassium (Tranxene®). *Gastrointest. Endoscopy,* 32:240.

46. Meldrum, B. S., and Chapman, A. G. (1986): Benzodiazepine receptors and their relationship to the treatment of epilepsy. *Epilepsia* 27 (Suppl. 1):S3–S13.

47. Mimaki, T., Tagawa, T., Ono, J., Tanaka, J., Terada, H., Itch, N., and Yabuuchi, H. (1984): Antiepileptic effect and serum levels of clorazepate on children with refractory seizures. *Brain Dev.,* 6:539–544.

48. Miribel, J., and Marinier, R. (1966): Résultats thérapeutique de quelques benzodiazepines en prise chronique dans l'epilepsie grave de l'enfant. *J. Med. Lyon.,* 47:1583–1589.

49. Möhler, H., and Okada, T. (1977): Benzodiazepine receptor: Demonstration in the central nervous system. *Science,* 198:849–851.

50. Moodley, P., Golombok, S., and Lader, M. (1985): Effects of clorazepate dipotassium and placebo on psychomotor skills. *Percept. Mot. Skills,* 61:1121–1122.

51. Naranjo, C. A., Sellers, E. M., Giles, H. G., and Abel, J. G. (1980): Diurnal variations in plasma diazepam concentrations associated with reciprocal changes in free fraction. *Br. J. Clin. Pharmacol.,* 9:265–272.

52. Norman, T. R., Fulton, A., Burrows, G. D., and Maguire, K. P. (1981): Pharmacokinetics of *N*-desmethyldiazepam after a single oral dose of clorazepate: The effect of smoking. *Eur. J. Clin. Pharmacol.,* 21:229–233.

53. Ochs, H. R., Greenblatt, D. J., Allen, M. D., Harmatz, J. S., Shader, R. I., and Bodem, G. (1979): Effect of age and Billroth gastrectomy on absorption of desmethyldiazepam from clorazepate. *Clin. Pharmacol. Ther.,* 26:449–456.

54. Ochs, H. R., Steinhaus, E., Locniskar, A., Knüchel, M., and Greenblatt, D. J. (1982): Desmethyldiazepam kinetics after intravenous, intramuscular, and oral administration of clorazepate dipotassium. *Klin. Wochenschr.,* 60:411–415.

55. O'Sullivan, G. F., and Wade, D. N. (1987): Flumazenil in the management of acute drug overdosage with benzodiazepines and other agents. *Clin. Pharmacol. Ther.,* 42:254–259.

56. Parker, J. L. (1979): Potassium clorazepate (Tranxene®)—Induced jaundice. *Postgrad. Med. J.,* 55:908–910.

57. Patel, D. A., and Patel, A. R. (1980): Clorazepate and congenital malformations. *J.A.M.A.,* 244:135–136.

58. Perchalski, R. J., and Wilder, B. J. (1978): Determination of benzodiazepine anticonvulsants in plasma by high-performance liquid chromatography. *Anal. Chem.,* 50:554–557.

59. Placidi, G. F., Tognoni, G., Pacifici, G. M., Cassano, G. B., and Morselli, P. L. (1976): Regional distribution of diazepam and its metabolites in the brain of cat after chronic treatment. *Psychopharmacology,* 48:133–137.

60. Post, C., Lindgren, S., Bertler, A., and Malmgren, H. (1977): Pharmacokinetics of *N*-desmethyldiazepam in healthy volunteers after single daily doses of dipotassium chlorazepate. *Psychopharmacology,* 53:105–109.

61. Preskorn, S. H., and Denner, L. J. (1977): Benzodiazepines and withdrawal psychosis. *J.A.M.A.,* 237:36–38.

62. Raihle, J. A., and Papendick, V. E. (1975): Clorazepate dipotassium. In: *Analytical Profiles of Drug Substances,* edited by K. Florey, pp. 91–112. Academic Press, New York.

63. Raisys, V. A., Friel, P. N., Graaff, P. R., Opheim, K. E., and Wilensky, A. J. (1980): High-performance liquid chromatographic and gas-liquid chromatographic determination of diazepam and nordiazepam in plasma. *J. Chromatogr.,* 183:441–448.

64. Raveux, R., and Briot, M. (1969): Étude du comportement du clorazépate dipotassique en solution. *Chim. Thér.,* 4:303–311.

65. Raveux, R., and Gros, P. (1969): Étude de l'excrétion du clorazépate dipotassique et de ses metabolites urinaires. III. Expérimentation chez l'homme après administrations en comparimés entériques et en gelules. *Chim. Thér.,* 4:481–487.

66. Raveux, R., Gros, P., and Navarro, J. (1969): Étude de l'excrétion du clorazépate dipotassique et de ses métabolites urinaires. II. Expérimentation chez le chien après administrations intraveineuse, intraduodénale et orale. *Chim. Thér.,* 4:357–360.

67. Rey, E., d'Athis, Ph., Giraux, P., de Lauture, D., Turquais, J. M., Chavinie, J., and Olive, G. (1979): Pharmacokinetics of clorazepate in pregnant and nonpregnant women. *Eur. J. Clin. Pharmacol.,* 15:175–180.

68. Rey, E., Giraux, P., d'Athis, Ph., Turquais, J. M., Chavinie, J., and Olive, G. (1979): Pharmacokinetics of the placental transfer and distribution of clorazepate and its metabolite nordiazepam in the feto-placental unit and in the neonate. *Eur. J. Clin. Pharmacol.,* 15:181–185.

69. Routledge, P. A., Kitchell, B. B., Bjornsson, T. D., Skinner, T., Linnoila, M., and Shand, D. G. (1980): Diazepam and *N*-desmethyldiazepam redistribution after heparin. *Clin. Pharmacol. Ther.,* 27:528–532.

70. Sangameswaran, L., Fales, H. M., Friedrich, P., and De Blas, A. L. (1986): Purification of a benzodiazepine from bovine brain and detection of

benzodiazepine-like immunoreactivity in human brain. *Proc. Natl. Acad. Sci. USA,* 83:9236–9240.

71. Scherkl, R., Kurudi, D., and Frey, H-H. (1988): Tolerance to the anticonvulsant effect of clorazepate and clonazepam in mice. *Pharmacol. Toxicol.,* 62:38–41.

72. Schmitt, J., Comoy, P., Suqunet, M., Callet, G., Le Muer, J., Clim, T., Brunaud, M., Salle, J., and Siou, G. (1969): Sur des nouvel les benzodiazépines hydrosolubles douées d'une puissante activité sur le systeme nerveux central. *Chim. Thér.,* 4:239–245.

73. Shader, R. I., Ciraulo, D. A., Greenblatt, D. J., and Harmatz, J. S. (1982): Steady-state plasma desmethyldiazepam during long-term clorazepate use: Effects of antacids. *Clin. Pharmacol. Ther.,* 31:180–183.

74. Shader, R. I., Georgotas, A., Greenblatt, D. J., Harmatz, J. S., and Allen, M. D. (1978): Impaired absorption of desmethyldiazepam from clorazepate by magnesium aluminum hydroxide. *Clin. Pharmacol. Ther.,* 24:308–315.

75. Shader, R. I., and Greenblatt, D. J. (1977): Clinical implications of benzodiazepine pharmacokinetics. *Amer. J. Psychiat.,* 134:652–656.

76. Shader, R. I., Greenblatt, D. J., Ciraulo, D. A., Divoll, M., Harmatz, J. S., and Georgotas, A. (1981): Effect of age and sex on disposition of desmethyldiazepam formed from its precursor clorazepate. *Psychopharmacology,* 75:193–197.

77. Simon, P. (1983): Antidepressants, benzodiazepines, and convulsions. *Biol. Psychiatr.,* 18:517.

78. Smyth, W. F., and Leo, B. (1975): A spectral and polarographic study of potassium clorazepate. *Analyt. Chim. Acta.,* 76:289–297.

79. Sokol, G. H., Greenblatt, D. J., Lloyd, B. L., Georgotas, A., Allen, M. D., Harmatz, J. S., Smith, T. W., and Shader, R. I. (1978): Effect of abdominal radiation therapy on drug absorption in humans. *J. Clin. Pharmacol.,* 18:388–396.

80. Staak, M., Moosmayer, A., Besserer, K., Speidel, K., and Kleinschmidt, A. (1982): Pharmakokinetische Untersuchungen nach oraler und parenteraler Applikation von Dikalium-chlorazepat. *Arzneim.-Forsch.,* 32:272–275.

81. Staak, M., Raff, G., and Strohm, H. (1980): Pharmacopsychological investigation of changes in mood induced by dipotassium clorazepate with and without simultaneous alcohol administration. *Int. J. Clin. Pharmacol. Ther. Toxicol.,* 18:283–291.

82. Stéru, L., Chermat, R., Millet, B., Mico, J. A., and Simon, P. (1986): Comparative study in mice of ten 1,4-benzodiazepines and of clobazam: Anticonvulsant, anxiolytic, sedative, and myorelaxant effects. *Epilepsia,* 27 (Suppl 1):S14–S17.

83. Troupin, A. S., Friel, P., Wilensky, A. J., Moretti-Ojemann, L., Levy, R. H., and Feigl, P. (1979): Evaluation of clorazepate (Tranxene®) as an anticonvulsant—A pilot study. *Neurology,* 29:458–466.

84. Wada, J. A. (1977): Pharmacological prophylaxis in the kindling model of epilepsy. *Arch. Neurol.,* 34:389–395.

85. Weber, L. W. D. (1985): Benzodiazepines in pregnancy—Academical debate or teratogenic risk? *Biol. Res. Preg.,* 6:151–167.

86. Wilensky, A. J., Levy, R. H., Troupin, A. S., Moretti-Ojemann, L., and Friel, P. (1978): Clorazepate kinetics in treated epileptics. *Clin. Pharmacol. Ther.,* 24:22–30.

87. Wilensky, A. J., Ojemann, L. M., Temkin, N. R., Troupin, A. S., and Dodrill, C. B. (1981): Clorazepate and phenobarbital as antiepileptic drugs: A double-blind study. *Neurology,* 31:1271–1276.

88. Wretlind, M., Pilbrant, Å., Sundwall, A., and Vessman, J. (1977): Disposition of three benzodiazepines after single oral administration in man. *Acta. Pharmacol. Toxicol.,* 40 (Suppl. 1):28–39.

Antiepileptic Drugs, Third Edition, edited by
R. Levy, R. Mattson, B. Meldrum,
J. K. Penry, and F. E. Dreifuss.
Raven Press, Ltd., New York © 1989.

59

Benzodiazepines

Clobazam

Simon David Shorvon

The first benzodiazepine drugs were synthesized by Sternbach and colleagues in 1933. Work on their development started in earnest in the mid 1950s, and by May 1958, the first patent applications had been made claiming that the 2-imino-1,4-benzodiazepine 4-oxides with various substitutions in the benzo and phenyl rings had important biological properties (74). Since then it has been generally recognized, in both animal and clinical work, that most if not all of these 1,4-substituted benzodiazepine drugs have marked antiepileptic activity. Pharmacokinetic differences exist among individual drugs, but the antiepileptic effect seems to be approximately equivalent. In animal experiments, the benzodiazepines have been shown to be effective against generalized seizures induced by pentylenetetrazol and maximal electroshock; against partial seizures induced by strychnine, alumina, or cobalt application; and against reflex epilepsy in the audiogenic mouse and photosensitive baboon. In man, the drugs have been shown to be effective in generalized tonic-clonic, myoclonic, and absence seizures, and against partial and reflex epilepsy. Of course, the two major drawbacks in clinical practice to their routine long-term use are the sedative effects and the fact that tolerance develops in the majority of patients. Thus, currently, their main clinical applications are as emergency or occasional treatment.

Clobazam is a benzodiazepine drug in which the imine group in the 4th and the 5th position of the diazepine ring is substituted by an amide group (48). This is the first so-called 1,5-benzodiazepine to be introduced into clinical practice, and it has properties that overlap but differ in degree from the 1,4-benzodiazepine drugs. The antiepileptic effects of clobazam were first reported in mice in 1973. Since then, considerable animal and clinical work on the drug, first in 1977 by Gastaut et al. (33), has been carried out, particularly in Europe, showing the drug to have clinical antiepileptic properties which single it out from the 1,4-benzodiazepines. Much is now known about its clinical effects, and its place in therapy is moderately well defined. Two symposia have been devoted to the anticonvulsant effects of clobazam (40,41), and one has been concerned with its pharmacology (39). Here I will concentrate on the antiepileptic effects of clobazam, but it should be noted that there is also a sizeable literature concerning its psychotropic, hypnotic, and muscle relaxant effects in animals and man.

CHEMISTRY

The structural formulae of clobazam and a reference 1,4-benzodiazepine (diazepam)

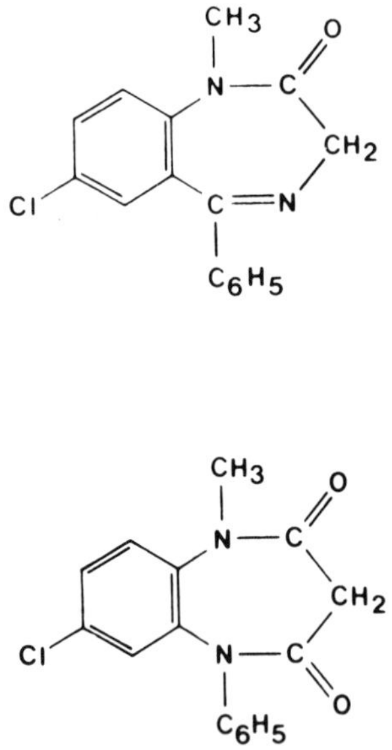

FIG. 1. Comparison of chemical structures of diazepam and clobazam. (A ring on left, B ring on right, C ring = C_6H_5).

are shown in Fig. 1. Following the introduction of diazepam and chlordiazepoxide, intensive studies of over 3,000 1,4-benzo- and heterodiazepines and their structure-activity relationships were carried out by Sternbach and colleagues (74). It was established that in the A ring, substitution in position 7 by electron-withdrawing groups (e.g., Cl, CF_3, NO_2) increased activity, and that substitution by electron-releasing groups and substitution in any position other than 7 decreased biological activity; in the B ring, large substitutions in position 1 decreased activity, and activity was increased by a methyl group; in the C ring, activity was increased by halogens in the 2' position and very strongly decreased by a substituent in the 4' position. It was only some years later that N substitution of the 5 position on the B ring, to produce 1,5-benzodiazepine compounds, was studied.

Clobazam is the only 1,5-benzodiazepine compound currently in general use. The molecule has an N atom in the 1 and 5 positions of the B ring, and a loss of the imine group (C = N double bond) at positions 4 and 5. Saturation of this imine group in the 1,4-benzodiazepines was early shown to be associated with loss of biological activity, but the activity of clobazam is clearly not dependent on this.

MECHANISMS OF ACTION

The mode of action of the benzodiazepines is discussed in Chapter 54. Most pioneering studies have been carried out on the 1,4-benzodiazepines, and it is now clear that all benzodiazepine drugs, including clobazam, act through the benzodiazepine receptors. At least three different receptors have been identified. A high affinity central receptor is linked to the GABA recognition site and acts by enhancing the inhibitory action of GABA. A lower affinity membrane binding site acts to limit repetitive firing, not through neurotransmitter mechanisms but perhaps by inactivating sodium ion exchange. A low affinity site in presynaptic terminals decreases Ca^{++} entry and therefore decreases neurotransmitter release.

The relationship of the benzodiazepine receptors to the treatment of epilepsy is well reviewed by Meldrum and Chapman (53). The mode of antiepileptic action of clobazam is probably largely analogous to that of diazepam and other 1,4-benzodiazepines, and Meldrum et al. (53) have proposed that differences between the various 1,4- and 1,5-benzodiazepines in terms of therapeutic efficacy and neurotoxicity are possibly due to the variation in degree of the agonist action at the high affinity receptor or to differing relative action at the high and low affinity receptors.

CLINICAL PHARMACOLOGY AND PHARMACOKINETICS

The oral absorption of clobazam, like that of all benzodiazepines, is fast and complete. The time to peak concentration ranges from

1 to 4 hr (66). The administration of food with the drug has variable effects, sometimes enhancing and sometimes retarding the speed of absorption (50). The drug is highly lipophilic and is rapidly distributed in fat and cerebral grey matter. Within 1 to 4 hr of administration it has accumulated in white matter and is then redistributed widely, and the volume of distribution is large (3,82).

Clobazam forms a number of metabolites (up to 12 in some species), but N-desmethylclobazam is the most important (Fig. 2). The half-life of N-desmethylclob-

azam is much longer (mean, 42 hr, range, 36–46 hr) than for clobazam (mean, 18 hr, range, 10–30 hr) (3), and N-desmethylclobazam reaches higher serum levels, especially with long-term administration (Fig. 3). In a multiple-dose study of clobazam (20) mg in 75 volunteers, the levels stabilized after 10 days and mean N-desmethylclobazam levels were approximately 10 times those of clobazam (66). As with other benzodiazepine drugs, the half-life of clobazam increases with the patient's age. Unlike 1,4-benzodiazepines, clobazam undergoes hydroxylation not at the 3 position of the het-

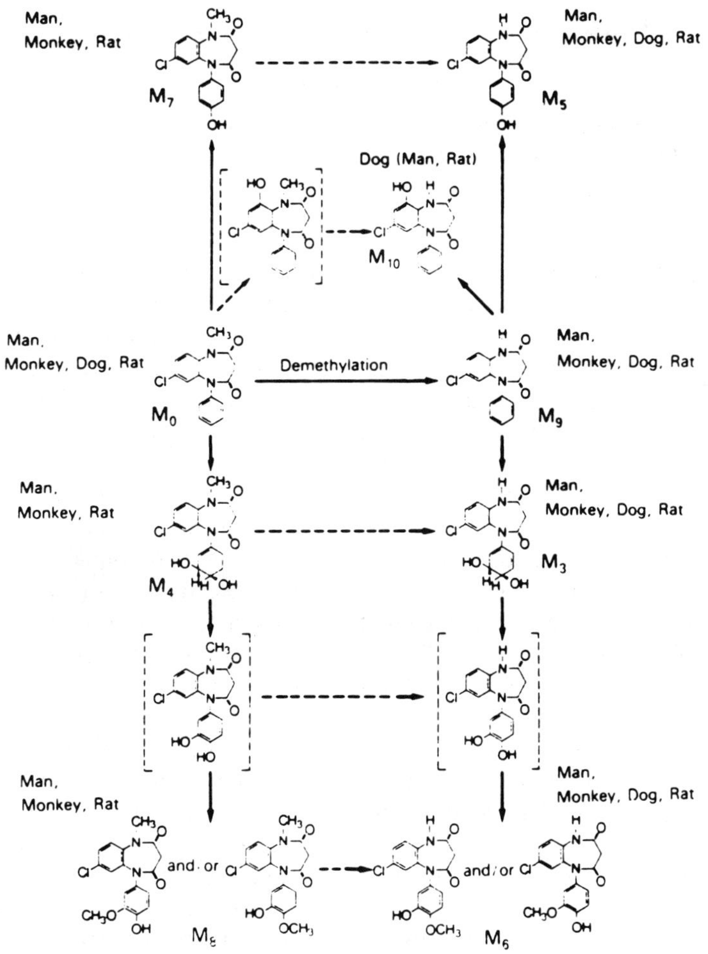

FIG. 2. Metabolism of clobazam in man, monkey, dog and rat (in man, N-desmethylclobazam is the most important metabolite). (From Volz et al., ref. 82, with permission.)

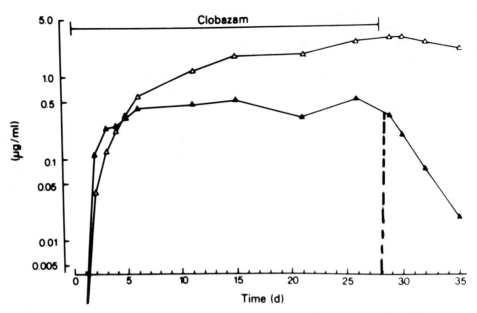

FIG. 3. Clobazam (▲) and *N*-desmethylclobazam (△) levels after 10 mg twice daily for 28 days (means of 10 subjects). (Reproduced from Rupp et al., ref. 66, with permission.)

erocyclic ring (82), but at the 4 position before conjugation. The drug is about 85% protein-bound, and so any factor altering plasma protein binding, may affect the total or free levels of the drug. Hepatic disease may alter both the metabolism of the drug and its protein binding, and so has a potentially profound effect on plasma clobazam levels.

The clinical pharmacokinetics of clobazam and its major metabolite (*N*-desmethylclobazam) have been investigated in different animal species (5,13,54,55,82) and also in man (3,11,17,28,36,42,66,77,81). Tedeschi et al. (77) administered a single 10-mg oral dose of clobazam to six healthy subjects and to 30 epileptic patients receiving long-term therapy with clobazam and other anticonvulsants. The time to peak concentration in the healthy controls varied from 0.5 to 2.0 hr (mean, 1.4 hr) and the mean elimination half life was 25.3 hours (range, 10.2–57.9). The mean AUC was 4,564 ng ml^{-1} h (range, 2,646–8,220). The peak serum levels varied from 164 to 325 ng/ml,

and the mg/kg dose bore a linear relationship to the level. In the epileptic patients, plasma clobazam levels varied from 20 to 290 ng/ml at different times of day, and the plasma level showed a linear relationship to dose only in adults, but even then there was a tenfold individual variability. In this study, children appeared to metabolize the drug faster than adults.

Meldrum and colleagues (13,54,55) noted that clobazam had a measurable antiepileptic effect for 5 to 6 hours after intravenous injection, by which time the plasma concentrations had fallen to low levels, and therefore suggested that an active metabolite of clobazam might be responsible for the antiepileptic effect. Meldrum and Croucher (55) then demonstrated that *N*-desmethylclobazam, the principal metabolite of clobazam, had antiepileptic activity in DBA/2 mice with audiogenic seizures and in the photosensitive epilepsy of *Papio papio* baboons. In the baboons, this effect was comparable with that of clobazam, and after an injection of clobazam, the blood levels of the derived *N*-desmethylclobazam exceeded those of clobazam within a few hours, and peaked at 6 hr. Since then, several studies have concentrated on the pharmacokinetics and efficacy of the derived *N*-desmethylclobazam in man.

Jawad et al. (42) studied the pharmacokinetics of a single dose of clobazam (30 mg) in six healthy volunteers and in six patients on long-term therapy with nonbenzodiazepine antiepileptic drugs. In both groups absorption was fast and complete, a peak level of clobazam was reached between 1 to 3 hr, and the time to peak levels of the derived *N*-desmethylclobazam was considerably longer. The mean area under the curve (AUC) for clobazam was 14,741 μg l^{-1} hr (range, 13,906–15,947) in the volunteers and was significantly smaller in the patients, and for *N*-desmethylclobazam was 21,227 μg l^{-1} hr in the volunteers (range, 13,886–38,537) and was significantly larger in the patients. The antipyrine half life in the volunteers was also longer. From these data, the authors concluded that clobazam is metabolized faster and more completely in patients on long-term antiepileptic therapy, presumably due to induced hepatic metabolism, and that as plasma *N*-desmethylclobazam levels are higher than those of clobazam in epileptic patients (but not the volunteers), it is likely that the derived *N*-desmethylclobazam contributes significantly to the antiepileptic activity of the drug. Further studies have followed, showing that the administration of *N*-desmethylclobazam was effective in the treatment of epilepsy (11,17,36). Indeed, it is now generally accepted that the antiepileptic effect of the orally administered drug in long-term therapy is predominantly due to the *N*-desmethylclobazam.

Clobazam is relatively insoluble, and is therefore not available for either intravenous or intramuscular injection. The rectal administration of clobazam was compared with the oral administration of a capsule in six normal volunteers (Fig. 4). The rectal solution was absorbed rapidly, with virtually no lag time and an initial rate of absorption exceeding that of the capsule. The period of time to peak levels and the peak levels, however, were similar for the rectal solution and the capsule. In contrast, diazepam also has a quicker initial absorption time, but higher peak levels after rectal than oral administration. Absorption from the clobazam suppository was slow. The AUC for all three preparations was similar. Plasma *N*-desmethylclobazam concentrations, peak concentrations, time to peak, and AUC were similar for all preparations. The variability in drug levels after rectal administration was smaller than after oral dosing, reflecting the simpler processes of absorption. The elimination half-lives after oral and rectal administration were equivalent.

The dose-to-serum level relationship in 34 chronic epileptic patients on oral clobazam therapy, studied on repeated occasions, showed a reasonable but not close correlation (84). As both clobazam and *N*-desmethylclobazam have anticonvulsant action and their pharmacokinetic relationship is variable and complex, it is perhaps not surprising that there is no clear correlation between the efficacy and plasma level of clobazam. All studies reporting serum levels and efficacy of clobazam have been cross-sectional, which is a poor method of demonstrating an effect, but none has shown any clear-cut correlation (23,68,71). Furthermore, no studies have clearly related the levels of *N*-desmethylclobazam to clobazam efficacy. Thus, the therapeutic range for plasma clobazam or *N*-desmethylclobazam levels has not been determined, but it is unlikely that any such range would be clinically useful.

INTERACTIONS WITH OTHER DRUGS

Most studies of the potential interactions of clobazam with other antiepileptic drugs have failed to demonstrate significant interactions with phenytoin, phenobarbital,

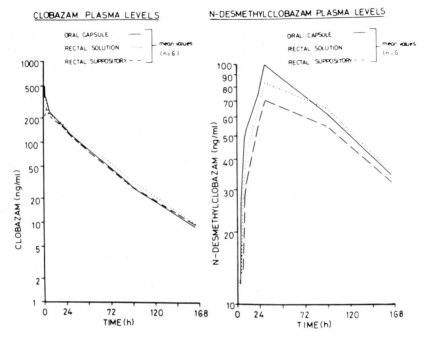

FIG. 4. Clobazam and N-desmethylclobazam plasma levels over 7 days after administration of 30 mg by capsule, rectal solution, and suppository in normal volunteers (mean values of 6 subjects). (From Davies et al., ref. 19, with permission.)

or carbamazepine (2,4,7,20,60,78,80,83). Goggin and Callaghan (34), however, noted that the addition of clobazam caused a 25% increase in serum drug levels in 29% of patients taking carbamazepine, 63% of patients taking phenytoin, 13% of those taking valproate, and 14% of those on phenobarbital. Cocks et al. (14) found that clobazam may elevate valproate levels, and recommended that a combination of valproate and clobazam, particularly at high doses, should be avoided as toxicity was common. Franceschi et al. (30) found that the addition of clobazam might elevate carbamazepine levels, and Wolf (84) reported one patient in which levels were "considerably increased." Koeppen et al. (45), in a large placebo-controlled, blinded study, found a "nonconsistent" trend of concomitant anticonvulsant levels to increase with the addition of clobazam. The contradictory findings in different studies are presumably due to variations in patient susceptibility, and although clinically significant interactions are unusual, they may occur. Alcohol may also significantly increase plasma clobazam levels (76).

PHARMACODYNAMICS

Experimental Studies

Clobazam was first shown to have antiepileptic activity in mice, where it was twice as effective as chlordiazepoxide against the tonic phase of seizures induced by pentylenetetrazol, and equiactive with chlordiazepoxide against maximal electroshock (6). The drug blocked audiogenic seizures in susceptible mice (DBA/2 audiogenic mice) for 1–2 hours at a dose of 1–4 mg/Kg i.p., and was effective against photic-induced seizures or myoclonus in photosensitive baboons *Papio papio* for 6 hours at the low dose of 2–12 mg/kg i.v. (13). Changes in the EEG were also noted, but behavioral changes were not marked. The antiepileptic effects of clobazam and diazepam (and also phenobarbital and valproate) in mice were then compared against a battery of well-standardized anticonvulsant test procedures (70). Clobazam, administered intraperitoneally, was effective against maximum electroshock and against seizures induced by strychnine, bicuculline, picrotoxin, and pentylenetetrazol, with protective indices that were superior to diazepam and the other anticonvulsants. A comparison of clobazam and diazepam in 5 NMRI mice showed that clobazam was less potent than diazepam in preventing clonic seizures, equiactive in antagonizing seizures elicited by maximal electroshock, and superior in preventing tonic seizures induced by bicuculline, pentylenetetrazol, and picrotoxin (46,47) (Fig. 5). The sedative and muscle relaxant effects, and the behav-

ioral side effects of clobazam were markedly less than those induced by diazepam. Thus, clobazam apparently inhibited both the spread of seizure activity and elevated the seizure threshold more effectively than diazepam, clonazepam, or phenobarbital. In all these studies, clobazam showed a broader spectrum of antiepileptic activity than diazepam or other 1,4-benzodiazepine drugs.

Other differences noted in early animal work concerned the sedative, relaxant, and neurotoxic effects of clobazam in comparison with the 1,4-benzodiazepines. Drugs without the imine group in positions 4 and 5 of ring B showed less sedative action (74), and clobazam had a relative absence of sedative or behavioral effects (13). In a study comparing the nonantiepileptic effects of clobazam, diazepam, and chlordiazepoxide in the mouse, cat, and dog, it was found that clobazam caused less sedation, behavioral depression, muscle relaxation, hyporeflexia, and ataxia than the other drugs (29).

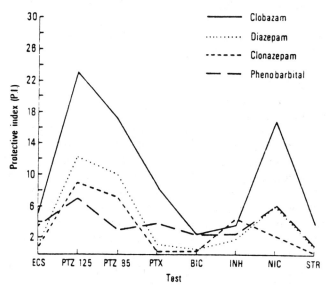

FIG. 5. Protective indices of clobazam, diazepam, clonazepam, phenobarbital (using the TD_{50} rotarod test/ED_{50} seizure test) against tonic extensor convulsions in NMR1 mice, induced by: electroshock (ECS), pentylenetetrazol (PTZ 125), picrotoxin (PTX), bicuculline (BIC), isoniazid (INH), nicotine (NIC), and strychnine (STR). Also, clonic seizures induced by pentylenetetrazol (PTZ 85). (From Kruse, ref. 47, with permission.)

Further, clobazam was found to be up to 10 times less potent than diazepam in causing sedation, ataxia, and muscle relaxation, or in inducing narcosis (47). In a study of the anxiolytic, sedative, antiepileptic, and muscle relaxant effects of different benzodiazepines in mice (75), a ratio of anticonvulsant to sedative action for clobazam was about five times greater than for diazepam and 20 times greater than for lorezepam and clonazepam. A similar ratio of anticonvulsant-to-muscle relaxant activity for clobazam was 2.5 times greater than for diazepam and four to eight times greater than for lorazepam and clonazepam.

In DBA/2 mice, the potency of *N*-desmethylclobazam appeared to be less than that of clobazam, but it had a longer duration of action (55), and in the baboon *Papio papio,* the metabolite (1–4 mg/kg, i.v.) had a protective action against photic-induced seizures similar to that of clobazam. The plasma concentrations of *N*-desmethylclobazam rapidly exceeded those of clobazam after administration of clobazam and reached a peak some 6 hr after injection. The authors concluded that in the baboon—and probably in man—the metabolite *N*-desmethylclobazam is responsible for a substantial part of the antiepileptic effect of clobazam.

These animal studies laid the foundations for the clinical work with clobazam. They demonstrated a potent broad-spectrum anticonvulsant effect, which like other benzodiazepine drugs was preferentially potent against pentylenetrazol-induced seizures rather than maximal electroshock, and was also evident in the audiogenic seizure mouse and in the myoclonus and seizures of the photosensitive *Papio papio*. The anticonvulsant effect, however, was more powerful than that of the 1,4-benzodiazepines and the sedative and muscle relaxant effects were less powerful.

CLINICAL USES

Clobazam was first used clinically as a nonsedative tranquilizer, and was available for several years before its antiepileptic activity was investigated in man. Gastaut et al. in Marseilles carried out the first clinical studies of clobazam in epilepsy, as indeed this group had been the first to report the clinical efficacy of diazepam in 1965 and had carried out pioneer work with subsequent benzodiazepines. Clobazam was first made available in October 1977 to the Marseilles group. It was initially tested in a two-stage procedure (33); first for a few days in 140 patients with frequent seizures, and then continued in those patients showing some response. The dosage used was 0.5–1 mg/kg/day. Several features were noted, which have been subsequently confirmed many times over. The drug had a rapid (sometimes within hours) and potent effect in a high proportion of these patients (76%) with severe epilepsy, although this effect was maintained in only 52% after a matter of months. Side effects were slight, and good results were obtained in patients with primary generalized seizures, partial seizures, Lennox-Gastaut syndrome, and reflex epilepsy. Following this report, there have been numerous investigations of the antiepileptic potential of clobazam.

Placebo-Controlled Studies

Seven double-blind, placebo-controlled trials of clobazam have been reported, four from the United Kingdom, one from France, one from Germany, and one multicenter European investigation. Critchley et al. (16) published the first study, involving 28 patients residing in an epilepsy center, who had mixed chronic uncontrolled epilepsy. The treatment periods were of 6 weeks duration with a 1-week washout period. Clobazam was added to existing therapy. Eighteen of 27 patients completing the two periods had significantly fewer seizures on clobazam (20 mg/day) than on placebo, six patients were entirely seizure-free on clobazam, and none were seizure-free in either the base-line or placebo periods. Evidence of rebound seizures following the withdrawal of clobazam was also noted.

Feely et al. (26,27) reported the effect of 20 to 30 mg of clobazam taken intermittently for 10 days each month for catamenial epilepsy. The results were analyzed by preference in a sequential procedure. Preference was defined as freedom from seizures in the 10-day period in patients having less than four seizures in a base-line period, or a greater than 50% reduction in those having four or more seizures in the base-line period. In 14 of 18 patients, clobazam was superior to placebo and in four cases no preference was established. This study therefore showed a highly significant effect in favor of clobazam in intermittent therapy. (It is worth noting the original and effective design of this study.)

Allen et al. (2) studied 26 patients from the Chalfont Centre who had intractable severe epilepsy and who were having four or more seizures a month. Subjects were given 30 mg of clobazam or placebo, in addition to their usual medication. The treatment periods were 9 weeks with a washout period of 8 weeks; this long period was chosen in light of the findings of Critchley et al. (16). Six patients withdrew from the study. A highly significant decrease in seizure frequency occurred during clobazam therapy ($p = 0.002$); three patients became seizure-free, and the effect on partial seizures was especially notable. The long-term follow-up of these patients was reported by Oxley (58), who observed the development of tolerence in many patients.

Dellaportas et al. (21) and Wilson et al. (83) compared clobazam and placebo in 31 patients with epilepsy who attended a general neurological outpatient clinic. Placebo or clobazam (10 or 20 mg a day) was added on a random basis to the patients' usual regimen. The seizure frequency over a 6-month period was compared with that of the previous 6 months. The clobazam-treated patients had significantly fewer seizures (median reductions, 30%) than did the placebo group. One patient became seizure-free

with the 10-mg clobazam therapy. No differences were noted in the effect on generalized and partial seizures. Aucamp (4) studied 12 institutionalized patients in a double-blind, crossover study with treatment periods of 9 weeks and a 5-week washout period. With clobazam (0.5 mg/kg/day) as adjunctive therapy, nine patients became seizure-free, and the others had significantly fewer ($p < 0.01$) and less severe ($p < 0.05$) seizures.

Schmidt et al. (68) studied 20 patients with therapy-resistant complex partial seizures. With treatment periods of 4 months, there was a highly significant reduction in seizure frequency during clobazam treatment. Koeppen et al. (45) reported a large multicenter study of 106 patients. The treatment periods were of 3 months, with a washout period of 1 month. With clobazam dosage varying from (10–40 mg/day) 19% of patients became seizure-free compared with none on placebo and the mean seizure frequency was more than halved compared with placebo (a result significant at the 0.05 level). A single-blind, placebo-controlled study has also been reported (22). With a treatment period of 10 weeks, patients were randomized to receive clobazam (20–50 mg/day), or placebo as adjunctive therapy. Clobazam was significantly superior to placebo.

In each of these studies, clobazam was highly efficacious in comparison with placebo. With the exception of the outpatient study (21,83), however, the drug was taken only for a short period (less than 3 months), as adjunctive therapy, and at a variety of doses (from 10 to 50 mg/day). In four studies, the patients had severe epilepsy and were institutionalized. Many patients had multiple seizure types, and the epilepsy was previously drug-resistant. Antiepileptic activity was noted against all seizure types. The results from these studies compare favorably with similar short-term studies of other benzodiazepines and other established antiepileptic drugs.

Open Studies

In addition to the controlled studies, many open studies of clobazam have been done since the early work of the Marseilles group (4,7–12,15,18,20,23,24,25,29,30, 32,35,37,38,49,51,52,59,60,62,63,65,69, 71,73,78,80,84,85). Koeppen (44) reviewed 21 open studies of 1,055 patients published between 1979 and 1983, and Trimble and Robertson (79) and Robertson (64) reviewed 22 studies of 880 patients published between 1979 and 1985 (Table 1). These studies reported patients aged 6 months to 69 years, with widely varying seizure types, differing etiologies, and epilepsy of variable severity. Two studies were of clobazam as monotherapy in children, some newly diagnosed and some previously treated (23,62), and the rest were of clobazam as adjunctive therapy in patients continuing to receive one or more other anticonvulsant drugs. The doses of the drug used varied from 10 to 80 mg per day.

The results of these clinical studies of clobazam are difficult to compare, not only because of the various designs, patient populations, and lengths of follow-up, but also because of different criteria for success or improvement. In studies giving figures, about 34% of patients treated were rendered seizure-free, albeit for a short period only in some reports, and perhaps a further 34% improved. In about 5% of all patients reported, seizure frequency appeared to worsen with the addition of clobazam. Patients of all ages, with various seizure types and epilepsies of various etiologies, showed improvement without any clear-cut differences. Certain authors noted a better response of partial seizures (2,37), especially in the absence of secondary generalization, but this trend was not clearly demonstrated (38). Conversely, other authors found clobazam particularly useful in secondary generalized seizures (4,32). Another suggestion is that symptomatic seizures seem particularly likely to respond (37), but this is an unconfirmed observation. In the largest double-blind, placebo-controlled study (45), no differences in efficacy of clobazam between seizure types was observed. Particularly emphasized is the efficacy of clobazam in patients with the notoriously difficult to treat Lennox-Gastaut syndrome (30,32,60), and clobazam is affirmed to be "without question, the benzodiazepine of choice for this form of epilepsy" (60).

Other Clinical Uses

As parenteral formulations are not routinely available, clobazam, unlike the 1,4-benzodiazepines, cannot be used as intravenous therapy in acute epilepsy (e.g., status epilepticus). Rectal administration, however, produces rapid and long-lasting plasma levels, and rectally administered clobazam is potentially useful in the emergency treatment of acute seizures or serial seizures. Formal studies of clobazam in acute therapy have not been undertaken, but it appears to have significant advantages (e.g., speed of action, duration of effect, reliability of plasma levels) over other compounds such as diazepam. For similar reasons, it would appear to have potential for the treatment of febrile convulsions, although there have been no reports of its use in this indication. Personal practice shows that clobazam is useful as occasional short-term prophylaxis, taken for instance on a day when it is particularly important to prevent a seizure (e.g., travel, interview, special occasions) in patients whose epilepsy is active or in remission. There have been no formal studies of the drug used in this way, although the rapid (often within an hour or so) and reliable short-term antiepileptic effect and the low incidence of side effects make it an ideal choice for such therapy. Clobazam has also been used successfully as intermittent therapy, for instance, in catamenial epilepsy (26,27).

Tolerance

The development of tolerance to the anti-epileptic effects of the 1,4-benzodiazepine drugs has been recognized for many years. Indeed, this is the primary reason for their limited role in the long-term therapy of epilepsy, in contrast to their primacy in acute treatment. The development of tolerance to antiepileptic drugs was the subject of a symposium held in 1985 (31).

It has been clear since the first clinical reports that tolerance to the effects of clobazam also develops. In the clinical studies reviewed above, the length of follow-up was noted to have an important influence by some authors. Gastaut (32), for instance, noted that 19% of patients were seizure-free after 6 months of treatment, but this result fell to 12% at 1 year and to 9% at 2 years. Similarly, Bianchi et al. (7) found 74% of 35 patients significantly improved (criteria not given) after 1 month, 51% after 3 months and 42% after 12 months of treatment. Schmidt et al. (68), in a double-blind trial, noted loss of efficacy in 56% of patients after 2 months of treatment and 73% after 3 months. During a 14-month follow-up of those who maintained improvement after the 3-month period, however, no further marked loss of efficacy was observed. Oxley (58), in a study of 52 patients with severe epilepsy at the Chalfont Centre, found that in 20 of the 26 patients (77%) who showed a significant improvement when clobazam was added to their usual regimen, the effects were lost within 1 to 8 months (median, 3.5 months). He also noted, as had become common clinical experience, that increasing the dose of clobazam in patients in whom tolerance develops does not circumvent the problem. Personal experience recalls a patient whose dose was increased to 90 mg a day, with the rapid development of tolerance to both the anticonvulsant and sedative effects at each dosage increment. Often, increasing the dosage of a drug will produce sedation without anticonvulsant ef-fect, and the development of tolerance to the anticonvulsant and sedative effects are not usually closely correlated.

The reported success of clobazam in intermittent therapy in catamenial epilepsy (26,27) implies that tolerance may be minimized by intermittent treatment, although the long-term follow-up of this group of patients has not been reported. For a small number of patients, however, this approach may prove useful. It has been suggested that drug holidays might avoid the development of tolerance, but there are no reports of clobazam used in this way. An alternative method has been to use the drug on alternative days, but personal experience shows that tolerance still develops. Theoretically, the use of very small doses of clobazam might possibly delay or avoid tolerance, but there are no reports of the drug used in this manner. Cross tolerance has not been well studied for clobazam; the use of treatment with alternating benzodiazepines might offer the prospect of prolonging their anticonvulsant efficacy. Tolerance is not related to changes in serum clobazam or *N*-desmethylclobazam levels. The drugs share the same receptor sites, but clinically at least have distinctive effects, and personal experience with one patient with alternating clobazam and nitrazepam therapy for myoclonic epilepsy suggests that this approach is worth further study.

Recently, it has been suggested that the use of flumazenil (a benzodiazepine antagonist) with a benzodiazepine drug may inhibit the development of tolerance without affecting the antiepileptic action of the benzodiazepine. This possible interaction will be the subject of future research. Finally, it is worth emphasizing that tolerance does not always develop, and clobazam is a drug worth trying in any suitable patient with intractable epilepsy. In a personal case, the addition of 10 mg of clobazam to the regimen of a patient with severe and intractable secondary generalized seizures completely abolished seizures for 2 years. The seizures

TABLE 1. *Summary of data from 22 open studies of clobazam in epilepsy*

Reference	No. of patients	Age (yr) (mean)	Daily dose	Seizure type	Efficiacy (% improvement)	No. of patients seizure-free	Incidence of tolerance (%)	Incidence of side effects (%)	Length of study or F/U
Allen et al. (1985)	52	16–69	10–30 mg	N/S	50	N/S	77	29	12 mo
Bianchi et al. (1980)	35	10–46	0.5 mg/kg	1° G 11, P 20, LG 4	74	N/S	43	N/S	1–12 mo
Bravaccio et al. (1979)	17	9–34	20–80 mg	G 7, P 6, G + P 3, LG 1	82	2	43	24	6 mo
Callaghan and Goggin (1984)	33	12–54 (25)	10–>40 mg	G 21, P 12	60	10 G (6 mo), 2 P (6 mo)	25	30	18 mo
Cano et al. (1981)	86	3–35 (16)	0.1–1.2 mg/kg	G, P	51	17 (>3 mo)	N/S	N/S	3 mo
Dalby (1985)	9	6–61	30–100 mg	G 7, P 1, LG 1, Atonic 1	78	5 (7 mo)	0	33	1–7 mo
Dehnerdt et al. (1980)	34	1.8–16 (29); 12–42 (29)	1.27 mg/kg, 0.55 mg/kg, 0.80 mg/kg	LG 15, P 9, G 4, Mixed 6	68	4	65	47	27 mo
Dulac et al. (1983)	24	0.5–16 (6)	0.5–1 mg/kg	P 21, Mixed 3	70	11	N/S	8	10 days–36 mo (mean, 9 mo)
Escobedo et al. (1979)	10	N/S	60 mg	Mixed	70	5	40	N/S	2
Farrell et al. (1984)	26	2–16	2–32 mg	LG, P, Infantile spasms	50	2	N/S	12	NS
Figueroa et al. (1984)	23	1–18 (9)	0.5–2 mg/kg	G 5, LG 7, P 11	70	11	21	52	6 mo (mean)

Study	No. patients	Age/wt range	Dose	Seizure type	No.	%				Duration
Franceschi et al. (1983)	18	16–45 (29) 3–10	0.3–0.7 mg/kg 0.5–1.0 mg/kg	TLE LG	11 7	89 —	N/S —	40 —	50 —	7–26 mo 7 days–14 mo
Gastaut (1981)	140	N/S	0.5–1 mg/kg	1° G 2° G LG P	27 2 69 42	76	35	33	33	>3 mo
Martin (1981) (1985)	54 48	8–65 (29)	0.1–0.75 mg/kg	Mixed		75–80	27 (6 mo) 17 (>1 yr) 13 (>2 yr) 6 (4 yr)	25	19	48 mo
Papini et al. (1980)	35	0.5–44	0.5–1.5 mg/kg	G LG P	11 6 18	83	11	11	69	1–4 mo
Péchadre et al. (1981)	26	3–30	up to 2.5 mg/kg	LG		58	2 (1 yr)	33	42	12 mo
Plouin and Jalin (1985)	15	0.5–23	0.5–1 mg/kg	P Mixed	12 3	87	6	23	N/S	12 mo
Ramos et al. (1981)	52	6–20	0.5–2 mg/kg	G P LG Mixed	10 24 8 10	71 57 50 38	N/S	N/S	N/S	8 mo
Scott and Moffett (1985)	60	(33)	20–40 mg	1° G P	23 37	95	N/S	N/S	N/S	4–6 mo (12 pts)
Shimizu et al. (1982)	36	1–16 (8)	0.2–1.82 mg/kg	G P	31 5	50	9	N/S	47	12 mo
Tondi et al. (1980)	36	0.75–13	1.4 mg/kg	Mixed		81	21	N/S	N/S	6 mo
Wolf (1985)	34	N/S	10–130 mg	P	27	41	7	N/S	N/S	30–63 mo

1° G, primary generalized seizures; P, partial seizures; LG, Lennox-Gastaut syndrome; G, generalized seizures; TLE, temporal lobe epilepsy; 2° G, secondary generalized seizures; N/S, not specified.
From Robertson, ref. 64, with permission.

recurred when the drug was discontinued for 3 days, and restarting it resulted again in seizure freedom, which has continued for 12 months. Why some patients develop tolerance and some do not is unclear.

Side Effects

The side effects of clobazam have been studied in several large series and reviews, many concerned with the anxiolytic rather than antiepileptic effect of the drug. Koeppen (43) reviewed 212 clinical trials of clobazam for anxiety and other psychiatric indications carried out between 1968 and 1981 involving 14,398 patients; 70 of these were double-blind comparisons with diazepam or placebo. The incidence of side effects was 33% for clobazam, 39% for diazepam, and 23% for placebo. The side effects could be classified as neurotoxic (drowsiness, dizziness, headache, nausea, ataxia, amnesia), anticholinergic (dry mouth, constipation, diarrhea, blurred vision), and paradoxical psychological (agitation, rage, confusion, irritability, insomnia) (Table 2). The double-blind studies showed a much higher incidence of side effects for diazepam (46%) compared with clobazam (26%). Koeppen noted that these studies, especially those from the United States, used high doses of clobazam (>30 mg a day) and diazepam (>15 mg a day). Furthermore, many of these studies were of patients with anxiety and psychiatric disturbances, for whom the reporting of side effects is higher than in patients with epilepsy. Personal practice shows that side effects are much less common with the use of smaller doses (10–20 mg).

Koeppen (44) also reviewed 23 open studies of clobazam in epileptic patients, in which 19 reported side effects. Where quantifiable data were available, the overall incidence of side effects was 33%, of which drowsiness, dizziness and fatigue were the most prominant (Table 3). Robertson (64)

TABLE 2. *Summary of reported side effects to clobazam, diazepam, and placebo in 70 double-blind studies (of the anxiolytic effects of clobazam)*

	Clobazam (N = 1690)	Diazepam (N = 1084)	Placebo (N = 889)
Drowsiness	25.8	45.5	9.9
Dizziness	7.0	12.0	2.8
Headache	2.1	3.2	2.9
Nausea	1.6	1.5	2.1
Dry mouth	3.0	2.3	0.9
Constipation	2.1	3.4	0.3
Diarrhea	0.4	1.4	0.3
Blurred vision	0.6	1.3	0.0
Agitation	0.8	1.7	0.3
Confusion	1.0	1.2	0.0
Irritability	0.5	1.2	0.3
Depression	1.7	2.2	0.3
Insomnia	1.8	1.6	0.6
Ataxia	0.2	1.4	0.0
Amnesia	0.3	0.5	0.1

Incidence as percentage of patients reporting side effects.

Reproduced from Koeppen, ref. 43, with permission.

reviewed 22 open studies of 880 patients with epilepsy, and found an overall incidence of side effects (where stated) of 38% (see Table 1). In general, these side effects were mild and transient, and the most common were sedative effects. Only 4% of patients were withdrawn from these studies because of side effects.

TABLE 3. *Adverse reactions of clobazam in 23 open studies in epileptic patients*

Adverse reactions	No. of studies
Drowsiness, dizziness, fatigue	19
Muscle weakness	7
Restlessness, aggressiveness	7
Weight increase	5
Ataxia	4
Unpleasant mood state	3
Atonic state	2
Hyperkinetic symptoms	2
Delusional state	2
Psychotic symptoms	2
Behavioral disturbances	2
Vertigo	2
Hypersalivation	2
Edema	2

Reproduced from Koeppen, ref. 45, with permission.

Various side effects were reported in placebo-controlled studies of epileptic patients. Del Pesce et al. (22) found drowsiness and impaired cognitive function (no incidence given) Critchley et al. (16) found no difference in side effects or behavior between clobazam and placebo, Allen et al. (2) found irritability, depression, and disinhibition in six patients on clobazam and two on placebo, Feely et al. (26) found sedation (four cases), depression (two cases), galactorrhea (one case), and nausea, diarrhea, tightness in the chest (one case) with clobazam, and Dellaportas et al. (21), using self-rating scales, found 50% of patients on clobazam and 20% on placebo reporting increased tiredness and lack of energy. In their carefully controlled investigation, Koeppen et al. (45) reported side effects in 28% of 106 patients taking clobazam, but these were usually mild and a significant problem in only 5% (compared with 2% of those on placebo). The only side effects reported with any frequency were drowsiness, dizziness, depressed mood, aggressiveness, blurred vision, and decreased motor activity. In a double-blind, placebo-controlled study of 10 healthy volunteers, clobazam (20–30 mg) had fewer side effects than lorazepam (2–3 mg) (67). Side effects tend to occur at high plasma levels of clobazam and *N*-desmethylclobazam.

The effects of clobazam on the EEG are similar in many respects to those of the 1,4-benzodiazepines. There is an increase in beta and theta and a reduction in alpha frequencies (67,72). Clobazam (10–20 mg) does not alter the total sleep time, the time to the first REM period, or the ratio of REM-to-non-REM sleep, but the latency to sleep onset and to stage 3 sleep, and the duration of stage 1 sleep are reduced (56,57). The hypnotic effects of clobazam are less satisfactory than those of nitrazepam, and this would bear out clinical practice. The effect of clobazam on epileptiform abnormalities has been reported in several clinical trials. The epileptiform EEG patterns are often but not always improved. A correlation between improvement in EEG and clinical efficacy was noted by some authors (9,31,33,45,51,59,60,62,69,71,78), but not others (11,20).

Clobazam appears to have no effect on hematological or serum or urinary biochemical measures or on blood pressure, pulse, respiration rate, body temperature, or the electrocardiogram (43,44). Apparently, no deaths attributable to clobazam treatment have been reported.

Withdrawal of Clobazam

As with all benzodiazepines, the withdrawal of clobazam may precipitate seizures. This effect was noted in the first studies of the drug in epilepsy (16,33) and has been confirmed by others, although the incidence of withdrawal seizures has not been estimated. Withdrawal seizures could possibly be avoided by slow withdrawal, and Allen et al. (1,2) noted more seizures in a double-blind study than in an open study in which clobazam was withdrawn more slowly. Symptoms in 17 of 106 patients during withdrawal of clobazam (compared with seven during withdrawal of placebo) included irritability, restlessness, and difficulty in concentration (45). No definite withdrawal seizures were observed. A case of possible psychosis occurred on withdrawal of clobazam in a patient with epilepsy (84). Two nonepileptic patients had a withdrawal syndrome with symptoms similar to those seen with the withdrawal of 1,4-benzodiazepines (61); the symptoms were severe insomnia, tension, restlessness, anxiety, panic attacks, hand tremor, profuse sweating, difficulty in concentration, nausea and dry retching, weight loss, photophobia, palpitations, muscle pains, and stiffness. The syndrome began as soon as the drug was stopped and lasted for 8 to 10 days. Both patients had been taking the drug to relieve anxiety, but the authors did not consider this reaction to be a return of the anxiety.

No other reports of a clobazam withdrawal syndrome have been published. Although it is recommended that clobazam be withdrawn slowly, no optimal rate of withdrawal has been calculated.

Dosage Regimens

The reported studies in epilepsy have used clobazam in a variety of doses (5–130 mg), some fixed and some on a mg/kg basis, and any dosage recommendations must be arbitrary. Earlier studies tended to use higher doses, and there is a strong clinical impression that the drug is as effective at a low dose (e.g., 10 mg/day in adults) as at a high dose (e.g., 40 mg/day in adults). In personal clinical practice, the usual initial dose is 10 mg given at night and increased to 20 to 30 mg given at night or in two divided doses if necessary. Few patients who fail to benefit with doses of 10 or 20 mg are improved at higher doses. Furthermore, increasing the dose does not usually overcome tolerance, if it has developed. Dose requirements are not consistently different in patients on co-medication with other antiepileptic drugs. Side effects are dose-related, and significant sedation is more frequent at doses in excess of 30 mg/day. The drug may also be usefully given at a dose of 10 mg for acute prophylaxis or as occasional therapy. The rectal administration of 20 to 30 mg of clobazam also will have rapid antiepileptic action and may be useful in acute seizures. Any reduction in clobazam should be carried out slowly in a staged incremental fashion.

SUMMARY

Clobazam is a 1,5-benzodiazepine with marked antiepileptic action. It binds to the benzodiazepine receptors, but the exact mechanism of its antiepileptic activity is un-

certain. The metabolite N-desmethylclobazam contributes significantly to the drug's action. No therapeutic range has been established for plasma levels of either clobazam or N-desmethylclobazam, and there is no clinical place for routine measurements of these plasma levels.

In animal studies, the drug has shown significant broad-spectrum antiepileptic efficacy, and also muscle relaxant, sedative, hypnotic, and other psychotropic properties. Clinically, the drug also has marked antiepileptic effects. There have been at least eight blind studies and 31 open studies of clobazam, and the findings are broadly similar. Clobazam is active against partial and generalized seizures, and in epilepsy of widely differing etiologies and in patients of all ages. The anti-epileptic effects of oral administration are greater than with other 1,4-benzodiazepines, but there have been no double-blind controlled comparisons of clobazam with other antiepileptic drugs. A major limitation to its long-term use is the development of tolerance. Clobazam seems to be a safe drug, and side effects, most commonly sedation, dizziness, and fatigue, are usually mild and transient. Seizures may be exacerbated by the abrupt withdrawal of clobazam.

REFERENCES

1. Allen, J. W., Jawad, S., Oxley, J., and Trimble, M. (1985): A long term study of the efficacy of clobazam as an antiepileptic drug. Short report. In: *Clobazam: Human Psychopharmacology and Clinical Applications,* edited by I. Hindmarch, P. D. Stonier, and M. R. Trimble, pp. 139–140. MR (eds). International Congress and Symposium Series, No. 74. Royal Society of Medicine, London.
2. Allen, J., Oxley, J., Robertson, M., Richens, A., and Jawad, S. (1983): Clobazam as adjunctive treatment in refractory epilepsy. *Br. Med. J.,* 286:1246–1247.
3. Aucamp, A. K. (1982): Aspects of the pharmacokinetics and pharmacodynamics of benzodiazepines with particular reference to clobazam. *Drug Development Research Supplement,* 1:117–126.
4. Aucamp, A. K. (1985): Clobazam as adjunctive therapy in uncontrolled epileptic patients. *Curr. Ther. Res.,* 37:1098–1103.

5. Ballabio, M., Caccia, S., Garattini, S., Guiso, G., and Zanini, M. G. (1981): Antileptazol activity and kinetics of clobazam and *N*-desmethylclobazam in the guinea pig. *Arch. Int. Pharmacodyn. and Ther.*, 253:192–199.

6. Barzaghi, F., Fournex, R., and Mantegazza, P. (1973): Pharmacological and toxicological properties of clobazam (1-phenyl-5-methyl-8-chloro-1,2,4,5,-tetrahydro-2,4-diketo-3H-1,5-benzodiazepines), a new psychotherapeutic agent. *Arzneim. Forsch.*, 23:683–686.

7. Bianchi, A., Bollea, A., and Sideri, G. (1980): L'emploi du clobazam dans l'epilepsie; Experience d'un an de traitement, Canger, R., Avanzini, G., Tassinari, C. A. (Hrsg) Progressi in Epilettologia. *Boll. Lega. Italiana contro l'Epilepsia*, 29–30:215–218.

8. Bonis, A. (1979): A clinical investigation into the usage of clobazam in the treatment of severe chronic epilepsy. *Unpublished report* (reported by Koeppen, 1985).

9. Bravaccio, F., Tata, M. R., Ambrosio, G. D., De Rosa, A., and Volpe, E. (1979): Sulle proprieta antiepilettiche di un diazepinico (clobazam). *Acta Neurol.*, 39:58–64.

10. Bun, H., Coassolo, P. H., Gouezo, F., Cano, J. P., Dravet, C., and Roger, J. (1985): Plasma levels and pharmacokinetics of clobazam and *N*-desmethylclobazam in epileptic patients. In: *Clobazam: Human psychopharmacology and clinical applications*, edited by I. Hindmarch, P. D. Stonier, and M. R. Trimble, pp. 159–161. International Congress Symposium Series No. 74. Royal Society of Medicine, London.

11. Callaghan, N., and Goggin, T. (1984): Clobazam as adjunctive treatment in drug resistant epilepsy—Report on an open prospective study. *Ir. Med. J.*, 77:240–244.

12. Cano, J. P., Bun, H., Iliadis, A., Dravet, C., Roger, J., and Gastaut, H. (1981): Influence of antiepileptic drugs on plasma levels of clobazam and desmethylclobazam: Application of research on relations between doses, plasma levels and clinical efficacy. In: *Clobazam*, edited by I. Hindmarch and P. D. Stonier, pp. 169–174. International Congress and Symposium Series, No. 43. Royal Society of Medicine, London.

13. Chapman, A. G., Horton, R. W., and Meldrum, B. S. (1978): Anticonvulsant action of a 1,5-benzodiazepine, clobazam, in reflex epilepsy. *Epilepsia*, 19:293–299.

14. Cocks, A., Critchley, E. M. R., Hayward, H. W., and Thomas, D. (1985): The effect of clobazam on the blood levels of sodium valproate. In: *Clobazam: Human Psychopharmacology and Clinical Applications*, I. Hindmarch, P. D. Stonier, and M. R. Trimble, pp. 155–157. International Congress and Symposium Series, No. 74. Royal Society of Medicine, London.

15. Courjon, J. (1979): Rapport sur l'action du clobazam sur l'epilepsie. *Unpublished report*, Lyon (reported by Koeppen 1985).

16. Critchley, E. M. R., Valil, S. D., Hayward, H. W., Owen, M. V. H., Cocks, A., and Freemantle, N.

P. (1981): Double-blind clinical trial of clobazam in refractory epilepsy. In: *Clobazam*, edited by I. Hindmarch and P. D. Stonier, pp. 159–163. International Congress and Symposium Series No. 43. Royal Society of Medicine, London.

17. Dailley, C., Feely, M., Gent, J. P., Haigh, J. R. M., and Pullar, T. (1986): A preliminary evaluation of *N*-desmethylclobazam in epilepsy (abstract). *Br. J. Pharmacol.*, 89:705P.

18. Dalby, M. A. (1985): Clobazam in resistant epilepsy—A retrospective survey. In: Clobazam: Psychopharmacology and Clinical Applications, edited by I. Hindmarch, P. D. Stonier, and M. R. Trimble, p. 188. International Congress and Symposium Series No. 74. Royal Society of Medicine, London.

19. Davies, I. B., McEwen, J., Pidgen, A. W., Robinson, J., Stonier, P. D. (1985): Comparison of *N*-desmethylclobazam and *N*-desmethyldiazepam: Two active benzodiazepine metabolites. In: Clobazam: psychopharmacology and clinical applications, edited by I. Hindmarch, P. D. Stonier, and M. R. Trimble, pp. 11–16. International Congress and Symposium Series, No. 74. Royal Society of Medicine, London.

20. Dehnerdt, M., Boenick, H. E., and Rambeck, B. (1980): Clobazam (Frisium) zur Behandlung komplizierter Epilepsien & *Epilepsie*, edited by H. Remschmidt, R. Rentz, and J. Jungmann, pp. 172–175. G. Thieme Verlag, Stuttgart.

21. Dellaportas, C. I., Wilson, A., and Clifford Rose, F. (1984): Clobazam as adjunctive treatment in chronic epilepsy. In: Advances in Epileptology: XVth Epilepsy International Symposium, edited by R. J. Porter, R. H. Mattson, A. A. Ward, Jr., and M. Dam, pp. 363–367. Raven Press, New York.

22. Del Pesce, M., Fua, P., Giuliani, G., Provinciali, L., Pigini, P., and Gamba, G. (1979): Clobazam as an antiepileptic drug. A controlled clinical trial of its efficacy, plasma levels and side effects in partial and secondary generalised epilepsy. In: *11th Epilepsy International Symposium, Florence;* abstract 423.

23. Dulac, O., Figueroa, D., Rey, E., and Arthuis, M. (1983): Monotherapie par le clobazam dans les epilepsies de l'enfant. *La Presse Medicale*, 12(17):1067–1069.

24. Escobedo, F., Otero, E., Chaparro, H., Flores, T., and Rubio, D. F. (1979): Experience with clobazam as another antiepileptic drug. *Rev. Inst. Nat. Nerv.*, 13:121–124.

25. Farrell, K., Jan, J. E., Julian, J. V., Betts, T. A., and Wong, P. K. (1984): Clobazam in children with intractable seizures. *Epilepsia*, 25:657.

26. Feely, M., Calvert, R., and Gibson, J. (1982): Clobazam in catamenial epilepsy. A model for evaluating anticonvulsants. *Lancet*, 2:71–73.

27. Feely, M., and Gibson, J. (1984): Intermittent clobazam for catamenial epilepsy: Avoid tolerance. *J. Neurol. Neurosurg. Psych.*, 47:1279–1282.

28. Fielding, S., and Hoffmann, I. (1979): Pharma-

cology of anti-anxiety drugs with special reference to clobazam. *Br. J. Clin. Pharmacol.,* 7:7s–15s.

29. Figueroa, D., Adlerstein, L., and Manterola, A. (1984): Clobazam en epilepsias refractarias del nino. *Rev. Child Pediatr.,* 55:401–405.

30. Franceschi, M., Ferini-Strambi, L., Mastrangelo, M., and Smirne, S. (1983): Clobazam in drug-resistant and alcoholic withdrawal seizures. *Clin. Trials J.,* 20:119–125.

31. Frey, H.-H., Froscher, W., Koella, W. P., Meinardi, H. (eds.) (1986): *Tolerance to Beneficial and Adverse Effects of Antiepileptic Drugs.* Raven Press, New York.

32. Gastaut, H. (1981): The effects of benzodiazepines on chronic epilepsy in man (with particular reference to clobazam). In: *Clobazam,* edited by I. Hindmarch and P. D. Stonier, pp. 141–150. International Congress and Symposium Series, No. 43. Royal Society of Medicine, London.

33. Gastaut, H., and Low, M. (1979): Antiepileptic properties of clobazam, a 1,5 benzodiazepine in man. *Epilepsia,* 20:437–446.

34. Goggin, T., and Callaghan, N. (1985): Blood levels of clobazam and its metabolites and therapeutic effect. In: *Clobazam: Human Psychopharmacology and Clinical Applications.* edited by I. Hindmarch, P. D. Stonier, and M. R. Trimble, pp. 149–153. International Congress and Symposium Series, No. 74. Royal Society of Medicine, London.

35. Grappe, G. (1982): Resultats du traitement de 61 epilepsies graves par le clobazam (thesis). University of Nancy (reported by Koeppen, 1985).

36. Haigh, J. R. M., Gent, J. P., and Calvert, R. (1984): Plasma levels of clobazam and its *N*-desmethyl metabolite: Protection against pentylenetetrazone-induced convulsions in mice. *J. Pharm. Pharmacol.,* 36:636–638.

37. Heller, A. J., Ring, H. A., and Reynolds, E. H. (1987): Clobazam for refractory epilepsy (letter). *Arch. Neurol.,* 44:578.

38. Heller, A. J., Ring, H. A., Reynolds, E. H. (1988): Factors relating to dramatic response to clobazam therapy in refractory epilepsy. *Epilepsy Research (in press).*

39. Hindmarch, I., Lal H., Stonier, P. D. (eds.) (1982): Pharmacology of clobazam. *Drug Development Research,* (Suppl.):1–186.

40. Hindmarch, I., and Sonier, P. D. (eds.) (1981): *Clobazam.* Royal Society of Medicine, International Congress and Symposium Series. Royal Society of Medicine, London; Academic Press, London; and Grune and Stratton, New York.

41. Hindmarch, I., Stonier, P. D., and Trimble, M. R. (eds.) (1985): *Clobazam: Human Psychopharmacology and Clinical Applications.* Royal Society of Medicine, London.

42. Jawad, S., Richens, A., and Oxley, J. (1984): Single dose pharmacokinetic study of clobazam in normal volunteers and epileptic patients. *Br. J. Clinic. Pharmacol.,* 18:873–877.

43. Koeppen, D. (1981): Clinical experience with clobazam (1968–1981). In: *Clobazam,* edited by I. Hindmarch and P. D. Stonier, pp. 193–198. Inter-

national Congress and Symposium Series, No. 43. Royal Society of Medicine, London.

44. Koeppen, D. (1985): A review of clobazam studies in epilepsy. In: *Clobazam: Human psychopharmacology and clinical applications,* edited by I. Hindmarch, P. D. Stonier, and M. R. Trimble, (eds) pp. 207–215. International Congress and Symposium Series, No. 74. Royal Society of Medicine, London.

45. Koeppen, D., Baruzzi, A., Capozza, M., Chauvel, P., Courgon, J., Favel, P., Harmant, J., Lorenz, H., Oller, F. V. L., Procaccianti, G., Rucquoy-Ponsar, M., Sallou, C., Sideri, G., Trottier, S., Weber, M., and Wolf, P. (1987): Clobazam in therapy resistant patients with partial epilepsy: A double blind placebo controlled crossover study. *Epilepsia,* 28:495–506.

46. Kruse, H. J. (1982): Clobazam: Induction of hyperlocomotion in a new nonautomatized device for measuring motor activity and exploratory behaviour in mice: Comparison with diazepam and critical evaluation of the results with an automatized hole-board apparatus. *Drug Devel. Res.,* 2 (Suppl. 1):145–151.

47. Kruse, H. J. (1985): Psychopharmacology of clobazam with special reference to its anitconvulsant activity. In: *Clobazam*—edited by I. Hindmarch, P. D. Stonier, and M. R. Trimble, pp. 113–120. Royal Society of Medicine, International Congress and Symposium Series, No. 74. Royal Society of Medicine Services, Limited, London.

48. Kuch, H. (1979): Clobazam: Chemical aspects of the 1,4 and 1,5 benzodiazepines. *Br. J. Clin. Pharmacol.,* 7 (Suppl. 1):17S–21S.

49. Loiseau, P. (1979a): Essai Clinique du Clobazam, I.3 mois. II. 1 an. Bordeaux (reported by Koeppen 1985).

50. Marcia Divoll, B. S., Greenblatt, D., Ciraulo, D., Surendra, K., Ho, I., and Shader, R. (1982): Clobazam kinetics: Intrasubject variability and effect of food on absorption. *J. Clin. Pharmacol.,* 22:69–73.

51. Martin, A. A. (1981): The antiepileptic effects of clobazam: A long term study in resistant epilepsy. In: *Clobazam,* edited by I. Hindmarch and P. D. Stonier, pp. 151–157. International Congress and Symposium Series, No. 43. Royal Society of Medicine, London.

52. Martin, A. A. (1985): Clobazam in resistant epilepsy—A long term study. In: *Clobazam: Human Psychopharmacology and Clinical Applications,* edited by I. Hindmarch, P. D. Stonier, and M. R. Trimble, pp. 137–138. International Congress and Symposium Series, No. 74. Royal Society of Medicine, London.

53. Meldrum, B. S., and Chapman, A. G. (1986): Benzodiazepine receptors and their relationship to the treatment of epilepsy. *Epilepsia,* 27 (Suppl. 1):S3–S13.

54. Meldrum, B. S., Chapman, A. G., and Horton, R. W. (1979): Clobazam: Anticonvulsant action in animal models of epilepsy. *Br. J. Clin. Pharmacol.,* 7:595–605.

55. Meldrum, B. S., and Croucher, M. J. (1982): An-

ticonvulsant action of clobazam and desmethyl-clobazam in reflex epilepsy in rodents and baboons. *Drug Devel. Res.,* (Suppl. 1):33–38.

56. Nicholson, A. N. (1979): Differential effects of the 1,4 and 1,5 benzodiazepines on performance in healthy man. *Br. J. Clin. Pharmacol.,* 7 (Suppl. 1):83S–84S.

57. Nicholson, A. N. (1981): Studies of the effects of 1,4 and 1,5 benzodiazepines on sleep in man. In: *Clobazam,* edited by I. Hindmarch, and P. D. Stonier, (eds.), pp. 67–72. Royal Society of Medicine and Academic Press, London.

58. Oxley, J. (1986): Tolerance to the antiepileptic effect of clobazam in patients with severe epilepsy. In: *Tolerance to Beneficial and Adverse Effects of Antiepileptic Drugs,* edited by H.-H. Frey, W. Froscher, W. P. Koella, and H. Meinardi. Raven Press, New York.

59. Papini, M., Pasquinelli, A., Rossi, L., Amantini, A., Zaccara, G., Fabiani, D., Favilla, A., and Lambruschini, L. (1980): Considerazioni preliminari sull 'ativita' antiepilettica del clobazam. *Riv. Ital. EEG Neurofis. Clin.,* 3:93–98.

60. Pechadre, J. C., Beudin, P., Devoize, J. L., and Gilbert, J. (1981): Rapports sur les effect antiepileptiques dans le syndrome de Lennox et Gastaut. *L'Encephale,* VII:181–190.

61. Petursson, H., and Lader, M. H. (1981): Withdrawal symptoms from clobazam. In: *Clobazam,* edited by I. Hindmarch, and P. D. Stonier pp. 181–183. International Congress and Symposium Series, No. 43. Royal Society of Medicine, London.

62. Plouin, P., and Jalin, C. (1985): EEG changes in epileptic children treated with clobazam as monotherapy. In: *Clobazam: Human Psychopharmacology and Clinical Applications,* edited by I. Hindmarch, P. D. Stonier, and M. R. Trimble pp. 191–107. International Congress and Symposium Series, No. 74. Royal Society of Medicine, London.

63. Ramos, P. R., Diez-Cvervo, A., Caro, J. S., Manrique, M., Serrano, J. P., and Coullant, J. (1981): Pharmacological action of clobazam in serious epileptic patients. In: *IIIrd World Congress of Biological Psychiatry,* Abstract F395, edited by G. Struwe, Stockholm.

64. Robertson, M. M. (1986): Current status of the 1,4 and 1,5 benzodiazepines in the treatment of epilepsy: The place of clobazam. *Epilepsia,* 27 (Suppl. 1):S27–S41.

65. Rucquoy-Ponsar, M., Harmant, J., and Sorel, L. (1979): *Étude Preliminaire des Effets Antiepileptiques du Clobazam (Frisium),* vortrag BCNBP, Luttich 11.

66. Rupp, W., Badian, M., Christ, O., Hajdu, P., Kulkarni, R., Taeuber, K., Uihlein, M., Bender, R., and Vanderbeke, O. (1979): Pharmacokinetics of single and multiple doses of clobazam in humans. *Br. J. Clin. Pharmacol.,* 7 (Suppl. 1):51S–57S.

67. Saletu, B., Grunberger, J., Berner, P., and Koeppen, D. (1985): On differences between 1,5 and 1,4 benzodiazepines: Pharmaco-EEG and psychometric studies with clobazam and lorazepam. In: *Clobazam: Human Psychopharmacology and Clinical Applications,* edited by I. Hindmarch, P. D. Stonier, and M. R. Trimble, pp. 23–46. International Congress and Symposium Series, No. 74. Royal Society of Medicine, London.

68. Schmidt, D., Rhode, M., Wolf, P., and Roeder-Wanner, U. (1986): Tolerance to the antiepileptic effect of clobazam. In: *Tolerance to Beneficial and Adverse Effects of Antiepileptic Drugs,* edited by H.-H. Frey, W. Froscher, W. P. Koella, and H. Meinardi, pp. 109–118. Raven Press, New York.

69. Scott, D. F., and Moffett, A. A. (1985): Clobazam as adjunctive therapy in chronic epilepsy: Clinical, psychological and EEG assessment. In: *Clobazam: Human Psychopharmacology and Clinical Applications,* edited by I. Hindmarch, P. D. Stonier, and M. R. Trimble, pp. 181–187. International Congress and Symposium Series, No. 74. Royal Society of Medicine, London.

70. Shenoy, A. K., Miyahara, J. T., Swinyard, E. A., and Kupferberg, H. J. (1982): Comparative anticonvulsant activity and neurotoxicity of clobazam, diazepam, phenobarbital and valproate in mice and rats. *Epilepsia,* 23 (4):399–408.

71. Shimizu, H., Abe, J., Futagi, Y., Onoe, S., Tagawa, T., Nimaki, T., Yamatodani, A., Kato, M., Kamio, M., Sumi, K., Sugita, T., and Yabuuchi, H. (1982): Antiepileptic effects of clobazam in children. *Brain and Development,* 4(1):57–62.

72. Sittig, W., Badian, M., Rupp, W., and Taeuber, K. (1981): The effect of clobazam and diazepam on computer EEG vigilance and psychomotor performance. In: *Clobazam,* edited by I. Hindmarch and P. P. Stonier, pp. 39–40.

73. Sorel, L., Kittirath, S. H., Rucquoy-Ponsar, M., and Harmant, J. (1982): *Étude de l'Action Antiepileptique du Clobazam (Frisium),* Ottingnies (reported by Koeppen, 1985).

74. Sternbach, L. H. (1980): The benzodiazepine story. In: *Benzodiazepines Today and Tomorrow,* edited by R. G. Priest, U. Vianna Filho, R. Amrein, and M. Skreta, pp. 5–18. MTP Press, Lancaster.

75. Stern, L., Chermot, R., Millet, B., Mico, J. A., and Simon, P. (1986): Comparative study in mice of ten 1,4 benzodiazepines and of clobazam: Anticonvulsant, anxiolytic, sedative and myorelaxant effects. *Epilepsia,* 27:S14–S17.

76. Taerber, K., Badian, M., Brettel, H. F., Royen, T. H., Rupp, W., Sittig, W., and Uilhein, M. (1979): Kinetic and dynamic interaction of clobazam and alcohol. *Br. J. Clin. Pharmacol.,* 7 (Suppl. 1):91S–97S.

77. Tedeschi, G., Riva, R., and Baruzzi, A. (1981): Clobazam plasma concentrations: Pharmacokinetic study in healthy volunteers and data in epileptic patients. *Br. J. of Clin. Pharmacol.,* 11:619–621.

78. Tondi, M., Mattu, B., Monaco, F., and Masia, G. (1980): Valutazione elettroclimica decli effetti antiepilettici del clobazam nell "eta evolutiva" *Riv. Ital. EEG Neurofis. Clin.,* 3:87–92.

79. Trimble, M. R., and Robertson, M. M. (1986): Clobazam. In: *New Anticonvulsant Drugs,* edited

by B. Meldrum and R. Porter, pp. 65–84. John Libby, London.

80. Vakil, S. D., Critchley, E. M. R., Cocks, A., and Hayward, H. (1981): The effect of clobazam on blood levels of phenobarbitone, phenytoin and carbamazepine (preliminary report). In: *Clobazam,* edited by I. Hindmarch and P. D. Stonier, pp. 165–167. International Congress and Symposium Series, No. 43. Royal Society of Medicine, London.

81. Vallner, J. J., Needham, T. E., Jun, H. W., Brown, W. J., Stewart, J. T., Kotzan, J. A., and Honigberg, I. L. (1978): Plasma levels of clobazam after three oral dosage forms in healthy volunteers. *J. Clin. Pharmacol.,* 18:319–324.

82. Volz, M., Christ, O., Kellner, H.-M., Kuch, H., Fehlhaber, H.-W., Gantz, D., Hajdu, P., and Cavagna, F. (1979): Kinetics and metabolism of clobazam in animals and man. *Br. J. Clin. Pharmacol.,* 7:41S–50S.

83. Wilson, A., Dellaportas, C. I., Clifford Rose, F. (1985): Low-dose clobazam as adjunctive therapy in chronic epilepsy. In: *Clobazam: Human Psychopharmacology and Clinical Applications,* edited by I. Hindmarch, P. D. Stonier, and M. R. Trimble, pp. 172–178. International Congress and Symposium Series, No. 74. Royal Society of Medicine, London.

84. Wolf, P. (1985): Clobazam in drug-resistant patients with complex focal seizures—Report of an open study. In: *Clobazam: Human Psychopharmacology and Clinical Applications,* edited by I. Hindmarch, P. D. Stonier, and M. R. Trimble, pp. 167–171. International Congress and Symposium Series, No. 74. Royal Society of Medicine, London.

85. Wolf, P., Beck-Mannagetta, G., Meencke, J., Roder, U. U., Rohland, C., and Schmidt, D. (1981): Erfahrungen mit der Anwendung von Clobazam (Frisium) als Antiepileptikum. In: *Epilepsie 1980,* edited by H. Remschmidt, R. Rentz, and J. Jungmann, pp. 164–171. Thieme, Stuttgart and New York.

Antiepileptic Drugs, Third Edition, edited by
R. Levy, R. Mattson, B. Meldrum,
J. K. Penry, and F. E. Dreifuss.
Raven Press, Ltd., New York © 1989.

60

Benzodiazepines

Lorazepam

Richard W. Homan and D. Hal Unwin

Lorazepam is becoming widely recognized as an effective medication for the treatment of status epilepticus (17,33,46,54, 65,67) despite the fact that, although approved by the FDA as an anxiolytic and preanesthetic agent by oral, intramuscular, and intravenous administration, lorazepam has not yet been approved for use as an anticonvulsant in general, or for the treatment of status epilepticus. Lorazepam is 7-chloro-5(*o*-chlorophenyl)-1,3-dihydro-3-dihydroxy-2H-1,4-benzoidazepin-2-one. Its structure is shown in Fig. 1. Lorazepam (Wy 4056) was developed by Wyeth Laboratories from oxazepam. The 2-chloro substitution resulted in a substantial increase in potency (12). Greenblatt and Shader (41) noted the high potency of lorazepam for prevention of seizures induced by pentylenetetrazol and maximal electroshock.

CHEMISTRY

Lorazepam was first synthesized by Bell et al. (12) in 1963. Lorazepam differs from other benzodiazepines by the presence of chloride substitutions at position 7 of the nucleus and the *ortho* position of the phenyl moiety, both of which serve to enhance potency as measured by prevention of pentylenetetrazol seizures. Like oxazepam, the 3-hydroxy group present on the nucleus fa-

cilitates conjugation and therefore allows for rapid elimination and prevention of accumulation (12,20).

Lorazepam has a molecular formula of $C_{15}H_{10}Cl_2N_2O_2$ with a molecular weight of 321.16. It is a white, odorless, crystalline powder with a melting point of approximately 168°C. It has pK_a values of 1.3 and 11.5, the former relating to protonation on the nitrogen at the 4 position of the nucleus and the latter relating to deprotonation of the hydroxyl group at the 3 position. It has also been suggested that the deprotonation occurring at pH 11.5 may occur on the nitrogen at the 1 position (73). Lorazepam is virtually insoluble in water (0.08 mg/ml) and virtually undissociated at physiologic pH.

METHODS OF DETERMINATION

An electron capture gas-liquid chromatography (GLC-ECD) method for determination of lorazepam has been described, but requires another 3-hydroxy benzodiazepine as an internal standard (38). Because lorazepam is not thermally stable under gas chromatographic conditions (73), this method assumes that the thermal-molecular rearrangement which occurs on the column is the same for both compounds. This method is capable of reliably measuring concentrations on the order of 1 ng/ml.

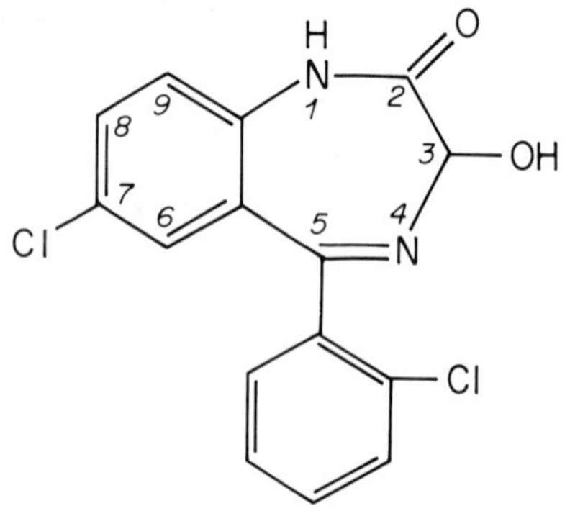

FIG. 1. Structure of lorazepam.

Howard et al. (47) used a single benzene extraction and GLC-ECD with acceptable variability at higher concentrations (>10–20 ng/ml). An added benefit of this method lies in the determination of a large number of samples (40) in less than 8 hr when compared to other methods which require more lengthy sample preparation. Egan and Abernethy (29) have described a high-performance liquid chromatographic technique for determination of lorazepam concentrations in plasma that is comparable to the GLC-ECD methods. Although this procedure requires a fairly complex extraction process it yields a sensitivity to 2.5 ng/ml.

CLINICAL PHARMACOLOGY AND PHARMACOKINETICS

Absorption and Distribution

Lorazepam is rapidly absorbed following oral dosing, with peak plasma levels occurring within 90–120 min (16,18). Sublingual dosing leads to higher peak levels more rapidly (within 60 min), but after 2 to 3 hr there is no significant difference in serum levels compared with oral dosing (18). Similarly, peak levels are attained within 90 min following intramuscular injection into the deltoid muscle (39). Approximately 90% of the total dose is absorbed through both oral and intramuscular routes (42).

Effects on oral absorption of lorazepam by other substances are primarily related to changes in gastric pH. By raising gastric pH above the dissocation constant (pK_a 1.3), the fraction of uncharged lorazepam increases, thereby facilitating absorption in the stomach. For example, a 400 mg dose of cimetidine enhances the rate of lorazepam absorption (59).

Lorazepam has an apparent volume of distribution (V_d) of approximately 1.0 L/kg (0.91–1.30 L/kg). Approximately 90% of the total drug is bound to plasma protein (14,26,63), a fraction that does not change when concentrations as high as 10,000 ng/ml are reached (63). It is this free fraction of drug which is biologically active and available for entry into the central nervous system (CNS). Cerebrospinal fluid (CSF) levels are 10% to 15% of serum levels, a value which approximates the unbound fraction in serum, suggesting that uptake occurs by passive diffusion and is limited by the serum free fraction (11,68). Age is positively correlated with free fraction, with elderly patients showing a small (0.7%) but significantly higher free fraction than younger subjects. Sex does not appear to affect protein binding (26).

Comer et al. (19) demonstrated the appearance of sleep spindles on EEG within 30 sec to 4 min following intravenous administration of a 2 or 5 mg dose to healthy volunteers, indicating a rapid penetration into CSF. Using anesthetized cats, Arendt et al. (11) found that lorazepam produced slow-wave activity on EEG a mean of 3.8 min following intravenous infusion of 0.5 mg/kg. This effect persisted for a mean of 28 min. Cerebrospinal fluid concentrations peaked within a mean of 7 min following infusion.

Plasma Level and Half-Life

Subjects receiving 50 μg/kg (2.5–3.5 mg) of lorazepam orally exceeded concentrations of 30 ng/ml after 30 min and obtained peak concentrations averaging 42.2 ng/ml within 90 min (16). Following a 4 mg oral dose, 10 patients yielded peak concentrations of approximately 58 ng/ml at 90 min following administration. Intramuscular administration to 20 patients yielded higher initial plasma levels, but a minimal difference between levels at 1 hr and no difference thereafter compared with oral administration. Though an initial higher concentration after intravenous administration is also observed, there is no significant difference between plasma levels after 2 hr regardless of route of administration (28). Lorazepam has little clinical effect at concentrations less than 10 ng/ml. Amnestic, anxiolytic, and sedative effects are noted above this level with the maximum effect on recall testing, anxiety, and sedative scores occurring at concentrations greater than 30 ng/ml (16).

The plasma half-life of lorazepam has a mean of 15 hr, (range, 8–25) in healthy individuals (42). Following intravenous administration, there is a rapid fall in blood levels with an apparent half-life ($t_{1/2\ \alpha}$) of 2 to 3 hours. This initial fall represents a redistribution phase followed by a second phase ($t_{1/2\ \beta}$) identical to the elimination rate following oral and intramuscular administration (28,42).

Greenblatt et al. (37) compared the kinetics of lorazepam in 15 healthy elderly patients to 15 healthy young subjects. The half-life of lorazepam in the elderly subjects was not significantly different from that in the nonsmoking young subjects (15.9 versus 14.1 hr). Abernethy et al. (3) studied the kinetics of lorazepam in obese subjects. Although volume of distribution (V_d) and clearance increased with increasing body weight, the elimination half-life, dependent on both V_d and clearance, was not significantly different.

Metabolism and Biotransformation

Lorazepam undergoes biotransformation to a glucuronide metabolite by conjugation on the 3-hydroxy group, the primary mechanism of clearance. Minor metabolites include a 2-quinazoline carboxylic acid and hydroxy-lorazepam. None of the metabolites of lorazepam has been found to possess any clinically important central nervous system (CNS) activity (42). Studies in man and animals have shown that the appearance of lorazepam-glucuronide in blood parallels the appearance of the free drug in serum. This rapid biotransformation leads to the appearance of lorazepam glucuronide in serum within 2 to 5 min following intravenous infusion (31). The liver is the primary organ for glucuronidation. Nevertheless, first-pass metabolism accounts for no more than 4% of the total oral dose failing to reach the systemic circulation (39).

Kraus et al. (52) studied the metabolism of lorazepam in 13 patients with alcoholic cirrhosis and nine patients with acute viral hepatitis. There was no difference in half-life in patients with acute viral hepatitis compared with normal controls. Four of the nine patients with hepatitis were restudied after clinical recovery with no difference in pharmacokinetic parameters compared with those measured during the course of the illness. The half-life of lorazepam in cirrhotics was increased by approximately 50% over normal controls. Clearance, however, was not significantly different and the increase in half-life could be explained on the basis of a concomitant increase in volume of distribution.

Excretion

A mean of 88% of the total dose of ^{14}C-lorazepam administered to eight healthy male subjects was recovered in the urine (78% as the glucuronide) and 7% was recovered in the stool (40). The renal clearance of lorazepam-glucuronide is 37 ml/min (42).

Morrison et al. (62) studied 10 patients with renal disease, four of whom were functionally anephric. There was no significant difference between the clearance of lorazepam in the renal-impaired patients compared with normal controls. The clearance of the lorazepam-glucuronide metabolite, however, was decreased markedly (clearance of 7 ml/min versus 37 ml/min). The resulting accumulation of the glucuronide metabolite is of little clinical significance since it possesses no known pharmacologic activity. Six-hr hemodialysis recovered approximately 40% of the total dose as the conjugate (62).

Relation of Plasma Levels to Seizure Control

Data concerning the relationship of plasma lorazepam levels to seizure control are derived primarily from two studies by Walker et al. (90,91). In the first of these, an open trial in status epilepticus (91), the investigators found that the minimum effective concentration of lorazepam at 15 and 120 min was approximately 30 ng/ml. Subsequently, this group confirmed the importance of a level of 30 ng/ml in an oral study (90). In this latter study, oral lorazepam was blindly adjusted to provide an "optimal" level (seizure reduction versus toxicity), which was found to be approximately 30 ng/ml.

PHARMACODYNAMICS

Studies of the pharmacodynamics of lorazepam show that it is an extremely potent anticonvulsant approximately equivalent to clonazepam. It appears to exert its effect primarily via binding with high affinity benzodiazepine (BZ) receptors, but may well have anticonvulsant effects via other mechanisms as well. Lorazepam has been found to be quite similar to clonazepam in its binding characteristics for BZ receptors (81). In a study of the ability of various benzodiazepines to displace ^{3}H-diazepam, Squires

and co-workers (66,82) found that the concentration causing 50% inhibition (IC_{50}) values for displacement of ^{3}H-diazepam were binding similar for lorazepam and clonazepam, and well below that of diazepam. Möhler et al. (61) noted a similar ranking of the benzodiazepines for ^{3}H-diazepam displacement with a wider discrepancy between clonazepam and lorazepam favoring clonazepam. Borea and Bonora (15) related inhibition of ^{3}H-diazepam binding to lipophilicity for several benzodiazepines. They found that 2-halogen–substituted benzodiazepine 2-one derivatives (including lorazepam) had very high receptor affinities. This finding correlates well with the increased potency of lorazepam over its parent compound oxazepam. Sieghardt and Schuster (79) demonstrated that a chloro substituent at positions 7 and 2′ of the BZ ring, and a hydroxy substituent at the 3 position all enhance affinity for the cerebellar, or BZ_1 receptors. Lorazepam has each of these features and had the lowest IC_{50} (highest affinity) for cerebellar receptors of any of the marketed compounds studied except triazolam.

Experimental Studies

Lorazepam has been found to be an effective anticonvulsant in a variety of animal models of epilepsy. Jensen et al. (49) employed audiogenic seizures in DBA/2 mice to study several compounds, including lorazepam. Lorazepam was found to be a more potent anticonvulsant in this model than triazolam, clonazepam, diazepam, oxazepam, or chlordiazepoxide. Interestingly, in the same study, the investigators found that clonazepam was a more potent inhibitor of ^{3}H-flunitrazepam binding than lorazepam. This suggests that the lorazepam anticonvulsant effect for this seizure model may depend on factors in addition to high affinity BZ receptor binding.

Steru et al. (83) found lorazepam and

clonazepam to be equally potent for prevention of maximal electroshock seizures in mice, and more potent than a series of other benzodiazepines including, but not limited to, clorazepate, diazepam, and oxazepam. Marcucci et al. (57) compared lorazepam and oxazepam for their effect on pentylenetetrazol-induced convulsions in mice. They found that, depending on the time of administration, lorazepam was from three to 12 times more potent than oxazepam with brain concentrations of lorazepam three to four times lower than oxazepam for the same degree of anticonvulsant activity. These findings were confirmed by Alps et al. (7). They evaluated the effect of lorazepam and several other benzodiazepines (clonazepam was not included) as well as phenobarbital, phenytoin, and trimethadione on maximal electroshock and pentylenetetrazol-induced convulsions. Lorazepam was the most potent of all the drugs tested in both seizure models.

The effect of lorazepam on myoclonus was studied in the photosensitive baboon, *Papio papio* (87). Lorazepam, administered intravenously at a dose of 0.5 mg/kg, effectively blocked myoclonic activity induced by the combination of DL-allyglycine and photic stimulation. Although lorazepam and clonazepam were approximately equivalent in their anticonvulsant efficacy in this model, the investigators noted that "differences exist between these drugs which cannot be predicted by studies on benzodiazepine receptors in general."

To summarize, testing in animal models has suggested that lorazepam would be effective for generalized tonic-clonic convulsions, absence seizures, and myoclonus.

Clinical Studies

The majority of clinical trials using lorazepam have been of the open variety. This is particularly understandable because the primary use of lorazepam in epilepsy has been for status epilepticus.

Status Epilepticus

There has been a question concerning the rapidity of onset of the effect of lorazepam on the CNS. Aaltonen et al. (1) found relatively slow penetration of the blood-brain barrier by lorazepam. The peak sedative effect of lorazepam activity is reported to occur 30 to 60 min following intravenous injection (20). Spindling was present in the EEG at 0.5 to 4 min following i.v. injection of 2 to 5 mg of lorazepam in patients, and peak CSF concentrations of lorazepam were found at 7 min following intravenous injection of 0.5 mg/kg of lorazepam in cats (11). Sorel et al. (80) treated seven patients with 5 mg of lorazepam intravenously for status epilepticus and found mean plasma lorazepam levels of 272, 237, 170, 106, and 80 ng/ml, at 0.5, 1, 2, 4, and 10 min, respectively. These findings correspond well with those reported by Comer et al. (20) who studied lorazepam kinetics in normal controls. Leppik et al. (55) reported the mean onset of action to be 3 min in 37 episodes of status epilepticus.

A possible advantage of lorazepam over diazepam is its longer duration of action. Following a single i.v. injection of 5 mg of lorazepam, Comer et al. (20) found that lorazepam levels remained above 30 ng/ml for approximately 18 hr (Fig. 2). In addition, Walker et al. (91) found mean lorazepam levels of 52 ng/ml 2 hr following a single intravenous injection of 4 mg of lorazepam in 10 patients successfully treated for status epilepticus. Walker et al. (90,91) also found that the optimal plasma concentration of lorazepam was approximately 30 ng/ml (Fig. 2).

We found a total of 157 reported episodes of clinical status epilepticus in adults treated with lorazepam in open trials (8,43,56,80,86,91,92). Leppik et al. (55) treated an additional 37 episodes of status epilepticus in a double-blind comparison of lorazepam with diazepam. Table 1 indicates

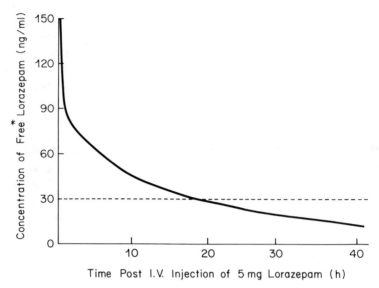

FIG. 2. Duration of action (*solid line*) and optional plasma concentration (*dashed line*) of lorazepam. The curve was calculated from data obtained from Comer et al. (20), and the effective plasma concentration was determined by Walker et al. (90, 91). *Free means non-conjugated, and does not refer to protein binding.

the results in the 194 episodes of status epilepticus in adults.

Of the open trials, two are particularly noteworthy. Sorel et al. (80) compared lorazepam and clonazepam in 50 adults with primary and secondary generalized epilepsy, partial epilepsy, and Lennox-Gastaut syndrome. Lorazepam (4 to 10 mg) and clonazepam (1 mg) were given intrave-nously, and doses were repeated if necessary. Thirty patients received each drug at different times, and 22 patients received lorazepam alone. The clinical results of lorazepam and clonazepam therapy were essentially identical. Improvement of 75% or better was obtained in 68% of the patients treated with lorazepam, and 69% of those treated with clonazepam. Lorazepam ap-

TABLE 1. *Treatment of status epilepticus in adults with lorazepam*

		Seizure type			
Reference	No. of patients or episodes	Primary and secondary generalized	Partial	Other	% Seizure control
Waltregny and Dargent (92)	10	4	4	2	100
Amand and Evrard (8)	8	6	1	1	75
Walker et al. (91)	21	7	12	2	90
Sorel et al. (80)	50	NA	NA	NA	63
Griffith and Karp (43)	9	3	6	—	100
Leppik et al. (55)	37	21	15	1	89
Levy and Krall (56)	20	7	13	—	60
Treiman et al. (86)	39	39	—	—	80
				Mean =	78

NA, Not available.

peared to be superior to clonazepam in EEG improvement; 53% of the lorazepam-treated patients had a 75% or greater improvement in the EEG, but clonazepam produced this degree of improvement in only 40% of the patients. The authors concluded that lorazepam produced either clinical or EEG improvement of 75% or better in 75% of the patients treated with this drug.

Treiman (86) compared lorazepam and phenytoin in 80 patients experiencing generalized tonic-clonic status epilepticus. Patients were randomized to receive either lorazepam (0.1 mg/kg) or phenytoin (18 mg/kg) intravenously as the initial drug, with 41 receiving phenytoin and 39 lorazepam. Thirty-one patients (80%) had status epilepticus corrected by lorazepam, while only 23 (56%) had resolution of status epilepticus with phenytoin. Lorazepam was found to be superior to phenytoin at the $p < .05$ level.

The only controlled study for the treatment of status epilepticus of which we are aware compared lorazepam with diazepam. Leppik et al. (55) treated 78 patients with 81 episodes of status epilepticus in a cooperative study employing a randomized double-blind protocol at three centers. Adult patients with generalized tonic-clonic, absence, elementary partial, or complex partial status epilepticus were included if they had received no prior anticonvulsant therapy for the specific episode of status being studied. Lorazepam (4 mg) or diazepam (10 mg) was given intravenously in a 2-ml volume injected over 2 min. The dose was repeated in 10 min if seizures persisted. After a 30 min delay, patients were given a loading dose of phenytoin even if seizures had not recurred following administration of the benzodiazepine. This precaution was deemed necessary because of the known short duration of diazepam action. Eleven episodes of status epilepticus were excluded from analysis for a variety of reasons, leaving 70 valid episodes, 37 of which were treated by lorazepam and 33 by diazepam. Of these, lorazepam was success-

ful in 78% and diazepam in 58% after the first injection, with 89% and 76%, respectively, following the second injection. This difference was not statistically significant. The latency of onset of action was 2 min for diazepam and 3 min for lorazepam, also a nonsignificant difference.

As with adults, experience with the use of lorazepam for the treatment of status epilepticus in children has been in open trials (Table 2). The main early experience in children was that of Amand and Evrard (8) who found a 79% success rate in 23 children with predominantly partial status epilepticus. Sorel et al. (80) had a 55% success rate in 11 children in a comparison of lorazepam and clonazepam.

Deshmukh et al. (24) studied lorazepam in the treatment of neonatal seizures in seven patients with severe hypoxic-ischemic encephalopathy. Loading doses of phenobarbital and phenytoin were given prior to administration of lorazepam. All patients had therapeutic levels of phenobarbital and five had therapeutic levels of phenytoin when lorazepam was given. The dose of lorazepam was 0.05 mg/kg given over 2 to 5 min. Seizures stopped in all seven patients, and remained under control for 24 hr in three. Seizures recurred at 12 hr in two patients, and with diminished frequency and severity at 8 hr in two others.

Lacey et al. (53) studied children and adolescents aged 2 to 18 years. In this open, multicenter study, 31 patients with elementary partial (seven patients), complex partial (three), generalized absence (eight), generalized convulsive (twelve), and myoclonic (one) status epilepticus were studied. Lorazepam was administered intravenously in a dose of 0.05 mg/kg at a rate of 1 ml/min. Second and third doses of the same amount were given at 15 min intervals if the seizures were not controlled. Lorazepam had an overall effectiveness of 81%, with generalized convulsive seizures (92%) and elementary partial seizures (86%) the most responsive. A particularly impressive

TABLE 2. *Treatment of status epilepticus in children with lorazepam*

Reference	No. of patients or episodes	Primary and secondary generalized	Partial	Other	% Seizure control
Waltregny and Dargent (92)	1		1		100
Amand and Evrard (8)	23	3	15	5	79
Walker et al. (91)	4	1	1	2	75
Sorel et al. (80)	11	NA	NA	NA	55
Levy and Krall (56)	1	1			100
Gilmore et al. (35)	13	NA	NA	NA	100
Deshmukh et al. (24)	7	NA	NA	NA	100
Lacy et al. (53)	31	20	10	1	81
Crawford et al. (22)	129	NA	NA	NA	79
				Mean =	80

NA, Not available.

finding was the duration of control, which was at least 3 hr in 83% of the patients, and 1 day or longer in nearly half of them. The latency to onset of control was 10 min. This was longer than in the study of Leppik et al. (55), which used an approximately equivalent dose and rate of administration in adults. It was also longer than the latency to onset noted by Amand and Evrard (8), who used a substantially higher dose in children. In this study, no adverse effects occurred. It appears that at this dose, the latency of onset may be longer in children than in adults.

The largest number of patients evaluated for the effectiveness of lorazepam in status epilepticus was surveyed by Crawford et al. (22). In a retrospective analysis, these workers found a total of 300 doses of lorazepam administered for status epilepticus over a nearly 3-year period. Of these, 129 were single or first doses, of which 79% were successful, i.e., clinical or electrical seizure activity ceased within 15 min of the injection. The median dose administered was 0.10 mg/kg in children aged <1 to 12 years, and 0.07 mg/kg in adolescents. Lorazepam was most effective for partial status epilepticus, with a success rate of 90%. An important finding of this study, not evaluated in other studies, was the absence of an effect of previously administered anticonvulsants on lorazepam. Lorazepam was equally effective regardless of whether previous acute treatment for that episode of status epilepticus had been phenobarbital, phenytoin, or diazepam. In patients who had been receiving long-term antiepileptic drug therapy, the effectiveness of lorazepam was equivalent to that of phenobarbital, phenytoin, carbamazepine, or valproic acid. However, lorazepam was significantly less effective for status epilepticus in patients who had been receiving long-term therapy with benzodiazepines (clonazepam or clorazepate). This finding may be related to down-regulation of the BZ receptor sites by long-term administration of benzodiazepines (78).

Postanoxic Myoclonus

Vincent and Vincent (89) reported six cases of continuous myoclonic activity following cardiac arrest, all of which responded to 4 mg of lorazepam given intravenously but not to phenytoin or phenobarbital. Latency of control of myoclonic activity was 4 min and the duration was permanent. However, the EEGs of four patients revealed a persistent burst-suppression pattern. Five of the patients died within 8 days of the onset of myoclonus, and one remained in a persistent vegetative state. Of importance is the occurrence of electroclinical dissociation. This has not been reported for lorazepam in any of the other studies noted above, and may be limited to this condition. Nevertheless, it suggests that EEG follow-up should be obtained as soon as possible following use of lorazepam (and other antiepileptic drugs) for the treatment of acute epileptic conditions, particularly if there is any delay of full recovery.

Chronic Epilepsy

Comparatively little work has been done on the effectiveness of lorazepam in chronic epilepsy. Two double-blind, placebo-controlled crossover trials have been conducted (60,90) and the effect of lorazepam on the interictal EEG has been studied (5,76). All of these investigations have demonstrated positive results.

Walker et al. (90) studied 10 patients with complex partial seizures (CPS) poorly controlled by therapeutic levels of standard antiepileptic drugs. Lorazepam was added to the base-line regimen. Lorazepam (or placebo) was initiated at a dose of 1 mg twice a day and adjusted to achieve maximum seizure control with minimum side effects ("optimal control"). Two patients experienced a substantial increase in seizures following crossover from lorazepam to placebo, and were withdrawn from the study. Of the eight patients who completed the study, seven had a reduction of seizure frequency while on lorazepam. Lorazepam was significantly superior to placebo at the $p < .01$ level. The therapeutic range for lorazepam at optimal control was found to be 20 to 30 ng/ml.

Moffett and Scott (60) used lorazepam to treat 24 patients with chronic epilepsy, eight with primary generalized seizures and 16 with partial seizures. Patients were treated with a small dose of lorazepam (1 mg/day) in comparison with the study of Walker et al. (90). Patients had extensive psychological testing to evaluate stress. In comparison with placebo, lorazepam resulted in significantly improved seizure control, especially for partial seizures. The investigators believed the lorazepam effect to be related to relief of stress. The low dose of lorazepam employed supports this concept, although the correlations presented between stress and seizure control also showed significant improvement with placebo.

Scott and Moffett (76) also evaluated the effect of lorazepam on interictal epileptiform discharges in the resting EEG. Lorazepam was administered intravenously at a dose of 0.0125 mg/kg (approximately 1 mg) to seven patients with primary generalized and 13 patients with partial seizures. Electroencephalographic spikes were counted before and after administration of lorazepam. For patients with primary generalized seizures, interictal discharges were markedly reduced within the first minute after administration, an effect which persisted for at least 90 min, except in one patient who experienced increased EEG abnormality. A similar, although less rapid and less prolonged effect, was found for focal spike discharges.

SIDE EFFECTS

Lorazepam, like most benzodiazepines, exerts its greatest toxicity on the central nervous system (32). The most common side effect of lorazepam is sedation. Anterograde amnesia, dysarthria, and impairment of psychomotor performance also occur at usual dosages (9,16,39). The sedative effects of lorazepam appear to be reversible with infusion of 1 mg/kg of aminophylline (93).

Transient global amnesia (74), alpha

coma (44), spindle coma (64) and orofacial dyskinesias (75) have been reported, but usually occur at toxic levels or in association with other drugs. Several case reports of delirium (13) and hallucinations (88) have also been published. The delirium appears reversible by physostigmine (13), although no reversal was observed in normal volunteers (70). All of these effects resolved when the drug was discontinued.

Treatment of status epilepticus with lorazepam has resulted in conversion of atypical absence associated with Lennox-Gastaut syndrome into tonic seizures (8,92). Withdrawal seizures occurred 24 to 60 hr following abrupt cessation of lorazepam in patients on long-term therapy (23,30,48, 50,90), confirming the danger of abrupt withdrawal of lorazepam.

Lorazepam does not appear to significantly suppress respiration at usual therapeutic doses (0.05 mg/kg) in normal volunteers (27,34,72). Cormack et al. (21) and Paulson et al. (72) have shown that concomitant administration of lorazepam with morphine and meperidine, respectively, tends to mitigate the depressant effects on respiration of these drugs. Patients who attempted suicide with lorazepam and who had plasma levels five to 15 times (300–600 ng/ml) the normal therapeutic levels did not show evidence of respiratory depression (6). However, respiratory depression has occurred in a small number of patients being treated for status epilepticus. This complication has been reported in 10 (5%) adults and five (2%) children, an overall incidence of 4%. Of these, five adults and two children had pre-existing severe medical illness including respiratory depression prior to lorazepam, although the remainder had no such history. Of interest is the fact that no case of respiratory depression has occurred with injections following the initial injection of lorazepam, a finding first noted by Crawford et al. (22) and confirmed in this review. Knapp and Fierro (51) found no significant decrease in cardiac output in 30 patients who received 5 mg of lorazepam prior to surgery.

Dilution of lorazepam into 20 ml of 5% dextrose or Ringer's lactate virtually eliminates the pain of injection or thrombophlebitis which is seen with diazepam (36). Prolonged use of undiluted lorazepam may lead to venous thrombosis, although this effect is not as common as with diazepam (45). Dilution with an equal amount of sterile water, normal saline, or 5% dextrose is recommended for intravenous infusion.

INTERACTIONS WITH OTHER DRUGS

Lorazepam, because of its independence of oxidative metabolic pathways, does not interact importantly with most other anticonvulsants. Aranko et al. (10) studied the effects of lorazepam when administered in combination with ethanol in nine healthy subjects. A greater impairment of psychomotor performance was seen in patients receiving the combination than with either drug alone. Abernethy et al. (2) found a marked increase in lorazepam half-life in nine subjects with concomitant administration of probenecid. Lorazepam clearance was decreased by 50% with a doubling of the elimination half-life. Probenecid was found to inhibit the glucuronidation of lorazepam with potential for accumulation and subsequent toxicity in patients on long-term therapy.

Propoxyphene (4), propranolol (69), oral contraceptives (84), and cimetidine (71,77), four commonly prescribed drugs, do not significantly interfere with the pharmacokinetics of lorazepam. The protein binding of lorazepam, unlike other benzodiazepines, is not altered by heparin (25).

TERATOGENICITY

Lorazepam does not appear to possess significant teratogenic potential, although it has been found to cross the placenta with equal serum levels in mother and fetus if given more than 10 min in advance of labor (58). Summerfield and Nielsen (85) found approximately 20% of the total maternal serum concentration of lorazepam measured in breast milk in four breast-feeding mothers. No significant neurobehavioral effects were noted in the infants, indicating the relative safety of this medication during breast feeding.

SUMMARY

Lorazepam is a potent anticonvulsant, the major use of which in epilepsy is for the treatment of status epilepticus. Pharmacokinetic characteristics indicate a rapid onset approximately equivalent to that of diazepam and a more prolonged duration of action than diazepam in this condition. Lorazepam is effective in approximately 80% of a variety of types of status epilepticus in both adults and children. The mechanism of action of lorazepam may involve binding to both high and low affinity benzodiazepine receptors. Lorazepam is not only highly effective for status epilepticus but a relatively safe drug to use in this condition, with respiratory depression the primary adverse effect seen in 4% of cases. Lorazepam is also effective in the long-term treatment of epilepsy in a small number of cases, perhaps via its anxiolytic action.

CONVERSION

Conversion factor:

$$CF = \frac{1000}{mol.\ wt.} = \frac{1000}{321.16} = 3.11$$

Conversion:

$$(\mu g/ml) \times 3.11 = (\mu moles/L)$$

$$(\mu moles/L) \div 3.11 = (\mu g/ml)$$

REFERENCES

1. Aaltonen, L., Kanto, J., and Salo, M. (1980): Cerebrospinal fluid concentrations and serum protein binding of lorazepam and its conjugate. *Acta Pharmacol. Toxicol. (Kbh.)*, 46(2):156–158.
2. Abernethy, D. R., Greenblatt, D. J., Ameer, B., and Shader, R. I. (1985): Probenecid impairment of acetaminophen and lorazepam clearance: Direct inhibition of ether glucuronide formation. *J. Pharmacol. Exper. Ther.*, 234(2):345–349.
3. Abernethy, D. R., Greenblatt, D. J., Divoll, M., and Shader, R. I. (1983): Enhanced glucuronide conjugation of drugs in obesity: Studies of lorazepam, oxazepam, and acetaminophen. *J. Lab. Clin. Med.*, 101(6):873–880.
4. Abernethy, D. R., Greenblatt, D. J., Morse, D. S., and Shader, R. I. (1985): Interaction of propoxyphene with diazepam, alprazolam and lorazepam. *Br. J. Clin. Pharmac.*, 19:51–57.
5. Ahmad, S., Perucca, E., and Richens, A. (1977): The effect of frusemide, mexiletine, (+)-propranolol and three benzodiazepine drugs on interictal spike discharges in the electroencephalograms of epileptic patients. *Br. J. Clin. Pharmac.*, 4:683–688.
6. Allen, M. D., Greenblatt, D. J., LaCasse, Y., and Shader, R. I. (1980): Pharmacokinetic study of lorazepam overdosage. *Am. J. Psychiatry*, 137(11):1414–1415.
7. Alps, B. J., Harry, T. V. A., and Southgate, P. J. (1973): The pharmacology of lorazepam, a broad-spectrum tranquillizer. *Curr. Med. Res. Opin.*, 1(5):239–261.
8. Amand, G., and Evrard, P. (1976): Le lorazepam injectable dans états de mal epileptiques. *Rev. Electroencephalogr. Neurophysiol. Clin.*, 6:532–533.
9. Ameer, B., and Greenblat, D. J. (1981): Lorazepam: A review of its clinical pharmacological properties and therapeutic uses. *Drugs*, 21:161–200.
10. Aranko, K., Seppala, T., Pellinen, J., and Mattila, M. J. (1985): Interaction of diazepam or lorazepam with alcohol: Psychomotor effects and bioassayed serum levels after single and repeated doses. *Eur. J. Clin. Pharmacol.*, 28:559–565.
11. Arendt, R. M., Greenblatt, D. J., de Jong, R. H., Bonin, J. D., Abernethy, D. R., Ehrenberg, B. L., Giles, H. G., Sellers, E. M., and Shader, R. I. (1983): *In vitro* correlates of benzodiazepine cerebrospinal fluid uptake, pharmacodynamic action and peripheral distribution. *J. Pharmacol. Exp. Ther.*, 227(1):98–106.
12. Bell, S. C., McCaully, R. J., Gochman, C., Childress, S. J., and Gluckman, M. I. (1968): 3-Substituted 1,4-benzodiazepin-2-ones. *J. Med. Chem.*, 11:457–461.
13. Blitt, C. D., and Petty, W. C. (1975): Reversal of lorazepam delirium by physostigmine. *Anesth. Analg.*, 54(5):607–608.
14. Bonati, M., Kanto, J., and Tognoni, G. (1982): Clinical pharmacokinetics of cerebrospinal fluid. *Clin. Pharmacokinet.*, 7:312–335.
15. Borea, P. A., and Bonora, A. (1983): Brain receptor binding and lipophilic character of benzodiazepines. *Biochem. Pharmacol.*, 32(4):603–607.
16. Bradshaw, E. G., Ali, A. A., Mulley, B. A., and Rye, R. M. (1981): Plasma concentrations and clin-

ical effects of lorazepam after oral administration. *Br. J. Anaesth.*, 53:517–521.

17. Browne, T. R. (1982): Therapy of status epilepticus. *Compr. Ther.*, 8(5):28–36.

18. Caille, G., Spenard, J., Lacasse, Y., and Brennan, J. (1983): Pharmacokinetics of two lorazepam formulations, oral and sublingual, after multiple doses. *Biopharm. Drug Dispos.*, 4:31–42.

19. Comer, W. H., Elliott, H. W., Nomof, N., Navarro, G., Kokka, N., Ruelius, H. W., and Knowles, J. A. (1973): Pharmacology of parenterally administered lorazepam in man. *J. Int. Med. Res.*, 1(4):216–225.

20. Comer, W. H., and Giesecke, A. H., Jr. (1982): Injectable lorazepam (Ativan). *Semin. Anesth.*, 1(1):33–39.

21. Cormack, R. S., Milledge, J. S., and Hanning, C. D. (1977): Respiratory effects and amnesia after premedication with morphine or lorazepam. *Br. J. Anaesth.*, 49:351–360.

22. Crawford, T. O., Mitchell, W. G., and Snodgrass, S. R. (1987): Lorazepam in childhood status epilepticus and serial seizures: Effectiveness and tachyphylaxis. *Neurology*, 37:190–195.

23. de la Fuente, J. R., Rosenbaum, A. H., Martin, H. R., and Niven, R. G. (1980): Lorazepam-related withdrawal seizures. *Mayo Clin. Proc.*, 55:190–192.

24. Deshmukh, A., Wittert, W., Schnitzler, E., and Mangurten, H. H. (1986): Lorazepam in the treatment of refractory neonatal seizures. *A.J.D.C.*, 140:1042–1044.

25. Desmond, P. V., Roberts, R. K., Wood, A. J. J., Dunn, G. D., Wilkinson, G. R., and Schenker, S. (1980): Effect of heparin administration on plasma binding of benzodiazepines. *Br. J. Clin. Pharmacol.*, 9:171–175.

26. Divoll, M., and Greenblatt, D. J. (1982): Effect of age and sex on lorazepam protein binding. *J. Pharm. Pharmacol.*, 34:122–123.

27. Dodson, M. E., Yousseff, Y., Maddison, S., and Pleuvry, B. (1976): Respiratory effects of lorazepam. *Br. J. Anaesth.*, 48:611–612.

28. Dundee, J. W., Lilburn, J. K., Toner, W., and Howard, P. J. (1978): Plasma lorazepam levels. *Anaesthesia*, 33:15–19.

29. Egan, J. M., and Abernethy, D. R. (1986): Lorazepam analysis using liquid chromatography: Improved sensitivity for single-dose pharmacokinetic studies. *J. Chromatogr.*, 380:196–201.

30. Einarson, T. R. (1980): Lorazepam withdrawal seizures. [Letter] *Lancet*, 1(8160):151.

31. Elliott, H. W., (1976): Metabolism of lorazepam. *Br. J. Anaesth.*, 48:1017–1023.

32. Elliott, H. W., Nomof, N., Navarro, G., Ruelius, H. W., Knowles, J. A. and Comer, W. H. (1971): Central nervous system and cardiovascular effects of lorazepam in man. *Clin. Pharmacol. Ther.*, 12(3):468–481.

33. Farrell, K. (1986): Benzodiazepines in the treatment of children with epilepsy. *Epilepsia*, 27 (Suppl.1):S45–S51.

34. Gasser, J. C., Kaufman, R. D., and Bellville, J. W. (1975): Respiratory effects of lorazepam, pentobarbital, and pentazocine. *Clin. Pharmacol. Ther.*, 18(2):170–174.

35. Gilmore, H. E., Veale, L. A., Darras, B. T., Dionne, R. E., Rabe, E. F., and Singer, W. D. (1984): Lorazepam treatment of childhood status epilepticus. *Ann. Neurol.*, 16:377.

36. Graham, C. W., Pagano, R. R., and Conner, J. T. (1978): Pain and clinical thrombophlebitis following intravenous diazepam and lorazepam. *Anaesthesia*, 33:188–191.

37. Greenblatt, D. J., Allen, M. D., Locniskar, A., Harmatz, J. S., and Shader, R. I. (1979): Lorazepam kinetics in the elderly. *Clin. Pharmacol. Ther.*, 26(1):103–113.

38. Greenblatt, D. J., Franke, J., Shader, R. I. (1978): Analysis of lorazepam and its glucuronide metabolite by electron-capture gas-liquid chromatography. Use in pharmacokinetic studies of lorazepam. *J. Chromatogr.*, 146(2):311–320.

39. Greenblatt, D. J., Joyce, T. H., Comer, W. H., Knowles, J. A., Shader, R. I., Kyriakopoulos, A. A., MacLaughlin, D. S., and Ruelius, H. W. (1977): Clinical pharmacokinetics of lorazepam: Intramuscular injection. *Clin. Pharmacol. Ther.*, 21(2):222–230.

40. Greenblatt, D. J., Schillings, R. T., Kyriakopoulos, A. A., Shader, R. I., Sisenwine, S. F., Knowles, J. A., and Ruelius, H. W. (1976): Clinical pharmacokinetics of lorazepam. Absorption and disposition of oral ^{14}C-lorazepam. *Clin. Pharmacol. Ther.*, 20(3):329–341.

41. Greenblatt, D. J., and Shader, R. I. (1974): *Benzodiazepines in Clinical Practice.* Raven Press, New York.

42. Greenblatt, D. J., Shader, R. I., Franke, K., MacLaughlin, D. S., Harmatz, J. S., Allen, M. D., Werner, A., and Woo, E. (1979): Pharmacokinetics and bioavailability of intravenous, intramuscular, and oral lorazepam in humans. *J. Pharm. Sci.*, 68(1):57–63.

43. Griffith, P. A., and Karp, H. R. (1980): Lorazepam in therapy for status epilepticus. *Ann. Neurol.*, 7(5):493.

44. Guterman, B., Sebastian, P., and Sodha, N. (1981): Recovery from alpha coma after lorazepam overdose. *Clin. Electroencephalogr.*, 12(4):205–208.

45. Hegarty, J. E., and Dundee, J. W. (1977): Sequelae after the intravenous injection of three benzodiazepines—Diazepam, lorazepam, and flunitrazepam. *Br. Med. J.*, 2:1384–1385.

46. Homan, R. W., and Walker, J. E. (1983): Clinical studies of lorazepam in status epilepticus. *Adv. Neurol.*, 34:493–498.

47. Howard, P. J., Lilburn, J. K., Dundee, J. W., Toner, W., and McIlroy, P. D. A. (1977): Estimation of plasma lorazepam by gas-liquid chromatography and a benzene extraction. *Anaesthesia*, 32:767–770.

48. Howe, J. G. (1980): Lorazepam withdrawal seizures. *Br. Med. J.*, 280(6224):1163–1164.

49. Jensen, L. H., Petersen, E. N., and Braestrup, C. (1983): Audiogenic seizures in DBA/2 mice discriminate sensitively between low efficacy ben-

zodiazepine receptor agonists and inverse agonists. *Life Sci.*, 33:393–399.

50. Kahan, B. B., and Haskett, R. F. (1984): Lorazepam withdrawal and seizures. *Am. J. Psychiatry*, 141(8):1011–1012.

51. Knapp, R. B., and Fierro, L. (1974): Evaluation of the cardiopulmonary safety and effects of lorazepam as a premedicant. *Anesth. Analg.*, 53(1):122–124.

52. Kraus, J. W., Desmond, P. V., Marshall, J. P., Johnson, R. F., Schenker, S., and Wilkinson, G. R. (1978): Effects of aging and liver disease on disposition of lorazepam. *Clin. Pharmacol. Ther.*, 24(4):411–419.

53. Lacey, D. J., Singer, W. D., Horwitz, S. J., and Gilmore, H. (1986): Clinical and laboratory observations: Lorazepam therapy of status epilepticus in children and adolescents. *J. Pediatr.*, 108(5):771–774.

54. Lederman, R. J. (1984): Status epilepticus. *Cleveland Clin. Q.* 51(2):261–266.

55. Leppik, I. E., Derivan, A. T., Homan, R. W., Walker, J., Ramsay, R. E., and Patrick, B. (1983): Double-blind study of lorazepam and diazepam in status epilepticus. *J.A.M.A.*, 249(11):1452–1454.

56. Levy, R. J., and Krall, R. L. (1984): Treatment of status epilepticus with lorazepam. *Arch. Neurol.*, 41:605–611.

57. Marcucci, F., Mussini, E., Airoldi, L., Guaitani, A., and Garattini, S. (1972): Brain concentrations of lorazepam and oxazepam at equal degree of anticonvulsant activity. *J. Pharm. Pharmac.*, 24:63–64.

58. McBride, R. J., Dundee, J. W., Moore, J., Toner, W., and Howard, P. J. (1979): Placental transfer of lorazepam. [Proceedings] *Br. J. Clin. Pharmacol.*, 7(4):420P.

59. McGowan, W. A. W., and Dundee, J. W. (1982): The effect of intravenous cimetidine on the absorption of orally administered diazepam and lorazepam. *Br. J. Clin. Pharmacol.*, 14:207–211.

60. Moffett, A., and Scott, D. F. (1984): Stress and epilepsy: The value of a benzodiazepine-lorazepam. *J. Neurol. Neurosurg. Psychiatry*, 47:165–167.

61. Möhler, H., Okada, T., Heitz, P., and Ulrich, J. (1978): Biochemical identification of the site of action of benzodiazepines in human brain by H-diazepam binding. *Life Sci.*, 22(11):985–988.

62. Morrison, G., Chiang, S. T., Koepke, H. H., and Walker, B. R. (1984): Effect of renal impairment and hemodialysis on lorazepam kinetics. *Clin. Pharmacol. Ther.*, 35(5):646–652.

63. Moschitto, L. J., and Greenblatt, D. J. (1983): Concentration-independent plasma protein binding of benzodiazepines. *J. Pharm. Pharmacol.*, 35:179–180.

64. Mouradian, M. D., and Penovich, P. E. (1985): Spindle coma in benzodiazepine toxicity: Case report. *Clin. Electroencephalogr.*, 16(4):213–218.

65. Niedermeyer, E., Froescher, W., and Fisher, R. S. (1985): Epileptic seizure disorders: Developments in diagnosis and therapy. *J. Neurol.*, 232:1–12.

66. Nielsen, M., Braestrup, C., and Squires, R. F. (1978): Evidence for a late evolutionary appearance of brain-specific benzodiazepine receptors: An investigation of 18 vertebrate and 5 invertebrate species. *Brain Res.*, 141:342–346.

67. Nourtsis, S. C. (1985): The use of lorazepam in the treatment of status epilepticus. *Hosp. Pharm.*, 20:463–466.

68. Ochs, H. R., Busse, J. Greenblatt, D. J., and Allen, M. D. (1980): Entry of lorazepam into cerebrospinal fluid. *Br. J. Clin. Pharmacol.*, 10:405–406.

69. Ochs, H. R., Greenblatt, D. J., and Verburg-Ochs, B. (1984): Propranolol interactions with diazepam, lorazepam, and alprazolam. *Clin. Pharmacol. Ther.*, 36(4):451–455.

70. Pandit, U. A., Kothary, S. P., Samra, S. K., Domino, E. F., and Pandit, S. K. (1983): Physostigmine fails to reverse clinical, psychomotor, or EEG effects of lorazepam. *Anesth. Analg.*, 62:679–685.

71. Patwardhan, R. V., Yarborough, G. W., Desmond, P. V., Johnson, R. F., Schenker, S., and Speeg, K. V., Jr. (1980): Cimetidine spares the glucuronidation of lorazepam and oxazepam. *Gastroenterology*, 79:912–916.

72. Paulson, B. A., Becker, L. D., and Way, W. L. (1983): The effects of intravenous lorazepam alone and with meperidine on ventilation in man. *Acta Anaesthiol. Scand.*, 27:400–402.

73. Rutgers, J. G., and Shearer, C. M. (1980): Lorazepam. In: *Analytical Profiles of Drug Substances*, Vol. 9, edited by K. Florey, pp. 397–421. Academic Press, New York.

74. Sandyk, R. (1985): Transient global amnesia induced by lorazepam. *Clin. Neuropharmacol.*, 8(3):297–298.

75. Sandyk, R. (1986): Orofacial dyskinesias associated with lorazepam therapy. *Clin. Pharm.*, 5:419–421.

76. Scott, D. F., and Moffett, A. (1981): Lorazepam: Its effect on the EEG paroxysmal activity in patients with epilepsy. *Acta Neurol. Scand.*, 64:353–360.

77. Sedman, A. J. (1984): Cimetidine-drug interactions. *Am. J. Med.*, 76:109–114.

78. Sher, P. K., Neale, E. A., Graubard, B. I., Habig, W. H., Fitzgerald, S. C., and Nelson, P. G. (1985): Differential neurochemical effects of chronic exposure of cerebral cortical cell culture to valproic acid, diazepam, or ethosuximide. *Pediat. Neurol.*, 1(4):232–237.

79. Sieghardt W., and Schuster, A: (1984): Affinity of various ligands for benzodiazepine receptors in rat cerebrum and hippocampus. *Biochem. Pharmacol.*, 33:4033–4038.

80. Sorel, L., Mechler, L., and Harmant, J. (1981): Comparative trial of intravenous lorazepam and clonazepam in status epilepticus. *Clin. Ther.* 4(4):326–336.

81. Speth, R. C., Wastek, G. J., Johnson, P. C., and Yamamura, H. I. (1978): Benzodiazepine binding in human brain: Characterization using [H] flunitrazepam. *Life Sci.*, 22(10):859–866.

82. Squires, R. F., and Braestrup, C. (1977): Benzo-

diazepine receptors in rat brain. *Nature,* 266:732–734.

83. Steru, L., Chermat, R., Millet, B., Mico, J. A., and Simon, P. (1986): Comparative study in mice of ten 1,4-benzodiazepines and of clobazam: Anticonvulsant, anxiolytic, sedative, and myorelaxant effects. *Epilepsia,* 27 (Suppl.1):S14–S17.

84. Stoehr, G. P., Kroboth, P. D., Juhl, R. P., Wender, D. B., Phillips, J. P., and Smith, R. B. (1984): Effect of oral contraceptives on triazolam, temazepam, alprazolam, and lorazepam kinetics. *Clin. Pharmacol. Ther.,* 36(5):683–690.

85. Summerfield, R. J., and Nielsen, M. S. (1985): Excretion of lorazepam into breast milk. *Br. J. Anaesth.,* 57(10):1042–1043.

86. Treiman, D. M., De Giorgio, C. M., Ben-Menachem, E., Gehret, D., Nelson, L., Salisbury, S. M., Barber, K. O., and Wickboldt, C. L. (1985): Lorazepam versus phenytoin in the treatment of generalized convulsive status epilepticus: Report of an ongoing study. *Neurology,* 35 (Suppl.1):284.

87. Valin, A., Cepeda, C., Rey, E., and Naquet, R. (1981): Opposite effects of lorazepam on two kinds of myoclonus in the photosensitive *Papio papio. Electroenceph. Clin. Neurophysiol.,* 52:647–651.

88. van den Berg, A. A. (1986): Hallucinations after oral lorazepam in children. [Letter]. *Anaesthesia,* 41(3):330–331.

89. Vincent, F. M., and Vincent, T. (1986): Lorazepam in myoclonic seizures after cardiac arrest. *Ann. Intern. Med.,* 104(4):586.

90. Walker, J. E., Homan, R. W., and Crawford, I. L. (1984): Lorazepam: A controlled trial in patients with intractable partial complex seizures. *Epilepsia,* 25(4):464–466.

91. Walker, J. E., Homan, R. W., Vasko, M. R., Crawford, I. L., Bell, R. D., and Tasker, W. G. (1979): Lorazepam in status epilepticus. *Ann. Neurol.,* 6(3):207–213.

92. Waltregny, A., and Dargent, J. (1975): Preliminary study of parenteral lorazepam in status epilepticus. *Acta Neurol. Belg.,* 75:219–229.

93. Wangler, M. A., and Kilpatrick, D. S. (1985): Aminophylline is an antagonist of lorazepam. *Anesth. Analg.,* 64:834–836.

Antiepileptic Drugs, Third Edition, edited by
R. Levy, R. Mattson, B. Meldrum,
J. K. Penry, and F. E. Dreifuss.
Raven Press, Ltd., New York © 1989.

61

Other Antiepileptic Drugs

Sulfonamides and Derivatives: Acetazolamide

Dixon M. Woodbury and John W. Kemp

The group of unsubstituted sulfonamides that inhibits the enzyme carbonic anhydrase has been shown to have anticonvulsant properties in experimental animals and to include useful antiepileptics in humans. These agents include acetazolamide (5-acetamido -1,3,4- thiadiazole -2- sulfonamide: Diamox), the most extensively studied drug of this group, and methazolamide (Neptazone), an agent little used at present. The usefulness of these agents is limited because of the rapid development of tolerance to their anticonvulsant effects. Their only well-documented biochemical effect is inhibition of carbonic anhydrase. Consequently, the anticonvulsant effect is thought to be mediated through inhibition of this enzyme, mainly in brain. Since this enzyme, which catalyzes the hydration and dehydration of carbon dioxide, is found in many tissues other than brain, inhibition of carbonic anhydrase in these tissues by acetazolamide causes disturbances of their function and thereby can cause side effects; it also can alter the distribution of acetazolamide and other drugs in the body.

It is important, therefore, to summarize the absorption, distribution, biotransformation, excretion, toxicity, mechanism of action, and therapeutic uses of acetazolamide and methazolamide. Maren (44) has written a comprehensive review of carbonic anhydrase and its inhibition by drugs, and

Woodbury (77) has reviewed the mechanism of the antiepileptic action of acetazolamide. Excellent discussions of carbonic anhydrase (CA) are found in the reviews by Carter (10) and Lindskog et al. (41) and discussions of its reactions with sulfonamides are by Coleman (15). The New York Academy of Sciences Monograph edited by Tashian and Hewitt-Emmett (71) is an excellent summary of the biology and chemistry of the carbonic anhydrases.

CHEMISTRY AND METHODS OF DETERMINATION

The structures of acetazolamide and methazolamide are shown in Fig. 1.

Acetazolamide is an unsubstituted sulfonamide with a pK_a of 7.4. The structure-activity relationships of the carbonic anhydrase inhibitors have been described by Maren (46). All unsubstituted aromatic sulfonamides (aryl-SO_2NH_2) inhibit CA, and no other class of organic compounds approaches these in activity. The K_1 for inhibition of CA in red cells and brain for acetazolamide is in the range of 1 to 6 $\times$ 10^{-8}M. Ability to inhibit CA also increases, in a homologous series, with lipid solubility of the undissociated sulfonamide molecule. Alkyl substitution in the SO_2NH_2 group confers only weak inhibitory activity to the

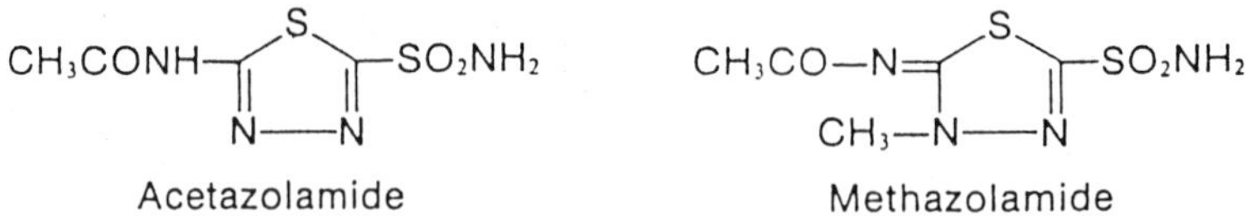

FIG. 1. Structures of acetazolamide and methazolamide.

molecule, whereas aromatic substitution yields high inhibitory activity, and resonating heterocyclic structures (e.g., acetazolamide, ethoxzolamide, benzolamide) confer very high activity on the SO_2NH_2 group. In benzene sulfonamides, ester or amide substitution in the *para* position yields far more active compounds than *ortho* or *meta* substitution. Very large or bulky fused-ring systems with multiple substituents seem to repress activity. Also, introduction of an acidic group appears to increase inhibitory activity in a degree relative to the strength of the acid group.

Methods for quantifying the concentrations of acetazolamide in body fluids utilize the carbonic anhydrase inhibition method of Maren et al. (48: see 31 for application of this method to epileptics), GLC with electron capture (73), and HPLC (7,13). Earlier workers (30) used a modification of the colorimetric procedure of Bratten and Marshall, but this is much less sensitive than the enzyme inhibition, gas-liquid chromatography (GLC) or high-performance liquid chromatography (HPLC) procedures. The GLC method is able to detect 10 ng/sample, the HPLC method is sensitive to 25 ng/ml plasma, and the enzyme assay 200 ng/ml. The molecular weight of acetazolamide is 222.

ABSORPTION

Acetazolamide is present in gastric juice (pH 2.0) predominantly in the un-ionized form. Since this form is adequately soluble in gastric juice, it is absorbed from the stomach to some extent. However, absorption occurs mainly in the duodenum and upper jejunum where the surface area is larger, the pH higher, and the solubility of the drug greater. The factors that affect the absorption of most weak acids also influence the absorption of acetazolamide, namely, pH, lipid and water solubility, and concentration in the gastrointestinal fluids.

Absorption is rapid, and peak levels in the plasma are reached 2 to 4 hr after oral ingestion of a single dose. In humans, oral doses in the range of 5 to 10 mg/kg appear to be completely absorbed (49), but at high doses, absorption is erratic and results in variable levels in the plasma (50). Absorption is complete within 2 hr in the dog (49). Wallace et al. (73) found that after oral administration of a single 250-mg dose to five volunteers, peak plasma water concentrations of acetazolamide of 10 to 18 μg/ml were reached 1 to 3 hr after the doses. Peak erythrocyte concentrations of 13 to 29 μg/ml were reached 1 hr later. Plasma levels declined thereafter more rapidly than erythrocyte levels (see below). Bayne et al. (7) found in humans that a single oral dose of 500 mg in the form of a tablet was absorbed more rapidly, reached a higher level (26 μg/ml), and fell off more rapidly than did a 500-mg timed release formulation. The peak time of absorption of the regular tablet was 3.5 hr, whereas for the timed release preparation, the plateau was reached at 3.5 hr but maintained a value of about 10 μg/ml until 10 hr. However, after this time, the plasma concentration fell off very slowly and at the same rate as that of the regular tablet, and at 45 hr after ingestion, significant levels were still present in the plasma.

DISTRIBUTION

Plasma Binding

Following absorption, acetazolamide is bound to plasma proteins to the extent of about 60% to 70% in rats, 50% to 60% in cats, 45% to 60% in dogs and 90% to 95% in humans (Table 1). Thus, the unbound levels are about 30% to 40% of the total except in humans in whom the value is 10% or less. The nature of the forces involved in the binding and the proteins to which the drug is bound have not been elucidated. Also, it is not known if other drugs compete with acetazolamide for binding to the protein although this appears to be the case for the increase in carbamazepine plasma concentrations induced by acetazolamide (21). The percentage of acetazolamide bound is dose-dependent (Table 1). This is evidence for saturation of the acetazolamide-binding proteins in plasma. The increased free levels at higher doses result in an increase in the rate of excretion in the urine and a decrease in the plasma half-life of acetazolamide. Since the PK_a of this drug is 7.4, at the pH of blood (7.4), half of the free level exists as the un-ionized, freely diffusible molecule. It is this molecule that penetrates into tissues and is available for binding to and subsequent inhibition of carbonic anhydrase (see below).

Plasma Half-Life and Volume of Distribution

The plasma half-life of acetazolamide varies markedly with the species (Table 1). The decay time, when plotted on semi-logarithmic paper, has two components: a very rapid one, of which the half-lives for various species are shown in Table 1, and a slow one. The rapid component represents movement of unbound diffusible acetazolamide into the total body water (50). After penetrating the cells, the drug also binds to the carbonic anhydrase present in tissues, including erythrocytes, renal cortex and medulla, stomach, salivary glands, pancreas, and brain. The slow component of the plasma decay curve, therefore, represents both the very low dissociation constant of the enzyme-inhibitor complex [EI] in the enzyme-containing tissues and the rate of renal excretion of acetazolamide that shifts the equilibrium, $[E_{free}] + [I_{free}] \rightleftharpoons [EI]$, to the left by removing free drug. The half-life of the slow component in the dog, for example, is about 2 days. This is in contrast to the half-life of the fast or mobile component of about 100 min (Table 1). After 24 hr, 90% of the drug in the body is bound to carbonic anhydrase in the various tissues as the enzyme-inhibitor [EI] complex. Of this amount, most is found in erythrocytes, kidney, and stomach, which contain very high concentrations of this enzyme. As seen in Fig. 2, erythrocytes contain very high concentrations of [^{3}H]acetazolamide as compared to other tissues (see also 12,13,31,39,73). The level of drug in the erythrocytes correlates with some of the pharmacological effects (e.g., ocular responses) and the toxicity of the drug, and can be expressed as a nonlinear pharmacokinetic model (12,39,40).

In a dog given 5 mg/kg (22 μmoles/kg) of acetazolamide, it was observed (44,47) that in the rapid phase of the plasma decay curve, 95% of the drug exists in the free form. Only 1.14 μmoles/kg were present as [EI], and this was mostly in red cells (1 μmole/kg), kidneys (0.1 μmole/kg), and stomach (0.04 μmole/kg); the amounts in the other carbonic anhydrase-containing tissues were negligible. The free level declined rapidly by first-order kinetics with a half-life of 100 min. The concentration of free acetazolamide was sufficiently high that for 4 hr more than 99.5% of the enzyme was inhibited. This is an amount sufficient to produce a therapeutic effect, e.g., prevention of seizures in epileptics and blockade of experimentally induced seizures in

TABLE 1. *Plasma binding, plasma total and free levels, brain levels, volume of distribution, and plasma half-life of acetazolamide in various species*

Species	Ref.	Dose (mg/kg) and route	% Bound in plasma	Concentration (µ/ml) Plasma Total	Plasma Free	Brain	RBC	Muscle	Saliva	CSF	Volume of distribution (liter/k)	Plasma half-life (hr)
Man Child	50	14 i.v.	90	46	46					0.6	0.2^a, 1.8^b	1.6 (fast phase)
Adult	44,50		95	10–20	0.5–1.0						0.1–0.2		
			90	25–50	2.5–5.0						0.3–0.5		
			83	75	13								
Adult	31, and personal communication	1.5 oral		6–9			22–29						10–12 (2nd phase)
Adult epileptics	31 and personal communication	2.5 oral		12–16			26–39						ca. 15
		5.0 oral		20–30			30–52						
		9.1–11.1 oral		30 (plateau) 19			52						
		(250 mg bid)		13			51–53						
				11									
	73,7,10	4 days / 1–2 wk / 1 mo / 2–8 mo (250 mg) oral	94	14 (10–18 at 1–3 hr)	0.6–1.1	18 (13–29) (2–7 h)			0.1–0.18			2 (fast phase) 13 (slow phase)
	7	7.2 (500 mg) oral	—	26 (3.5 hr)								
Dog Adult	51	5 i.v.	60	12	4.8					0.1–0.15 / 0.5–1.0 / 1.25–2.5	0.4^a, 1.0^b	1.7 (fast phase) 48 (slow phase)
	44		60	2.3	0.8–1.2							
			45	10–20	5.5–11.0							
			33	15–20	16–33							
Cat Adult	44	i.v.	63	2–3	0.7–1.1					0.2–0.3		2
	53		51	10–20	4.9–9.8					1–2		
Rat Adult	44	i.v.	69	2–3								1.1
	44		67	10–20								
			60	25–50								
			36	70–100								
			24	260–350								
	44	20 oral	67	101 (0.5 hr)	33	4.8	112	56				
				32 (2.0 hr)	11	3.5	101	42				
				11 (3 hr)		12 (3 hr)	40 (3 hr)					
	31	20 i.p.	65									
Mouse Adult	44	i.p.	16	2–3								
	44		5	10–20								0.2

^{a} Volume of distribution based on total concentration of acetazolamide in plasma early after administration.
^{b} Volume of distribution based on unbound concentration of acetazolamide in plasma early after administration.

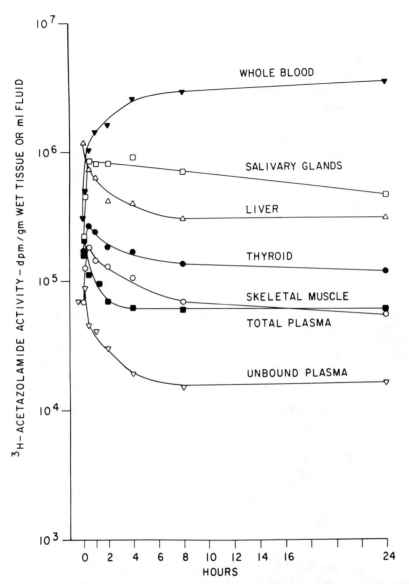

FIG. 2. Distribution of ³H-acetazolamide into various tissues of adult rats with time after i.p. administration.

animals (see 57, for example). By 8 hr, the free concentration in plasma was small, and the therapeutic effect was finished. At this time, of the 22 μmoles/kg injected into the animal, less than 1 μmole was free drug and all of the remaining drug was bound to carbonic anhydrase. The total molar concentration of acetazolamide found in the tissues 24 to 48 hr after ingestion of the drug was found to be a measure of the molar concentration of carbonic anhydrase, because it was almost all bound as [EI] (44,47).

The apparent volumes of distribution of acetazolamide in humans and in dogs in doses from 5 to 20 mg/kg are shown in Table 1. In humans, the value based on total plasma concentration is 0.2 liter/kg (20%) (50), and in the dog, 0.4 liter/kg (40%) (51). The difference between human and dog results mainly from differences in plasma binding of these two species (Table 1). If the volume of distribution in humans is calculated from the free level in the plasma, it is 1.8 liter/kg (180%), a value that indicates accumulation or binding in tissues even during the early phase of the distribution of acetazolamide in the body. Most of the excess over the amount in total body water is bound to erythrocyte carbonic anhydrase, as described above. The volume of distribution in dogs based on the free plasma level is also greater than can be accounted for in total body water (1.0 liter/kg).

Distribution into Tissues and Transcellular Fluids

As just described, acetazolamide rapidly diffuses into tissue water as the free form and then binds to tissue carbonic anhydrase. In these tissues, its concentration is higher than in plasma. Thus, in the rat (Fig. 2), the concentration of [^{3}H]acetazolamide is higher in erythrocytes, salivary glands, liver, and thyroid gland than the total concentration in plasma, and considerably higher than the concentration of the free drug in plasma. The highest concentration is found in erythrocytes which also contain the most carbonic anhydrase. These tissues are carbonic anhydrase-containing tissues, and the high concentrations undoubtedly reflect the high affinity of acetazolamide for this enzyme.

It has also been shown (see 47 for a summary) that the concentration of the drug is higher in stomach, kidney, cortex and medulla, pancreas, choroid plexus, ciliary process, and inner ear tissues, all of which are secretory organs in which carbonic anhydrase is present and involved in the secretory process. The concentration of the drug in noncarbonic anhydrase-containing tis-

sues such as smooth muscle and heart is about the same as that of the free drug in the plasma.

The concentration of acetazolamide in various tissues of 3-day-old rats has also been assessed. The concentration relative to plasma is lower than in the same tissues in adult rats, with the exception of muscle in which the concentration is the same as the free level in plasma. These tissues (liver, salivary glands, thyroid, erythrocytes) in 3-day-old rats have a lower activity of carbonic anhydrase and also a lower concentration of acetazolamide than do the corresponding adult tissues. This is further evidence that the binding is to carbonic anhydrase.

Acetazolamide penetrates into all transcellular fluids (44). The levels in cerebrospinal fluid (CSF), aqueous humor, saliva (31,73), and gastric juice are generally lower than the free level in plasma. The level in bile is higher than the free level in plasma, and acetazolamide is probably actively excreted in bile, as are many other drugs that are weak acids. The concentration in milk also appears to be higher than that in plasma (49); further experimentation should reveal if acetazolamide is actively secreted into this fluid. The low level in saliva relative to the free drug concentration in plasma suggests that this drug may be actively reabsorbed across the ducts of the salivary gland. Acetazolamide crosses the placenta and enters the fetal bloodstream and tissues; large doses cause teratogenic effects.

CSF and Brain Distribution

The concentration of acetazolamide in the CSF in various species of animals (humans, dog, cat) is lower than the free level in the plasma. This can be explained either by removal of the drug by bulk flow of CSF, similar to the process by which inulin is removed, by active secretion out of the CSF across the choroid plexus, or by both processes, after its slow entrance into the CSF via the cerebral capillaries across the blood-brain barrier. Since the concentration of acetazolamide in CSF can be increased by large doses of acetazolamide to a greater extent than the increase in plasma concentration, it appears that the drug obeys saturation kinetics in its movement across the choroid plexus. This suggests that it is actively transported out of the CSF and that saturation of the transport system blocks this transport and increases CSF (and brain) levels of the drug (see 78 for a summary). Further evidence for active transport out of CSF could be obtained by determining if the concentration in the CSF is increased by probenecid, a drug that blocks the transport of weak acids out of CSF.

The concentration of acetazolamide in brain of adult rats is lower than the total concentration in plasma but higher than that of CSF; however, in 3-day-old rats the CSF concentration is higher than that of brain (Table 1). When the brain concentration in adult rats is compared with that in the CSF (or free plasma concentration since it is the same as that in CSF), the concentration is much higher in brain (Fig. 3). This is to be expected since glial cells in brain contain carbonic anhydrase and since CSF is in equilibrium with the interstitial fluid of the brain and serves as the source of drug for this tissue. The brain-to-CSF ratio for [³H]acetazolamide in adult rats at equilibrium (24 hr) is 2.0, and in 3-day-old rats it is 1.1 (Fig. 3). The concentration of acetazolamide starts to increase in the brain relative to the CSF and approaches the adult

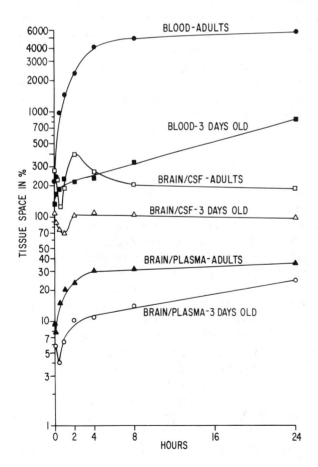

FIG. 3. Tissue-to-plasma and tissue-to-CSF ratio in percent of ³H-acetazolamide in adult and 3-day-old rats. Note that there are higher spaces of blood, brain/plasma, and brain/CSF in adult than in 3-day-old rats.

values about the 10th day after birth, a time when glial cells begin to proliferate in the brain. Since glial cells are the main carbonic anhydrase-containing cells in the brain (22, see 77,79,80 for reviews), the acetazolamide found in the brain is localized to these cells. However, studies by Rogers and Hunt (62) on the distribution of carbonic anhydrase-II messenger RNA in chick brain by the method of *in situ* hybridization demonstrated that the most intense carbonic anhydrase-II hybridization was to the choroid plexus, Bergmann glia of the cerebellum, to the Müller cells in the retina, but that it was also present in cells identifiable as neurons in hyperstriatum, tectum, and thalamus. Thus, this enzyme may have a function in some central neurons in some species.

Studies on the subcellular distribution of carbonic anhydrase in brain have demonstrated that this enzyme is found predominately (75–80%) in the cytoplasm (supernatant fraction) and in crude mitochondria (20–25%) (32). However, the crude mitochondrial fraction in brain contains synaptosomes and myelin, as well as mitochondria. Subsequent studies (3,9,17,65–67,89) have demonstrated that carbonic anhydrase is also found in myelin and cell membranes. Its presence in brain cell mitochondria is still debatable (see 17), although data from this laboratory (3,18) have demonstrated its presence in these subcellular organelles. Thus, Anderson et al. (3) showed that mitochondria in oligodendrocytes of C57 (audiogenic seizure-resistant) and DBA (audiogenic seizure-sensitive) mice contain carbonic anhydrase whereas mitochondria in astrocytes do not. They also demonstrated that in astrocytes carbonic anhydrase is present in the cytoplasm, on the outer surface of intracellular vesicles, and on the inner surface of the plasma membrane. In oligodendrocytes this enzyme is also present in the cytoplasm and in the myelin, but not in other membranes. DBA mice had more enzyme in both cell types than did C57 mice. Also oligodendrocytes

had more carbonic anhydrase than did astrocytes. When acetazolamide is given, carbonic anhydrase activity in the cytoplasmic myelin and membrane fractions, but not that in mitochondria, is inhibited. Thus, this drug does not appear to penetrate into this organelle (83,84). The relation between the inhibition of this enzyme in the various subcellular fractions by acetazolamide to its anticonvulsant effects is discussed below.

The concentration of acetazolamide in brain and CSF can be influenced by many factors. In anticonvulsant doses, the carbonic anhydrase in the choroid plexus is inhibited and its activity reduced. This results in a reduction of CSF production and flow. Since some of the drug in the CSF of humans is undoubtedly removed by bulk flow of CSF, the reduced CSF flow produced by acetazolamide will decrease its outflow and thereby increase the concentration of this drug in the CSF and in the brain. This will result in increased inhibition of the brain enzyme. Drugs such as digitalis glycosides and the high-ceiling saluretics—ethacrynic acid and furosemide—that inhibit CSF production and decrease flow can also increase the concentration of acetazolamide in CSF and brain. Also, drugs such as probenecid that inhibit active transport of drugs out of CSF could also increase the level of acetazolamide in CSF and brain by blocking its transport out of CSF.

The acid-base status of the patient can alter the distribution of acetazolamide in the body and in the CSF and brain. Since it is a weak acid with a pK_a of 7.4, alteration of pH of the extracellular or cellular fluids affects the percentage of drug in the un-ionized form. It is in this form that the drug freely diffuses across cell membranes. The potentiation by CO_2 and ammonium chloride of the inhibitory effect of acetazolamide on experimental seizures in animals can be explained, at least in part, as a result of the acidosis produced by these agents increasing the concentration of un-ionized drug in the plasma (23,56,87). This would increase the level of drug in the brain and hence its anticonvulsant effect.

BIOTRANSFORMATION

In humans, 100% of a single orally administered dose of acetazolamide is recovered in the urine in 24 hr (44); there is no evidence that it is metabolized to another substance in the liver (44). In dogs, the average total amount recovered in the urine is 70%, all present as acetazolamide. Some is secreted in the bile and lost in feces, but the fate of the remainder is not known (44). In rats, only 30% of acetazolamide is recovered as such in urine, but a large fraction is excreted in the bile and presumably in the feces (44). No evidence has been found that metabolism of the drug occurs in rats. Only unchanged drug is found in the urine of cats; hence, it is also not metabolized in this species (1).

EXCRETION

As is the case with certain other sulfonamides that are acetylated on the amino nitrogen, acetazolamide is secreted by renal tubular cells in humans (43,50); about 80% of the drug is excreted by tubular secretion. In the dog, clearance of unbound acetazolamide is equal to or slightly below that of creatinine (49); however, Weiner et al. (74) have shown that probenecid decreases this clearance, a fact suggesting that in addition to reabsorption, tubular secretion also occurs in this species. Thus, as for many weak acids, the excretion of acetazolamide is dependent both on passive tubular reabsorption as the un-ionized molecule and on tubular secretion as the anionic species. Tubular secretion is restricted to the unbound fraction in plasma (12). The elderly have a reduced capacity to clear unbound acetazolamide from plasma and this correlates with their age-related reduction in creatinine clearance. They also have a reduced

plasma protein binding which offsets the reduced unbound clearance of acetazolamide resulting in similar excretory rates as in younger persons and children (12).

High doses of the drug inhibit renal carbonic anhydrase which results in increased urinary excretion of bicarbonate and alkalinization of the urine. This results in systemic metabolic acidosis. The increased pH of the urine decreases the percentage of the drug in the un-ionized form. This, therefore, decreases the amount reabsorbed and increases urinary excretion. However, the systemic metabolic acidosis decreases the amount in the ionized form: hence, less is available for tubular secretion, but more of the un-ionized species is available for penetration into cells. The net effect of the high doses, therefore, depends on which of these processes predominates when the pH is changed and on what happens to intracellular pH in renal tubule cells as compared with cells in other tissues.

INTERACTIONS WITH OTHER DRUGS

Since acetazolamide is not metabolized by the liver, its level in the body cannot be affected by drugs that either induce or inhibit the drug-metabolizing enzymes in the liver. However, it is actively excreted in the bile and in the feces. Consequently, drugs that either decrease or accelerate bile flow or inhibit the transport of weak acids into bile can alter the level of the drug in the plasma. Although no such effects have been reported in humans, such changes are theoretically possible and should be kept in mind.

The absorption of drugs from the intestinal tract is also altered by acetazolamide (69). This effect appears to be related to inhibition of carbonic anhydrase in isolated loops of duodenum and ileum in rats. For example, Schnell and Miya (69) found that the absorption in the ileum of *d*-amphetamine was decreased and that of salicylic acid was increased by acetazolamide. Plasma levels reflected the effect on absorption; the pH of the ilial contents was decreased. In the duodenum, acetazolamide increased the absorption of *d*-amphetamine and decreased that of salicylic acid; the pH of the contents was not changed. It has not been determined if this drug affects absorption of other drugs from the intestinal tract in humans, but this remains a real possibility.

Probenecid, which blocks renal tubular secretion of acids, has been shown to decrease the excretion of acetazolamide in urine. This increases the level in the plasma and also in the CSF and brain and thereby can affect its anticonvulsant activity.

The interaction of acetazolamide with drugs that affect CSF production and with factors that alter acid-base balance in the body are discussed in a previous section. In rats, acetazolamide has been shown to enhance the degree of central depression produced by pentobarbital, to increase the duration of pentobarbital-induced sleep time, and to increase the brain pentobarbital space (59). This last effect is probably a result of the ability of acetazolamide to decrease CSF flow (60) and thereby decrease the bulk removal of pentobarbital from the brain. It is likely that this effect occurs in humans not only for pentobarbital but also for other sedatives and anticonvulsants.

Since acetazolamide is bound to plasma proteins to an extent greater than 90% in humans, it is likely that many drugs that are bound to the same proteins can compete with this drug for the binding sites. Although this has not been demonstrated clinically, it, too, remains a theoretical possibility. Inui et al. (31) found that some other anticonvulsants given in various combinations with acetazolamide did not alter the plasma or erythrocyte concentrations of acetazolamide in epileptic patients. However, acetazolamide has been reported to increase carbamazepine plasma concentrations when given to children resistant to carbamazepine (21).

Acetazolamide also influences the activity of other drugs because of the many effects in the body that result from inhibition of carbonic anhydrase. Thus, alkalinization of urine and production of a saluresis, production of a systemic acidosis, inhibition of CSF production, decreased secretion of ocular fluids, and other changes that result from carbonic anhydrase inhibition can all produce effects on the penetration of other drugs into various fluids and tissues and on the level of other drugs in the plasma. Most of the effects are in the direction of increasing the concentration of weak acids in the tissues. In the case of anticonvulsants, most of which are weak acids, this is an advantage because adequate concentrations of the anticonvulsant in brain can be obtained with lower doses, with the consequent reduction in side effects caused by the anticonvulsant. It is reasonable, therefore, to use acetazolamide in combination with other anticonvulsants, particularly in patients refractory to these drugs and in those in whom side effects may be troublesome, as was demonstrated by Forsythe et al. (21) in carbamazepine-resistant epilepsy in children. Complete remission of seizures for 2 years was obtained in nine of 22 children when acetazolamide (10 mg/kg) was added to carbamazepine (20 mg/kg) and six had more than 75% reduction, whereas increasing the dose of carbamazepine alone without addition of acetazolamide (from 20 to 25 mg/kg) impaired seizure control by more than 75% in only three of 25 children. Thus, acetazolamide allowed reduction of carbamazepine dosage with consequent reduction of side effects and better seizure control.

PHARMACOLOGICAL EFFECTS

Acetazolamide is a potent anticonvulsant agent in both laboratory animals and epileptic patients (5,20,42,43,52,57,82,83,88). In experimental animals, it abolishes the tonic extensor component of the maximal electroshock (MES) seizure, as does CO_2, and it potentiates this effect of CO_2 on seizure pattern (82,83). The anticonvulsant action of acetazolamide is not abolished by nephrectomy; hence, this action is independent of the systemic acidosis it produces from inhibition of renal CA.

Falbriard and Gangloff (20) noted that acetazolamide slightly increased the threshold voltage for stimulation of the cortex and markedly increased the threshold of the diencephalon. This drug also prevents audiogenic seizures (19). It protects against seizures produced by inhalation of 30% CO_2 or by withdrawal from 50% CO_2 (88). In addition, acetazolamide protects against seizures evoked by various pharmacological agents. It reduces the intensity of spinal discharges induced by convulsive doses of strychnine, and it antagonizes pentylenetetrazol- and picrotoxin-induced seizures, but in doses higher than those necessary to protect against MES seizures. It thus possesses, as does CO_2, a wide spectrum of anticonvulsant action. Also, as is the case with CO_2, acetazolamide selectively depresses monosynaptic pathways in the spinal cord without affecting synaptic recovery or posttetanic potentiation (see 82 for summary). Thus, both acetazolamide and CO_2 have the same spectrum of effects on the nervous system and probably act in the same manner, by causing an accumulation of CO_2 in the brain, as discussed below.

These data have been interpreted to mean that acetazolamide and CO_2 affect some neuronal process that is more critically concerned in the spinal cord monosynaptic pathway than in polysynaptic circuits. The most outstanding difference between the component synapses of these two systems is that the safety factor with which transmission occurs is lower for monosynaptic than for polysynaptic pathways. It is suggested, therefore, that acetazolamide and CO_2 decrease the safety factor of transmis-

sion and that depression is produced by the drug at all synapses in which the safety factor is low, as in the spinal monosynaptic pathways.

Further evidence that carbonic anhydrase is involved in the spread of discharges was presented by Davenport (16) who observed that in rabbits treated with a carbonic anhydrase inhibitor, thiophene-2-sulfonamide, local stimulation of the cerebral cortex did not affect the general electrical activity of the stimulated area.

Carbonic anhydrase inhibitors other than acetazolamide have also been shown to affect the nervous system. Sulfanilamide abolishes the tonic extensor component of the MES in experimental animals and possesses a weak antiepileptic effect in man. Methazolamide and ethoxzolamide, congeners of acetazolamide, also exhibit anticonvulsant activity in experimental animals (26,27).

Millichap et al. (53–55) have presented convincing evidence that carbonic anhydrase is of functional significance in the development of the electroshock seizure pattern in maturing rats and guinea pigs. They suggested that this enzyme was important in the development of the ability to exhibit maximal tonic convulsions in which a generalized spread of the seizure discharge is probably involved, but that the enzyme probably was not involved in the capacity to exhibit clonic seizures, which involves localized neuronal discharges. This suggestion was supported by their observations that the hyperkinetic behavior induced by electroshock in rats not over 10 days old was refractory to acetazolamide, that the clonic seizures induced by electroshock in 10- to 20-day-old rats were abolished only by very large doses of this drug, and that the tonic type of seizures seen in 21-day or older rats was abolished by low doses of acetazolamide. However, in mice, acetazolamide elevates the minimal electroshock clonic seizure threshold in doses that also block tonic extension induced by electroshock and also block pentylenetetrazol-induced clonic seizures (4) (see below).

There is much experimental and clinical evidence (see 83 for summary) that tolerance develops to the anticonvulsant activity of acetazolamide. If the anticonvulsant activity of acetazolamide results from a localized increase in P_{CO_2} in neuronal cells, it follows logically that the tolerance that is known to develop to the anticonvulsant effect of acetazolamide should be accompanied by tolerance to the anticonvulsant effect of CO_2. That this assumption is correct was demonstrated by Koch and Woodbury (35) who found that tolerance developed to the repeated administration of acetazolamide and that cross-tolerance concurrently developed to CO_2. These data provide further strong evidence for a common mode of action of CO_2 and acetazolamide.

MECHANISM OF ACTION OF ACETAZOLAMIDE

Since the only well-documented biochemical effect of acetazolamide is inhibition of carbonic anhydrase, it has been demonstrated that the mechanism of its anticonvulsant action (as well as the other sulfonamide CA inhibitors) is through inhibition of this enzyme in the brain (26,27,57). The consequence of inhibition of brain carbonic anhydrase is CO_2 accumulation, which appears to cause the anticonvulsant effect of this drug, and, as mentioned above, acetazolamide and CO_2 have identical actions as far as their effect on the central nervous system are concerned. However, in higher doses, acetazolamide produces a greater effect on the brain by causing a retention of CO_2 in the body secondary to inhibition of red cell carbonic anhydrase (see summary in 44).

Summaries of the mechanism of action of this drug on the CNS and its relationship to carbonic anhydrase have been provided by Woodbury and colleagues (76,77,79,80, 81,82–85), and summaries of the role of carbonic anhydrase in the CNS are given by Sapirstein et al. (68).

Because the primary anticonvulsant effect of acetazolamide is mediated through an effect on brain carbonic anhydrase, it is pertinent to discuss the distribution of this enzyme in brain. Studies originally carried out by Giacobini (22) and subsequently by other investigators (33,64,65,72) have demonstrated that carbonic anhydrase is located in the glial cells of the brain and also appears to be located in the glial product, myelin (9,33,65–67,89). Roussel et al. (65) have demonstrated by the indirect immunoperoxidase technique that the carbonic anhydrase II isoenzyme is specifically localized in the cytoplasm of oligodendrocytes and astrocytes and that it is also present in the cytoplasmic areas of the myelin sheath but does not appear in the compact myelin. No reaction was found in neuronal cell bodies. These workers also noted a strong positive reaction to the antiserum in the choroid plexus (see also 62). Subcellular distribution studies show that the enzyme is located in the cytosolic, membrane (mitochrondria, microsomes), and myelin fractions of brain cells, predominantly glia, as discussed above.

The role of carbonic anhydrase in myelin is not clear, but it appears to be concerned with enhancing CO_2 transfer across the myelin sheath and/or formation of myelin, since the carboxylation of acetyl CoA, a step in fatty acid synthesis, to malonyl CoA by the biotin-requiring enzyme acetyl CoA carboxylase requires HCO_3^- and not CO_2 as one of its substrates. Whether acetazolamide inhibits formation of myelin has not been ascertained, but data in this laboratory have demonstrated that in rat cerebral cortex, the fixation of $^{14}CO_2$ into the acid-soluble and combined protein and lipid fractions is inhibited by acetazolamide. Also, DBA mice, which are susceptible to audiogenic seizures, have increased activity of this enzyme in this myelin fraction, as well as increased amounts of myelin (18,70). Acetazolamide appears to inhibit CO_2 fixation in brain by inhibiting carbonic anhydrase, thereby reducing the HCO_3^- in the cell available for synthesis into fatty acids. The experiments of Anderson et al. (4) demonstrated a role for carbonic anhydrase in myelin in the electroshock seizure clonic threshold-elevating effects of acetazolamide. They found that elevation of the electroshock seizure threshold by acetazolamide in mice correlated both in time-course and dose with the degree of inhibition of carbonic anhydrase activity in the myelin fraction of the cerebral cortex. Also, tolerance to this effect of acetazolamide on the clonic seizure threshold developed *pari passu* with an increase in the activity and total amount of carbonic anhydrase II in the myelin fraction of the cerebral cortex (2).

When acetazolamide is given, the carbonic anhydrase in the brain is inhibited to the extent of >99.0%. This results in an accumulation of total CO_2 in the brain (36,63,83). This CO_2 accumulation is sufficient to account for the prevention of the tonic extensor component of the maximal electroshock, since the effects on the brain of CO_2 itself are identical to those of acetazolamide (82,83). In high doses, acetazolamide inhibits erythrocyte carbonic anhydrase (see below) and causes some CO_2 accumulation which may contribute to the anti-MES effect of the drug (26,27). The mechanism of the increase in total CO_2 in the brain induced by acetazolamide appears to be due to inhibition of carbonic anhydrase in the cytosolic fraction of the glial cells in brain. This enzyme is involved in the transfer of H^+ and/or HCO_3^- from neurons to glial cells and interference with this process by acetazolamide causes CO_2 to back up in neurons in amounts sufficient to block the spread of a seizure discharge and result in an anticonvulsant effect. Anderson et al. (4) have shown that the anti-MES effect of acetazolamide in mice is correlated both in time-course and dose with the de-

gree of inhibition of carbonic anhydrase in the cytosolic fraction of the brainstem. Tolerance to the anti-MES effect of prolonged administration of acetazolmide developed in parallel with an increase in the activity and total amount of carbonic anhydrase II in the cytosolic fraction of the brainstem (3).

Other evidence for a role of glial cell carbonic anhydrase in the regulation of brain excitability comes from studies on cobalt-induced focal epileptogenic lesions in the frontal cortex of rats (see 77,80,81,85,86 for summaries). Such lesions caused an increase in glial cell carbonic anhydrase in the regions of increased polyspike activity in the EEG (around primary focus in frontal cortex, secondary focus on opposite side, parietal cortex) but not in areas in which polyspike activity was not present (occipital cortex). The increase in carbonic anhydrase was accompanied by a decrease in total brain CO_2 and an increase in CO_2 fixation. These effects are opposite to those produced by acetazolamide and suggest that the glial carbonic anhydrase response to increased neuronal activity enhances the ability of these cells to handle the greater metabolic production of CO_2 caused by the increased neuronal activity. Since acetazolamide given in either single doses or for prolonged periods to cobalt-implanted rats inhibits carbonic anhydrase in the glial cells, increases polyspike activity on the electroencephalogram, and enhances clinical seizure activity in such rats, it is evident that this glial enzyme response is a protective mechanism to the increased neuronal activity that, by maintaining K^+ and acid-base homeostasis, delimits the spread of seizure activity. Thus, acetazolamide has two anticonvulsant effects on seizure properties: the anti-MES effect, which measures spread of seizure activity and effectiveness against generalized tonic-clonic seizures in epileptic patients and appears to be directly related to CO_2 accumulation as a result of inhibition of carbonic anhydrase in the cytoplasm of the cell, and elevation of the seizure threshold for initiation of seizures, which appears to be related to inhibition of the enzyme in myelin. In addition, this drug has an excitatory effect (decrease in electroshock seizure threshold and enhanced seizure and polyspike activity), generally with higher doses, that appears to be related to blockade of a glial anion (Cl^-, HCO_3^-) transport system that requires this enzyme and occurs only when the enzyme in glia has been induced in response to increased excitability, as is the case in cobalt-induced focal seizures or in DBA audiogenic seizure mice. In this case acetazolamide blocks the adaptive effect of this enzyme in glia to protect against the increase in excitability (see 79–81).

As mentioned below, experimental animals develop tolerance to the anti-MES effects of prolonged administration of acetazolamide (35). Epileptic patients also develop tolerance with long-term treatment (5,31,42,43,52). The development of tolerance to the anticonvulsant effects of acetazolamide results from the induction both of increased activity and amount of enzyme in glial cells (2,6,19) and the production of more glial cells. Thus, the glial cells play an active role, mediated via carbonic anhydrase, in regulating excitability of the brain as well as in maintaining anion homeostasis. The development of tolerance to acetazolamide, which is the main cause of its limited use in epileptic patients, is thus the result of induction of carbonic anhydrase in glial cells and proliferation of glia. Therefore, a higher dose of acetazolamide is required to produce the same degree of inhibition achieved initially.

These data support a fundamental role of carbonic anhydrase in glial cell metabolism such that any drug, hormone, injury, or other insult that compromises the rate at which this enzyme can catalyze the hydration of CO_2 to form HCO_3^- for anion transport into glial cells and for CO_2 fixation reactions involving synthesis of fatty acids for myelin formation, synthesis of neurotrans-

mitters, synthesis of carbamylphosphate for pyrimidine synthesis or urea cycle amino acids, and formation of oxalacetate for utilization in the Krebs cycle will immediately set in motion the machinery for activation and synthesis of new carbonic anhydrase to relieve these compromised vital functions of the cell (see 2).

In addition to the carbonic anhydrase inhibitor drugs and cobalt implantation, as described above, increases of carbonic anhydrase activity in glial cells can be observed during maturation and aging (18,38,53–55,86), in audiogenic seizure mice (18,86), in mice given several subconvulsive doses of strychnine which also induces tolerance to the convulsant effects of this drug, and in animals subjected to multiple electroshock seizures (*unpublished observations*).

The development of tolerance to the anticonvulsant effect of acetazolamide proceeds by two mechanisms that are dose-dependent: (a) increase in the total amount of carbonic anhydrase II, changes that suggest increased synthesis of this enzyme, and (b) activation of existing molecules of carbonic anhydrase II, a process that appears to involve phosphorylation (2). Both these processes probably are mediated by cyclic AMP. Thus, it is of particular interest that Kimelberg and colleagues (14,34,58) have shown *in vitro* that both norepinephrine and dibutyryl cyclic AMP induce an increase in the carbonic anhydrase activity found in the soluble but not in the membrane fraction of cultured astrocytes obtained from 1- to 3-day-old rat brains and that this increase parallels the rate of process extension of these astrocytes. There was also an induced increase in Na^+, K^+-ATPase, but the increase did not parallel growth of the fibers. The stimulation by norepinephrine was blocked by propanolol. Norepinephrine also increased the phosphorylation of carbonic anhydrase, an effect also blocked by propanolol. Thus, the norepinephrine-induced increase in cyclic AMP levels in brain results in activation of astroglial carbonic anhydrase because of cyclic AMP-stimulated phosphorylation of the enzyme (14). Such experiments provide direct evidence for a role of adrenergic stimulation and cyclic AMP in regulation of carbonic anhydrase activity and growth of glial cells and in regulation of brain excitability.

The regulation of excitability may be due to the transmitter-induced increase in carbonic anhydrase as a normal response. Thus Church et al. (14) have proposed that the activation of astroglial carbonic anhydrase by putative transmitters may be involved in specific ion-transport responses of these cells, which, under certain conditions, can lead to astroglial swelling. Further evidence is that the anticonvulsant effect of acetazolamide is blocked by reserpine which depletes biogenic amines, particularly the catecholamines (28,37). How or whether this is related to effects on carbonic anhydrase is still unclear.

Effects of acetazolamide and other inhibitors of this enzyme on neurotransmitters have been little studied (see 76 for summary). Acetazolamide, similarly to CO_2, increases γ-aminobutyric acid (GABA) levels in the brain (82), which may account for some of its anticonvulsant effects. Whether this is related to its inhibition of carbonic anhydrase is not known. Effects on other neurotransmitters are also unknown.

CLINICAL USE

Many reports attest to the efficacy of acetazolamide and other sulfonamide carbonic anhydrase inhibitors against various types of epilepsy. Acetazolamide was first introduced for the therapy of epilepsy by Bergstrom et al. (8), and subsequent reports (5,21,24,31,42,45,52) confirmed its effectiveness in most types of epilepsy (generalized tonic-clonic, absence, and complex partial seizures). However, the value of these carbonic anhydrase inhibitors is lim-

ited because of the rapid development of tolerance to their anticonvulsant effects (5,42,43,52). This shortens their effectiveness to a time period of rarely longer than 3 to 6 months. They are however, useful for longer periods of time when used as adjuncts to primary antiepileptic drugs such as ethosuximide, carbamazepine, or phenytoin. In many cases tolerance does not develop when acetazolamide is used in this manner (see, e.g., 21). Once tolerance has developed, withdrawal of the drugs for a period of time restores susceptibility to their antiepileptic effects. Acetazolamide has also proved of value as an adjunct drug used intermittently in the therapy of catamenial epilepsy. In such patients water retention occurs, and this drug causes a saluretic effect. Hydrochlorothiazide is also used but does not have an antiepileptic effect. Hence, it is not known whether the antiepileptic effect of acetazolamide also contributes to the control of seizures in such patients. Acetazolamide is probably most useful in absence attacks (24), particularly in combination with ethosuximide. Tolerance development, however, limits its period of usefulness even in this condition.

Toxicity, as described below, is particularly low and is mainly related to tingling of hands and feet, an effect that disappears in a few days, and alteration of taste sensation. Transient somnolence also is occasionally present.

Onset of the antiepileptic effect of acetazolamide is rapid, and seizures in patients with absences may cease within 3 to 4 hr. However, recurrence may also occur within 24 hr of ceasing administration of the drug. Since the half-life is 10 to 12 hr in humans, steady-state plasma levels are reached only after 40 to 48 hr. The usual dose is 250 mg given one to three times a day (250 to 750 mg/day). Doses larger than this do not produce any greater effects, since inhibition of brain carbonic anhydrase has occurred to the maximal extent possible. High doses increase erythrocyte drug levels to about 50 μg/ml (31), a level sufficient to cause the side effects discussed above which appear to result from CO_2 retention as a result of inhibition of CO_2 exchange across the erythrocyte membrane. Hence, erythrocyte levels of acetazolamide appear to be a better indicator of toxicity than do plasma levels (31).

Relation of Plasma Acetazolamide Levels to Therapeutic Effect

The plasma acetazolamide levels in humans in effective antiepileptic doses (250 mg three times daily or about 10 mg/kg per day) are 10 to 14 μg/ml. Inui et al. (31) found that four of eight patients given 500 mg/day (250 mg twice daily) were free of focal motor or generalized tonic-clonic seizures when their plasma acetazolamide concentrations reached 8 to 14 μg/ml; the other four had reduced frequencies of attacks at plasma concentrations in the same range. Erythrocyte concentrations in these patients ranged from 49 to 53 μg/ml. Except for brain, the levels of acetazolamide in carbonic anhydrase-containing tissues, as discussed above, are considerably higher than those in the plasma. In muscle, which contains a carbonic anhydrase that is resistant to inhibition by acetazolamide and does not bind this drug (61), the concentration in the blood-free tissue is nearly the same as in an ultrafiltrate of plasma and varies with the plasma concentration.

Development of Tolerance

Tolerance to the anticonvulsant effects of acetazolamide develops with long-term administration to animals (2,6,19,35,83,87) or humans (5,31,42,43,52). This is the main limitation to its therapeutic use. Inui et al. (31) showed that with long-term use of the

drug, the initially high plasma levels (see Table 1) decrease after 1 to 2 months to a plateau value about 60% of the initial steady-state concentration. This is paralleled by a tolerance to its anticonvulsant effects, and an increased dose is required to obtain the same effect. The decrease in plasma level is not accompanied by a decrease in the concentration of acetazolamide in the erythrocytes, an observation that suggests that the drug in the plasma has moved into the erythrocytes and other carbonic anhydrase-containing tissues, including brain, because its presence in the body has induced the synthesis of more carbonic anhydrase to combat the inhibition imposed by the drug. The increased amount of carbonic anhydrase would then allow more binding of acetazolamide as the [EI] complex. The only source of the drug to move into the cells is the plasma. Data from the effects of prolonged acetazolamide treatment of rats with cobalt-induced focal epileptogenic lesions support this postulate, since this drug increased activity of this enzyme in the primary and secondary focal areas of such rats, and this was accompanied by tolerance to the CNS effects of the acetazolamide (see 79,80,85,86 for summaries). Also, prolonged administration of acetazolamide induces increased activity and amount of carbonic anhydrase in normal and audiogenic seizure-susceptible mice with development of tolerance to the anticonvulsant effect of the drug in the normal but not the audiogenic-seizure susceptible mice (3,6,19).

Toxicity

Very large doses of acetazolamide can be tolerated without significant side effects. In fact, it is one of the least toxic of the antiepileptic drugs. All effects would seem to be related to inhibition of carbonic anhydrase with the exception of the hypersensitivity reactions. Several subjective complaints have been noted, such as drowsiness and paresthesias. The most severe objective reactions are skin rashes, abdominal distention, and cyanosis. Reactions similar to those produced by other sulfonamides have also been reported (see 11 for summary). An interesting side effect of acetazolamide is its ability to alter taste sensation in at least 90% of patients (25,29, cited in 75 with a partial English translation in 25). It totally eliminates the tingle or prickly feeling of carbonation, and hence gives a flat taste to such beverages. The effect is specific for carbonic anhydrase inhibitors and is localized in the taste buds, which contain carbonic anhydrase (see 75).

Inui et al. (31) have described the time sequence of the appearance of side effects with acetazolamide on administration of 5 mg/kg to four healthy adults, correlated with the concentration of the drug in the erythrocytes. In these four subjects, the concentration of acetazolamide in the erythrocytes rapidly rose to values greater than 40 µg/ml, and all four developed symptoms attributable to the drug as follows: 1 hr after administration: face paresthesia, numbness of the extremities, hyperpnea, all of which lasted for 24 hr; 3 to 4 hr: dizziness, nausea, and perspiration; 6 hr.: weakness of hands and numbness of fingers. Most symptoms disappeared in 8 to 24 hr. In hepatic cirrhosis, episodes of disorientation

may be induced by acetazolamide. It has been postulated that alkalinization of the urine diverts ammonia of renal origin from the urine into the systemic circulation and produces the disorientation. Calculus formation and ureteral colic have been attributed to the marked reduction in urinary citrate produced by acetazolamide and associated with either no change or even a rise in urinary calcium.

Teratogenic effects of acetazolamide have been described in experimental animals, and it is recommended that this drug not be given to women in early pregnancy (45).

METHAZOLAMIDE

Methazolamide has a pK_a of 7.2 and, like acetazolamide, is a weak acid whose movement across cells is dependent on the unionized form; hence, it is pH dependent. It is similar to acetazolamide in many respects but is more readily diffusible into tissues, and the free levels in the tissues are the same as the free levels in plasma. The pertinent data for this drug are summarized in Table 2. Plasma binding is approximately equal in all species (55–70%) except the mouse. Brain and CSF levels are generally higher relative to plasma than with acetazolamide, and the drug penetrates into brain much faster than does acetazolamide. The

TABLE 2. *Plasma binding, plasma total and free levels, brain levels, and plasma half-life of methazolamide in various species[a]*

Species (adult)	Dose (mg/kg) and route	5 Bound in plasma	Concentration (µg/ml)						Plasma half-life (min)
			Plasma		Brain	RBC	Muscle	CSF	
			Total	Free					
Man	oral	55	2–50	2.9–23				0.3–7.5	300
Dog	i.v.	55	2–50						150
Cat	i.v.	68	2–50						180
Rat	20 oral	55	103	46	20	110	35		—
			76	34	3	120	45		
Mouse	i.v.	5	2–50						66

[a] Compiled from Maren, ref. 43.

CSF-to-plasma ratio is 0.15 for methazolamide.

In humans, after an oral dose the plasma half-life is as long as 10 hr. Excretion in the urine of the unchanged drug is by glomerular filtration and tubular reabsorption. In humans, about 20% to 30% of methazolamide is removed as such in urine; the remainder 70% to 80% is metabolized to an as yet unknown compound.

Functionally, a lower dose of methazolamide than of acetazolamide is required to inhibit carbonic anhydrase because higher levels in the tissues can be obtained for the same dose.

As with acetazolamide, binding of methazolamide to tissue carbonic anhydrase does occur. The pharmacology of this drug is summarized elsewhere by Maren (44). Its pharmacological effects and mechanism of action are like those of acetazolamide, as discussed above.

SUMMARY

Acetazolamide is rapidly absorbed, becomes effective within hours, and is rapidly eliminated in the urine as the unchanged drug. Metabolism by the liver does not occur. Binding to plasma proteins is high (90% in humans), and only the free form is available for diffusion into tissues. This process is pH-dependent. Soon after administration, the drug is present in total body water as the free drug, which is present in sufficient concentrations to inhibit carbonic anhydrase in brain and other tissues and to produce its anticonvulsant and other effects. Binding occurs to tissue carbonic anhydrase to form the enzyme-inhibitor complex [EI], and after 24 hr, almost all of the drug is present in tissue in this form. This complex has a low dissociation constant; hence, the drug is released from the tissues only slowly as it is excreted in the urine. This is a slow process with a half-life of several days.

Acetazolamide penetrates into the brain and CSF slowly and reaches a concentration much lower than the total level in the plasma. The concentration in the brain, however, is higher than that in the CSF, and the brain level is dependent on its concentration in this fluid. The concentration in brain and CSF is dependent on many factors such as the rate of CSF flow, the rate of transport of the drug out of the CSF, and the permeability of the blood-brain barrier. Most of the bound drug in the body is found in the erythrocytes which contain a high amount and activity of carbonic anhydrase.

Renal excretion of acetazolamide is by tubular reabsorption and secretion. Biliary excretion of the drug also occurs, particularly in dogs and rats.

Few drug interactions with acetazolamide have been described, but many theoretical possibilities for interaction exist.

The toxicity of acetazolamide is low, and generally minor side effects result from its use.

Acetazolamide exerts its anticonvulsant action by inhibiting carbonic anhydrase in myelin, in cytoplasm, and in membranes of glial cells. This results in CO_2 accumulation in brain and blockade of anion transport, effects that block spread of seizure activity and elevate seizure threshold.

CONVERSION

Acetazolamide

Conversion factor:

$$CF = \frac{1000}{\text{mol. wt.}} = \frac{1000}{222} = 4.50$$

Conversion:

$$(\mu g/ml) \times 4.50 = (\mu moles/liter)$$

$$(\mu moles/liter) \div 4.50 = (\mu g/ml)$$

ACKNOWLEDGMENTS

This work was supported in part by U.S. Public Health Service Grants #5R01-

NS21255 and #1R01-NS21834 from the National Institute of Neurological and Communicative Disorders and Stroke. D. M. Woodbury is a Research Career Awardee (5-K06-NS-13838) of the NINCDS.

REFERENCES

1. Achor, L. B., and Roth, L. J. (1957): Metabolic fate of acetazolamide-S^{35} (Diamox) in the cat. *Fed. Proc.*, 16:277.
2. Anderson, R. E., Chiu, P., and Woodbury, D. M. (1989): Mechanisms of tolerance to the anticonvulsant effects of acetazolamide in mice: Relation to the activity and amount of carbonic anhydrase in brain. *Epilepsia* 30:208–216.
3. Anderson, R. E., Engstrom, F. L., and Woodbury, D. M. (1984): Localization of carbonic anhydrase in the cerebrum and cerebellum of normal and audiogenic seizure mice. In: *Biology and Chemistry of the Carbonic Anhydrases,* edited by R. E. Tashian and D. Hewitt-Emmett, Ann. N.Y. Acad. Sci., 249:502–504.
4. Anderson, R. E., Howard, R. A., and Woodbury, D. M. (1986): Correlation between effects of acute acetazolamide administration to mice on electroshock seizure threshold and maximal electroshock seizure pattern, and on carbonic anhydrase activity in subcellular fractions of brain. *Epilepsia*, 27:504–509.
5. Ansell, B., and Clarke, E. (1956): Acetazolamide in treatment of epilepsy. *Br. Med. J.*, 1:650–661.
6. Banks, D. A., Anderson, R. E., and Woodbury, D. M. (1986): Induction of new carbonic anhydrase II following treatment with acetazolamide in DBA and C57 mice. *Epilepsia*, 27:510–515.
7. Bayne, W. F., Rogers, G., and Crisologo, N. (1975): Assay for acetazolamide in plasma. *J. Pharm. Sci.*, 64:402–404.
8. Bergstrom, W. H., Garzoli, R. F., Lombroso, C., Davidson, D. T., and Wallace W. M. (1952): Observations on metabolic and clinical effects of carbonic anhydrase inhibitors in epileptics. *Am. J. Dis. Child.*, 84:71–73.
9. Cammer, W., Fredman, T., Rose, A. L., and Norton, W. T. (1976): Brain carbonic anhydrase: Activity in isolated myelin and the effect of hexachlorophene. *J. Neurochem.*, 27:165–171.
10. Carter, M. J. (1972): Carbonic anhydrase: Isoenzymes, properties, distribution, and functional significance. *Biol. Rev.*, 47:465–513.
11. Chao, D. H. C., and Plumb., R. L. (1961): Diamox in epilepsy: A critical review of 178 cases. *J. Pediatr.*, 58:211–228.
12. Chapron, D. J., Sweeney, K. R., Feig, P. U., and Kramer, P. A. (1985): Influence of age on the disposition of acetazolamide. *Brit. J. Clin. Pharmac.*, 19:363–371.
13. Chapron, D. J., and White, L. B. (1984): Determination of acetazolamide in biological fluids by reverse-phase high performance liquid chromatography. *J. Pharmaceutical Sci.*, 73:985–989.
14. Church, G. A., Kimelberg, H. K., and Sapirstein, V. S. (1980): Stimulation of carbonic anhydrase activity and phosphorylation in primary astroglial cultures by norepinephrine. *J. Neurochem.*, 34:873–879.
15. Coleman, J. E. (1975): Chemical reactions of sulfonamides with carbonic anhydrase. *Annu. Rev. Pharmacol.*, 15:221–242.
16. Davenport, H. W. (1946): Carbonic anhydrase in the nervous system. *J. Neurophysiol.*, 9:41–46.
17. Dodgson, S. J., Forster, R. E. II, Storey, B. T., and Mela, L. (1980): Mitochondrial carbonic anhydrase. *Proc. Natl. Acad. Sci.*, 77:5562–5566.
18. Engstrom, F. L., Kemp, J. W., and Woodbury, D. M. (1984): Subcellular distribution of carbonic anhydrase and Na^+, K^+- and HCO_3^--ATPases in brains of DBA and C57 mice. *Epilepsia*, 25:759–764.
19. Engstrom, F. L., White, H. S., Kemp, J. W., and Woodbury, D. M. (1986): Acute and chronic acetazolamide administration in DBA and C57 mice: Effects of age. *Epilepsia*, 27:19–26.
20. Falbriard, A., and Gangloff, H. (1955): Action d'un inhibiteur de la carboanhydrase l'acetazolamide, sur l'excitabilité du cortex, du thalamus et du rhinencephale. *Experientia*, 11:234–235.
21. Forsythe, W. I., Owens, J. R., and Toothill, C. (1981): Effectiveness of acetazolamide in the treatment of carbamazepine-resistant epilepsy in children. *Develop. Med. Child Neurol.*, 23:761–769.
22. Giacobini, E. (1962): A cytochemical study of the localization of carbonic anhydrase in the nervous system. *J. Neurochem.*, 9:169–177.
23. Goldberg, M. A., Barlow, C. F., and Roth, L. J. (1961): The effects of carbon dioxide on the entry and accumulation of drugs in the central nervous system. *J. Pharmacol. Exp. Ther.*, 131:308–318.
24. Golla, F. L., and Sessions, H. R. (1957): Control of petit mal by acetazolamide. *J. Ment. Sci.*, 103:214–217.
25. Graber, M., and Kelleher, S. (1988): Side effects of acetazolamide: The champagne blues. *Am. J. Med.*, 84:979–980.
26. Gray, W. D., Maren, T. H., Sisson, G. M., and Smith, F. H. (1957): Carbonic anhydrase inhibition VII. Carbonic anhydrase inhibition and anticonvulsant effect. *J. Pharmacol. Exp. Ther.*, 121:160–170.
27. Gray, W. D., and Rauh, C. E. (1967): The anticonvulsant action of inhibitors of carbonic anhydrase: Site and mode of action in rats and mice. *J. Pharmacol. Exp. Ther.*, 156:383–396.
28. Gray, W. D., and Rauh, C. E. (1971): The relation between monoamines in brain and the anticonvulsant action of inhibitors of carbonic anhydrase. *J. Pharmacol. Exp. Ther.*, 177:206–218.
29. Hansson, H. P. J. (1961): On the effect of carbonic anhydrase inhibition on the sense of taste; an unusual effect of a medication. (Translated by Jane Dennis Vigertz, quoted in 25). *Nord. Med.*, 65:566–567.
30. Harke, W., Schirren, C., and Wehrmann, R.

(1959): Experimentelle Untersuchungen zur Bestimmung der Acetazolamid-Ausscheidung im menschlichen Harn mittels eines Diazotier-und Kupplungsverfahrens. *Klin. Wochenschr.*, 37:1040–1044.

31. Inui, M., Azuma, H., Nishimura, T., and Hatada, N. (1982): The concentration of acetazolamide in blood and saliva. In: *The XIIIth Epilepsy International Symposium,* edited by H. Akimoto, H. Kazamatsuri, M. Seino and A. A. Ward, Jr. *Advances in Epileptology,* 13:307–309. Raven Press, New York.

32. Karler, R., and Woodbury, D. M. (1960): Intracellular distribution of carbonic anhydrase. *Biochem. J.,* 75:538–543.

33. Kimelberg, H. K., Biddlecome, S., Narumi, S., and Bourke, R. S. (1978): ATPase and carbonic anhydrase activities of bulk-isolated neuron, glia, and synaptosome fractions from rat brain. *Brain Res.,* 141:305–323.

34. Kimelberg, H. K., Narumi, S., Biddlecome, S., and Bourke, R. S. (1978): $(Na^+ + K^+)ATPase$, $^{86}Rb^+$ transport and carbonic anhydrase activity in isolated brain cells and cultured astrocytes. In: *Dynamic Properties of Glia Cells,* edited by E. Schoffeniels, G. Franck, L. Hertz, and D. B. Tower, pp. 347–357. Pergamon Press, Oxford.

35. Koch, A., and Woodbury, D. M. (1958): Effects of carbonic anhydrase inhibition on brain excitability. *J. Pharmacol. Exp. Ther.,* 122:335–342.

36. Koch, A., and Woodbury, D. M. (1960): Carbonic anhydrase inhibition and brain electrolyte composition. *Am. J. Physiol.,* 198:434–440.

37. Koslow, S. H., and Roth, L. J. (1971): Reserpine and acetazolamide in maximum electroshock seizure in the rat. *J. Pharmacol. Exp. Ther.,* 176:711–717.

38. Koul, O., and Konungo, M. S. (1975): Alterations in carbonic anhydrase of the brain of rats as a function of age. *Exp. Gerontol.,* 10:273–278.

39. Kunka, R. L., and Mattocks, A. M. (1979): Nonlinear model for acetazolamide. *J. Pharm. Sci.,* 68:342–346.

40. Kunka, R. L., and Mattocks, A. M. (1979): Relationship of pharmacokinetics to pharmacological response for acetazolamide. *J. Pharm. Sci.,* 68:347–349.

41. Lindskog, S., Henderson, L. E., Kannan, K. K., Liljas, A., Nyman, P. O., and Standberg, B. (1971): Carbonic anhydrase. In: *The Enzymes, Vol. 5.,* 3rd edition, edited by P. D. Boyer, pp. 587–665. Academic Press, New York.

42. Lombroso, C. T., Davidson, D. T., Jr., and Gross-Bianchi, M. L. (1956): Further evaluation of acetazolamide (Diamox) in treatment of epilepsy. *J.A.M.A.,* 160:268–272.

43. Lombroso, C. T., and Forsythe, I. (1960): A long-term follow-up of acetazolamide (Diamox) in the treatment of epilepsy. *Epilepsia,* 1:493–500.

44. Maren, T. H. (1967): Carbonic anhydrase: Chemistry, physiology and inhibition. *Physiol. Rev.,* 47:595–781.

45. Maren, T. H. (1971): Editorial. Teratology and carbonic anhydrase inhibition. *Arch. Ophthalmol.,* 85:1–2.

46. Maren, T. H. (1976): Relations between structure and biological activity of sulfonamides. *Annu. Rev. Pharmacol. Toxicol.,* 16:309–327.

47. Maren, T. H. (1963): The binding of inhibitors to carbonic anhydrase *in vivo:* Drugs as markers for enzyme. In: *Proc. 1st International Pharmacology Meeting,* pp. 39–48. Pergamon Press, New York.

48. Maren, T. H., Ash, V. I., and Bailey, E. M. (1954): Carbonic anhydrase inhibition. II. A method for determination of carbonic anhydrase inhibitors, particularly of Diamox. *Bull. Johns Hopkins Hosp.,* 95:244–249.

49. Maren, T. H., Mayer, E., and Wadsworth, B. C. (1954): Carbonic anhydrase inhibition. I. The pharmacology of Diamox (2-acetylamino-1,2,4-thiadiazole-5-sulfonamide). *Bull. Johns Hopkins Hosp.,* 95:199–243.

50. Maren, T. H., and Robinson, B. (1960): The pharmacology of acetazolamide as related to cerebrospinal fluid and the treatment of hydrocephalus. *Bull. Johns Hopkins Hosp.,* 106:1–24.

51. Maren, T. H., Wadsworth, B. C., Yale, E. K., and Alonso, L. G. (1954): Carbonic anhydrase inhibition. III. Effects of Diamox on electrolyte metabolism. *Bull. Johns Hopkins Hosp.,* 95:277–321.

52. Millicap, J. G. (1956): Anticonvulsant action of Diamox in children. *Neurology (Minneap.),* 6:552–559.

53. Millicap, J. G. (1957): Development of seizure patterns in newborn animals. Significance of brain carbonic anhydrase. *Proc. Soc. Exp. Biol. Med.,* 96:125–129.

54. Millicap, J. G. (1958): Seizure patterns in young animals. II. Significance of brain carbonic anhydrase. *Proc. Soc. Exp. Biol. Med.,* 97:606–611.

55. Millicap, J. G., Balter, M., and Hernandez, P. (1958): Development of susceptibility to seizures in young animals. III. Brain water, electrolyte and acid-base metabolism. *Proc. Soc. Exo. Biol. Med.,* 99:6–11.

56. Millicap, J. G., Thatcher, L. D., and Williams, P. M. (1955): Anticonvulsant action of acetazolamide, alone and in combination with ammonium chloride. *Fed. Proc.,* 14:370.

57. Millicap, J. G., Woodbury, D. M., and Goodman, L. S. (1955): Mechanism of the anticonvulsant action of acetazolamide, a carbonic anhydrase inhibitor. *J. Pharmacol. Exp. Ther.,* 115:251–258.

58. Narumi, S., Kimelberg, H. K., and Bourke, R. S. (1978): Effects of norepinephrine on the morphology and some enzyme activities of primary monolayer cultures from rat brain. *J. Neurochem.,* 31:1479–1490.

59. Reed, D. J. (1968): The effects of acetazolamide on pentobarbital sleeptime and cerebrospinal fluid flow of rats. *Arch. Int. Pharmacodyn. Ther.,* 171:206–215.

60. Reed, D. J., and Woodbury, D. M. (1962): Effect of urea and acetazolamide on brain volume and cerebrospinal fluid pressure. *J. Physiol. (Lond.),* 164:265–273.

61. Register, A. M., Koester, M. K., and Noltman, E.

A. (1978): Discovery of carbonic anhydrase in rabbit skeletal muscle and evidence for its identity with "basic muscle protein". *J. Biol. Chem.,* 253:4143–4152.

62. Rogers, J. H., and Hunt, S. P. (1987): Carbonic anhydrase-II messenger RNA in neurons and glia of chick brain: Mapping by *in situ* hydridization. *Neuroscience,* 23:343–361.

63. Rollins, D. E., Withrow, C. D., and Woodbury, D. M. (1970): Tissue acid-base balance in acetazolamide-treated rats. *J. Pharmacol. Exp. Ther.,* 174:535–540.

64. Rose, S. P. R., and Sinha, A. K. (1971): Bulk separation of neurones and glia: A comparison of techniques. *Brain Res.,* 33:205–217.

65. Roussel, G., Delaunoy, J. P., Nussbaum, J. L., and Mandel, P. (1979): Demonstration of a specific localization of carbonic anhydrase C in the glial cells of rat CNS by an immunohistochemical method. *Brain Res.,* 160:47–55.

66. Sapirstein, V. S., and Lees, M. B. (1978): Purification of myelin carbonic anhydrase. *J. Neurochem.,* 31:505–511.

67. Sapirstein, V. S., Lees, M. B., and Trachtenberg, M. C. (1978): Soluble and membrane bound carbonic anhydrases from rat CNS: Regional development. *J. Neurochem.* 31:283–287.

68. Sapirstein, V. S., Strocchi, P., and Gilbert, J. M. (1984): Properties and function of brain carbonic anhydrase. In: *Biology and Chemistry of the Carbonic Anhydrases,* edited by R. E. Tashian and D. Hewitt-Emmett. *Annals N.Y. Acad. Sci.,* 429:481–493.

69. Schnell, R. C., and Miya, T. S. (1970): Altered absorption of drugs from the rat small intestine by carbonic anhydrase inhibition. *J. Pharmacol. Exp. Ther.,* 174:177–184.

70. Seyfried, T. N., Glaser, G. H., and Yu, R. K. (1978): Cerebrum, cerebellum and brainstem gangliosides in mice susceptible to audiogenic seizures. *J. Neurochem.,* 31:21–28.

71. Tashian, R. E., and Hewitt-Emmett, D. (eds.) (1984): *Biology and Chemistry of the Carbonic Anhydrases. Annals N.Y. Acad. Sciences,* 429:640.

72. Tower, D. B., and Young, G. M. (1973): The activities of butyrylcholinesterase and carbonic anhydrase, the rate of anaerobic glycolysis, and the question of a constant density of glial cells in cerebral cortices of various mammalian species from mouse to whale. *J. Neurochem.,* 20:269–278.

73. Wallace, S. M., Shah, V. P., and Riegelman, S. (1977): GLC analysis of acetazolamide in blood, plasma, and saliva following oral administration to normal subjects. *J. Pharm. Sci.,* 66:527–530.

74. Weiner, I. M., Washington, J. A., and Mudge, G. H. (1959): Studies on the renal excretion of salicylate in the dog. *Bull. Johns Hopkins Hosp.,* 105:284–297.

75. Wistrand, P. J. (1984): The use of carbonic anhydrase inhibitors in ophthalmology and clinical medicine. *Ann. N.Y. Acad. Sci.* 429:609–619.

76. Woodbury, D. M. (1977): Pharmacology and mechanisms of action of antiepileptic drugs. In: *Scientific Approaches to Clinical Neurology,* edited by E. S. Goldensohn and S. H. Appel, pp. 693–726. Lea and Febiger, Philadelphia.

77. Woodbury, D. M. (1980): Carbonic anhydrase inhibitors. *Adv. Neurol.,* 27:617–633.

78. Woodbury, D. M. (1983): Pharmacology of anticonvulsant drugs in CSF. In: *Neurobiology of Cerebrospinal Fluid, Vol. II.,* edited by J. Wood, chap. 38, pp. 615–628. Plenum Press, New York.

79. Woodbury, D. M., Anderson, R. E., Chiu, P., and Engstrom, F. (1988): Role of glial cell carbonic anhydrase in seizures. In: *The Biochemical Pathology of Astrocytes,* edited by M. D. Norenberg, L. Hertz, and A. Schousboe, pp. 503–517. Alan R. Liss, Inc., New York.

80. Woodbury, D. M., Engstrom, F. L., McQueen, J. K., Anderson, R. E., White, H. S., and Yen-Chow, Y. C. (1986): Role of glial carbonic anhydrase in focal and generalized tonic-clonic seizures. In: *Dynamic Properties of Glia Cells II. Cellular and Molecular Aspects,* edited by T. Grisar, G. Franck, L. Hertz, W. T. Norton, M. Sensenbrenner, and D. M. Woodbury. *Advances in the Biosciences, Vol. 61,* pp. 329–341. Pergamon Press, New York.

81. Woodbury, D. M., Engstrom, F. L., White, H. S., Chen, C. F., Kemp, J. W., and Chow, S. Y. (1984): Ionic and acid-base regulation of neurons and glia during seizures. *Ann. Neurology,* 16 (suppl.):S135–S144.

82. Woodbury, D. M., and Esplin, D. W. (1969): Neuropharmacology and neurochemistry of anticonvulsant drugs. *Proc. Assoc. Res. Nerv. Ment. Dis.,* 37:24–56.

83. Woodbury, D. M., and Karler, R. (1960): The role of carbon dioxide in the nervous system. *Anesthesiology,* 21:686–703.

84. Woodbury, D. M., and Kemp, J. W. (1970): Some possible mechanisms of action of antiepileptic drugs. *Pharmakopsychiatr. Neuropsychopharmakol.,* 3:201–226.

85. Woodbury, D. M., and Kemp, J. W. (1977): Basic mechanisms of seizures: Neurophysiological and biochemical etiology. In: *Psychopathology and Brain Dysfunction,* edited by C. Shagass, S. Gershon, and A. J. Friedhoff, pp. 149–182. Raven Press, New York.

86. Woodbury, D. M., and Kemp, J. W. (1979): Initiation, propagation and arrest of seizures. In: *Patholophysiology of Cerebral Energy Metabolism,* edited by B. B. Mrsulja, L. M. Rakic, I. Klatzo, and M. Spatz, pp. 313–351. Plenum Press, New York.

87. Woodbury, D. M., and Rollins, L. T. (1954): Anticonvulsant effects of acetazolamide, alone and in combination with CO_2, on experimental seizures in mice. *Fed. Proc.,* 13:418.

88. Woodbury, D. M., Rollins, L. T., Gardner, M. D., Hirschi, W. L., Hogan, J. R., Rallison, M. L., Tanner, G. S., and Brodie, D. A. (1958): Effects of carbon dioxide on brain excitability and electrolytes. *Am. J. Physiol.,* 192:79–90.

89. Yandrasitz, J. R., Ernst, S. A., and Salganicoff, L. (1976): The subcellular distribution of carbonic anhydrase in homogenates of perfused rat brain. *J. Neurochem.,* 27:707–715.

Antiepileptic Drugs, Third Edition, edited by
R. Levy, R. Mattson, B. Meldrum,
J. K. Penry, and F. E. Dreifuss.
Raven Press, Ltd., New York © 1989.

62

Other Antiepileptic Drugs

Bromides

Fritz E. Dreifuss

Bromide was first used, unsuccessfully, in the early 1800s for the treatment of tuberculous abscesses in place of iodides. By 1850 it was recognized that the bromide ion had pharmacological actions resembling sedation. Because epilepsy was thought to be related to masturbation and also to hysteria, and because bromide preparations were soon recognized as having antiaphrodisiac properties, bromide was introduced by Locock (6) in 1857 for the treatment of catamenial seizures. For half a century, until the introduction of phenobarbital in 1912, it was the principal anticonvulsant.

ABSORPTION, DISTRIBUTION, AND EXCRETION

All the inorganic salts of bromine are water-soluble and rapidly absorbed from the intestinal tract. The distribution of bromide is similar to that of chloride, and it is thought that the bromide space is similar to that of the chloride space (4). Body tissues do not distinguish between chloride and bromide and thus the total halide concentration in the extracellular fluid remains relatively constant. Chloride and bromide tend to displace each other according to the intake and excretion of each ion. The drug is not protein-bound, is freely diffusible, and has a volume of distribution similar to that of chloride, although there is some difference in the distribution of bromide and chloride ions in some tissues, such as the gastric mucosa (9). The biological half-life of bromide ions in human blood is around 12 days (10).

Bromide is excreted via the urine. Excretion is quite slow and to some extent dependent on the rate of ingestion of other halides and can be hastened by a sodium load. Small amounts of bromide are also excreted in tears, sweat, and unswallowed saliva, and the concentration in saliva is 1.5 times that in plasma. Bromide that is swallowed in saliva is reabsorbed from the gastrointestinal tract. Cerebrospinal fluid concentrations of bromide are somewhat less than those of plasma, possibly as a result of choroid plexus secretion of the ion rather than passive diffusion (8).

The slowness of bromide excretion accounts for the long half-life. Steady state is reached very slowly but to some extent is influenced by chloride intake, and the lower the chloride intake the more rapid the accumulation of bromide. Bromide readily crosses the placenta. In general, iodide is the most rapidly excreted halogen, followed by bromide and then chloride, although the rapidity of excretion is to some extent concentration-dependent.

A recent study on the pharmocokinetics of bromides (11) added some valuable information concerning their bioavailability. A dose equivalent of 30 mg/kg of bromide was administered orally and intravenously, and the bioavailability, clearance, and elimination half-life were calculated. Bioavailability with the oral dose was 75% to 118%, and there was no significant difference between the serum concentration curves for oral or intravenous administration for any of the time points measured. The elimination half-life was 11.9 ± 1.4 days with oral administration and 9.4 ± 1.5 days with the intravenous route. The log-linear regressions of the concentration-time curves were excellent, indicating first-order elimination. Variation of volume distribution between subjects was minimal due to the distribution of bromide into the extracellular water space. Renal clearance was 267 ± 1.7 mg/kg/day. It was calculated that high chloride loads would increase bromide clearance and shorten the half-life and, conversely, a salt-deficient diet would have the opposite effect. The length of the half-life determines the steady-state concentration time with long-term drug exposure. Under these circumstances, four to five elimination half-lives would have to elapse before a steady-state concentration of bromide is reached, which means that 40 to 50 days would have to elapse for this estimate to be valid. Obviously, the complete bioavailability of the bromide ion with the oral route of administration can prove useful for calculation of extracellular body fluid.

MECHANISMS OF ACTION

A possible mode of action of bromide in the nervous system is anion potentiation of benzodiazepine receptors. γ-Aminobutyric acid (GABA) receptors appear to be coupled with a chloride channel, and the bromide effect on the benzodiazepine binding might be related to the GABA ionophore, which is normally a chloride channel (7). Since bromide has a smaller hydrated diameter than chloride, its passive movement across cell membranes is faster and therefore tends to hyperpolarize the postsynaptic membrane, which is activated by inhibitory neurotransmitters (12). It has also been found that anions which can substitute for chloride synaptically can inhibit strychnine binding (3). Moreover, it is possible that long-term administration of bromide induces plasticity in dendrites as has been shown in the superior cervical ganglia and in mouse neuroblastoma cells, where continuous bromide administration appears to promote synaptogenesis (3).

CLINICAL USE

The drug is usually administered as triple bromide elixir containing 1,200 mg per 5 ml delivered as equal quantities of potassium, sodium, and ammonium salts. The usual dosage in children under 6 years of age ranges from 300 mg twice a day to 600 mg three times a day; over 6 years of age, a dose of 300 mg to 1 g is given three times a day. The therapeutic blood bromide concentration is approximately 75 to 125 mg/100 ml (10–15 mEq/liter), and the concentration should be carefully monitored, as toxic effects may occur when it exceeds 150 mg/100 ml. The physical condition of the patient, the presence of food in the stomach or the fasting state and salt intake, dehydration, and vomiting, as well as impaired renal function, all affect the blood bromide concentration.

The toxic effects of bromides are vividly described in the quotation from Hammond (5): "As you see, he is broken down in appearance, has large abscesses in his neck, and is altogether in a bad condition. But this is better than to have epilepsy." Chronic bromide intoxication occurs when toxic doses of bromide are given over a prolonged period. Because of the slow excretion of bromide from the body, its accumulation is insidious. Chronic bromism usually occurs in older or elderly persons, particularly when renal function is somewhat impaired.

Symptoms of mild bromism are weakness, tiredness, lack of concentration, loss of appetite, and memory. In more severe cases, symptoms include restlessness, headache, insomnia, disorientation and depression, memory loss, and increasing dementia, occasionally with hallucinations. Incoordination, diminution of deep tendon reflexes, and ultimately loss of pupil reflexes may occur. The mucous membranes are dry, the tongue is dry and coated, there is loss of appetite, and there may be emaciation. Vasomotor disturbances may occur. Bromide intoxication rarely occurs with blood bromide levels below 200 mg/100 ml, but the levels are usually considerably higher.

Skin rashes may occur, but are not always present. The most common is an acneiform eruption on the face that may spread over the neck, chest, and arms and become more generalized. A nodular type of rash, vesicles, or pustules also may be seen. The skin rash is frequently found in younger persons, and the mental changes are more likely to occur in older persons.

Bromide intoxication is treated by stopping the medication and enhancing its urinary excretion by the administration of large amounts of fluid and, if necessary, by the infusion of saline and administration of 3 to 7 g of sodium chloride or 5 to 8 g of ammonium chloride in fractional doses daily. Bromide displaces chloride in the extracellular fluid, and with bromide intoxication, approximately 40% of chloride has been replaced by bromide. Ammonium chloride is the drug of choice in cases of congestive heart failure, where an undue amount of sodium chloride is contraindicated. Hemodialysis will quite rapidly lower the bromide level.

Although bromide was the drug of choice for the treatment of epilepsy for many years, present-day use of this drug has become extremely restricted by the development of less toxic anticonvulsants. It has been said that the success rate of the treatment of certain types of epilepsy has not increased greatly since the days of bromide therapy, but the modern drugs are considerably less toxic, which is their main advantage over the bromides.

Dreifuss and Bertram (2) treated various types of seizures with bromide when other anticonvulsants were unsuccessful. Only generalized tonic-clonic seizures responded well to bromide therapy, which was considerably less effective in complex partial seizures and absence seizures. Similar findings were reported by Boenick et al. (1), who recommended a trial of bromides in therapy-resistant tonic-clonic seizures.

REFERENCES

1. Boenick, H. E., Lorenz, J. H., and Jurgens, U. (1985): Bromide-hute als Antiepileptische Substanzen noch nutzlich? *Nervenarzt,* 10:579–582.
2. Dreifuss, F. E., and Bertram, E. H. (1986): Bromide therapy for intractable seizures. *Epilepsia,* 27:593.
3. Eins, S., Spoerri, P. E., and Heyder, E. (1983): Plasticity in dendrites by continuous bromide or GABA administration in superior cervical ganglion and in mouse neuroblastoma cells. *Cell. Tissue Res.,* 229:475–460.
4. Gamble, J. J., Jr., Robertson, J. S., Hanningan, C. A., Foster, C. G., and Farr, L. E. (1953): Chloride, bromide, sodium and sucrose spaces in man. *J. Clin. Invest.,* 32:483–489.
5. Hammond, W. A. (1874): *Clinical Lectures on Diseases of the Nervous System.* TMB Cross, New York.
6. Locock, C. (1857): Discussion of paper by E. H. Sieveking: Analysis of 52 cases of epilepsy observed by author. *Lancet,* 1:527.
7. Palachios, J. M., Nieholt, D. L., and Kuhar, M. J. (1979): Ontogeny of GABA and benzodiazepine receptors: Effects of Triton x-100, bromide and muscimal. *Brain Res.,* 179:390–395.
8. Patrick, S. I., and Eadie, G. S. (1952): Bromides in spinal fluid and serum. *Ann. J. Physiol.,* 168:254–259.
9. Söremark, R. (1960): Excretion of bromide ions by human urine. *Acta Physiol. Scand.,* 50:306–310.
10. Söremark, R. (1960): The biological half-life of bromide ions in human blood. *Acta Physiol. Scand.,* 50:119–123.
11. Vaiseman, N., Koren, G., and Pencharz, P. (1986): Pharmacokinetics of oral and intravenous bromide in normal volunteers. *Clin. Toxicol.,* 23:403–413.
12. Woodbury, D. M., and Pippenger, C. E. (1982): Bromides. In: *Antiepileptic Drugs,* 2nd edition, edited by D. M. Woodbury, J. K. Penry, and C. E. Pippenger, pp. 791–801. New York, Raven Press.

Antiepileptic Drugs, Third Edition, edited by
R. Levy, R. Mattson, B. Meldrum,
J. K. Penry, and F. E. Dreifuss.
Raven Press, Ltd., New York © 1989.

63

Other Antiepileptic Drugs

Paraldehyde

Lawrence A. Lockman

Paraldehyde (Paraacetaldehyde) has been in clinical use since 1882 when it was introduced by Cervello (7); its use as a general hypnotic was advocated by Strahan in 1885 (28). It has been recommended for the treatment of status epilepticus in both children (11) and adults (34,35). The antiepileptic effect occurs at somewhat lower doses than the hypnotic effect, though the margin is small. Paraldehyde has also been widely used in the treatment of delirium tremens (15); however, diazepam may be equally effective and safer (29). Though relatively easy to manufacture, paraldehyde is unstable, making storage and administration difficult; it also interacts with plastics which further complicates administration. Unfortunately, the intravenous preparation has been withdrawn by the manufacturer in the United States for economic rather than medical reasons. A preparation suitable for rectal use is still widely available.

CHEMISTRY AND METHODS OF DETERMINATION

Paraldehyde (2,4,5-trimethyl-1,3,5-trioxane) is the condensation product of acetaldehyde and is prepared by the polymerization of acetaldehyde catalyzed by HCl and H_2SO_4 at medium to high temperature. The molecular weight of paraldehyde is 132.16, and with specific gravity of 0.994, 1 ml is essentially equal to 1 g. The solubility in water is temperature-dependent; the maximum solubility (12.8%) occurs at 12°C. At 37°C the solubility in water is 7.8% (25); the solubility in blood has not been studied. However, intravenous administration of solutions of greater than 10% concentration may exceed the solubility and lead to droplets of pure paraldehyde in the blood.

Paraldehyde can be measured by chemical or gas chromatographic methods. In one chemical method, the drug is converted to acetaldehyde by treatment with heat and acid, and acetaldehyde is then assayed. This technique can be linked to an enzymatic assay using DPNH (30). In another method, paraldehyde and acetaldehyde are measured simultaneously by reaction at room temperature with hydroxylamine hydrochloride to form an aldoxime (12). Free acetaldehyde is measured, then hydroxylamine-HCl is added with heating. Paraldehyde is depolymerized to acetaldehyde which then forms the oxime, which is measured. Paraldehyde is measured directly with gas chromatography. Because ethanol and acetaldehyde elute separately, this method is advantageous when there is the possibility that alcohol may interfere with the assay (1).

Paraldehyde decomposes in the presence of light and air to acetaldehyde, with further conversion to glacial acetic acid. The drug is incompatible with many plastics, including polystyrene and styrene-acrylonitrile copolymer, as well as with rubber (9). Glass syringes are usually recommended. However, it has been demonstrated that 5 ml Plastipak and Glaspak syringes (Becton-Dickinson) may be stable in the presence of paraldehyde for up to 3 hr. Another suggested alternative is the use of polyvinyl chloride tubing of Butterfly infusion sets (Abbott Hospital Products, North Chicago, IL; No. 4506) with a polyethylene catheter (Clay Adams Intramedic Polyethylene Tubing, ID 0.015 inch, PE-20) (13).

ABSORPTION, DISTRIBUTION, AND EXCRETION

Paraldehyde, although readily absorbed after oral or intramuscular administration, is usually administered rectally or intravenously. The strong odor and taste of the drug renders the oral route unacceptable for most patients. Intramuscular use has been associated with sterile abscess formation, although this complication may be due to decomposition during storage. Injury to the sciatic nerve has also been reported. Rectal absorption is essentially complete when the drug is administered in an equal volume of mineral or vegetable oil. Peak absorption occurs 2 to 4 hr after the dose. Absorption after intravenous administration is, of course, complete.

Paraldehyde is rapidly distributed to the brain. Drowsiness or anesthesia occurs within 2 to 5 min after i.v. injection. Peak concentration in the cerebrospinal fluid (CSF) is found 20 to 60 min after oral or intramuscular administration. In adults, the steady-state volume of distribution (V_d) is 0.89 liter/kg. In infants, the mean apparent V_d was 3.8 ± 1.8 liter/kg (range, 2.0 to 7.7). Brain concentrations are about 25% to 30% lower than blood concentrations.

The distribution of ^{14}C-paraldehyde has been studied in rats (31). After a 0.1 ml/kg slow bolus injection, the serum distribution half-life was 6.7 ± 4.6 min and the elimination half-life was 8.2 ± 1.8 hr. The drug was found not be protein-bound. Drug was concentrated two-fold to three-fold more in fat than in the body organs. Paraldehyde entry into brain was largely determined by the rate of cerebral blood flow (31).

Paraldehyde readily crosses the placenta; cord blood levels are almost equal to maternal levels (12).

Although the pungent odor of paraldehyde is unmistakable in the exhaled breath of patients who have received the drug, only a small proportion is actually excreted by the pulmonary route. In normal subjects given 60 mg/kg orally, about 7% of the administered dose was exhaled in the first 4 hr. Paraldehyde was the only detectable exhaled excretion product. Excreted percentages did not depend on dose, and concentrations of drug in the exhaled air were unaffected by changes in minute volume, although the amounts excreted per unit time were proportional to volume of respiration (20). In mice, the rate of pulmonary excretion was a function of dose but it did not exceed 14%; the rate was higher in animals with livers damaged by the prior administration of carbon tetrachloride (17). On the other hand, up to 100% pulmonary excretion has been reported in rats (23).

Thurston et al. (30) found that after intramuscular administration, clinical effects of paraldehyde were seen long before maximal serum levels were reached. Sedation occurred by 3 min and sleep by 5 to 15 min although maximal serum levels were not reached until 20 to 60 min after injection. CSF fluid levels averaged 75% of serum levels 1 hr after injection.

BIOTRANSFORMATION

Biotransformation occurs in the liver where paraldehyde is first depolymerized to acetaldehyde which is then oxidized to acetic acid (Fig. 1) (36). It takes place in microsomes and requires an intact cytochrome P-450 system (37). The rate of the oxidation step is at least fourfold that of the depolymerization step (17); therefore acetaldehyde does not accumulate to measurable levels. At lower concentrations, the rate of transformation is dose-dependent; it is constant at higher concentrations.

In nine full-term human infants infused with paraldehyde at the rate of 150 mg/kg/hr in a 5% solution in 5% dextrose, the disposition rate constant was 0.0680 ± 0.0071 hr^{-1}, and the half-life 10.2 ± 1.0 hr; volume of distribution was 1.73 ± 0.20 liter/kg; and clearance was 0.121 ± 0.023 liter/hr/kg (13). These half-lives are significantly greater than the 6.13 hr reported in adults (1) and higher than the 7.4 hr in children reported by Thurston et al. (30). Interestingly, phenobarbital administration decreased both paraldehyde clearance and volume of distribution in a manner linearly related to the logarithm of the phenobarbital dose (13). The authors attributed this effect to competitive inhibition of the cytochrome P-450 oxidase system.

In another study of newborn infants, 10 received an intravenous bolus of 200 mg/kg followed by an infusion of 16 mg/kg/hr and four received a 400 mg/kg bolus (19). Total body clearance was 154.6 ± 71.5 ml/kg/hr (range, 61.1 to 316). The mean apparent volume of distribution was 3.8 ± 1.8 liter/kg (range, 2.0 to 7.7), and the elimination half-life ($T_{1/2}$) was 18.1 ± 5.5 hr (range, 8 to 27). The elimination half-life inversely correlated with the paraldehyde total body clearance (TBC) according to the formula:

$$T_{1/2} = 26.79 - 0.06 \text{ TBC}$$

$$(r = 0.69, p < 0.01)$$

There was no correlation between the half-life and volume of distribution. Total body clearance was not affected by barbiturates, phenytoin, or renal failure (19).

CLINICAL USE

Before safer and more effective medications became available, paraldehyde was used as a sedative and hypnotic and also for obstetrical anesthesia. It was also widely used in treating the alcohol withdrawal syndrome, but has been completely supplanted by more effective agents, such as the benzodiazepines. Its sole remaining use is in the treatment of status epilepticus or ongoing seizures (5), particularly in infants and children. With the unavailability of the parenteral form, this indication also may disappear.

The drug is usually administered intravenously or rectally. If used intravenously, the paraldehyde is diluted with normal saline to a concentration not to exceed 10%. It is then infused slowly in a dose of about 0.3 ml/kg (i.e., 3 ml/kg of the 10% solution). The dose may be repeated in 15 to 20 min, and a maintenance antiepileptic drug must also be administered.

The rectal dose is also about 0.3 ml/kg diluted with an equal volume of mineral or vegetable oil. If needed, the dose can be

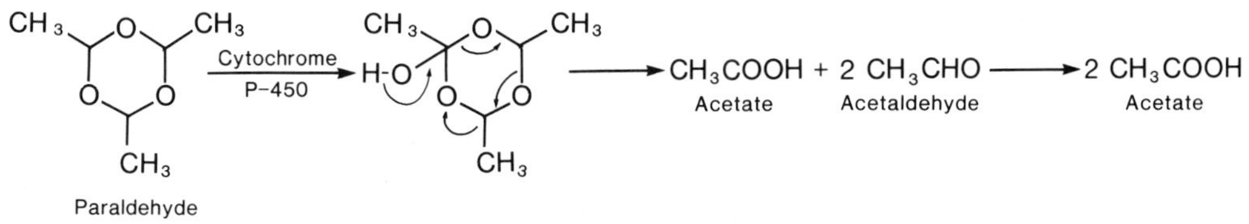

FIG. 1. Paraldehyde metabolism.

repeated in 15 or 20 min; before repeating the dose, the characteristic odor should be present in the expired air to ensure that the first dose was absorbed and to preclude the rapid absorption of a double dose. The drug should never be administered intra-arterially, and it should not be administered without proper dilution.

Relation of Plasma Concentration to Seizure Control

There are few studies of the antiepileptic efficacy and plasma concentrations of paraldehyde. Anesthesia usually can be obtained with concentrations of 120 to 330 mg/liter (12), but Thurston et al. (1968) did not achieve the third stage of anesthesia with levels as high as 300 mg/liter (30). In early studies in humans (8) it was found that intravenous injections of 1 to 3 ml of undiluted paraldehyde did not influence pulse, blood pressure, or consciousness, although intense coughing occurred for 2 to 5 min after the injection; 6 ml caused some diminution of consciousness and slight decrease in blood pressure; 9 to 12 ml led to sleep, slight decrease in blood pressure, but no cough.

The determination of blood paraldehyde levels to monitor the drug's efficacy and toxicity has not been routine. The dose effective in halting status epilepticus in experimental animals is about 100 to 200 mg/kg (8); it has been calculated that this dose would yield serum levels of 150 to 200 mg/liter in humans (3). In the newborn, levels above 100 mg/liter were associated with an antiepileptic effect (19). Paraldehyde was administered either as a 200 mg/kg intravenous bolus, followed by an infusion of 16 mg/kg/hr (in 10 infants) or as a 400 mg/kg bolus (in four infants) to achieve these levels.

Toxicity

The safety margin for paraldehyde may be quite narrow. The minimal anesthetic dose for dogs, cats, and rabbits is 0.3 mg/kg; the mean lethal dose is 0.45 ml/kg for cats and rabbits and 0.5 ml/kg for dogs (6). One newborn infant survived a serum paraldehyde level of 1,744 mg/liter (3), but death has occurred with levels as low as 543 mg/L (10).

Direct injury from arterial injection leading to both arterial and venous thrombosis has been reported in a postterm newborn with respiratory distress treated with two doses (0.15 mg/kg) of undiluted paraldehyde, the first intramuscularly and the second, inadvertently, via the umbilical artery (14). Post-mortem examination showed thrombosis of the arterioles and venules of the lower limbs, and arterioles of the liver, kidneys, and lungs. Direct injection of undiluted paraldehyde at a dose of 0.3 ml/kg into an umbilical artery catheter in another newborn infant led to multiple vesicular lesions over the lower trunk and lower limbs; several toes sloughed and there were full thickness wounds; the injury was attributed to microembolization (32).

Pulmonary edema has been reported following the administration of parenteral paraldehyde in adults (22). Cyanosis, cough, and hypotension thought to be due to pulmonary edema have been reported following administration of 2.0 ml of undiluted paraldehyde in a 2-year-old child; they recurred on readministration of a reportedly appropriate saline dilution (26). The mechanism is not known, but is speculated to be due to direct injury of the capillary-alveolar membrane. Other deaths have been related to pulmonary compromise with acute right-sided heart failure, often in association with high doses or direct administration of undiluted drug (6).

Because of the large volume needed, intramuscular injection into the gluteal regions is recommended, but may lead to sciatic nerve injury.

The conversion of paraldehyde to glacial acetic acid in the presence of light and air has led to some samples containing as much as 40% to 98% acetic acid (4,16), which is very toxic and may cause death if injected. Outdated paraldehyde has also been reported to cause severe chemical proctitis when administered rectally (27).

Severe metabolic acidosis may be seen in long-term users (33) and after overdose (2). Significant lactic acidosis has occurred following a single exposure (40 ml intramuscularly) in a 30-year-old man (21).

MECHANISM OF ACTION

The mechanism of paraldehyde's antiepileptic drug action is unknown. Paraldehyde has a depressant action on all levels of the nervous system, but exerts its strongest influence on the cerebral cortex, where it may abolish all signs of electrical activity (8). Paraldehyde may block neuromuscular transmission in the peripheral nervous system (24). The central mechanisms are less clear. Paraldehyde has a variable effect on serotonin metabolism, principally by inhibiting monoamine oxidase activity (18).

CONVERSION

Conversion factor:

$$CF = 1000/\text{mol. wt.} = 1000/132.16 = 7.57$$

Conversion:

$$(\mu g/ml) \times 7.57 = (\mu moles/L)$$

$$(\mu moles/L)/5.43 = (\mu g/ml)$$

REFERENCES

1. Anthony, R. M., Andorn, A. C., Sunshine, I., and Thompson, W. L. (1977): Paraldehyde pharmacokinetics in alcohol abusers. *Fed. Proc.,* 36:285.
2. Beier, L. S., Pitts, W. H., and Conick, H. C. (1963): Metabolic acidosis occurring during paraldehyde intoxication. *Ann. Intern. Med.,* 58:155–158.
3. Bostrom, B. (1982): Paraldehyde toxicity during treatment of status epilepticus. *Am. J. Dis. Child.,* 136:414–415.
4. Bowles, G. C. (1964): Tighter system of drug control needed to prevent drug thefts. *Mod. Hosp.,* 103:120–127.
5. Browne, T. R. (1983): Paraldehyde, chlormethiazole, and lidocaine for treatment of status epilepticus. *Advances Neurol.,* 34:509–517.
6. Burstein, C. L. (1943): The hazard of paraldehyde administration: Clinical and laboratory studies. *J.A.M.A.* 121:187–190.
7. Cervello, V. (1884): Reschesches cliniques et physiologiques sur la paraldehyde. *Arch. Ital. Biol.,* 6:113.
8. de Elio, F. J., de Jalon, P. G., and Obrador, S. (1949): Some experimental and clinical observations on the anticonvulsive action of paraldehyde. *J. Neurol. Neurosurg. Psychiat.,* 12:19–24.
9. Evans, R. J. (1961): Effect of paraldehyde on disposable syringes and needles. *Lancet,* 2:1451.
10. Figot, P., Hine, C., and Way, E. (1952): The estimation and significance of paraldehyde levels in blood and brain. *Acta Pharmacol. Toxical.,* 8:290–304.
11. Foreman, P. M. (1974): Therapy of seizures in children. *Am. Fam. Phys.,* 10:144–148.
12. Gardner, H. L., Levine, H., and Bodansky, M. (1940): Concentration of paraldehyde in the blood following its administration during labor. *Am. J. Obstet. Gynec.,* 40:435–439.
13. Giacoia, G. P., Gessner, P. K., Zaleska, M. M., and Boutwell, W. C. (1984): Pharmacokinetics of paraldehyde disposition in the neonate. J. Pediatr., 104:291–295.
14. Gooch, W. M., 3d, Kennedy, J., Banner, W., Jr., and McGuire, H. J. (1979): Generalized arterial and venous thrombosis following intra-arterial paraldehyde. *Clin. Toxicol.,* 15:39–44.
15. Hart, W. T. (1961): A comparison of promazine and paraldehyde in 175 cases of alcohol withdrawal. *Am. J. Psychiatry,* 118:323–327.
16. Hayward, J. N., and Boshell, B. R. (1957): Paraldehyde intoxication with metabolic acidosis. *Am. J. Med.,* 23:965–976.
17. Hitchcock, P., and Nelson, E. E. (1943): The metabolism of paraldehyde. II. *J. Pharmacol. Exp. Ther.,* 79:286–294.
18. Huff, J. A., Davis, V. E., Brown, H., and Clay, M. M. (1971): Effects of chloral hydrate, paraldehyde, and ethanol on the metabolism of [^{14}C]-serotonin in the rat. *Biochem. Pharmacol.,* 20:476–482.
19. Koren, G., Butt, W., Rajchgot, P., Mayer, J., Whyte, H., Pape, K., and MacLeod, S. M. (1986): Intravenous paraldehyde for seizure control in newborn infants. *Neurology,* 36:108–111.
20. Lang, D. W., and Borgstedt, H. H. (1968): Rate of pulmonary excretion of paraldehyde in man. *Toxicol. Applied Pharm.,* 15:269–274.
21. Linter, C. M., and Linter, S. P. K. (1986): Severe lactic acidosis following paraldehyde administration. *Brit. J. Psychiatr.,* 149:650–651.
22. Mountain, R., Ferguson, S., Fowler, A., Hyers, T. (1982): Noncardiac pulmonary edema following administration of parenteral paraldehyde. *Chest,* 82:371–372.
23. Nitzescu, I. I., Georgescu, I. D., and Timus, D.

(1936): Le dosage de paraldehyde dans l'air respiratoire chez les animaux anesthesies avec la paraldehyde. *Compt. Rend. Soc. Biol.,* 121:1660–1661.

24. Quilliam, J. P. (1955): Action of hypnotic drugs on frog skeletal muscle. *Br. J. Pharmacol.,* 10:133–146.

25. Robinson, L. J. (1938): Intravenous paraldehyde narcosis for pneumoencephalography. *N. Eng. J. Med.,* 219:114–117.

26. Sinal, S. H., and Crowe, J. E. (1976): Cyanosis, cough, and hypotension following intravenous administration of paraldehyde. *Pediatrics,* 57:158–159.

27. Stanley, J. H. (1980): Rectal disease in a patient with delirium tremens. *J.A.M.A.,* 243:1749–1750.

28. Strahan, S. A. K. (1885): Action of paraldehyde, the new hypnotic. *Lancet,* i:220.

29. Thompson, W. L., Johnson, A. D., Maddrey, W. L., and Osler Medical Housestaff (1975): Diazepam and paraldehyde for treatment of severe delirium tremens. A controlled trial. *Ann. Int. Med.,* 82:175–180.

30. Thurston, J. H., Liang, H. S., Smith, J. S., Valentini, E. J. (1968): New enzymatic method for measurement of paraldehyde: Correlation of ef-

fects with serum and CSF levels. *J. Lab. Clin. Med.,* 72:699–704.

31. Treiman, D. M., and Chelberg, R. D. (1983): Pharmacokinetics of paraldehyde in rat blood and brain. *Neurology,* 33 (Suppl. 2):233.

32. Wait, R. B., Greenhalgh, D., and Gamelli, R. L. (1984): Vascular injury in the neonate associated with intra-arterial injection of paraldehyde. *Clin. Pediat.,* 23:324.

33. Waterhouse, C., and Stern, A. E. (1957): Metabolic acidosis occurring during ingestion of paraldehyde. *Am. J. Med.,* 23:987–989.

34. Wechsler, I. S. (1940): Intravenous injection of paraldehyde for the control of convulsions. *J.A.M.A.,* 114:2198.

35. Wolfe, C. R., Buscemi, J. H., and Branch, C. E., Jr. (1979): Anticonvulsant therapy with oral paraldehyde. *Ann. Neurol.,* 6:554.

36. Zaleska, M. M., and Gessner, P. K. (1982): Metabolism of [^{14}C]paraldehyde in mice *in vivo,* generation and trapping of acetaldehyde. *J. Pharmacol. Exp. Therap.,* 224:614–619.

37. Zera, R. T., and Nagasawa, H. T. (1981): Metabolism of paraldehyde to acetaldehyde by rat liver microsomes. *Res. Comm. Chem. Path. Pharmacol.,* 34:531–541.

Antiepileptic Drugs, Third Edition, edited by
R. Levy, R. Mattson, B. Meldrum,
J. K. Penry, and F. E. Dreifuss.
Raven Press, Ltd., New York © 1989.

64

Other Antiepileptic Drugs

Progabide

Paolo L. Morselli, Kenneth G. Lloyd, and Raffaele Palminteri

GABA (γ-aminobutyric acid) is the major known inhibitory neurotransmitter in the central nervous system. Several recent findings support the theory that an impairment in the function of GABA-containing neurons may play an important role in the genesis or maintenance of ictal discharges (56,58,59,61,63,71,74). Furthermore, neurochemical findings indicate an alteration in the function of GABAergic neurons in epileptogenic brain tissue specimens of epileptic patients suffering from drug-refractory temporal lobe epilepsy (56,58,59,72). Thus, pharmacodynamic and neurochemical data suggest that GABAmimetic drugs acting directly at GABA receptors (GABA agonists) may be effective anticonvulsants.

On the basis of these findings, a new class of compounds (benzylidene series) with high specificity for GABA receptors were developed for studies in models of epilepsy (6,7). As one of these compounds, progabide has undergone extensive investigations and represents the first GABA agonist developed for clinical use.

CHEMISTRY

Progabide, 4-[{(4-chlorophenyl)(5-fluoro-2-hydroxyphenyl)methylene} amino] butanamide, is a synthetic compound defined as the Schiff's base obtained from γ-aminobutyramide and a substituted benzophenone. The compound was synthetized by Kaplan and collaborators in 1976 (46). Progabide ($C_{17}H_{16}ClFN_2O_2$) (Fig. 1) has a molecular weight of 334.78 and a melting point of 138°C to 142°C. It appears as a nonhygroscopic microcrystalline yellow powder and is not light sensitive. The compound is easily soluble in alcohols, acetone, toluene, and chloroform, but its solubility is very limited in ether and water (<0.5%). Its log P (partition coefficient octanol/water at pH 7.4) of 3.19 suggests a good penetration across biological membranes (99). The UV spectra, when measured in ether solution, show an absorption maximum at 331 nm. In more polar solvents, the main peak at 331 nm diminishes while a new maximum appears at 415 nm, suggesting the existence of the molecule in an *ortho*-quinoid form (99). Progabide is an amphoteric molecule; in acid medium it can be present in protonated form, and in base an anion can be generated. Two pK_a values can hence be observed: 3.35 for the transition immonium cation-neutral form and 12.80 for the transition neutral form-phenolate anion. In solution in strongly acidic medium the compound is relatively instable, whereas useful hydrolytic stability is observed at neutral or basic pH (up to 8.09).

SL 75.102, 4-[{(4-chlorophenyl)(5-fluoro-2-hydroxyphenyl)methylene}amino]butan-

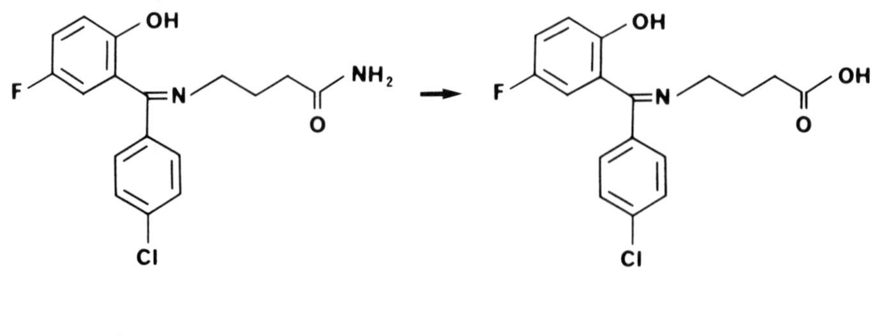

PROGABIDE   SL 75 102 (PGA)

FIG. 1. Chemical structures of progabide and its acid metabolite SL 75.012 (PGA).

oic acid is the carboxylic acid analog of progabide and represents its main active metabolite in animals and man. As monosodium salt ($C_{17}H_{14}ClFN_2O_2$), it has a molecular weight of 357.75 and a melting point of 231°C. It appears as a nonhygroscopic microcrystalline yellow powder and is not light sensitive. The compound is soluble in alcohols and water (5%) as well as in less polar solvents. Like progabide, it is instable in acid solutions, slowly decomposing to yield GABA and an *ortho*-hydroxy-benzophenone. The log P is 0.84, suggesting a reduced penetration across biological membranes (99).

METHODS OF DETERMINATION

The determination of progabide (PGB), SL 75.102 (PGA), and the corresponding benzophenone in biological fluids and tissues can be performed by gas-liquid chromatography (GLC) (17,38) and high-pressure liquid chromatography (HPLC) (3,4,81,101).

Gas-Liquid Chromatography

The GLC technique was the first method developed (38). Plasma samples or tissue homogenates are extracted with 5 ml of toluene. The organic phase is brought to dry-

ness. The dry residue is then reacted with heptafluorobutyric anhydride. The dry residue is redissolved in *n*-hexane and an aliquot of the solution is injected into a gas-chromatograph equipped with a ^{63}N ECD. Operating conditions are: oven temperature 230°C; injection port 250°C; detector temperature 275°C; nitrogen gas flow, 40 ml/min. The column is packed with OV-17 3% on GaschromQ (80–100 mesh). 4-[{(4-Chlorophenyl-5-chloro-2-hydroxyphenyl)methylene}amino]butanamide is used as internal marker. Under the conditions described, retention times are 2.4 min for progabide and 4.2 min for the internal marker. The minimal detectable amount (injected) is of the order of 10 pg, corresponding to a sensitivity of 10 to 20 ng per sample. A variant to the above method permitting the quantification of PGA and the benzophenone following reduction of the imine bond has been described (17).

High-Pressure Liquid Chromatography

The instability of the imine bond presents the main difficulty in the quantification of PGB. An improvement is represented by the method described by Yonekawa et al. (102) in which the reduction of the imine bond with sodium borohydride leads to a stable reduced compound which can then be purified and back-extracted in acidic conditions. However, this did not allow the determination of PGB and PGA in blood and tissue samples.

The procedure was further improved by Padovani et al. (81), allowing simultaneous determination of PGB, PGA, and the benzophenone in total blood and tissue samples. One ml of biological matrix is added to 0.5 ml of 2M acetate buffer pH 4.5. The mixture is then extracted with 8 ml of toluene, and 0.5 ml of 0.5% sodium borohydride in ethanol is added to the organic phase. The reduced compounds PGB and PGA are then back-extracted with 2 ml of 0.25 M citrate buffer pH 1.8, while the benzophenone remains in the organic layer. The aqueous phase is adjusted to pH 6.5–7.7 with 200 μl of methanol-0.015M phosphate buffer pH 7.1 (4:6 v/v), and 100 μl are injected into the chromatograph. In order to quantify PGB and PGA together with the benzophenone in one single chromatographic run, the two organic extracts were pooled prior to the HPLC separation. The internal marker was 4-[{(4-chlorphenyl)(5-chloro-2-hydroxyphenyl)methylene}amino]butanamide. Separation is carried out on a Hypersil ODS 3 μm (150 × 4.6 mm) reversed-phase column packed according to the technique described by Broquaire (15). The mobile phase consists of a quaternary solvent mixture of methanol-acetonitrile-phosphate buffer (0.033M, pH 5.5)-sodium chloride (1.5M) (30:30:40:9 v/v). The column effluent is monitored electrochemically at an oxidation potential of +850 mV versus an Ag/AgCl reference electrode. The retention times are 3.1 min for PGA, 4.1 min for PGB, 5.9 min for their internal marker, and 5.0 and 7.0 min, respectively, for the benzophenone and its internal marker. The minimum detectable concentration is 1 ng/ml (three times the base-line noise), and the practical limit is around 10 ng/ml. No chromatographic interferences are usually observed with samples containing other antiepileptic drugs up

to 2 to 5 μg. This HPLC method was compared with the GLC procedure and a good correlation between the two methods was observed.

A more rapid and simple method suitable for the determination of PGB and PGA (but not the benzophenone) in human biological samples (blood, plasma, urine) has recently been proposed by Ascalone et al. (3). The assay involves a single rapid (5 min) extraction of PGB and PGA into 5 ml of toluene from 1 ml of biological matrix buffered at pH 4.8 with 0.5 ml 2M acetate buffer. Following gentle evaporation of the organic phase, the residue is dissolved into a suitable volume of HPLC mobile phase and chromatographed onto a silica column with UV detection. The analytical column was 30 × 0.39 cm I.D. filled with 10 μm μPorasil. The mobile phase was methanol-acetic acid-water (2.6:0.3:0.15) diluted to 100 ml with methylene chloride (v/v). Flow rate was 1.5 ml/min. The chromatographic system consists of a constant flow pump (Kontron-Model 414-T) coupled to a Model PU 4020 UV spectrophotometric liquid chromatography detector operated at a wavelength of 340 nm and at a sensitivity of 0.02 a.u.f.s. Retention times were 4 min for PGA, 6.2 min for the internal marker 4[{(5-chloro-2-hydroxy-3methyl-phenyl)(4-chlorophenyl)methylene}amino]butanamide and 8.5 min for PGB. According to the authors, the addition of water to the mobile phase is very important, increasing separation and peak symmetry. The detection limit is about 30 ng/ml of plasma or blood with a signal-to-noise ratio of 3 to 1 for both compounds.

A comparison with the previous HPLC method yielded identical results, with a good correlation between the two techniques (r = 0.985 for PGB and 0.979 for PGA). The procedure appears suitable for routine determination of PGB and PGA in a large number of blood samples. Co-administered antiepileptic drugs or theophylline do not interfere with the assay (4).

ABSORPTION

Experimental Studies

In the rat, intraperitoneally administered PGB is rapidly absorbed, with dose-related maximal plasma concentrations attained within 20 to 40 min. Higher doses (200 mg/kg) are generally followed by a plateau, suggesting a relatively slow absorptive process compatible with the physicochemical properties of the drug (101,73). Balance studies indicate that the molecule is nearly completely absorbed. However, it undergoes an extensive first-pass effect and in the rat at 20 mg/kg, the estimated bioavailability is 10% to 15%. It may increase up to 35% to 40% at 100 mg/kg (18).

The same absorption profile with dose-related peak plasma PGB levels has been observed in mice (36%), hamsters (49%), cats, dogs, and baboon (*Papio anubis*) (10%) (18,73). In the rhesus monkey (*Macaca mulatta*), the estimated bioavailability is 30% to 60% (44,54).

Clinical Studies

Peak plasma PGB concentrations are attained 1 to 3 hr after oral administration and are proportional to the dose in the range of 600 to 1,500 mg. The estimated bioavailability of PGB is 40% to 65% for the commercially available micronized formulation (54,73,91). Studies with [^{14}C]-labeled progabide have shown that 84% of the orally administered radioactivity is absorbed and recovered in the 48-hr urine and 96-hr feces (82).

DISTRIBUTION AND ELIMINATION

Experimental Studies

Autoradiographic and quantitative studies in the rat with [^{14}C]-labeled progabide have shown that the drug and its metabolites distribute extensively to various organs and tissues with a rapid brain penetration of the unchanged molecule (33,100). Brain PGB concentrations are 1.5 to 2-fold higher than those in plasma, and their rate of decay is about three times slower than in plasma. Brain PGA concentrations are about one-tenth of the plasma concentrations up to 3 to 4 hr after administration (33,100). Data on the distribution of progabide and PGA in the rat brain indicate that the two compounds are present at higher concentrations in areas such as cortex, hippocampus, thalamus, and cerebellum (33,36). It is interesting to note that these areas are usually involved in the genesis and/or spread of seizure activity.

Specific studies on biliary excretion indicate that 77% of the radioactivity is eliminated in the bile in 7 hr with more than 50% of the dose being excreted within the first hour. This finding, together with excretion in the feces of 10% of the dose following intravenous administration, suggests the possibility of extensive enterohepatic recycling (32). In all the species studied, PGB was found to be present only in traces in the urine, whereas free and conjugated metabolites accounted for 75% to 80% of the dose (33).

The decay of plasma PGB concentrations can be described by a one-compartment open model with an apparent plasma half-life of about 40 min in the hamster, 60 min in the mouse, 90 min in the rat, 2 to 3 hr in the dog, 60 min in the baboon (73), and 3 to 4 hr in the cat. Total body clearance values (liter/kg/hr) are 7.5 in the mouse, 15.9 in the hamster, 2.8 in the rat, and 2.7 in the baboon (18). In the rhesus monkey, after intravenous administration the rate of disappearance of progabide also follows first-order kinetics (44), and is described by a one-compartment open model. The apparent plasma half-life is 0.5 to 0.8 hr and the volume of distribution about 2 liters/kg, with a plasma clearance of 5 to 9 liters/hr, suggesting a high (0.5) extraction ratio. Steady-state levels were rapidly attained and maintained during a 7-day constant infusion without modification of plasma clearance values (54).

The apparent plasma half-life of PGA is about 1 hr in the mouse and 3.6 hr in the rat (18). No data are available for other species.

Clinical Studies

Progabide is about 96% bound to plasma proteins, and PGA is 98% bound. The binding of both compounds remains constant over a wide range of concentrations exceeding those found in plasma or blood during repeated treatment (42,43,54). The binding of progabide to human serum albumin (HSA) is characterized by one saturable class of sites ($N = 3.8 \pm 0.2$ and $K = 2.5 \times 10^4 M^{-1}$). The binding to alpha-1-acid glycoprotein (AGP) is also saturable ($N = 1.7 \pm 0.2$ and $K = 3.1 \pm 10^4 M^{-1}$). PGA shows two saturable classes of binding sites to HSA: (a) $N = 0.8 \pm 0.1$ and $K_1 = 10^6 M^{-1}$; and (b) $N = 7.9 \pm 0.2$ and $K_2 = 8.1 \times 10^3 M^{-1}$). The binding to alpha-1-acid glycoprotein was also shown to be saturable ($N = 0.7 \pm 0.1$ and $K = 1.6 \times 10^4 M^{-1}$). Progabide and PGA are bound to a lesser extent to red blood cells, lipoprotein, and gamma globulins.

The blood-to-plasma ratio is about 0.62 to 0.73 for progabide and 0.53 to 0.55 for PGA. Progabide has been found to be present in cerebrospinal fluid (CSF) and neurosurgical brain specimens of epileptic patients treated with the drug at concentrations in good agreement with its physicochemical profile. Brain PGB concentrations were 2.5 times those in plasma, while CSF levels were 3% to 4% (Morselli and Loiseau, *unpublished data*).

In healthy volunteers, the apparent plasma half-life after a single dose of micronized PGB tablets varied from 2 to 4 hr and was not modified after repeated treat-

ment. The estimated total body clearance varied from 0.7 to 1.1 liter/hr/kg (54,73,90,91). Furthermore, PGB did not modify the urinary excretion of D-glucaric acid (90). The apparent plasma PGA half-life ranged from 6 to 10 hr (90,91). In infants and children, progabide is generally rapidly absorbed with peak blood concentrations attained between 1 and 2 hr (5,30,71). In a study of 14 children with epilepsy, aged 1.6 to 14 years, the apparent elimination half-life of progabide was in the range (2–4 hr) of that found in adult epileptic patients. However, the apparent total body clearance values were about 60% to 100% higher than in adult epileptic (mean, 1.7 l/hr/kg versus 1.1 liter/hr/kg respectively) (5). The elimination half-life of PGA ranged from 4 to 10 hr.

In contrast, a definite reduction of the progabide elimination rate has been found in cirrhotic patients (11,91) and in neonates (1,2), and the PGA elimination rate was found to be considerably prolonged in chronic renal insufficiency (11,91). No significant modifications were noted in hemodialyzed patients and in elderly subjects (11,73,91). During repeated administration, steady-state levels of either PGB or PGA were reached within 2 to 4 days and maintained over the observation period (54,90).

BIOTRANSFORMATION

Experimental Studies

In animals, progabide is metabolized through four major routes of biotransformation (32,33) leading to 10 metabolites, as indicated in Fig. 2. The major pathways are the following: (a) hydrolysis of the amide group on the GABAmide side chain leading to the formation of acid derivates; (b) hydrolysis of the imine bond leading to benzophenone derivates; (c) hydroxylation on C-3 of the 5-fluoro-2-hydroxyphenyl ring leading to *ortho*-dihydroxy compounds; and

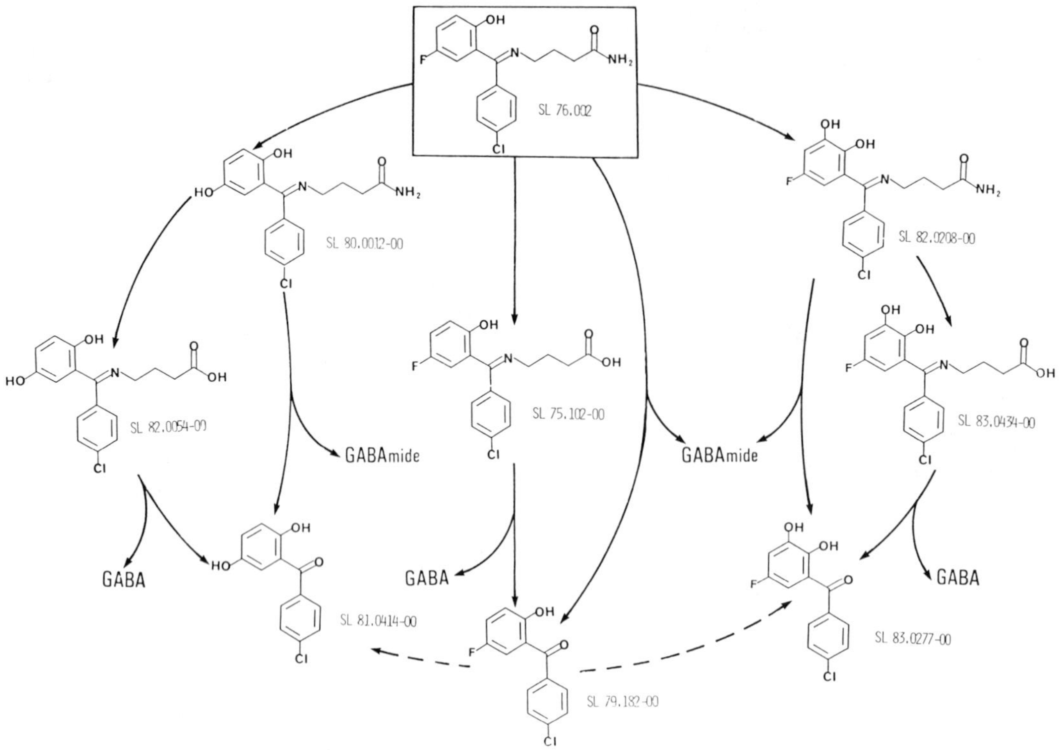

FIG. 2. Metabolic pathways of progabide in animals and man.

(d) hydroxylation on C-5 of the 5-fluoro-2-hydroxyphenyl ring leading to *para*-dihydroxy compounds. All of these metabolites are eliminated mainly as glucuronide derivatives but SL 79.182-00 was also found as the sulfoconjugate. Unchanged progabide is eliminated only in trace amounts. After intravenous administration, *ortho*-dihydroxy metabolites acount for 47%, 43%, and 29% of the administered dose in the hamster, rat, and baboon, respectively, whereas after oral treatment, these metabolites are less important (30%, 8%, and 8%, respectively). In contrast, the benzophenone resulting from the hydrolysis of the imine bond is more abundant in the glucuro- and sulfoconjugated form after oral dosing (respectively 38% and 15% in the hamster; 67% and 31% in the rat, and 55% and 32% in the baboon). C-5 hydroxylation appears to be a minor route of biotransformation.

Clinical Studies

The metabolic pathways of progabide in man are qualitatively and quantitatively similar to those observed in animal species. Progabide and PGA are present in plasma in concentrations of the same order of magnitude, whereas the levels of the benzophenone (SL 79.182-00) are 30% to 50% of those of progabide. The major metabolites found in urine result from the hydrolysis of the imine bond and account for 55.6% to 75% of the administered dose (SL 79.182-00, SL 81.0414-00, SL 83.0434-00, SL 83.0277-00) (33,81).

DRUG INTERACTIONS

Effects of Progabide on Other Drugs

A recent study (12) in healthy volunteers indicates that during co-treatment with progabide, a rise in carbamazepine (CBZ) epoxide concentrations and reduced clearance of phenytoin (PHT) and phenobarbital (PB) can be observed in some subjects. These data suggest that progabide may have an inhibitory effect on the clearance of other drugs. It is not clear, however, if this effect is exerted at the hepatic or renal level. In fact, the antipyrine kinetic profile is not modified following repeated dosing with progabide (12,90).

The effect of PGB on other antiepileptic drugs appears to be similar to the competitive inhibition described with PB and sulthiame (50,51,86). That is a situation where the inhibition is exerted only toward drugs metabolized through the same enzymatic system, is concentration-dependent, and occurs in a limited number of cases. The effect on PHT clearance is in favor of a competitive, concentration-dependent inhibition at the hepatic microsomal level, partially reduced or masked by a concomitant displacing effect of PGB and PGA on PHT binding (98) and consequent increased excretion of PHT. An alternative hypothesis could be reduced renal excretion of conjugated 5HPPH (5-(*p*-hydroxyphenyl)-5-phenylhydantoin) with consequent feedback inhibition on the hydroxylation of PHT. The same type of reasoning can be put forward for PB, where both hepatic and renal mechanisms may play a role in reducing the total clearance of the drug, as already observed during concomitant administration of PHT (51,76) and valproate (VPA) (67).

Data from epileptic patients receiving progabide indicate the same type of modification in plasma levels of associated antiepileptic drug. Kutt et al. (52) reported that in epileptic patients progabide may cause an increase of CBZ epoxide and CBZ transdiol levels without modifying CBZ concentrations. According to the authors, the mechanism behind the phenomenon could be both a reduction of epoxy-hydrase activities and reduced renal excretion of the trans-

diol. Other authors (16,20,37,60,65,66, 69,97) indicate that plasma CBZ concentrations are not modified by progabide, but a significant reduction in plasma CBZ levels has been described by Dam et al. (25) and Van Parys et al. (94). Brundage et al. (16) reported a significant increase of plasma PHT levels in 69% of the patients receiving combined treatment with progabide (versus 12% during placebo). Other available data on PHT levels in epileptic patients are rather conflicting. Several authors (20,25,89,93,94) have described significant elevation of PHT in 40% to 80% of the cases following PGB co-administration, and others (66,97) have reported only moderate increases in 5% to 10% of the patients or no variations at all (37,69,78). The same holds true for phenobarbital. A moderate increase in plasma PB concentrations has been observed by some authors (69,78,89) but not others (25,37,66,97).

The available data do not permit a clear definition of the above-mentioned interactions. The clinical relevance of the increase in CBZ epoxide and plasma PB concentrations appears to be rather limited, but the elevation in plasma PHT concentrations during associated treatment with progabide may be of real clinical importance because of the peculiar saturation kinetics of PHT and of the possibly severe side effects of PHT.

No pharmacokinetic interactions have been observed between progabide and clonazepam (96) and between progabide and alcohol (92). However, the possibility of potentiation of clonazepam's sedative effects should be considered (96).

Effect of Other Antiepileptic Drugs on Progabide

The pharmacokinetic profile of progabide may be significantly altered by CBZ, which significantly increases the clearance of both progabide and PGA (9,90). An interaction at the plasma protein binding level has been described with VPA, which may increase significantly the free fraction of both progabide and PGA (42).

RELATION OF PLASMA CONCENTRATION TO SEIZURE CONTROL

Blood levels of progabide and PGA in epileptic patients treated concomitantly with progabide and other antiepileptic drugs are apparently unrelated to the daily dose administered. A daily oral dose of 20 to 45 mg/kg yielded trough blood levels of 300 to 3,500 ng/ml, with a fivefold to sixfold interindividual variability for the same dose (9). However, in three recent studies (8,10,49), blood levels of progabide and PGA associated with a satisfactory therapeutic response (50% reduction in seizure frequency) were significantly higher than blood levels in patients not responding to the drug. Furthermore, a significant difference in therapeutic blood concentrations of both PGB and PGA was observed in a comparison of monotherapy versus polytherapy. The apparent therapeutic thresholds were 600 to 800 ng/ml for progabide and 900 to 1,400 for PGA in polytherapy and 1,000 to 1,200 ng/ml for progabide and 1,900 to 2,400 for PGA in monotherapy. Better therapeutic responses were also observed in those patients whose blood PGB and PGA levels were constantly within the above values. No relationship has yet been established between drug levels and side effects or toxic signs.

TOXICITY

Experimental Studies

Progabide shows a similarly low acute toxicity in the mouse and in the rat with an LD$_{50}$ of 1,350 and 4,000 mg/kg by the oral and intraperitoneal routes, respectively

(34). In subacute (4 weeks) preliminary studies with daily doses ranging from 100 to 1,000 mg/kg, increases in liver weight without changes in biochemical parameters were observed in the rat. In the dog, doses of 500 mg/kg were associated in three out of four animals with a twofold increase in SGPT levels without microscopic abnormalities. A modest increase in liver weight (unaccompanied by biochemical changes) was observed in baboons at 800 mg/kg/day. Subchronic (14 and 13 weeks) and chronic (26 and 52 weeks) studies performed in rats, hamsters, dogs, and baboons indicated that progabide is devoid of major toxicity (34). In all the above mentioned studies, no significant modification of behavior, clinical chemistry, or hormonal parameters were evident at daily doses of up to 250 to 350 mg/kg. Furthermore, no treatment-related changes were detected histologically in any of the tissues examined. High daily doses of progabide ($\geq$500 mg/kg for 13 to 52 weeks) induced lethargy, unsteady gait, and other nonspecific signs of sedation and/or myorelaxation in the rat, dog, and baboon. A decrease in food consumption was also observed together with an increase in thyroid (rat) and liver weight (rat and baboons) without microscopic abnormalities.

Administered to pregnant rats and rabbits in a daily oral dose of up to 100 mg/kg and 600 mg/kg, respectively, progabide had no effect on either litter size or litter weight. Similarly no effects on fertility were observed in the rat at daily doses of up to 1,000 mg/kg.

Carcinogenicity and mutagenicity studies concluded that progabide has no mutagenic potential and does not present any carcinogenic risk to man (34). In a study conducted on prepubertal rats, progabide did not modify testicular or seminal vesicle weights (28).

Clinical Studies

Available data in man include studies in healthy volunteers (single doses up to 2,500 mg and repeated doses up to 60 mg/kg) and in patients with syndromes other than epilepsy, such as movement disorders, depression, spasticity, or schizophrenia (doses up to 40 mg/kg), with a treated population of more than 2,800 subjects.

In general, progabide is well tolerated. The adverse events most frequently observed are drowsiness, mood changes, irritability, gastrointestinal disturbances, dizziness, and fatigue. Relative frequency of side effects ranges from 5% to 20% and the described events are transient and moderate in most cases (21,71). The percentage of drop-outs for clinical adverse events in the controlled clinical trials to date has been rather low. In the epileptic population, it ranges from 2% to 7.8% in patients receiving progabide in polytherapy and from 1.5% to 3% in patients treated with progabide only (9, 21, 23, 25, 37, 49, 55, 66, 69, 71, 78, 93, 94, 95,97). Three acute psychotic episodes with confusion and hallucinations and paranoid ideation were observed during treatment with progabide or on progabide withdrawal (37,41). The responsibility of the drug, however, is uncertain.

The main cause for concern is represented by an increase in liver aminotransferase levels which, for abnormalities equal or higher than twice the upper limit of normal, are detected in about 9% of patients (21,71,83,84). Aminotransferase abnormalities were associated with jaundice and/or other signs or symptoms in 0.64% of the patients. Four cases developed encephalopathy. The hepatic injury was mainly cytolytic and, as with other drugs causing cytolytic damage (e.g., isoniazide, iponiazide, valproic acid), the fatality rate was about 10% (77,83).

The occurrence of abnormal liver function tests is limited mainly to the first 6 months of progabide treatment, and, therefore, in this period regular and frequent monitoring of liver function is mandatory. More precisely, data suggest that monitoring during the first 4 months would detect about 75% of patients with elevated aminotransferase levels and almost all of those who may have overt hepatic injury. In about 50% to 80% of the cases, normalization of liver function tests was observed without discontinuing the treatment (83,84). In four cases of massive overdose (from 6 to 24 grams, or 10 to 40 times the average unitary dose), the most prominent clinical sign was central nervous system depression ranging from drowsiness to stage II coma. Respiratory depression or signs of cardiovascular impairment were not observed in any of the patients. Laboratory tests, including liver function tests, were normal in all subjects. All patients recovered without sequelae within 30 hr with the use of supportive therapy only (39).

PHARMACODYNAMICS

Laboratory Studies

Neuropharmacological Results

The anticonvulsant spectrum of progabide is remarkably wide. The compound is active in models related to or apparently unrelated to impairment of GABAergic transmission (56,58,100,103). Progabide has a protective anticonvulsant effect in models based on (a) blockade of the GABA receptor by bicuculline, (b) inactivation of the GABA receptor-coupled chloride ion channel by systemic administration of picrotoxinin or by intracortical injection of penicillin, and (c) the decrease of synaptic GABA concentrations by allylglycine, an inhibitor of glutamic acid decarboxylase (100,103). In the penicillin-induced focal seizures model in the cat, the activity of progabide is comparable to that of PHT (100). In other models apparently unrelated to impairment of GABAergic transmission, progabide displayed an anticonvulsant spectrum similar to that of VPA (63,64,100,103).

Most of the models mentioned above and

used to characterize the anticonvulsant profile of progabide are widely accepted for the evaluation of new antiepileptic drugs (48). Progabide has been shown to be active in all models studied to date, including the photosensitive baboon (*Papio papio*) (19,80), the convulsions induced by kainic acid (100), and amygdala kindling in rats (45,65).

The anticonvulsant activity is usually present with doses that are lower than those inducing sedation and/or impairment of motor performance (100). Altogether the available data demonstrate that stimulation of GABA receptors by progabide and PGA protects not only from seizures mediated by an impairment of GABAergic transmission, but also from those related to other mechanisms, as for instance blockade of glycine receptors by strychnine or stimulation of glutamate receptors by kainic acid. On the basis of these findings, it has been proposed that GABA receptor stimulation by progabide and PGA should be effective in a wide range of human epilepsies irrespective of the underlying, unknown, pathogenetic mechanism.

Neurophysiological Results

GABA receptor agonists have, by definition, the same neurophysiological effects as GABA itself in model systems for GABA receptors. Progabide injected intravenously causes a potent reduction in the firing rate of neurons in the rat dorsal Deiters' nucleus. However, the low solubility of the compound does not allow it to be used in microiontophoresis. The acid metabolite PGA, which has an anticonvulsant spectrum parallel to that of progabide (100) and is more potent in displacing [³H]GABA from its binding sites on rat and human brain membranes (57), causes depolarization associated with increased chloride conductance in the rat dorsal root ganglion preparation (29). The depolarizations induced by PGA or by GABA itself have the same off-rate, show cross-desensitization, are bicuculline- and picrotoxinin-sensitive and, most importantly, have the same reversal potential, indicating that both compounds act at the same recognition site controlling the chloride ionophore (13,14,29). It may also be of interest to emphasize that administration of progabide may lead to reduced glucose utilization in various structures of the central nervous system (24).

Neurochemical Results

Both progabide and PGA displace [³H]GABA and [³H]muscimol from their binding sites in rat and human brain membrane preparations (13,14,57). Furthermore, progabide displaces specific [³H]muscimol binding to $GABA_A$ receptors in *in vivo* models (40,47). These effects are observed at concentrations that do not inhibit GABA uptake, metabolism (via GABA-T), or synthesis (GAD activity). Furthermore, progabide and PGA have no activity at recognition sites for alpha or beta adrenoceptors, histamine receptors, muscarinic receptors, and binding sites for kainic acid (53,57). However, progabide, as for other GABAmimetics, indirectly modulates other neurotransmitter systems. Progabide and PGA decrease the biochemical indices of dopamine neuron activity as well as the activation of dopamine neurons induced by neuroleptics (62,88); they may also increase striatal acetylcholine levels, suggesting a decrease in acetylcholine turnover (87,103,104). With a single injection, progabide induces an enhancement of norepinephrine (NE) turnover, which is blocked by picrotoxin, whereas repeated administration leads to reduction of the enhanced NE turnover (88). The effect on NE systems probably occurs via an indirect mechanism, since iontophoretic administration of GABA on locus coeruleus cells results in a reduction of their firing rate (35).

Serotoninergic neurons are also affected. Single-dose and repeated administration of progabide reduces 5HT turnover with supersensitivity of the postsynaptic target cells (88,104).

Clinical Studies

Single doses of 600 to 2,500 mg of progabide administered to healthy volunteers of various ages did not induce any evident effects on performance (visual and acoustic reaction times, critical flicker fusion, tracking and short-term memory), waking or sleep EEG patterns, blood pressure, or heart rate (22,68,92). In the course of treatment with daily doses of 1,800–2,400 mg, sedation and hypotonia were occasionally observed, and minor gastric distress was present during the first 7 to 10 days of treatment. In general, the drug appeared to be very well tolerated at both clinical and biological (clinical chemistry) levels. Administration of progabide (1,200 mg/day) for 7 days to healthy volunteers did not induce any endocrine modifications involving plasma prolactin, follicle-stimulating hormone, luteinizing hormone cortisol, androgens, thyroid-stimulating hormone (basal and after thyrotropin hormone), T^4, T^3 uptake, FT and thyroxin-binding globulin (68). The only exception was the growth hormone response to hypoglycemia, which was inhibited by the compound. Moderate inhibition of domperidone-induced hyperprolactinemia has been reported in healthy volunteers. However, no such effect could be noticed on haloperidol-induced hyperprolactinemia (70). Recent findings in psychotic patients under neuroleptic treatment confirm the lack of effect of progabide on prolactin levels (F. Brambilla, *personal communication*).

PROPOSED MECHANISM OF ACTION

It appears that progabide and its acidic metabolite PGA are highly specific agonists for both $GABA_A$ and $GABA_B$ receptors (14,57). It is generally assumed that $GABA_A$ receptor agonist activity is mainly responsible for the anticonvulsant profile, since baclofen (prototypic $GABA_B$ agonist) has only very limited anticonvulsant activity (101). However, combined $GABA_{A+B}$ agonists (such as progabide) have a wider anticonvulsant spectrum than do pure $GABA_A$ agonists (56).

Binding techniques have shown that progabide and PGA displace various [^{3}H]-ligands (GABA, muscimol, isoguvacine) from $GABA_A$ receptors in various brain membrane preparations. These results have been confirmed by autoradiographic studies (14). The agonist activity of PGA and progabide has been further confirmed by the inhibition of GABA release from tissue slices and by the enhancement of [^{3}H]diazepam binding *in vitro* (13,57). The specificity of progabide and PGA for GABA receptors demonstrated *in vitro* is reflected by their activity *in vivo*. *In vivo*, progabide displaces [^{3}H]muscimol binding to GABA receptors in the mouse brain (40) and increases [^{3}H]diazepam binding (47). Furthermore, within the $GABA_A$ receptor macromolecular complex, progabide exerts its activity independently of the ω_1 subunit "recognition site for benzodiazepines." A specific antagonist for this site, RO-15-1788, does not influence the anticonvulsant activity of progabide (60). Thus, *in vitro* and *in vivo* data provide evidence that progabide and PGA act via direct stimulation of postsynaptic GABA receptors, which increases chloride conductance across the membrane. This leads to a diminution in cell firing and to a decrease in the hyperexcitable state of the brain.

CLINICAL USE

Adults

Progabide was introduced for clinical use in France in 1985. The drug is indicated for the treatment of complex partial seizures, elementary partial seizures, generalized tonic-clonic seizures, atonic seizures, and myoclonic seizures. Absence seizures do not appear to benefit from progabide. Because of its potential liver toxicity, the use of the drug is currently restricted to patients whose seizures are difficult to control with other antiepileptic drugs and/or patients experiencing marked side effects of the other drugs. In adults, therapy with progabide is usually initiated with the administration of three 300-mg tablets every 8 hr. The daily dose is then gradually increased to 30 to 35 mg/kg within the first 2 weeks of treatment, and it may be increased to 40 to 45 mg/kg after the first month if no disturbing side effects are present. In order to avoid peak-related side effects and to reduce daily fluctuations in progabide and PGA concentrations, the drug should be administered three or four times a day.

An improvement in seizure control, in responders, is usually appreciable within 1 to 2 months at full doses. In general, the therapeutic effect is maintained over time without a tolerance phenomenon. The degree and rate of improvement appears to be related to the severity of the syndrome and to the dose administered (71,72). Several controlled clinical trials have shown that the addition of progabide to existing regimens may be beneficial in about 30% to 50% of drug-resistant epilepsies, with differences in percentages of responders varying according to the type of the epilepsy and the severity of the syndrome. These results have been obtained in a population in which 48% of the patients had one or more daily seizures (71). Progabide also has been found superior to placebo in six individual trials (37,49,66,69,93,97), but in three others (25,55,80), there were no significant differences in the treatments. The observed differences could be explained by an unusually high rate of placebo responders or the low doses employed, which were rarely greater than 30–35 mg/kg a day. Two studies have compared the clinical effectiveness of progabide and VPA. In the first (23), the activity of progabide was inferior to that of VPA, while in the second (79), the therapeutic results of the drugs were comparable, with a better safety profile for progabide.

Several open long-term studies were conducted in patients suffering from less severe epilepsies and in responders from the double-blind trials (9,37,75,78,94). Progabide was added to existing regimens for 5 to 12 months or more and showed a therapeutic benefit in 60% to 70% of the patients. In several instances, the benefit appeared to improve over time, and about 25% of the patients were seizure-free after 12 months of treatment.

Two recent studies (9,37) evaluated the possibility of achieving progabide monotherapy in moderate to severe forms of epilepsy responding unsatisfactorily to other antiepileptic drugs. Gradual withdrawal of pre-existing therapies was possible in about 30% to 40% of the patients, who responded positively during the addition of progabide, and a therapeutic benefit was maintained with progabide alone over 6 to 12 months of observation. In further studies, progabide was used alone in newly treated patients presenting with more than two seizures in the preceding month. The available information on the patients treated so far for 8 to 12 months or more indicates a positive result in 76% of the patients, with about 70% of them being seizure-free (26,27; Giusti et al, *personal communication*). These findings are in good agreement with the recent studies of Gerstle et al. (37) and Benassi et al. (9), who used progabide as the only therapeutic agent in patients with a minimal response to CBZ or PHT.

Children

In children, progabide has been shown to be active in all types of seizures, with the exception of absences. According to a recent review by Dulac (30), the drug is useful in primary generalized epilepsies, (tonic-clonic and myoclonic), secondary generalized epilepsies, and resistant partial epilepsies with or without a focal deficit. Even if the drug is only minimally active in "pure absences," it may be of benefit in myoclonic absences. The compound does potentiate the effects (toxic and therapeutic) of benzodiazepines, without evidence of tolerance. As in adults, the safety of the drug in children is satisfactory; somnolence and irritability have been described in about 10% of the cases. In some cases of partial seizures with secondary generalization, reduction or full control of partial seizures may be accompanied by an increase in generalized seizures.

The available information on the activity of progabide in pediatric patients concerns four studies in children and one study in neonates (1,2,27,31,49,95). In a study of more than 300 children with severe epilepsies who were treated with progabide for 3 to 12 months or more, 65% of the patients appeared to respond favorably to the drug (71). The good results obtained in focal partial epilepsy and severe myoclonic epilepsy should be emphasized (30,31,49). Furthermore, the antiepileptic activity of progabide is associated with a favorable effect on alertness, mood, and school performance in children with behavioral disturbances.

The pediatric formulation consists of a 150-mg powdered preparation and 300-mg tablets. As in adults, the daily intake should be given in three divided doses, with a gradual increase of the daily dose to 30 mg/kg in 10 days. The dose can then be further increased up to 50 mg/kg a day or more if CBZ is associated. In case of association with benzodiazepines, it may be useful to increase the dose more gradually because potentiation of the benzodiazepine side effects may occur. Liver transaminases should be monitored every 15 days for the first 3 months, and then on a monthly basis up to 6 months. Further monitoring every 3 months appears to be satisfactory.

Recent observations in newborns suffering from postasphyxic neonatal convulsions indicate that progabide is a very useful addition to the very limited therapeutic armamentarium for these seizures. In 15 neonates suffering from either status epilepticus or frequent convulsions not responding to PHT, PB, or clonazepam, progabide given as an aqueous suspension of 60 mg/kg a day (t.i.d.) had a rapid and sustained anticonvulsant effect in 13 out of 15 cases (1,2).

CONCLUSIONS

The findings reported above represent the information available as of January 1988 from more than 2,500 patients treated with progabide for periods ranging from 1 month to more than 5 years. The available data indicate that in selected patients, both adults and children, progabide administered at full doses provides a significant and sustained reduction in seizure frequency. Because of the possibility of hepatic injury, its use should be accompanied by close monitoring of biochemical parameters during the first 6 months of treatment. The therapeutic action appears to be present in three major types of epilepsy: primary generalized epilepsy, secondary generalized epilepsy, and partial epilepsy. Progabide appears to be useful in epileptic patients responding minimally to the available antiepileptic drugs. The wide spectrum of action at the clinical level confirms the observations from pharmacological models and supports the hypothesis of an impairment of the GABAergic system in epilepsy.

ACKNOWLEDGMENTS

The authors wish to thank Miss Marie-Pierre Vignaud for the careful preparation of the manuscript.

CONVERSION

Conversion factor:

$$CF = \frac{1000}{\text{mol. wt.}} = \frac{1000}{334.78} = 2.99$$

Conversion:

$$(\mu g/ml) \times 2.99 = (\mu moles/liter)$$

$$(\mu moles/liter) \div 2.99 = (\mu g/ml)$$

REFERENCES

1. André, M., Boutroy, M. J., Bianchetti, G., Padovani, P., Vert, P., and Morselli P. L. (1989): Therapeutic action and pharmacokinetics of progabide in neonates suffering from convulsive syndromes (submitted).
2. André, M., Boutroy, M. J., Vert, P., and Morselli, P. L. (1985): Therapeutic effect of Progabide in neonatal convulsions. In: *16th Epilepsy International Congress*, Hambourg, Sept. 6–9, 1985 (Abstract no. 15).
3. Ascalone, V., Catalani, B., DalBô, L. (1985): Determination of progabide and its acid metabolite in biological fluids by HPLC on silica column and UV detector. *J. Chromat. Biomed. Applic.*, 344:231–239.
4. Ascalone, V., and DalBô, L. (1986): Chromatographic selectivity and maintenance of column efficiency during the high-performance liquid chromatographic analysis of progabide and its acid metabolite. *J. Chromat. Biomed. Appl.*, 382:412–414.
5. Assael, B. M., Viani, F., Thénot, J. P., Bianchetti, G., Padovani, P., and Morselli, P. L. (1989): Pharmacokinetics of progabide in epileptic children (*submitted*).
6. Bartholini, G., Scatton, B., Zivkovic, B., and Lloyd, K. G. (1979): On the mode of action of SL 76002, a new GABA receptor agonist. In *GABA neurotransmitters*, edited by P. Krogsgaard-Laarsen, J. Scheel-Kruger and H. Kofod, pp. 326–339. Munksgaard, Copenhagen.
7. Bartholini, G., Scatton, B., Zivkovic, B., Lloyd, K. G., Depoortere, H., Langer S. Z., and Morselli, P. L. (1985): GABA receptor agonists as a new therapeutic class. In: *Epilepsy and GABA receptor agonists—Basic and therapeutic research*, L.E.R.S. vol. 3, edited by G. Bartholini, L. Bossi, K. G. Lloyd, and P. L. Morselli, pp.1–30. Raven Press, New York.
8. Benassi, E., Besio, G., Bianchetti, G., Loeb, C., and Morselli, P. L. (1988b): Blood levels of Progabide and its active metabolite (PGA) in epileptic patients: Relationships to the therapeutic outcome. *J. Clin. Pharm. Res.* VIII:609–613.
9. Benassi, E., Besio, G., Bo, G. P., Cocito, L.,
10. Maffini, M., Mainardi, P., and Loeb, C. (1988a): Observations on the activity of Progabide as monotherapy in complex partial seizures. *J. Clin. Pharm. Res.* VIII:353–361.
11. Benassi, E., Besio, G., Fonrazi, M., Mainardi, P., and Loeb, C. (1984): Preliminary results on the effects of progabide on partial complex seizures. *Clin. Neuropharmacol.*, 7 (Suppl. 1): 394–395.
11. Bianchetti, G., Padovani, P., Miquet, P., Thiercelin, J. F., Larribaud, J., Bouchet, J. L., Thénot, J. P., Trocherie, S., and Morselli, P. L. (1984): Pharmacokinetic profile of progabide in patients with hepatic cirrhosis and renal insufficiency. In: *Biopharmaceutics and Pharmacokinetics, vol. II: Experimental Pharmacokinetics*, edited by J. M. Aiache and J. Hirtz, pp. 454–459. Clermont Ferrand University Publ., Clermont Ferrand.
12. Bianchetti, G., Padovani, P., Thénot, J. P., Thiercelin, J. F., and Morselli, P. L. (1987): Pharmacokinetic interactions in progabide with other antiepileptic drugs. *Epilepsia*, 28:68–73.
13. Bowery, N. G., Hill, D. R., and Hudson, A. L. (1982): Evidence that SL 75102 is an agonist at GABA_B as well as GABA_A receptors. *Neuropharmacol.*, 21:391–395.
14. Bowery, N. G., Hill, D. R., Hudson, A. L., and Price, G. W. (1985): GABAmimetic action of SL 75.102 at neuronal receptors. In: *Epilepsy and GABA receptor agonists—Basic and Therapeutic Research*, L.E.R.S. vol. 3, edited by G. Bartholini, L. Bossi, K. G. Lloyd, and P. L. Morselli, pp. 63–80. Raven Press, New York.
15. Broquaire, M. (1979): Simple method of packing high-performance liquid chromatographic columns with high-reproducibility. *J. Chromat.*, 170:43–52.
16. Brundage, R. C., Cloyd, J. C., Leppick, I. E., Graves, N. M., and Welty, T. E. (1987): Effect of Progabide on serum phenytoin and carbamazepine concentrations. *Clin. Neuropharm.*, 10:545–554.
17. Burke, J. T., and Thénot, J. P. (1985): Determination of antiepileptic drugs. *J. of Chromat. Biomed. Appl.*, 340:199–241.
18. Burke, J. I., Durand, A., Ferrandes, B., and Morselli, P. L. (1984): Plasma levels of Progabide and related metabolites in four animal species. In: *Biopharmaceutics and Pharmacokinetics: II. Experimental Pharmacokinetics*, edited by J. M. Aiache and J. Hirtz, pp. 493–500. Clermont Ferrand University Publ., Clermont Ferrand.
19. Cepeda, C., Worms, P., Lloyd, K. G., and Naquet, P. (1982): Action of progabide in the photosensitive baboon *Papio papio*. *Epilepsia*, 24:463–470.
20. Cloyd, J. C., Brundage, R. C., Leppick, I. E., Graves, N. M., and Welty, T. E. (1985): Effect of progabide on serum phenytoin and carbamazepine concentrations: A preliminary report. In: *Epilepsy and GABA Receptor Agonists—Basic and Therapeutic Research*, L.E.R.S. vol. 3, edited by G. Bartholini, L. Bossi, K. G. Lloyd, and

P. L. Morselli, pp. 271–277. Raven Press, New York.

21. Coquelin, J. P., Krall, R., Bossi, L., Musch, B., and Morsellli, P. L. (1985): Drug safety profile of progabide. In *Epilepsy and GABA Receptor Agonists—Basic and Therapeutic Research,* L.E.R.S. vol. 3, edited by G. Bartholini, L. Bossi, K. G. Lloyd, and P. L. Morselli, pp. 431–440. Raven Press, New York.

22. Court, L. A., Thébault, J. J., and Trocherie, S. (1985): Quantitative pharmaco-electroencephalography of the effect of progabide. In: *Epilepsy and GABA Receptors Agonists—Basic and Therapeutic Research,* L.E.R.S. vol. 3 edited by G. Bartholini, L. Bossi, K. G. Lloyd, and P. L. Morselli, pp. 303–309. Raven Press, New York.

23. Crawford, P., and Chadwick, D. (1986): A comparative study of Progabide, valproate and placebo as add-on therapy in patients with refractory epilepsy. *J. Neurol. Neurosurg. Psychiat.,* 49:1251–1257.

24. Cudennec, A., Duverger, D., Lloyd, K. G., MacKenzie, E. T., McCulloch, J., Motohashi, N., Nishikawa, T., and Scatton, B. (1987): Effects of the GABA receptor agonist, progabide, upon local cerebral glucose utilization. *Brain Research,* 423:162–172.

25. Dam, M., Gram, L., Philbert, A., Hansen, B. S., Blatt-Lyon, B., Christiensen, J. M., and Angelo H. R., 1983): Progabide: A controlled trial in partial epilepsy. *Epilepsia,* 24:127–135.

26. Dandelot, J. B., Bossi, L., Poulain, D. J., Musch, B., and Morselli, P. L. (1984): Progabide monotherapy in previously untreated epileptic patients. *Neurology,* 34 (Suppl. 1):266.

27. Dandelot, J. B., Mignard, C., Mignard, D., Bousquet, C., Choucair, Y., Nakache, P., Poulain, D., and Bossi, L. (1985): Progabide monotherapy in naïve epileptic patients in La Réunion Island. In *Epilepsy and GABA Receptor Agonists—Basic and Therapeutic Research,* L.E.R.S. vol. 3, edited by G. Bartholini, L. Bossi, K. G. Lloyd, and P. L. Morselli, pp. 409–414. Raven Press, New York.

28. Debeljuk, L., Diaz, M. D. C., Maines, V. M., and Seilicovich, A. (1983): Prolonged treatment with gamma-amino-butyric-acid-mimetic substances in prepuberal male rats. *Archives of Andrology,* 10:239–244.

29. Desarmenien, M., Feltz, P., Headley, P. M., and Santangelo, F. (1981): SL 75102 as a gamma-aminobutyric acid agonist: Experiments on dorsal root ganglion neurons "in vitro". *Br. J. Pharmacol.,* 72:355–364.

30. Dullac, O. (1987): Traitement des épilepsies de l'enfant et du nourrisson. *Revue Internationale de Pédiatrie,* 171:5–23.

31. Dulac, O., Bossi, L., Régnier, F., Poulain, D., Battin, J., Drossart, F., Dandelot, J. B., Bertsch, M., and Arthuis, M. (1985): Long-term open trial of progabide in epileptic children. In: *Epilepsy and GABA Receptor Agonists—Basic and Therapeutic Research,* L.E.R.S. vol. 3, edited by G.

32. Ferrandes, B., Durand, A., Fraisse-André, J., and Morselli, P. L. (1984): Metabolic studies of progabide (SL 76002) in the rat. In: *Metabolism of Antiepileptic Drugs,* edited by R. H. Levy et al., pp. 183–190. Raven Press, New York.

33. Ferrandes, B., Durand, A., Padovani, P., Burke, J. T., Garrigou, D., Fraisse-André, J., Hermann, P., and Allen, J. (1985): Metabolism of progabide in four animal species and in man. In: *Epilepsy and GABA Receptor Agonists—Basic and Therapeutic Research,* L.E.R.S. vol. 3, edited by G. Bartholini, L. Bossi, K. G. Lloyd, and P. L. Morselli, pp. 217–229. Raven Press, New York.

34. Friedmann, J. C., and Prenez, A. (1985): Safety evaluation of progabide. In: *Epilepsy and GABA Receptor Agonists—Basic and Therapeutic Research,* L.E.R.S. vol. 3, edited by G. Bartholini, L. Bossi, K. G. Lloyd, and P. L. Morselli, pp. 203–215. Raven Press, New York.

35. Gallager, D. W., and Aghajanian, G. K. (1976): Effects of antipsychotic drugs on the firing of dorsal raple cells. II. Reversal by picrotoxin. *Eur. J. Pharmacol.,* 39:357–364.

36. Garrigou-Gadenne, D., Durand, A., Ferrandes, B., and Morselli, P. L. (1988): Kinetics of the distribution of Progabide and related metabolites in various areas of the rat brain (*submitted*).

37. Gerstle de Pasquet, E., Scaramelli, A., Pineyrùa de Caceres, M., L'Héritier, C., Feldman, S., Santana, R., Aguilar, J. et al. (1989): A double blind placebo controlled cross-over tiral on Progabide as add-on therapy in epileptic patients (*submitted*).

38. Gillet, G., Fraisse-André, J., Lee, C. R., Dring, G., and Morselli, P. L. (1982): Gas chromatographic method for the determination of progabide (SL 76002) in biological fluids. *J. Chromatogr. Biomed. Applic.,* 230:154–161.

39. Girad, M., Poulain, D., and Bossi, L. (1987): Tentatives de suicide au progabide. *La Presse Médicale,* 16:681.

40. Guidotti, A., and Ferrero, P. (1985): *Ex vivo* binding of ^{3}H muscimol to $GABA_A$ recognition sites: A tool to characterize GABA receptor agonists. In: *Epilepsy and GABA Receptor Agonists—Basic and Therapeutic Research,* L.E.R.S. vol. 3, edited by G. Bartholini, L. Bossi, K. G., Lloyd, and P. L. Morselli, pp. 31–41. Raven Press, New York.

41. Gutierrez, A., Dreifuss, F. E., and Santilli, N. (1984): Psychiatric symptoms associated with Progabide therapy. *Epilepsia,* 25:657.

42. Hamberger, C., Barre, J., Brandebourger, M., Urien, S., Taillet, A., Thénot, J. P., and Tillement, J. P. (1987): Progabide and SL 75.102 binding to plasma proteins and red blood cells in humans. *Int. J. Clin. Pharm. Therap. and Toxicol.,* 25:178–184.

43. Hamberger, C., Barre, J., and Tillement, J. P. (1985): Binding of progabide and SL 75102 to human serum proteins: Intractions with other antiepileptic drugs. In: *Epilepsy and GABA Re-*

ceptor Agonists—Basic and Therapeutic Research, L.E.R.S. vol. 3, edited by G. Bartholini, L. Bossi, K. G. Lloyd, and P. L. Morselli, pp. 243–251. Raven Press, New York.

44. Johno, I., Ludwick, B. T., and Levy, R. H. (1982): Pharmacokinetic profile of progabide, a new gamma-aminobutyric acid mimetic drug, in rhesus monkey. *J. Pharm. Sci.,* 71:633–636.

45. Joy, R. M., Albertson, T. F., and Starek, L. G. (1984): Analysis of the action of progabide, a specific GABA receptor agonist, on kindling and kindling seizures. *Exp. Neurol.,* 83:144–154.

46. Kaplan, J. P., Raizon, B. M., Desarmenien, M., Feltz, P., Headley, P. M., Worms, P., Lloyd, K. G., and Bartholini, G. (1980): New anticonvulsants: Schiff bases of GABA and GABAmide. *J. Med. Chem.,* 23:702–704.

47. Koe, B. K. (1983): Enhancement of benzodiazepine binding by progabide (SL 76.002) and SL 75.103. *Drugs in Development and Research,* 3:421–432.

48. Krall, R. L., Penry, J. K., White, B. G., Kupferberg, H. J., and Swinyard, E. A. (1978): Antiepileptic drug development. II. Anticonvulsant drug screening. *Epilepsia,* 19:409–428.

49. Kulakowsky, S., Meynckens, M., and Coupez-Lopinot, R. (1985): Double-blind study of a new antiepileptic drug, progabide, in severe childhood patients. In: *Epilepsy and GABA Receptor Agonists—Basic and Therapeutic Research,* L.E.R.S. vol. 3, edited by G. Bartholini, L. Bossi, K. G. Lloyd, and P. L. Morselli, pp. 377–387. Raven Press, New York.

50. Kutt, H. (1974): Interactions with antiepileptic drugs involving multiple mechanisms. In: *Drug Interactions,* edited by P. L. Morselli, S. Garattini, and S. N. Cohen, pp. 211–222. Raven Press, New York.

51. Kutt, H., and Kutt, H. P. (1982): Phenobarbital interactions with other drugs. In: *Antiepileptic Drugs,* 2nd edition, edited by D. M. Woodbury, J. K. Penry, and C. E. Pippenger, pp. 329–340. Raven Press, New York.

52. Kutt, H., Solomon, G. E., Dhar, A. K., Resor, S. R., Krall, R. L., and Morselli, P. L. (1984): Effects of progabide on carbamazepine epoxide and carbamazepine concentrations in plasma. Proceeding of Annual Meeting of the American Epilepsy Society, San Francisco, California, November 8 and 9, 1984. *Epilepsia,* 25:674.

53. Langer, S. G., Arbilla, S., Scatton, B., Zivkovic, B., Galzini, A. M., Lloyd, K. G., and Bartholini, G. (1985): Progabide and SL 75.102 interaction with gamma-aminobutyric-acid receptors and effects on neurotransmitters and receptors systems. In: *Epilepsy and GABA Receptor Agonists—Basic and Therapeutic Research,* L.E.R.S., vol. 3, edited by G. Bartholini, L. Bossi, K. G., Lloyd, and P. L. Morselli, pp. 81–90. Raven Press, New York.

54. Levy, R. H., Johno, I., Wilensky, A. J., Pitlick, W. H., Friel, P. N., and Anderson, G. D. (1985): Pharmacokinetics of progabide in rhesus monkey and normal man. In: *Epilepsy and GABA Recep-tor Agonists—Basic and Therapeutic Research,* L.E.R.S. vol. 3, edited by G. Bartholini, L. Bossi, K. G. Lloyd, and P. L. Morselli, pp. 231–241, Raven Press, New York.

55. Leppick, I. E., Dreifuss, F. E., Porter R. J., Bowman, J., et al. (1987): A controlled study of Progabide in partial seizures: Methodology and results. *Neurology,* 37:963–968.

56. Lloyd, K. G. (1986): La théorie GABAergique de l'épilepsie. *La Revue du Praticien,* 36:243–254.

57. Lloyd, K. G., Arbilla, S., Beaumont, K., Briley, M., DeMontis, G., Scatton, B., Langer, S. Z., and Bartholini, G. (1982): Gamma-aminobutyric acid (GABA) receptor stimulation. II. Specificity of progabide (SL 76 002) and SL 75 102 for the GABA receptor. *J. Pharmacol. Exp. Ther.,* 220:672–677.

58. Lloyd, K. G., Bossi, L., Morselli, P. L., Munari, C., Rougier, M., and Loiseau, H. (1986): Alterations of GABA mediated transmission in human epilepsy. In: *Advances in Neurology—Basic Mechanisms of the Epilespies, Vol. 44,* edited by A. V. Delgado Escueta, A. A. Ward, D. M. Woodbury, and R. Porter, pp. 1033–1044. Raven Press, New York.

59. Lloyd, K. G., Bossi, L., Morselli, P. L., Rougier, M., Loiseau, P., and Munari, C. (1985): Biochemical evidence for dysfunction of GABA neurons in human epilepsy. In: *Epilepsy and GABA Receptor Agonists—Basic and Therapeutic Research,* L.E.R.S. vol. 3, edited by G. Bartholini, L. Bossi, K. G. Lloyd, and P. L. Morselli, pp. 43–51. Raven Press, New York.

60. Lloyd, K. G., Bovier, P., Broekkamp, C. L. E., and Worms, P. (1981): Reversal of the antiaversive and anticonvulsant actions of diazepam but not progabide by a selective antagonist of benzodiazepine receptors. *Eur. J. Pharmacol.,* 75:77–78.

61. Lloyd, K. G., and Morselli, P. L. (1987): Psychopharmacology of GABAergic drugs. In: *Psychopharmacology—Third Generation of Progress,* edited by H. Y. Meltzer, pp. 183–195. Raven Press, New York.

62. Lloyd, K. G., Worms, P., Zivkovic, B., Scatton, B., and Bartholini, G. (1980): Interaction of GABA mimetics with nigro-striatal dopamine neurons. *Brain Research Bulletin,* 5 (Suppl. 2):439–445.

63. Loescher, W. (1985a): GABAmimetic in animal models of seizures states. In: *Epilepsy and GABA Receptor Agonists—Basic and Therapeutic Research,* L.E.R.S. vol. 3, edited by G. Bartholini, L. Bossi, K. G. Lloyd, and P. L. Morselli, pp. 109–119. Raven Press, New York.

64. Loescher, W. (1985b): Influence of pharmacological manipulation of inhibitory and excitatory neurotransmitter systems on seizure behavior in the mongolian gerbil. *J. Pharmacol. Exp. Ther.,* 233:204–213.

65. Loescher, W., and Schwark, W. S. (1985): Evaluation of different gamma-amino-butyric acid receptor agonists in the kindled amygdala seizure model in rats. *Experimental Neurol.,* 89:454–460.

66. Loiseau, P., Bossi, L., Guyot, M., Orofiamma, B., and Morselli, P. L. (1983): Double blind cross-over trial of progabide versus placebo in severe epilepsies. *Epilepsia,* 24:703–715.

67. Loiseau, P., Orgogozo, J. M., Brachet-Liermain, A., and Morselli, P. L. (1978): Pharmacokinetic studies on the interaction between phenobarbital and valproic acid. In: *Advances in Epileptology,* edited by H. Meinardi and A. J. Rowan, pp. 261–265. Swets & Zeitliner B. V., Amsterdam.

68. London, D. R., Menon, V. J., Loizou, L., Horrocks, P. M., Butt, W. R., and Gomeni, R. (1985): Neuroendocrine effects of Progabide in comparison with other gamma-amino-butyric acid agonists. In: *Epilepsy and GABA Receptor Agonists—Basic and Therapeutic Research,* L.E.R.S. vol. 3, edited by G. Bartholini, L. Bossi, K. G. Lloyd, and P. L. Morsellli, pp. 295–302. Raven Press, New York.

69. Martinez-Lage, J. M., Bossi, L., Morales, G., Martinez-Vila, E., Orofiamma, B., and Viteri, C. (1984): Progabide treatment in severe epilepsy: A double-blind cross-over trial versus placebo. *Epilepsia,* 25:586–593.

70. Menon, V. J., Butt, W. R., Thiercelin, J. F., Gomeni, R., Morselli, P. L., and London, D. (1984): Effects in man of Progabide on prolactin release induced by haloperidol or domperidone. *Psychoneuroendocrinology,* 9:141–146.

71. Morselli, P. L., Bartholini, G., and Lloyd, K. G. (1986a): Progabide. In: *New Anticonvulsant Drugs,* edited by B. S. Meldrum and R. J. Porter, pp. 237–252. John Libbey & Co. Ltd., London.

72. Morselli, P. L., and Bossi, L. (1986b): GABAergic drugs for intractable epilepsies. In: *Intractable Epilepsy: Experimental and Clinical Aspects,* edited by D. Schmidt and P. L. Morselli, pp. 209–217. Raven Press, New York.

73. Morselli, P. L., Burke, J., Padovani, P., Bianchetti, G., Ferrandes, B., and Thenot, J. P. (1984): Pharmacokinetic profile of progabide in 5 animal species and man. In: *Metabolism of Antiepileptic Drugs,* edited by R. H. Levy, et al., pp. 191–197. Raven Press, New York.

74. Morselli, P. L., and Lloyd, K. G. (1985): Mechanism of action of antiepileptic drugs. In: *The Epilepsies,* edited by R. J. Porter and P. L. Morselli, pp. 40–81. Butterworths, London.

75. Morselli, P. L., Loiseau, P., Martinez-Lage, J. M., and Bossi, L. (1984): Long-term follow up with progabide in resistant epilepsies. In: *Advances in Epileptology: XVth Epilepsy International Symposium,* edited by R. J. Porter, R. H. Mattson, A. A. Ward, and M. Dam, pp. 177–180. Raven Press, New York.

76. Morselli, P. L., Rizzo, M., and Garattini, S. (1971): Interaction between phenobarbital and diphenylhydantoin in animals and in epileptic patients. *Proc. N.Y. Acad. Sci.* (USA), 179:88–107.

77. Munoz, S. J., Fariello, R., and Maddrey, W. C. (1987): Submassive necrosis associated with the use of progabide: A GABA receptor agonist. *Dig. Dis. Sci.,* 33:375–380.

78. Musch, B., Cambier, J., Loiseau, P., Fournier, V., Bossi, L., Beausart, M., Benoît, C., Chatel, M., Deville, M. C., Favel, P., Ferrière, G., Geets, W., Goas, J. Y., Kulakowski, S., Louette, N., Martinez-Lage, M., and Remy, C. (1986): Open long-term multicenter trial with progabide in epileptic patients. *Eur. Neurol.,* 26:113–119.

79. Musch, B., Courjon, J., Vercelletto, P., Loiseau, P., Kurz, P., Meaulle, F., Beaussart, M., Goffaux, P., and Jaburian, P. (1989): A comparative controlled study of the antiepileptic effect of valproic acid and Progabide (*submitted*).

80. Naquet, R., Valin, A., and Bryère, P. (1985): Progabide, benzodiazepines, and myoclonus in *Papio papio.* In: *Epilepsy and GABA Receptor Agonists—Basic and Therapeutic Research,* L.E.R.S. vol. 3, edited by G. Bartholini, L. Bossi, K. G. Lloyd, and P. L. Morselli, pp. 159–171. Raven Press, New York.

81. Padovani, P., Deves, C., Bianchetti, G., Thénot, J. P., and Morselli, P. L. (1984): Determination of progabide and its main acid metabolite in biological fluids using HPLC and electrochemical detection. *J. Chromatogr.,* 308:229–239.

82. Padovani, P., Thénot, J. P., Warrington, S., Hermann, P., Fraisse-André, F., Thiercelin, J. F., Larribaud, J., and Morselli, P. L. (1983): Metabolism of progabide in man. In: *Advances in Epileptology, XVth Epilepsy International Symposium,* edited by R. J. Porter, R. H. Mattson, A. A. Ward, and M. Dam, pp. 169–175. Raven Press, New York.

83. Palminteri, R., Krall, R., and Zimmerman, H. J. (1989): Hepatic injury associated with the investigational use of the GABA-receptor agonist progabide *Hepatology* (*in press*).

84. Palminteri, R., L'Héritier, C., and Bossi, L. (1985): Progabide and liver function tests. *16th Epilepsy International Congress,* Hamburg, Sept. 6–9, 1985. (Abstract no. 363).

85. Pascard, C., Kaplan, J. P., Raizon, B., and Mompon, B. (1982): Structure of 4[(4-chlorophenyl) (5-fluoro-2-hydroxyphenyl)methylamino]butanamide: Progabide (SL 76.002). *Acta. Crystallogr.,* 33b:3131–3132.

86. Patsalos, P. M., and Lascelles, P. T. (1977): *In vitro* hydroxylation of diphenylhydantoin and its inhibition by other commonly used anticonvulsant drugs. *Biochem. Pharm.,* 26:1629–1633.

87. Scatton, B., and Bartholini, G. (1982): GABA receptor stimulation IV. Effect of progabide (SL 76.002) and other GABAergic agents on acetylcholine turnover in rat brain areas. *J. Pharmacol. Exp. Ther.,* 220:689–695.

88. Scatton, B., Zivkovic, B., Dedek, J., Lloyd, K. G., Constantinidis, J., Tissot, R., and Bartholini, G. (1982): GABA receptor stimulation III. Effect of progabide (SL 76.002) on norepinephrine, dopamine and 5-hydroxytryptamine turnover in rat brain areas. *J. Pharmacol. Exp. Ther.,* 220:678–688.

89. Schmidt, D., and Utech, K. (1986): Progabide for refractory partial epilepsy: A controlled add-on trial, *Neurology,* 36:217–221.

90. Thénot, J. P., Bianchetti, G., Abriol, C., Feuer-

stein, J., Lambert, D., Thébault, J. J., Warrington, S. J., and Rowland, M. (1985): Interactions between progabide and antiepileptic drugs. In: *Epilepsy and GABA Receptor Agonists—Basic and Therapeutic Research,* L.E.R.S. vol. 3, edited by G. Bartholini, L. Bossi, K. G. Lloyd, and P. L. Morselli, pp. 259–269. Raven Press, New York.

91. Thiercelin, J. F., Bouchet, J. L., Miguet, J. P., Martin-Dupont, C., Thénot, J. P., and Larribaud, J. (1985): Pharmacokinetics of progabide in renal and hepatic insufficiency: Comparison with data obtained in healthy subjects. In: *Epilepsy and GABA Receptor Agonists—Basic and Therapeutic Research,* L.E.R.S. vol. 3, edited by G. Bartholini, L. Bossi, K. G. Lloyd, and P. L. Morselli, pp. 253–258. Raven Press, New York.

92. Vandel, B., Trocherie, S., Padovani, P., Thiercelin, J. F., Orofiamma, B., Larribaud, J., and Bianchetti, G. (1985): Research on interaction between progabide and alcohol in man. In: *Epilepsy and GABA Receptor Agonists—Basic and Therapeutic Research,* L.E.R.S. vol. 3, edited by G. Bartholini, L. Bossi, K. G. Lloyd, and P. L. Morselli, pp. 287–294. Raven Press, New York.

93. Van der Linden, G. J., Meinardi, H., Meijer, J. W. A., Bossi, L., and Gomeni, C. (1981): A double-blind cross-over trial with progabide (SL 76 002) against placebo in patients with secondary generalized epilepsy. In: *Advances in Epileptology: XIIth Epilepsy International Symposium,* edited by M. Dam, L. Gram, and J. K. Penry, pp. 141–144. Raven Press, New York.

94. Van Parys, J. A. P., Van der Linden, G. J., Goedhart, D. M., Meijer, J. W. A., and Meinardi, H. (1985): Clinical experience with progabide in severe in- and out-patients. In: *Epilepsy and GABA Receptor Agonists—Basic and Therapeutic Research,* L.E.R.S. vol. 3, edited by G. Bartholini, L. Bossi, K. G. Lloyd, and P. L. Morselli, pp. 343–351. Raven Press, New York.

95. Viani, F., and Romeo, A. (1985): Effect of progabide on seizures and behavior in therapy-resistant epileptic children. In: *Epilepsy and GABA Receptor Agonists—Basic and Therapeutic Research,* L.E.R.S. vol. 3, edited by G. Bartholini, L. Bossi, K. G. Lloyd, and P. L. Morselli, pp. 369–375. Raven Press, New York.

96. Warrington, S. J., O'Brien, C., Thiercelin, J. F., Orofiamma, B., and Morselli, P. L. (1985): Evaluation of pharmacodynamic interaction between progabide and clonazepam in healthy man. In: *Epilepsy and GABA Receptor Agonists—Basic and Therapeutic Research,* L.E.R.S. vol. 3, edited by G. Bartholini, L. Bossi, K. G. Lloyd, and P. L. Morselli, pp. 279–286. Raven Press, New York.

97. Weber, M., Verspignani, H., Rémy, M. C., Regnier, F., and Bossi, L. (1985): Controlled trial of progabide versus placebo in severe therapy resistant epilepsies. In: *Epilepsy and GABA Receptor Agonists—Basic and Therapeutic Research,* L.E.R.S. vol. 3, edited by G. Bartholini, L. Bossi, K. G. Lloyd, and P. L. Morselli, pp. 353–361. Raven Press, New York.

98. Wedzikowska, T., Durand, A., Ferrandes, B., and Morselli, P. L. (1984): Protein binding of Progabide and its acid metabolite: Interactions with four antiepileptic drugs in the rat. In: *Proceedings of the IXth European Congress on Drug Metabolism,* Pont-à-Mousson, June 84, edited by A. Siest, pp. 70–71.

99. Wick, A. E., Mompon, B., and Rossey, G. (1985): Chemistry of progabide. In: *Epilepsy and GABA Receptor Agonists—Basic and Therapeutic Research,* L.E.R.S. vol. 3, edited by G. Bartholini, L. Bossi, K. G. Lloyd, and P. L. Morselli, pp. 53–62. Raven Press, New York.

100. Worms, P., Depoortere, H., Durand, A., Morselli, P. L., Lloyd, K. G., and Bartholini, G. (1982): Gamma-aminobutyric acid (GABA) receptor stimulation. I. Neuropharmacological profiles of progabide (SL 76002) and SL 75102, with emphasis on their anticonvulsant spectra. *J. Pharmacol. Exp. Ther.,* 220:660–671.

101. Worms, P., and Lloyd, K. G. (1981): Functional alterations of GABA synapses in relation to seizures. In: *Neurotransmitters, seizures and epilepsy,* edited by P. L. Morselli, K. G. Lloyd, W. Löscher, B. Meldrum, and E. H. Reynolds, pp. 37–46. Raven Press, New York.

102. Yonekawa, W., Kupferberg, H. J., and Lambert, T. (1983): Measurement of Progabide and its deaminated metabolite in plasma by high performance liquid chromatography and electrochemical detection. *Journal Chromat.,* 276:103–110.

103. Zivkovic, B., Lloyd, K. G., and Bartholini, G. (1985): Anticonvulsant spectrum of action of progabide in laboratory models of convulsant disorders. In: *Epilepsy and GABA Receptor Agonists—Basic and Therapeutic Research,* L.E.R.S. vol. 3, edited by G. Bartholini, L. Bossi, K. G. Lloyd, and P. L. Morselli, pp. 101–108. Raven Press, New York.

104. Zivkovic, B., Scatton, B., Dedek, J., and Bartholini, G. (1982): GABA influence on noradrenergic and serotoninergic transmissions: Implications in mood regulation. In: *New Vistas in Depression,* edited by S. Z. Langer, R. Jakahashi, J. Segawa, and M. Briley, pp. 195–201. Pergamon Press, New York.

Antiepileptic Drugs, Third Edition, edited by
R. Levy, R. Mattson, B. Meldrum,
J. K. Penry, and F. E. Dreifuss.
Raven Press, Ltd., New York © 1989.

65

Other Antiepileptic Drugs

Adrenocorticotropic Hormone (ACTH)

O. Carter Snead, III

The effect of oral steroids on the convulsive state was first reported in 1942 when McQuarrie et al. (41) observed the exacerbation of seizures by deoxycorticosterone. Subsequently, Hoefer and Glaser (19) demonstrated that adrenocorticotropic hormone (ACTH) and cortisone produced slowing in the EEG. Some authors (8,70) expressed concern that ACTH might be proconvulsant in adult seizure patients, whereas others (13,47) came to the opposite conclusion: that ACTH and cortisone treatment was associated with normalization of the EEG.

The first report of the therapeutic efficacy of ACTH in childhood seizures came in 1950, when Klein and Livingston (31) observed a beneficial effect of the steroid in four of six children, aged 4.5 to 16 years, with various types of intractable seizures. In 1958, Sorel and Dusaucy-Bauloye (62) reported a dramatic response to ACTH therapy in a series of children with infantile spasms who showed normalized behavior, controlled seizures, and improved EEG. This finding was confirmed the following year (10,15,63), and the benefit of oral steroids in this condition also was established (10,37). Since those initial reports, a bewildering array of studies concerning the use of oral steroids and/or ACTH in infantile spasms has been published. Most of the studies were uncontrolled, and all used a

hodgepodge of dosage regimens (for reviews see 1,20,26,28,32). In fact, the only commonality among these various works is the seizure type studied, infantile spasms.

The first, and still unsurpassed, clinical description of infantile spasms was made in 1841 by West (71) in a poignant letter to the *Lancet*. In this correspondence, Dr. West described a mysterious malady afflicting his son, which was characterized by "bobbings of the head" and "bowings and relaxings" in clusters of "from ten to twenty or more times at each attack" and a progressive deterioration of intellect such that "he . . . never smiles or takes any notice, but looks placid and pitiful." The clinical presentation of infantile spasms, so lucidly described by West, has now been carefully studied and further characterized by continuous monitoring with EEG-videotelemetry (29). The spasms may be divided into flexor, extensor, and mixed, with the latter being the most common, and extensor spasms the least common. Flexor spasms consist of flexion of the neck, trunk, arms, and legs. Abdominal flexion may be massive, giving rise to the "jack-knife" or "salaam" seizures that are the hallmark of infantile spasms. During extensor spasms, there is abrupt extension of the neck, trunk, and legs. The mixed flexor-extensor spasms are characterized by flexion of the neck, trunk, and arms, and extension of the legs.

Infantile spasms usually occur in clusters many times daily, but particularly upon awakening, and are often associated with a cry. The doubling over and crying seen with massive abdominal flexor spasms may lead to a misdiagnosis of colic.

The EEG abnormality classically associated with infantile spasms was described as hypsarrythmic by Gibbs and Gibbs (16). This term refers to high voltage choatic slowing, multifocal spikes, and marked asynchrony. The definition was expanded by Hrachovy et al. (24) to include areas of focal abnormality, synchrony, asymmetries, and/or burst suppression.

Infantile spasms are associated with mortality of 10% to 20% and morbidity of 75% to 90% (26,27,32). The morbidity consists of generally moderate to severe mental retardation. The spasms are quite age-specific, usually occurring within the first 6 months of life, but the incidence drops off rapidly after 12 months. The spasms rarely, if ever, occur after the age of 4 years (20). The term West's syndrome refers to those children who have infantile spasms, a hypsarrythmic EEG, and mental retardation (27).

EFFICACY IN INFANTILE SPASMS

There are only a few accepted canons regarding the treatment of infantile spasms. First, the spasms are almost always intractable to treatment with standard anticonvulsant drugs. Second, ACTH or oral steroid therapy will significantly reduce seizures in 50% to 65% of patients. Third, there may be an inverse relation between response to treatment and age, with younger patients responding better (42,75). Fourth, the prognosis of most patients is dismal and depends heavily on the etiology of the spasms, the pre-existing neurologic and developmental status, the presence or absence of other seizures, and the age of the patient at the onset of the seizures

(27,36). The best prognosis is found in patients who are older than 3 months but less than 12 months of age and neurologically normal at the onset, who have no other kind of seizures, and who lack a demonstrable etiology for the spasms. Finally, natural ACTH is preferable to the synthetic form of the drug, since the former seems to have fewer side effects.

There are several controversial questions regarding the treatment of infantile spasms that engender little agreement: Which is the most effective therapy, ACTH or oral steroids? What is the optimal dose of these drugs? How long should the patient be treated? Does it make a difference in the ultimate outcome whether the patient is treated early or late in regard to onset of the spasms? Does it make any difference in the outcome of a patient with pre-existing mental retardation and an abnormal brain whether the spasms are treated at all? There is no definitive answer to any of these questions. Various reports of the efficacy of different regimens and the relation of treatment to outcome are difficult to compare because no standard regimen has been used. With one exception (23), all studies have been either retrospective (48,54,55) or open, prospective trials. Only one author (36) has looked carefully and prospectively at the cryptogenic group, those children who are normal at the onset of the spasms and in whom no etiology can be found. Since this is the group with the best prognosis (27,36), it is the most important one in which to define a standard treatment regimen.

Although some reports (26,27) have shown no difference in the efficacy of ACTH or oral steroids and no long-term benefit in treating spasms, the most compelling confirmation of these findings is found in the study of Hrachovy et al. (23). In this double-blind study, patients were randomized to receive either 20 units of ACTH a day plus prednisone placebo or prednisone (2 mg/kg/day) plus ACTH placebo for 2 weeks. If seizure control was achieved, a 1 week taper was carried out, or if not, the patient was crossed over to the other regimen. There was no difference in the response rate between the two groups and no relation between the duration of spasms before treatment and outcome. An all-or-none treatment response was observed. No attempt was made to control for other anticonvulsant drugs or to analyze the cryptogenic group separately.

The evidence in favor of early ACTH treatment of infantile spasms comes from several prospective open trials, two of which were published by Hrachovy et al. (21,22) prior to the study described above. Lombroso (36), using a dose of ACTH standardized for body surface area (110 units/m²/day) found no short-term difference between ACTH and prednisone (2 mg/kg/day), but observed that ACTH was superior in the cryptogenic group over the long term in regard to a better developmental outcome and decreased frequency of other seizure types. In addition, children treated with ACTH within 1 month of the onset of spasms fared better than those in whom ACTH therapy was delayed, a conclusion also reached by Singer et al. (54,55) in a retrospective study. Another open trial (59,60) achieved control of spasms in 90% of patients treated with ACTH in a dose standardized for body surface area (150 units/m²/day) compared with 40% of patients treated with prednisone (2 mg/kg/day).

TABLE 1. *ACTH protocol*

I. Diagnosis
  A. Clinical history
  B. EEG
  C. EEG-videotelemetry monitoring
II. Admission to hospital
  A. Height, weight, blood pressure, estimation of body surface area.
  B. Base-line laboratory data: CBC, electrolytes, calcium, phosphorus, serum cortisol (early morning), thyroid function, renal function, fasting and 2-hour postprandial glucose, urinalysis.
  C. Diagnostic workup as indicated (usually includes CT scan).
III. Nursing and parent instruction
  A. Daily weight and urine glucose screening.
  B. Blood pressure measurement every shift.
  C. Parent education for administration of ACTH, screening urine, and keeping seizure calendar.
IV. ACTH schedule
  A. Use ACTH gel (80 units/cc) and record all lot numbers
  B. All doses are in units/m² surface area and given I.M. as follows:

Week		
1		75 b.i.d.
2		75 q.d.
3–4		75 q.o.d.
5–6		50 q.o.d.
7–8		40 q.o.d.
9–10		20 q.o.d.
11–12		10 q.o.d.

V. Follow-up
  A. Weekly visits the first month, then biweekly visits.
  B. EEG at 1, 2, and 4 weeks after starting ACTH.
  C. Blood pressure daily the first week, then three times weekly; parents check urine three times daily at home.
  D. Electrolytes, calcium, phosphorus, and urinalysis at each visit, and serum glucose if urine is positive for sugar.

TREATMENT OF INFANTILE SPASMS

These conflicting data create a real dilemma for the physician trying to decide the best course of action for a child with infantile spasms. Although clearly there is a lack of consensus for the best way to treat this disorder, the preferred approach is an aggressive one in which a high dose of ACTH is used as soon as the diagnosis is made.

There are two reasons for this action. First, in the retarded child who develops spasms, one can never be sure that the retardation and incidence of later debilitating seizures will not be made worse if the spasms are allowed to continue unabated. When this reasoning is applied to the cryptogenic group of patients, the evidence is more compelling (36). Second, the regimen described in Table 1 has yielded a very good success rate in over 200 children (59,60).

The diagnosis of infantile spasms is established by a clinical description of the seizures, an EEG, and EEG-videotelemetry for 6 to 12 hr. Once the diagnosis is made, the child is admitted to the hospital in order to begin the ACTH and to teach the parents to give the injection, measure urine glucose, and recognize spasms so they can keep an accurate seizure calendar. In addition, any diagnostic work-up indicated by clinical circumstances is performed at this time. An endocrine profile, complete blood-cell count, and urinalysis are obtained and electrolytes, base-line renal function, and serum calcium, phosphorus, and glucose levels are measured before the ACTH is started. The drug is not begun if any of these studies are abnormal.

The initial dose of ACTH is 150 units/m²/day of ACTH gel, 80 units/ml i.m., in two divided doses, for 1 week. The second week the dose is 75 units/m²/day in one daily dose. The third and fourth weeks the dose is 75 units/m² every other day. Then over the next 8 weeks the ACTH is gradually tapered, as outlined in Table 1. The lot number of the ACTH gel is carefully recorded. Usually a treatment response is seen within the first 7 days, but if no response is seen in 2 weeks, the lot is changed.

The patient is discharged on day three of therapy and arrangements are made for daily blood pressure measurement the first week, then three times weekly after that. If hypertension occurs, attempts are made to control it with salt restriction and diuretic therapy rather then stopping the ACTH. The patient is followed in the outpatient clinic weekly for the first month and then biweekly. A waking and sleeping EEG is obtained at 1, 2, and 4 weeks after the start of ACTH to determine the treatment response. It has been suggested (23,28) that the only way to determine the therapeutic response is by remonitoring the patient because the parents do not recognize the spasms. However, since the treatment response is all or none (23,29), a positive

treatment response is suggested when parents trained to recognize spasms say that there are no seizures in a child in whom the waking and sleeping EEG has normalized. A high relapse rate (50%) can occur during the tapering period, particularly in the symptomatic patients. When this occurs, the dose is increased to the previously effective dose for 2 weeks and then another taper is begun. If the seizures continue despite the dosage increase, the dose is increased to 150 units/m²/day and the regimen restarted.

Adrenocorticotropic hormone is a dangerous drug, particularly at these high doses; however, the morbidity and mortality reported by Riikonen and Donner (50) seem exceptionally high, perhaps because synthetic ACTH was used. Virtually all children will develop cushingoid features. Many will show extreme irritability early in the course, and a few will develop hypertension. However, one should be constantly alert for sepsis, glucosuria, metabolic abnormalities involving electrolytes, calcium, and phosphorus (52), and congestive heart failure. An additional reversible side effect of ACTH is cerebral ventriculomegaly (6,35). The etiology of this effect is obscure, but it emphasizes the importance of doing diagnostic computerized tomographic (CT) scans in children with infantile spasms before the initiation of ACTH.

EFFICACY IN OTHER SEIZURE TYPES

Adrenocorticotropic hormone also has been found to be useful in younger children with multiple seizure types that are severe and intractable, particularly atypical absence, myoclonic, tonic, and atonic seizures in varying combinations (7,31,33,34, 45,57,59,60,74). This also includes patients with Lennox-Gastaut syndrome, a disorder characterized by slow spike-wave, atypical absence, myoclonus, and frequent ictal falls (57,61). Again, several uncontrolled, prospective studies suggest that ACTH is superior to oral steroids against these types of seizures (33,34,59). The same regimen for ACTH described in Table 1 is used for these severe mixed seizures. It should be stressed that ACTH is a drug of last resort for these types of seizures and should be employed only after an aggressive, logical trial of the standard anticonvulsant drugs has failed. The ACTH generally offers only temporary relief, since 70% to 90% of patients with multiple seizure types will suffer a relapse of seizures during the ACTH taper.

MECHANISM OF ACTION

The anticonvulsant mechanism of action of ACTH can only be speculated upon (5,49,61). If one accepts the point of view that there is no difference in efficacy between ACTH and oral steroids, it follows that the mechanism of action of ACTH relates to some effect of cortisol on the brain, mediated perhaps by steroid receptors in the central nervous system (40). Indeed, corticosteroids have been shown to reduce the excitability of hippocampal pyramidal cells *in vitro* (68). Alternatively, cortisol could be selectively neurotoxic (53) to the excess of excitatory glutaminergic neurons that is unique to the developing brain (18).

Adrenocorticotropic hormone might work through some extra adrenal mechanism. In support of this thesis are the data suggesting superior efficacy of ACTH as well as other studies showing that ACTH is effective against infantile spasms in adrenal-suppressed patients (4,12,73). There are now substantial electrophysiologic data to support a direct effect of ACTH on the electrical activity of the brain (44,67), an activity that resides in fragments of the peptide that are devoid of corticotropic activity (65,66). However, therapeutic trials of these fragments in children with seizures have been disappointing (46,72,73).

Adrenocorticotropic hormone in brain is intimately associated with endogenous opiate peptides (2,3,69), some of which have potent epileptogenic properties (58). Theoretically, ACTH could suppress seizure activity by acting via these opiatergic systems. Alternatively, corticotropin releasing factor (CRF), another peptide which is quite epileptogenic (11), might play a role in the pathogenesis of infantile spasms. If so, ACTH could act by inhibiting CRF release. Adrenocorticotropic hormone also has the ability to increase GABAergic tone (30), a property shared by corticosteroids (38,39). Such an effect would be expected to raise the seizure threshold. The latter data may explain why the benzodiazepine nitrazepam is reported to have an efficacy equal to that of ACTH against infantile spasms (9).

Riikonen (49) has reviewed the developmental characteristics of infantile spasms and the hypothesis that these patients have a discrepancy between brain development and age. The idea is that something occurs in the eventual developmental schema of brain that leads to cessation of seizures. This would explain why infantile spasms rarely occur after 18 months of age. Adrenocorticotropic hormone might speed up the process of brain development, perhaps through its effect on protein synthesis, myelination, or dendritic development (25,43). The therapeutic effect of ACTH could be mediated through adrenal steroids other than cortisol. Glaser (17) suggested that mineralocorticoids might be important in this regard and more recently, Riikonen and Perheentupa (51) have reported that ACTH responders may be identified by high serum dehydroepiandrosterone/androstanedione ratios.

A final possibility is that there are other peptides in the ACTH gel that may play a role in the therapeutic effect observed. The commercial ACTH gel used is a porcine pituitary extract that may well contain many other peptides. Conceivably, one or more of these, such as dynorphin (14,64), could contribute to the anticonvulsant effect of the drug.

CONCLUSIONS

Adrenocorticotropic hormone is useful against infantile spasms and, to a lesser degree, other severe, intractable, mixed seizures in children. However, 30 years after the utility of ACTH in the treatment of infantile spasms was first reported, controversy still rages about the dose, duration of therapy, effectiveness relative to oral steroids, and long-term benefit of this mode of therapy. In addition, the anticonvulsant mechanism of action of ACTH remains completely unknown. One of the major reasons for the lack of knowledge about how ACTH works and the empirical way in which this drug is used in infantile spasms is that there is no known animal model for this type of seizure. Until such a model is found (56), the pathogenesis of this terrible disorder and the mechanism by which ACTH alleviates these seizures will remain a mystery.

ACKNOWLEDGMENT

This work was supported in part by grant No. F06 TWO 1277 from the Fogarty International Center.

REFERNCES

1. Aicardi, J. (1986): *Epilepsy in Children*, pp. 17–38. Raven Press, New York.
2. Akil, H., Watson, S. T., Young, G., Lewis, M. E., Khachaturian, H., and Walker, J. M. (1984): Endogenous opioids: Biology and function. *Ann. Rev. Neurosci.*, 7:223–255.
3. Axelrod, J., and Reisine, T. D. (1984): Stress hormones: Their interaction and regulation. *Science*, 224:452–459.
4. Crosley, C. J., Richman, R. A., and Thorpy, M. J. (1980): Evidence for cortisol-independent anticonvulsant activity of adrenocorticotropic hormone in infnatile spasms. *Ann. Neurol.*, 8:220.
5. Dazord, A. (1983): Mécanisme d'action de l'ACTH. *Ann. Endocrinol. (Par.)*, 44:15–28.
6. Deonna, T., and Voumard, C. (1979): Reversible cerebral atrophy and corticotrophin. *Lancet*, 2:207.
7. Dobbs, J. M., and Baird, H. W. (1960): The use of corticotropin and a corticosteroid in patients with minor motor seizures. *Amer. J. Dis. Child.*, 100:584–585.
8. Dorfman, A., Apter, N. S., Smull, K., Bergenstal, D. M., and Richter, R. B. (1951): Status epilepticus coincident with the use of pituitary adrenocorticotropic hormone; report of three cases. *J. Amer. Med. Assoc.*, 146:25–29.
9. Dreifuss, F., Farwell, J., Holmes, G., Joseph, C., Lockman, L., Madsen, J. A., Minarcik, C. J., Rothner, A. D., and Shewmon, A. (1986): Infantile spasms. Comparative trial of nitrazepam and corticotropin. *Arch. Neurol.*, 43:1107–1110.
10. Dumermuth, G. (1959): Über die Blitz-Nick-Salaam-Krämpfe und ihre Behandlung mit ACTH und Hydrocortison: Vorläufige Mitteilung. *Helv. Ped. Acta*, 14:250–270.
11. Ehlers, C. L., Henriksen, S. J., Wang, M., Rivier, J., Vale, W., and Bloom, F. E. (1983): Corticotropin releasing factor produces increases in brain excitability and convulsive seizures in rats. *Brain Res.*, 278:332–336.
12. Farwell, J., Milstein, J., Opheim, K., Smith, E., and Glass, S. (1984): Adrenocorticotropic hormone controls infantile spasms independently of cortisol stimulation. *Epilepsia*, 25:605–608.
13. Friedlander, W. J., and Rottgers, E. (1951): The effects of cortisone on the electroencephalograph. *Electroencephalogr. Clin. Neurophysiol.*, 3:311–320.
14. Garant, D. S., and Gale, K. (1985): Infusion of opiates into substantia nigra protects against maximal electroshock seizures in rats. *J. Pharmacol. Exp. Ther.*, 234:45–48.
15. Gastaut, H., Salfiel, J., Raybaud, C., Pitot, M., and Meynadier, A. A. (1959): À propos du traitement par l'ACTH des encéphalites myoclonique de la premiére enfance avec majeure—(Hypsarythmia). *Pediatrie*, 14:35–45.
16. Gibbs, F. A., and Gibbs, E. L. (1952): *Atlas of Electroencephalography, Vol. 2: Epilepsy*. Addison-Wesley, Cambridge, Massachusetts.
17. Glaser, G. H. (1953): On the relationship between adrenal cortical activity and the convulsive state. *Epilepsia*, 2:7–14.
18. Greenamyre, T., Penny, J. B., Young, A. B., Hudson, C., Silverstein, F. S., and Johnston, M. V. (1987): Evidence for transient perinatal glutaminergic innervation of globus pallidus. *J. Neurosci.*, 7:1022–1030.
19. Hoefer, P. F. A., and Glaser, G. H. (1950): Effects of pituitary adrenocorticotrophic hormone therapy: Electroencephalographic and neuropsychiatric changes in 15 patients. *J. Amer. Med. Assoc.*, 143:620–624.
20. Holmes, G. L. (1987): *Diagnosis and Management of Seizures in Children*, pp. 212–225. W.B. Saunders, Philadelphia.
21. Hrachovy, R. A., Frost, J. D., Kellaway, P., and Zion, T. E. (1979): A controlled study of prednisone therapy in infantile spasms. *Epilepsia*, 20:403–407.
22. Hrachovy, R. A., Frost, J. D., Kellaway, P., and

Zion, T. E. (1980): A controlled study of ACTH therapy in infantile spasms. *Epilepsia*, 21:631–636.

23. Hrachovy, R. A., Frost, J. D., Kellaway, P., and Zion, T. E. (1983): Double-blind study of ACTH vs. prednisone therapy in infantile spasms. *J. Pediatr.*, 103:641–645.

24. Hrachovy, R. A., Frost, J. D., and Kellaway, P. (1984): Hypsarythmia: Variations on the theme. *Epilepsia*, 25:317–325.

25. Huttenlocher, P. R. (1974): Dendritic development in neocortex of children with mental defect and infantile spasms. *Neurology*, 24:203–210.

26. Jeavons, P. M., and Bower, B. D. (1964): *Infantile Spasms: A Review of the Literature and a Study of 112 Cases.* Heineman, London.

27. Jeavons, P. M., Bower, B. D., and Dimitrakoudi, M. (1973): Long term prognosis of 150 cases of "West Syndrome." *Epilepsia*, 14:153–164.

28. Kellaway, P. R., Frost, J. D., and Hrachovy, R. A. (1983): Infantile spasms. In: *Antiepileptic Drug Therapy in Pediatrics*, edited by P. L. Morselli, C. E. Pippenger, and J. K. Penry, pp. 115–136. Raven Press, New York.

29. Kellaway, P., Hrachovy, R. A., Frost, J. D., and Zion, T. (1979): Precise characterization and quantification of infantile spasms. *Ann. Neurol.*, 6:214–218.

30. Kendall, D. A., McEwen, B. S., and Enna, S. J. (1982): The influence of ACTH and corticosterone on the [^{3}H]-GABA receptor binding in rat brain. *Brain Res.*, 236:365–374.

31. Klein, R., and Livingston, S. (1950): The effect of adrenocorticotrophic hormone in epilepsy. *J. Pediatr.*, 37:733–742.

32. Lacy, J. R., and Penry, J. K. (1976): *Infantile Spasms.* Raven Press, New York.

33. Lagenstein, I., Willig, R. P., and Iffland, E. (1978): Behandlung frühkindlicher Anfälle mit ACTH und Dexamethasone unter standardisierten Bedingungen. I. Klinische Ergebnisse. *Mschr. Kinderheilk.*, 126:492–499.

34. Lagenstein, I., Willig, R. P., and Iffland, E. (1978): Behandlung frühkindlicher Anfälle mit ACTH und Dexamethasone unter standardisierten Bedingungen. II. Elektroencephalographische Beobachtungen. *Mschr. Kinderheilk.*, 126:500–506.

35. Lagenstein, I., Willig, R. P., and Kühne, D. (1979): Cranial computed tomography (CCT) findings in children treated with ACTH and dexamethasone: First results. *Neuropädiatrie*, 10:370–384.

36. Lombroso, C. T. (1983): A prospective study of infantile spasms: Clinical and therapeutic correlations. *Epilepsia*, 24:135–158.

37. Low, N. L. (1958): Infantile spasms with mental retardation: I. Treatment with cortisone and adrenocroticotropin. *Pediatrics*, 22:1165–1169.

38. Majewska, M. D., Bisserbe, J. C., and Eskay, R. L. (1985): Glucocorticoids are modulators of GABA$_A$ receptors in brain. *Brain Res.*, 339:178–182.

39. Majewska, M. D., Harrison, T. L., Schwartz, R. D., Barker, J. E., and Paul, S. M. (1986): Steroid hormone metabolites are barbiturate-like modulators of the GABA receptor. *Science*, 232:1004–1008.

40. McEwen, B. S., DeKloet, E. R., and Rostene, W. (1986): Adrenal steroid receptors and actions in the nervous system. *Physiol. Rev.*, 66:1122–1187.

41. McQuarrie, I., Anderson, J. A., and Ziegler, M. R. (1942): Observations on the antagonistic effects of posterior pituitary and cortico-adrenal hormones in the epileptic subject. *J. Clin. Endocrinol.*, 2:406–410.

42. Millichap, J. G., and Bickford, R. G. (1962): Infantile spasms, hypsarythmia, and mental retardation. *J. Amer. Med. Assoc.*, 182:125–129.

43. Oda, M. A. S., and Huttenlocher, P. R. (1974): The effect of corticosteroids on dendritic development in the rat brain. *Yale J. Biol. Med.*, 3:155–165.

44. Olpe, H. R. and Jones, R. S. G. (1982): Excitatory effects of ACTH on noradrenergic neurons of the locus coeruleus in the rat. *Brain Res.*, 251:177–179.

45. Paul, L., O'Neal, R., Ybanez, M., and Livingston, S. (1960): Minor motor epilepsy: Treatment with corticotropin (ACTH) and steroid therapy. *J. Amer. Med. Assoc.*, 172:1408–1412.

46. Pentella, K., Bachman, D. S., and Sandman, C. A. (1982): Trial of an ACTH 4-9 analog (ORG 2766) in children with intractable seizures. *Neuropediatrics*, 13:59–62.

47. Pine, I., Engel, F. L., and Schwartz, T. B. (1951): The electroencephalogram in ACTH and cortisone treated patients. *Electroencephalogr. Clin. Neurophysiol.*, 3:301–310.

48. Pollack, M. A., Zion, T. E., and Kellaway, P. (1979): Long term prognosis of patients with infantile spasms following ACTH therapy. *Epilepsia*, 20:255–260.

49. Riikonen, R. (1983): Infantile spasms: Some new theoretical aspects. *Epilepsia*, 24:159–168.

50. Riikonen, R., and Donner, M. (1980): ACTH therapy in infantile spasms: Side effects. *Arch. Dis. Child.*, 55:664–672.

51. Riikonen, R., and Perheentupa, J. (1986): Serum steroids and success of corticotropin therapy in infantile spasms. *Acta Paediatr. Scand.*, 75:598–600.

52. Riikonen, R., Simell, O., Jääskeläinen, J., Rapola, J., and Perheentupa, J. (1986): Disturbed calcium and phosphate homeostasis during treatment with ACTH of infantile spasms. *Arch. Dis. Child.*, 61:671–676.

53. Sapolsky, R. M., Krey, L. C., and McEwen, B. S. (1984): Prolonged glucocorticoid exposure reduces hippocampal neuron number: Implications for aging. *J. Neurosci.*, 5:1222–1227.

54. Singer, W. D., Haller, J. S., Sullivan, L. R., Wolpert, S., Mills, C., and Rabe, E. (1982): The value of neuroradiology in infantile spasms. *J. Pediatr.*, 100:47–50.

55. Singer, W. D., Rabe, E. F., and Haller, J. S. (1980): The effect of ACTH therapy on infantile spasms. *J. Pediatr.*, 96:485–489.

56. Snead, O. C. (1984): Neuropeptides and infantile spasms: Search for an animal model. In: *Advances in Epileptology: XVth Epilepsy International Sym-*

posium, edited by R. J. Porter, R. H. Mattson, A. A. Ward, and J. K. Penry, pp. 193–196. Raven Press, New York.

57. Snead, O. C. (1987): Pharmacology of epileptic falling spells. *Clin. Neuropharmacol.*, 10:205–214.

58. Snead, O. C., and Bearden, L. J. (1982): The epileptogenic spectrum of opiate agonists. *Neuropharmacology*, 21:1137–1144.

59. Snead, O. C., Benton, J. W., and Myers, G. J. (1983): ACTH and prednisone in childhood seizure disorders. *Neurology*, 33:966–970.

60. Snead, O. C., Hosey, L. C., Swann, J. W., Spink, D., and Martin, D. (1986): High dose ACTH in infantile spasms and mixed seizure disorders of children: Efficacy of plasma ACTH and cortisol levels. *Ann. Neurol.*, 20:419.

61. Snead, O. C., and simonato, M. (1989): Opiate peptides and seizures. In: *Neurotransmitters and Epilepsy*, edited by R. J. Fisher and J. T. Coyle. Allan R. Liss, New York (*in press*).

62. Sorel, L., and Dusaucy-Bauloye, A. (1958): À propos de cas d'hypsarythmia de Gibbs: Son traitement spectulaire par l'ACTH. *Acta Neurol. Belg.*, 58:130–141.

63. Stamps, F. W., Gibbs, E. L., Rosenthal, I. M., and Gibbs, F. A. (1959): Treatment of hypsarythmia with ACTH. *J. Amer. Med. Assoc.*, 171:408–411.

64. Tortella, F. C., Robles, L., and Holaday, J. W. (1985): Seizure threshold studies with dynorphin (1–13) in rats: Possible interactions among κ-, μ-, and δ-opioid binding sites. *Pharmacologist*, 27:179.

65. Urban, I., and DeWeid, D. (1976): Changes in excitability of the theta generating substrate by ACTH 4-10 in the rat. *Exp. Brain Res.*, 24:325–334.

66. Urban, I., Lopes de Silva, F. H., Storm van Leeuwen, W., and DeWeid, D. (1974): A frequency shift in the hippocampal theta activity: An electrical correlate of central action of ACTH analogues in the dog? *Brain Res.* 69:361–365.

67. Van Delft, A. M. L., and Kitay, J. I. (1972): Effect of ACTH on single unit activity in the diencephalon of intact and hypophysectomized rats. *Neuroendocrinology*, 9:188–196.

68. Vidal, C., Jordan, W., and Zieglgansberger, W. (1986): Corticosterone reduces the excitability of hippocampal pyramidal cells *in vitro. Brain Res.*, 383:54–59.

69. Watson, S. J., Richard, C. W., and Barchas, J. D. (1978): Adrenocorticotrophin in rat brain: Immunocytochemical localization in cells and axons. *Science*, 200:1080–1082.

70. Wayne, H. S. (1954): Convulsive seizures complicating cortisone and ACTH therapy: Clinical and electroencephalographic observations. *J. Clin. Endocrinol. Metab.*, 14:1039–1045.

71. West, W. J. (1941): On a peculiar form of infantile convulsions. *Lancet*, 1:724–725.

72. Willig, R. P., and Lagenstein, I. (1980): Therapiever such mit einem ACTH-Fragment (ACTH 4-10) bei frühkinklichen Anfällen. *Mschr. Kinderheilk.*, 128:100–103.

73. Willig, R. P., and Lagenstein, I. (1982): Use of ACTH fragments in children with intractable seizures. *Neuropediatrics*, 13:55–58.

74. Willig, R. P., Lagenstein, I., and Iffland, E. (1977): Cortisoltagesprofile unter ACTH- und Dexamethason-Therapie frühkindlicher Anfälle (BNS- und Lennox-Syndrom). *Mschr. Kinderheilk.*, 126:191–197.

75. Willoughby, J. A., Thurston, D. L., and Holowach, J. (1966): Infantile myoclonic seizures: An evaluation of ACTH and corticosteroid therapy. *J. Pediatr.*, 69:1136–1138.

Antiepileptic Drugs, Third Edition, edited by
R. Levy, R. Mattson, B. Meldrum,
J. K. Penry, and F. E. Dreifuss.
Raven Press, Ltd., New York © 1989.

66

Potential Antiepileptic Drugs

Oxcarbazepine

Mogens Dam and Peder Klosterskov Jensen

INTRODUCTION

Oxcarbazepine (OXC) is chemically related to the antiepileptic drug carbamazepine (CBZ). It was synthesized as a follow-up compound for CBZ and has a similar therapeutic profile but improved tolerability. Oxcarbazepine is effective against electrically and chemically induced seizures in animals (e.g., electroshock test, pentylenetetrazol test). Experimentally induced seizures are considered to be the most reliable method for the detection of potential antiepileptic agents as there is a fairly good correlation between experimental anticonvulsant activity *in vivo* and therapeutic antiepileptic efficacy as far as the most important clinically used antiepileptic drugs are concerned.

In man, OXC is almost immediately and completely metabolized to 10,11-dihydro-10-hydroxyCBZ (DH-OH-CBZ). The antiepileptic effects of OXC and DH-OH-CBZ are comparable in both animals and man.

CHEMISTRY

Oxcarbazepine is 10,11-dihydro-10-oxo-CBZ (molecular weight of 252.28). With CBZ it shares the dibenzazepine nucleus bearing the 5-carboxamide substituent, but is structurally different in the 10,11-position

(Fig. 1). This molecular variation results in differences in metabolism. From its physicochemical properties OXC can be classified as a neutral lipophilic compound. The solubility of OXC in aqueous media is very low.

EXPERIMENTAL PHARMACOLOGY

The information in this section is based in part on unpublished data from tests conducted by or for Ciba-Geigy Ltd., Basle, Switzerland, where all reports are on file.

Effects on the Cardiovascular System

In anesthetized cats OXC caused a slight and transient decrease of blood pressure at the high dose of 10 mg/kg i.v. In contrast to OXC, DH-OH-CBZ produced a slight and not dose-dependent increase in blood pressure at the dose range of 0.1 to 10 mg/kg.

The blood pressure responses to adrenaline, noradrenaline, and acetylcholine were hardly affected by OXC or DH-OH-CBZ. In conscious, trained dogs OXC and DH-OH-CBZ, 100 mg/kg p.o., had no clear effect on blood pressure or heart rate. In dogs with a normal base-line–ECG no changes appeared after administration of 100 mg/kg p.o. of either compound.

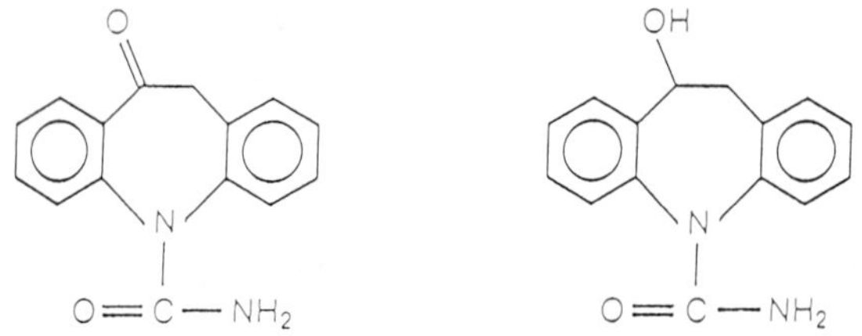

OXC
10,11-dihydro-10-oxo-
carbamazepine

DH-OH-CBZ
10,11-dihydro-10-hydroxy-
carbamazepine

FIG. 1. Structure of oxcarbazepine (10,11-dihydro-10-oxo-carbamazepine) and its metabolite 10,11-dihydro-10-hydroxy-carbamazepine.

Oxcarbazepine was without significant effects on rate and force of contraction of the isolated guinea-pig atrium, up to a concentration of 10 μg/ml. The concentration of 100 μg/ml was toxic and led to atrial standstill.

Renal Effects in the Rat

In water-loaded rats, OXC, 100 mg/kg p.o., had no effects on urine and electrolyte (sodium, potassium, and chloride) excretion or on urine osmolality during the first 2 hr following administration. Oxcarbazepine, 300 mg/kg p.o., caused a slight decrease in electrolyte excretion, a marked reduction in urine volume, and a distinct increase in urine osmolality. Subsequently (2–4 hr after administration), both doses (100 and 300 mg/kg p.o.) increased electrolyte excretion and urine osmolality without affecting urine volume.

DH-OH-CBZ, 100 and 300 mg/kg p.o., affected electrolyte excretion and urine osmolality over 4 hr similarly to equal doses of OXC after 2 to 4 hr. DH-OH-CBZ, like OXC, was transiently antidiuretic. The antidiuretic effects occurring after high doses of OXC and DH-OH-CBZ could not be reproduced in rats with hereditary diabetes insipidus. The antidiuretic activity of OXC and DH-OH-CBZ may therefore be ascribed to stimulation of vasopressin release.

Effects on the Nervous System

Observation Tests

In mice and rats, unwanted effects such as decreased motility, ataxia, and muscular hypotonia are seen at OXC doses of 100 mg/kg p.o. and above. The threshold dose for sedation is considered to be 30 mg/kg p.o. (DH-OH-CBZ, 100 mg/kg p.o.) in mice and 100 mg/kg p.o. (as DH-OH-CBZ) in rats (1). In dogs and tupaias OXC does not lead to unwanted effects in doses up to 300 and 200 mg/kg p.o., respectively. When OXC, 100 mg/kg p.o., is given to rhesus monkeys, moderate sedation, slight ataxia, decreased motility, and motor retardation are observed.

Central Damping Effects

In mice, OXC inhibits orientation motility, prolongs anesthesia, and impairs performance in the traction test and the rotorod test at doses of 100 mg/kg and higher, i.e., at doses well above the ED_{50} for protection against electroshock-induced convulsions (10–20 mg/kg p.o.). Up to 800 mg/kg p.o., the compound does not impair the behavior of rats on the nonrotating inclined cylinder.

Effect on Sleep-Waking Behavior and EEG

Oxcarbazepine, 3, 10, and 30 mg/kg p.o., has no significant effects on slow-wave and paradoxical sleep, nor on behavior and EEG, in freely moving cats.

Hypothalamic Rage Reaction

Oxcarbazepine, 100 mg/kg p.o., and DH-OH-CBZ, 30 mg/kg, produce an increase of 10% to 15% in the threshold current required to elicit a rage reaction in freely moving cats with chronically implanted electrodes in the hypothalamic area. This slight, though definite effect of the compounds may indicate a potential psychotropic effect in man, akin to, yet weaker than, that described for CBZ (1).

Fighting Reaction

Oxcarbazepine does not influence the foot-shock-induced fighting reaction, up to 100 mg/kg. It inhibits fighting in five of eight pairs of mice at the dose of 200 mg/kg p.o.

Interaction with 5-hydroxytryptophan, tetrabenazine and physostigmine

Oxcarbazepine does not potentiate the effect of 5-hydroxytryptophan in mice or antagonize catalepsy following injection of tetrabenazine, 20 mg/kg i.p., in rats nor death following 0.8 mg/kg i.v. of physostigmine (mice) at doses up to 100 to 300 mg/kg p.o.

Reflex Studies

Inhibition of the patellar and flexor reflexes in the anesthetized cat is observed only at OXC doses of 10 mg/kg i.v. and above. The less specific linguomandibular reflex is diminished by this drug in a dose-dependent manner after doses of 0.1 mg/kg i.v. and above.

Peripheral Nerves in Diabetic Rats

Oxcarbazepine, 300 mg/kg p.o., shows a tendency to increase the excitability threshold of the tail nerves in five of nine streptozotocin diabetic rats following a 15 day treatment period. Such an effect is not observed with DH-OH-CBZ, but is more pronounced with CBZ, 100 mg/kg p.o. This finding is of interest since increases in excitability threshold may underlie the effects of OXC against convulsions and trigeminal neuralgia.

Antiepileptic Properties

Electroshock and Pentylenetetrazol Tests in Mice and Rats

Oxcarbazepine and DH-OH-CBZ inhibit the hind-limb extension elicited by a supramaximal electroshock (ED_{50}, 10–20 mg/kg p.o.) in rats and mice (1). This effect lasts about 8 hr in the rat. No loss of efficacy in this test system is noted in rats treated daily with OXC for 4 weeks (13). In the pentylenetetrazol test in mice, OXC is approximately two to three times less active than in the electroshock test (ED_{50}, 23–30 mg/kg p.o.). The ED_{50} of DH-OH-CBZ is 52 mg/kg p.o. under these experimental conditions (1).

Picrotoxin and Strychnine Tests in Mice

The picrotoxin and strychnine tests in mice are based on antagonism of the inhibitory neurotransmitters GABA and glycine. In both systems, the anticonvulsive activity of OXC and DH-OH-CBZ is relatively weak, with ED_{50} values ranging from 150 to

250 mg/kg p.o. (1). When the dose of picrotoxin is increased from 7.5 to 12 mg/kg i.p., OXC is without anticonvulsant effect up to 200 mg/kg p.o.

Chronic Aluminum Foci in Rhesus Monkey

Rhesus monkeys made epileptic by implantation of aluminum gel in the motor cortical area are considered to be a model of posttraumatic and partial (Jacksonian type) epilepsies in man (2,3). In single-dose studies, OXC showed complete seizure suppression at 50 mg/kg p.o. and very marked reduction of seizure severity at 20 mg/kg i.m. DH-OH-CBZ was less effective than OXC under these experimental conditions, as seizures were not completely abolished following 50 and 100 mg/kg p.o. and were less markedly inhibited at 20 mg/kg i.m.

In multiple-dose studies, daily doses of OXC, 30 to 60 mg/kg i.m. for 7 days, abolished or markedly reduced seizures. With oral administration, it was less potent, as 100 mg/kg was needed to reduce seizure frequency by 50% to 99%. Again, DH-OH-CBZ was less effective than OXC in that it abolished seizures only at a daily dose of 150 mg/kg i.m. and lead to a mild reduction of seizure frequency at 200 mg/kg p.o. However, all data were obtained with only one to four animals per dose group.

TOXICOLOGY

The information in this section is based on unpublished data from tests conducted by or for Ciba-Geigy Ltd., Basle, Switzerland, where all reports are on file.

OXC in Animals

In acute toxicity studies in mice and rats, extremely high doses of OXC were tolerated. The oral LD_{50} was estimated to be higher than 5,000 mg/kg in both species.

In 3-month oral toxicity studies, OXC did not cause any treatment-related deaths in either rats (100–3,000 mg/kg) or dogs (60–600 mg/kg). In the rat, doses of 300 mg/kg or above were associated with increased liver weight as a consequence of a reversible hypertrophy of the centrilobular hepatocytes. In the dog, increases in liver weight were only observed at the highest dose.

In 6-month oral toxicity studies in rats, doses of approximately 100, 300, and 1,000 mg/kg caused no fatalities. Body weight and food consumption were adversely affected at the two highest doses. As in the 3-month study, reversible dose-dependent hepatic changes were observed. These findings could be explained by enzyme induction. In the male rat, these morphological changes were correlated with decreased ALP and increased serum glutamate pyruvate transaminase (SGPT) activity. Blood urea nitrogen values were increased in all treated groups. Minor kidney changes were also present in all treated groups and consisted mainly of dilated cortical tubules.

In a 12-month oral toxicity study of OXC (60, 200, 400 mg/kg) in dogs, food intake was reduced in the females at the highest dose during the first 6 months and three out of four dogs showed slight atrophy of the thymic tissue after 6 months of treatment. There was no evidence of treatment-related effects, and 200 mg/kg/day represented a "no toxic effect level" for dogs.

DH-OH-CBZ in Animals

In acute toxicity studies in mice, rats, and Chinese hamsters, very high doses of DH-OH-CBZ were tolerated (LD_{50}: rats, 4,520 mg/kg p.o.; Chinese hamsters, >6,000 mg/kg p.o.; mice, 1,240 mg/kg p.o.).

In 3-month oral toxicity studies of DH-OH-CBZ, doses of 200, 600, and 2,000 mg/

kg were administered to rats by gavage once daily for 3 months. In all groups, a highly significant dose-related increase in liver weight was seen and at the highest dose a slight but significant increase in SGPT levels. Microscopically, there was centrilobular hepatocyte hypertrophy (marked at 2,000 mg/kg) with some scattered hepatocyte necrosis in the two highest dose-groups. These changes were considered to represent enzyme induction. In the recovery period, the retarded growth rates in both sexes at 2,000 mg/kg and in females at 600 mg/kg normalized. The liver weights were increased relative to body weight only in females in both groups and in males at 2,000 mg/kg. The slight hepatocyte hypertrophy found at 600 and 2,000 mg/kg was much less pronounced.

In dogs, DH-OH-CBZ was administered in gelatine capsules once daily for 3 months at doses of 60, 200, and 600 mg/kg (the highest dose was reduced to 400 mg/kg on day 13). At 400 and 200 mg/kg, dose-related clinical symptoms included lethargy, ataxia, muscular tremor, vomiting, and salivation. At 200 and 400 mg/kg, growth rates were adversely affected in the majority of animals, and mild to marked anemia occurred in some. At autopsy in the highest dose-group, atrophic thymus was present and heart weight was reduced in three out of six dogs. No special histological changes were found. During the recovery period, no clinical symptoms occurred and body weight improved. Autopsy and histological examination showed no changes related to DH-OH-CBZ.

A 6-month toxicity study was performed in Sprague-Dawley rats to which DH-OH-CBZ was administered in doses of about 50 to 600 mg/kg. Body weight was depressed in a dose-dependent manner. There was a positive trend toward an increase in SGPT in the high-dose group compared with the control group, but SGPT returned to normal after 1 month's recovery period.

Two groups of beagles were treated with DH-OH-CBZ for 6 months and 12 months, each with doses of 30, 100, and 300 mg/kg p.o. (reduced to 200 mg/kg after 4 weeks). Treatment-related clinical signs were noted in dogs from all groups. Emesis, salivation, ataxia, depression, decreased activity, tremor, and opisthotonos were noted in the high-dose group and to a lesser extent after 100 mg/kg. With 30 mg/kg, ataxia and tremor were rarely seen. Slight to moderate anorexia and marked weight loss were noted for the animals given 300 mg/kg during the first 4 weeks. There was a slight increase in the absolute and relative liver weights of the medium and high-dose groups. After 1 month's recovery period, clinical findings were incidental. No treatment-related changes were found with respect to urine analysis, ophthalmologic and auditory examinations, ECG findings, heart rate, and gross and microscopic pathology. Daily treatment at 30 mg/kg was considered a nontoxic-effect level.

Carcinogenicity

Oxcarbazepine was administered in the diet to 60 male and 60 female rats at doses of 25, 75, and 250 mg/kg/day for 104 weeks. Gross necropsy findings were generally comparable in nature and frequency between control and treated groups. Histological liver changes included vacuolar degeneration and a dose-related hepatic centrilobular megalocytosis and cystic degeneration in treated males and females. Histopathological examination of tissues revealed no compound-related increases in the frequency of neoplasms in the animals that died or were sacrificed before the end of the study. However, the incidence of hepatocellular carcinomas was significantly increased in females of the medium and high-dose groups that completed 2 years of treatment. Hepatic neoplastic nodules (considered to be benign) also occurred with greater frequency in all treated groups.

Focal hepatocellular alteration, being consistent with so-called preneoplastic changes, occurred with increased incidence in both females and males treated with the highest dose of OXC.

In comparison to the corresponding results of an earlier study with CBZ, the results of the present study indicate that there are no fundamental differences between these two compounds as to carcinogenic potential in rats. Carcinogenicity studies in mice showed no difference in the number of hepatocellular carcinomas between the control and the treated animals. With regard to hepatic neoplastic nodules, similar findings in mice and rats were observed.

Teratogenicity

In a study in rats with doses up to 150 mg/kg p.o., OXC had no effects on the fertility and overall reproductive performance of the parents F0 and F1 generations. No malformations or anomalies were recorded for the F1 and F2 fetuses or F1 pups. Teratogenicity studies in mice and rats, even at maternally toxic doses (250 mg/kg and 300 mg/kg, respectively), showed no evidence of teratogenic potentials of OXC. In a perinatal and postnatal study of OXC, female rats received 25, 75, or 150 mg/kg p.o. from day 15 of pregnancy until weaning of the pups. Oxcarbazepine did not show any adverse effects on the growth and development of the progeny.

Mutagenicity

No mutagenic potential of OXC or DH-OH-CBZ was detected in the Ames test. In the nucleus anomaly test, no evidence of mutagenic effects was seen in somatic interphase nuclei from Chinese hamsters treated with OXC. Chromosome studies were performed on somatic cells of Chinese hamsters, on spermatogonia of mice, and

spermatocytes of mice. No evidence of a mutagenic effect was seen.

PHARMACOKINETICS

Experimental Studies

Absorption and Elimination

Single-dose radiotracer studies in the rat, dog, and baboon (4) demonstrate complete bioavailability of OXC after oral administration. In the rat, complete absorption is suggested by the extent of urinary excretion of radioactive material, which is about the same after intravenous and oral dosing (45.8% versus 47.2% of dose). Bioavailability in the dog is equal, since the areas under the plasma concentration curves of unchanged substance are virtually the same after both modes of administration. In the baboon, 97% of the oral dose of radiotracer appears in the urine, demonstrating complete absorption from the gastrointestinal tract.

Total radioactivity is completely excreted within 120 to 144 hr, the bulk appearing within 48 hr. There are species differences as to the route of elimination: in the baboon the renal route is predominant, whereas in the rat and dog renal excretion approximately equals fecal recovery. Independent studies with bile-fistula rats revealed a high extent of biliary elimination of radioactivity in this species (78.7% of an oral dose).

Protein Binding

The binding of OXC to serum proteins in the rat, rabbit, and dog, determined by equilibrium dialysis (37°C) at concentrations of 1 and 10 µg/ml, accounts for $57.7 \pm 4\%$, $63.5 \pm 1.6\%$, and $65.6 \pm 1.9\%$, respectively. The metabolite, DH-OH-CBZ, is bound to a minor extent in all three animal species studied, viz. 27% to 28% of serum concentration.

Metabolism

Differences are observed in the metabolic handling of OXC after oral administration of single doses to different animal species and to healthy volunteers (4). In urine (after β-glucuronidase treatment) only small amounts of total radioactivity are attributable to intact ^{14}C-OXC (<5%), indicating extensive biotransformation in the rat, dog, and baboon. In the baboon ^{14}C-DH-OH-CBZ covers as much as 55% of total urinary radioactivity, but in the rat and dog only 12% and 3%, respectively. The second metabolite, 10,11-dihydro-10,11-*trans*-dihydroxy-CBZ (DH-*trans*-DOH-CBZ), does not account for more than 5% of the urinary excretion in any of the animal species (4). In man OXC is largely converted to DH-OH-CBZ. In this respect only cats, baboons and rhesus monkeys are reliable metabolic models for humans (Fig. 2) (4,15).

Enzyme Induction

In rats, in contrast with the findings in man, OXC shows an inducing potency on hepatic drug-metabolizing enzymes comparable to that of CBZ when tested with 80 mg/day for four consecutive days (19).

Clinical Studies

Absorption and Distribution

Oxcarbazepine is almost completely absorbed, as 96% of a single dose of 400 mg ^{14}C-OXC in two healthy volunteers was excreted in the urine within 10 days, 85% within 48 hr (4).

Oxcarbazepine and its main metabolite, DH-OH-CBZ, are both lipophilic compounds and therefore able to pass rapidly through biological membranes. The distribution volume of DH-OH-CBZ, as estimated by renal clearance values and renal elimination rates, is 0.3 liter/kg (4,5,16).

About 50% of DH-OH-CBZ is bound to

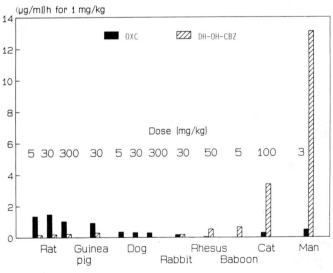

FIG. 2. Areas under the plasma concentration curves (AUC), calculated to the dose unit of 1 mg/kg, following single oral administration of oxcarbazepine to different animal species and to healthy volunteers.

plasma proteins, Kristensen et al. (8) found the free fraction to be 53.1 ± 14.4 (SD) % in their investigation of DH-OH-CBZ in serum and saliva.

Metabolism

Oxcarbazepine is a pro-drug for the active metabolite, DH-OH-CBZ. After a single dose of 400 mg ^{14}C-OXC to healthy volunteers, peak plasma concentration of OXC was about 0.4 µg/ml during the first 4 hr, compared with a plasma peak concentration of DH-OH-CBZ of about 5 µg/ml and that of DH-*trans*-DOH-CBZ of about 0.3 µg/ml (4). The dose-dependence of the plasma kinetics of OXC was thus studied on the basis of the plasma concentrations of DH-OH-CBZ in six volunteers treated with single oral doses in a three-period change-over design. The AUC (0–72 hr) of OXC amounted to only 1% to 2% of the AUC for DH-OH-CBZ. The plasma concentration of the other metabolite, DH-*trans*-DOH-CBZ, could only be determined in a few samples. It was therefore not possible to calculate AUC for this substance.

The elimination half-life of DH-OH-CBZ in healthy volunteers is 8 to 10 hr and the elimination is mono-exponential. Both OXC and the other metabolite, DH-*trans*-DOH-CBZ, accounted for less than 1% of the plasma concentration of DH-OH-CBZ. Repeated oral doses of OXC or DH-OH-CBZ (200 mg t.i.d. in nine volunteers) gave nearly identical trough plasma levels of DH-OH-CBZ, independent of which drug was given (5). The concentration of OXC and the other metabolite, DH-*trans*-DOH-CBZ, were both negligible. There were no indications of autoinduction or accumulation, as no changes in plasma levels of DH-OH-CBZ were observed during the 10 days.

Steady-state plasma concentration of OXC was studied in 23 patients with epilepsy (11 females, aged 10–55 years) who had their CBZ replaced by a 30% to 50% higher dose of OXC. The individual doses ranged from 600 to 1,600 mg/day (mean: 1,130 mg/day). Blood samples drawn 2 weeks after reaching the individual therapeutic level of OXC showed the amount of OXC to be very low, as in the volunteers. The mean plasma DH-OH-CBZ level was 9.3 µg/ml. DH-*trans*-DOH-CBZ levels were higher than in the volunteers, which may be due to induction of the biotransformation of DH-OH-CBZ to DH-*trans*-DOH-CBZ during long-term treatment (11).

These findings were confirmed in another study of steady-state concentrations in 10 patients (two females), who were treated with 800 to 1,600 mg OXC a day. The plasma OXC levels were low (0–2.1 µg/ml) compared with the levels of DH-OH-CBZ (2.1-9-9 µg/ml). The concentration of DH-*trans*-DOH-CBZ was also higher than expected from data in volunteers (0.9–3.0 µg/ml).

The 10-hour daytime profile of DH-OH-CBZ was studied in nine patients treated with OXC administered t.i.d. and b.i.d. C_{max}, C_{min}, and AUC were all reduced during the b.i.d. period, but only C_{min} showed a statistically significant reduction (9.7%). The mean fluctuation index was increased by 24%, which was statistically significant.

A first indication of clinically important interactions with OXC was observed in a clinical trial comparing OXC with CBZ. After 12 weeks the treatment was changed to CBZ or OXC, respectively, for another 2 weeks. All patients were already being treated with at least one other antiepileptic drug. Statistically significant increases in the steady-state plasma levels of valproate (27%) were observed in all patients receiving only valproate during OXC treatment. In 17 out of 19 patients treated concomitantly with valproate and phenytoin, co-medication plasma levels increased by 21% and 25%, respectively, during OXC treatment. Recent studies seem to confirm that substituting OXC for CBZ results in decreased enzyme induction, causing an increase in serum levels of concomitant antiepileptic drugs (9,14).

This indication of a reduced induction potential of OXC was confirmed in another study using antipyrine as a test compound for the induction properties. Eight patients treated with CBZ in monotherapy in a b.i.d. regimen for at least 6 months received a single dose of antipyrine (600 mg). Plasma antipyrine levels were measured during 24 hr. Carbamazepine was gradually replaced by OXC and the treatment was stabilized in a b.i.d. regimen for 6 to 8 weeks. After a similar dose of antipyrine the level was measured. The mean elimination half-life of antipyrine increased during treatment with OXC to 10.8 ± 5.1 hr, compared with 7.5 ± 2.0 hr during CBZ treatment. These findings are a strong indication of decreased enzyme induction during OXC treatment, compared with CBZ treatment.

Elimination

About 96% of ^{14}C-OXC is excreted in the urine within 10 days (4). About 71% of the total urinary radioactivity is attributed to DH-OH-CBZ, about 50% being present as the free compound and the rest as glucuronide conjugate. Only 0.6% is due to unchanged OXC and about 9% to its direct glucuronide. The other metabolite, DH-*trans*-DOH-CBZ, covered about 3% of the total urinary radioactivity (15).

This indicates that in addition to the main route of biotransformation of OXC, i.e., reduction to the hydroxy-metabolite, a minor pathway is a direct glucuronidation of OXC and to an even lesser extent the formation of a sulfate conjugate (about 4%).

CLINICAL EFFICACY

A total of 791 patients have been included in the clinical trial program. Of these, 581 patients were exposed to either OXC or its primary metabolite, DH-OH-CBZ; 326 patients were treated in monotherapy. The duration of treatment varied from 8 to 52 weeks; 143 patients were treated for more than 1 year.

Therapeutic Efficacy

In a Scandinavian double-blind, multicenter study in which 235 patients with newly diagnosed epilepsy were randomly allocated to treatment with either OXC or CBZ (17), 165 patients (82 on CBZ, 83 on OXC) were evaluated in the analysis of efficacy. There was no difference in the number of seizures between the two treatment groups (mean, 0.4 ± 3.0 for OXC and 0.3 ± 1.4 for CBZ). More than 80% of the patients experienced at least a 50% reduction in seizure frequency in both treatment groups. A global evaluation of efficacy was made by the physician at the end of the treatment. The efficacy was judged as either excellent or good in 96% of the patients receiving OXC and in 97% of those treated with CBZ. No differences in EEG recordings could be detected between the treatment groups.

Another double-blind, between-patient study compared the efficacy of CBZ and OXC in 118 patients who were not well controlled with previous antiepileptic drugs or who had tolerability problems (18). No difference in the mean number of seizures was observed between the two treatment groups (mean $\pm$ SD, 1.0 ± 2.1 for OXC and 1.0 ± 2.5 for CBZ). A comparison between the mean number of seizures per month before treatment with OXC or CBZ showed a reduction in both treatment groups (mean $\pm$ SD, 4.4 ± 10.4 versus 1.0 ± 2.1 for OXC and 3.3 ± 4.9 versus 1.0 ± 2.5 for CBZ).

In a double-blind, crossover study comparing OXC and CBZ in 48 patients not well controlled on a minimum of two and a maximum of four antiepileptic drugs, an overall decrease in seizure frequency (9%) was seen during the OXC period compared with the CBZ period; a significant decrease of tonic-clonic (20%) and tonic (31%) seizures was observed (6). Similar results were found by Reinikainen et al. (12) in a double-blind study of 40 ambulatory epileptic patients.

The therapeutic effect of OXC and DH-OH-CBZ was compared in a double-blind, between-patient study in patients treated with CBZ in monotherapy but either not well controlled or with tolerability problems; 59 patients (43 males) were available for the efficacy analysis.* No difference in the number of seizures was observed between the two treatment groups. This result indicates no difference between the efficacy of OXC and its primary metabolite, DH-OH-CBZ, which is in line with the pharmacokinetic experience that the active compound is in fact DH-OH-CBZ, whether the patient is treated with OXC or DH-OH-CBZ itself.

Overall, OXC has been shown to be as effective as CBZ for the treatment of generalized tonic-clonic seizures and partial seizures, with and without secondary generalization, in both monotherapy and polytherapy. The equivalent dose is about 50% higher than that of CBZ. A simplification of the dose regimen (from three times a day to twice a day) may be possible in some patients.

Tolerability

The tolerability of OXC was studied by evaluating its effect on a number of laboratory tests (white blood count, platelet count, red blood count, liver function tests, and urine analysis), as well as pulse rate, blood pressure, and adverse effects.

In the Scandinavian multicenter trial in patients with newly diagnosed epilepsy (17), a total of 190 patients (98 treated with CBZ and 92 treated with OXC) were included in the analysis of tolerability. The number of patients with side effects (74%

* Internal report, CIBA–GEIGY.

versus 68%) and the mean number of side effects per patient (3.5 versus 2.8) tended to be lower during treatment with OXC. Any side effect classified as severe led to immediate discontinuation of the treatment. Thirty-eight patients experienced severe side effects, 25 on CBZ and 13 on OXC; the difference was statistically significant in favor of OXC ($p = 0.04$). The major reason for stopping the treatment was allergic reaction in both treatment groups. In the Scandinavian multicenter trial in patients who were not well controlled on previous medication or with tolerability problems (18), no difference was observed in either the number of patients with side effects or the severity of the side effects.

The side effects of OXC were compared with those of its metabolite, DH-OH-CBZ, in a double-blind, between-patient study in patients already treated with CBZ in monotherapy, but either not well controlled or with tolerability problems.* No difference was observed in the number of patients with side effects during treatment with OXC or DH-OH-CBZ.

The nature of the adverse reactions is very similar in the different studies. The most commonly reported side effects are tiredness, headache, dizziness, and ataxia. The laboratory tests show some fluctuation of white blood count and liver function tests, independently of the treatment. Only two patients were withdrawn from the studies, both on CBZ. One had leukopenia and the other a sudden increase in the liver parameters. In both these patients the abnormal values returned to normal after discontinuation of the treatment. Electrolytes were not included in the regular test battery in most trials.

In 1987 Johannessen and Nielsen (7) reported a case of hyponatremia with water intoxication due to OXC. They suggested a direct or indirect effect on the kidneys, as the arginine-vasopressin values were found to be low. Houtkooper et al. (6) reported a significant decrease in serum sodium during treatment with OXC (mean ± SD, 135 ± 6 mmol/liter versus 138 ± 6 mmol). In a cross-sectional study, 21 of 41 patients on OXC were hyponatremic (serum sodium levels <135 mmol/liter). Patients treated with doses higher than 30 mg/kg/day had a significantly higher risk of becoming hyponatremic (10).

Oxcarbazepine was gradually substituted for CBZ in 55 children with an average age of 12.5 years (3–20 years), while concomitant antiepileptic treatment was kept constant. Before the start of the trial all patients had been treated with at least two antiepileptic drugs, including CBZ. Forty-two patients were available for the analysis of tolerability. Severe side effects were recorded in one patient who had nausea and vomiting after 6 weeks' treatment with 1,200 mg OXC a day, and 36% of the patients experienced side effects during the trial. Two children experienced aggressiveness, and two had fever of unknown origin. Some minor changes and fluctuations in white blood count, platelets, red blood count, and liver function tests were seen. However, all the changes in laboratory test values were reversible and did not result in any discontinuation of the treatment.

SUMMARY

Oxcarbazepine is well absorbed after oral administration. In humans it is rapidly and largely metabolized to DH-OH-CBZ, to which its antiepileptic effect is closely related. The efficacy of OXC, in a 50% higher dose, is comparable to that of CBZ. It is at least as well tolerated as CBZ. Allergic skin reactions seem to be less frequent during treatment with OXC than with CBZ. Severe side effects of OXC are significantly less frequent than those of CBZ. No clinically relevant changes in laboratory test values have been observed except for hyponatremia, which needs further investigation to establish its clinical role. Oxcarbazepine

has been shown to be a weaker inducer of the liver enzymes than CBZ, which may be important for the development of chronic side effects such as vitamin D deficiency and for the metabolism of hormones (i.e., during treatment with oral contraceptives). In addition, the lower enzyme induction will improve the treatment of patients on polytherapy.

Oxcarbazepine thus seems to be a valuable alternative to CBZ in patients suffering from generalized tonic-clonic convulsions and partial seizures with or without secondary generalization.

ACKNOWLEDGMENTS

The authors wish to thank Dr. J. W. Faigle, Dr. H. Fritz, Dr. J. Kraetz, and Dr. M. Schmutz for contributing to the sections Pharmacokinetics, Toxicology, and Animal Pharmacology.

CONVERSION

Conversion factor:

$$CF = \frac{1000}{mol.\ wt.} = \frac{1000}{252.3} = 3.96$$

Conversion:

$$(\mu g/ml) \times 3.96 = (\mu moles/liter)$$

$$(\mu moles/liter) \div 3.96 = (\mu g/ml)$$

REFERENCES

1. Baltzer, V., and Schmutz, M. (1978): Experimental anticonvulsive properties of GP 47 680 and of GP 47 779, its main human metabolite; Compounds related to carbamazepine. In: *Advances in Epileptology, 1977*, edited by H. Meinardi and A. J. Rowan, pp. 295–299. Swets and Zeitlinger, Amsterdam/Lisse.
2. David, J., and Grewal, R. S. (1976): Effect of carbamazepine (Tegretol) on seizure and EEG-patterns in monkeys with aluminia-induced local motor and hippocampal foci. *Epilepsia*, 17:415–422.
3. David, J., and Grewal, R. S. (1977): Time course

and development of electro-clinical features in relation to pentylenetetrazol thresholds in monkeys with focal seizures. *Life Sci.*, 21:1109–1116.

4. Feldmann, K. F., Brechbühler, S., Faigle, J. W., and Imhof, P. (1978): Pharmacokinetics and metabolism of GP 47 680, a compound related to carbamazepine in animals and man. In: *Advances in Epileptology, 1977*, edited by H. Meinardi and A. J. Rowan, pp. 290–294. Swets and Zeitlinger, Amsterdam/Lisse.

5. Feldmann, K. F., Dörhöfer, G., Faigle, J. W., and Imhof, P. (1981): Pharmacokinetics and metabolism of GP 47 779, the main human metabolite of oxcarbazepine (GP 47 680) in animals and healthy volunteers. In: *Advances in Epileptology: XIIth Epilepsy International Symposium*, edited by M. Dam, L. Gram, and J. K. Penry. Raven Press, New York.

6. Houtkooper, M. A., Lammertsma, A., Meyer, J. W. A., Goedhart, D. M., Meinardi, H., von Oopchat, C. A. E. H., Blom, G. F., Höppener, R. J. E. A., and Hulsman, J. A. R. J. (1987): Oxcarbazepine (GP 47 680): A possible alternative to carbamazepine? *Epilepsia*, 28:693–698.

7. Johannessen, A. C., and Nielsen, O. A. (1987): Hyponatremia induced by oxcarbazepine. *Epil. Res.*, 1:155–156.

8. Kristensen, O., Klitgaard, N. A., Jönsson, B., and Sindrup, S. (1983): Pharmacokinetics of 10-OH-carbamazepine, the main metabolite of the antiepileptic oxcarbazepine, from serum and saliva concentrations. *Acta Neurol. Scan.*, 68:145–150.

9. Kuyk, J., Schelvis, A. J., Jougeneel, R. S., Scheeper, N., and Alpherts, W. C. J. (1985): CBZ versus oxcarbazepine (GP 47 680): Influence of some psychological functions and behaviour variables. Poster presented at the 16th Epilepsy International Congress, Hamburg.

10. Nielsen, O. A., Johannessen, A. C., and Bardum, B. (1988): Oxcarbazepine induced hyponatremia, a cross-sectional study. *Epil. Res.* (*in press*).

11. Rai, P. V., Egli, M., and Wad, N. (1979): Serum levels studies of oxcarbazepine and its metabolites in clinically effective dosage. 11th Epilepsy International Symposium, Florence.

12. Reinikainen, K. J., Keränen, T., Halonen, T., Komulainen, H., and Riekkinen, P. J. (1987): Comparison of oxcarbazepine and carbamazepine: A double-blind study. *Epil. Res.*, 1:284–289.

13. Schmutz, M., David, J., Grewal, R. S., Bernasconi, R., and Baltzer, V. (1986): Pharmacological and neurochemical aspects of tolerance. In: *Tolerance to Beneficial and Adverse Effects of Antiepileptic Drugs*, edited by H. Frey et al., pp. 25–34. Raven Press, New York.

14. Schobben, F., and Willemse, J. (1985): Substitution of carbamazepine by oxcarbazepine in epileptic children. Poster presented at the 16th Epilepsy International Congress, Hamburg.

15. Schütz, H., Feldmann, K. F., and Faigle, J. W. (1986): The metabolism of ^{14}C-oxcarbazepine in man. *Xenobiotica*, 16:769–778.

16. Theisohn, M., and Heinmann, G. (1982): Disposition of the antiepileptic oxcarbazepine and its metabolites in healthy volunteers. *Eur. J. Clin. Parmacol.*, 22:545–551.

17. The Scandinavian Oxcarbazepine Study Group (Running committee: Dam, M., Ekberg, R., Löyning, Y., Waltimo, O., and Jacobsen, K.) (1988): A double-blind study comparing oxcarbazepine and carbamazepine in patients with newly diagnosed, previously untreated epilepsy. *Epil. Res.*, (*in press*).

18. The Scandinavian Oxcarbazepine Study Group (Running committee: Dam, M., Ekberg, R., Löyning, Y., Waltimo, O., and Jacobsen, K.) (1988): Oxcarbazepine versus carbamazepine in previously unsatisfactorily treated epilepsy. *Acta Neurol. Scan.*, (*in press*).

19. Wagner, J., and Schmid, K. (1987): Induction of microsomal enzymes in rat liver by oxcarbazepine, 10,11-dihydro-10-hydroxy-carbamazepine and carbamazepine. *Xenobiotica*, 17:951–956.

Antiepileptic Drugs, Third Edition, edited by
R. Levy, R. Mattson, B. Meldrum,
J. K. Penry, and F. E. Dreifuss.
Raven Press, Ltd., New York © 1989.

67

Potential Antiepileptic Drugs

Gabapentin

B. Schmidt

INTRODUCTION

Gabapentin is a new amino acid molecule, 1-(aminomethyl) cyclohexane-acetic
acid, synthesized by Gödecke/Parke-Davis
Laboratories in Freiburg, Germany. It is
structurally unrelated to any anticonvulsant
in current therapeutic use. It was designed
to mimic the steric conformation of the inhibitory neurotransmitter GABA and, in
contrast to GABA, to penetrate the blood-
brain barrier.

Gabapentin has shown antiepileptic activity in man in a series of controlled and
open-label studies of its efficacy in partial
and generalized seizures. The mechanism
of action has not yet been clarified. The initial hypothesis of a direct GABAmimetic
action can be excluded. Gabapentin is active not only in seizures evoked by an impairment of inhibition but also in a wide variety of other models of epilepsy.

Clinical and laboratory investigations are
currently in progress worldwide to establish
the role of gabapentin in the treatment of
epilepsy.

CHEMISTRY

Gabapentin, an amino acid, was tailored
as a structural analog to the inhibitory
amino-acid neurotransmitter γ-aminobu-

tyric acid (GABA) (13). Unlike GABA, it
penetrates the blood-brain barrier due to its
physicochemical properties. At the isoelec-
tric point (IEP = 7.14), gabapentin exists
as a zwitterion together with the un-ionized
form. Near this pH, its partition coefficient
(log P between *n*-octanol and aqueous pH
7.4 buffer) is −1.10. Its aqueous solubility
at pH 7.4 exceeds 10%.

Gabapentin has a molecular weight of
171.24, forms colorless crystals, has a melting point of 165° to 167°C, and pK_{a1} of 3.68
and pK_{a2} of 10.70 at 25°C (4).

As confirmed by X-ray structure analysis, the pseudo ring conformation of the
GABA molecule is integrated into a lipophilic cyclohexane system (Fig. 1).

Gabapentin can be determined down to
the submicrogram and nanogram range in
plasma and urine by means of high-performance liquid chromatography. The method
is based on the detection of amino acids by
pre-column derivatization with 2,4,6-trini-
trobenzenesulfonic acid utilizing ultraviolet
photometric detection (9).

ANIMAL PHARMACOLOGY AND
MECHANISM OF ACTION

Animal Models

Validated standard animal models of seizures, including rodents and monkeys, have

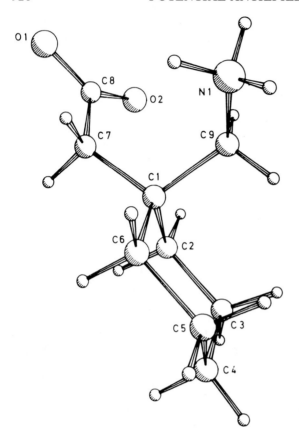

FIG. 1. Conformation of gabapentin in the unit cell. The completely folded conformation comprising C(7)–C(1)–C(9) brings the carboxyl and ammonium groups close together (bond distances to N(1): O(1)4.28, C(8)3.57, O(2)3.90). (From Bartoszyk et al., ref. 4, with permission.)

been used to screen the anticonvulsant activity of gabapentin. Tables 1 and 2 summarize activity in chemically, genetically, and electrically induced seizures. Details of experimental conditions are given in (4).

Gabapentin was further investigated in animal seizures provoked by excitatory amino acids and electrical kindling of the ventral hippocampus.

Gabapentin, given 90 min pretest in doses of 30 to 240 mg/kg (3), had no effect on seizures provoked by kainic acid (0.5 mmol/kg i.p.), but prolonged the latency to onset of clonic convulsions and tonic extension following *N*-methyl-D-aspartic acid 1 mmol/kg i.p.

In the hippocampal kindling rat model, gabapentin had no effect on the threshold for after-discharge 30 to 120 min following administration of doses up to 316 mg/kg i.p. (4).

Electrophysiological Studies

Paired-pulse orthodromic stimulation of rat hippocampal pyramidal cells has been used for the evaluation of GABAergic mechanisms. Gabapentin decreased GABAergic inhibition at doses of 3 mg/kg i.p. and above. These doses are lower than those exhibiting anticonvulsant effects in the animal models described above. A decrease of the recurrent inhibition was also observed at anticonvulsant doses of phenytoin. It is concluded that gabapentin and

TABLE 1. *Gabapentin activity in chemical convulsion models*

Convulsant	ED$_{50}$ values (mg/kg) p.o.	
	Gabapentin	Sodium Valproate
Bicuculline	32	—[a]
Picrotoxin	57	131
3-Mercaptopropionic acid	31	71
Isonicotinic acid	20	325
Semicarbazide	5	76
Strychnine	34	251
Pentylenetetrazol	52	155
Pentylenetetrazol, subcutaneous	147	83

Oral ED$_{50}$ values for protection from seizures for gabapentin given 60 to 120 min before seizure provocation or sodium valproate given 30 min before the test.

[a] Not tested.

phenytoin affect GABAergic inhibition in the rat hippocampus in a manner opposite to that of diazepam and pentobarbital (7).

Haas and Wieser (8) tested gabapentin in several paradigms on hippocampal slices of the rat in order to clarify its mechanism of action. No specific interaction with inhibition due to chloride or potassium channel activation could be observed. These results exclude a direct interaction with GABA-A or GABA-B receptors and a short-term potentiating effect on GABA actions, making

inhibition of GABA uptake or a change in postsynaptic sensitivity to GABA unlikely.

Biochemical Investigations

In order to test the hypothesis of a direct GABAmimetic action of gabapentin, a series of ligand-binding and GABA-turnover experiments was carried out using mostly valproate or tritiated ligands, respectively, as positive controls (4). The conclusion to be drawn from the results displayed in Table 3 is that, although gabapentin is a structural GABA analog, it shows no direct GABA-mimetic action.

Prominent effects on monoamine neurotransmitter release were observed with concentrations of gabapentin which are even lower than those measured in the brain after moderate *in vivo* doses (11,14). Gabapentin significantly reduced the stimulation-evoked neurotransmitter release from slices preincubated with monoamines (Fig. 2).

The release of acetylcholine was not altered by gabapentin, thus indicating a lack of generalized neuronal depression. The effects of gabapentin were not antagonized by the GABA$_A$ receptor antagonist bicuculline. Interaction experiments with gabapentin and GABA$_B$ agonists showed that the

TABLE 2. *Gabapentin activity in reflex-induced seizure models and maximal electroshock*

Model	Stimulus	Reaction	Protection by gabapentin
Audiogenic seizures: DBA/2 J mice	10.9 KHz/30 sec	clonic convulsions	ED$_{50}$ 16 mg/kg p.o. (60 min pretest)
		tonic extensions	ED$_{50}$ 3 mg/kg p.o. (60 min pretest)
Reflex epilepsy: Mongolian gerbil	Spontaneous on automatic shaker	tonic-clonic convulsions myoclonic	Min. effective dose 10 mg/kg p.o. (30 min pretest)
Photosensitive seizures: baboon (Meldrum 1984, *unpublished*)	Photically induced	myoclonic response	No effect up to 240 mg/kg i.v.
Maximal electroshock seizures: rat and mouse	Electrically induced	tonic-clonic convulsions	ED$_{50}$ 9.4 mg/kg p.o. (120 min pretest) (rat) No effect up to 2,000 mg/kg (mouse)

TABLE 3. *Biochemical pharmacology related to GABA*

Investigation of	Test system	Gabapentin effect
GABA$_A$-binding	^{3}H-muscimol	no effect
GABA$_B$-binding	^{3}H-baclofen	no effect
Glycine-binding	^{3}H-strychnine	no effect
Dopamine-binding	^{3}H-spiroperidol	no effect
GABA-transaminase activity	Gabaculine control IC$_{50}$ 95 mmol/l	weak inhibition 6 mmol/l
Neuronal GABA uptake	rabbit caudate nucleus synaptosomes	no effect up to 1 mmol/l
Total GABA content	mouse nerve terminals Valproate control	no effect

effects of gabapentin were additive to the effects of the GABA$_B$ agonists by a different, as yet unidentified mode of action (4).

General Pharmacology

Gabapentin does not exhibit influence on the cardiovascular system at therapeutic doses. Even at the highest doses tested in anesthetized dogs (128 mg/kg i.v.), only a slight deterioration of ECG, heart rate, arterial blood pressure, cardiac contractility, right ventricular and end-diastolic pressures, and femoral flow were measured.

Sedation occurred in mice after gabapentin, 400 mg/kg p.o., with a 40% to 48% decrease in spontaneous motility. Hexobarbital-induced sleep in mice was prolonged. Besides a nondose-dependent, unspecific inhibition of nictitating membrane contraction in the cat, no other alpha-blocking properties of gabapentin have been observed. Catalepsy induced by haloperidol

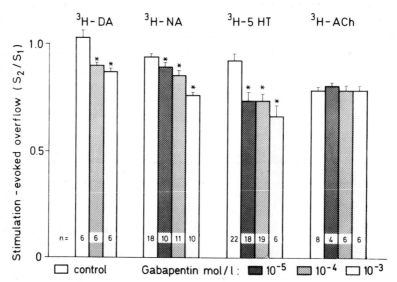

FIG. 2. Effect of gabapentin on the stimulation-evoked tritium overflow from rabbit caudate nucleus slices preincubated with ^{3}H-dopamine (^{3}H-DA) or ^{3}H-choline (^{3}H-ACh) or from rat cerebral cortex slices preincubated with ^{3}H-noradrenaline (^{3}H-NA) or ^{3}H-serotonin (^{3}H-5HT). After preincubation, slices were superfused and stimulated electrically for two periods (S$_1$, S$_2$). Gabapentin was added before S$_2$. Values represent means $\pm$ SEM of the numbers of experiments indicated in the columns. Significant differences from corresponding controls, $p < 0.05$.

was dose-dependently potentiated by gabapentin. Gabapentin showed neither antiaggressive nor analgesic effects.

In animal models, gabapentin exhibits strong antispastic potency. Etonitazene-induced muscle rigidity was antagonized in rats starting from 30 mg/kg p.o. The dose-dependent reduction of rigidity indicates a supraspinal site of action (4). No interference with transmission on neuromuscular endplate in cats has been seen up to 16 mg/kg i.v.

TOXICOLOGY

The acute toxicology of gabapentin was evaluated in mice and rats, both sexes, and adults and 3-week-old animals. Even at the highest doses tested, 8,000 mg/kg p.o., 4,000 mg/kg s.c., and 2,000 mg/kg i.v., no deaths occurred within the 2-week observation period. Weight gain was normal in the treated and control groups. Autopsies performed at the end of the observation period showed no substance-related damage to internal organs. The intoxication pattern showed ataxia and labored breathing in some animals in the highest dose groups.

In 6-month, long-term dosing in rats, a slight impairment of hepatic function, with recovery at 3 weeks postdosing and with no histomorphological changes of the liver, has been noted after gabapentin, 1,500 mg/kg daily. In beagle dogs, in whom gabapentin is metabolized to a greater extent than in rats, initial sedation and repeated vomiting occurred in some animals in the highest dose group (2,000 mg/kg daily for 6 months).

Alkaline phosphatase and glutamate transaminase were slightly elevated and occasionally albumin and the albumin-to-globulin ratio were slightly lowered. Liver weight was elevated, and in two cases hepatocellular hydropic enlargement was noted histologically. These phenomena were reversible within weeks after dosing.

No mutagenic activity was observed in the standard Ames-Salmonella-Test and Chinese hamster chromosome-metaphase as well as bone marrow micronuclei systems. A daily dose of up to 1,500 mg/kg of gabapentin given to pregnant rats and rabbits during organogenesis did not result in malformations of fetuses.

The generally very low toxicity in acute and chronic animal experiments is confirmed by the safety profile seen in volunteers and patients.

Phase I human safety data obtained from 14 healthy volunteers and more than 70 spastic patients out of placebo-controlled monotherapy studies, indicated no dose-related adverse reactions, or clinical or laboratory abnormalities associated with gabapentin treatment in daily doses up to 3,600 mg/day. Fatigue, dizziness, and disturbances of accommodation were reported in the treatment and placebo groups. Single nondose-related instances of nystagmus, arterial hypotension, diarrhea, muscle weakness, dry mouth, and sleep disturbance have been reported (4).

PHARMACOKINETICS

Absorption, metabolism, and excretion of gabapentin was investigated in rats, dogs, and healthy volunteers following oral administration of ^{14}C-labeled substance. In all three species, maximum blood levels were attained within 2 to 4 hr. The elimination half-life of gabapentin ranged from 2 to 3 hr in rats, 3 to 4 hr in dogs, and 5 to 7 hr in man.

Following intravenous administration to rats, similar blood and brain concentrations of gabapentin were observed after a short distribution phase (Table 4).

More than 93% of the radioactivity administered to rats was eliminated renally as unchanged substance after 32 hr. In dogs, 35% of total urinary radioactivity was excreted as *N*-methyl-gabapentin. In man, no metabolite was observed either in plasma

TABLE 4. *Gabapentin concentrations in various tissues following intravenous administration of 25 mg/kg ^{14}C-gabapentin-HCl to rats*

Tissue	Concentration (μg/g fresh tissue) (means + SD, N = 5)			
	15 min	1 hr	2 hr	4 hr
Cerebrum	8.55 ± 0.96	11.78 ± 2.21	4.99 ± 0.88	2.06 ± 0.53
Cerebellum	11.02 ± 2.24	11.92 ± 0.80	5.18 ± 0.78	1.92 ± 0.49
Medulla oblongata	8.79 ± 1.04	10.53 ± 0.67	4.86 ± 0.90	1.84[a] ± 0.75
Blood	21.16 ± 1.75	13.22 ± 0.61	6.64 ± 0.98	2.25 ± 0.48
Adipose tissue	6.88 ± 3.68	4.11 ± 1.81	1.67[a] ± 0.12	0.68[a] ± 0.18
Pancreas	185.88 ± 25.71	91.37 ± 11.58	48.19 ± 13.08	14.74 ± 4.86
Liver	25.31 ± 2.55	14.96 ± 1.28	8.01 ± 1.15	2.93 ± 0.45
Kidneys[b]	81.36 ± 42.24	56.97 ± 4.83	25.54 ± 8.68	10.76 ± 1.76

[a] N = 4.
[b] Values vary with varying amounts of urine in the kidneys.
In rats renal ^{14}C-recovery was 99.8%.
From Vollmer et al., ref. 17, with permission.

or in urine. No binding of gabapentin to human plasma proteins or human serum albumin occurred over a concentration range from 10^{-8} to 10^{-3} mol/liter (18).

The pharmacokinetic parameters following i.v., oral solution, and a capsule formulation used in clinical trials have been investigated in 12 healthy male volunteers in a randomized three-way crossover study using 150 mg i.v., 300 mg oral solution, and a 300 mg capsule.

The plasma concentration data following i.v. administration can best be described by a three-compartment model. The contribution of the terminal elimination phase is 80% to 90% of the total plasma AUC which amounts to 21.0 ± 2.4 μg hr/ml. Mean half-life of the γ-phase is 5.3 ± 0.7 hr (N = 12). Half-life values for the α- and β-phases are 0.1 hr and 0.6 hr, respectively.

The β-phase may be of significance for the penetration of the blood-brain barrier. This is deduced from rat organ distribution experiments in which maximum brain levels are expected approximately 1 hr following i.v. administration. The mean transit time was approximately 7 hr. The volume of distribution at steady state was calculated to be approximately 50 liters. Gabapentin is found to be completely eliminated un-

changed in the urine, thus renal clearance equals total clearance amounting to 120 to 130 ml/min.

Table 5 and Fig. 3 give the mean values for pharmacokinetic parameters following p.o. administration of 300 mg gabapentin in solution and in a soft gelatine capsule (N = 12). The capsule formulation and the solution are equivalent in bioavailability, the AUC being 60% of the respective intravenous AUC (15).

Within the range of 25 to 300 mg single doses, there is a linear correlation between 2 hr plasma levels of gabapentin and the dose administered to patients on gabapentin monotherapy (18).

TABLE 5. *Pharmacokinetic parameters following p.o. administration of 300 mg gabapentin in solution or capsule*

	Solution		Capsule	
	Mean	SD	Mean	SD
$t_{1/2}$ (hr)	6.0 ± 1.4		5.9 ± 1.0	
AUC (μg[a] hr/ml)	25.1 ± 5.6		24.6 ± 4.4	
C_{max} (μg/ml)	2.7 ± 0.8		2.7 ± 0.8	
T_{max} (hr)	2.3 ± 1.2		3.0 ± 1.4	
A_e (u)[a] (mg)	193 ± 31		203 ± 51	
Cl (ml/min)	131.6 ± 26.5		137.3 ± 22.8	

[a] Amount excreted with urine.
N = 12.

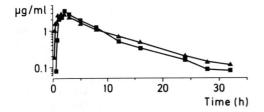

FIG. 3. Individual plasma concentration time profile following oral administration of 300 mg gabapentin as solution (▲—▲) and capsule (■—■) to a healthy volunteer.

In a three-way crossover dose proportionality study in fasting, healthy volunteers, the disposition parameters following 100 mg, 300 mg, and 900 mg single doses are independent of the dose administered (16). The pharmacokinetics of gabapentin 400 mg single dose as well as 400 mg t.i.d. for 8 days was investigated in epileptic patients on stable phenytoin monotherapy. The parameters obtained are not different from those of various studies in volunteers or patients where gabapentin was the only drug.

Co-administration of gabapentin with phenytoin did not result in clinically significant interference with the phenytoin plasma levels in epileptic patients (2).

To investigate a possible influence of prolonged gabapentin administration on liver enzyme activity, a double-blind, phenytoin-controlled parallel group trial in healthy volunteers was carried out using antipyrine clearance as a model for enzyme induction properties. From day 15 to day 29, either 400 mg gabapentin t.i.d. or 100 mg phenytoin t.i.d. was given. Base-line values on day 1 compare well to the values after 2-week dosing (day 29) and 2 weeks after last dose (day 43).

Administration of gabapentin does not affect any of the antipyrine parameters measured. No enzyme induction had occurred. Administration of phenytoin, a well-known, enzyme-inducing anticonvulsant, resulted in increased antipyrine clearance ($p < 0.05$), decreased antipyrine AUC ($p < 0.05$) and decreased elimination half-life ($p < 0.05$) (1).

THERAPEUTIC EFFICACY

In a double-blind, placebo-controlled study, the encephalotropic and psychotropic properties of gabapentin were studied in 10 healthy subjects by means of quantitative pharmaco-EEG and psychometric analyses. The subjects received randomized single oral doses of 50 mg, 100 mg, 200 mg, and 400 mg gabapentin as well as placebo at weekly intervals. EEG recordings were carried out after 0, 1, 2, 4, 6, and 8 hours; psychometric tests were done at the same time except for the first hour.

Computer-assisted spectral analysis of the EEG shows moderate though significant central effects of gabapentin in doses of 200 to 400 mg compared to placebo, which are maximally pronounced in the 2nd hour post-drug. These alterations are generally characterized by an attenuation of total power, augmentation of delta and theta activity and a decrease of alpha activity, indicating central nervous system (CNS)-inhibitory properties. Only at the late hours is there a shift toward a vigilance promotion.

Psychometric and psychophysiological evaluation demonstrates subtle psychotropic effects compared to placebo, characterized mostly by an improvement in concentration, numerical memory, complex reaction, and performance in the alphabetical reaction test (12).

A dose-related antiepileptic effect was observed in an 8-month randomized double-blind, crossover trial on 25 patients with severe partial or generalized epilepsies carried out in the United Kingdom. Gabapentin was added in randomized sequence to a one to two anticonvulsant base-line treatment in daily doses of 300 mg, 600 mg, and 900 mg for 2 months each, after a 2-month base-line period.

The median frequency of all seizures was significantly reduced from 3.3 to 2.1/week (45%) on 900 mg/day of gabapentin compared to base-line period ($p < 0.0001$). The 300 mg and 600 mg doses did not differ significantly from base line. The 900 mg dose was significantly better than 600 mg ($p = 0.05$) and 300 mg ($p = 0.01$). Nine patients (43%) had seizure frequency reduced by at least 50% when receiving 900 mg/day gabapentin. Seven and three patients, respectively, experienced 50% reduction in seizure frequency while receiving 600 mg and 300 mg gabapentin. One patient was entirely seizure-free for the full 2-month treatment period while receiving 600 mg per day.

There is no evidence that gabapentin had significant interactions with other antiepileptic drugs. Psychometric testing failed to reveal any changes between base-line and active treatment or between different doses of gabapentin, indicating no impairment of performance.

One patient was dropped from the study due to serial absence seizures within the titration phase. Eight out of 25 patients reported one or more adverse events when taking 300 mg daily dose, 15 out of 25 on one or more occasions taking 600 mg/day and 11 out of 25 taking 900 mg/day. Six patients reported adverse events from base-line therapy only when admitted to the study. Most reports under active treatment concerned drowsiness (eight reports with base-line anticonvulsants, 11 when gabapentin was added), tiredness, and dizziness. In no cases were the side effects sufficient to warrant premature withdrawal of the drug. No clinically relevant laboratory value changes have been noted in either of the 2-month treatment intervals compared to base line (5).

Gabapentin proved to be effective in re-ducing the number of partial seizures compared to placebo in a further double-blind, parallel group design. A total of 127 patients with severe refractory partial epilepsy was randomized after a 3-month base-line period either to 3-month gabapentin 1,200 mg daily dose (400 mg t.i.d.) or placebo added to mostly one to two anticonvulsants at constant doses.

The efficacy analysis involved 110 patients. Both treatment groups were comparable with respect to population characteristics and severity of the disease. Adding gabapentin resulted in a responder rate (50% reduction in seizure frequency) of 26% compared to 10% when placebo was added. This difference is statistically significant ($p = 0.042$). Comparing the base-line seizure frequencies (B) with treatment seizure frequencies (T), the response ratio (T − B:T + B) is −0.204 (adjusted mean) under gabapentin (which is equivalent to a 34% mean reduction in seizure frequency) and −0.061 under placebo (11% mean reduction) which is significantly different ($p = 0.004$). Figure 4 gives the distribution of patients with a certain change in seizure frequency compared to base line displayed in 25% categories.

Overall 10 patients were dropped (six in the gabapentin group, four in the placebo group), nine of them because of adverse events and one (placebo) for nonmedical reasons. When gabapentin or placebo was added, 57% of the patients reported adverse events mostly rated mild to moderate in the gabapentin group, compared to 38% in the placebo group. Severe adverse events occurred in five patients, three in the gabapentin group and two in the placebo group. The distribution of the most frequent side effects is given in Table 6.

On the basis of the plasma samples taken throughout the study, no influence of gabapentin was observed on the plasma levels of concomitant anticonvulsants. Deviations of laboratory parameters were comparable in both treatment groups and not clinically relevant (10).

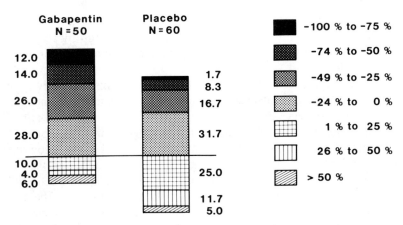

FIG. 4. Percentage change of number of partial seizures—distribution. Efficacy sample N = 110.

The spectrum of anticonvulsant activity in different seizure types was subjected to further preliminary investigation in a multicenter, base-line–controlled open study, conducted in the German-speaking area on previously drug-resistant epileptic patients with a minimum of four seizures per month during the 3-month base-line period.

Previous therapy with marketed anticonvulsants had to have been unsuccessful even at the highest tolerated doses and polytherapy up to three base-line drugs indicated for the type of epilepsy. Target for an individual titration was 400 mg t.i.d., to be increased in exceptional cases up to 1,800 mg daily. Once the final optimal dose within the given range was reached, a 2-month observation period with gabapentin added was compared to the last 2 months of the baseline period. Of the 70 patients enrolled, five were excluded from the efficacy analysis because of side effects, and 13 were not evaluable for nonmedical reasons.

Taking all seizure types together, there was a reduction in seizure frequency of more than 50% in 28% of the patients (N = 52), a reduction in seizure frequency of some degree in 71% of the patients, and an increase in seizures in 28% of the patients. The respective numbers for the different seizure types are as follows: partial seizures (N = 29 patients) 31%, 79%, and 21%; generalized tonic-clonic seizures (N = 20) 35%, 70%, and 30%; absences (N = 10) 50%, 90%, and 10%. A reduction in seizure frequency of 75% to 100% is seen in 15% of all seizures together, 25% in generalized tonic-clonic, 17% in partial seizures, and 20% in absences. Six patients were free of seizures during the observation period and beyond for at least 75 to a maximum of 219 days. None of these seizure-free patients received more than 1,200 mg daily, two received only 600 mg daily.

The incidence of subjective complaints

TABLE 6. *Side effects in patients receiving gabapentin and placebo*

	Gabapentin group (N = 61)	Placebo group (N = 66)
Somnolence	13%	3%
Fatigue	12%	—
Dizziness	7%	5%
Weight increase	5%	—
Ataxia	5%	—
Headache	3%	11%
Nausea	3%	3%
Diplopia	3%	—
Acne	—	3%
Rash	—	3%

was 51% (mainly fatigue and dizziness) of all 70 patients entered; 49% reported no side effects. Of these adverse events, 1% was definitely gabapentin-related, and 23% were possibly related to the addition of gabapentin. Only five of the patients had to discontinue the study because of side effects: 1st patient—staggers when walking; 2nd patient—nausea, gastric pain, dizziness, alopecia; 3rd patient—low white blood count, fatigue; 4th patient—fatigue, dizziness, lack of concentration; 5th patient—fatigue, dizziness, dysarthria. In the remaining patients, side effects were mild and/or transient. Plasma levels of the other concomitant antiepileptic drugs were not changed by gabapentin (6).

SUMMARY

Gabapentin has consistently shown antiepileptic activity in patients previously considered drug-resistant (according to the definition of the ILAE) throughout clinical studies when added to the existing unsuccessful drug regimen. This has been established for partial seizures with or without secondary generalization in well-controlled, double-blind trials for daily doses between 900 and 1,200 mg. A broader spectrum extending into primary generalized epilepsies is suggested from pilot trials (to be confirmed in formal proof of efficacy studies currently underway). In a review of hundreds of patients records, there was little evidence of side effects except for transient, mostly mild to moderate somnolence in some patients, when gabapentin was given as add-on therapy. In monotherapy in spastic patients, these types of side effects were in the placebo range. In long-term treatment over 1 year, no signs of chronic toxicity (laboratory values included) have been observed, nor any loss of efficacy over time. In all clinical studies and in a pharmacokinetic trial versus phenytoin, there was no evidence of clinically significant in-

teraction with other anticonvulsants. This finding is backed up by the fact that gabapentin is not metabolized in man, does not bind to plasma proteins, and does not change liver enzyme activity as demonstrated by the antipyrine model.

Due to its low acute and chronic toxicity (nonteratogenic in three species), its pharmacokinetic and pharmacodynamic properties, and its efficacy in previously drug-resistant patients, gabapentin will likely be a significant addition to the treatment armamentarium for the epilepsies once its development has been extended to include less severe cases and monotherapy.

CONVERSION

Conversion factor:

$$CF = \frac{1000}{mol.\ wt.} = \frac{1000}{171.24} = 5.84$$

Conversion:

$$(\mu g/ml) \times 5.84 = (\mu moles/liter)$$

$$(\mu moles/liter) \div 5.84 = (\mu g/ml)$$

REFERENCES

1. Allen, E., Javad, B., Wroe, B., and Richens, A. (1987): Does the anticonvulsant gabapentin lack enzyme inducing properties? 17th Epilepsy International Congress, Jerusalem.
2. Anhut, H., Leppik, I., Schmidt, B., and Thomann P. (1988): Drug interaction study of the new anticonvulsant gabapentin with phenytoin in epileptic patients. *Naunyn Schmiedeberg's Arch. Pharmacol. Suppl. Vol. 337*, 29. Spring Meeting of the German Pharmacological Society, Mainz.
3. Bartoszyk, G. D. (1983): Gabapentin and convulsions provoked by excitatory amino acids. *Naunyn-Schmiedeberg's Arch. Pharmacol.*, 324:R24.
4. G. D. Bartoszyk, N. Meyerson, W. Reimann, G. Satzinger, and A. von Hodenberg (1986): In: *New Anticonvulsant Drugs*, edited by B. S. Meldrum and R. J. Porter. John Libbey & Company Ltd., London.
5. Crawford, P., Ghadiali, E., Lane, R., Blumhardt, L., and Chadwick, D. (1987): Gabapentin as an antiepileptic drug in man. *Neurol. Neurosurg. and Psych.*, 50:682–686.
6. Deisenhammer, E., et al. (Austrian, German,

Swiss Study Group) (1987): Gabapentin in the treatment of drug resistant epileptic patients. 17th Epilepsy International Congress, Jerusalem.

7. Dooley, D.-J., Bartoszyk, G. D., Rock, D. M., Satzinger, G. (1985): Preclinical pharmacology of gabapentin. 16th Epilepsy International Congress, Hamburg.

8. Haas, H. L., and Wieser, H.-G. (1986): Gabapentin: Action on hippocampal slices of the rat and effects in human epileptics. Northern European Epilepsy Meeting, York.

9. Hengy, H., and Kölle, E.-U. (1985): Determination of gabapentin in plasma and urine by high-performance liquid chromatography and precolumn labelling for ultraviolet detection. *J. Chromat.*, 341:473–478.

10. Patterson, V., et al. (UK Study Group) (1988): Gabapentin as an anticonvulsant in partial epilepsy. 40th Meeting of the American Academy of Neurology, Cincinnati.

11. Reimann, W. (1983): Inhibition by GABA, baclofen and gabapentin of dopamine release from rabbit caudate nucleus: Are there common or different sites of action? *Eur. J. Pharmacol.*, 94:341–344.

12. Saletu, B., Grünberger, J., and Linzmayer, L. (1986): Evaluation of encephalotropic and psychotropic properties of gabapentin in man by pharmaco-EEG and psychometry. *Int. Clin. Pharmacol., Ther., and Toxicol., Vol. 24*, 7:362–373.

13. Satzinger, G., Hartenstein, J., Herrmann, M., and Heldt, W. (1974): DP 2,460,891; US 4,024,175.

14. Schlicker, E., Reimann, W., and Göthert, M. (1985): Gabapentin decreases monoamine release without affecting acetylcholine release in the brain. *Arzneimittel-Forsch./Drug Res.*, 35:1347–1349.

15. Vollmer, K.-O., Anhut, H., Thomann, F., Wagner, F., and Jähnchen, D. (1987): Pharmacokinetic model and the absolute bioavailability of the new anticonvulsant gabapentin. 17th Epilepsy International Congress, Jerusalem.

16. Vollmer, K.-O., Thomann, P., Most, M., von Hodenberg, A., Meyerson, N., and Schmidt, B. (1986): Pharmacokinetics of the new anticonvulsant gabapentin in man. Golden Jubilee Conference and Northern European Epilepsy Meeting, University of York, UK.

17. Vollmer, K.-O., von Hodenberg, A., and Kölle, E.-U. (1986): Pharmacokinetics and metabolism of gabapentin in rat, dog and man. *Arzneimittel-Forsch./Drug Res.*, 36:830–839.

18. Von Hodenberg, A., Kölle, E.-U., and Vollmer, K.-O. (1986): Comparative metabolism studies in rat, dog and man. 16th Epilepsy International Congress, Hamburg.

Antiepileptic Drugs, Third Edition, edited by
R. Levy, R. Mattson, B. Meldrum,
J. K. Penry, and F. E. Dreifuss.
Raven Press, Ltd., New York © 1989.

68

Potential Antiepileptic Drugs

Vigabatrin

Alan Richens

INTRODUCTION

The importance of γ-aminobutyric acid (GABA) as an inhibitory transmitter in the central nervous system is now well established (23). By activating GABA$_A$ receptors, the transmitter opens up chloride channels in the postsynaptic membrane resulting in electrical stabilization. It follows that activation of these receptors, either by a direct agonist effect or by increasing the synaptic concentration of GABA, will inhibit neuronal activity.

GABA is synthesized from glutamate by the activity of glutamic acid decarboxylase (GAD) in presynaptic nerve terminals. The GABA released during neurotransmission either is taken up by glial cells or re-enters the presynaptic terminal by a re-uptake mechanism. It is then converted by GABA-aminotransferase (GABA-T) into glutamate and succinic semialdehyde. This synthetic pathway is called the GABA-shunt because it provides an alternative pathway for conversion of ketoglutarate to succinate in the tricarboxylic acid cycle (see Chapter 4).

It has been speculated that epilepsy might be caused by a deficiency of GABA in the brain but so far there is little support for this hypothesis. A derangement of glutamate transmission, the main excitatory system in the brain, is an alternative possibility. Nevertheless, pharmacological enhance-

ment of GABA transmission is one means of reducing neuronal excitability and this approach has been used with success. Benzodiazepine drugs, for instance, are known to enhance GABA transmission by activating receptors adjacent to the GABA$_A$ receptor. Preventing the breakdown of GABA is an alternative means of increasing inhibitory transmission, and vigabatrin in known to act in this way. It acts as an enzyme-activated suicide inhibitor of GABA-aminotransferase.

CHEMISTRY

Vigabatrin (γ-vinyl GABA; 4-amino-hex-5-enoic acid) is a synthetic derivative of the neurotransmitter GABA (Fig. 1). It exists as a racemic mixture of two enantiomers. The $S(+)$-enantiomer possesses pharmacological activity, whereas the $R(-)$-enantiomer is inactive. Selective synthesis of the $S(+)$-enantiomer would reduce the dose and possibly the cost, and this might be feasible in the future. With few exceptions (25), the pharmacological work on the drug to date has been carried out on the racemic mixture. Vigabatrin is freely water-soluble and has a molecular weight of 129.16.

METHODS OF DETERMINATION

As vigabatrin is an amino acid, it is possible to measure plasma and urine concen-

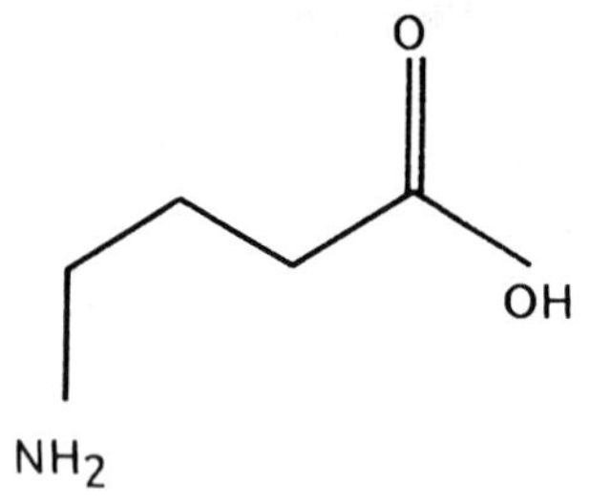

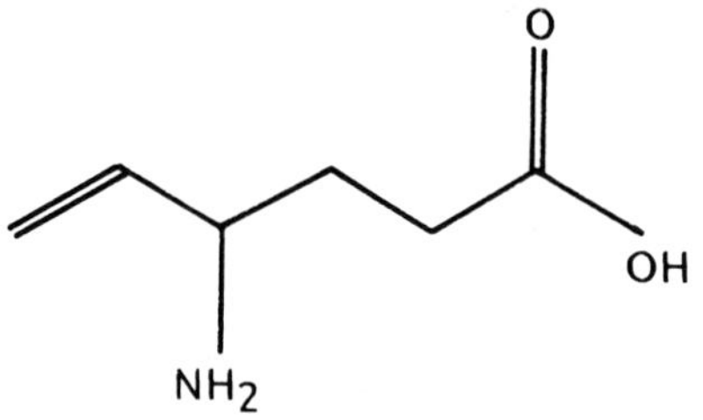

FIG. 1. Structures of GABA (**top**) and vigabatrin (γ-vinyl-GABA) (**bottom**).

trations with an amino acid analyzer (10), but this is time consuming. Methods for measuring GABA are applicable to analyzing vigabatrin, and these include ion-exchange high-performance liquid chromatography (HPLC) with post-column derivatization and fluorescence detection of the dansylated derivative of the drug with a fluorometric detector (40). The latter method involves the use of copper chloride which complexes with the endogenous amino acids thereby enhancing the specificity of the assay. It is possible to separate the $S(+)$ and $R(-)$-enantiomers using a chiral capillary gas chromatographic column coupled to a mass spectrometer (11), but this technique is too complex for routine use. However, methods that do not distinguish between the two enantiomers may be of limited value because only a proportion

of the assayed substance is in the pharmacologically active form.

PHARMACOKINETICS

Experimental Studies

In rat and dog, the absorption of orally administered vigabatrin is almost complete, with peak plasma concentrations being reached within an hour, but in monkey the absorption is less complete. First-pass metabolism is minimal. Vigabatrin distributes into total body water but there is evidence of tissue binding in the rat because its volume of distribution exceeds total body water. Penetration into the cerebrospinal fluid (CSF) occurs readily but steady-state CSF concentrations achieved in the dog are much higher than in other species. Renal excretion is the major route of elimination in all species, biotransformation accounting for less than 20% of the dose. Vigabatrin is not bound to plasma proteins and does not influence cytochrome P-450–dependent drug metabolizing enzyme activity in rat liver, therefore interactions with other antiepileptic drugs would not be anticipated from these studies.

Clinical Studies

As vigabatrin is freely water-soluble, dissolution of oral formulations is rapid and is not significantly affected by food. Peak plasma concentrations are reached about 1 hour after dosing (2) and the plasma concentrations of $R(-)$-enantiomer are almost double those of the pharmacologically active $S(+)$-enantiomer following administration of the racemate to healthy volunteers. It is possible that the bioavailability of the $R(-)$-enantiomer is greater than that of the $S(+)$-enantiomer. Although absolute bioavailability studies have not yet been performed, a minimum 80% of an oral dose is recovered in the urine with no evidence of dose-dependency.

A single 1.5-g dose of the racemate will produce a peak concentration of the $S(+)$-enantiomer of 50 to 100 mmol/liter. The terminal elimination half-lives of the two enantiomers are similar at about 7 to 8 hr, giving a renal clearance of 1.3 ml·min^{-1}·kg^{-1}. When pharmacokinetic parameters of the $S(+)$-enantiomer obtained after dosing with the racemate are compared with those obtained after dosing with pure $S(+)$-γ-vinyl GABA at half the dose of the racemate, no significant differences are found (12). Thus, co-administration of the $R(-)$-enantiomer has no influence on the pharmacokinetics of the $S(+)$-enantiomer. No chiral inversion takes place since no $R(-)$-enantiomer is identified in the plasma on oral administration of the $S(+)$-enantiomer.

Vigabatrin is eliminated largely by renal excretion of the unchanged drug; about 50% of an oral dose of the $S(+)$-enantiomer is excreted in the urine in the first 48 hr in subjects with normal renal function, but the proportion of the $R(-)$-enantiomer recovered is higher (about 65%). It has been found that the extrarenal clearance of this $S(+)$-enantiomer is greater than for the $R(-)$-enantiomer. The renal clearance of both enantiomers shows a good correlation with creatinine clearance. A reduced creatinine clearance results in a reduced renal clearance for both enantiomers, but because of the greater extrarenal clearance of the $S(+)$-enantiomer, the R to S ratio will increase in renal failure. When used in the elderly or in patients with renal failure, the maintenance dose may need to be reduced.

PHARMACODYNAMICS

Experimental Studies

Biochemistry

Vigabatrin is an enzyme-activated, irreversible inhibitor of GABA-T. It is thought to bind covalently to the active site of the enzyme as it undergoes catalytic conversion. Lippert et al. (20) suggested that it forms a Schiff base with pyridoxal phosphate in the active site of GABA-T. The enzyme abstracts the labilized proton at C-4 from this aldimine Schiff base and the charge stabilization by the pyridine ring induces the aldimine to ketimine tautomerism, which is characteristic of the normal mechanism of conversion. This reactive (C-5, C-6) ketimine forms a stable adduct with a nucleophilic residue in the enzyme active site resulting in irreversible inhibition.

Vigabatrin does not inhibit GABA-T from nonmammalian sources, GAD, or aspartate transaminase, but alanine aminotransferase is slowly inhibited. Other compounds can inhibit GABA-T, such as γ-acetylenic GABA, ethanolamine-o-sulfate, aminooxyacetic acid and, to a lesser extent, valproic acid.

Biochemical Pharmacology

Single doses of vigabatrin injected intraperitoneally into mice cause a rapid decrease in GABA-T activity to about 20% of control activity within 3 to 4 hr (18). Recovery to control levels takes several days because new enzyme has to be synthesized; in the mouse the half-life of GABA-T was found to be 3.4 days. A small reduction in the activity of GAD is also seen but this is thought to a be a consequence of feedback inhibition caused by high concentrations of GABA. Whole brain GABA concentration increases with a similar time course to the reduction in GABA-T activity. Repeated dosing causes a more profound and sustained elevation of GABA concentration (30).

The changes in GABA-T activity and GABA concentration occur in all areas of the brain that have been assayed, although to differing extents, as might be expected from the uneven distribution of GABAergic neurons in the brain. A disproportionately greater increase in synaptosomal compared to nonsynaptosomal GABA in rat cortex is seen after vigabatrin treatment. Furthermore, when GABAergic nerve terminals are destroyed by unilateral section in rat substantia nigra, vigabatrin has less effect on the denervated side than on the innervated side (17). This evidence indicates that an increase in a releasable, functional pool of GABA is caused by vigabatrin. With the use of cultured mouse neurons and astrocytes, it has been shown that only the $S(+)$-enantiomer can be actively transported and the neurons, but not astrocytes, have a high affinity uptake system, in line with the observation that neuronal GABA-T is more sensitive than astrocytic GABA-T to vigabatrin (38).

Cerebrospinal fluid concentrations of both free and conjugated GABA in rats have been shown to rise after vigabatrin administration (3). An increase in plasma GABA concentration reflects an effect on peripheral sites of GABA synthesis.

Anticonvulsant Effect

The effect of vigabatrin in modifying experimental seizures is variable. Audiogenic and strychnine-induced seizures in rodents are antagonized (37) as are photically induced seizures in primates (24), but seizures caused by the GABA-receptor antagonists, bicuculline and picrotoxin, are less readily blocked. The reason for this is unclear but may relate to the fact that the increase in GABA concentration is predominantly in the glial compartment rather than the nerve terminals. Electroshock seizures (17) and amygdala-kindled seizures (19) in the rat, but not pentylenetetrazol seizures, are also antagonized by vigabatrin. The time course of seizure protection relates closely to the increase in synaptosomal GABA concentration rather than whole brain GABA (16). Midbrain injection of vigabatrin in rats pro-

duces a broad spectrum of anticonvulsant activity (17). The anticonvulsant activity observed in these studies is associated with the $S(+)$-enantiomer only (25).

Other Pharmacological Actions

In general behavioral terms, the increase in brain GABAergic function produced by vigabatrin causes a decrease in locomotor activity, general sedation, hypothermia, moderate antinociception (27), and reduces food intake. When given intravenously, it produces sustained falls in blood pressure in rats, cats, and dogs.

Experimental Toxicology

Toxicological studies in rodents indicate that vigabatrin can cause central nervous system depression and convulsions in high single doses. The LD_{50} values in rats and mice are about 60 times higher than the maximum daily dose used in patients.

Repeated administration in doses of 300 mg/kg/day can cause alopecia and reduced weight gain in rodents. This dose in dogs caused anorexia, weight loss, and anemia. Monkeys given 500 mg/kg/day developed diarrhea, thought to be due to dose-dependent absorption in this species.

Toxicity studies of long-term vigabatrin administration in mice, rats, and dogs have shown that intramyelinic edema occurs in the white matter of the brain at doses of 50 to 100 mg/kg/day (7). Microscopically, the primary change consists of microvacuoles of 20 to 80 μm in diameter which are characterized by separation of the outer lamellar sheaths of myelinated axons. The area of the rat brain most affected by the intramyelinic edema is the cerebellum; the other affected areas include the reticular formation, optic tract, anterior commissure, columns of fornix, colliculus, and hippocampus. These changes show lack of progression despite continuing therapy and are reversible when vigabatrin is stopped, although some residual changes, namely eosinophilic spheroids, swollen axons or dendrites, and corpora amylacea have been observed in the cerebellum of rats.

In monkeys given 300 mg/kg/day occasional microvacuoles can be noted, but arguably no more than in control animals.

The exact mechanism by which the microvacuolation arises is unclear, but it is known to be associated with the active and not the inactive enantiomer. Other GABA-transaminase inhibitors have also been shown to have this effect. Although the histological appearances resemble those caused by hexachlorophene, triethyltin and isoniazid, they differ in that they are generalized rather than limited to a few sites, show no clear dose relationship, and are reversible.

The functional significance of these lesions is uncertain. However, studies of evoked potentials in dogs have shown that a dose of 300 mg/kg/day given for 12 weeks significantly slowed the central conduction time of the somatosensory but not the auditory evoked potential (1). These changes, and the microvacuolation accompanying them, fully recovered after 17 weeks off vigabatrin.

Reproduction studies have shown only a low incidence of cleft palate in the rabbit. Mutagenicity and carcinogenicity studies have been negative (27). Vigabatrin also reduces food intake, and when given intravenously, it produces sustained falls in blood pressure in rats, cats, and dogs.

Clinical Studies

In man, orally administered vigabatrin increases the concentration of free and conjugated GABA in the CSF, indicating that the drug penetrates the central nervous system (36). Vigabatrin concentrations of around 2 nmol·l^{-1} have been measured in lumbar CSF 24 hr after a single oral dose of 50 mg/kg (2). Cerebrospinal fluid concentrations of excitatory amino acids are not changed by prolonged treatment with vigabatrin (13), but plasma GABA concentration is increased by the drug. GABA-T is present in platelets and measurement of the inhibition of this enzyme has been proposed as a marker of the pharmacodynamic effect of vigabatrin in man (33). The time course of the inhibition of platelet GABA-T in man and experimental animals is similar to the change in brain GABA-T activity in animal studies (4). Brain GABA-T activity has not been measured in man following vigabatrin administration.

Cerebrospinal fluid and plasma β-alanine may be increased by vigabatrin, but this is to be expected because this amino acid is normally degraded by GABA-T (36).

CLINICAL TRIALS

Efficacy

Double-blind, placebo-controlled studies in epilepsy were undertaken at a very early stage of the clinical assessment of vigabatrin, and it quickly became known that the compound had a significant antiepileptic effect. Six European trials (Table 1) have used the add-on crossover technique in patients with drug-resistant epilepsy (8,22,34,41,42,43). A total of 153 patients were recruited and efficacy was evaluated in 131. All suffered from drug-resistant epilepsy and experienced at least four seizures per month. The majority had complex partial seizures with or without secondary generalization. The daily dose of vigabatrin varied from 1.5 to 3 g and the duration of treatment varied from 7 to 12 weeks.

Two patients had complete remission of seizures during the study period. A total of 98 patients, all with complex partial seizures with or without secondary generalization, demonstrated a reduction in seizure frequency when compared to the placebo

Table 1. *Efficacy of vigabatrin compared with placebo in six European double-blind, crossover trials*

Reference	No. of patients who entered study	No. of patients completing study		Duration of treatment (weeks)	Dose of vigabatrin (g/day)	Reduction in seizure frequency		Mean weekly seizure frequency		
		All seizure types	Partial seizures only			>50%	>75%	P	V	(p)
33	24	22	22	9	3	14	6	6.4	3.8	(<0.01)
8	21	18	18	12	3	8	3	2.2	1.3	(<0.01)
22	23	19	17	9	3	11	2	10.7	6.3	(<0.01)
41	23	20	19	7	1.5–3	12	4	6.7	5.4	(NS)
42	31	30	26	12	2–3	9	2	12.7	14.7	(NS)
43	23	17	11	12	3	1	0	7.2	8.3	(NS)

P, placebo; V, vigabatrin; p, significance of difference; NS, not significant.

period. Forty-five (46%) had a 50% or greater reduction in seizure frequency (Table 2). Mean seizure frequency during vigabatrin treatment in these six trials was reduced to about 50% to 60% per cent of the frequency during administration of placebo. In each of the trials a significant effect in favor of vigabatrin was found when complex partial seizures with or without secondary generalization were considered (Table 2). The less favorable response in patients suffering from other types of seizure resulted in statistical significance being lost in three of the trials (41–43) when the analysis included these patients (Table 1).

The least favorable of these trials (43) was performed on inpatients, whereas the other trials were on outpatients; the former were also on a larger number of psychoactive drugs, perhaps accounting for their less satisfactory response. There was no relationship, however, between the type of other antiepileptic drug and efficacy. Overall, better results were obtained in patients with 10 or fewer seizures per week. A small number of children were included in these trials and their responses were less favorable.

A preliminary report (32) of a parallel group study in which vigabatrin was replaced by placebo has also shown a result in favor of vigabatrin. Thirty-one adult patients with resistant tonic-clonic and partial seizures were first given vigabatrin in doses of up to 3 g/day in an open manner. Nine-

Table 2. *Mean weekly seizure frequency for complex partial seizures with or without secondary generalization in six Europen double-blind, crossover trials*

Reference	Number of patients	Reduction in seizure frequency		Seizure frequency		
		>50%	>75%	P	V	(p)
33	22	14	6	6.4	3.8	(<0.01)
8	18	7	4	2.1	1.3	(<0.01)
22	17	9	1	10.6	6.5	(<0.01)
41	15	9	3	3.0	1.5	(<0.02)
42	15	5	2	3.6	1.8	(<0.02)
43	11	1	0	4.0	2.5	(<0.05)
	TOTAL	45(46%)	16(16%)			

P, placebo; V, vigabatrin; p, significance of difference.

teen patients who showed a 50% or greater reduction in seizure frequency were then randomized either to continue vigabatrin or to substitute the active drug with placebo in a double-blind parallel group study. Those continuing on vigabatrin maintained their good response (a median fall of 56% in seizure frequency compared with the base-line period), but those who were changed to placebo experienced a 22% increase in seizure frequency.

A dose reduction study performed in Finnish patients with complex partial seizures (39) showed that 3 g of vigabatrin daily appeared to be superior to 1.5 g daily. Of 75 patients entered into an open trial, 41 showed a 50% or greater reduction in seizure frequency. Twenty-eight of these were randomized either to continue on 3 g daily or to reduce to 1.5 g daily. Seizures remained better controlled on the higher dose although even with the reduced dose the seizure frequency was significantly lower than in the base-line period.

Additional evidence for a dose-related antiepileptic effect comes from a preliminary single-blind trial (9). In successive 4-week periods the dose of vigabatrin was increased in 1 g increments to 3 g daily in 15 patients with therapy-resistant epilepsy (mostly complex partial seizures). The median seizure frequency fell from eight per 4-week period during the base-line placebo treatment to five on 1 g daily, five on 2 g daily, and two on 3 g daily.

A North American multicenter, single-blind, add-on trial of vigabatrin in refractory complex partial seizures (5) included 89 patients with a minimum of three seizures per month. The drug was titrated in each patient up to a maximum dose of 4 g/day or 50 mg/kg/day (whichever was the less) and continued for a 12-week maintenance period. Of the 84 patients who completed the maintenance period, 51% had a 50% or greater reduction in complex partial seizure frequency, and 7% had complete seizure control. Twenty patients also had secondary generalized tonic-clonic seizures, and of these 15 experienced a 50% or greater reduction of the frequency of these seizures. In 66 (74%) of the patients, the therapeutic response rates judged on seizure frequency and severity warranted continued administration of vigabatrin in an open-label, follow-up study. Over the next 4 to 25 months, 26 patients discontinued vigabatrin, 13 from seizure breakthrough or adverse effects.

In a Danish long-term study (29) involving a mean follow-up period of 9.3 months, 20 out of 36 patients experienced a 50% or greater reduction in seizure frequency. Most of the patients studied had complex partial seizures, but three of the responders had juvenile myoclonic epilepsy. No signs of tolerance to the antiepileptic effects were observed.

The only published trial of vigabatrin in children (21) involved 135 patients with refractory epilepsy, including partial and generalized seizures, Lennox-Gastaut syndrome, and West syndrome. The drug was added to existing treatment in a dose of 40 to 80 mg/kg/day in an open study. Eleven patients became seizure-free and 37% of the children had a greater than 50% reduction in seizures. High doses (above 100 mg/kg/day) were not associated with a greater efficacy. Partial seizures responded best, with good to excellent results in 49%.

Adverse Reactions and Toxicology

In general, adverse events associated with vigabatrin therapy have been mild and infrequent (Table 3). Drowsiness and fatigue are the most commonly reported effects, particularly in the European double-blind studies in which a fixed dose of drug was started abruptly. A psychosis or confusion was induced in a few patients. Weight gain has been noted occasionally in long-term studies; it is not certain whether this is a pharmacological effect of vigabatrin, although there is evidence in animal

Table 3. *Adverse events in patients receiving vigabatrin*[26]

Adverse event	% of people experiencing adverse event	
	European double-blind studies (*N* = 131)	All patients (*N* = 1,147)
Drowsiness	27.2	13.6
Fatigue	7.6	8.9
Irritability/ nervousness	5.4	3.5
Dizziness	5.4	5.2
Weight gain	NR	4.0
Headache	4.1	3.7
Confusion	3.4	1.9

NR, not recorded.

studies that GABA is involved in weight maintenance. Cohort analyses have failed to show any late emergence of adverse events from prolonged treatment up to 3 years in duration.

This clinical experience is reassuring considering the adverse central nervous system toxicity in animal screening tests discussed earlier. However, the clinician faces difficulties in devising screening methods for detecting a similar type of microvacuolation in patients. Computerized tomography scans have been performed in a number of patients before and after some months of vigabatrin therapy and have shown no change, but this technique is limited in its quantitative differentiation of tissue density. Magnetic resonance imaging scanning, which is particularly sensitive to changes in brain water content, has also demonstrated no change in the few patients studied so far.

In view of the involvement of the visual pathways in animal toxicological tests and the fact that somatosensory evoked potentials in dogs are affected by vigabatrin therapy (1), visual, somatosensory, and brain stem evoked potentials have been recorded in epileptic patients treated with the drug (5,6,14). No significant effects of vigabatrin were observed. The limited amount of postmortem brain material which has become

available has not shown intramyelinic edema (15,28). Soluble proteins in the CSF have not been altered in vigabatrin-treated patients, although changes associated with reduced protein synthesis have been shown in rats (31).

At the time of writing, there is no evidence to suggest that vigabatrin has a neurotoxic effect in man as it does in experimental animals.

Drug Interactions

As vigabatrin is not metabolized by the microsomal oxidase enzymes in the liver and is not bound to plasma proteins, interactions leading to alteration in the kinetics of vigabatrin would not be expected. When this drug is used in patients on phenytoin, however, a 20% to 40% reduction in steady-state serum phenytoin levels is seen (5,34). The mechanism of this interaction is unclear because no change in phenytoin binding occurs and the ratio of the HPPH metabolite to parent drug is not altered, ruling out an effect on the major metabolic pathway for phenytoin (35). Furthermore, vigabatrin does not induce liver enzymes when antipyrine is used as the test substrate (35).

Small but significant decreases in serum phenobarbitone and primidone concentrations were also seen in the North American single-blind study (5), but this has not been observed in other trials, perhaps because of the less frequent use of these two drugs. No interaction with carbamazepine has been noted.

CONCLUSION

Vigabatrin is a promising new antiepileptic compound whose mode of action is understood. Clinical trials to date are most encouraging in resistant epilepsy but it has yet to be evaluated as monotherapy. Concern that the CNS toxicity seen in animal experiments may also occur in humans has so far been unfounded, but more clinical experience is required.

CONVERSION

Conversion factor:

$$CF = \frac{1000}{\text{mol. wt.}} = \frac{1000}{129.16} = 7.74$$

Conversion:

$$(\mu g/ml) \times 7.74 = (\mu moles/liter)$$

$$(\mu moles/liter) \div 7.74 = (\mu g/ml)$$

REFERENCES

1. Arezzo, J. C., Schroeder, C. E., Litwak, M. S., and Steward, D. L. (1989): Effects of vigabatrin on evoked potentials in dogs. *Br. J. Clin. Pharmac.*, (Suppl.)27:53–60.
2. Ben Menachem, E., Persson, L. I., Schechter, P. J., Haegele, K. D., Huebert, N., Hardenberg, J., Dahlgren, L., and Mumford, J. P. (1989): The effect of different vigabatrin treatment regimens on CSF biochemistry and seizure control in epileptic patients. *Br. J. Clin. Pharmac.*, (Suppl.)27:79–85.
3. Bohlen, P., Huot, S., and Palfreyman, M. G. (1979): The relationship between GABA concentrations in brain and cerebrospinal fluid. *Brain Res.*, 167:297–305.
4. Bolton, J. B., Rimmer, E., Williams, J., and Richens, A. (1989): The effect of vigabatrin on brain and platelet GABA-transaminase activities. *Br. J. Clin. Pharmac.*, (Suppl.)27–42.
5. Browne, T. R., Mattson, R. H., Penry, J. K., Smith, D. B., Treiman, D. M., Wilder, B. J., Ben-Menachem, E., Napoliello, M. J., Sherry, K. M., and Szabo, G. K. (1987): Vigabatrin for refractory complex partial seizures: Multicentre single-blind study with long term follow up. *Neurology*, 37:184–189.
6. Cosi, V., Callieco, R., Galimberti, C. A., et al. (1989): Effect of vigabatrin (gamma-vinyl-GABA) on visual, brain stem auditory and somatosensory evoked potentials in epileptic patients. *Eur. Neurol.*, (in press).
7. Graham, D. G., (1989): Neuropathology of vigabatrin. *Br. J. Clin. Pharmac.*, (Suppl.)27:43–45.
8. Gram, L., Klosterskov, P., and Dam, M. (1985): Gamma-vinyl GABA: A double blind placebo-controlled trial in partial epilepsy. *Clin. Neurol.*, 17:262–266.
9. Gram, L., Lyon, B. B., and Dam, M. (1983): Gamma-vinyl-GABA: A single blind trial in patients with epilepsy. *Acta Neurol. Scand.*, 68:34–39.
10. Grove, J., Fozard, J. R., and Mamout, P. S. (1981): Assay of α-difluoro-methylornithine in body fluids and tissue by automatic amino-acid analysis. *J. Chromatogr.*, 223:409–416.
11. Haegele, K. D., Schoun, J., and Alken, R. G. (1983): Determination of the $R(-)$ and $S(+)$ enantiomers of γ-vinyl-aminobutyric acid in human body fluids by gas chromatography–mass spectrometry. *J. Chromatogr.*, 274:103–110.
12. Haegele, K. D., and Schechter, P. J. (1986): Kinetics of the evaluations of vigabatrin after an oral dose of the racemate or the active *S*-enantiomer. *Clin. Pharmac. Ther.*, 40:581–586.
13. Halonen, J., Lehtinen, M., Pitkanen, A., Ylinen, A., and Riekkinen, P. J. (1989): Inhibitory and excitatory amino acids in CSF of patients with complex partial seizures during chronic treatment with γ-vinyl GABA (vigabatrin). *Epilepsy Research*, 2:246–252.
14. Hammond, E. J., Ranger, R. J., and Wilder, B. J. (1988): Evoked potential monitoring of vigabatrin patients. *Br. J. Clin. Prac.*, 42 Symposium (Suppl.)61:16–23.
15. Hauw, J. J., Trottier, S., Boutry, J. M., Sun, P., Sazpovitch, V., and Duyckaerts, C. (1988): The neuropathology of vigabatrin. *Br. J. Clin. Prac.*, 42(Suppl.)61:10–13.
16. Iadarola, M. J., and Gale, K. (1981): Cellular compartments of GABA in brain and their relationship to anticonvulsant activity. *Mol. Cell Biochem.*, 39:305–330.
17. Iadarola, M. J., and Gale, K. (1982): Substantia nigra: Site of anticonvulsant activity mediated by gamma-aminobutyric acid. *Science*, 218:1237–1240.
18. Jung, M. J., Lippert, B., Metcalf, B. W., Bohlen, P., and Schechter, P. J. (1977). γ-Vinyl GABA (4-amino-hex-5-enoic acid), a new selective irreversible inhibitor of GABA-T: Effects on brain GABA metabolism in mice. *J. Neurochem.*, 29:797–802.
19. Kalichman, M. W., Burnham, W. M., and Livingstone, K. E. (1982): Pharmacological investigation of gamma-aminobutyric acid (GABA) and fully developed generalized seizures in the amygdala-kindled rat. *Neuropharmacol.*, 21:127–131.
20. Lippert, B., Metcalf, B. W., Jung, M. J., and Casara, P. (1977): 4-Amino-hex-5-enoic acid, a selective catalytic inhibitor of 4-aminobutyric-acid aminotransferase in mammalian brain. *Europ. J. Biochem.*, 74:441–445.
21. Livingston, J. H., Beaumont, D., Arzimanoglou, A., and Aicardi, J. (1989): Vigabatrin in the treatment of epilepsy in children. *Br. J. Clin. Pharmac.*, (Suppl.)27:109–112.
22. Loiseau, P., Hardenberg, J. P., Pestre, M., Guyot, M., Schechter, P. J., and Tell, G. P. (1986): Double-blind placebo controlled study of vigabatrin (gamma-vinyl GABA) in drug-resistant epilepsy. *Epilepsia*, 27:115–120.
23. Meldrum, B. (1982): Pharmacology of GABA. *Clin. Neuropharmacol.*, 5:293–316.
24. Meldrum, B., and Horton, R. (1978): Blockade of epileptic responses in the photosensitive baboon, *Papio papio*, by two irreversible inhibitors of GABA-transaminase, gamma-acetylenic GABA

(4-amino-hex-5-ynoic) and gamma-vinyl GABA (4-amino-hex-5-enoic acid). *Psychopharmacol. (Berlin),* 59:47–50.

25. Meldrum, B. S., and Murugaiah, K. (1983): Anticonvulsant action in mice with sound-induced seizures of the optical isomers of gamma-vinyl GABA. *Europ. J. Pharmacol.,* 89:149–152.

26. Mumford, J. P. (1988): A profile of vigabatrin. *Br. J. Clin. Prac.,* 42(Suppl.)61:7–9.

27. Palfryman, M. G., Schechter, P. J., Buckett, W. R., Tell, G. P., and Koch-Weser, J. (1981): The pharmacology of GABA-transaminase inhibitors. *Biochem. Pharmacol.,* 30:817–824.

28. Pedersen, B., Hojgaard, K., and Dam, M. (1987): Vigabatrin: No microvacuoles in a human brain. *Epilepsy Res.,* 1:74–76.

29. Pedersen, S. A., Klosterskov, P., Gram, L., and Dam, M. (1985): Long-term study of gamma-vinyl GABA in the treatment of epilepsy. *Acta Neurol. Scand.,* 72:295–298.

30. Perry, T. L., Kish, S. J., and Hansen, S. (1979): Gamma-vinyl GABA: Effects of chronic administration on the metabolism of GABA and other amino compounds in rat brain. *J. Neurochem.,* 32:1641–1645.

31. Persson, L. I., Ronnback, L., and Ben-Menachem, E. (1989): Changes in CSF and brain soluble proteins following vigabatrin treatment in rats. *Br. J. Clin. Pharmac.,* (Suppl.)27:73–77.

32. Reynolds, E. H., Ring, H., and Heller, A. (1988): A controlled trial of gamma-vinyl-GABA (vigabatrin) in drug resistant epilepsy. *Br. J. Clin. Pharmac.,* (Suppl.)4261:33.

33. Rimmer, E., Kongola, G., and Richens, A. (1988): Inhibition of the enzyme, GABA-aminotransferase, in human platelets by vigabatrin, a potential antiepileptic drug. *Br. J. Clin. Pharmac.,* 25:251–259.

34. Rimmer, E. M., and Richens, A. (1984): Double-blind study of gamma-vinyl GABA in patients with refractory epilepsy. *Lancet,* 1:189–190.

35. Rimmer, E. M., and Richens, A. (1988). Interaction between vigabatrin and phenytoin. *Br. J. Clin. Pharmac.,* (Suppl.)27:27–33.

36. Schechter, P. J., Hanke, N. F. J., Grove, J., Huebert, N., and Sjoerdsma, A. (1984): Biochemical and clinical effects of γ-vinyl GABA in patients with epilepsy. *Neurology,* 34:182–186.

37. Schechter, P. J., and Tranier, Y. (1978): The pharmacology of enzyme activated inhibitors of GABA-transaminase. In: *Enzyme-Activated Irreversible Inhibitors,* edited by N. Seiler, M. J. Jung, J. and Koch-Weser, pp. 149–162. Elsevier, Amsterdam.

38. Schousboe, A., Larsson, O. M., and Seiler, N. (1986): Stereoselective uptake of the GABA-transaminase inhibitors gamma-vinyl GABA and gamma-acetylenic GABA into neurons and astrocytes. *Neurochem. Res.,* 11:1497–1505.

39. Sivenius, M. R. J., Ylinen, A., Murros, K., Matilainen, R., and Riekkinen, P. (1987): Double-blind dose reduction study of vigabatrin in complex partial epilepsy. *Epilepsia,* 28:688–692.

40. Smithers, J. A., Lang, J. F., and Okerholm, R. A. (1985): Quantitative analysis of vigabatrin in plasma and urine by reversed-phase high-performance liquid chromatography. *J. Chromatogr.,* 341:232–238.

41. Tartara, A., Manni, R., Galimbert, C. A., Hardenberg, J., Orwin, J., and Perruca, E. (1986): Vigabatrin in the treatment of epilepsy: A double-blind, placebo-controlled study. *Epilepsia,* 27:717–723.

42. Tassinari, C. A., Michelucci, R., Ambrosetto, G., and Salvi, F. (1987): Double-blind study of vigabatrin in the treatment of drug-resistant epilepsy. *Arch. Neurol.,* 44:907–910.

43. Tell, G. P., and Hardenberg, J. (1985): Double-blind, placebo-controlled study of 3 g/day oral gamma vinyl GABA (GVG) in the treatment of therapy resistant epileptic patients. Merrell-Dow Project Report 85-LP-ST-0607.

Antiepileptic Drugs, Third Edition, edited by
R. Levy, R. Mattson, B. Meldrum,
J. K. Penry, and F. E. Dreifuss.
Raven Press, Ltd., New York © 1989.

69

Potential Antiepileptic Drugs

Lamotrigine

Lennart Gram

INTRODUCTION

Several of the major antiepileptic drugs, for example, phenytoin, phenobarbital, and primidone, exhibit an antifolate effect. This fact prompted Reynolds et al. (27) to formulate the so-called folate hypothesis, which suggests that the antiepileptic effect of these drugs is caused by their antifolate properties. However, a number of controlled studies supplementing the therapeutic regimen of epileptic patients with either folate or placebo, failed to confirm this hypothesis. No deterioration in seizure control was observed during folate treatment (5,10,14,17,19,26).

However, since research workers, including those at Wellcome Laboratories, were able to demonstrate that folic acid and other folates exhibited convulsant properties in experimental animals (1,15), the idea of developing a new antiepileptic drug from antifolate compounds was pursued. Lamotrigine possesses potent anticonvulsant activity, but has only weak antifolate activity. In the phenyltriazine series, from which lamotrigine was developed, no correlation was found between antifolate and anticonvulsant activities. Recent studies of the mechanism of action of lamotrigine, investigating the release of endogenous amino acids from slices of rat cerebral cortex, seem to suggest that the therapeutic effect of lamotrigine may be due to inhibition of the release of the excitatory transmitter glutamate (18). Two reviews of lamotrigine have appeared (11,22).

CHEMISTRY AND METHODS OF DETERMINATION

The chemical formula of lamotrigine is 3,5-diamino-6-(2,3-dichlorophenyl)-1,2,4-triazine (Fig. 1). The molecular weight is 256.09, with a pK_a of 5.5. It is a white powder, which is chemically stable. The solubility in water and in ethanol is low, in the range of 1 mg/ml. Plasma concentrations of lamotrigine can be determined by high-performance liquid chromatograpphy (HPLC).

EXPERIMENTAL PHARMACOLOGY

The anticonvulsant action of lamotrigine has been investigated in the maximal electroshock test in mice and rats and in the pentylenetetrazol infusion test in mice (23). Comparing the values for the abolition of hindleg extension in the electroshock test to that of phenytoin, phenobarbital, diazepam, carbamazepine, valproate, and ethosuximide, lamotrigine exhibited the most potent and persistent action in both animal species with oral ED_{50} values of 2.6 and 1.9

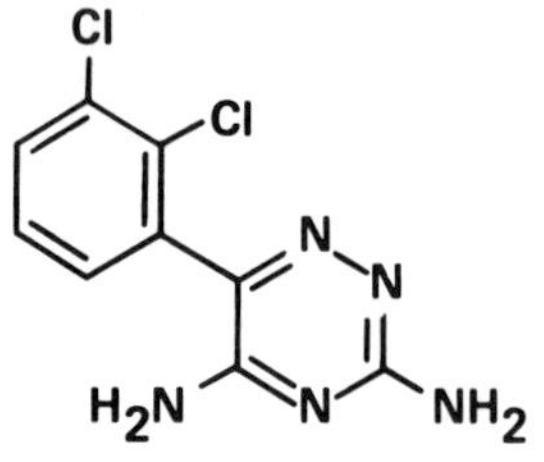

LAMOTRIGINE

FIG. 1. 3,5-Diamino-6-(2,3-dichlorophenyl)-1,2,4-triazine.

mg/kg in mice and rats, respectively. In the pentylenetetrazol test lamotrigine, phenytoin, and carbamazepine demonstrated comparable efficacy (ED_{50} approximately 8 mg/kg), in abolition of the hindleg extension, and were less potent than diazepam (ED_{50} 3.9 mg/kg). None of the drugs prolonged the latency of onset of pentylenetetrazol-induced clonus. However, very high doses of lamotrigine, 160 mg/kg, and of phenytoin reduced the clonus latency. Consequently, the anticonvulsant profile of lamotrigine in these tests seems to be similar to that of phenytoin and carbamazepine. However, differences were found in the visual-evoked after-discharge test in rats, suggesting a wider profile for lamotrigine. In contrast to phenytoin and carbamazepine, which were ineffective, lamotrigine was effective at doses similar to those in the electroshock test.

TOXICOLOGY

Experimental Studies

Lamotrigine has received extensive toxicological evaluation in several animal species (22). In rats and mice the acute lethality of lamotrigine following oral administration demonstrates a 40 to 100-fold separation between anticonvulsant ED_{50} and LD_{50}. Subchronic toxicity (30-day studies) has been investigated in rats and marmosets, using doses of lamotrigine up to 50 mg/kg per day. In marmosets, lamotrigine, 22.5 to 50 mg/kg per day, induced salivation and mild ataxia. Chronic toxicity (3 to 6 months treatment) has been demonstrated in rats and monkeys at doses up to 25 and 20 mg/kg per day, respectively. No toxicity that would preclude oral administration to man was demonstrated. Miller et al. (23) studied behavioral toxicity in mice and found no signs of toxicity with a dose of 80 mg/kg, which corresponds to approximately 30 times the ED_{50}. Doses of 160 mg/kg, however, resulted in signs of acute neurological toxicity (ataxia and jitteriness).

Clinical Studies

A double-blind, placebo-controlled comparative study of the acute central nervous system effects of orally administered lamotrigine, phenytoin, and diazepam in healthy volunteers has been published (6). Diazepam, 10 mg, impaired adaptive tracking, increased body sway, affected saccadic velocity, and smooth pursuit of the eyes, and caused sedation. Phenytoin, 1,000 mg, had similar effects, while 500 mg caused only an insignificant trend toward deterioration. Lamotrigine, 120 mg, failed to differ from placebo in any of these tests. The only effect of lamotrigine, 240 mg, was a significant increase in body sway. The effect of lamotrigine on evoked responses has been compared to that of phenytoin in a double-blind, placebo-controlled study (22). No effect of lamotrigine, 120 and 240 mg, was observed, whereas both 500 and 1,000 mg of phenytoin induced changes in the evoked responses.

Carcinogenicity and Teratogenesis

No mutagenic effects of lamotrigine have been observed in the Ames test and in an *in vitro* cytogenic study in cultured peripheral human lymphocytes (22). No carcino-

TABLE 1. *Pharmacokinetics of lamotrigine*

Absorption	2–4 hr
Protein binding	55%
Volume distribution	1.1 liter/kg
Half-life	15–60 hr[a]
Elimination	first-order
Enzyme induction	0
Proposed therapeutic blood level	1–3 µg/ml

[a] Valproate prolongs the half-life of lamotrigine.

genic effects have been seen in lifetime studies in rats and mice. In rats, mice, and rabbits, lamotrigine has not demonstrated any teratogenic potential when administered orally in doses of 25, 125, and 30 mg/kg per day, respectively, during the period of organogenesis (22).

PHARMACOKINETICS

Investigation of the disposition of lamotrigine in several animal species has demonstrated that the drug is well absorbed after oral ingestion, that it distributes widely throughout the body, that the major route of elimination is via the urine, that considerable variation in plasma half-life exists in different animals, ranging from 2 to 5 hr in dogs to up to 52 hr in monkeys. In addition there seems to be species variation in the metabolism of lamotrigine. In monkeys and in humans it is extensively metabolized and excreted predominantly as a glucuronide conjugate, whereas in rats the metabolism is less extensive, the major metabolic products being an *N*-oxide and a glucuronide conjugate (25). Lamotrigine did not cause enzyme induction with regard to cytochrome P-450 after 30 days of treatment in rats.

Major pharmacokinetic variables of lamotrigine in humans are shown in Table 1. In normal volunteers single-dose and repeated administration of lamotrigine in doses up to 240 mg/day has indicated rapid absorption, time of peak concentration (T_{max}) of 2.75 ± 1.29 hr (mean $\pm$ SD), a

volume of distribution of 1.1 ± 0.12 liter/kg, a protein binding of 55%, linear kinetics, and a half-life of 24 ± 5.7 hr (7,8). No signs of auto-induction of metabolism were detected following 7 days of treatment.

Single-dose pharmacokinetics of lamotrigine has also been studied in epileptic patients during treatment with concomitant antiepileptic medication. Comedication with enzyme-inducing drugs such as carbamazepine and phenytoin reduced the half-life of lamotrigine to 15 hr (range, 7.8–33.3 hr), and concomitant treatment with valproate prolonged the half-life ($T_{1/2}$) to 59 hr (range, 30.5–88.8 hr) (3). Seven days of treatment with lamotrigine in epileptic patients demonstrated a volume of distribution of 1.28 liter/kg ($\pm$ 0.24), a T_{max} of 2.0 hr ($\pm$ 1.2) and a half-life of 14.3 hr ($\pm$ 6.9) in patients being treated with enzyme-inducing antiepileptic drugs. Patients receiving valproate together with enzyme-inducing drugs exhibited a $T_{1/2}$ of 29.6 hr ($\pm$ 10), and blood levels of lamotrigine ranged from 0.8 to 5.2 µg/ml on daily doses of 75 to 250 mg (16).

CLINICAL EFFICACY

Three single-dose or short-term clinical studies of lamotrigine are summarized in (Table 2). Initial testing of the clinical efficacy of lamotrigine in humans involved evaluation, in an open-label study, of the effect of single doses of the drug on photosensitivity (3). All six patients showed a reduction of photosensitivity. Peak blood levels of lamotrigine ranged from 2.1 to 3.45 µg/ml. The side effects were mild and transitory.

Jawad et al. (16) investigated patients with severe epilepsy, irrespective of seizure type, in an open, 1-week dosing study. The doses of lamotrigine were 75 to 250 mg/day, depending upon pretrial determination of the half-life in each patient. A significant reduction ($p < 0.01$) in complex partial sei-

TABLE 2. *Single-dose and short-*

Reference	Subjects and seizure types[a]	Design
Binnie et al., 1986	6 pts. with photosensitive epilepsy (various seizure types)	Open-label trial of LTG, single-dose add-on
Jawad et al., 1987	23 (20) pts. with severe epilepsy (various seizure types)	Open-label trial of LTG, base line & 1 week add-on
Binnie et al., 1987	10 pts. with various seizure types	Double-blind trial of LTG vs placebo crossover, base line & 2 × 1 week add-on

zures was observed, although the decrease in generalized tonic-clonic seizures failed to reach significance. Blood levels of concomitant antiepileptic drugs remained unchanged during lamotrigine treatment. Mean trough lamotrigine levels were 1.7 and 1.8 µg/ml in responders (≥50% reduction) and nonresponders (<50% reduction), respectively. Side effects were mild and consisted mainly of drowsiness.

The first double-blind, placebo-controlled clinical evaluation of lamotrigine was reported in 1987 (2). The design involved crossover and 2 × 1 week of treatment. The trial involved patients with therapy-resistant epilepsies, exhibiting different seizure types, who received lamotrigine, 125 to 300 mg/day, depending upon individual pretrial determination of the half-life of the drug. The seizure frequency was reduced in seven of 10 patients, which represents a strong trend ($p = 0.055$) toward improvement. Blood lamotrigine levels ranged from 0.75 to 3.18 µg/ml, and concentrations of concomitant drugs remained unchanged during the trial. The most frequently observed side effects were drowsiness, ataxia, and headache, resulting in a dose reduction in two patients.

Three long-term controlled trials of lamotrigine have been performed (Table 3). Binnie et al. (4) investigated 34 outpatients with refractory partial epilepsies. The treatment period was 12 weeks and the dose of lamotrigine ranged from 50 to 400 mg/day.

Doses were adjusted by an unblinded investigator with the aim of obtaining trough blood lamotrigine levels of 0.5 to 3.0 µg/ml. The number of partial seizures was reduced in 19 out of 30 patients completing the study ($p < 0.02$). However, only two patients experienced a 50% or greater reduction in seizure frequency. The median reduction in seizure frequency during lamotrigine therapy was 17%. Generalized seizures occurred too infrequently to allow a statistical analysis. Blood levels of concomitant drugs were unchanged throughout the study. The estimated mean trough concentration of lamotrigine in patients responding to the drug was 1.74 µg/ml. There was no significant difference between the frequency of side effects during treatment with placebo or with lamotrigine. Clinical laboratory tests showed no changes attributable to lamotrigine. Only one patient was withdrawn from the trial for a drug-related side effect, a rash occurring during lamotrigine treatment.

Richens et al. (29) studied 24 outpatients with therapy-resistant partial epilepsies. Doses of lamotrigine ranged from 75 to 400 mg/day and were adjusted to obtain a trough lamotrigine level of 1.5 to 2.5 µg/ml. The seizure frequency was reduced in 18 patients ($p < 0.02$), and 14 patients experienced more than a 50% reduction. The median reduction in seizures attributable to lamotrigine was 59%. The incidence of side effects did not differ between placebo and lamotrigine treatment periods. Laboratory *term studies of lamotrigine (LTG)*

Dose	Concomitant treatment	Results	Side effects
120 or 240 mg	Unchanged	Photosensitivity reduced in all pts. (abolished in 2)	Diplopia, drowsiness
75–250 mg/ day	Constant blood levels	Reduction in complex partial seizures[b]	Drowsiness, dizziness, nausea
125–300 mg/ day	Constant blood levels	Seizures reduced in 7 pts.[c] (6 pts. ≥50%)	Ataxia, dizziness, headache

[a] Numbers in parentheses are patients who completed the study.
[b] $p < 0.01$ (Wilcoxon)
[c] $p = 0.055$ (Sign test)

screening demonstrated no abnormalities that could be ascribed to lamotrigine. Of the three drop-outs, only one was directly related to the test drug. However, the side effects observed in this patient during treatment with lamotrigine (ataxia, tiredness, and diplopia) may have been caused by a malignant disease, which proved fatal shortly afterwards. It was not considered to be drug-related.

In the study of Oxley and Sander (24), the dose of lamotrigine ranged from 100 to 300 mg/day and was adjusted to obtain a trough blood level of 0.5 to 3.0 μg/ml. Seizures were reduced in 12 patients ($p > 0.20$). The median reduction amounted to 18%. Only two patients experienced more than a 50% reduction. Blood levels of concomitant antiepileptic drugs remained constant during the study. The incidence of side effects did not differ during lamotrigine treatment compared with the placebo periods. Clinical laboratory test values showed no abnormalities. Eight patients were withdrawn from

TABLE 3. *Controlled clinical trials of lamotrigine*

Reference	Patients and seizure types[a]	Dose	Results	Side effects
Binnie et al., 1988	34 (30) outpts. with refractory partial seizures, some secondarily generalized	50–400 mg/day	Seizure frequency reduced in 19 pts.[b] (2 pts. ≥50%)	Diplopia, drowsiness, dizziness, headache, tiredness
Richens et al., 1988	24 (21) outpts. with refractory partial seizures, some secondarily generalized	75–400 mg/day	Seizure frequency reduced in 18 pts.[b] (14 pts. ≥50%)	Diplopia, drowsiness, tiredness, ataxia, headache
Oxley and Sanders, 1988	26 (18) inpts. with refractory epilepsy (various seizure types)	100–300 mg/day	Seizure frequency reduced in 12 pts.[c] (2 pts. ≥50%)	Diplopia, dizziness, ataxia, headache

[a] Numbers in parentheses are patients who completed the study.
[b] $p < 0.02$ (Wilcoxon)
[c] $p > 0.20$
All studies were double-blind, crossover trials comparing lamotrigine and a placebo as add-on therapy, placebo base line and 2 × 12 weeks.

the study, but none provided clear-cut evidence of lamotrigine-induced toxicity.

CONCLUSIONS

Lamotrigine seems to be an important innovative antiepileptic compound with an interesting mechanism of action. For many years, development of new antiepileptic drugs has focused on augmenting inhibition, mainly through the GABA system (20). Recently, however, there is recognition that decreasing excitation might be a fruitful alternative (21). In epileptic animals, blocking excitatory transmission results in an anticonvulsant response (9,21). Lamotrigine is the first drug in which clinical studies indicate that the antiepileptic effect may be caused by a decrease in excitation (18).

Studies of the clinical efficacy of lamotrigine seem to substantiate the effect, even in the treatment of therapy-resistant epilepsy. The apparent inconsistency between the results of the three controlled trials may be ascribed to the fact that one study (24) recruited only inpatients with refractory epilepsies, and the other two studies involved outpatients with intractable epilepsy. The difference in severity of epilepsy may explain the nonsignificant result of the former study, since it must be assumed that it contained the most severe cases of epilepsy. Furthermore, in comparison with other antiepileptic drugs, it may indicate an inferior antiepileptic potency of lamotrigine, proportional to that of carbamazepine and valproate, both of which have been demonstrated to reduce seizure frequency significantly, even in inpatients with severe epilepsies (12,13,28,30). However, the studies of other antiepileptic drugs were all conducted during the 1970s and involved patients not receiving either valproate or carbamazepine. Clearly, lamotrigine was tested in a patient population already receiving these drugs as part of their concomitant medication. However, despite the small though significant seizure reduction in the Dutch study (4) and the presence of only a nonsignificant trend toward efficacy in the Chalfont investigation (24), lamotrigine appears to have an antiepileptic effect combined with apparently limited toxicity. The presence of only mild to moderate side effects raises the question of whether the doses used in the clinical trials might be suboptimal. It seems desirable to pursue further the efficacy of this drug in the treatment of less severe cases of epilepsy, involving more flexible dosing, with the aim of comparing lamotrigine to standard antiepileptic drugs. Information on the antiepileptic profile of lamotrigine with regard to different seizure types and/or epileptic syndromes is not currently available and should be investigated.

CONVERSION

Conversion factor:

$$CF = \frac{1000}{mol. \ wt.} = \frac{1000}{256.09} = 3.90$$

Conversion:

$$(\mu g/ml) \times 3.90 = (\mu moles/liter)$$

$$(\mu moles/liter) \div 3.90 = (\mu g/ml)$$

REFERENCES

1. Baxter, M. G., Miller, A. A., and Webster, R. A. (1973): Some studies on the convulsant action of folic acid. *Brit. J. Pharmacol.*, 48:350.
2. Binnie, C. D., Bientema, D. J., Debets, R. M. C., van Emde Boas, W., Meijer, J. W. A., Meinardi, H., Peck, A. W., Westendorp, A.-M. and Yuen, W. C. (1987): Seven day administration of lamotrigine in epilepsy: placebo-controlled add-on trial. *Epilepsy Res.* 1:202–208.
3. Binnie, C. D., van Emde Boas, W., Kasteleijn-Nolste-Trenite, D. G. A., de Korte, R. A., Meijer, J. W. A., Meinardi, H., Miller, A. A., Overweg, J., Peck, A. W., van Wieringen, A., and Yuen, W. C. (1986): Acute effects of lamotrigine (BW 430C) in persons with epilepsy. *Epilepsia*, 27:248–254.
4. Binnie, C. D., van Wieringen, A., Debets, R. M. C., Engelsman, M., and Overweg, J. (1988): A randomised double blind placebo controlled crossover

trial of lamotrigine in patients with treatment resistant partial epilepsy. Wellcome Research Laboratories, *internal report.*

5. Bowe, T. R., Cornish, E. J., and Dawson, M. (1971): Evaluation of folic acid supplements in children taking phenytoin. *Dev. Med. Child. Neurol.*, 13:343–354.

6. Cohen, A. F., Ashby, L., Crowley, D., Land, G. S., Peck, A. W., and Miller, A. A. (1985): Lamotrigine (BW 430C), a potential anticonvulsant. Effect on the central nervous system in comparison with phenytoin and diazepam. *Br. J. Clin. Pharmacol.*, 20:619–629.

7. Cohen, A. F., Fowle, A. S. E., Land, G. S., and Bye, A. (1985): BW 430C—A new anticonvulsant. Pharmacokinetics in normal man. *Epilepsia*, 25:656.

8. Cohen, A. F., Land, G. S., Breimer, D. D., Yuen, W. C., Winton, C., and Peck, A. W. (1987): Lamotrigine, a new anticonvulsant: Pharmacokinetics in normal humans. *Clin. Pharmacol. Ther.*, 42:535–541.

9. Croucher, M. J., Collins, J. F., and Meldrum, B. S. (1982): Anticonvulsant action of excitatory amino acid antagonists. *Science,* 216:899–901.

10. Gibberd, F. B., Nicholls, A., and Wright, M. G. (1981): The influence of folic acid on the frequency of epileptic attacks. *Europ. J. Clin. Pharmacol.*, 19:57–60.

11. Gram, L. (1987): Lamotrigine. In: *Epilepsy: Progress in Treatment,* edited by M. Dam, S. I. Johannessen, B. Nilsson, and M. Sillanpää, pp. 269–271. John Wiley and Sons, Chichester.

12. Gram, L., Flachs, H., Würtz-Jørgensen, A., Parnas, J., and Andersen, B. (1979): Sodium valproate, serum levels and clinical effect. A controlled study. *Epilepsia*, 20:303–312.

13. Gram, L., Rasmussen, K. E., Flachs, H., Würtz-Jørgensen, A., Sommerbeck, K. W., and Løhren, V. (1977): Valproate sodium: A controlled clinical trial including monitoring of serum levels. *Epilepsia*, 18:141–148.

14. Grant, R. H. E., and Stores, O. P. R. (1970): Folic acid and folate-deficient patients with epilepsy. *Br. Med. J.*, 4:644–648.

15. Hommes, O. R., and Obbens, E. A. M. T. (1972) The epileptogenic action of na-folate in the rat. *J. Neurol. Sci.,* 16:271–281.

16. Jawad, C. D., Yuen, W. C., Peck, A. W., Hamilton, M. J., Oxley, J. R., and Richens, A. (1987): Lamotrigine: Single-dose pharmacokinetics and initial 1 week experience in refractory epilepsy. *Epilepsy Res.*, 1:194–201.

17. Jensen, O. N., and Olesen, O. V. (1970): Subnormal serum folate due to anticonvulsive therapy. *Arch. Neurol.*, 22:181–182.

18. Leach, M., Harden, C. M., and Miller, A. A. (1986): Pharmacological studies of lamotrigine, a novel potential antiepileptic drugs: II. Neurochemical studies of the mechanism of action. *Epilepsia*, 27:490–497.

19. Mattson, R. H., Gallagher, B. B., Reynolds, E. H., and Glas, D. (1973): Folate therapy in epilepsy. *Arch. Neurol.*, 29:78–81.

20. Meldrum, B. S. (1978): Gamma-aminobutyric acid and the search for new anticonvulsant drugs. *Lancet,* 2:304–306.

21. Meldrum, B. S. (1984): Amino acid neurotransmitters and new approaches to anticonvulsant drugs. *Epilepsia*, 25 (Suppl. 2):S140–S149.

22. Miller, A. A., Sawyer, D. A., Roth, B., Peck, A. W., Leach, M. J., Wheatley, P. L., Parsons, D. N., and Morgan, R. J. I. (1986): Lamotrigine. In: *New Anticonvulsant Drugs,* edited by B. S. Meldrum and R. J. Porter. pp. 165–177. John Libbey, London.

23. Miller, A. A., Whetley, P. L., Sawyer, D. A., Baxter, M. G., and Roth B. (1986): Pharmacological studies on lamotrigine, a novel potential antiepileptic drug: I. Anticonvulsant profile in mice and rats. *Epilepsia*, 27:483–489.

24. Oxley, J., and Sander, J. (1988): A randomised double blind placebo controlled crossover add-on trial of lamotrigine in patients with treatment resistant seizures. Wellcome Research Laboratories, *internal report.*

25. Parson, D. M., and Miles, D. W. (1984): Metabolic studies with BW 430C. *Epilepsia*, 25:655.

26. Ralston, A. J., Snaith, R. P., and Hinley, J. B. (1970): Effect of folic acid on fit frequency and behaviour in epileptics on anticonvulsants. *Lancet,* 1:867–868.

27. Reynolds, E. H., Milner, G., Matthews, D. M., and Chanarin, I. (1966): Anticonvulsant therapy, megaloblastic haemopoiesis and folic acid metabolism. *Quart. J. Med.,* 35:521–537.

28. Richens, A., and Ahmad, S. (1975): Controlled trial of sodium valproate in severe epilepsy. *Br. Med. J.,* 4:255–256.

29. Richens, A., Jawad, S., and Wroe, S. (1988): A randomised double blind placebo controlled crossover add-on trial of lamotrigine in patients with treatment resistant seizures. Wellcome Research Laboratories, *internal report.*

30. Rodin, E. A., Rim, C. S., and Rennick, P. M. (1974): The effect of carbamazepine on patients with psychomotor epilepsy: Results of a double-blind study. *Epilepsia*, 15:547–561.

Antiepileptic Drugs, Third Edition, edited by
R. Levy, R. Mattson, B. Meldrum,
J. K. Penry, and F. E. Dreifuss.
Raven Press, Ltd., New York © 1989.

70

Potential Antiepileptic Drugs

Stiripentol

Pierre Loiseau and Bernard Duche

INTRODUCTION

A study of the sedative and anticonvul-sant properties of a series of 38 1-alkoxy-aryl-3-alkyl-1-alkene-3-ol, and of the cor-responding ketones enabled Astoin et al. (1978) to select five compounds whose psy-chopharmacological effects were further studied. One of them, 4,4-dimethyl-1-[(3,4 methylenedioxy) phenyl]-1-penten-3-ol, demonstrated important anticonvulsant properties in rodents and a low level of tox-icity. This substituted phenol, stiripentol (STP), is structurally unrelated to other antiepileptic drugs. Stiripentol anticonvul-sant activity was documented in several an-imal models. An old-fashioned clinical trial was performed in France in the 1970s. It was an open study, without rigorous guide-lines, without knowledge of the peculiar pharmacokinetic profile of the drug, and with too low a daily dosage (300 mg/day). Nonetheless, the addition of STP to stan-dard anticonvulsant therapy in 135 outpa-tients was well tolerated and improved some patients.

Extensive pharmacokinetic studies have been done since 1982, allowing better uti-lization of the drug in complex partial and refractory absence seizures.

CHEMISTRY AND METHODS OF DETERMINATION

Stiripentol is 4,4-dimethyl-1-(3,4 methy-lenedioxy) phenyl]-1-penten-3-ol (Fig. 1). It has a molecular weight of 234. It is obtained by reduction of the corresponding ketone by means of potassium borohydride. The ketone is obtained by condensing piperonal and pinaclone (3,3-dimethyl-2-butanone) in a basic medium. Stiripentol is soluble in ethanol and acetone, moderately soluble in chloroform, and insoluble in water. The molecule is stable under normal conditions.

A high-performance liquid chromatogra-phy HPLC method is used to assay STP in blood. After extraction with ether, the chro-matographic separation is achieved with a reversed-phase column and detection with an ultraviolet detector at a wavelength of 254 nm (9).

ANIMAL PHARMACOLOGY

The general pharmacological properties have been reported by Astoin et al. (1). In the anesthetized dog receiving STP, 2.5 or 5 mg/kg i.v., no significant changes were seen in the different hemodynamic param-eters of the systemic circulation. After in-

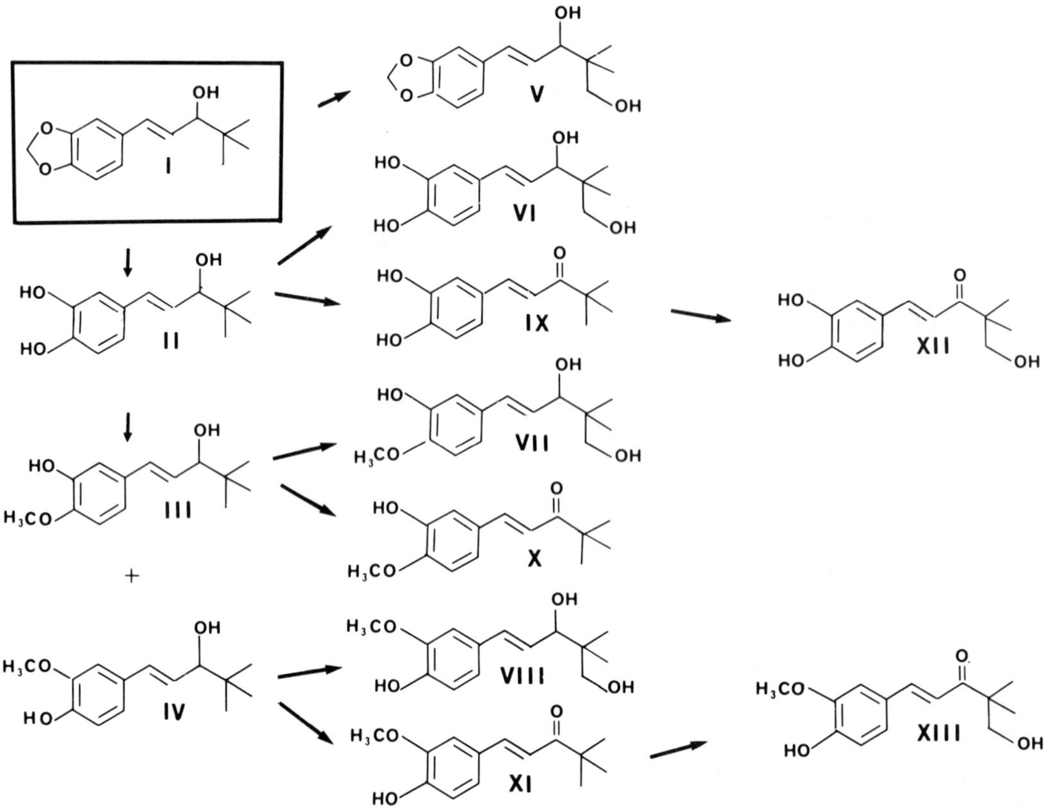

FIG. 1. Metabolites (II–XIII) and metabolic pathways of stiripentol (1).

traperitoneal administration of 100 mg/kg, bleeding and clotting times were unaffected. Capillary permeability and capillary resistance were also unaffected by intraperitoneal injection of 200 mg/kg.

Oral administration of 200 mg/kg for 4 days in the prepubertal male and female rat was followed by a very slight decrease in weight of the thyroid gland in males and a slight decrease in adrenal weight in females; these changes were not physiologically significant. There was no significant change in urine output in the rat following STP 50, 100, or 200 mg/kg i.p. or 250 or 750 mg/kg p.o. There was no action on bile flow following intraduodenal administration of 100 mg/kg. There was no development of gastric ulceration in the rat following administration of 200 mg/kg p.o. Finally, there was no

anti-inflammatory action on the paw induced by carrageenan in the rat receiving STP, 600 mg/kg p.o.

Study of STP actions on the central nervous system show that 200 mg/kg administered intraperitoneally in mice or rats increased the duration of barbiturate narcosis, decreased the amount of spontaneous movements, and rendered mice less aggressive. Rotorod-test and traction-test performances remained unchanged.

Anticonvulsant Activity

The anticonvulsant activity of STP was first demonstrated in mice after injection of pentylenetetrazol (PTZ) and in rats with supramaximal electroshock (1). Further studies were performed in different species. Stiripentol produces a dose-related inhibition of electrically induced convulsions in rats (21). The ED_{50} of injected STP was approximately 240 mg/kg intraperitoneally. The recovery time was much lower in treated rats than in controls and was dose-related (controls, 278 sec; STP, 170 sec at 250 mg/kg).

Stiripentol antagonizes chemically induced convulsions. Administered after intraperitoneal injection of PTZ in mice it produced a dose-related protection against death. The ED_{50} of intraperitoneally injected STP for PTZ-induced convulsions was 200 mg/kg and at this dose the mean time before death was 2.5 times longer than in the control animals (21).

Stiripentol given orally in rabbits 30 min after a first i.v. injection of PTZ reduced the formation of PTZ-specific paroxysmal waves and the paroxysms did not increase after a second and third injection. Almost all of the control animals experienced motor reactions after the second or third injection. In contrast, none of the STP-treated animals developed convulsions or tonic spasms (21). Stiripentol efficacy was investigated in intravenous PTZ-infusion seizures in the rat. Anticonvulsant response was expressed by the ratio of threshold doses of PTZ required to elicit forelimb clonus after administering STP to it during the predrug state. Stiripentol exhibited definite anticonvulsant properties in this seizure model, and 200 mg/kg protected 45% of mice against death due to bicuculline (21). Stiripentol has little effect on strychnine-induced convulsions. Only 20% of mice were protected against death with 200 mg/kg of STP (21).

Acute efficacy tests of STP were conducted in an alumina-gel rhesus monkey model of partial epilepsy (12,14). The paradigm consisted of a challenge to the convulsant 4-deoxypyridoxine hydrochloride (4-DP). A 150 mg/kg dose of 4-DP activating the epileptogenic focus in the model elicited a series of secondarily generalized tonic-clonic seizures with a 5 to 35 min interseizure interval. In different sequential treatments, the convulsant was challenged after the first seizure with either the solvent (propylene glycol and ethanol) or one of three doses of STP. The data were compared with those obtained with valproate. Stiripentol at the highest dose (resulting in a plasma level of 35 µg/ml) performed comparably to valproate by delaying the onset of seizures but did not eliminate them as had phenytoin, carbamazepine, phenobarbital, and diazepam in similar earlier studies. Rhesus monkeys were rendered epileptic by alumina-gel cortical injections. They presented infrequent spontaneous seizures but frequent interictal paroxysmal discharges. In two separate prolonged-dose studies (13,14), STP was given in a multiple-dose regimen by gastric catheter for 4 weeks at different doses to test the drug effectiveness against EEG interictal spikes. The doses of STP were adjusted to bring its plasma concentrations to 24 to 28 µg/ml in one study and 12 to 14 µg/ml in the other study. Stiripentol at 12 to 14 µg/ml significantly reduced EEG interictal spike rates, strongly with the higher dose, similarly but to a lesser extent with the low dosage. An irreversible pharmacological effect (carry-over effect) was found, the postdrug discharge rates being lower than the predrug base-line frequencies.

Mechanism of Action

The anticonvulsant activity of STP might involve a direct or indirect GABAergic mechanism (23). In the rat brain, the drug stimulates certain enzymes specifically (beta-hydroxybutyrate dehydrogenase) and inhibits other ones (GABAtransaminase, sulfatase) (24). ^{3}H-labeled STP has a distribution similar to that of endogenous GABA, i.e., in peripheral molecular layer and pyramidal cells of the cortex and in the cerebellum (Purkinje cells, neuroglial cells, and Golgi cells) (25). The hypothesis was tested using ratioactive binding (21). Stiripentol showed no affinity for GABA$_A$, GABA$_B$, glycinergic, or benzodiazepine receptors. On the other hand, it inhibited the synaptosomal uptake of glycine and GABA in concentrations of STP compatible with pharmacological activity. The inhibition might be responsible for the increase in cerebral concentration of GABA in the mouse brain 30 min after intraperitoneal administration of 300 mg/kg of STP (24).

These neurochemical studies suggest that the anticonvulsant activity of STP is not due to a direct activation of the two main inhibitor neurotransmitters or of benzodiazepine receptors. Stiripentol increases the cerebral GABA concentration by inhibition of its synaptosomal uptake and its metabolic turnover. The mechanism of action of STP is clearly different from that of valproic acid, but in view of experimental data (14,22) it could share the same antiabsence activity.

TOXICOLOGY

Toxicity in Animals

After a single dose of STP the initial determination of LD$_{50}$ was done on male Swiss mice and male Wistar rats (1). Stiripentol was injected intraperitoneally in the form of a suspension in 1% carboxymethyl cellulose aqueous solution. Further determinations were done in the male and female mouse and rat, using the oral or intravenous route (21). The toxicity of single-dose administration of STP is very low after oral administration, >5,000 mg/kg in mouse and >3,000 mg/kg in rat, i.p. route; 15,000 mg/kg in rat and mouse and 75 mg/kg in mouse when given intravenously.

The chronic oral toxicity of STP was studied in the male and female rat. (M. Maillet, D. A. Albert, 1974, document on file).

A daily dose of 30, 60, or 300 mg/kg was administered for 6 months. Animals receiving this treatment did not show any abnormalities other than a slightly reduced weight gain in the females treated with the higher doses.

In a long-term toxicology study, beagle dogs were subjected to daily administration of 25, 62.5, or 156.25 mg/kg STP for 13 months. No difference was seen between the control animals and the dogs treated with the low dose. Slight changes were seen in liver function with the higher doses, although no notable corresponding histological abnormalities were observed. Some microhemorrhages were seen with the highest dose.

In the pregnant mouse at doses of 50, 200, or 800 mg/kg/day, there was no evidence of fetal toxicity nor any effect on the internal and skeletal morphology of the fetus (M. Maillet, D. A. Albert, 1974, document on file). At the same doses in the pregnant rabbit, no teratogenic effect was seen and STP had no toxic influence on the fetus; at the two highest doses there was a certain degree of toxicity for the mothers with an abortifacient action but with no feto-toxic effect.

The only effects on peri- and postnatal development in the rat were a reduction in weight gain of the mothers in the highest-dose group (800 mg/kg/day) and in the mean weight of the newborn at the time of littering. After treatment was stopped, growth in the offspring of this group occurred normally. It can be concluded that STP has no toxic effect during the peri- and postnatal period in the rat.

The potential mutagenic effect of STP was evaluated by means of two tests, the Ames test using *Salmonella typhimurium in vitro* and the micronucleus technique in the mouse. Stiripentol showed no sign of any genetic activity in either of the two tests. It can be considered free of any mutagenic potential under the conditions of these two tests. The chemical structure of the molecule does not suggest any carcinogenic potential (i.e., absence of nitrogen in the molecule) and the mutagenicity studies revealed no problem.

Toxicity in Man

Without double-blind trials of STP, a precise evaluation of its adverse effects is very difficult. More than 100 patients received the drug during the last 5 years, sometimes for long periods (maximum, 4 years). In general, symptoms or signs of toxicity were seldom observed and, to the best of our knowledge, only six patients dropped out because of apparent toxicity.

Neurotoxicity

Stiripentol usually had a beneficial psychotropic effect, but a few patients developed adverse reactions. Six normal adult men received STP for 14 days (15). They performed memory and attentional tasks at day 1 and day 14 (Rey test, Violon and Seyll battery for learning and retrieval, Zazzo test for attention). No detrimental effect was found except for a mild (7%) reduction in verbal learning score. Furthermore, the performance in the more complex task of attention improved significantly after STP treatment.

During a pharmacokinetic study on polymedicated patients, five subjects underwent memory and attentional tasks before and after 30 days of exposure to STP (5). No significant change was noted in scores for the memory tasks and for the one-sign Zazzo attentional task. This result was somewhat surprising in light of the fact that the plasma level of other anticonvulsants rose during the trial. For example, phenytoin levels in three patients were 8, 8.5, and 12.5 μg/ml at day 1, and 18, 17, and 24.5 μg/ml, respectively, at day 30. Furthermore, a significant improvement was noted for the more complex two-sign attention task. This task involves both memory and

attention. An improvement due to retesting (practice effect) was unlikely since the one-sign-task score remained unaffected.

A neuropsychological evaluation of STP was undertaken in 11 patients with either drug-resistant epilepsy (nine patients) or toxic effects of anticonvulant drugs (two patients) (15). Several motor, perceptual, and attentional tasks were performed before and after STP administration for 2 months. Stiripentol was added to previous drugs, which were maintained at constant plasma levels. Pretrial side effects (mainly drowsiness) decreased or disappeared in seven of nine patients who became more alert. An improvement in the performances of two tasks requiring sustained attention was noted. No significant difference was found in the other tasks.

At the end of a pilot study (18), each patient was asked which therapeutic regimen he or she preferred. Stiripentol in monotherapy was preferred by 19 out of 21 patients and by all the patients in bitherapy for reasons of subjective well-being and feelings of improvement in affective and cognitive functions. Similar remarks were made by patients and patients' relatives after long-term STP administration (17).

In normal subjects as well as epileptic patients, the most frequent symptom reported has been a mild dose-dependent insomnia. Drowsiness has rarely been noted except in comedicated patients. In these cases, it was due to a rise of phenytoin or phenobarbital levels. However, three acute psychotic reactions have been reported (17,18). One female patient presented acutely with visual hallucinations, delirium, and agitation with self-inflicted injury when she was taking 500 mg of carbamazepine and 2,700 mg of STP daily (levels of 8.4 μg/ml and 8.7 μg/ml, respectively). This patient had antecedents of mild psychiatric disturbances. Another patient, after 30 weeks of therapy with 2,700 mg/day of STP and 150 mg/day of phenytoin developed visual hallucinations and delirium. The plasma phenytoin level was 41 μg/

ml but there were no cerebellar or vestibular signs. The third patient developed a manic agitation after 9 weeks of STP exposure at a daily dose of 1,800 mg. In all three patients, STP was stopped and normality regained in a few days.

Digestive and Cardiovascular Toxicity

Gastric or abdominal discomfort, anorexia, nausea, and vomiting have been reported in a few patients. They usually occur within the first few days of STP administration and are of a benign, dose-related nature. However, STP had to be stopped in some patients.

In normal volunteers and epileptic patients, STP administration caused no detectable effect on the cardiovascular system as measured by blood pressure, heart rate, or EKG. Each patient had repeated laboratory tests (hematology, blood chemistry, urinalysis) during STP exposure. No significant treatment-related alteration was noted.

PHARMACOKINETICS

Absorption

The kinetics of STP were investigated after oral and intraperitoneal administration in rhesus monkeys (9). Stiripentol was dissolved in 100% polyethylene glycol 400 at a concentration of 100 mg/ml for oral administration. A suspension was prepared in 2% carboxymethylene cellulose at a concentration of 40 mg/ml for intraperitoneal use. Absorption of STP was incomplete by both routes of administration. The mean ($\pm$ SD) fraction of the dose absorbed was 0.21 ($\pm$ 0.15) after oral administration and 0.28 ($\pm$ 0.13) by the intraperitoneal route with a 40 mg dose. There was no difference in bioavailability between the two routes at 80 mg. This low bioavailability suggested either insolubility or a hepatic first-pass ef-

fect. The latter was demonstrated, but there also appears to be a solubility problem.

Distribution

Single-Dose Studies in Animals and Man

An i.v. administration of ^{3}H-STP was performed in Wistar rats (20). In the blood, the concentration-time curve demonstrated a two-phased elimination. In a first phase, radioactivity decreased rapidly ($T_{1/2}$ = 1 hr). A much slower decrease was noted during a second phase lasting more than 24 hr ($T_{1/2}$ = 13 hr).

The kinetic behavior of STP after i.v. administration was more extensively established in the rhesus monkey (10). Stiripentol was dissolved in 100% polyethylene 400 at a concentration of 100 mg/ml. Following discrete i.v. doses (40, 80, and 120 mg), the disappearance of STP from plasma was multiphasic in all monkeys at all three dose levels. These data did not fit equations corresponding to usual compartment models. Noncompartmental methods were therefore used to determine the plasma clearance (Cl), the volume of distribution at steady state (V_{dss}), and the mean residence time (MRT). Mean plasma Cl ($\pm$ SD) at 40, 80, and 120 mg were 1.10 ($\pm$ 0.07), 0.92 ($\pm$ 0.08), and 0.86 ($\pm$ 0.15) liters/hr/kg, respectively. The differences among Cl values obtained at the three doses were statistically significant, suggesting dose dependency in the elimination of STP. Mean ($\pm$ SD) V_{dss} values at 40, 80, and 120 mg were 1.10 ($\pm$ 0.35), 1.01 ($\pm$ 0.30), and 1.01 ($\pm$ 0.32) liter/kg, respectively. Obviously, there was no dose dependency in this parameter. Neither was there any dose dependency for MRT, which was 0.32, 0.29, and 0.35 hr, respectively. The large volume of distribution indicated that STP distributes extravascularly with a high degree of tissue binding. The decrease of Cl with dose provided evidence of nonlinearity.

The pharmacokinetics of STP after single-dose oral administration was investigated in six healthy men (2). Each subject received one dose of 300, 600, or 1,200 mg STP in powder form and another 600 mg in solution. Plasma concentration-time curves showed a multiphasic elimination as observed in monkeys, with a much slower decrease after 8 hr. The average oral clearance was 1.3 to 1.8 liter/hr/kg and the average mean residence time was 4 hr, without any significant difference among the three doses. The average peak concentrations ($\pm$ SD) were 0.83 $\pm$ 0.39, 1.60 $\pm$ 0.57, and 3.43 $\pm$ 0.77 after single doses of 300, 600, or 1,200 mg, respectively. The corresponding mean peak times ($\pm$ SD) were 1.25 $\pm$ 0.87, 1.5 $\pm$ 0.77, and 1.58 $\pm$ 1.27. The bioavailability of the solution form relative to the same dose in powder form was 21 $\pm$ 9%. This incomplete absorption can be explained by precipitation of STP in a crystalline form in the aqueous environment of the gastrointestinal tract. No metabolite was detectable in the plasma.

Multiple-Dose Kinetics in Normal Man

Each of six healthy male volunteers received a 300 mg oral dose on day 1, and four daily doses of STP (1,200 mg/day) from day 2 to day 8 (2). There was a nearly eightfold decrease in oral clearance of STP between day 1 and day 8, indicating that STP accumulated in a nonlinear fashion during multiple dosing. The fraction of dose metabolized through conjugation and methylenedioxy-ring opening increased 183% and 49%, respectively, but the formation clearance for all pathways decreased. These findings suggested that the steady-state plasma- level–to–dose ratio of STP will increase with the daily dose and that the time to reach steady state will also increase with dose.

In another study (4), Michaelis-Menten kinetic parameters for STP were assessed in six other healthy men. Stiripentol was administered p.o. incrementally three times a day in doses of 200, 400, and then 600 mg for consecutive periods of 3, 4, and 7 days, respectively. Stiripentol steady-state concentration at the three administration levels increased more than proportionally with dosage. An increase from 600 to 1,200 mg/day resulted in a 309% increase in average C_{SS}, and from 1,200 to 1,800 mg/day in a 79% increase in average C_{SS}. The mean oral clearance of STP $\pm$ SD at 600 mg/day (1.090 $\pm$ 624 liter/day) was significantly greater than at 1,200 mg/day (506 $\pm$ 219 liter/day) or 1,800 mg/day (405 $\pm$ 151 liter/day). Average steady-state concentrations predicted from individually determined V_m (average velocity of conversion of STP to its metabolites) and K_m (Michaelis constant) parameters were in good agreement with experimentally observed levels, indicating that the kinetics of STP are of the Michaelis-Menten type. The mean ($\pm$ SD) V_m, K_m, and V_m-to-K_m ratio were 2.299 $\pm$ .490 mg/day, 2.20 $\pm$ 1.28 mg/liter, and 1.24 $\pm$ .837 liter/day, respectively.

Multiple-Dose Kinetics in Epileptic Patients

Since clinical use of STP would involve its administration in polytherapy, it was necessary to characterize its kinetics in comedicated epileptic patients. Six adult patients with an uncontrolled localization-related epilepsy and treated with a combination of two or more antiepileptic drugs received STP in a thrice daily regimen with six dosage increments: 600, 1,200, 1,500, 1,800, 2,100, and 2,400 mg/day (5). Steady-state levels at 600, 1,200, and 2,400 mg/day increased in a nonlinear fashion, indicating Michaelis-Menten kinetics. An increase in dosing rate from 600 to 1,200 mg/day resulted in a 253% rise in C_{SS} and from 1,200 mg/day to 2,400 mg/day in a 397% rise in C_{SS}. Average oral clearance of STP ($\pm$ SD) at 600 mg/day was 41.5 $\pm$ 23.4 liter/

day/kg, greater than that at 1,200 mg/day (20.3 ± 8.8 liter/day/kg) or 2,400 mg/day (8.5 ± 3.8 liter/day/kg). A large intersubject variability in clearance at all dosages was noted (300% to 400%). The apparent *in vivo* Michaelis-Menten parameters were determined from three mean steady-state concentrations. The average (± SD) V_m, K_m, and V_m-to-K_m were 49.3 ± 13.1 mg/kg/day, 1.35 ± 1.08 mg/liter, and 50.2 ± 27.5 liter/day, respectively, with less intersubject variability in V_m (coefficient of variation: 27%) than in K_m (coefficient of variation: 80%). These figures differ notably from those obtained in healthy volunteers. The metabolism of STP is induced by the conventional antiepileptic drugs (phenytoin, carbamazepine, phenobarbital). The mean oral clearance of STP (± SD) at 1,200 mg/day was 300% those reported in normal subjects receiving the same dose (0.85 ± 0.37 liter/kg/hr vs 0.28 ± 0.08 liter/kg/hr). V_m was larger and K_m smaller in comedicated patients than in normal subjects. The values of V_m suggest that the maximal elimination rate for STP in comedicated epileptic patients is approximately 3,000 mg/day.

Protein Binding and STP in Tissues

The plasma protein binding of STP, measured by equilibrium dialysis, was very high—more than 99% in monkeys and in man—and was concentration-dependent in monkeys (9).

The radioactive constituents were measured in the liver, lung, kidney, and central nervous system of Wistar rats following i.v. administration of ^{3}H-STP (20). The liver accumulated very rapidly (peaking at 30 min) the highest radioactivity, followed by the kidneys. So, STP appears to be rapidly metabolized in the liver and excreted by the kidney. In the central nervous system, a maximum radioactivity was noted in the cerebellum.

Metabolism

In the study by Pieri et al. (20), two main metabolites were identified in urine of rats. The metabolites resulted from a break of the methylenedioxy ring. Only one of these metabolites (methoxyl metabolite) had anticonvulsant activity [on the electroshock but not the pentylenetetrazol (PTZ) seizure model].

In monkeys (9), less than 2% of the drug was found unchanged in urine, suggesting that STP is eliminated by metabolism. The mean fraction of the dose excreted as glucuronide was 32% to 35%. Glucuronidization of STP represents a significant elimination pathway. The other metabolic pathways resulting from the opening of the methylenedioxy ring are minor. Two percent of the dose was excreted as a *p*-hydroxy metabolite and 2% as an *m*-hydroxy metabolite. These last two metabolites were not detectable in plasma. The *p*-hydroxy metabolite does not contribute significantly to the pharmacological activity.

In healthy men (2), only traces of STP were excreted unchanged in urine. Around 20% of the dose was excreted in urine in 12 hr as conjugate, without significant differences among the three oral doses (300, 600, and 1,200 mg). However, for the minor metabolites resulting from the ring opening of the methylenedioxy moiety (*p*-hydroxy and *m*-hydroxy metabolites), also excreted as conjugates, a significant difference was found between the 300 and 1,200 mg doses, suggesting dose dependency in the metabolism of STP by this pathway.

Two studies were undertaken to elucidate the metabolic fate of STP in man (8,19). Thirteen metabolites were detected in urine and identified by gas chromatography-mass spectrometry (GC-MS) analysis. The structures of nine metabolites were confirmed subsequently by synthesis. Their nature revealed five distinct metabolic pathways (Fig. 1).

1. Conjugation with glucuronic acid (metabolite I, 22% to 30% of the dose)
2. Opening of the methylenedioxy ring, giving a dihydroxy compound (II, 11% to 14%) which is further metabolized
3. *O*-methylation of catechol metabolites at the 3 and 4 positions (III and IV, 17–24%)
4. Hydroxylation of the *t*-butyl group, minor direct pathway (V, 1%) or further metabolism of the hydroxy compound (VI, 3–6%) or of metabolites III and IV (VII and VIII, 5%)
5. Conversion of the allylic alcohol sidechain to the isomeric 3-pentanone structure (IX, 7–9%) or of metabolites III and IV (X and XI, 0.4%).

Two additional metabolites were found which result from a combination of methylenedioxy-ring opening, gamma-butyl-hydroxylation and isomerization of the 3-pentanone (XII and XIII, 5–9%). Metabolites of STP excreted into urine over 12 hr accounted for the majority (73%) of an acute dose, whereas a further 18% was recovered in feces as the unchanged drug.

It has been established that several methylenedioxyphenyl derivatives inhibit the microsomal oxidation of drugs. The opening of the methylenedioxy ring to generate catechol derivatives probably accounts for the inhibitory effects of STP upon the oxidative metabolism of other antiepileptic drugs.

Drug Interactions

Stiripentol is a broad-spectrum inhibitor of drug metabolism. It decreases the clearance and therefore increases the plasma level of simultaneously prescribed drugs, but with an interdrug and intersubject variability.

Phenytoin

Stiripentol had a marked effect on phenytoin (PHT) levels in all five subjects who received it (5). Symptoms of PHT toxicity occurred in the first two patients. In the three other subjects who received PHT, its dosage was systematically reduced to prevent toxicity. Despite this reduction in dosage, plasma PHT concentrations rose. A dose-dependent inhibitory effect by STP was hypothesized: a 38% reduction in PHT clearance occurred at 1,200 mg/day and a 78% reduction occurred at 2,400 mg/day. However, determinations at 1,200 mg were made after only 9 days of STP intake, and a new steady state was probably not achieved. In subsequent clinical trials, the daily dosage of PHT had to be reduced in all the patients to maintain approximately constant plasma PHT levels. An interindividual variability was noted, necessitating a wide range of dosage reductions (from 25–57%, mean, 45%) (16).

Carbamazepine

In the above-mentioned study (5), STP reduced the clearance of carbamazepine (CBZ) in the two patients taking this drug. In one of them, it fell from 209 liter/day on day 1 to 60.8 liter/day on day 30. Plasma CBZ content rose from 3.83 μg/ml on day 1 to 6.26 μg/ml on day 9 and, although the dose of CBZ was decreased to 600 mg/day on day 11, its level reached 9.86 μg/ml on day 30. The STP-CBZ interaction was investigated by measuring the clearance of CBZ. In eight patients before and after 10 weeks of STP treatment (2,400–3,000 mg/day). Mean ($\pm$ SD) CBZ clearance decreased from 6.1 ($\pm$ 1.1) to 2.0 ($\pm$ 0.7)/liter/hr (8). An interindividual variability in the increase in plasma content was also noted. A 12.5% to 50% reduction of CBZ was necessary to maintain a constant plasma content (16).

Stiripentol acts by inhibiting the formation of carbamazepine epoxide. In monkeys, the CBZ epoxide-to-CBZ ratio decreased from 0.26 to 0.06 when STP was added and increased to 0.26 when STP was removed (11). In man, a low-value of the CBZ epoxide-to-CBZ ratio (mean $\pm$ SD, 0.06 ± 0.016) was found (7,8). Two studies were undertaken to determine whether STP affects the formation and/or the elimination of the epoxide (6). In study I, STP was administered (1,000–3,000 mg/day) to four adult epileptic patients on CBZ monotherapy. After 2 weeks of STP treatment, CBZ clearance was reduced from 120 ± 28 to 55.8 ± 7.3 liter/day and the ratio of CBZ-10,11-epoxide (EPO) to CBZ in plasma decreased from 0.137 ± 0.025 to 0.072 ± 0.012. The CBZ dose-to-plasma concentration ratio and EPO-to-CBZ plasma ratio each required an equilibration time of 7 to 10 days following initiation of STP. Study II focused on the effect of STP on EPO elimination. Six normal adult volunteers each received two single oral doses of EPO (100 mg suspension). Stiripentol did not have a significant effect on EPO half-life ($5.89 \pm .55$ hr control, 5.65 hr with STP) or plasma clearance ($1.78 \pm .24$ ml/min/kg control, $1.98 \pm .24$ ml/min/kg with STP). These two studies lead to the following conclusions: (a) epoxide hydrolase is not affected by short-term STP therapy; and (b) changes in EPO-to-CBZ plasma ratio in Study I were entirely due to inhibited formation of EPO.

Phenobarbital

Stiripentol decreases the clearance of phenobarbital (PB). In the study by Levy et al. (5), it fell from 3.84 liter/day on day 1 to 2.25 liter/day on day 30 in one patient and from 5.06 on day 1 to 3.42 liter/day on day 30 in another patient. The data on plasma levels were inconclusive because the period of observation in this study was shorter than that required for PB levels to rise from one steady state to another. However, a rise in plasma level was noted in the three patients who received the drug. A reduction of PB dosage ranging from 10% to 43% (mean,

30%) was necessary to maintain a constant plasma level in seven patients (15).

Primidone

Scarce unpublished data tend to demonstrate that STP inhibits the metabolism of primidone (PRM) into PB. Stiripentol increased plasma PRM levels to a point where toxic signs appeared in all four patients. A concomitant decrease of PB level was noted.

Valproic Acid

During clinical trials, no significant rise in plasma valproic acid (VPA) levels was observed. However, wide daily fluctuations in VPA concentrations and isolated sampling did not allow a clear opinion. The interaction of STP-VPA was investigated in normal subjects (3). Eight healthy volunteers received VPA (1,000 mg/day for 11 days) without and with STP (1,200 mg/day). The mean ($\pm$ SD) VPA plasma level at steady state increased from 62.6 ± 10 to 68 ± 12 μg/ml. C_{max} and C_{min} increased by 14% and 13%, respectively. The smallness of STP's impact was completely explained by a lack of effect on major metabolic pathways of VPA (glucuronidation and beta oxydation). However, a pronounced inhibition of cytochrome P-450–mediated pathways was found. The formation and clearance of the hepatotoxic delta-4-VPA was reduced by 32%.

THERAPEUTIC EFFICACY

Seizures were monitored throughout a pharmacokinetic study on six patients with uncontrolled localization-related symptomatic epilepsy (4). The study was designated as a kinetic evaluation rather than an efficacy trial and no conclusion was drawn concerning efficacy: the period of STP treatment (30 days) was insufficient to permit an accurate assessment of efficacy and rise in plasma levels of concomitant antiepileptic drugs (Table 1). Nonetheless, an improvement in seizure frequency was apparent in four patients. Three of them were seizure-free during the study and one of them has remained controlled for more than 4 years (Patient F).

A bicenter pilot efficacy study in refractory partial epilepsy was carried out in Bordeaux (France) and Pamplona (Spain). Preliminary results were published (18). Its aim was to replace all existing therapy by STP as a one-drug treatment in outpatients. The study design was as follows: (a) Period I: an 8-week base line with constant daily dosage of conventional antiepileptic drugs at a so-called therapeutic level; (b) Period II: a crossover period with introduction of STP (600 mg/day the first week, 1,200 mg/day the next 3 weeks, and 1,800 mg/day thereafter) and withdrawal of other antiepileptic drugs over 4 weeks (when only one drug) or 8 weeks (when two drugs, one of them withdrawn over 4 weeks); (c) Period III: monotherapy period, with STP dosage increased when possible to 2,400 mg/day over 2 weeks, then maintained constant; (d) Period IV: bitherapy period. In case of STP monotherapy failure, one of the drugs of the base line was reintroduced. Forty-three patients entered the study, 22 dropped out during Period II (16 for increased number or intensity of seizures, four for poor compliance, two for adverse events). Twenty-one reached Period III. Eighteen went on to Period IV before the scheduled end of Period III. The three others remained totally seizure-free for periods of 27, 44, and 47 days for the first time in their illness. But it became necessary to return to bitherapy in these patients. Seventeen patients reached Period IV, receiving STP with one of the base-line drugs (CBZ in 10, PB in 4, PHT in 3). Twelve experienced a seizure reduction of 50% to 75% during at least 3 months of follow-up. Mean ($\pm$ SD) STP daily dose was 38 mg/kg $\pm$ 10 (range, 27–46 mg/kg) during Period III and Period IV. The plasma level of the associated antiepileptic drug was, in Period IV, inferior to the base-line level in 10 patients, superior in seven patients. The associated drug's dose was inferior in 14 patients, unchanged in three patients.

The following conclusions may be suggested: obviously, STP was not more active than PB, PHT, or CBZ in the majority of these patients. However, they had very resistant epilepsies with frequent seizures, more than one type of seizure, and a mean

TABLE 1. *Open study of stiripentol in six epileptic patients*

Patient	Sex	Duration of disease (yr)	Monthly seizure frequency		Comedication	Levels		
			Base line	+ STP		Base line		+ STP
A	F	10	>4	0	PHT + CLB	PHT:	7.9	20.4
B	F	13	1.5	4	PHT + PB	PHT:	9.6	29.4
						PB:	20.6	44.1
C	M	14	4–28	20	PHT + PRM + NZP	PHT:	3.4	13.5
						PB:	21.5	15.6
D	M	20	3–10	4	PHT + CBZ	PHT:	12.9	7.3
						CBZ:	3.6	9.7
E	M	4	>30	0	CBZ + PB	CBZ:	5.1	8.2
						PB:	17.6	28.6
F	M	16	4–28	0	PHT + PB	PHT:	12.5	29.8
						PB:	34.4	46.1

CBZ, carbamazepine; CLB, clobazam; NZP, nitrazepam; PB, phenobarbital; PHT, phenytoin.

epilepsy duration of 18 years. Stiripentol was presumably less active than conventional antiepileptic drugs, since several patients experienced an exacerbation of seizures during the crossover period, when a partly active drug was withdrawn. However, the reduction rate was too fast, as shown in some patients by the appearance of generalized convulsive attacks (i.e., withdrawal seizures) and not their usual partial seizures. As for the improved patients, the study design did not allow excluding a role of higher plasma levels of the previous drugs.

A long-term, open trial was performed in refractory patients with a severe localization-related symptomatic epilepsy (17). Its design was as follows: (a) an 8-week baseline period; (b) introduction of STP, a dose of 1,800 to 3,000 mg/day, t.i.d., being reached in about 10 days, (c) adjustment of the other drug(s) over 8 to 16 weeks, i.e., a withdrawal of one drug, then two, and a decrease in the daily dosage of the unique or the remaining drug, according to its plasma level; (d) an 8-week evaluation period. Thirty patients entered the study. Twenty-six completed the 8-week evaluation period. During this period, three patients were seizure-free, seven had an over 50% reduction in seizure frequency, 13 were slightly improved, and seizures increased in six patients. Plasma STP levels were not clearly correlated with the clinical response. Ten patients dropped out after 9 to 52 weeks of STP bitherapy because of a relapse. However, 16 subjects were still on trial with a follow-up ranging from 20 to 75 weeks (mean, 46 weeks) and had developed no tolerance. The authors concluded that STP is a nontoxic agent, efficacious in 16 of 26 patients although increased plasma levels of the concomitant antiepileptic drugs remain an obstacle to a definitive interpretation of the results. The reported benefit of STP is certainly not due to the rise in plasma level of other drugs. Some patients had previously presented CBZ levels similar to those achieved by STP inhibitory action with more frequent seizures.

In a neurospychological and efficacy evaluation of STP (15), 10 patients with a localization-related symptomatic epilepsy and one patient with an idiopathic generalized epilepsy were administered STP during 2 months as comedication. The base-line dose of other drugs was reduced to maintain plasma levels unchanged. Six of the nine uncontrolled patients experienced a decrease in seizure frequency greater than or equal to 50%. Two patients were completely controlled but experienced an isolated seizure, one after 6 months and the other after 17 months of treatment.

A preliminary report of STP efficacy in refractory absence seizures has been published (16). The updated results are as follows. Stiripentol was given as comedication to 20 patients ranging in age from 13 to 46 years. All 20 suffered from an idiopathic generalized epilepsy (absence + generalized tonic-clonic seizures, 16; juvenile absence epilepsy, absence status, myoclonic + atonic + GTC seizures, myoclonic + GTC seizures, one each). They were uncontrolled with antiabsence and other anticonvulsant drugs (Table 2). Stiripentol doses ranged from 21 to 68 mg/kg/day. Plasma STP levels remained low when in combination with inducing agents. Plasma levels of other drugs were maintained constant, with a dosage reduction for PB, PRM, and CBZ. Trial duration ranges now from 1 to 15 months. Only six patients experienced mild side effects (gastric, 4; insomnia, 2). Stiripentol was stopped in four patients because of an unchanged seizure frequency. Two initially improved patients relapsed without change in the drug regimen. For this reason, only 15 patients having at least a 3-month trial duration will be considered. Five patients achieved a sustained seizure control and six other patients maintained an over 50% reduction of seizure frequency. However, three of the controlled patients relapsed when VPA was withdrawn. Stiri-

TABLE 2. *Stiripentol in absence seizures*

Patient			Seizure type and age at onset	Resistant to	Stiripentol trial			
No.	Sex	Age			Duration (month)	Dose mg/kg	Level μg/ml	Result
1	M	26	Myocl. Abs. (5 yr) + GTCS (6 yr)	VPA, VPM, ESM, TMO, PB, PRM, CZP, DZP, PGB	2	30		No efficacy
2	F	13	Abs. Status (5 yr)	VPA, ESM, PB, CBZ, PGB, CZP, NZP	15	68	17.0	Efficacy: 50%
3	M	38	Abs. (22 yr) + GTCS (16 yr)	VPA, VPM, PB, PHT, PGB, CBZ	14	29	6.1	Efficacy: 62%
4	M	37	Abs. (10 yr) + GTCS (13 yr)	VPA, PB, PRM, PHT, CBZ	15	32	2.6	90% efficacy 3 months. Relapse
5	F	14	Abs. (12.5 yr)	VPA	2	28		Efficacy: 75%. Lost for follow-up
6	F	19	Myocl. Abs. (8 yr) + GTCS (11 yr)	VPA, PB, CLB, Trinuride	1/2	36		No efficacy
7	F	46	Abs. (18 yr) + GTCS (18 yr)	VPA, PB, CBZ, CZP, PGB	15	29		Complete control
8	M	39	Abs. (7 yr) + GTCS (11 yr)	VPA, PB, PHT, CBZ	15	33	2.5	Complete control with VPA + STP
9	F	41	Atonic, Myocl. Abs. (9 yr) + GTCS (12 yr)	VPA, PB, PHT, CBZ, CLB	13	21	4.0	Efficacy: 75%
10	M	17	Abs. (9 yr) + GTCS (16 yr)	VPA, ESM, PB, PGB	11	28		No efficacy
11	F	29	Abs. (12 yr) + GTCS (19 yr)	VPA, PB, GVG	11	27	7.1	Complete control
12	F	26	Abs. (20 yr) + GTCS (11 yr)	VPA, PB, CZP	11	63	6.5	90% efficacy 2 months. Relapse
13	F	27	Myocl. Sz. (2 yr) + GTCS (2 yr)	VPA, PB, PHT	8	40	8.1	Control with VPA + STP
14	M	33	Awakening GM + Abs. (14 yr)	VPA, PB, PHT	8	21	13.7	Control with VPA + STP
15	F	23	Abs. (21 yr) + GTCS (17 yr)	VPA, CBZ	5	55	5.4	Efficacy: 50%
16	F	27	Abs. (10 yr) + GTCS (13 yr)	VPA, VPM, ESM, CZP, PB	5	55	22.7	No efficacy
17	M	29	Abs. (6 yr) + GTCS (11 yr)	VPA, ESM, TMO, PHT, PB, PRM, CBZ	7	32	3.9	Efficacy: 75%
18	M	28	Abs. (15 yr) + GTCS (12 yr)	VPA, DZP, CZP, CBZ, PB, PHT	3	46		Efficacy: 50%

Myocl. Abs., myoclonic absence; GTCS, generalized tonic-clonic seizure; Abs., absence; Awakening GM Abs., awakening grand mal absence.

CBZ, carbamazepine; CLB, clobazam; CZP, clonazepam; DZP, diazepam; ESM, ethosuximide; GVG, vigabatrin; NZP, nitrazepam; PB, phenobarbital; PGB, progabide; PHT, phenytoin; PRM, primidone; TMO, trimethadione; VPA, valproate; VPM, valpromide; STP, stiripentol.

pentol is a very promising drug in the treatment of refractory absence seizures, but its efficacy in monotherapy in this condition is not clear.

SUMMARY

Stiripentol has demonstrated a marked antiepileptic activity in animal studies against PTZ-induced and electrically induced seizures. In the alumina-gel–rhesus monkey model, it performed comparably to VPA by delaying the onset of seizures and by reducing EEG interictal spike rates. An indirect GABAergic mechanism may be involved. Much is known of STP's pharmacokinetic properties. Its Michaelis-Menten–type kinetics are nonlinear. The steady-state plasma level-to-dose ratio increases with the daily dose, and the time to reach steady state also increases with dose. Only a part of oral doses reaches the systemic circulation because of poor solubility and a hepatic first-pass effect. Stiripentol is very strongly protein-bound. Elimination is mostly by biotransformation. Thirteen metabolites have been identified in urine. Stiripentol metabolism is induced by the major antiepileptic drugs. It is a potent inhibitor of phenytoin, carbamazepine, phenobarbital, and primidone metabolism. Of particular interest is the inhibition of toxic metabolites of these drugs, such as carbamazepine epoxide and delta-4-valproic acid. Combination drug therapy with STP may result in a decreased exposure to arene oxide metabolism of other anticonvulsants. Daily dosages up to 50 mg/kg are usually well tolerated, as are plasma levels up to 20 μg/ml. The plasma level-to-dose ratio is variable. Phase II trials in Spain and France demonstrated STP's efficacy in difficult-to-treat partial epilepsies. The role of the drug itself and of its action on the other drugs is under evaluation. A constant interaction with CBZ, PHT, or PB hindered both the management and the interpretation of the trials. Stiripentol is probably not as potent as major anticonvulsants. However, given as comedication, it alleviates the adverse reactions and potential risks of other antiepileptic drugs. In keeping with its properties in animals, STP is probably a potent therapeutic agent in absence seizures and possibly also in tonic-clonic seizures of generalized idiopathic epilepsies.

CONVERSION

Conversion factor:

$$CF = \frac{1000}{\text{mol. wt.}} = \frac{1000}{234} = 4.27$$

Conversion:

$$(\mu g/ml) \times 4.27 = (\mu moles/liter)$$

$$(\mu moles/liter) \div 4.27 = (\mu g/ml)$$

REFERENCES

1. Astoin J., Marivain, A., Riveron, A., Crucifix, M., Lapotre, M., and Torrens, Y. (1978). Action de nouveaux alcools alpha-ethyléniques sur le système nerveux central. *Eur. J. Med. Chem. Chim. Ther.*, 13:41–47.
2. Levy, R. H., Lin, H. S., Blehaut, H., and Tor, J.A. (1983): Pharmacokinetics of stiripentol in normal man: Evidence of nonlinearity. *J. Clin. Pharmacol.*, 23:523–533.
3. Levy, R. H., Loiseau, P., Guyot, M., Acheampong, A., Tor, J., and Rettenmeir, A. W. (1987): Effects of stiripentol on valproate plasma level and metabolism. *Epilepsia*, 28:605.
4. Levy, R. H., Loiseau, P., Guyot, M., Blehaut, H., Tor, J., and Moreland, T. A. (1984a): Michaelis-Menten kinetics of stiripentol in normal humans. *Epilepsia*, 25:486–491.
5. Levy, R. H., Loiseau, P., Guyot, M., Blehaut, H., Tor, J., and Moreland, T. A. (1984b): Stiripentol kinetics in epilepsy: Nonlinearity and interactions. *Clin. Pharmacol. Ther.*, 36:661–669.
6. Levy, R. H., Martinez-Lage, M., Kern, B. M., and Viteri, C. (1987): Effect of stiripentol on the formation and elimination of carbamazepine-epoxide. *Abstracts, 17th Epilepsy International Congress,* Jerusalem, Israel, Sept. 6–11, p. 71.
7. Levy, R. H., Martinez-Lage, M., Tor, J., Blehaut, H., Gonzalez, I., and Baindridge, G. (1986): Stiripentol level-dose relationship and interactions with carbamazepine in epileptic patients. *Epilepsia*, 26:584.

8. Levy, R. H., Moreland, T. A., Baillie, T. A., Astoin, J., and Lepage, F. (1985). Metabolic fate of stiripentol in man. *Abstracts, 16th Epilepsy International Congress,* Hamburg, Sept. 6–9.

9. Lin, H. S., and Levy, R. H. (1983): Pharmacokinetic profile of a new anticonvulsant, stiripentol, in the rhesus monkey. *Epilepsia,* 24:692–702.

10. Lin, H. S., Levy, R. H., Blehaut, H., and Tor, J. (1984): Pharmacokinetic properties and metabolic profile of stiripentol in primates. In: *Metabolism of Antiepileptic Drugs,* edited by R. H. Levy, W. H. Pitlick, M. Eichelbaum, and J. Meijer, pp. 199–207. Raven Press, New York.

11. Lockard, J. S., and Levy R. H. (1986): EEG effects of stiripentol in add-on with carbamazepine in monkey model. *Epilepsia* 27:648.

12. Lockard, J. S., Levy, R. H., Maris, D. O., and Rhodes, P. H. (1983): Stiripentol in alumina-gel monkeys: 4-Deoxypyridoxine hydrochloride paradigm. *Epilepsia,* 24:252.

13. Lockard, J. S., Levy, R. H., Rhodes, P. H., and Moore, D. F. (1984): Stiripentol and EEG spike rate in acute/chronic tests in monkeys model. *Epilepsia,* 25:667.

14. Lockard, J. S., Levy R. H., Rhodes, P. H., Moore D. F. (1985): Stiripentol in acute/chronic efficacy test in monkey model. *Epilepsia* 26:704–712.

15. Loiseau, P., Strube, E., Tor, J., Levy, R. H., and Dodrill, C. (1988): Evaluation neuropsychologique et thérapeutique du stiripentol dans l'épilepsie. Résultats préliminaires. *Rev. Neurol (Paris),* 144:165–172.

16. Loiseau, P., and Tor, J. (1987a): Stiripentol in absence seizures. *Epilepsia,* 28:579.

17. Martinez-Lage, M., Levy, R. H., Gonzalez, I., Viteri, C., Tor, J., and Blehaut, H. (1987): Stiripentol in therapy-resistant and severe epileptic patients: A long-term open trial in bitherapy. In: *Advances in Epileptology, Vol. 16,* edited by P. Wolf, M. Dam, D. Janz, and F. E. Dreifuss, pp. 541–546. Raven Press, New York.

18. Martinez-Lage, M., Loiseau, P., Levy, R. H., Gonzalez, I., Strube, E., Tor, J., and Blehaut, H. (1984): Clinical antiepileptic efficacy of stiripentol in resistant partial epilepsies. *Epilepsia,* 25:673.

19. Moreland, T. A., Astoin, J., and Lepage, F. (1986): The metabolic fate of stiripentol in man. *Drug Metab. Disp.,* 14:654–662.

20. Pieri, F., Wegmann, R., and Astoin, J. (1982): Etude pharmacocinétique du ^{3}H-stiripentol chez le rat. *Eur. J. Drug Metab. Pharmacokinet.,* 7:5–10.

21. Poisson, M., Huguet, F., Savatier, A., Bakri-Logeais, F., and Narcisse, G. (1984): A new type of anticonvulsant, stiripentol. *Arzneimittelforsch,* 34:199–204.

22. Shen, D. D., Levy, R. H., Savitch, J. L., and Bainbridge, B. (1987): Pharmacodynamic profile of stiripentol (STP) in a pentylenetetrazol (PTZ) threshold seizure rat model. *Abstracts, 17th Epilepsy International Congress,* Jerusalem, Israel, Sept. 6–11, p. 71.

23. Vincent, J. C. (1986): Stiripentol. In: *New Anticonvulsant Drugs,* edited by B. S. Meldrum and R. J. Porter, pp. 255–263. John Libbey, London.

24. Wegman, R., Ilies, A., and Aurousseau, M. (1978): Enzymologie pharmaco-cellulaire du mode d'action du stiripentol au cours de l'épilepsie cardiazolique. III: Les métabolismes protidique, nucléoprotidique, lipidique et des protéoglycans. *Cell. Mol. Biol.,* 23:455–480.

25. Wegman, R., Ilies, A., Aurousseau, M., and Patte, F. (1979): Enzymologie pharmaco-cellulaire du mode d'action du stiripentol au cours de l'épilepsie cardiazolique. IV: Répartition cellulaire et tissulaire du ^{3}H-stiripentol. *Cell Mol. Biol.,* 24:51–60.

Antiepileptic Drugs, Third Edition, edited by
R. Levy, R. Mattson, B. Meldrum,
J. K. Penry, and F. E. Dreifuss.
Raven Press, Ltd., New York © 1989.

71

Potential Antiepileptic Drugs

Flunarizine and Other Calcium Entry Blockers

C. D. Binnie

INTRODUCTION

A characteristic feature of epileptogenesis is burst firing of individual neurons. The burst comprises a slow paroxysmal depolarizing ion shift (PDS) upon which is superimposed a train of action potentials (8,54). Bursting depends largely on influx of Ca^{++}, although other ionic currents are also involved (55,83).

In epileptic foci induced by cortical application of penicillin the extracellular activity of calcium ions decreases during epileptic discharges (14,33). Intracellular injection of the experimental calcium antagonist D890 reduces the amplitude of PDSs (80). Similarly, intraventricular application of verapamil reversibly reduces the amplitude of depolarization shifts and the rate of occurrence of epileptiform discharges (73). These drugs do not suppress excitatory postsynaptic potentials (79) or somatosensory-evoked potentials (72). Following application of pentylenetetrazol to hippocampal slices, addition of flunarizine to the bathing medium suppresses spontaneous rhythmical burst activity without producing any change in amplitudes or rates of occurrence of postsynaptic potentials, excitability, or action potentials of CA3 neurons (11). By contrast, Bay K8644, which stimulates calcium entry, increases liability to tonic-clonic convulsions in DBA/2 mice (27).

These findings suggest that calcium currents may play an important role in epileptogenesis and that calcium entry blockers deserve consideration as potential antiepileptic drugs.

CHEMISTRY AND METHODS OF DETERMINATION

Flunarizine (molecular weight = 477.42) is a difluorinated piperazine derivative: (E)-1-[*bis*(4-fuorophenyl)methyl]-4-(3-phenyl-2-propenyl) piperazine dihydrochloride (Fig. 1). It is a cream-colored hygroscopic powder that is highly lipophilic and insoluble in water. Solutions of 0.5 mg/ml can be prepared by the addition of 2% hydroxypropyl-β-cyclodextrin.

Flunarizine is marketed as Sibellium by Janssen Pharmaceutica, and is available as red and gray capsules of 5 mg.

High-performance liquid chromatography (HPLC) and gas-liquid chromatography assays are available (81,82).

EXPERIMENTAL PHARMACOLOGY

Desmedt et al. (28) demonstrated the anticonvulsant activity of flunarizine against

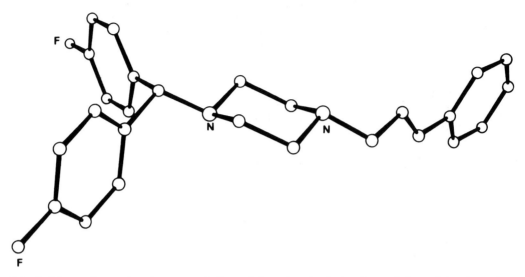

FIG. 1. Three dimensional representation of the chemical structure of flunarizine based on the crystal structure conformation of cinnarizine.

maximal pentylenetetrazol-induced seizures in rats and maximal electroshock seizures in mice. In these models flunarizine suppressed only tonic seizures, a profile of activity shared by carbamazepine and phenytoin. Activity against tonic seizures was demonstrated in other models, including D,L-allylglycine (5), and intravenous bicuculline in rats and mice (75). A similarity between flunarizine, phenytoin, and carbamazepine was also shown in the bicuculline seizure threshold test (3). These drugs antagonized tonic forepaw seizures, not by producing a progressive threshold increase, but rather by total suppression so that increased doses of bicuculline failed to produce tonic seizures. Clonic seizures are antagonized by flunarizine, phenytoin, and carbamazepine in amygdaloid-kindled rats and dogs (6,77). Flunarizine was also effective in genetic models of epilepsy, suppressing audiogenic tonic seizures in DBA/2 mice and reducing mortality, but having no effect on agitation and clonic seizures (75). Flunarizine also suppresses photomyoclonus in photosensitive baboons, *Papio papio* (26).

These findings may offer some evidence concerning the mode of action of flunarizine. GABAergic compounds exhibit a dose-related elevation of seizure threshold (43,44,49,59). This may be contrasted with the antagonism of tonic seizures by flunarizine, carbamazepine, and phenytoin which shows an all or none effect. Experimental evidence that flunarizine does not increase GABAergic inhibition was reported by Ashton et al. (4) using the paired-pulse stimulation technique in hippocampal slices described by Ashton and Wauquier (7). At separations of 12 to 30 msec the population spike response to the second pulse normally shows facilitation which is converted into inhibition by GABAergic agents. Flunarizine in biologically significant concentrations did not show this effect. An anticonvulsant profile similar to those of phenytoin and carbamazepine raises the possibility of an analogous mechanism of action, namely on voltage-sensitive sodium channels (78). Direct evidence of a possible sodium channel blockade may be inferred from the study of Ashton et al. (4) showing that flunarizine and carbamazepine at biologically relevant concentrations similarly inhibited the binding of batrachotoxinin A 20-alpha-benzoate, which implicates binding site II of the sodium channel (10). It remains at present uncertain whether flunarizine, despite being a potent calcium entry blocker, owes its anticonvulsant action to an effect on sodium channels.

The ED_{50} of flunarizine in those models where it is effective is typically in the range 6 to 40 mg/kg (67). The duration of action ranges from 3 to 24 hr, being greatest in the amygdaloid kindling model.

By means of blocking calcium entry, flunarizine inhibits various calcium-dependent mechanisms:

1. Vascular smooth muscle contraction due to various agents is inhibited, although normal vascular tone is not (1,37,68).
2. Endothelial cells contraction due to calcium overload (20).
3. Membrane rigidity due to calcium influx in anoxic erythrocytes (30).
4. Anoxic brain damage (69) and, possibly by a related mechanism, spreading depression (76).

It also depresses vestibular function and nystagmus in the rabbit (50).

EXPERIMENTAL TOXICOLOGY

In the rotorod ataxia test (mice) disequilibrium appears at 300 mg/kg of flunarizine, some 10 to 20 times the ED_{50} (60). In mice the LD_{50} after 7 days is 815 mg/kg for males and >1,280 mg/kg for females.

In rats, prolonged administration of flunarizine, 5 or 20 mg/kg daily for 18 months, did not produce significant toxic effects. Doses of 80 mg/kg produced weight loss, increased mortality, and serological changes. In dogs 12 months' administration of up to 20 mg/kg had no toxic effects, but 40 mg/kg was lethal due to central nervous system (CNS) depression and weight loss.

Mutagenicity and carcinogenicity tests (18 months mouse and 24 months rats) were

negative (56). Flunarizine did not affect the fertility of male or female rats in doses up to 160 mg/kg and showed no teratogenicity or increased fetal loss in rats and rabbits.

CLINICAL PHARMACOKINETICS

Normal Subjects

Peak plasma concentrations of flunarizine are reached within 2 to 4 hr of a single 10 mg oral dose in fasting normal subjects (35), and their subsequent decay can be described by a three-exponential equation, with sequential distribution half-lives of 3.1 hr and 17 hr and a terminal half-life of 22 days. Heykants and Van Peer (36) therefore proposed a three-compartment model. The absolute bioavailability is 86% (25). The comparative bioavailability of a capsule formulation is equivalent to that of an aqueous solution (70); that of tablets is 10% less (35). The distribution volume of flunarizine is of the order of 78 liter/kg (36), probably reflecting the high uptake of the drug in lipoid structures due to its marked lipophilic properties. Flunarizine is 99.1% protein-bound at concentrations of 0.5 μg/ml (46).

At a daily dose of 10 mg, 8 weeks are required to approach dynamic steady state (2). This is less than might be predicted from the drug's terminal half-life and is due to the considerably shorter half-lives of distribution. Plasma levels show considerable interindividual variations with an interquartile range of approximately 30 to 100 ng/ml at 10 mg daily (34). Within any individual steady-state level is proportional to dose (34, 16). After administration of flunarizine is discontinued, plasma levels of the drug decay with a terminal half-life of 19 days (36).

Patients with Epilepsy

In patients receiving flunarizine as add-on therapy to antiepileptic medication

(12,31,52,65), flunarizine steady-state concentrations were four to five times lower than those reported in patients receiving the same doses in monotherapy (34). Mean plasma flunarizine concentrations at 10 and 20 mg daily were 18.1 and 59.3 ng/ml, respectively (12). These findings indicate that antiepileptic drugs such as carbamazepine and phenytoin induce flunarizine liver metabolism. Although not confirmed by Treiman et al. (65), a trend may be that an increase in the number of enzyme-inducing antiepileptic drugs administered (i.e., more than one drug) further reduces the plasma flunarizine concentrations (12).

After increasing oral dosages and varying between 5 and 105 mg daily, Treiman et al. (65) found almost linearly increasing steady-state plasma concentrations within individual patients. Kinetics of flunarizine administered as add-on therapy are therefore linear in the therapeutic dose range.

Metabolism

Only limited data on human metabolism of flunarizine are available. Less than 0.01% of a single oral dose of 30 mg was excreted unchanged in the urine within 48 hr in eight normal subjects, and less than 5% of the administered dose appeared in the feces (17). Heykants et al. (34) suggested first-pass metabolism of flunarizine in the liver as a source of interindividual variation in plasma levels. Some 5% of administered flunarizine is found in urine or feces as *P*-hydroxyflunarizine and flunarizine-*N*-oxide. Other metabolites are unknown, but in animals the major metabolic pathway involves *N*-dealkylation (45).

Drug Interactions

There is no evidence from clinical trials of enzyme induction or inhibition by flunarizine nor of any other pharmacokinetic influence of flunarizine on other antiepilep-

tic drugs (12,22,31,42,52). Flunarizine in plasma is strongly bound to proteins (99.1%), but does not affect plasma binding of comedication (31).

CLINICAL EFFICACY AND SAFETY

Twelve open trials of add-on flunarizine therapy in patients with intractable epilepsy have been reported (Table 1). In all trials the seizure frequency during at least 2 months of flunarizine administration was compared with that over a base-line period of not less than 2 months. At least a 50% reduction in seizure frequency was considered clinically significant. In 11 of the trials, 74 of 197 patients (38%) showed a seizure reduction by this criterion, and 11 (6%) had a similar increase in seizures while on flunarizine. Eight patients became seizure-free. In the twelfth trial, 22 of 30 patients achieved the criterion of 50% seizure reduction, but the possible number showing an increase was not reported. Three trials included both adults and an unspecified number of children, and three were based only on patients under 17 years of age (*N* = 38). The results in these studies were similar to those obtained overall (50% seizure reduction in 41 (46%) of 98 children and adults, and 12 (32%) of 38 children and adolescents).

In adults, 15 mg of flunarizine per day was generally the optimal dose for efficacy and avoiding adverse reactions in patients already receiving enzyme-inducing drugs.

Two single-blind and eight double-blind trials (Table 2) have been performed using a two-period crossover design. An additional planned crossover study was terminated after the first period due to logistic problems and therefore could only be analyzed as a parallel design (22,23). Three studies compared only mean seizure incidence during the two treatments and found that seizure incidence on flunarizine was significantly lower than on placebo (the dif-

TABLE 1. Open trials of flunarizine

| Reference | No. | | Age | | Seizure types | | | | | Flunarizine, dosage mg/day | Dosing period, mths | 50% Change in seizure frequency | | Withdrawals | |
| | Patients | Evaluated | Mean | Range | Partial | Generalized | | | Other or not specified | | | | | | |
						Abs	T-C	Other				Decrease	Increase	Number	Reason
Binnie et al., 1985	A	47	35	17–64	47		6		4	10–25	6–12	16	6	5	2, wanted pregnancy; 2, noncompliant; 1, lost aura
Debandt et al., 1985	A	8	33	25–38	3	5	6			10–25	4	2	2	2	1, too few seizures in base line; 1, intercurrent illness
Sorel, 1987	A	20	31	20–51	18	1	2	1	1	10–20	4	10	2	—	—
De Domenico et al., 1987	A	11	28	18–71	6		3	1		>70 kg: 15; ≤70 kg: 10	3	1	0	—	—
Curatolo et al., 1986	C + Ado	21	5	0.5–17	12				9	>10 kg: 5; ≤10 kg: 2.5	3	8	1	5	5, drowsiness
Giroud et al., 1987	C	10	12	18–15	6		4			5–10	3	3	0	—	—
Pothmann et al., 1986	C + Ado + A	21	12	1–20					21	5–20	<3	10	0	3	1, noncompliant; 2, moved away
Declerk et al., 1986	C + A	14	?	5–36					14	10		1	0	—	—
Tata et al, 1987	A	30	?	18–50	13		2	15		10–20	<6	22	?	—	—
Takahashi, 1978	A	13	36	17–53	12			1		10	7	4	0	—	—
Umezawa, 1987	A + C	25	?	10–54					25	10	<22	15	0	1	1, depressed
Konishi, 1987	C + Ado	7	?	6–16					7	4–10	1	4	0	—	—

A, adult 17 years old or more; C, child not more than 13 years old; Ado, adolescent 13 to 17 years old; Abs, absence; T-C, tonic-clonic.

TABLE 2. *Controlled trials of flunarizine*

Reference	No. Patients	No. Evaluated	Age Mean	Age Range	Seizure types Partial	Generalized Abs	Generalized T-C	Generalized Other	Other or not specified	Flunarizine, dosage mg/day	Dosing period, mths	50% Change in seizure frequency Decrease	Increase	Withdrawals Number	Reason
Overweg et al., 1984	Ado + A	30	33	15–56	29		8	3		10	3	7	0	3	1, drowsy 1, intercurrent illness 1, too few seizures in base line
Touquet et al., 1985	Ado + A	5	21	15–27	4		1			10 after loading	2	2	0	—	—
Fröscher et al., 1988	Ado + A	22	32	14–51	22		2			15 after loading	4	2	3	8	all noncompliance or protocol violation
Mancia, 1987	Ado + A	29	34	16–57	22		5	1	1	>70 kg: 15 ≤70 kg: 10	3	20% mean seizure reduction on flunarizine		—	—
Moglia et al., 1986	Ado + A	20	36	15–73	17				3	>70 kg: 15 ≤70 kg: 10	3	33% mean seizure reduction on flunarizine		—	—
Bergamasco et al., 1987	A	27	33	17–64	21	1	1		5	>70 kg: 15 ≤70 kg: 10	3	34% mean seizure reduction on flunarizine		3	?
Cavazzuti et al., 1986	Ado + C	14	13	3–17	0		2	2	10	>12 yr: 10 ≤12 yr: 5	3	5	0	—	—
Curatolo et al., 1986	C	16	5	0.5–13	6				10	>10 kg: 5 ≤10 kg: 2.5	3	1	0	—	—
Starreveld et al., 1987	A	25	32	17–47	25	1	5	5		15	4	7	2	9	4, hospitalized 1, died (before FLN) 3, noncompliant 1, too few seizures
Keene et al., 1987	C Ado A	29	11	0.2–24					29	≤20 kg: 5 20–40 kg: 10 >40 kg: 15	4	6	1	5	3, did not start Phase I 1, side effects (on placebo) 1, progressive degenerative disorder
Declerck and Wauquier, 1978/1983	Ado + C	PS F7	12	9–17	3				9	10	3	PO/5 F3/7		8	8, protocol violation

A, adult 17 years old or more; C, child not more than 13 years old; Ado, adolescent 13 to 17 years old; Abs, absence; T-C, tonic-clonic.

ference being in the 20% to 34% range). The other seven studies employed the criterion of a 50% difference in the seizure frequency between treatments. Thirty patients (21%) were improved on flunarizine versus six (9%) on placebo. Overall this effect is highly significant, although it achieved statistical significance in only two individual trials. In the parallel study, three of seven patients receiving flunarizine showed a 50% reduction of seizures by comparison with base line, and none of five met this criterion on placebo. Two studies were concerned exclusively with children under 17 years of age (N = 30) and in these, six patients (20%) showed a 50% difference in seizure frequency in favor of flunarizine, and none showed a similar reduction in seizures on placebo. Doses employed were 10 to 15 mg daily in adults, 2.5 to 5 mg in children up to puberty, and 10 mg in adolescence. The period of active dosing was 3 months or longer with one exception (2 months).

A majority of patients studied had partial seizures and flunarizine appears to have shown efficacy in both partial and generalized seizures and in both partial and secondary generalized epilepsy. A more detailed analysis of the effects of seizure type and epilepsy syndrome is not possible due to inconsistencies in the classifications employed. Thus the only reports of so-called absence seizures concern adults in whom these attacks, it may be presumed, were in most instances complex partial seizures. Some authors appear to have regarded generalized tonic-clonic convulsions in patients with known partial epilepsy as being presumptive partial seizures with secondary generalization. Others appear not to have distinguished such attacks from tonic-clonic convulsions in primary generalized epilepsy.

In long-term therapy from 6 to over 22 months, there is no evidence of tolerance (32,66,71).

Human Safety

Flunarizine has been taken continuously for up to 14 years for indications other than epilepsy, notably migraine and vertigo. Drug-related changes in hematological, biochemical, renal, or hepatic variables have not been found. In trials in epilepsy where flunarizine was added to antiepileptic comedication, there have been no flunarizine-related changes in laboratory values over 1 year (51). Many patients exhibited elevated liver enzymes prior to addition of flunarizine due to induction by the other medication, but this was not increased by the drug.

Adverse Reactions

Add-on therapy with flunarizine was generally well tolerated. Drowsiness was reported in 26% of patients in open trials, but in only 8% under placebo-controlled conditions. This effect was closely related to blood levels and dosage, sharply increasing in frequency at above 50 ng/ml or 20 mg/day (12). In 16 patients who showed a 50% seizure reduction, this could be maintained without concomitant drowsiness in all but two after dose adjustment (12). Ten of the 12 patients in a tolerability study by Treiman et al. (64) developed symptoms of sedation, but eight did so only at plasma levels above 100 mg/ml. The second most common adverse experience was weight gain (3%). Extrapyramidal symptoms and depression have been occasionally reported during flunarizine therapy for other indications, although a causal relationship has not been established. In the trials of flunarizine in epilepsy reviewed here, only one case of depression and no instances of extrapyramidal symptoms have been reported. Treiman et al. (65) increased blood flunarizine levels to 120 ng/ml without producing these side effects.

TABLE 3. *Adverse reactions during flunarizine treatment and probably related to flunarizine*

Reference	N[a]	Drowsiness	Weight gain	Others
Binnie et al., 1985	47	15	8	2, memory impairment 1, aggression
Debandt et al., 1985	8		2	
Sorel, 1987	20	2	3	1, memory impairment
De Domenico, 1987	6	—	—	
Curatolo et al., 1986	26	5		
Giroud et al., 1987	10	3		
Pothmann et al., 1986	21	5	1	
Declerck et al., 1986	14	—	—	
Tata et al., 1987	30	—	—	
Overweg et al., 1987	31	1	—	
Touquet et al., 1985	5	—	—	
Fröscher et al., 1988	22	1	—	1, more alert
Mancia et al., 1987	22	—	—	6, asthenia
Moglia et al., 1986	20	9	—	1, dizziness
Bergamasco et al., 1987	27	6	—	
Cavazutti et al., 1986	14	1	—	2, torpor and apathy
Curatolo et al., 1986	16	—	—	
Starreveld et al., 1987	25	—	—	
Keene et al., 1987	29	—	—	
Declerk and Wauquier, 1983	12	—	—	
Takahashi, 1987	13	4	7	
Umezawa, 1987	26	—	—	1, depression
Konishi, 1987	7	3	3	

[a] Patients completing trial or withdrawn because of adverse reactions.

OTHER CALCIUM ENTRY BLOCKERS

Leaving aside the issue of whether the antiepileptic action of flunarizine is in fact due to blockade of calcium entry, it is of interest that other calcium entry blockers also suppress paroxysmal depolarization shifts. The possible therapeutic value in epilepsy of other known members of this class of drugs is uncertain, however. Several, such as verapamil, tiapamil, and diltiazem, do not readily penetrate the blood-brain barrier. Some, including nifedipine and nitrendipine, are effective against bicuculline-induced seizures in rats (74). Meyer et al. (47) found nimodipine to be effective against pentylenetetrazol and bicuculline-induced seizure activity, and Dolin et al. (29) demonstrated both nimodipine and nitredipine to be effective against pentylenetetrozol-induced convulsions but not against NMDA induced convulsions. Wauquier et al. (74) did not find any effect of

nimodipine against bicuculline-induced hindpaw extension. De Sarro et al. (27) found the dihydropyridines, nifedipine, nicardipine, nimodipine, and nitrendipine to be effective in intraperitoneal doses of the order of 40 to 160 μmol/kg against all phases of audiogenic seizures in DBA/2 mice. Diltiazem was also effective but verapamil was not active even with intraventricular administration. None of these drugs shows the unique characteristic of flunarizine in preventing pathological calcium overload without affecting the normal function of voltage-dependent calcium channels, and hence synaptic transmission. In theory such calcium antagonists might be expected, therefore, to produce CNS side effects more readily than flunarizine.

A trial of verapamil as add-on therapy in epilepsy (41) had to be abandoned before any conclusions about efficacy could be made, as the drug inhibited carbamazepine metabolism, rapidly producing intoxication. Diltiazem also caused carbamazepine intoxication, but nifedipine did not (13). An open trial of nifedipine add-on therapy showed 50% seizure reduction in four of nine patients, without elevation of carbamazepine levels (40). Clearly no conclusion about the value of calcium entry blockers other than flunarizine is possible until further clinical testing has been undertaken.

SUMMARY

Flunarizine as add-on therapy produces a clinically significant reduction in seizure frequency in a third of therapy-resistant patients with epilepsy. It is effective in both adults and children and no particular type of epilepsy has yet been shown to be especially sensitive or resistant to this drug. Long-term safety is good; side effects are generally mild, dose-related, and avoidable by dose reduction without loss of therapeutic effect. In adults the optimal blood level for seizure control without side effects is about 50 ng/ml. In the presence of enzyme-inducing comedication this will generally be achieved at a daily dose of 15 to 20 mg. Without enzyme-inducing comedication 10 mg daily will probably suffice. In children weighing less than 20 mg, 5 mg is a suitable daily starting dose. Because of the long terminal half-life, a single daily dose may be given.

The more general value of flunarizine as an antiepileptic drug in patients who are not therapy-resistant can be assessed only when monotherapy trials are available.

CONVERSION

Conversion factor:

$$CF = \frac{1000}{\text{mol. wt.}} = \frac{1000}{477.42} = 2.09$$

Conversion:

$$(\mu g/ml) \times 2.09 = (\mu moles/liter)$$
$$(\mu moles/liter) \div 2.09 = \mu g/ml$$

REFERENCES

1. Amery, W. K., Wauquier, A., Van Nueten, J. M., and De Clerck, F. (1981): The anti-migrainous pharmacology of flunarizine (R14 950), a calcium antagonist. *Drugs Under Experimental and Clinical Research*, 7:1–10.
2. Araki, G., Saito, T., Ishii, A., and Deguchi, T. (1982): Phase I study of KW-3149 (flunarizine hydrochloride). *Kiso to Rinsho*, 16:171–177.
3. Ashton, D. (1983): Bicuculline seizure thresholds, actions of diazepam, pentobarbital and etomidate isomers alone and in combination with Ro 15-1788, picrotoxin and (±) DMBB. *Eur. J. Pharmacol.*, 94:319–325.
4. Ashton, D., Marrannes, R., Pauwels, P. J., Van Belle, H., Reid, K., and Wauquier A. (1986): Possible mechanisms of flunarizine's anticonvulsant activity. *Health Science Review:* International Workshop on Flunarizine in Epilepsy, Beerse, May 24, 1985, p. 45–59.
5. Ashton, D., and Wauquier, A. (1979a): Effects of some anti-epileptic, neuroleptic and GABAminergic drugs on convulsions induced by D,L-allyglycine. *Pharmacol. Biochem. Behav.*, 11:221–226.
6. Ashton, D., and Wauquier, A. (1979b): Behavioural analysis of the effects of 15 anticonvulsants in amygdaloid kindled rats. *Psychopharmacology*, 65:7–13.
7. Ashton, D., and Wauquier, A. (1985): Modulations of a GABA-ergic inhibitory circuit in the *in vitro* hippocampus by etomidate isomers. *Anaesthesia and Analgesia*, 64:975–980.
8. Ayala, G. F., Dichter, M., Gumnit, R. Z., Matsumoto, H., and Spencer, W. A. (1973): Genesis of epileptic interictal spikes: New knowledge of cortical feedback systems suggest a neurophysiological explanation of brief paroxysms. *Brain Res.*, 211:227–234.
9. Bergamasco, B., Cantello, R., and Riccio, A. (1987): Utilita della flunarizina come coordiuvante nel trattamento dell'epilessia (confronto in doppio cieco con un placebo in disegno cross over) (*unpublished report*).
10. Bidard, J. N., Vijverberg, H. P. M., Frelin, C., Chungue, E., Legrand, A.-M., Bagnis, R., and Ladunski, M. (1984): Cignatoxin is a novel type of Na^+ channel toxin. *J. Biol. Chem.*, 259:8253–8357.
11. Bingmann, D., and Speckmann, E. J. (1984): Paroxysmal depolarization shifts in neurons of hippocampal slices: Depression by calcium antagonists. *Pflügers Arch.*, S402,R29.
12. Binnie, C. D., de Beukelaar, F., Meijer, J. W. A., Meinardi, H., Overweg, J., Wauquier, A., and van Wieringen, A. (1985): Open dose-ranging trial of

flunarizine as add-on therapy in epilepsy. *Epilepsia*, 26:424–428.

13. Brodie, M. J., and Macphee, G. J. A. (1986). Carbamazepine neurotoxicity precipitated by diltiazem. *Br. Med. J.*, 292:1170–1171.

14. Caspers, H., Speckmann, E. J., and Lehmenkühler, A. (1980): Electrogenesis of cortical DC potentials. In: *Motivation Motor and Sensory Processes of the Brain: Electrical Potentials, Behaviour and Clinical Use*, edited by H. H. Kornhuber and L. Deecke, pp. 3–15. *Prog Brain Res., Vol. 54*. Elsevier, Amsterdam, New York, Oxford.

15. Cavazzuti, G. B., Galli, V., and Benatti, A. (1986): The use of flunarizine in pediatric epilepsy. *Functional Neurology*, 1(4):551–554.

16. Chaikin, P., Flor, S. C., Marriott, T. B., and Weintraub, H. S. (1982b): A clinical evaluation of the pharmacokinetics and pharmacological effects of flunarizine on myocardial conduction: A single blind multiple dose study. *Ortho Pharmaceutical Corporation*. Raritan, New Jersey.

17. Chaikin, P., Soledad, C. F., Marriott, T. B., and Weintraub, H. S. (1982a): The pharmacokinetics of single doses of flunarizine in normal volunteers. *Ortho Pharmaceutical Corporation*. Raritan, New Jersey.

18. Curatolo, P., Bruni, O., Brindesi, I., Pruna, D., and Cusmai, R. (1986): La flunarizina nelle epilessie formaco-resistenti dell'infanzia e dell'adolescenza. *Rivista di Neurologica*, 56:25–38.

19. Debandt, R., De Smedt, R., Jorens, H., Leysen, M., Rodrigus, E., and Van Eycken, L. (1985): Flunarizine as 'add-on' therapy in institutionalized patients with refractory epilepsy. Effect on seizure incidence and behaviour. *Janssen Research Product Information Service*, CRR R 14950/65.

20. De Clerck, F., De Brabander, M., Neels, H., and Van de Velde, V. (1981): Direct evidence for the contractile capacity of endothelial cells. *Thrombosis Research*, 23:505–520.

21. Declerck, A. C., Oei, L. T., and Wauquier, A. (1986): Flunarizine in mentally retarded children with therapy-resistant epilepsy. *Health Science Review: International Workshop of Flunarizine in Epilepsy*. Beerse, May 24, 1985, p. 68.

22. Declerck, A. C., and Wauquier, A. (1978): Double-blind study on the effectiveness of flunarizine in therapy-resistant epilepsy in mentally retarded children. *10th Epilepsy International Symposium, Abstract*, p. 169.

23. Declerck, A. C., and Wauquier, A. (1983): Flunarizine, a double-blind study in therapy resistant mentally retarded epileptic children. *Suppl. del Bolletino Chimico Farmaceutico*, 122:9CL–16CL.

24. De Domenico, P., Gallitto, G., Musolino, R., and Di Perri, R. (1987): Saggio dell 'Utilita' condiuvante della flunarizina in epilettia gravi (*unpublished report*).

25. De Rood, M., Vandesteene, R., Gasparini, R., Van Peer, A., Woestenborghs, R., Heykants, J., Geets, T., and de Beukelaar, F. (1984): Preliminary study on the intravenous pharmacokinetics

of flunarizine (0.1 mg/kg) in man. *Janssen Pharmaceutica, Clinical Research Report*, R14 950/62.

26. De Sarro, G. B., Nisticó, G., and Meldrum, B. (1986): Anticonvulsant properties of flunarizine on reflex and generalised models of epilepsy. *Neuropharmacology*, 25:695–701.

27. De Sarro, G. B., Meldrum, B. S., and Nisticó, G. (1988): Anticonvulsants effects of some calcium entry blockers in DBA/2 mice. *Br. J. Pharmacol.*, 93:247–256.

28. Desmedt, L. K. C., Niemegeers, C. J. E., and Janssen, P. A. J. (1975): Anticonvulsant properties of cinnarizine and flunarizine in rats and mice. *Arzneim Forsch*, 25:1408–1413.

29. Dolin, S. J., Grant, A. J., Hunter, A. B., and Little, H. J. (1986): Anticonvulsant profile and whole brain concentrations of nitrendipine and nimodipine. *Brit. J. Pharmacol.*, 89:866P.

30. Flameng, W., Verheyen, F., Borgers, M., De Clerck, F., and Brugmans, J. (1979): The effect of flunarizine treatment on human red blood cells. *Angiology*, 31:516–525.

31. Fröscher, W., Bülau, P., Burr, W., Kiefer, H., Kreiten, K., Penin, H., Rao, M. L., and de Beukelaar, F. (1988): Double-blind, placebo-controlled trial in flunarizine in therapy-resistant persons with epilepsy. *Clin. Neuropharm. (in press)*.

32. Giroud, M., Nivelon, J. L., and Dumas, R. (1987): Antiepileptic activity of flunarizine in 10 therapy-resistant children with epilepsy. *La Presse Médicale*, 16:18:913.

33. Heinemann, U., Lux, H. A., and Gutnick, M. J. (1977): Extracellular free calcium and potassium during paroxysmal activity in the cerebral cortex of the rat. *Exp. Brain Res.*, 27:237–243.

34. Heykants, J., De Cree, J., and Hörig, C. (1979): Steady-state plasma levels of flunarizine in chronically treated patients. *Arzneim. Forsch./Drug Research*, 29(11):1168–1171.

35. Heykants, J., Michielsen, L., Lorreyne, W., Woestenborghs, R., Scheijgrond, H., and Reyntjens, A. (1981): Bioequivalence study of two flunarizine formulations (a 5 mg capsule and a 10 mg tablet) in a group of 6 healthy subjects. (*unpublished report*). (Janssen, Sept. 1981).

36. Heykants, J., and Van Peer, A. (1983): Steady-state pharmacokinetic of flunarizine in man are predictable from single-dose kinetics. *Janssen Pharmaceutica, Clinical Research Report*, R14950/58, June 1983.

37. Kato, H., Kurihara, J., Ishii, K., and Kassuya, Y. (1981): Vasodilating effect of flunarizine in anaesthetized dogs. *Archives Internationales de Pharmacodynamie et de Therapie*, 249:257–263.

38. Keene, D., Whiting, S., Humphreys, P., Findlay, H. P., and Cumming, B. (1987): Flunarizine, an add-on drug in the treatment of refractory childhood epilepsy. *XXIInd Canadian Congress of Neurological Sciences*, Vancouver, June 1987.

39. Konishi, T., Murakami, M., Yamatani, M., Koda, O., Okada, T., Seto, H., and Nitani, T. (1987): Efficiency of flunarizine (a calcium entry blocker in therapy resistant epileptic children with partial

epilepsy. *The 20th Congress of the Japanese Society of Epilepsy, Abstract Book*, p. 131.

40. Larkin, J. G., Butler, E., and Brodie, M. J. (1978): Nifedipine for epilepsy? *17th Epilepsy International Congress, Jerusalem. Book of Abstracts*, p. 15.

41. Macphee, G. J. A., Thompson, G. G., Gordon, T., McInnes, and Brodie, M. J. (1986): Verapamil potentiates carbamazepine neurotoxicity: A clinically important inhibitory interaction. *Lancet*, 700–703.

42. Mancia, D. (1987): La flunarizina come coordiuvante della terapia di base nel trattamento dell'epilessia (Studio clinico controllato) (*unpublished report*).

43. Meldrum, G. S. (1979): Convulsant drugs, anticonvulsants and GABA-mediated neuronal inhibition. In: *Gaba-neurotransmitters*, edited by P. Krogsgaard-Larsen, J. Scheel-Kruger, and H. Kofod, pp. 390–405. Munksgaard, Copenhagen.

44. Meldrum, B. S. (1983): Convulsants and anticonvulsant drug mechanisms. In: *Current Problems in Epilepsy*, edited by M. Baldy-Moulinier, D. H. Ingvar, and B. S. Meldrum, pp. 324–336. John Libbey, London.

45. Meuldermans, W., Hendricks, J., Hurkmans, R., Swysen, E., Woestenborgs, R., Lauwers, W., and Heykants, J. (1983): Excretion and metabolism of flunarizine in rats and dogs. *Arzneim. Forsch./Drug Res.*, 33:1142–1151.

46. Meuldermans, W., Hurkmans, R., and Heykants, J. (1978): A comparative study of the plasma protein binding and the distribution of flunarizine and cinnarizine in human blood. *Clinical Research Report No. R14 950/30*. Janssen Research Product Information Service.

47. Meyer, F. B., Anderson, R. E., Sundt, T. M., and Sharborough, F. W. (1986): Selective central nervous system calcium channel blockers—A new class of anticonvulsant agents. *Mayo Clin*, 61:239–247.

48. Moglia, A., Bergamasco, B., Di Perri, R., and Mancia, D. (1986): Flunarizine as add-on therapy in epilepsy, cross over study versus placebo. *Furet. Neurol.*, 1:547–550.

49. Olsen, R. W. (1982): Drug interactions at the GABA-receptor ionophore complex. *Annu. Rev. Pharmacol. Toxicol.*, 22:245–277.

50. Oosterveld, W. J. (1974): Vestibular pharmacology of flunarizine compared to that of cinnarizine. *Journal for Oto-Rhino-Laryngology and its Borderlands*, 36:157–164.

51. Overweg, J. (1987): Safety evaluation of flunarizine after long-term 'add-on' administration in epileptic patients. *Clinical Research Report R14 950/71*, Janssen Research Product Information Service.

52. Overweg, J., Binnie, C. D., Meijer, J. W. A., Meinardi, H., Nuijten, S. T. M., Schmaltz, S., and Wauquier, A. (1984): Double-blind placebo-controlled trial of flunarizine as add-on therapy in epilepsy. *Epilepsia*, 25 (2):217–222.

53. Pothmann, R., Braumann, G., and Kröger, T. (1986): Calciumeintrittsblockade als Zusatz-Behandlung bei therapieresistenten kindlichen epilepsien. *Deutsche Sektion der Internationalen Liga gegen Epilepsis*: 26, abstract p. 56. Jahrestagung, Münster.

54. Prince, D. A. (1978): Neurophysiology of Epilepsy. *Annu. Rev. Neurosci.*, 1:395–415.

55. Prince, D. A. (1982): Epileptogenesis in hippocampal and neocortical neurones. In: *Physiology and Pharmacology of Epileptogenic Phenomena*, edited by M. R. Klee, H. D. Lux, and E. J. Speckman, pp. 151–161. Raven Press, New York.

56. Ray, J. A., and Van Caurteren, H. (1986): Flunarizine—A review of nonclinical toxicity data available by March 1986. *Nonclinical Research Report N 49 721*, Janssen Research Product Information Service.

57. Sorel, L. (1987): La flunarizine dans l'épilepsie: Evaluation d'un traitment "additif" de quatre nous chez des patients resistant an traitment antiépileptique existant. *Acta Neurol. Belg.*, 87:140–147.

58. Starreveld, E., et al. (1987): Flunarizine in epilepsy (*report to be written*).

59. Study, R. E., and Barker, J. L. (1981): Diazepam and (−) pentobarbital: Fluctuation analysis reveals different mechanisms for the potentiation of GABA responses in cultured central neurones. *Proc. Natl. Acad. Sci. USA*, 78:7180–7184.

60. Swinyard, E. A., Wolf, H. H., Franklin, M. R., White, H. S., Woodhead, J. H., Kupferberg, H. J., and Stables, J. P. (1987): The profile of anticonvulsant activity and acute toxicity of flunarizine (59076) and some prototype antiepileptic drugs in mice and rats. The early evaluation of anticonvulsant drugs. (*Contract No. NO1-NS-4-2361*). January 5, 1987.

61. Takahashi, T. (1978): An open trial of flunarizine hyrochloride as add-on treatment in therapy-resistant epileptics.

62. Tata, M. R., Guizzaro, A., Giudici, S., Parisi, A., and Bravaccio, F. (1987): Flunarizine in pharmacoresistant epilepsies: Preliminary experiences in 30 cases. *Internatioinal Symposium on Calcium Antagonists, Pharmacology and Clinical Research*, p. 113. New York City, February 10–13, 1987.

63. Touquet, G., and Van Cappel, F. (1985): Flunarizine as adjunvans in therapy resistant epilepsy, a double-blind placebo-controlled trial. *Clinical Research Report No. 14950/64*, Janssen Research Product Information Service.

64. Treiman, D. M., De Giorgia, C. M., Cornish, J. W., and Cereghino, J. J. (1986): Efficacy and toxicity of flunarizine in partial onset seizures at concentrations of 30, 60, 120 ng/ml. *Epilepsia*, 27 (5):649–650.

65. Treiman, D. M., Tsay, J.-Y., Whitley, L. P., Seaman, C. A., Kupferberg, H. J., Pledger, G. W., and Cereghino, J. J. (1987): Final report of flunarizine open tolerability study. *Epilepsy Research*, NINCDS, Bethesda.

66. Umezawa, Y., Amano, K., Kawamurah, H., Tanigawa, T., Kawashima, H., Nagao, T., Kurosu, A., Arai, T., Murao, N., and Kitamura, K. (1987): Add-on therapy of flunarizine in therapy-resistant

epilepsy. *The 20th Congress of the Japanese Society of Epilepsy, Abstract Book*, p. 92.

67. Van Bever, W. (1974): Acute oral toxocity (LD$_{50}$) of flunarizine dihydrochloride in mice, rats and guinea pigs. *Janssen Pharmaceutica, Preclinical Research Report R14950/1*, December 1974.

68. Van Neuten, J. M., and Janssen, P. A. J. (1973): Comparative study of the effect of flunarizine and cinnarizine on smooth muscles and cardiac tissues. *Archives Internationales de Pharmacodynamie et de Therapie*, 204:37–35.

69. Van Reempts, J., Borgers, M., Van Dael, L., Van Eyndhove, J., Van de Ven, M. (1983): Protection with flunarizine against hypoxic-ischaemic damage of the rat cerebral cortex. A quantitative morphologic approach. *Archives Internationales de Pharmacodynamie et de Therapie*, 262:76–78.

70. Van de Velde, V., Van Peer, A., Timmerman, P., Woestenborghs, R., Van Rooy, P., Amery, W., and Heykants, J. (1987): Bioavailability of flunarizine capsules relative to a reference solution of dueterium-labelled flunarizine. *Janssen Pharmaceutica, Clinical Research Report, R 14 950/72.*

71. Van Wieringen, A., Ashton, D. De Beukelaar, F., Binnie, C. D., Overweg, J., and Vauquier, A. (1986): Flunarizine in the treatment of epilepsy. In: *Epilepsy and Calcium*, edited by H. Schalse, and J. Walden, pp. 387–399. Urban and Schwartzenberg.

72. Walden, J., Speckmann, E. J., Witte, O. W. (1984): Effects of the calcium antagonist verapamil on spontaneous and evoked bioelectric activity on the cerebral cortex. *Pflügers Arch.*, 402:R36.

73. Walden, J., Speckmann, E. J., Witte, O. W. (1985): Suppression of focal epileptiform discharges by intracerebroventricular perfusion of a calcium antagonist. *Electroenceph. Clin. Neurophysiol.*, 61:299–309.

74. Wauquier, A., Ashton, D., Clincke, G., and Fransen, J. (1985): "Calcium entry blockers" as cerebral protecting agents: Comparative activity in tests of hypoxia and hyperexcitability. *Japan J. Pharmacol.*, 38:1–7.

75. Wauquier, A., Ashton, D., Clincke, G., Fransen, J., Gillardin, J. M., and Janssen, P. A. J. (1986): Anticonvulsant profile of flunarizine. *Drug Dev. Res.*, 7:49–60.

76. Wauquier, A., Ashton, D., Clincke, G., and Van Reempts J. (1982): Pharmacological protection against brain hypoxia: The efficacy of flunarizine, a calcium entry blocker. In: *The Role of Hypoxia in the Pathogenesis of Migraine*, edited by F. Clifford-Rose, and W. K. Amery, pp. 139–154. Pitman, London.

77. Wauquier, A., Ashton, D., and Melis W. (1979): Behavioural analysis of amygdaloid kindling in Beagle dogs and the effects of clonazepam, diazepam, phenobarbital, diphenylhydantoin and flunarizine on seizure manifestation. *Exp. Neurology.*, 64:579–586.

78. Willow, M., and Catterall, W. A. (1982): Inhibition of binding of [^{3}H] batrachotoxin in A-20-α-benzoate to sodium channels by the anticonvulsant drugs diphenylhydantoin and carbamazepine. *Mol. Pharmacol.*, 22:627–635.

79. Witte, O. W., Speckmann, E. J., and Walden, J. (1984): Contribution of calcium and calcium-dependent membrane currents to epileptic discharges in neocortical neurons of the rat. *Cell Calcium*, 5:311.

80. Witte, O. W., Walden, J., Speckmann, E. J., and Elger, C. E. (1983): Reduction of penicillin-induced paroxysmal depolarization shifts in neurons of rat cerebral cortex by intracellular injection of calcium channel blocker. *Neurosci. Lett. Suppl.*, 14:S405.

81. Woestenborgs, R., Michielsen, L., Lorreyne, W., and Heykants, J. (1982): Sensitive gas chromatographic method for the determination of cinnarizine and flunarizine in biological samples. *J. Chromatogr.*, 232:85–91.

82. Woestenborgs, R., Timmerman, P., Van Peer, A., and Heykants, J. (1988): The use of stable-isotope methodology in pharmacokinetic studies involving flunarizine. In: *Methodological surveys in biochemistry and analysis*. Vol. 18.

83. Wong, R. K. S., Prince, D. A., and Basbaum, A. I. (1979): Dendritic mechanisms underlying penicillin induced epileptiform activity. *Science*, 204:1228–1231.

Antiepileptic Drugs, Third Edition, edited by
R. Levy, R. Mattson, B. Meldrum,
J. K. Penry, and F. E. Dreifuss.
Raven Press, Ltd., New York © 1989.

72

Potential Antiepileptic Drugs

Felbamate

Ilo E. Leppik and Nina M. Graves

Felbamate (W-554; AD-03055) was developed at Wallace Laboratories (Cranbury, New Jersey) in the context of an extensive program that also developed meprobamate and carisoprodol. Its chemical structure is similar to that of meprobamate, an antianxiety agent, but it is much more potent in animal models of epilepsy than its nearest chemical relative.

Extensive studies of its anticonvulsant profile in animal models of epilepsy indicate that felbamate is effective in blocking seizures induced by maximal electroshock (MES), pentylenetetrazol, and picrotoxin, but it is relatively ineffective against biculline- and strychnine-induced seizures. Its major advantage appears to be its low toxicity. In studies involving rats, doses of up to 1 gram per day were given for up to 3 months, with the only effect noted being crystalluria. These doses are far in excess of amounts required for protection against seizures in animal models, and thus the protective index of felbamate is considerably higher than the observed for other antiepileptic drugs. No teratogenic or behavioral effects have been found in reproductive or teratology studies in rats and rabbits.

Although clinical studies are still limited, felbamate appears to have little neurotoxicity in humans. However, felbamate does inhibit the metabolism of phenytoin (PHT), and some of the neurotoxicity observed in clinical studies may have been due to increases in PHT concentrations rather than to felbamate itself. This promising novel agent is currently undergoing more extensive clinical trials to determine its efficacy and safety in treatment of epilepsy.

CHEMISTRY AND METHODS OF DETERMINATION

Felbamate (2-phenyl-1,3-propanediol dicarbamate)* is a dicarbamate with the empirical formula $C_{11}H_{14}N_2O_2$ and a molecular weight of 238.24 (Fig. 1). It is a white, odorless powder which is very slightly soluble in water, sparingly soluble in methanol and acetone, slightly soluble in ethanol and chloroform, and quite soluble in dimethyl sulfoxide, 1-methyl-2-pyrrolidinone, and *N,N*-dimethyl formamide.

Felbamate can be analyzed by high-performance liquid chromatography (HPLC) using a 39% methanol/water mobile phase and a C18 column. Concentrations in the ranges of 0.5 to 100 µg/ml can be detected with this methodology (4). However, carbamazepine (CBZ) metabolites may cause interference when the methanol/water mobile phase is employed. A modification of

---

* Chemical abstract service registry number: 25451-15-4.

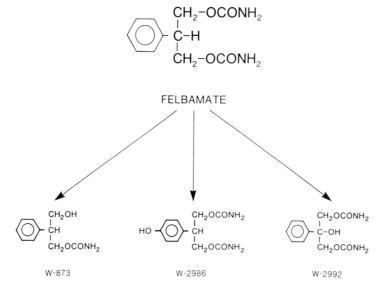

FIG. 1. Structures of felbamate and its major metabolites.

the HPLC assay using a 20% acetonitrile/water mobile phase and a C18 column has been developed (14). These assays have a coefficient of variation of less than 5% over the concentration range of 0.5 to 100 mg/liter.

ANIMAL STUDIES

Extensive studies of the anticonvulsant profile of felbamate in animals have been conducted by Wallace Laboratories, the University of Washington (6), and the Epilepsy Branch of the NINCDS (11).

The potency of felbamate compared to standard antiepileptic drugs is described in Table 1. In the MES seizure model, PHT is most potent, followed by phenobarbital and then by felbamate. Ethosuximide confers no protection in this model. The MES model is thought to be predictive of drugs effective for partial seizures. In contrast, the subcutaneous pentylenetetrazol seizure threshold model has been used to identify antiabsence drugs. In this model PHT confers no protection, whereas valproate and

ethosuximide are both potent. Felbamate also has some potency in this model, thus felbamate has a spectrum broader than PHT and ethosuximide in these two widely used tests. In other tests, however, the spectra are somewhat different (see Table 1). Phenobarbital and valproate exhibit efficacy in the subcutaneous bicuculline and strychnine models, but felbamate and PHT are not effective. In the subcutaneous picrotoxin model, felbamate is more potent than valproate and ethosuximide, but PHT is ineffective. Thus, felbamate possesses a unique spectrum of activity in these standard tests for seizure activity. It has been stated that felbamate seems to increase seizure threshold and prevent seizure spread (12).

Felbamate also has demonstrated activity in rhesus monkeys with aluminum hydroxide lesions in the pre- and postcentral gyri. Felbamate, in doses of 60 to 105 mg/kg, produced a significant decrease in seizures after the first hour of dosing, but the effect was transient (6).

The protective index of a substance is calculated by dividing the TD_{50}, the median

TABLE 1. *Anticonvulsant potency of felbamate, phenytoin, phenobarbital, ethosuximide, and valproate in rodents*

	Felbamate	Phenytoin	Phenobarbital	Valproate	Ethosuximide
ED_{50}					
MES					
Mouse					
PO	81.1	9.0	20.1	665	—[a]
Rat					
PO	47.8	29.8	9.1	490	—[a]
S.C. PTZ					
Mouse					
PO	548	—[a]	12.6	388	193
Rat					
PO	238	—[a]	11.6	180	54
S.C. Bic	—[a]	—[a]	37.7	360	459
S.C. Pic	156	—[a]	27.5	387	243
S.C. Strych	—[a]	Max 50%[b]	95.3	293	Max 62.5%[b]

[a] No protection.
[b] ED_{50} cannot be calculated because of the maximal dose, only the percent indicated were protected.
ED_{50}, the dose of drug required to produce the end point at which 50% of the animals are protected from seizures; MES, maximal electroshock; S.C. PTZ, subcutaneous pentylenetetrazol seizure threshold; S.C. Bic, subcutaneous bicuculline seizure threshold; S.C. Pic, picrotoxin seizure threshold; S.C. Strych, strychnine seizure pattern tests.
From Swinyard et al., 1986.

toxic dose, by the ED_{50}, the median effective dose. The TD_{50} is measured by the rotorod test. The higher this number, the greater the difference between effective doses and toxic doses. The ideal antiepileptic substance would have a very high protective index. A substance that is very potent but also has significant toxicity would have a protective index of 1 or less than 1 and would not be a clinically useful compound. In the MES seizure test, both felbamate and PHT have very high protective indices, with PHT being greater than 100 in the rat and felbamate greater than 62 (Table 2). In contrast, valproate and ethosuximide have protective indices of less than 1 in the rat MES test. In the subcutaneous pentylenetetrazol test, felbamate has a much higher protective index than PHT and is similar to that of the other three medications. However, because felbamate is ineffective for bicuculline and strychnine seizures, protective indices for it cannot be calculated (see Table 2).

The safety ratio for a substance can be calculated by taking the TD_3, which is the minimal toxic dose, and dividing by the ED_{97}, a dose at which 97% of the animals will be protected. This measurement gives a degree of separation between toxicity and efficacy. Again, felbamate has a very high safety ratio in comparison to the other medications, especially in the rat. Perhaps the most unusual feature of felbamate is its relative lack of lethality. Mice and rats could tolerate single doses of 3,000 mg/kg without significant side effects. Doses higher than 3,000 mg/kg were limited by technical problems of administering that quantity of medication. In contrast, the LD_{50}, the median lethal dose, was 230 mg/kg for PHT and 265 mg/kg for phenobarbital. Valproate and ethosuximide had LD_{50} values of 1,205 mg/kg and 1,752 mg/kg, respectively.

Safety studies of felbamate with long-term treatment in rats, dogs, and rabbits have been completed. Female rats receiving 600 mg/kg and both male and female rats receiving 1,200 mg/kg per day had decreased food consumption and reduction in

TABLE 2. *The protective index of felbamate, phenytoin, phenobarbital, ethosuximide, and valproate in rodents*

	Felbamate	Phenytoin	Phenobarbital	Valproate	Ethosuximide
PI (TD_{50}/ED_{50})					
MES					
Mouse					
PO	19.1	9.59	4.82	1.90	<0.44
Rat					
PO	>62.8	>100	6.68	0.57	>0.84
S.C. PTZ					
Mouse					
PO	2.82	<0.29	7.69	3.26	4.56
Rat					
PO	>12.6	N.A.	5.29	1.56	18.8
S.C. Bic	—[a]	<0.65	1.83	1.18	0.96
S.C. Pic	5.23	<0.65	2.51	0.72	
S.C. Strych	—[a]	<0.65	0.72	1.45	—[a]

[a] PI cannot be calculated.

PI, protective index; MES, maximal electroshock; S.C. PTZ, subcutaneous pentylenetetrazol seizure threshold; S.C. Bic, subcutaneous bicuculline seizure threshold; S.C. Pic, picrotoxin seizure threshold; S.C. Strych, strychnine seizure pattern tests.

From Swinyard et al., 1986.

body weight. Drug-related changes were not seen in any of the blood parameters studied or on microscopic evaluation of the tissues. Beagle dogs given up to 1,000 mg/kg per day were found to have weight loss, but no drug-related changes were seen on microscopic evaluation of tissues from these dogs. In rabbits some hepatic cell liposis and/or necrosis was observed with doses exceeding 100 mg/kg. These changes appeared to be dose-related. To date, studies of reproductive toxicity in the rat and rabbit have not shown any fetal anomalies or alterations in reproductive performance (13).

Animal studies thus indicate that felbamate is a potent antiepileptic compound in many of the standard models. However, its uniqueness lies in a very high margin of safety in those models in which it is effective. Felbamate thus appears to be less toxic than antiepileptic compounds currently available, and this experimental finding, if confirmed in human studies, would place it in a category of highly desirable compounds for the treatment of epilepsy.

BIOTRANSFORMATION

Profiles of metabolites of felbamate in blood, bile, and urine have been analyzed for the rat, dog, and rabbit. Major metabolites have been identified by Carter-Wallace by means of HPLC and mass spectral analysis, using both electron impact and chemical ionization techniques. In the rat, approximately 20% of the metabolites were conjugated. After enzymatic hydrolysis, 81% of the products were accounted for as 27% felbamate, 31% W-2986, and 23% W-2992. In the dog, an additional metabolite, eventually identified as W-873, was isolated (see Fig. 1). These three metabolites have not shown significant anticonvulsant activity or neurotoxic properties (13).

CLINICAL PHARMACOKINETICS

Pharmacokinetic data on felbamate are available from three studies: one involving volunteers and two using patients with epilepsy. One of the studies in patients with epilepsy was primarily a pharmacokinetic study (14), and the other was the NIH-sponsored study of felbamate's safety and efficacy, which also permitted estimation of some pharmacokinetic parameters.

In the study reported by Perhatch et al. (8), single and multiple doses of felbamate were given to healthy volunteers. Five volunteers each received a single 600-mg dose. This dose produced a mean maximal serum concentration (Cp_{max}) of 9.9 $\mu g/ml$ and a mean elimination half-life of 20.2 hr. Following a single 800-mg dose, the Cp_{max} was 14.4 + 1.5 $\mu g/ml$ and the mean elimination half-life was 19.4 hr. Multiple dosing of 600 mg twice daily for a few weeks led to a mean elimination half-life of 19.9 hr and a mean steady-state concentration of 29.0 $\mu g/ml$. Mean peak and trough concentrations were 31.8 $\mu g/ml$ and 22.6 $\mu g/ml$, respectively. In these volunteers, at doses of up to 1,200 mg/day, the pharmacokinetics appeared linear.

Wilensky et al. (14) studied the pharmacokinetics of felbamate in patients with epilepsy. Eight patients receiving either PHT or CBZ were given a single 200-mg dose of felbamate and then given an ascending dose schedule of 200 mg b.i.d., 400 mg b.i.d., 600 mg b.i.d., and 800 mg b.i.d. through day 21. Serial blood samples for the pharmacokinetic analysis were obtained after the single 200-mg dose and after the last 800-mg dose. Peak concentrations after a single 200-mg dose ranged from 2.65 to 4.10 $\mu g/ml$. These

occurred 1 to 4 hr after the doses. Single dose median half-life was 13.3 hr (range, 11.2 to 16.1 hr). Following chronic doses of 800 mg twice daily, the median half-life was 14.6 hr. The half-life in this study was shorter than the half-life determined in normal volunteers, possibly from enzyme induction by PHT or CBZ. Six of eight patients also exhibited a decrease in apparent clearance after long-term administration, although in general the decreases were less than 40% (Table 3). This decrease in apparent clearance, plus an observed trend for trough serum concentrations to increase slightly during long-term dosing of 800 mg twice daily led to the suggestion of possible nonlinearity in the dose-level relationship. The median apparent volume of distribution after the single dose was 0.822 liter/kg and after long-term dosing was 0.73 liter/kg.

During the double-blind safety and efficacy trial of felbamate in patients receiving both PHT and CBZ, blood was obtained biweekly at approximately the same time after a dose to measure felbamate concentrations. In 32 patients from the University of Minnesota, the maximum dose of felbamate was 2,600 mg/day, given in three divided doses. The mean dose received was 2,400 mg/day (range, 2,400 to 2,600 mg/day). The mean serum felbamate concentration achieved following these doses was 32.4 $\mu g/ml$ (range, 21.5 to 44.8 $\mu g/ml$). The

TABLE 3. *Pharmacokinetic parameters of felbamate in humans*

Study	Patients	$T_{1/2}$ (hr)	Apparent clearance (liters/hr)	V_d (liters/kg)
Volunteers (ref. 8)				
Single 600-mg dose	$N = 5$	20.2		
Long-term 600-mg b.i.d. dose	$N = 5$	19.9		
Pharmacokinetic (ref. 14)[a]				
Single 200-mg dose	$N = 8$	13.3	3.5	0.82
Long-term 800-mg b.i.d. dose	$N = 8$	14.6	2.8	0.73
Efficacy study[b]				
Long-term 2,600 mg/day	$N = 32$		2.8	0.70

[a] Patients receiving PHT or CBZ.
[b] Patients receiving both PHT and CBZ.

apparent clearance was 3.2 liter/hr (range, 2.4 to 3.9 liter/hr). There was considerable variability in concentrations achieved (Fig. 2). A population pharmacokinetic analysis using NONMEM (9) was performed on the data from this study. With the routinely collected clinical data, the apparent clearance was 2.86 liter/hr.

INTERACTIONS WITH OTHER ANTIEPILEPTIC DRUGS

A significant drug interaction exists between felbamate and PHT. During the initial pharmacokinetic study in patients, a significant increase in PHT concentrations was noted in three out of four patients (14). In two of these patients, the PHT dose had to be decreased because of toxicity. In pilot studies prior to the large scale safety and efficacy evaluation, PHT concentrations rose in all four patients, necessitating a 20% decrease in PHT doses (10). In the double-blind efficacy study, PHT dose decreases of 10% to 30% were required to maintain stable serum PHT concentrations in all 32 patients. There is evidence that felbamate may be a competitive inhibitor of PHT metabolism, since PHT concentrations increased primarily at higher doses of felbamate (>20 mg/kg) (1).

Although PHT concentrations increased with concomitant felbamate treatment, CBZ concentrations decreased. During the safety and efficacy evaluation, CBZ concentrations decreased slightly but significantly (3). The mean decrease was 1.3 µg/ml and occurred in 30 out of 32 patients. Apparent CBZ clearance increased 28% during felbamate treatment (2).

At present, felbamate has been given only to patients taking PHT and CBZ, so that interactions with other drugs are not known at this time.

CLINICAL EFFICACY

Only phase 1 and phase 2 studies of felbamate have been performed in humans to date (Table 4). The initial reports of clinical efficacy of felbamate can be found in a pharmacokinetic study, the primary goal of which was to identify pharmacokinetics in eight patients (15). Nevertheless, some information was gathered regarding seizure control. In six of the eight subjects, there was a "moderate to marked reduction in seizure frequency." Three patients also had "less severe seizures." However, one of these patient's PHT level had increased, thus it was not clear whether felbamate or increased levels of PHT were responsible

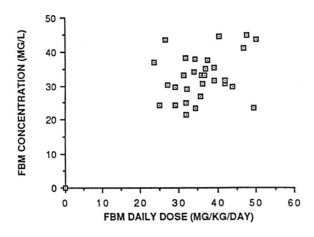

FIG. 2. Felbamate (FBM) dose-concentration relationship in 32 patients from the University of Minnesota sample receiving phenytoin and carbamazepine. Patients had received felbamate for 10 weeks and had steady-state plasma felbamate levels.

TABLE 4. *Summary of clinical trials investigating the efficacy of felbamate in patients with partial seizures*

Study description (reference no.)	No. of patients	Maximum dose (mg/day)	Outcome
Open-label, add-on pharmacokinetic study: U. of WA (14)	8	1,600	6 patients improved
Open-label pilot; U of MN and U of VA (10)	4	2,400	3 patients improved
Double-blind, placebo crossover, add-on to PHT and CBZ; U of MN and U of VA[b]	56	2,600	Statistically significant difference favoring felbamate over placebo
Double-blind, 3-period crossover, add-on to CBZ; NIH (7)[a]	28	3,000	13 patients improved
Open-label, add-on in patients withdrawn from other antiepileptic drugs for monitoring; U of MN[a]	10	3,600	8 patients improved

[a] Study in progress.
[b] Data analysis in progress.

for the improvement. Doses of felbamate in these patients ranged up to 1,600 mg per day.

In the NIH sponsored open-label pilot study at two centers involving four male patients, felbamate was titrated to a maximum dose of 2,400 mg. Three of the four patients showed improvement in seizure control either by reduction of seizure frequency or by change in seizure type from complex partial to simple partial (10).

A double-blind, placebo-controlled trial of felbamate as add-on treatment to PHT and CBZ in 56 patients has been completed. This study followed essentially the same protocol as in the two-center progabide study (5). The results of this felbamate study are still being analyzed. However, preliminary results indicate a statistically significant difference between felbamate and placebo. These results have been sufficiently encouraging for Carter-Wallace to begin a series of additional studies.

A study at NIH of 28 inpatients with epilepsy is still in progress (7). This study involves a triple crossover of felbamate or placebo in patients receiving only CBZ. Of 27 patients completing the study to date, 13 had sufficient reduction in seizure frequency to continue on felbamate after the study (Theodore, *personal communication*).

TOXICITY

Definite neurotoxicity of felbamate has not been observed in patients independent of PHT or CBZ. In the NIH sponsored placebo-controlled, double-blind study, some toxicity was observed, but in almost all cases it was reversed by reducing PHT doses and bringing the PHT levels back into the target range. In this study of 56 patients, preliminary review of laboratory data indicated no significant hepatotoxicity or hematological toxicity. Thus, data from clinical studies suggest that felbamate may have a better therapeutic index than standard antiepileptic drugs. A study in which the dose is titrated rapidly to 3,600 mg/day after partial withdrawal of standard antiepileptic drugs is in progress and should give some indication of the tolerability of these higher doses.

ACKNOWLEDGMENTS

This work was supported in part by NINCDS grant #P50-NS-16308-08. We are grateful to Carter Wallace for providing access to their preclinical data. We thank Theresa Vikla for word processing.

CONVERSION

Conversion factor:

$$CF = \frac{1000}{mol.\ wt.} = \frac{1000}{238.24} = 4.20$$

Conversion:

$$(\mu g/ml) \times 4.20 = (\mu moles/liter)$$

$$(\mu moles/liter) \div 4.20 = (\mu g/ml)$$

REFERENCES

1. Fuerst, R. H., Graves, N. M., Leppik, I. E., Brundage, R. C., and Holmes, G. B. (1988): Felbamate increases phenytoin but decreases carbamazepine concentrations. *Epilepsia*, 29:488–491.
2. Graves, N. M., Holmes, G. B., Fuerst, R. H., and Leppik, I. E. (1989): Effect of felbamate on phenytoin and carbamazepine serum concentrations. *Epilepsia*, 30:225–229.
3. Holmes, G. B., Leppik, I. E., and Fuerst, R. H. (1987): Felbamate: Bidirectional effects on phenytoin and carbamazepine serum concentrations. *Epilepsia*, 28:578 (abstract).
4. Kelton, E. (1982): Determination of W-554 in human plasma over the concentration range 100.0 to 0.5 μg/ml by high performance liquid chromatography. Wallace Laboratories, Cranbury, New Jersey.
5. Leppik, I. E., Dreifuss, F. E., Porter, R., et al.
6. Lockard, J. S. (1984): Final Report: Major efficacy study in primates (rhesus) of Wallace ADD 03055 (W-554). Department of Neurosurgery, University of Washington, June 1984. Data on file at Wallace Laboratories.
7. Nice, F., Raubertas, R., and Porter, R. (1986): New methodology for clinical trials of drugs in patients with partial epileptic seizures. United States Public Health Service Professional Association 21st Annual Meeting, Washington, DC, June 15–18, 1986 (abstract).
8. Perhatch, J. L., Weliky, I., Newton, J. J., Sofia, R. D., Romanyshyn, W. M., and Arndt, W. F. (1986): Felbamate. In: *New Anticonvulsant Drugs*, edited by B. S. Meldrum and R. J. Porter, pp. 117–125. John Libbey and Company.
9. Sheiner, L. B., Rosenberg, B., and Marathe, V. (1977): Estimation of population characteristics of pharmacokinetic parameters from routine clinical data. *J. Pharmacokin. Biopharm.*, 5:445–479.
10. Sheridan, P. H., Ashworth, M., Milne, K., et al. (1986): Open pilot study of felbamate in partial seizures. *Epilepsia*, 27:649.
11. Swinyard, E. A., and Kupferberg, H. J. (1982): The profile of anticonvulsant activity and acute toxicity of 03046, 03055 and some prototype antiepileptic drugs in mice and rats. Epilepsy Branch, NINCDS, NIH, Bethesda, Maryland.
12. Swinyard, E. A., Sofia, R. D., and Kupferberg, H. J. (1986): Comparative anticonvulsant activity and neurotoxicity of felbamate and four prototype antiepileptic drugs in mice and rats. *Epilepsia*, 27:27–34.
13. Wallace Laboratories. W-554 Investigational Drug Brochure, October 1984, Carter Wallace, Inc., Cranbury, New Jersey.
14. Wilensky, A. J., Fuel, P. N., Ojemann, L. M., Kupferberg, H. K., and Levy, R. H. (1985): Pharmacokinetics of W-554 (ADD 03055) in epileptic patients. *Epilepsia*, 26:602–606.

(1987): A controlled study of progabide in partial seizures: Methodology and results. *Neurology*, 37:963–968.

Antiepileptic Drugs, Third Edition, edited by
R. Levy, R. Mattson, B. Meldrum,
J. K. Penry, and F. E. Dreifuss.
Raven Press, Ltd., New York © 1989.

Appendix

Chemical Structures of Antiepileptic Drugs

René H. Levy and David Thomassen

1. List of drugs represented:

Acetazolamide	Metharbital
ACTH	Methazolamide
Bromides	Methsuximide
Carbamazepine	Methylphenobarbital
Clobazam	Nitrazepam
Clonazepam	Oxcarbazepine
Clorazepate	Paraldehyde
Diazepam	Phenobarbital
Ethosuximide	Phenytoin
Ethotoin	Primidone
Felbamate	Progabide
Flunarizine	Stiripentol
Gabapentin	Trimethadione
Lamotrigine	Valproic acid
Lorazepam	Vigabatrin
Mephenytoin	

2. Carbon atoms are not shown explicitly, but are depicted symbolically, and attached hydrogen atoms are implied, e.g., partial structure

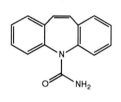

Acetazolamide

H₂N—Ser–Tyr–Ser–Met–Glu–His–Phe·Arg
Lys–Lys–Gly–Val–Pro–Lys–Gly·Trp
Arg–Arg·Pro–Val–Lys–Val–Tyr·Pro
Ala–Leu·Gln·Asp·Glu–Ala·Gly–Asp
Glu—Ala·Phe·Pro–Leu·Glu–Phe——COOH

ACTH

Br ⁻ ⁺X

(⁺X = ⁺Na, ⁺K)

Bromides

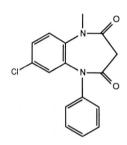

Carbamazepine

Clobazam

Clonazepam

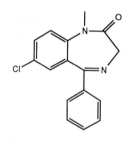

Clorazepate dipotassium

Diazepam

Ethosuximide

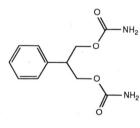

Ethotoin

Felbamate

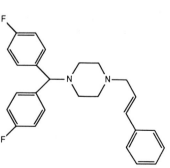

Flunarizine

Gabapentin

Lamotrigine

Lorazepam

Mephenytoin

Metharbital

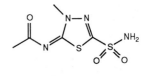

Methazolamide

Methsuximide

Methylphenobarbital

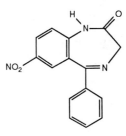

Nitrazepam

Oxcarbazepine

Paraldehyde

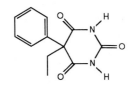

Phenobarbital

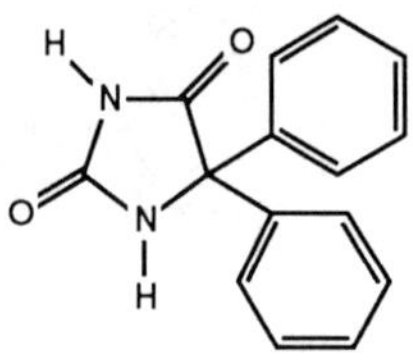

Phenytoin

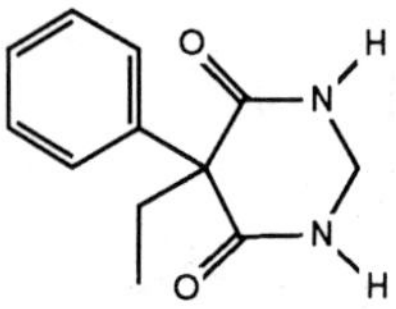

Primidone

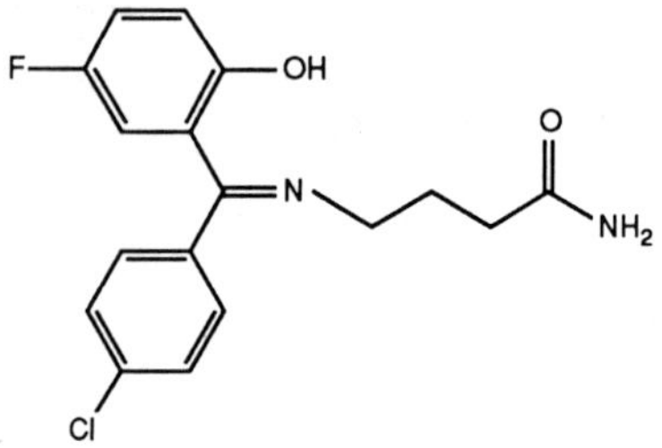

Progabide

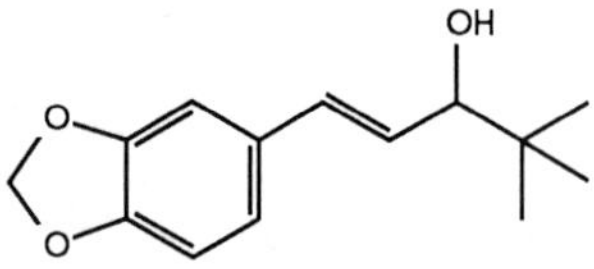

Stiripentol

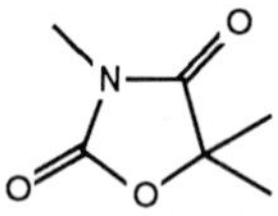

Trimethadione

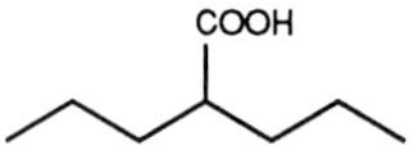

Valproic Acid

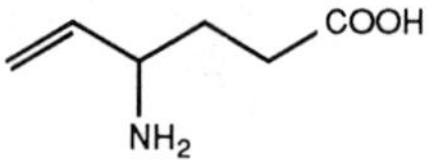

Vigabatrin

Author Index

Anderson, G. D., 305
Baillie, T. A., 601
Baruzzi, A., 785
Binnie, C. D., 971
Booker, H. E., 715
Bourgeois, B. F. D., 401, 633
Browne, T. R., 197, 707
Cereghino, J. J., xxiii
Chang, T., 197, 663, 671, 679
Cloyd, J. C., 391, 439
Cramer, J. A., 341, 621
Dam, M., 913
Dean, J. C., 133
De Lorenzo, R. J., 143
Dodson, W. E., 293
Dreifuss, F. E., 643, 699, 877
Duche, B., 533, 955
Eadie, M. J., 357
Faigle, J. W., 491
Fariello, R., 567
Feldmann, K. F., 491
Ferrendelli, J. A., 653
Fincham, R. W., 413
Franklin, M. R., 85
Friel, P. N., 805
Glazko, A. J., 159

Gram, L., 555, 947
Graves, N. M., 983
Haefely, W., 721
Holland, K. D., 653
Homan, R. W., 841
Jensen, P. K., 555, 913
Johannessen, S. I., 283
Kemp, J. W., 855
Kerr, B. M., 505
Kupferberg, H. J., 257, 577
Kutt, H., 215, 313, 457
Leppik, I. E., 391, 439, 983
Levy, R. H., 1, 505, 521, 583
Lloyd, K. G., 887
Lockman, L. A., 881
Loiseau, P., 533, 955
Macdonald, R. L., 59, 447
Mattson, R. H., 103, 341, 621
Meldrum, B. S., 59
Michelucci, R., 785
Morselli, P. L., 473, 887
Painter, M. J., 329
Palminteri, R., 887
Penry, J. K., 133
Perucca, E., 23
Pitlick, W. H., 521
Plaa, G. L., 49

Porter, R. J., 117
Prichard, J. W., 267
Rangel, R. J., 233
Ransom, B. R., 267
Rettenmeier, A. W., 601
Reynolds, E. H., 241
Richens, A., 23, 937
Rust, R. S., 293
Sato, S., 765
Schäfer, H., 379
Shen, D. D., 583
Sherwin, A. L., 685
Schmidt, B., 925
Schmidt, D., 735
Schottelius, D. D., 413
Shorvon, S. D., 821
Smith, D. B., 423
Smith, M. C., 567
Snead, O. C., III, 905
Swinyard, E. A., 85
Tassinari, C. A., 785
Unadkat, J. D., 1
Unwin, D. H., 841
White, H. S., 85
Wilder, B. J., 233
Wilensky, A. J., 805
Woodbury, D. M., 177, 855
Woodhead, J. H., 85

Subject Index

Absence seizures, 686–688
  acetazolamide, 869
  atypical, 686–687
  characteristics, 685–688
  clonazepam, 771
  diagnosis, 687
  diazepam, 753
  drug selection principles, 103–105
  drug withdrawal prognosis, 136
  ethosuximide, 688–696
  methsuximide, 712
  pathophysiological characteristics, 687–688
  prognostic factors, 694–695
  stiripentol, 966–968
  trimethadione, 716–718
  valproate, 633, 691
Absence status, 687
Absolute bioavailability, 583
Absorption, 1–21
  acetazolamide, 856
  bromides, 877–878
  carbamazepine, 471–472
  clobazam, 825
  clorazepate, 809–810
  diazepam, 735–737
  drug interactions, 56
  and drug selection, 113
  ethosuximide, 671–673
  ethotoin, 261–262
  general principles, 1–21
  lamotrigine, 949
  lorazepam, 842
  methsuximide, 708–709
  methylphenobarbital, 358–359
  nitrazepam, 787–788
  oral administration, 6–9
  oxcarbazepine, 918–920
  paraldehyde, 882
  phenobarbital, 293–295, 313–314
  phenytoin, 177–181, 216–217
  primidone, 391–392
  progabide, 890
  stiripentol, 960
  trimethadione, 717
  valproate, 583–585
  vigabatrin, 938
Absorption rate constant, 7
Absorption ratio, 100
aca system, 667
ACCULEVEL technique
  carbamazepine, 461

phenobarbital, 289–290
  phenytoin, 169–170
Acenocoumarol, 34
Acetaminophen
  phenobarbital and, 320, 323
  phenytoin and, 225
Acetazolamide, 855–871
  absence seizures, 104
  absorption, 856
  acidosis and, 862–863
  d-amphetamine and, 863–864
  biotransformation, 863
  carbamazepine and, 864
  carbon dioxide and, 865–867
  chemistry, 855–856
  in children, 858
  clinical use, 869–871
  conversion, 872
  distribution, 857–863
  excretion, 863
  half-life, 857–860
  interactions with other drugs, 863–864
  mechanism of action, 866–869
  methods of determination, 855–856
  pentobarbital and, 864
  pharmacological effects, 864–866
  phenobarbital and, 319
  plasma levels, therapeutic effect, 870
  primidone and, 393, 433
  probenecid and, 864
  protein binding, 857
  structure, 856, 992
  teratogenesis, 871
  tolerance, 866, 868–870
  toxicity, 870–871
Acetone, 382
Acetophenetidin, 323
Acetylation
  general principles, 27
  nitrazepam, 791
Acetylcholine
  carbamazepine action, 452
  phenobarbital, 275
  phenytoin effects, 154
  progabide action, 896
Acetylsalicylic acid; *see also* Salicylic acid
  phenytoin and, 218
Acidosis
  acetazolamide and, 862–863
  paraldehyde and, 885
9-Acridinecarboxaldehyde, 456
  gas chromatography, 506–507

Acroparesthesias, 794
ACTH, 905–910
    cerebral ventriculomegaly, 908
    efficacy, 905–909
    in infantile spasms, 905–908
    mechanism of action, 909
    nitrazepam and, 797
    prednisone comparison, efficacy, 906–908
    protocol, 907–908
    structure, 992
    synthetic versus natural form, 906, 908
    toxicity, 908
    West syndrome, 106, 797
Action potentials
    carbamazepine action, 447–451
    phenobarbital action, 274–275
Activated charcoal
    phenobarbital, 294–295, 313
    phenytoin, 217
Acute cholangitis, 557
Acute intermittent porphyria, 560
Acute toxicity tests, 90–91
Adenosine system
    carbamazepine, 451–452
    benzodiazepine receptor ligands, 731
    drug action, 73–74
    drug evaluation, 90, 96
Adrenal cortical function, 558–559
Adverse effects, see Side effects
Affinity, 725
Afterhyperpolarization, 63
Age at onset, 134
Age factors
    carbamazepine dosage, 548
    drug kinetics, 15–16
    drug metabolism, 29–31
    drug selection, 111
    phenobarbital enzyme induction, 316
    primidone, 405, 434
    valproate metabolism, 609
Aged
    clorazepate, 811–812
    diazepam binding, 739, 741
    drug disposition, 16
    drug metabolism, 30–31
    glucuronidation, 31
    nitrazepam, 788–790, 795
    primidone, 434
    valproate, 593
Agranulocytosis
    ethosuximide, 702
    phenytoin, 250
Ah receptor, 36–37
Albumin, 181
Albutoin, 257
Alcohol, see Ethanol interactions
Alcohol consumption, and phenobarbital, 316
Alcohol withdrawal syndrome, 637

Alcoholic epilepsy, 109
Alcoholism, and diazepam, 740
Allergic drug reactions, 51
3-Allyl-5-isobutyl-2-thiohydantoin, 257
Alopecia
    and drug selection, 110
    valproate, 644
Alpha$_1$ acid-glycoprotein, 473
"Alpha coma," 795
Alumina lesions, 568–569
Ambulatory EEG monitoring, 127
Amenorrhea, 645
Ames Seralyzer, 169
Amidopyrine, 319–320
γ-Aminobutyrate acid, see GABA entries
γ-Aminobutyrate transaminase, see GABA-
    transaminase
δ-Aminolevulinic acid synthase, 349
2-Amino-5-phosphonovalerate, 72
Aminophylline, 745
Aminotransferase levels, 895
Amiodarone, 221
d-Amphetamine, 864
Amygdala
    nitrazepam, 796
    phenytoin distribution, 189
    phenytoin effects, 146
Analgesics
    phenobarbital and, 317–320
    phenytoin and, 218–219, 224–225
Androgens, phenytoin toxicity, 248
Anemia, see Aplastic anemia; Megaloblastic
    anemia
Anesthesia, 270–271
Animals, experimental
    drug testing, 86, 100
    human correlation, 100
Antacids
    clorazepate and, 812
    phenytoin and, 216
    primidone and, 393
Anterior dorsal thalamic nucleus, 146
Antiasthma agents
    phenobarbital and, 320
    phenytoin and, 225
Antibiotics
    phenobarbital and, 318, 320
    phenytoin and, 225
Antibodies, phenytoin and, 250–251
Anticoagulants
    phenobarbital and, 320
    phenytoin and, 219, 225
Antiepileptic Drug Development Program, 86
Antidiuretic effect, carbamazepine, 558
Antidiuretic hormone
    carbamazepine and, 558
    phenytoin and, 248
Antidiuretics, phenytoin and, 225

Antifungal agents, phenytoin and, 220
Antimicrobial agents, phenytoin and, 219–220
Antineoplastic agents, phenytoin and, 220
Antipyretics
    phenobarbital and, 317–320
    phenytoin and, 218–219, 224–225
Antipyrine clearance
    drug effects, 38
    gabapentin and, 931
    phenobarbital and, 319–320
Antiulcer agents
    phenobarbital and, 320
    phenytoin and, 221
Aplastic anemia
    carbamazepine, 557
    ethosuximide, 702
    phenytoin, 250
Apoenzyme Reactive Immunoassay System
    (ARIS), 168–169, 289–290
Apparent oral clearance, 8–9
Appetite increase, 111
Area under the curve, 5–6, 8, 12–13
Arene oxide
    phenytoin metabolism, 25–26, 197–199
    structure, 26
    teratogenicity role, 199
Arene oxide–N.I.H. shift pathway, 199
Arginine vasopressin levels, 558
ARIS test, 168–169, 289–290
Arylhydrocarbon hydroxylase, 36–37
Aspartate
    drug mechanisms, 76–77
    ethosuximide action, 656
    valproate effect, 572
Asphyxia, 299
Aspiration pneumonia, 794
Asterixis, 644
Astrocytes, phenobarbital and, 274
Astrogliosis, 189–190
Ataxia
    clobazam, 827
    clonazepam, 774–775
    phenytoin, 241–242
    primidone, 441
Attention effects
    carbamazepine, 542–543
    phenobarbital, 344–345
    primidone, 429
    stiripentol, 959
Atypical absence seizure, see Lennox-Gastaut
    syndrome
Autoimmune thyroiditis, 702
Autoinduction
    carbamazepine, 38–39, 475, 523
    phenobarbital, 310
Autoreceptors, 73
Azaserine, 76

Barbital, conversion, 376
Barbiturates
    calcium channels, 67–68
    carbamazepine comparison, 108
    enzyme induction, 38–39
    GABA$_A$ receptor, 70–71
Basal ganglia, ethosuximide, 702
Bayesian forecasting, 20–21
Behavioral effects
    carbamazepine, benefits, 541–544
    clonazepam, 774–775
    phenobarbital, 333–335, 342–343, 429
    phenytoin, 243–244
    primidone, 429
Benzodiazepine agonists
    receptor action, 725–730
    tolerance, 729, 732
Benzodiazepine antagonists, 745
Benzodiazepine binding; see also Benzodiazepine
    receptor
    ethosuximide, 655
    neurotransmitter systems, 655–657
Benzodiazepine receptor, 721–732; see also
    GABA$_A$ receptor
    agonist effects, 728–731
    bromide action, 878
    and calcium influx, 731–732
    clonazepam action, 768–770
    endogenous ligands, 732
    ligand pharmacology, 724–730
    phenytoin and, 154–155
    potassium conductance, 732
    sodium channels, 732
    structure, 722–728
    tolerance and, 729, 732
    typology, 723
Benzodiazepines; see also Benzodiazepine
    receptor; GABA$_A$ receptor
    absence seizures, 104–105
    antiepileptic potential, evaluation, 96–100
    GABA release, 76
    mechanisms of action, 721–732
    valproate interactions, 626
Benzylmalonate methylester monoamide, 458
Beta-carbolines, 745
Bicuculline seizure threshold test, 86–87, 89,
    96–100
Bilirubin
    and enzyme induction, 40
    phenobarbital effect, 323
Bioavailability, 7–9
Biotransformation, 23–45
    acetazolamide, 863
    drug interactions and, 56
    ethotoin, 262
    felbamate, 986
    general principles, 23–45
    kinetic principles, 11–13

Biotransformation (*contd.*)
    lorazepam, 843
    mephenytoin, 259
    methylphenobarbital, 362–365
    nitrazepam, 791
    oxcarbazepine, 919–921
    paraldehyde, 882–883
    phenobarbital, 305–311
    phenytoin, 197–209, 217–218
    primidone, 401–410
    progabide, 891–892
Bipolar disorder, valproate and, 637
Bishydroxycoumarin
    phenobarbital and, 320
    phenytoin and, 219
Bleomycin, phenytoin and, 220
Blepharospasm, 773
Blood-brain barrier
    ethosuximide, 674
    valproate, 586–588
Blood dyscrasias, 702
Blood flow, 42–43
Body fat
    clorazepate, 810–811
    ethosuximide, 673–674
    phenytoin, 186–187
Body weight, 20
Bone disease
    phenobarbital, 348
    phenytoin, 246–247
    primidone, 443
Bone marrow suppression
    ethosuximide, 702
    valproate, 645
Bradycardia, 559
Bradykinesia, 702
Brain distribution
    acetazolamide, 860–863
    carbamazepine, 472–473, 498–499
    carbamazepine 10,11-epoxide, 498–499
    diazepam, 738
    ethosuximide, 673–674
    phenobarbital, 295–296
    phenylethylmalonamide, 393
    phenytoin, 186–190
    primidone, 393
    valproate, 585–589
Brain growth, 331, 347
Brain Uptake Index, 587–588
Breast milk
    acetazolamide, 860
    carbamazepine, 477, 548
    diazepam, 751
    ethosuximide, 675, 694
    lorazepam, 851
    methylphenobarbital, 372
    nitrazepam, 789
    phenobarbital, 296

Bromides, 877–879
    absorption and distribution, 877–878
    clinical use, 878–879
    excretion, 877–878
    mechanisms of action, 878
    structure, 992
    toxicity, 878–879
Bromism, 878–879
Bromosulphalein, 57
Bronchial hypersecretion, 794
Burst firing
    carbamazepine effect, 451
    cellular mechanisms, 62–64

CA_1 pyramidal cells, 63, 451
CA_2 pyramidal cells, 63–64
CA_3 pyramidal cells, 63–64
Cable telemetry, 127
Caffeine, 452
Calcium
    phenobarbital and, 272–274
    phenytoin and, 149–151
Calcium channels
    benzodiazepine receptor ligands, 731–732
    burst firing, 63
    drug mechanisms, 65, 67–69
    ethosuximide, 654–655
    phenytoin and, 150–152
Calcium-containing fillers, 216
Calcium entry blockers, 971–979
    carbamazepine and, 525
Calcium valproate, 584
Calmodulin systems, 151–153
L-Canaline, 76
Carbamazepine, 447–565
    absorption, 471–472
    in animals, 500–502
    autoinduction, 38–39, 475, 523
    barbiturates comparison, efficacy, 108
    biotransformation, 491–502
    cardiac toxicity, 559
    chemistry, 455–456
    in children, 477–478, 533–549, 556
    classification, action, 61
    clinical use, 533–549
    clonazepam comparison, efficacy, 540
    clonazepam interactions, 524, 776
    conversion, 426
    distribution, 472–474
    dosage choice, 544–546
    doxycycline and, 524
    drug interactions, 521–528
    enzyme induction, 38–39
    ethosuximide and, 524
    half-life, 120–121, 474–475, 501, 522
    hematological toxicity, 557–558
    hepatotoxicity, 557

hypersensitivity reactions, 556–557
initiation of, 118–119, 545
intake intervals, 120
mechanisms of action, 447–453
metabolites, 491–502
    anticonvulsant action, 498–500
    chemistry, 491–496
metabolism, 491–502
methods of determination, 456–466
neurotoxicity, 555–556
overdosage, 560
oxcarbazepine comparison, 920–922
phenobarbital comparison, efficacy, 335–336,
    539–541
phenobarbital interactions, 319, 321
phenytoin comparison, efficacy, 233–235,
    539–541
phenytoin interactions, 222, 225–226, 237,
    523–524
plasma levels, 122
    drug interactions, 526–527
    effectiveness, 122, 547–548
pregnancy, 31, 476–477
primidone comparison, efficacy, 429, 539–541
primidone interactions, 419, 523
progabide interactions, 893
psychotropic effects, 541–544
and seizure type, efficacy, 104–109
side effects, and selection, 109–112
sodium channel, 64–66
structure, 448, 456, 491, 992
synaptic actions, 451–452
toxicity, 548, 555–561
valproate comparison, efficacy, 540, 636
valproate interactions, 523–525, 549, 625–628
Carbamazepine-diol
    structure, 448
    sustained repetitive firing, 449
Carbamazepine, 10,11-epoxide
    absorption, 471
    anticonvulsant action, 499–500
    biotransformation, 509–512
    chemistry, 456, 493, 505–507
    clearance, 497, 512–513
    conversion, 466
    distribution, 473
    dosage, and kinetics, 480–481
    drug interactions, 513–517, 527
    elimination, 474–476
    and enzyme inhibition, 41
    half-life, 512
    metabolism, 493–498
    methods of determination, 462–466, 505–507
    neurotoxicity, 508–509, 555
    pharmacokinetics, 512–513
    pharmacology, 507–509
    phenobarbital and, 515
    phenytoin and, 226, 515

pregnancy, 477
progabide and, 893
structure, 448, 492
sustained repetitive firing, 449
teratogenicity, 500
toxicology, 500
valproic acid and, 515–516, 625–626
valpromide and, 498, 500, 508, 515–516
Carbamazepine 10,11-*trans*-dihydrodiol
    chemistry, 457
    elimination, 475–476, 511
    metabolism, 496, 506, 509–510
    methods of determination, 462–465, 506–507
    pharmacology, 507–508
    structure, 509
Carbon dioxide, acetazolamide and, 865–867
Carbonic anhydrase
    acetazolamide inhibition, 864, 866–869
    brain excitability role, 869
    and seizures, 865
    tolerance role, 868
Carbonic anhydrase inhibition method, 856
Carbonic anhydrase inhibitors, 865
Carcinogenicity, 53
Cardiac failure, carbamazepine, 479, 559
Cardiovascular effects
    carbamazepine, 559
    phenobarbital, 331
Carnitine, 603
Carnitine deficiency, valproate, 645
Cat
    acetazolamide distribution, 858
    phenytoin metabolism, 183–184, 209
Catamenial epilepsy
    acetazolamide, 869
    clobazam, 831
Catechol metabolites, phenytoin, 206–209
Catecholamines, 452
Caudate nucleus, 570
Cerebellar syndrome, phenytoin, 241–242
Cerebral cortex
    carbamazepine, 473
    phenytoin distribution, 188
    phenytoin effects, 146
Cerebral ventriculomegaly, ACTH, 908
Cerebrospinal fluid
    acetazolamide, 860–863
    carbamazepine, 473–474, 499
    carbamazepine 10,11-epoxide, 499
    ethosuximide, 674
    lorazepam, 842
    nitrazepam, 789
    phenobarbital, 295–296
    phenytoin, 186–190
    primidone, 393–394
    vigabatrin, 941
CFF (critical flicker fusion), 792
Charcoal, *see* Activated charcoal

Chemically induced convulsions, 86–87
Chemistry
    acetazolamide, 855–856
    carbamazepine, 455–456
    clobazam, 821–822
    clonazepam, 765
    clorazepate, 805–806
    diazepam, 735
    ethosuxidime, 663
    ethotoin, 261
    felbamate, 983–984
    flunarizine, 971
    gabapentin, 925
    lamotrigine, 947
    lorazepam, 841
    mephenytoin, 257–258
    metharbital, 357
    methsuxidime, 707–708
    methylphenobarbital, 357
    nitrazepam, 785
    oxcarbazepine, 913
    phenobarbital, 283–291
    phenytoin, 159–172
    primidone, 379–381
    progabide, 888
    stiripentol, 955
    valproate, 577–581
    vigabatrin, 937
Childhood absence epilepsy, 104
Children
    drug kinetics, 15–16
    drug metabolism, 29–30
    drug selection, 111
    drug withdrawal studies, 134–135, 138, 140
    side effects, 111
Chloramphenicol
    phenobarbital and, 318, 320
    phenytoin and, 219, 225
Chlordiazepoxide, 223
Chloride channels; see also GABA$_A$ receptor
    phenytoin, 152
Chlorpromazine
    phenobarbital and, 319, 322
    phenytoin and, 224, 228
Cholangitis, 557
Cholecalciferol, 227
Cholesterol, 323
Cholinergic system; see also Acetylcholine
    carbamazepine action, 452
Chorea, and clonazepam, 773
Chromatography, see Gas chromatography-mass
        spectrometry; Gas-liquid chromatography;
        High-performance liquid chromatography;
        Thin-layer chromatography
Chromosomes, see Mutagenicity
Chronic liver disease, 14–15
Chronopharmacokinetics, 18–19

Cigarette smoking
    clorazepate elimination, 812
    enzyme induction and, 37
Cimetidine
    carbamazepine and, 525, 549
    clorazepate and, 812
    diazepam and, 744
    nitrazepam and, 792
    phenobarbital and, 314, 320
    phenytoin and, 221
Circadian rhythm
    carbamazepine elimination, 474
    drug metabolism, 31–32
Cirrhosis
    phenobarbital effect, 337
    valproate elimination, 594
Classification, seizures, 103–104
Clearance
    concepts, 4–6
    in disease states, 13–14
    and half-life, 6
Cleft lip/palate, 751
Clinical use; see also Seizure control
    acetazolamide, 869–871
    bromides, 878–879
    carbamazepine, 533–549
    clobazam, 830–836
    clonazepam, 828–836
    clorazepate, 813–815
    diazepam, 752–756
    ethosuximide, 685–696
    lamotrigine, 949–951
    lorazepam, 844–849
    nitrazepam, 796–799
    oxcarbazepine, 921–923
    paraldehyde, 883–884
    progabide, 897–899
    stiripentol, 964–968
    valproate, 633–639
Clobazam, 821–836
    absorption, 825
    chemistry, 821–822
    clinical use, 825–836
    diazepam comparison, efficacy, 827
    dosage regimens, 836
    drug interactions, 825–826
    mechanisms of action, 822
    neurotoxicity, 827–828, 834
    pharmacodynamics, 826–830
    pharmacology and kinetics, 822–825
    rectal administration, 825, 830
    side effects, 834–835
    structure, 822, 992
    tolerance, 831, 834
    withdrawal, 835–836
Clonazepam, 765–777
    absence seizures, 771
    absorption, 766

antiepileptic potential, 96–100
biotransformation, 766–767
carbamazepine comparison, efficacy, 540
carbamazepine interactions, 524
chemistry, 765
in children, 767–768, 773–775
classification, 61
complex partial seizures, 771
distribution, 766
drug interactions, 776
excretion, 766
half-life, 767–768
infantile spasms, 772
Lennox-Gastuat syndrome, 772
lorazepam comparison, efficacy, 846–847
mechanism of action, 768–771
methods of determination, 765–766
myoclonic seizures, 772–773
partial agonist properties, 729
phenobarbital interactions, 319
phenytoin interactions, 223
photosensitive seizures, 773
plasma levels, seizure control, 767–768
primidone interactions, 421
side effects, 773–776
simple partial seizures, 772
status epilepticus, 773
structure, 766, 992
teratogenicity, 776
tolerance, 771
tonic-clonic seizures, 771
toxicity, 773–776
valproate interactions, 626, 644
Clorazepate, 805–817
absorption, 809–810
adverse effects, 816
alcohol interactions, 812
biotransformation, 807–809
chemistry, 805–806
conversion, 817
distribution, 810–811
drug interactions, 812–813
elimination, 811–812
mechanisms of action, 813
teratogenicity, 816
tolerance, 816–817
Coagulation defects, 246
Coenzyme A, 603–604
Cognitive effects
and drug selection, 110–111
folic acid, 246
phenobarbital, 333–335, 343–344
phenytoin, 243–244
Colorimetric procedures, *see* Spectrophotometric
methods
Coma, valproate and, 644
Competitive benzodiazepine antagonists, 726–730

Complex partial seizures, 107–109
carbamazepine, 544
clobazam, 829
clonazepam, 771
clorazepate, 814–815
drug selection, 107–109
lorazepam, 849
methsuximide, 712–713
phenobarbital, 335–336
valproate, 635
vigabatrin, 942–943
Compliance, 125–126
Computed tomography, 129
Congestive heart failure, 479, 559
Conjugation reactions
age factors, 30–31
general principles, 26–27
induction of, 40
inhibition of, 41
Connective tissue disorders
and drug selection, 110
phenobarbital, 348
primidone, 443
Contraceptives, *see* Oral contraceptives
Conversion
acetazolamide, 872
barbital, 376
carbamazepine, 466
carbamazepine 10,11-epoxide, 466
clonazepam, 777
clorazepate, 817
diazepam, 757
dimethadione, 719
ethosuximide, 667
ethotoin, 263
felbamate, 990
flunarizine, 979
gabapentin, 934
lamotrigine, 952
lorazepam, 851
mephenytoin, 263
metharbital, 376
methsuximide, 713
methylphenobarbital, 376
nitrazepam, 799
oxcarbazepine, 923
paraldehyde, 885
stiripentol, 968
trimethadione, 718
vigabatrin, 945
Cord blood, *see* Umbilical cord serum
Corpus callosotomy, 129
Corticosteroid treatment; *see also* ACTH
hypersensitivity reaction, 556
West syndrome, 106
Corticothalamic transmission, *see* Thalamocortical
system

Cortisol
  carbamazepine effect, 558
  enzyme induction, 40
  phenytoin effect, 227, 247
Critical flicker fusion, 792
Crystalluria, 441–442
Cyclic nucleotide regulation
  brain excitability, 869
  phenytoin, 152–153
Cyclohexyl adenosine, 451
Cyclosporin
  phenobarbital and, 320
  phenytoin and, 225
Cytochrome P-450 isozymes
  carbazepine metabolism, 496–497
  genes, 24–25
  oxidation role, 24
  phenobarbital induction, 314, 316
Cytochrome P450dbl gene, 28
Cytochrome, P450mp gene, 29

Danazol, carbamazepine and, 526
Darvon, *see* Propoxyphene
Debrisoquine hydroxylator phenotype, 28, 498
Delta-4 VPA, 549
Delta wave, 136
Demeclocycline, 558
Denzimol, 526
Dependence
  clobazam, 835–836
  clorazepate, 816–817
  diazepam, 750
  nitrazepam, 793–794
  partial benzodiazepine agonists, 729
  phenobarbital, 345–346
Depression
  carbamazepine, benefits, 541–544
  phenobarbital side effect, 334, 343
  primidone, 440
Dermatitis bullosa, 443
Desipramine, 322
N-Desmethylclobazam, 823–826, 828
N-Desmethyldiazepam
  bioavailability, 810
  biotransformation, 742–744, 806–807
  clinical use, 813–815
  distribution, 810–811
  elimination, 811–812
  mechanism of action, 813
  methods of determination, 806–807
  pharmacokinetics, 739–742
  plasma levels, 750
  structure, 800
N-Desmethylmethsuximide, 709–710
Dexamethasone, 227
Dextropropoxyphene, 317
Dialysis, valproate and, 594

Diamox, *see* Acetazolamide
Diazemul, 752
Diazepam, 735–757
  absorption, 735–738
  age-dependent metabolism, 30
  biotransformation, 742–744
  chemistry, 735
  in children, 739, 741
  conversion, 756
  distribution, 738–742
  dose and plasma concentration, 745–746
  emergency treatment, 750, 752–756
  excretion, 742
  GABA receptor, 70–72
  GABA release, 76
  habituation, 750
  half-life, 738, 740, 742
  interactions with other drugs, 744–745
  intramuscular administration, 738, 750
  intravenous administration, 737–738, 752–754
  lorazepam comparison, efficacy, 752–753
  methods of determination, 735
  oral administration, 735–736, 750–751, 756
  phenobarbital comparison, efficacy, 338
  phenobarbital interactions, 319, 744
  phenytoin interactions, 223, 744
  plasma concentration, seizure control, 745–754
  in pregnancy, 741, 751
  prophylaxis, 755, 756
  rectal administration, 738, 750, 755
  respiratory depression and, 748
  structure, 7, 992
  teratogenesis, 751
  therapeutic use, 752–756
  tolerance, 749–750
  toxicity, 748–749, 751–752
    plasma levels, 748–749
  valproate interactions, 626, 744
Diazoxide, phenytoin and, 221
Dicoumarol, phenytoin and, 225
Diet, drug metabolism, 31–32
Diethylphenylxanthine, 451
Differential pulse polarography, 170
Digitoxin, 225
Dihydrodiol, 201–202
  metabolic pathways, 201, 308–309
  phenobarbital and, 308–309
  phenytoin metabolism, 26, 197–202, 209
  stereoselective formation, 202
  structure, 26, 201, 307
10,11-Dihydro-10-hydroxy-carbamazepine, 913–923
4,4′-Dihydroxy metabolites, phenytoin, 209
3,4-Dihydroxyphenylacidic acid, 452
Dilantin, *see* Phenytoin
Dilantin Infatabs, 159
Dilantin Sodium Kapseals, 159
Dilantin-125 Suspension, 159

Diltiazem
  carbamazepine and, 525
  clinical use, 978
Dimethadione
  calcium channels, 67
  conversion, 719
  excretion, 717
  mechanism of action, 716–717
  methods of determination, 715–716
  plasma levels, 718
  structure, 715–716
5,5-Diphenylimidazolin-4-one, 257
Discontinuation of antiepileptic drugs, 133–141
Disopyramide, 225
Displacement, drug interactions, 56
Distribution, 1–21
  acetazolamide, 857–863
  bromides, 877–878
  carbamazepine, 472–474
  carbamazepine epoxide, 512
  clonazepam, 766
  clorazepate, 810–811
  diazepam, 738–742
  ethosuximide, 673–675
  ethotoin, 261–262
  general principles, 1–21
  lamotrigine, 949
  lorazepam, 842
  methsuximide, 708–709
  methylphenobarbital, 360–361
  nitrazepam, 788–789
  paraldehyde, 882
  phenobarbital, 295–297
  phenytoin, 144, 181–190
  physiological basis, 3–6
  primidone, 393–394
  progabide, 890–891
  stiripentol, 960–962
  trimethadione, 717
  valproate, 585–590
Disulfiram
  diazepam and, 744
  phenytoin and, 224
Dizziness, 110
Dogs
  acetazolamide distribution, 857–860
  carbamazepine metabolism, 501–502
  diazepam pharmacokinetics, 740–741
  phenytoin metabolism, 183–184, 209
DON (6-diazo-5-oxo-l-norleucine), 76
Dopamine
  carbamazepine and, 452
  clonazepam action, 768
  ethosuximide action, 656
  phenytoin interactions, 228
  progabide action, 896
Dosage
  biotransformation and, 32–35
  carbamazepine, 544–545

changes in, timing, 120–121
  diazepam, 745–746
  ethosuximide, 692–694
  initiation of therapy, 118–119
  methsuximide, 710–711, 713
  phenobarbital, 331–332, 335
  phenytoin, 235–236
  primidone, 431–434
  valproate, 637–639
Dose-dependent kinetics, 17–18
Dose-response relationships, 54–55
Dosing interval, 10–11
Dosing ratio, 10
Doxenitoin, 257
Doxycycline
  carbamazepine and, 524
  phenobarbital and, 320
  phenytoin and, 225
Driving impairment, nitrazepam and, 794
Drooling, nitrazepam and, 794
Drowsiness, see Sedation
Drug interactions, see Interactions, drug
Drug withdrawal, 133–141
  clobazam, 835–836
  clorazepate, 816–817
  EEG prediction, 136–137
  general principles, 133–141
  lorazepam, 850
  phenobarbital, 345–346
  and plasma drug levels, 138
  protocol, 139
  research recommendations, 140
  risk-benefit ratio, 139–140
  seizure type indicator, 136–137
  timing of, 138
Dry-phase immunology, 168
Dupuytren's contracture, 110
  phenobarbital, 348
  primidone, 443
Duration of drug effect, 95
Duration of epilepsy, 134–136
Dynorphin, 909
Dyskinesias, phenytoin and, 242

Eclamptic convulsive attacks, 773
EEG (electroencephalography)
  absence seizures, 686–687
  carbamazepine, 556
  clobazam, 835
  clonazepam, 770
  diazepam plasma levels, 746–747
  drug withdrawal prognosis, 136–137
  intractable epilepsy monitoring, 126–127
  lorazepam, 842, 849
  nitrazepam, 796
  phenobarbital, 271
  primidone, 427–428, 441
  surgery evaluation, 129

Elderly, *see* Aged
Electroencephalography, *see* EEG
Electron capture gas chromatography, 787
  acetazolamide, 856
  clorazepate, 806
  lorazepam, 841–842
Electroshock seizure tests, 86–87, 92
Elimination; *see also* Excretion
  carbamazepine, 474–476
    species differences, 501
  carbamazepine epoxide, 512
  clorazepate, 811–812
  diazepam, 742
  drug metabolites, 11–13
  ethosuximide, 675–676
  felbamate, 987
  general principles, 1–21
  lamotrigine, 949
  methylphenobarbital, 361–362
  oxcarbazepine, 918–921
  phenobarbital, 297–300
  physiological basis, 3–6
  primidone, 392–398
  progabide, 890–891
  valproate, 590–595
  vigabatrin, 938–939
Elimination clearance, 12
Elimination rate, 9–10
Elimination rate constant, 7, 10
EMIT, *see* Enzyme multiplied immunoassay
  technique
Encephalopathy, 243
Enzyme immunoassay
  phenytoin, 165–166
  valproate, 580
Enzyme immunochromatography
  phenobarbital, 289–290
  phenytoin, 169–170
Enzyme induction, 35–40, 42
Enzyme inhibition, 40–42
Enzyme-inhibitor complex, 857
Enzyme-linked immunosorbent assay (ELISA),
  165–166
Enzyme multiplied immunoassay technique (EMIT)
  barbiturates, 358–359
  carbamazepine, 460
  ethosuximide, 667
  phenobarbital, 287
Enzyme saturation
  general principles, 32–33
  phenytoin, 184
Epilepsia partialis continua, 772
Epilepsy centers, 127–128
Epilepsy Foundation of America, 128
Epoxide hydrolase
  dihydrodiol formation, 201–202
  teratogenicity role, 199, 201
  valpromide inhibition, 41–42

Epoxide phenobarbital
  metabolism, 208–309
  structure, 307
Erythema multiforme
  ethosuximide, 701
  phenytoin, 249
Erythrocytes
  acetazolamide, 860, 870
  carbamazepine, 474
Erythromycin, 521, 526, 548
Estrogens
  carbamazepine and, 559
  phenytoin and, 248
Eterobarb, spectrum of action, 268
Ethanol interactions, 57
  antiepileptic drugs, 57
  clorazepate, 812
  lorazepam, 850
  phenobarbital, 350
  phenytoin, 224
Ethosuximide, 653–705
  absence seizures, 685–687
  absorption, 671–673
  antiepileptic potential, evaluation, 96–100
  basal ganglia involvement, 702
  behavioral effects, 693, 700
  biotransformation, 679–683
  blood dyscrasias, 702
  brain enzyme activity and, 654
  calcium channels, 67, 69
  carbamazepine and, 524
  central metabolism effect, 653–654
  chemistry, 663
  in children, 675, 688–696
  classification, 61
  clinical use, 685–696
  conversion, 667
  distribution, 673–675
  dosage effects, absorption, 671–673
  drug interactions, 703
  excretion, 675–676
  fraction, 679
  half-life, dosage, 120–121, 675
  idiosyncratic reactions, 701
  initiation of, 119
  marrow depression, 702
  mechanisms of action, 653–658
  metabolites, 679–683
  methods of determination, 663–667
  pharmacokinetic modeling, 676–677
  plasma levels, 122
    and dose, 692–694
    effectiveness, 122, 688–694
  primidone and, 379, 419
  protein binding, 673
  seizure type, efficacy, 104–105
  structure, 664, 680, 992
  systematic lupus erythematosus, 701

teratogenicity, 694, 703
therapeutic specificity, 653
toxicity, 699–704
    acute, 699
valproate comparison, efficacy, 691
valproate interactions, 625
Ethotoin, 261–263
    absorption and distribution, 261–262
    biotransformation, 262
    chemistry, 261
    clinical efficacy, 262–263
    conversion, 263
    excretion, 261–262
    methods of determination, 261
    structure, 992
    toxicity, 262–263
7-Ethoxycoumarin deethylase, 37
7-Ethoxyresorufin-*O*-deethylase, 37
Ethylacetate, 382
Ethylphenacemide, 421
5-Ethyl-5-phenylhydantoin (Nirvanol), 257–258
Evoked potentials
    nitrazepam, 796
    phenobarbital, 271
    vigabatrin, 944
Excitatory amino acids, 656
Excretion; *see also* Elimination
    acetazolamide, 863
    bromides, 877–878
    carbamazepine, 474–476
    clonazepam, 766
    diazepam, 742
    dimethadione, 717
    drug interactions, 56–57
    ethosuximide, 675–676
    ethotoin, 261–262
    kinetics, 9
    lorazepam, 843–844
    methsuximide, 708–709
    nitrazepam, 789–791
    paraldehyde, 882
    phenytoin, 190–191
    primidone, 397–398
    valproate, 595
Experimental animals, 86
Extraction ratio, 4–5, 8

Facial changes, phenytoin toxicity, 249
Fast acetylation, 28, 220
Febrile illnesses, 186
Febrile seizures
    diazepam prophylaxis, 755–756
    nitrazepam, 798
    phenobarbital, 333
    primidone, 434
    valproate, 636–637
Feed-back inhibition, 63
Feed-forward excitation, 63–64

Feed-forward inhibition, 63
Felbamate, 983–990
    animal studies, 984–986
    biotransformation, 986
    chemistry, 983–984
    clinical efficacy, 988–989
    conversion, 990
    dose-concentration relationship, 987–988
    drug interactions, 223, 988
    methods of determination, 983–984
    pharmacokinetics, 986–988
    phenytoin and, 223, 988
    structure, 984, 992
    toxicology, 985–986, 989
Fetal anticonvulsant syndrome, 251
Fetal development
    side effects, 111–112
    toxicity detection, 52–53
Fibrinogen depletion, 645
First-pass effect, 8
Flash methylation
    phenobarbital 285–286
    p-HPPH, 171
Flow-dependent clearance, 5
Flumazenil
    diazepam and, 745
    receptor antagonist properties, 729
Flunarizine, 971–979
    adverse reactions, 977–978
    chemistry, 971
    clinical efficacy, 974–977
    conversion, 979
    drug interactions, 223, 226–227, 319, 322, 974
    experimental pharmacology, 971–973
    metabolism, 974–975
    methods of determination, 971
    pharmacokinetics, 973–974
    phenobarbital interactions, 319, 322
    phenytoin interactions, 223, 226–227
    structure, 972, 992
    toxicology, 973, 977–978
Fluorescence polarization immunoassay (FPIA)
    carbamazepine, 461
    ethosuximide, 667
    phenobarbital, 287–288
    phenytoin, 167–168
    primidone, 386
    valproate, 580
Fluorometry
    carbamazepine, 457
    nitrazepam, 785
    phenytoin, 161
Fluphenazine, 656
Fluroxene, 323
Focal epilepsy
    diazepam, plasma levels, 747–748
    drug selection, 107–109
    phenobarbital, 269–270
    valproate, 568–569

Focal neurological deficit, 134
Folate deficiency
    enzyme induction mechanism, 39
    phenobarbital, 323, 347–348
    primidone, 442
Folic acid
    antiepileptic mechanisms, 245–246
    neuropsychiatric disorders, 246
    phenytoin and, 224, 227, 244–246
Folic acid deficiency, 244–246
Follicle-stimulating hormone, 248
Food intake effects
    carbamazepine, 472
    clobazam, 822
    clorazepate, 811
    nitrazepam, 788
    phenytoin, 216–217
    valproate, 584
Formation clearance, 12
Free drug levels, 122–123
Free fatty acids, 628
Free fraction in plasma, 14
Frequency of seizures, 134–135
Frozen shoulder, 110
    phenobarbital, 348
    primidone, 443
Full agonists, 726–730
Full inverse receptor antagonists, 730
Furosemide
    phenobarbital and, 323
    phenytoin and, 217, 225

G-proteins, 69
GABA; see also GABA receptor; GABA_A receptor
    clonazepam action, 768–770
    ethosuximide action, 655
    inhibitory action, 68–69, 730
    metabolism, 74–76
    phenobarbital, 272
    phenytoin, 153
    receptor agonist action, 730–731
    release of, 76
    structure, 938
    uptake, 76
    valproate and, 569–570
    vigabatrin effect, 76, 939–941
GABA agonists, see Progabide
GABA receptor; see also GABA_A receptor
    bromide action, 878
    drug action, 63–65, 69–72
    drug evaluation studies, 89–90, 96
    ethosuximide action, 655–656
    inhibitory mechanism, 68–72, 730–731
    phenobarbital effect, 274
    progabide action, 896–897
GABA_A receptor, 721–732
    carbamazepine, 452

drug action, 69–72
    ligand pharmacology, 724–731
    progabide effect, 897
    structure, 69, 722, 725
    typology, 723
GABA-transaminase
    GABA metabolism, 74–75
    vigabatrin inhibition, 74, 939, 941
Gabapentin, 925–934
    animal pharmacology, 925–929
    antipyrine effects, 931
    chemistry, 925
    conversion, 934
    electrophysiology, 926–927
    GABA effects, 927
    mechanism of action, 925–929
    pharmacokinetics, 929–931
    side effects, 932–934
    structure, 926, 993
    therapeutic efficacy, 931–934
    toxicology, 929
Gait, neurotoxicity test, 91
β-Galactosidase, 167
Galactoxyl umbelliferone, 167
Gas chromatography
    diazepam, 735
    ethosuximide, 663–666
Gas chromatography-mass spectrometry
    carbamazepine, 458
    carbamazepine epoxide, 506
    clonazepam, 765–766
    diazepam, 735
    ethosuximide, 665
    methsuximide, 708
    methylphenobarbital, 358
    phenobarbital, 287
    primidone, 385–386
    valproate, 609
Gas-liquid chromatography
    carbamazepine, 457–459
    clonazepam, 765–766
    diazepam, 735
    dimethadione, 716
    flunarizine, 971
    lorazepam, 841–842
    methylphenobarbital, 358
    nitrazepam, 787
    phenobarbital, 285–286, 290
    phenytoin, 161–164
    primidone, 381–385
    progabide, 888
    trimethadione, 716
    valproate, 577–579
Gastrointestinal distress
    and drug selection, 110, 112
    methsuximide, 711
    phenobarbital, 350
    valproate, 643

Generalized absence seizures
  drug classification, 61
  pathways, propagation, 62
  sodium channel blockade, 67
Generalized idiopathic epilepsies, 103–106
Generalized tonic-clonic seizures
  diazepam, 753
  drug classification, 61
  drug selection, efficacy, 107–108
  drug withdrawal prognosis, 136
  phenobarbital, 335–336
  phenytoin, 233–235
  sodium channel blockade, 67
  valproate, 633–634
Generic preparations
  absorption, 120
  carbamazepine, 549
  primidone, 392, 431
Genetic factors
  carbamazepine metabolism, 498
  drug metabolism, 28–29, 34–35, 316–317
  phenobarbital enzyme induction, 316–317
Gilles de la Tourette syndrome, 773, 776
Gingival hypertrophy, 144
Glial cells
  carbonic anhydrase, 866–868
  phenobarbital, 274
D-Glucaric acid excretion, 38
1-β-D-Glucopyranosyl phenobarbital
  phenobarbital metabolism, 308
  structure, 307
Glucose metabolism, 248
β-Glucuronidase, 171, 495
Glucuronidation
  carbamazepine, 495–497
  enzyme induction, 40
  ethosuximide, 681
  general principles, 26–27
  valproate, 602–603
N-Glucuronide of phenytoin, 209
Glusulase, 171
Glutamate
  carbamazepine action, 452
  drug mechanisms, 76–77
  excitation effect, 71
Glutamate decarboxylase, 74–75
Glutamic acid, 572
Glutaminase, 76
Glutamine, 76
Glutaminic acid decarboxylase, 654
Glycine
  clonazepam action, 770
  nitrazepam action, 796
  valproate conjugation, 603–604
Glycosuria, phenytoin and, 248
Graft survival, 702
Grand mal epilepsy, *see* Generalized tonic-clonic
  seizures
Granulocytopenia, 110, 702
Griseofulvin, 313–314, 320

Guinea pigs, diazepam and, 740–741, 744
Gum hypertrophy, phenytoin and, 248–249

Habituation; *see also* Dependence
  diazepam, 750
  phenobarbital, 345–346
Hair changes, valproate and, 644
Half-life, antiepileptic drug
  acetazolamide, 857–860
  in aged, 16
  carbamazepine, 120–121, 474–475
  carbamazepine epoxide, 512
  clonazepam, 767–768
  clorazepate, 807–808
  diazepam, 738, 740
  and drug intake intervals, 120
  ethosuximide, 121, 675
  lamotrigine, 949
  lorazepam, 842–843
  methsuximide, 710
  methylphenobarbital, 361
  nitrazepam, 788–790
  pharmacokinetic principles, 2, 6
  phenobarbital, 120–121, 297–299, 332
  phenytoin, 121, 182–186, 204–205, 208
  primidone, 120–121, 394–395, 404, 427
  and steady-state levels, 10–11, 120–122
  valproate, 120–121, 595
Haloperidol
  carbamazepine and, 524
  phenobarbital and, 322
HD_{50}/TD_{50} ratio, 99
head growth, phenobarbital and, 347
"Head-space" technique, 578
Heart, ethosuximide distribution to, 673–674
Heart failure, carbamazepine and, 479
Heart rate, neonates, 331
Hematological toxicity
  carbamazepine, 557–558
  phenobarbital, 347
  phenytoin, 249–250
  primidone, 442
  valproate, 645
Heme biosynthesis, 560
Hemifacial spasm, 773
Hemopoietic reactions, phenytoin, 249–250
Heparin, 812
Hepatic clearance
  carbamazepine, 522
  concepts, 4, 8–9
Hepatic disease
  carbamazepine kinetics, 479
  diazepam kinetics, 739–741
  drug kinetics, 14–15
  drug metabolism, 43–44
  phenobarbital effect, 337, 349–350
  valproate elimination, 594
  valproate metabolism, 611

Hepatic function
  drug evaluation tests, 93–94
  experimental design, 100
Hepatic toxicity
  carbamazepine, 557
  and drug selection, 110
  primidone, 442
  progabide, 895
  valproate, 613–614, 645–647
Hepatitis
  carbamazepine, 557
  phenobarbital, 337
  phenytoin, 250
  primidone, 405–406
  valproate, 594
Heroin, phenobarbital and, 350
Hexobarbital, stereoselectivity, 34
Hexobarbital sleep time test, 92–93
Hiccups, intractable, 637
High-performance liquid chromatography
  acetazolamide, 856
  carbamazepine, 461–464
  carbamazepine epoxide, 506
  clonazepam, 766
  clorazepate, 806–807
  dimethadione, 716
  ethosuximide, 665–666
  flunarizine, 971
  p-HPPH, 171–172
  lorazepam, 842
  mephenytoin, 258
  methsuximide, 708
  nitrazepam, 787
  phenobarbital, 286–287, 290
  phenytoin, 164–165
  primidone, 381–384
  progabide, 888–889
  stiripentol, 955
  trimethadione, 716
  valproate, 579–580
Hindleg tonic extension, 87
Hippocampal neurons
  burst firing, 62–63
  carbamazepine, 449–451
  phenobarbital, 269, 276
Hippocampus
  carbamazepine distribution, 473
  phenytoin distribution, 189
  phenytoin effect, 146
Hirsutism, phenytoin and, 144, 249
Homogeneous enzyme immunoassay, *see* Enzyme
    multiplied immunoassay technique
Homovanillic acid
  carbamazepine and, 452
  valproate and, 587
m-HPPH, 171, 209
p-HPPH, 163–165
  assay, 171–172

excretion, 190
metabolic pathways, 201
phenytoin inhibition, feedback, 34
phenytoin metabolite, 26, 170–172, 197–202, 209
species differences, 209
stereoselective formation, 202
structure, 26, 170, 198
valproate interactions, 624
Humans, drug toxicity, 54
Hydrolysis, 26
Hydroxybutyrate, 654–656
2-Hydroxycarbamazepine
  anticonvulsant activities, 499–500
  carbamazepine metabolism, 494
3-Hydroxycarbamazepine, 494, 499–500
25-Hydroxycholecalciferol, 322
6-Hydroxycortisol, 247
5-(1-Hydroxyethyl)-5-phenylbarbituric acid, 307, 309
5-Hydroxyindoleacetic acid, 587
10-Hydroxyl-11-methylsulfonyl-10,11-
    dihydrocarbamazepine, 510
9-Hydroxymethyl-10-carbamoyl acridan, 476
  anticonvulsant activities, 499–500
  carbamazepine metabolism, 509–510
  epoxide pathway, 493–494
2-Hydroxyphenetidin, 323
p-Hydroxyphenobarbital, 306–309, 402
5-(4-Hydroxyphenyl)-5-phenylhydantoin, *see*
    p-HPPH
2-Hydroxy-valproate, 606
3-Hydroxy-valproate, 604–605
Hyperactivity
  clonazepam and, 774–775
  phenobarbital and, 333–334, 342–343
Hyperammonemia, 645
Hyperbilirubinemia, 349–350
Hyperglycemia, phenytoin and, 248
Hyperglycinemia, 645
Hyperglycinuria, 645
Hypersensitivity reactions
  carbamazepine, 556–557
  diazepam, 752
  phenobarbital, 350–351
  phenytoin, 249
  primidone, 443
Hyperventilation, 688
Hyponatremia
  carbamazepine, 558
  oxcarbazepine, 922–923
Hypotension, 748
Hypothermia, 794
Hypothyroidism
  carbamazepine and, 558
  phenytoin and, 248
Hypsarrhythmia, *see* West syndrome
  definition, 906

Ibuprofen, 219
"Ictal" events, 62–63
Idiopathic benign childhood epilepsy, 107
Idiopathic generalized epilepsy
  carbamazepine, 544
  drug selection, 103–106
Idiosyncratic drug reactions
  classification, 50
  monotherapy versus polytherapy, 124
Iminodibenzyl, 455–456
Iminostilbene
  elimination, 475
  gas chromatography, 458–459
  high-pressure liquid chromatography, 464
Iminostilbene epoxide, 511
Iminostilbene-10,11-*trans*-dihydrodiol, 511
Imipramine
  carbamazepine similarity, 456
  phenytoin and, 224
Immunoassay methods
  carbamazepine, 459–461
  clonazepam, 766
  ethosuximide, 666–667
  methylphenobarbital, 351–359
  nitrazepam, 785–786
  phenobarbital, 287–291
  phenytoin, 165–170
  primidone, 386
Immunoglobulins, 250–251
Immunosuppressants
  phenobarbital and, 320
  phenytoin and, 225
Impotence
  and drug selection, 110–111
  phenobarbital, 346
  phenytoin and, 248
  primidone and, 440
Inactive conformation, channels, 66
Individualization of dose, 19–21
Infantile spasms
  ACTH, 905–908
  brain development hypothesis, 909
  clinical description, 905
  clonazepam, 772
  morbidity and mortality, 906
  nitrazepam, 797
  phenobarbital, 329–335
  prognosis, 906
Infants
  drug kinetics, 15–16
  drug selection, 111
  side effects, 111
Inferior colliculus, 189
Infusion rate, 9–10
Inhibitory mechanisms, *see* Synaptic inhibition
Inhibitory postsynaptic potential, 152
Initiation of therapy, 118–119
  carbamazepine, 545

general principles, 118–119
  phenytoin, 235–236
  primidone, 432
  and side effects, 110
Insomnia
  nitrazepam, 793–794
  phenobarbital, 342
  stiripentol, 959
Intellectual function
  ethosuximide, 700
  phenobarbital, 333–335, 343–345
  phenytoin, 243
Interactions, drug
  acetazolamide, 863–864
  biotransformation effect, 56–57
  carbamazepine, 521–528
  clobazam, 825–826
  clonazepam, 776
  clorazepate, 812–813
  diazepam, 744–745
  ethosuximide, 703
  experimental testing, 94
  liver parameters, 93–94
  lorazepam, 850
  methsuximide, 710
  methylphenobarbital, 365–367
  nitrazepam, 791–792
  phenobarbital, 313–323
  phenytoin, 215–228
  polytherapy risk, 124
  primidone, 413–421
  progabide, 892–894
  toxicity, 55–58
  valproate, 621–630
  vigabatrin, 944
Interictal epileptiform discharges, 849
"Interictal" events, 62–63
International classification of epilepsies and
    epileptic syndromes, 104
International classification of epileptic seizures,
    104
Intractable hiccups, 637
Intractable seizures, *see* Refractory seizures
Intravenous administration, 2–6
Intrinsic clearance, 4–5, 9, 12–14
  carbamazepine, 522
  disease states, 13–15
Intrinsic efficacy, 725–726, 729
Inverse benzodiazepine agonists, 725–730
Involuntary movements, 242
Isobolograms, 94
Isoniazid
  carbamazepine and, 548
  phenytoin and, 219–220
  primidone and, 419

Josamycin, 548

Kainate receptor, 71
Kainic acid, 656
Kidney disease, *see* Renal disease
Kindling
    drug evaluation, 90
    partial inverse agonists, 730
    phenobarbital, 270
    valproate, 569

L channel, 67–68
Lactose excipient, 179, 216
Lamotrigine, 947–952
    chemistry, 947
    clinical efficacy, 949–951
    conversion, 952
    experimental pharmacology, 947–948
    methods of determination, 947
    pharmacokinetics, 949
    phenobarbital and, 319
    phenytoin and, 223, 227
    structure, 948, 993
    teratogenesis, 948–949
    toxicology, 948–951
Late onset epilepsy, 134
Lateral geniculate body, 657
Learning behavior, phenobarbital and, 344
Left temporal abnormalities, 636
Lennox-Gastaut syndrome
    ACTH, 908
    clonazepam, 772, 830, 832–833
    clorazepate, 815
    drug selection, 106–107
    nitrazepam, 798
    valproate, 634–635
Lethality, 54–55
Leukopenia
    carbamazepine, 557–558
    clonazepam, 774–775
    diazepam, 751
    and drug selection, 110
    methsuximide, 711
    nitrazepam, 795
    phenytoin, 250
    primidone, 442
Levonantradol, 745
Libido
    and drug selection, 110–111
    phenobarbital, 346
    primidone, 440
Light exposure, clonazepam and, 771
Limbic seizures, 62
Lipid meals, 216
Lithium carbonate, 744
Liver
    acetazolamide, 859–860
    ethosuximide distribution, 673–674
    phenytoin distribution, 186–187

primidone biotransformation, 403
    progabide effect on, 895
Liver disease, *see* Hepatic disease
Liver enzyme studies, 93–94, 100
Liver microsomes, 309
Liver toxicity, *see* Hepatic toxicity
Loading dose
    general principles, 118–119
    methylphenobarbital, 372–373
    phenytoin, 235
    and steady-state levels, 10–11, 122
Long-term memory, 345
Lorazepam, 841–851
    absorption and distribution, 842
    chemistry, 841
    in children, 847–848
    clonazepam comparison, efficacy, 846–847
    conversion, 851
    diazepam comparison, efficacy, 847
    drug interactions, 850
    duration of action, 845
    excretion, 843–844
    half-life, 842–843
    metabolism and biotransformation, 843
    methods of determination, 841–842
    pharmacodynamics, 844–849
    phenytoin comparison, efficacy, 847
    plasma levels, 842–844
    postanoxic myoclonus, 848–849
    side effects, 849–850
    status epilepticus, 752–753, 845–848
    structure, 842, 993
    teratogenicity, 850
    withdrawal, 850
Low-incidence toxic reactions, 55
Low-threshold calcium current, 655, 658
Lung, ethosuximide distribution, 673–674
Luteinizing hormone, 248
Lymphadenopathy
    carbamazepine, 556
    phenytoin, 250
    primidone, 442

M proteins, 70
Macrocytic anemia, 442
Macrocytosis, 245
Macrolide antibiotics
    carbamazepine and, 548
    enzyme inhibition, 41
Magnetoencephalography, 129
Malnutrition syndrome, 480
Manic-depressive illness, 544
Manic reactions
    carbamazepine, 559
    stiripentol, 960
Marrow suppression, *see* Bone marrow
    suppression

Mass balance, 491–493
Mass spectrometry, *see* Gas chromatography-mass spectrometry
Maternal serum, valproate, 589
Maximal threshold tests, 86–88, 92, 94
Maximum velocity
  clearance concepts, 4
  nonlinear kinetics, 17–18
Mechanisms of action, 59–78
  acetazolamide, 866–869
  ACTH, 909
  benzodiazepines, 721–733
  bromides, 878
  clobazam, 822
  clorazepate, 813
  ethosuximide, 653–658
  general principles, 59–78
  phenytoin, 143–156
  progabide, 897
  stiripentol, 957–958
  trimethadione, 716–717
Median effective dosage, 55, 91–92, 96–100
Median hypnotic dose, 96–100
Megaloblastic anemia
  carbamazepine, 557
  phenobarbital, 347
  phenytoin, 245
  primidone, 442
Membrane stabilization, 150
Membranous glomerulopathy, 559
Memory
  phenobarbital and, 334, 343–345
  primidone, 440
Menstruation, 184
Mental retardation, and prognosis, 134
Mental symptoms; *see also* Psychotic reactions
  carbamazepine and, 541–544
  phenytoin and, 243
Meperidine
  phenobarbital and, 320
  phenytoin and, 224–225
Mephenytoin, 257–261
  biotransformation, 259
  chemistry, 257
  clinical efficacy, 260–261
  conversion, 263
  methods of determination, 258
  polymorphic metabolism, 259–260
  stereoselectivity, 259
  structure, 258, 993
  toxicity, 260–262
Mephenytoin hydroxylator phenotype
  definition, 29
  stereoselectivity, 34–35
Mephobarbital
  mechanisms of action, 268
  stereoselectivity, 35
meta-HPPH, 171, 209

Metabolic bone disease, 246–247
Metabolites, kinetics, 11–13
Metahydroxyphenobarbital, 308
Methadone
  phenobarbital and, 320
  phenytoin and, 225
Metharbital, 357–376
  biotransformation, 362–365
  chemistry, 357
  conversion, 376
  hepatic metabolism, 362
  methods of determination, 357–359
  pharmacodynamics, 374–375
  structure, 358, 993
  therapeutic use, 375
  toxicity, 374
Methazolamide, 871–872, 993
Methobarbital, 334
Methods of determination
  acetazolamide, 855–856
  carbamazepine, 456–466
  carbamazepine epoxide, 462–466, 506–507
  carbamazepine 10,11-*trans*-diol, 506–507
  clonazepam, 765–766
  diazepam, 735
  ethosuximide, 663–667
  ethotoin, 261
  felbamate, 983–984
  flunarizine, 971
  lorazepam, 841–842
  mephenytoin, 258
  metharbital, 357–359
  methylphenobarbital, 357–359
  phenobarbital, 283–291
  phenytoin, 143–156
  primidone, 381–387
  progabide, 888–889
  stiripentol, 955
  valproate, 577–581
  vigabatrin, 937–938
Methsuximide, 707–713
  absorption and distribution, 708–709
  biotransformation, 709–710
  chemistry, 707–708
  conversion, 713
  dosage and administration, 713
  dose-related side effects, 710–711
  drug interactions, 710
  excretion, 709
  methods of determination, 707–708
  phenobarbital interactions, 319, 321–322
  phenytoin interactions, 223, 226
  primidone interactions, 419
  structure, 708, 993
  therapeutic use, 712–713
  toxicity, 711–712
9-Methylacridine, 456
N-Methyl-D-aspartate, 63–64

3-*O*-Methyl catechol metabolites, 206–209
3-Methylcholanthrene, 35–36
Methylfolate treatment, 246
N-Methyloxazepam, 743–744
Methylparatyrosine, 656
Methylphenidate
   phenytoin and, 224
   primidone and, 421
Methylphenobarbital, 357–376
   absorption, 359–360
   biotransformation, 362–365
   chemistry, 357
   conversion, 376
   distribution, 360
   dosage guidelines, 373–374
   elimination, 361–362
   interactions with other drugs, 365–367
   methods of determination, 357–359
   pharmacodynamics, 374–375
   phenobarbital derivation, plasma, 367–370
   plasma levels, 365, 367–374
     and toxicity, 370–371
   in pregnancy, 372
   renal excretion, 361–362
   stereoselectivity, 363
   structure, 358, 993
   therapeutic use, 375
   tolerance, 371
   toxicity, 374
   valproate and, 367
5-(4-Methylphenyl)-5-phenylhydantoin, 161
3-Methylsulfonylcarbamazepine, 499–500
Metoprolol, 35
Metrazol-induced seizures, 86–88, 90–100
Metronidazole, 220
Metyrapone, 217
Michaelis constant
   clearance concepts, 4
   nonlinear kinetics, 17–18
Michaelis-Menten equation
   clearance concepts, 4
   enzyme saturation, 33
Miconazole, 220
Microvacuoles, 940–941, 944
Milacemide, 223, 227
Minimal threshold tests, 85, 90
Misonidazole, 227
MK-801, 72
Modulated receptor hypothesis, 66
Monoamine oxidase inhibitors, 57
Monoexponential decay, 13
Monotherapy
   drug withdrawal advantage, 137
   polytherapy comparison, 123–125
   rationale, 123–125
Mood effects, carbamazepine, 541–544
"Morning set-up" plan, 126
Motor cortex, phenobarbital and, 269, 276

Motor endplate potentials, 154
Movement disorders
   carbamazepine, 555
   phenytoin, 242
MPPH, 161, 164
Multicompartment kinetic models, 11
Multiple-dose kinetics, 9–11
Multiple-drug regimens, 123–125
Muscle
   ethosuximide distribution, 673–674
   phenytoin distribution, 186–187
Muscle spindle discharges, 448–449
Muscle tone test, 91
Mutagenicity, 53–54
   diazepam, 752
   oxcarbazepine, 918
   primidone, 435
   stiripentol, 958
   testing for, 53–54
Myelin, carbonic anhydrase, 866–868
Myelomeningocele, 648
Myoclonic seizures
   clonazepam, 772–773
   drug classification, 61
   drug selection principles, 105
   nitrazepam, 797
   progabide, 899
   valproate, 634

N channel, 67–68
NADPH-linked aldehyde reductase, 654
Nafimidone
   carbamazepine and, 526
   phenytoin and, 223
Neocortex, burst finding, 62–63
Neonatal withdrawal syndrome, 345–346
Neonates, *see* Newborns
Nephelometric inhibition immunoassay
   phenobarbital, 288
   primidone, 386
Neuropathy, phenytoin and, 244
Neuropsychological tests, 541–543
Neurotoxicity
   animal tests, 90–91
   carbamazepine, 555–556
   carbamazepine epoxide, 508–509, 555
   clobazam, 827–828, 834
   clonazepam, 774–775
   detection, 94–100
   and drug selection, 109–112
   lorazepam, 849–850
   nitrazepam, 794
   phenobarbital, 341–346, 407–409
   primidone, 407–409, 439–441
   stiripentol, 959–960
   trimethadione, 718
   valproate, 644
   vigabatrin, 940–941, 943–944

Neurotransmitters
  drug effects, 74–77
  ethosuximide action, 655–657
  phenytoin, 153–154
Neutropenia, valproate and, 645
Newborns; see also Infantile spasms
  drug kinetics, 15–16
  drug metabolism, 29–31
  drug selection, 111
  side effects, 111
Nicotinamide
  carbamazepine and, 525
  primidone and, 419–421, 433
Nifedipine
  calcium channels, 68
  clinical use, 978
Nightmares, nitrazepam and, 794
"N.I.H. shift" technique, 197–198
Nimodipine, 978
Nipecotic acid, 76
Nirvanol, 35, 257–258
Nitrazepam, 785–799
  absorption, 787–788
  ACTH comparison, 797
  bioavailability, 787–788
  biotransformation, 791
  chemistry, 785
  in children, 794–798
  conversion, 799
  dependence, 793–794
  distribution, 788–789
  in elderly patients, 795
  excretion, 789–791
  interactions with other drugs, 791–792
  metabolic pathways, 786
  methods of determination, 785–787
  overdose, 795
  pharmacodynamics, 795–796
  plasma concentration, clinical effects, 792–794
  side effects, 794–795
  in status epilepticus, 798–799
  structure, 785–786, 993
  teratogenicity, 795
  therapeutic use, 796–799
  tolerance, 793
  toxicity, 794–795
Nitrendipine, 978
Nitrogen-phosphorus detector, 286
NMDA, burst firing mechanism, 63–64
NMDA receptor, 71–72
Noncompliance, 125–126
Nonlinear Mixed Effect Modeling (NON-MEM), 19–20
Nonlinear pharmacokinetics, 17–21
NON-MEM (Nonlinear Mixed Effect Modeling), 19–20
Norepinephrine
  brain excitability role, 869

  carbamazepine and, 452
  phenytoin and, 153–154
  progabide action, 896
Nortriptyline, 322
Nuclear magnetic resonance, 129
Nutritional factors, 31–32
Nystagmus
  clonazepam, 774–775
  phenytoin, 241–242
  primidone, 440–441

Obesity, 788, 790
Oligodendrocytes, 274
Once-a-day administration, 120
Oncogenicity, 350
One-compartment pharmacokinetic model, 2–3
Open channels, 66
Ophthalmoplegia, 441
Oral administration
  drug absorption, 99–100
  experimental studies, 95, 99–100
  kinetics, 6–11
Oral clearance, 8–9
Oral contraceptives
  carbamazepine effect, 559
  nitrazepam clearance, 792
  phenobarbital and, 322
  phenytoin and, 227, 248
Oral dose/intraperitoneal dose ratio, 99–100
Ornithine transcarbamylase deficiency, 645
Osteomalacia, 39
  carbamazepine, 559
  methsuximide, 712
  phenobarbital, 348
  phenytoin, 246–247
Overdoses
  carbamazepine, 560
  diazepam, 749
  methsuximide, 711
  nitrazepam, 795
  phenobarbital, 345
  primidone, 392–393, 441–442
  progabide, 895
Oxazepam
  diazepam biotransformation, 743–744
  pharmacokinetics, 740–741
Oxazolidinediones, 105
Oxcarbazepine, 913–923
  absorption, 918–920
  carbamazepine comparison, 920–922
  carcinogenicity, 917–918
  cardiovascular effects, 913–914
  chemistry, 913
  in children, 923
  clinical efficacy, 921–923
  conversion, 923
  elimination, 918, 921

Oxcarbazepine (*contd.*)
　enzyme induction, 919–921
　experimental pharmacology, 913–916
　metabolism, 919–921
　nervous system effects, 914
　protein binding, 918–919
　renal effects, 914
　structure, 914
　teratogenicity, 918
　toxicology, 916–918, 922–923
Oxidation, 24–26
Oxidative procedures, phenytoin, 161
3-Oxo-valproate, 604–605, 607, 610–611, 614
4-Oxo-valproate, 606–607

Pancreas
　ethosuximide distribution, 674
　phenytoin effect, 248
Pancreatitis
　carbamazepine, 557
　valproate, 647–748
Pancytopenia
　ethosuximide, 702
　methsuximide, 712
Papio papio, 773, 796, 827, 845
para-HPPH, *see* *p*-HPPH
Paraldehyde, 881–885
　absorption and distribution, 882
　biotransformation, 882–883
　chemistry, 881
　clinical use, 883–884
　conversion, 885
　excretion, 882
　mechanism of action, 885
　methods of determination, 881–882
　and plastics, 882
　pulmonary edema and, 884
　structure, 883, 993
　toxicity, 884–885
Paranoia, primidone and, 440
Parkinsonian syndrome, 702
Paroxysmal awakenings, 773
Paroxysmal bursting, *see* Burst firing
Paroxysmal depolarization shift
　calcium entry blockers, 978
　cellular mechanisms, 62–63
Partial benzodiazepine agonists
　pharmacologic consequences, 729
　receptor action, 725–730
　tolerance, 729, 732
Partial seizures
　carbamazepine, 544
　clonazepam, 771–772
　clorazepate, 814–815
　diazepam, 753, 756
　drug selection, 107–109
　drug withdrawal prognosis, 136

　lamotrigine, 950–951
　lorazepam, 849
　methsuximide, 712–713
　nitrazepam, 798
　phenobarbital, 335–336
　phenytoin, 233–235
　progabide, 898–899
　surgery, 128–129
　valproate, 635–636
　vigabatrin, 942–943
Peak time, 7
Pediatric Dilantin-30 Suspension, 159
4-Pentenoic acid, 613, 647
Pentobarbital, 67–68
Pentylenetetrazol, *see* Metrazol-induced seizures
Perceptual-motor performance
　diazepam, 748
　phenobarbital, 334, 344
　primidone, 440
Performance impairment, nitrazepam, 794
Perinatal asphyxia, 299
Peripheral neuropathy
　carbamazepine, 555–556
　phenytoin, 244
Personality changes, clonazepam, 774–775
pH
　oral administration kinetics, 6–7
　phenobarbital and, 277, 295–296, 299, 306
Pharmacodynamics
　clobazam, 826–830
　diazepam, 752
　nitrazepam, 795–796
　primidone, 406–410
　vigabatrin, 939–941
Pharmacokinetics, 1–21
　age effects, 15–16
　in disease states, 13–15
　and drug selection, 112–113
　drug withdrawal relevance, 137–138
　general principles, 1–21
　intravenous administration, 2–6
　linear phenomena, 1–17
　nonlinear phenomena, 17–21
　oral administration, 6–11
Pheneturide, 223
Phenindione, 219
Phenobarbital, 267–355
　absorption, 293–295, 313–314
　action potentials, 274–275
　age-dependent changes, 30
　autoinduction, 310
　biotransformation, 305–311
　calcium channels, 67–68
　carbamazepine comparison, efficacy, 335–336,
　　539–541
　carbamazepine epoxide interactions, 515
　carbamazepine interactions, 321
　chemistry, 283–291

in children, 297–298, 331–335
chromatography, 285–287
classification, action, 61
clinical use, 329–338
clonazepam interactions, 776
conversion, 291
dependence, 345–346
diazepam comparison, efficacy, 338
diazepam interactions, 744, 753
distribution, 276–277, 295–297
efficacy, 233–235
elimination, 297–300
energy metabolism effect, 275–276
enzyme induction, 38–39, 270
epoxidation, 308–309
excretion, 305–306
in febrile seizures, 333
focal epileptic discharge, 269–270
folate deficiency and, 347–348
GABA receptor, 70–72
N-glucosidation, 308
half-life, dosage, 120–121, 297–299, 332
hepatic toxicity, 349–350
hydrolysis, 309
hydroxylation, 306–309
hyperexcitable axons and, 270
hypersensitivity, 350–351
immunoassays, 287–289
induction of drug metabolism, 314–317
infants and children, 331–335
initiation of, 119
interactions with other drugs, 313–323
kindling effect, 270
mechanisms of action, 267–277
metabolic pathways, 306–308
methobarbital and, side effects, 334
methods of determination, 283–291
in neonatal seizures, 329–331
phenytoin comparison, efficacy, 235, 269,
    335–336, 338
phenytoin interactions, 180, 221–222, 226, 237,
    315, 318–319, 321
plasma levels, 122
in pregnancy, 31
primidone comparison, efficacy, 335–336,
    428–431
primidone interactions, action, 268, 406–410,
    413–415
progabide interactions, 319, 893
and seizure type, efficacy, 107–109
side effects, and selection, 109–112
stereoselectivity, 34
structure, 60, 284, 380, 993
synaptic transmission, 271–274
synthesis, 284
toxicity, 341–352
    cognitive, 333–335, 343–344
    hematological, 347

neurotoxicity, 341–346
sedation, 341–342
valproate interactions, 318–319, 321, 526–527,
    610, 621–623, 627–628
valproate toxicity and, 344
vitamin D and, 322, 348
vitamin K and, 337, 348
Phenobarbital N-glucopyranoside, 307
Phenobarbital-to-primidone ratio, 404–405,
    416–418, 426–433
Phenothiazines
    phenobarbital and, 319
    phenytoin and, 224
Phenprocoumon
    nitrazepam and, 791
    phenytoin and, 219
Phenylbutazone
    phenytoin, 218–219
    valproate and, 628
Phenylethylacetyluria, 319
Phenylethylmalonamide
    chemistry, 379–381
    clearance, 395–396
    conversion, 387
    distribution, brain, 393
    elimination, 398
    interactions with primidone and phenobarbital,
        413–415
    metabolic pathways, 401–402
    methods of determination, 381–387
    neurotoxicity, pharmacodynamics, 407–409
    primidone and, 396–397, 405–410, 413–415
    structure, 380
Phenylethylmalonamide-to-phenobarbital
    relationship, 405, 416–418, 426–433
Phenytoin, 159–255
    absorption, 177–181
        formulation effect, 179
    antacids and, 216, 221
    anticoagulants and, 219
    antiepileptic potential, evaluation, 96–100
    assay, 160–170
    ataxia, 242
    biotransformation, 197–209, 217–218
    calcium channel effect, 150–151
    calcium systems, 151–152
    carbamazepine comparison, efficacy, 233–235,
        538–541
    carbamazepine epoxide interactions, 515
    carbamazepine interactions, 222, 225–226, 237,
        523
    chemistry, 159–172
    in children, 180, 184–185
    chloramphenicol and, 219
    chloride permeability, 152
    classification, 61
    clinical use, 233–238
    clonazepam and, 223, 776

Phenytoin (*contd.*)
  conversion, 172
  cyclic nucleotide metabolism, 152–153
  diazepam and, 223, 744, 753
  distribution, 181–190
  dose-dependent absorption, 178–180
  dose-dependent kinetics, 185, 203–208
  elimination kinetics, 204–205
  enzyme induction, 38–39
  ethanol and, 224
  excretion, 190–191
  felbamate interactions, 223, 988
  half-life, 121, 183–186, 204–205, 208
  hydroxylation, 200
  induction, metabolism, 217–218
  inhibitors, 217–218
  initiation of, 118, 235–236
  interactions with other drugs, 215–228, 237
  intravenous administration, 235–236
  isoniazid and, 219–220
  long-term administration, 206
  maintenance, 235–236
  mechanisms of action, 143–156
  metabolic pathways, 197–209
  metabolites, 170–172
  methylphenidate and, 224
  neuronal excitability, 145–147
  neurophysiological effects, 147–149
  neurotransmitters, 153–154
  nonlinear kinetics, 17–18, 179–180, 185, 202–209
  phenobarbital comparison, efficacy, 235,
       335–336, 338
  phenobarbital interactions, 180, 221–222, 226,
       237, 315, 318–319, 321
  phenylbutazone and, 218–219
  physiological effects, 147–149
  plasma, 181–184
    bindings, 181–184
    distribution, 186–188
    effectiveness, 122
    half-life, 184–186
  in pregnancy, 31–32
  primidone comparison, efficacy, 429, 433
  primidone interactions, 227, 415–418
    plasma levels, 433
  progabide interactions, 223–224, 893
  propoxyphene and, 218
  protein binding, 181–184, 217
  rats versus mice, absorption, 178–179
  receptor molecules, 154–155
  salicylates and, 217–218
  saturation kinetics, implications, 32–33, 40
  seizure type, efficacy, 104–109
  serum concentration, 203–206
  side effects, 109–112
  sodium channel, 64–66
  stereoselective hydroxylation, 202
  structure, 60, 159–160, 994

  sulthiame and, 223
  teratogenicity, 251
  toxicity, 144, 237, 241–251
    chronic aspects, 243–249
    prevention, 251
  valproate comparison, efficacy, 233–235, 634
  valproate interactions, 222–223, 226, 623–625,
       627–628
  vitamins and, 227
Phenytoin hydroxylator phenotype, 29
Photosensitive seizures
  clobazam, 827
  clonazepam, 773
  lamotrigine, 950–951
  nitrazepam, 796
Physical activity, and metabolism, 31–32
Picrotoxin seizure threshold test, 86–87, 89,
       96–100
Placental transfer, *see* Pregnancy
Plasma binding, *see* Protein binding
Plasma drug levels
  effectiveness range, 122
  monitoring, 122
  and withdrawal, 138
Plasma free fraction, 14
Plasma volume, 3
Plastics, paraldehyde incompatibility, 882
Plateau principle, 9–10
cis-Platinum, 220
Polycyclic hydrocarbons, 36–37
Polyradiculitis, 441
Polytherapy, 123–125
Population pharmacokinetics, 19–21
Porphyria
  clonazepam, 776
  phenobarbital, 349
Positional sense test, 91
Positron emission tomography, 129
Postanoxic myoclonus, 634, 848–849
Postsynaptic potential field potential, 451
Posttetanic potentiation
  carbamazepine, 448–449, 451
  phenytoin, 147–148
Potassium conductance
  benzodiazepine receptor agonists, 732
  ethosuximide, 655
  valproate, 571
Pregnancy
  carbamazepine, 476–477, 548
  clorazepate, 811
  diazepam, 741, 751
  drug metabolism, 31
  drug selection, 111–112
  ethosuximide, 674–675, 694
  methylphenobarbital, 372
  nitrazepam, 789
  pharmacokinetics, 16–17
  phenobarbital, 336–337

primidone, 398, 405, 434–435
side effects, 111–112
valproate, 593–594, 611
Premature infants, 29
Presynaptic effects, 73
Primary tonic-clonic seizures
drug selection, 105–106
valproate, 634
Primidone, 379–445
absorption, 391–392
acetazolamide interactions, 393, 433
behavioral toxicity, 429
biotransformation, 401–410
carbamazepine comparison, efficacy, 429, 433, 539–541
carbamazepine interactions, 419–523
plasma levels, 433
chemistry, 379–381
in children, 419, 434
clearance, 395–396
clinical use, 423–435
conversion, 387
distribution, 393–394
drug interactions, 413–421
elimination, 394–398
enzyme induction, 38–39
ethosuximide and, 419
excretion, 397–398
formulation effect, 392
half-life, 120–121, 394–395, 404, 427
hypersensitivity reactions, 443
initiation of, 119, 432
mechanisms of action, 406–410
metabolism, 401–406
methods of determination, 381–387
overdose, 392–393, 441–442
phenobarbital comparison, efficacy, 335–336, 428–431
phenobarbital interactions, 396–397, 403–410, 413–415
phenylethylmalonamide and, 396–397, 405
phenytoin comparison, efficacy, 429
phenytoin interactions, 226, 415–418
plasma concentrations, efficacy, 122, 426–433
in pregnancy, 31, 398, 405
pro-drug controversy, 423–435
and seizure type, efficacy, 107–109
side effects, 109–112, 429
solubility and stability, 380
structure, 380, 994
teratogenicity, 434–435, 443
toxicity, 429, 439–441
hematological, 442
hepatic and renal, 442
nervous system, 407–409, 439–441
valproate interactions, 419, 625
Probenecid
acetazolamide and, 864
lorazepam and, 850

Prochlorperazine, 319
Progabide, 887–900
absorption, 890
biotransformation, 891–892
carbamazepine epoxide effect, 508, 515–516, 893
chemistry, 887–888
in children, 898–899
clinical use, 897–899
conversion, 900
distribution, 890–891
drug interactions, 892–894
elimination, 890–891
endocrine effects, 897
GABA receptor action, 895–897
liver toxicity, 895
mechanism of action, 897
methods of determination, 888–889
pharmacodynamics, 895–897
phenobarbital and, 319, 893
phenytoin and, 223–224, 893
structure, 888, 994
therapeutic levels, 894
toxicity, 894–895
valproate and, 894, 898
Progesterone, 248
Prolactin
phenytoin and, 248
progabide and, 897
"Prompt release" preparations, 120
Propionic acid, 605
Propoxyphene
carbamazepine and, 521, 526
carbamazepine epoxide and, 513
enzyme inhibition, 41
phenytoin and, 218
2-*n*-Propylglutaric acid, 607
2-*n*-Propylsuccinic acid, 607
Protective index, 94–100
Protein binding
acetazolamide, 857
carbamazepine, 473, 527–528
clorazepate, 810
diazepam, 739–742
drug biotransformation and, 42–43
drug interactions, 56, 217
methylphenobarbital, 361
nitrazepam, 789
oxcarbazepine, 918–919
phenobarbital action, 314
phenobarbital effect, neonates, 331
phenytoin, 181–184, 217
stiripentol, 962
valproate, 585–588
and brain uptake, 588
Prothrombin, 337
Psoralen, 227
Psychomotor seizures
carbamazepine, 538–540
nitrazepam, 798

Psychotic reactions
  carbamazepine, 559
  ethosuximide, 693
  phenytoin, 144
  stiripentol, 959–960
Psychotropic drugs
  phenobarbital and, 319, 322
  phenytoin and, 224
Psychotropic effects, carbamazepine, 541–544, 559
Pulmonary edema, paraldehyde, 884
"Pulse dose," 609
Pyknolepsy, 104

Quinidine, 225
Quisqualate receptor, 71–72

Rabbits
  carbamazepine, 501–502
  carbamazepine epoxide, 501–502, 512–514
  diazepam kinetics, 740–741
  nitrazepam metabolism, 791
Radial partition immunoassay, 288–289
Radiculitis, 441
Radioimmunoassay, *see* Immunoassay methods
Radiotelemetry, 127
Rafampin, 219
Rage reactions, clorazepate, 816
Ramsay-Hunt syndrome, 773
Ranitidine
  carbamazepine and, 525
  phenytoin and, 221
Rashes, *see* Skin rashes
Rats
  acetazolamide distribution, 857–861
  carbamazepine epoxide, 510–514
  carbamazepine metabolism, 500–501
  diazepam, 740–741, 744
  nitrazepam biotransformation, 791
  phenytoin kinetics, 178–179, 183
  phenytoin metabolites, 209
Rebound insomnia, 793–794
Receptor binding, 89–90
Reduction, 25
Referrals, refractory epilepsy, 127–128
Refractory seizures, 126–128
Relapse rates
  studies, 134
  and withdrawal duration, 138
Remission, 133–134
Renal clearance
  carbamazepine, 476
  general principles, 9
  phenobarbital, 298–299, 306
Renal disease
  carbamazepine kinetics, 479
  drug kinetics, 13–14
  drug metabolism, 43–44

phenobarbital effect, 337
  primidone metabolism, 406
Renal toxicity
  carbamazepine, 559
  primidone, 442
Respiratory depression
  diazepam, 748
  lorazepam, 850
  nitrazepam, 794
Resting channel conformation, 66
Restless legs, clonazepam, 773
Restrictive clearance, 4–5
Reticular formation
  ethosuximide action, 657
  phenobarbital action, 269
Reticulocytosis, 442
Retinotoxicity, 560
Rhesus monkey, 501–502, 510–514
Rickets
  phenytoin toxicity, 246–247
  vitamin D_3 metabolism, 39
Righting test, 91, 96–99
RO-15-1788, 897
RO-15-4513, 745
Rotorod test, 91, 94–99, 508

Saccades, 793
"Safety ratio," 99
Salicylates, 184, 217–218
Salicyclic acid
  acetazolamide and, 864
  valproate and, 628
Saliva
  carbamazepine, 465–466, 474
  ethosuximide, 675
  phenobarbital, 296, 332
  phenytoin, 186–187
  primidone, 393–394
  valproate, 589
Salivary glands, 859–860
Salivary hypersecretion, 794
Saturation kinetics
  implications, 32–33
  phenytoin, 184
Schizoaffective disorder, 637
Scleroderma, 701
Sedation
  clobazam, 827, 834–835
  clonazepam, 774–775
  clorazepate, 816
  diazepam, 748
  and drug selection, 110
  lorazepam, 849–850
  phenobarbital, 341–342
Seizure classification, 103–104
Seizure control; *see also* Clinical use
  acetazolamide, 869–871
  bromides, 878–879

carbamazepine, 533–549
clobazam, 826–836
clonazepam, 767–768
diazepam, 745–757
ethosuximide, 688–696
felbamate, 988–989
lorazepam, plasma levels, 844
methylphenobarbital, 367–374
nitrazepam, 796–799
paraldehyde, 883–884
phenobarbital, 335–338
primidone, 423–435
progabide, 894, 898
trimethadione, 718
valproate, 633–639
Seizure excerbation
carbamazepine, children, 556
clonazepam, 771, 774
ethosuximide, 700
lorazepam, 850
nitrazepam, 794
"Seizure index," 689
Seizure initiation, 61–62
Seizure propagation, 62
Seizure spread
drug action, 61–62
drug testing, 85
phenobarbital, 269
Seizure threshold
drug testing, 85–87
phenytoin, 146–147
Selected ion monitoring, 459
Serial seizures, 756
Serotonin
carbamazepine action, 452
clonazepam action, 768
nitrazepam, 796
progabide, 896
Severity of epilepsy, 134–136
Sex behavior, phenobarbital and, 346
Sex factors
carbamazepine half-life, 501
drug metabolism, 31
enzyme induction, phenobarbital, 316
nitrazepam distribution, 788
side effects, 111–112
Sex hormone binding protein, 323
Sex hormones
carbamazepine and, 559
phenytoin and, 248
Short-term memory, 345
Sick sinus syndrome, 559
Side effects; see also Toxicity
acetazolamide, 870–871
carbamazepine epoxide, 508–509
classification, 50–51
clobazam, 834–835
clonazepam, 773–776

clorazepate, 816
diazepam, 748
and drug selection, 109–112
ethosuximide, 699–702
flunarizine, 977–978
lamotrigine, 951
lorazepam, 849–850
methsuximide, 710–711
monotherapy versus polytherapy, 123–124
nitrazepam, 794–795
oxcarbazepine, 922–923
phenobarbital, children, 334–335
primidone versus phenobarbital, 429, 439
valproate, 639, 643–648
Simple partial seizures
clonazepam, 772
clorazepate, 814–815
valproate, 635
Single-ion monitoring chromatography, 385
Single seizures, 117–118
SKF525A, 407, 425–426
Skin rashes
bromides, 879
carbamazepine, 548, 556
ethosuximide, 701
methsuximide, 712
phenobarbital, 350
phenytoin, 249
primidone, 443
SL 75 102, 888–889, 896
Sleep
clobazam and, 835
nitrazepam and, 796
phenobarbital action, 270–271
Sleep time tests, 92–93
Slow acetylation, 28, 220
Slow-release carbamazepine, 546
Smoking, see Cigarette smoking
Sodium bromide, 57–58
Sodium channels
benzodiazepine receptor agonists, 732
burst firing, 63
carbamazepine, 447–451
drug mechanisms, 64–67
ethosuximide, 655
phenytoin, 149–150
use-dependent inhibition, 150
Sodium conductance, 149–150
Sodium hydrogen divalproate, 584
Sodium-potassium ATPase, 149
Sodium-potassium transport, 149–150
Sodium valproate; see also Valproate
bioavailability, 584
Sound-induced seizures, 62
Spacing of drug administration, 120
Sparse data, 19
Sparteine oxidation, 498

Spectrophotometric methods
nitrazepam, 785
phenobarbital, 285
phenytoin, 160
Speech rate, 334
Sperm, phenytoin and, 191, 248
Spinal trigeminal nucleus, 451
Spleen, ethosuximide distribution, 673–674
SSA-dehydrogenase, 75
Stance test, 91
Starvation effects, 299
Status epilepticus
clonazepam, 773
diazepam clinical use, 752–756
diazepam, plasma levels, 747–748
and drug withdrawal, 139–140
lorazepam, 845–848
nitrazepam, 798–799
paraldehyde, 883–884
phenobarbital, 337–338
phenytoin, 236–237, 243
Steady state
and dosage, 120–122
drug metabolites, 12–13
pharmacokinetics, 9–10
Stereoselectivity
drug metabolism, 34–35
methylphenobarbital, 363
Steroids
phenobarbital and, 322–323
phenytoin and, 227, 247–248
Stevens-Johnson syndrome
ethosuximide, 701
phenytoin toxicity, 249
Stiff man syndrome, 773
Stiripentol, 955–968
in absence seizures, 966–968
absorption, 960
animal pharmacology, 955–958
carbamazepine and, 526, 963–964
carbamazepine epoxide and, 513–514
chemistry, 955
conversion, 968
distribution, 960–962
drug interactions, 963–964
mechanism of action, 957–958
metabolic pathways, 956
metabolism, 962–963
methods of determination, 955
phenobarbital and, 319, 964
phenytoin and, 224, 963
protein binding, 962
structure, 956, 994
teratogenicity, 958
therapeutic efficacy, 964
toxicology, 958–960
valproate and, 964
Stokes-Adams attacks, 559

Structures of antiepileptic drugs, 992–994; *see also*
under specific drugs
Strychnine seizure pattern test, 86–87, 89, 96–100
Stupor, 644
Substantia nigra, 770
Substrate-labeled fluorescent immunoassay
(SLFIA)
carbamazepine, 460–461
phenobarbital, 288
phenytoin, 166–167
primidone, 386
valproate, 580
Succinic semialdehyde dehydrogenase, 569
Succinimides; *see also* Ethosuximide;
Methsuximide
primidone and, 419
"Suicide inhibitors," 42
Sulfinpyrazone, 35
Sulfonamides, 855–879; *see also* Acetazolamide;
Methazolamide
phenytoin and, 219–220
Sulthiame, 223
Superior colliculus, 189
Supramaximal tests, 85–87
Surgery, 128–129
Sustained attention, 344–345
Sustained repetitive firing
carbamazepine, 447–451
phenytoin effect, 148–149, 450
sodium channel, 64–66
valproate, 450
Swallowing impairment, 794
Sweat, phenobarbital and, 296
Sydenham's chorea, 637
Symptomatic epilepsies
carbamazepine, 544
characteristics, 107
Synaptic inhibition
carbamazepine, 451–452
drug action, 67–71
phenytoin, 154
valproate, 571–572
Systemic clearance, 5–6, 8
Systemic lupus erythematosus
carbamazepine, 556
ethosuximide, 701
phenobarbital, 351–352
phenytoin, 250
primidone, 443

T channel, 67–69
Tardive dyskinesia
clonazepam, 773
valproate, 637
Taste sensation, 871
TCPO (1,3-epoxy-3,3,3-trichloropropane), 199
TD$_{50}$/ED$_{50}$ ratio, 99

TD$_3$/ED$_{97}$ ratio, 99
Tears
  carbamazepine, 466
  ethosuximide, 675
  phenobarbital, 296
  valproate, 589
Temporal lobe abnormalities, 636
Temporal lobe lesions, 129
Teratogenicity
  acetazolamide, 871
  arene oxide, 199
  carbamazepine, 559–560
  carbamazepine 10,11-epoxide, 500
  clonazepam, 776
  clorazepate, 816
  diazepam, 751
  ethosuximide, 694, 703
  ethotoin, 262
  lorazepam, 850–851
  methylphenobarbital, 372
  monotherapy versus polytherapy, 124
  nitrazepam, 795
  oxcarbazepine, 918
  phenobarbital, 336–337, 351–352
  phenytoin, 251
  primidone, 434–435, 443
  stiripentol, 958
  testing for, 53
  trimethadione, 718
  valproate, 648
  valproate metabolites, 613
Test systems, 60–61
Testosterone
  carbamazepine and, 559
  phenytoin and, 248
Tetramethylammonium hydroxide, 161–162
Thalamocortical system
  ethosuximide, 657–658
  trimethadione, 717
  valproate, 571
Thalamus, carbamazepine and, 473
Theophylline
  carbamazepine and, 451
  phenobarbital and, 320
  phenytoin and, 225
Thin-layer chromatography
  clonazepam, 766
  clorazepate, 806–807
  nitrazepam, 786
  phenobarbital, 285, 290
Thioridazine, 319, 322
"Three-state" hypothesis, 727–728
Thrombocytopenia
  carbamazepine, 558
  ethosuximide, 702
  phenytoin, 250
  primidone, 442
  valproate, 110, 645

Thyroid function
  drug metabolism effect, 44
  phenytoin toxicity, 248
Thyroid gland, acetazolamide and, 859–860
Thyroid hormones, carbamazepine and, 558
Thyroid stimulating hormone, 248
Thyrotropin, 181
Thyroxine
  carbamazepine and, 558
  phenytoin displacement, 181, 248
Tiapamil, 978
Time-dependent kinetics, 18–19
Time of onset, 95
Time of peak effect, 87, 91, 95
Timing of drug administration, 119–121
TMAH (tetramethylammonium hydroxide),
  161–162
TMPAH (trimethylphenylammonium hydroxide),
  161
Tolbutamide, 224
Tolerance
  acetazolamide, 866, 868–870
  carbonic anhydrase role, 868
  clobazam, 831, 834
  clonazepam, 771
  diazepam, 749–750
  drug evaluation tests, 92–93
  methylphenobarbital, 371
  nitrazepam, 793
  partial benzodiazepine agonists, 729
  phenobarbital, 342
  primidone, 409–410, 440–441
Tonic-clonic seizures
  carbamazepine, 544
  clonazepam, 771
  drug selection principles, 105–108
  drug withdrawal prognosis, 136
  phenobarbital, 335–336
  phenytoin, 146–147, 233–235
  primidone versus phenobarbital, 425, 429, 431
  valproate, 633–634
Tonic seizure phase, 146–147
Toxic dose, 91–92, 95–100
Toxicity, 49–58
  acetazolamide, 870–871
  ACTH, 908
  acute, 90–91
  animal tests, 90–91
  bromides, 878–879
  carbamazepine metabolites, 499–500
  classification, 49–51
  clonazepam, 773–776
  detection, 52–55, 94–100
  diazepam, 748–749, 751–752
  drug interactions, 55–58
  and drug selection, 109–112
  ethosuximide, 699–704
  felbamate, 985–986, 989

Toxicity (*contd.*)
  flunarizine, 973, 977–978
  gabapentin, 929
  general principles, 49–58
  incidence, 51
  lamotrigine, 948–949
  methylphenobarbital, 370–371, 374
  nitrazepam, 794–795
  oxcarbazepine, 916–918
  paraldehyde, 884–885
  phenobarbital, 341–352
  progabide, 894–895
  stiripentol, 958–960
  vigabatrin, 940–941
Trans-carbamazepine diol, *see* Carbamazepine
  10,11-*trans*-dihydrodiol
Transient leukopenia, 557
Trazodone, 224
Tremor, valproate and, 644
Triacetyloleandomycin, 521, 526
Tricyclic antidepressants
  drug interactions, 57
  phenobarbital and, 322
  phenytoin and, 224
Trifluoroethanol, 323
Trigeminal complex, 571
Trigeminal neuralgia
  carbamazepine epoxide, 508
  clonazepam, 773
Triiodothyronine, 181, 248
Trimethadione, 715–719
  absence seizures, 105, 715–718
  calcium channels, 67
  chemistry, 715–716
  conversion, 718
  methods of determination, 715–716
  pharmacokinetics, 717
  plasma levels, seizure control, 718
  structure, 60, 715–716, 944
  teratogenicity, 105, 111–112, 718
  toxicity, 718
Trimethylphenylammonium hydroxide (TMPAH),
  161
Troleandomycin, 548
Twins, enzyme induction, 316–317
Two-compartment model, 11
Two-stage approach, 19–20
"Two-state" hypothesis, 727–728

Ultraviolet absorbance
  carbamazepine, 457
  phenytoin, 160
Umbilical cord serum
  diazepam, 751
  ethosuximide, 675
  nitrazepam, 789
  valproate, 589

Uremia
  drug metabolism effect, 44
  valproate and, 594, 629
Urinary excretion, kinetics, 9
Urine, phenytoin metabolites, 209

Valproate, 567–651
  absorption, 583–585
  administration, 637–638
  age-dependent metabolism, 30
  antiepileptic potential, evaluation, 96–100
  benzodiazepine interactions, 626, 746
  biotransformation, 601–614
  carbamazepine comparison, efficacy, 540, 636
  carbamazepine epoxide interactions, 515–516,
    549, 625–626
  carbamazepine interactions, 523–525, 610,
    625–628
    toxicity, 549
  chemistry, 577–581
  in children, 592–593, 609–610
    efficacy, 636–639
  classification, 61
  clearance, 590–595
  clinical use, 636–639
  clonazepam interactions, 626, 644
  concentration-effect relationship, 637–639
  conversion, 581
  distribution, 585–590
  dose effects, metabolism, 609
  elimination, 590–595
  enzyme induction, 38–39
  enzyme inhibition, 41
  ethosuximide comparison, efficacy, 691
  ethosuximide interactions, 625
  half-life, 120–121, 595
  hepatotoxicity, 645–647
  intake intervals, 120
  mechanisms of action, 567–573
  metabolism, 602–608
    species differences, 612
  metabolites
    assays, 608–609
    pharmacological activity, 612–613
    plasma and brain, 588–589
    urinary, 607–608
  methods of determination, 577–581, 608–609
  overdosage, 643
  β-oxidation, 604–605
  ω-oxidation, 605–606, 611
  pancreatitis, 647–648
  phenobarbital comparison, efficacy, 627–638
  phenobarbital interactions, 318–319, 321,
    526–527, 610, 621–623, 627–628
    mechanism, 318
  phenytoin comparison, efficacy, 234, 634
  phenytoin interactions, 222–223, 226, 623–625,
    627–628

plasma levels, 122
  and brain levels, 586–587
  effectiveness, 122
pregnancy, 31, 593–594
primidone interactions, 419, 625
progabide comparison, efficacy, 898
protein binding, 585
and seizure type, efficacy, 103–109
side effects, and drug selection, 109–112
sodium channel, 64
structure, 578
sustained repetitive firing effect, 450
teratogenicity, 648
toxicity, 639, 643–648
uremia and, 594
Δ^2-Valproate, 612–613
Δ^4-Valproate, 613
δ-^{2}-Valproate, 588–589
Valproate coenzyme A, 603–604
Valproate glucuronide, 602–603
Valpromide
  bioavailability, 584–585
  carbamazepine and, 498, 500, 508, 515–516, 525
  enzyme inhibition, 41–42
  in febrile seizures, 637
Valproylcarnitine, 603
Valproylglycine, 603–604
Ventilatory requirements, 331
Ventrolateral thalamus
  ethosuximide and, 657
  valproate and, 571
Verapamil
  carbamazepine and, 525
  carbamazepine epoxide and, 513
  clinical efficacy, 978–979
Veratridine, 450–451
Verbal learning, 334
Video monitoring, 126–127
Vigabatrin, 937–945
  chemistry, 937
  in children, 943
  clinical trials, 941–944
  conversion, 945
  dose-related efficacy, 943
  drug interactions, 944
  GABA-release, 76, 939–941
  GABA-T inhibition, 74, 939, 941

methods of determination, 937–938
microvacuoles, 940–941
pharmacodynamics, 939–941
pharmacokinetics, 938
phenytoin interactions, 944
structure, 938, 994
toxicity, 940–941, 943–944
Vigilance, 334, 344
Viloxazine, 548
Vinblastine, 220
Vitamin B_{12} deficiency, 245
Vitamin D
  carbamazepine toxicity, 559
  phenobarbital effects, 322, 348
  phenytoin toxicity, 247
Vitamin D_3 metabolism, 39
Vitamin K-dependent coagulation
  factors, 227, 246
  phenobarbital and, 337, 348
  primidone and, 442
Vitamins, phenytoin and, 227
Volume of distribution, 3–4, 6, 11

Warfarin
  phenobarbital and, 320
  phenytoin and, 219, 225
  stereoselectivity, 35
  valproate and, 628
Water balance, 558
Water retention, 558
Weight gain
  clonazepam, 774–775
  and drug selection, 111
  valproate, 644
  vigabatrin, 943–944
West syndrome
  definition, 906
  drug selection, 106
  nitrazepam, 797
White matter tissues, 189–190
Withdrawal, *see* Drug withdrawal

Zonisamide
  phenobarbital and, 319
  phenytoin and, 224, 227